5th edition

comprehensive pharmacy review

EDITORS

Leon Shargel, PhD, RPh
Alan H. Mutnick, PharmD, FASHP, RPh
Paul F. Souney, MS, RPh
Larry N. Swanson, PharmD, FASHP, RPh

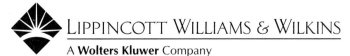

LIPPINCOTT WILLIAMS & WILKINS
A **Wolters Kluwer** Company

Philadelphia · Baltimore · New York · London
Buenos Aires · Hong Kong · Sydney · Tokyo

Editor: David B. Troy
Managing Editor: Matthew J. Hauber
Marketing Manager: Samantha Smith
Production Editor: Jennifer Ajello
Designer: Risa Clow
Compositor: Graphic World
Printer: Data Reproductions Corp.

351 West Camden Street
Baltimore, MD 21201

530 Walnut Street
Philadelphia, PA 19106

Printed in the United States of America

Library of Congress Cataloging-in-Publication Data is available. ISBN: 0-7817-4486-5
The publishers have made every effort to trace the copyright holders for borrowed material. If they have inadvertently overlooked any, they will be pleased to make the necessary arrangements at the first opportunity.

To purchase additional copies of this book, call our customer service department at **(800) 638-3030** or fax orders to **(301) 824-7390**. International customers should call **(301) 714-2324**.

Visit Lippincott Williams & Wilkins on the Internet: http://www.LWW.com. Lippincott Williams & Wilkins customer service representatives are available from 8:30 am to 6:00 pm, EST.

04 05 06 07 08
1 2 3 4 5 6 7 8 9 10

Contents

Contributors

Loyd V. Allen, Jr, PhD
Editor-in-Chief
International Journal of Pharmaceutical
  Compounding
Edmond, Oklahoma
Professor Emeritus
College of Pharmacy
University of Oklahoma
Oklahoma City, Oklahoma

Anton H. Amann, PhD, RPh
Executive Vice President
Operations and Research & Development
Andrx Corporation
Ft. Lauderdale, Florida

Connie Lee Barnes, PharmD, RPh
Associate Professor
Director, Drug Information Center
Department of Pharmacy Practice
Campbell University School of Pharmacy
Buies Creek, North Carolina

Faith L. Barnett, PharmD
Clinical Pharmacist
Department of Pharmacy
Cherry Hospital
Goldsboro, North Carolina

Lawrence H. Block, PhD, RPh
Professor of Pharmaceutics
Director, Center for Biotechnology
Division of Pharmaceutical Sciences
Mylan School of Pharmacy
Duquesne University
Pittsburgh, Pennsylvania

Riccardo L. Boni, PhD
Assistant Professor of Pharmaceutics
Division of Pharmaceutical Sciences
Mylan School of Pharmacy
Duquesne University
Pittsburgh, Pennsylvania

Donald F. Brophy, PharmD, BCPS
Assistant Professor
School of Pharmacy
Virginia Commonwealth University
Richmond, Virginia

Todd A. Brown, MHP, RPh
Associate Clinical Specialist
Department of Pharmacy Practice
School of Pharmacy
Bouve College of Health Sciences
Northeastern University
Boston, Massachusetts

Judy L. Chase, PharmD, FASHP
Clinical Pharmacy Coordinator
Division of Pharmacy
M.D. Anderson Cancer Center
Houston, Texas

Carolyn L. Dabirsiaghi, PhD
Professor
Natural and Physical Sciences
Baltimore City Community College
Baltimore, Maryland

Steven M. Davis, PharmD, BCPS
Associate Professor
Department of Pharmacy Practice
Campbell University School of Pharmacy
Buies Creek, North Carolina
Clinical Coordinator
Department of Pharmacy
Wake Forest University Baptist Medical
  Center
Winston-Salem, North Carolina

Ronald J. DeBellis, PharmD, RPh
Associate Professor, Pharmacy Practice
Department of Pharmacy Practice
Massachusetts College of Pharmacy and
    Health Sciences
Clinical Specialist, Critical Care
Pulmonary, Allergy, and Critical Care
University of Massachusetts Memorial
    Medical Center
Worcester, Massachusetts

Stephen C. Dragotakes, RPh, BCNP
PET Nuclear Pharmacy
Mass General Hospital
Boston, Massachusetts

Alice C. Engelbrecht, RPh, CP
Drug Information Center
Presbyterian Hospital
Oklahoma City, Oklahoma

Janet Espirito, PharmD
Oncology Pharmacy Practice Resident
M.D. Anderson Cancer Center
Division of Pharmacy
Houston, Texas

Maria Evasovich, MD
Assistant Professor of Surgery/General
    Surgery
Surgical Critical Care/Head and Neck
    Surgery
Department of Surgery
Medical School
University of Minnesota
Minneapolis, Minnesota

John Fanikos, RPh, MBA
Clinical Assistant Professor
Pharmacy Practice
Northeastern University
Assistant Director of Pharmacy
Pharmacy Department
Brigham and Women's Hospital
Boston, Massachusetts

Godwin W. Fong, PhD
Department of Research and Development
Pharmaceutical Development Consulting
Westborough, Massachusetts

Stephen H. Fuller, PharmD, BCPS, CPP, RPh
Associate Professor
Department of Pharmacy Practice
Campbell University School of Pharmacy
Buies Creek, North Carolina
Clinical Pharmacist
Cary Healthcare Associates
Cary, North Carolina

Gail Goodman-Snitkoff, PhD
Associate Professor
Basic and Pharmaceutical Sciences
Albany College of Pharmacy
Albany, New York

James B. Groce III, PharmD, CACP, RPh
Associate Professor
Department of Pharmacy Practice
Campbell University School of Pharmacy
Clinical Pharmacy Specialist—
    Anticoagulation
Moses Cone Health System
Greensboro, North Carolina

Tina M. Harrison, PharmD, FASCP, CGP, RPh
Assistant Professor
Department of Pharmacy Practice
Campbell University School of Pharmacy
Buies Creek, North Carolina

Marc W. Harrold, PhD
Professor of Medicinal Chemistry
Division of Pharmaceutical Sciences
Mylan School of Pharmacy
Duquesne University
Pittsburgh, Pennsylvania

John E. Janosik, PharmD, RPh
Medical Liaison
Medical Affairs
Roche Laboratories
Hudson, Ohio

Brian G. Katona, PharmD, RPh
Medical Affairs Director
AstraZeneca LP
Wayne, Pennsylvania

Alan F. Kaul, RPh, MS, MBA, FCCP
Adjunct Professor of Pharmacy
Pharmacy Practice
University of Rhode Island College of
    Pharmacy
Kingston, Rhode Island
President
Medical Outcomes Management, Inc.
Foxborough, Massachusetts

Kevin P. Keating, MD
Assistant Professor of Surgery
Director, Surgical Critical Care
Director, Nutritional Support Service
Hartford Hospital
Hartford, Connecticut

Teresa Bailey Klepser, PharmD
Associate Professor
Director of Managed Care
Pharmacy Practice Residency
Ferris State University College of Pharmacy
Kalamazoo Center for Medical Studies
Michigan State University
Kalamazoo, Michigan

John D. Leary, PhD, RPh
Massachusetts College of Pharmacy and
    Allied Health Sciences
Boston, Massachusetts

Charles Lee, MS, RAC
Senior Specialist
Regulatory Affairs
Amgen, Inc.
Thousand Oaks, California

Pui-Kai Li
Associate Professor of Medicinal Chemistry
College of Pharmacy
Ohio State University
Columbus, Ohio

Scott F. Long, RPh, PhD
Associate Professor of Pharmacology and
    Toxicology
Department of Pharmaceutical Sciences
School of Pharmacy
Southwestern Oklahoma State University
Weatherford, Oklahoma

Michelle A. Long, PharmD
Medical Information Specialist, GI
AstraZeneca LP
Durham, North Carolina

D. Byron May, PharmD, BCPS, RPh
Associate Professor
Department of Pharmacy Practice
Campbell University School of Pharmacy
Buies Creek, North Carolina
Clinical Pharmacist
Duke University Medical Center
Durham, North Carolina

David I. Min, MS, PharmD
Associate Professor
Division of Clinical and Administrative
    Pharmacy
University of Iowa, College of Pharmacy
Clinical Pharmacy Specialist
Department of Pharmaceutical Care
University of Iowa Hospitals and Clinics
Iowa City, Iowa

J. Edward Moreton, PhD
Professor
Pharmacology and Toxicology
Department of Pharmaceutical Sciences
University of Maryland School of Pharmacy
Baltimore, Maryland

Alan H. Mutnick, PharmD, RPh, FASHP
Adjunct Associate Professor
Clinical and Administrative Practice
University of Iowa, College of Pharmacy
Iowa City, Iowa

Jeffrey P. Norenberg, MS, BCNP, FASHP
Chair, Radiopharmacy Graduate
    Concentration
College of Pharmacy
University of New Mexico Health Sciences
    Center
Cancer Research and Treatment Center
University of New Mexico Health Sciences
    Center
Albuquerque, New Mexico

Robert C. Pavlan, Jr, BS Pharm, JD
School of Pharmacy
Bouve College of Health Sciences
Northeastern University
Boston, Massachusetts
Pavlan & Associates
Attorneys at Law
Belmont, Massachusetts

Beth Bryles Phillips, PharmD, BCPS
Assistant Professor (Clinical)
Division of Clinical and Administrative
   Pharmacy
College of Pharmacy
University of Iowa, College of Pharmacy
Clinical Pharmacy Specialist, Ambulatory
   Care
Department of Pharmaceutical Care
University of Iowa Hospitals and Clinics
Iowa City, Iowa

John J. Ponzillo, PharmD
Critical Care
Clinical Pharmacy
St. John's Mercy Medical Center
St. Louis, Missouri

Robert A. Quercia, MS, RPh
Associate Clinical Professor
University of Connecticut, School of
   Pharmacy
Storrs, Connecticut
Director, Drug Information Service
Director, Total Parenteral Nutrition Service
Department of Pharmacy
Hartford Hospital
Hartford, Connecticut

Azita Razzaghi-Hedayat, PharmD
Manager—Pharmacovigilance & Medical
   Information
Genzyme Corporation
Cambridge, Massachusetts

**Gerald E. Schumacher, PharmD, PhD,
   RPh**
Professor of Pharmacy
School of Pharmacy
Bouve College of Health Sciences
Northeastern University
Boston, Massachusetts

Mollie Ashe Scott, PharmD, BCPS, CPP
Director
Department of Pharmacotherapy
Mountain AHEC
Asheville, North Carolina
Clinical Associate Professor
UNC School of Pharmacy
Assistant Professor of Family Medicine
UNC School of Medicine

Leon Shargel, PhD, RPh
Vice President, Biopharmaceutics
Eon Labs, Inc.
Laurelton, New York
Adjunct Associate Professor
School of Pharmacy
University of Maryland
Baltimore, Maryland

Penny S. Shelton, PharmD, BCPP, RPh
Clinical Assistant Professor
Department of Pharmacy Practice
Campbell University School of Pharmacy
Buies Creek, North Carolina
MEDS Program Director
Resources for Seniors
Raleigh, North Carolina

Mark K. Sorenson, RPh
Adjunct Instructor
University of Iowa College of Pharmacy
Clinical Pharmacy Specialist/Pediatrics
University of Iowa Hospitals and Clinics
Iowa City, Iowa

Paul F. Souney, RPh, MSc
Senior Director Medical Affairs
AstraZeneca LP
Wayne, Pennsylvania

Larry N. Swanson, PharmD, FASHP

Professor and Chairman
Department of Pharmacy Practice
Campbell University School of Pharmacy
Buies Creek, North Carolina

Barbara A. Szymusiak-Mutnick, BSPharm, RPh, MHP

Adjunct Assistant Professor
Division of Clinical and Administrative
   Practice
University of Iowa College of Pharmacy
Clinical Pharmacist
Department of Pharmaceutical Care
University of Iowa Hospitals and Clinics
Iowa City, Iowa

Mona Gold Tsoukleris, PharmD, RPh, BCPS

Pharmacy School Associate Professor
Pharmacy Practice and Science
University of Maryland School of Pharmacy
Clinical Pharmacist and Asthma Educator
Pediatrics
University of Maryland Hospital for
   Children
Baltimore, Maryland

Ashiwel S. Undie, PhD

Associate Professor
Neuropharmacology and
   Pharmacogenomics
School of Pharmacy
University of Maryland
Department of Pharmaceutical Sciences
Baltimore, Maryland

Andrew L. Wilson, PharmD, FASHP

Associate Professor
School of Pharmacy
Virginia Commonwealth University
Director, Pharmacy Services
Medical College of Virginia Hospitals
Richmond, Virginia

Peter K. Wong, PhD, MBA, MS, RPh

Adjunct Assistant Professor
Community Health/Health System
   Management
School of Medicine
Wright State University
Vice President, Clinical Effectiveness and
   Performance Improvement
Administration/Medical Affairs
Good Samaritan Hospital
Dayton, Ohio

Margaret C. (Peggy) Yarborough, PharmD, MS, BC-ADM, CDE

Professor
Department of Pharmacy Practice
Campbell University School of Pharmacy
Buies Creek, North Carolina
Pharmacist Clinician
Wilson Community Health Center
Wilson, North Carolina

Nelson S. Yee, MD, PhD, RPh

Instructor
Medicine
University of Pennsylvania School of
   Medicine
Attending Physician
Medicine
University of Pennsylvania Health System
Philadelphia, Pennsylvania

Anthony E. Zimmermann, PharmD, RPh

Associate Professor of Pharmacy Practice
Department of Pharmacy Practice
Massachusetts College of Pharmacy
Worcester, Massachusetts
Critical Care Specialist
Pharmacy
Mercy Medical Center
Springfield, Massachusetts

Preface

This new edition of *Comprehensive Pharmacy Review* reflects the continuing evolution of pharmacy practice and educational requirements. Career opportunities for pharmacists are greater than ever before. Pharmaceutical education, including pharmaceutical science and practice, must prepare pharmacy practitioners for the future. Pharmacists now work in academic pharmacy, community pharmacy, long-term care and consulting pharmacy including hospice and home care, pharmaceutical and health care distributors, pharmaceutical industry, professional trade organizations, uniformed (public health) services, U.S. and state governments, hospital and institutional practice settings, and managed care pharmacy. Pharmacists are taking a more active role in health care, including counseling and medication therapy, disease-state management, screening programs such as diabetes or high cholesterol, as well as the more traditional role of dispensing medication and educating patients.

This new edition of *Comprehensive Pharmacy Review* has been revised to reflect the current educational requirements for a successful career in pharmacy. The main objective of the *Comprehensive Pharmacy Review* is to provide a comprehensive study guide for pharmacy students and other candidates who are preparing for the North American Pharmacist Licensure Examination™ (NAPLEX®). The *Comprehensive Pharmacy Review* contains topic outlines and practice questions according to the pharmacy school curriculum. This review publication, along with the separate booklet of simulated NAPLEX® exams and CD-ROM that supplements this review, provides both guidance and test practice for NAPLEX® candidates.

While the principal market for *Comprehensive Pharmacy Review* remains NAPLEX® candidates, the Comprehensive Pharmacy Review is also intended for a broader audience of pharmacy undergraduates and health professionals who seek detailed summaries of pharmacy subjects. Encompassed by the review is a range of topics central to the study of pharmacy—chemistry, pharmaceutics, pharmacology, pharmacy practice, drug therapy—organized to parallel the pharmacy curriculum and presented in outline form for easy use. It can therefore be used as a quick review (or preview) of essential topics by a diverse group of readers, including:

- Matriculating pharmacy students. The organization and topical coverage of *Comprehensive Pharmacy Review* are such that many pharmacy students will want to purchase it in their first professional year and use it throughout their pharmacy education to prepare for course examinations.
- Instructors and preceptors. *Comprehensive Pharmacy Review* also functions as an instructor's manual and a reference for teachers and tutors in pharmacy schools. Chapter outlines can be used to organize courses and to plan specific lectures.
- Professional pharmacists. *Comprehensive Pharmacy Review* offers practitioners a convenient handbook of pharmacy facts. It can be used as a course refresher and as a source of recent information on pharmacy practice. The appendices include prescription dispensing information, common prescription drugs, and general pharmacy references.

The organization of the fifth edition has been revised to reflect the current changes in the undergraduate pharmacy curriculum. Part I, Pharmaceutical Sciences, contains subject matter pertaining to the basic science of pharmacy. Part II, Pharmacy Practice, contains subject matter for the practice of pharmacy with emphasis on pharmaceutical care.

This volume represents the contributions of more than two dozen specialists, each delivering a current summary of his or her field to a review guide that is not only accurate and up-to-date, but also comprehensible to students, teachers, and practitioners alike.

Taking a Test

One of the least attractive aspects of pursuing an education is the necessity of being examined on the material that has been presented. Instructors do not like to prepare tests, and students do not like to take them.

However, students are required to take many examinations during their learning careers, and little if any time is spent acquainting them with the positive aspects of tests and with systematic and successful methods for approaching them. Students perceive tests as punitive and sometimes feel that they are merely opportunities for the instructor to discover what the student has forgotten or has never learned. Students need to view tests as opportunities to display their knowledge and to use them as tools for developing prescriptions for further study and learning.

While preparing for any exam, class and board exams as well as practice exams, it is important that students learn as much as they can about the subject they will be tested on as well as prepare to discover just how much they may not know. Students should study to acquire knowledge, not just to prepare for tests. For the well-prepared student, the chances of passing far exceed the chances of failing.

Materials Needed for Test Preparation

In preparing for a test, most students collect far too much study material, only to find that they simply do not have time to go through all of it. They are defeated before they begin because either they cannot get through all the material, leaving areas unstudied, or they race through the material so quickly that they cannot benefit from the activity.

It is generally more efficient for the student to use materials already at hand; that is, class notes, one good outline to cover and strengthen all areas and to quickly review the whole topic, and one good text as a reference for complex material that requires further explanation.

Also, many students attempt to memorize far too much information, rather than learning and understanding less material and then relying on that learned information to determine the answers to questions at the time of the examination. Relying too heavily on memorized material causes anxiety, and the more anxious students become during a test, the less learned knowledge they are likely to use.

Attitude and Approach

A positive attitude and a realistic approach are essential to successful test taking. If the student concentrates on the negative aspects of tests or on the potential for failure, anxiety increases and performance decreases. A negative attitude generally develops if the student concentrates on "I must pass" rather than on "I can pass." "What if I fail?" becomes the major factor motivating the student to run from failure rather than toward success. This results from placing too much emphasis on scores. The score received is only one aspect of test performance. Test performance also indicates the student's ability to use differential reasoning.

In each question with five alternatives, of which one is correct, there are four alternatives that are incorrect. If deductive reasoning is used, the choices can be viewed as having possibilities of being correct. The elimination of wrong choices increases the odds that a student will be able to recognize the correct choice. Even if the correct choice does not become evident, the probability of guessing correctly increases. Eliminating incorrect choices on a test can result in choosing the correct answer.

Answering questions based on what is incorrect is difficult for many students since they have had nearly 20 years of experience taking tests with the implied assertion that knowledge can be displayed only by knowing what is correct. It must be remembered, however, that students can display knowledge by knowing something is wrong, just as they can display it by knowing something is right.

Preparing for the Examination

1. Study for yourself. Although some of the material may seem irrelevant, the more you learn now, the less you will have to learn later. Also, do not let the fear of the test rob you of an important part of your education. If you study to learn, the task is less distasteful than studying solely to pass a test.
2. Review all areas. You should not be selective by studying perceived weak areas and ignoring perceived strong areas. Cover all of the material, putting added emphasis on weak areas.
3. Attempt to understand, not just to memorize, the material. Ask yourself: To whom does the material apply? When does it apply? Where does it apply? How does it apply? Understanding the connections among these points allows for longer retention and aids in those situations when guessing strategies may be needed.

4. Try to anticipate questions that might appear on the test. Ask yourself how you might construct a question on a specific topic.
5. Give yourself a couple days of rest before the test. Studying up to the last moment will increase your anxiety and cause potential confusion.

Taking the Examination

1. Be sure to pace yourself to use the test time optimally. You should use all of your allotted time; if you finish too early, you probably did so by moving too quickly through the test.
2. Read each question and all the alternatives carefully before you begin to make decisions. Remember, the questions contain clues, as do the answer choices.
3. Read the directions for each question set carefully. You would be amazed at how many students make mistakes in tests simply because they have not paid close attention to the directions.
4. It is not advisable to leave blanks with the intention of coming back to answer questions later. If you feel that you must come back to a question, mark the best choice and place a note in the margin. Generally speaking, it is best not to change answers once you have made a decision. Your considered reaction and first response are correct more often than changes made out of frustration or anxiety.
5. Do not let anxiety destroy your confidence. If you have prepared conscientiously, you know enough to pass. Use all that you have learned.
6. Do not try to determine how well you are doing as you proceed. You will not be able to make an objective assessment, and your anxiety will increase.
7. Do not become frustrated or angry about what appear to be bad or difficult questions. You simply do not know the answers; you cannot know everything.

Specific Test-Taking Strategies

Read the entire question carefully, regardless of format. Test questions have multiple parts. Concentrate on picking out the pertinent key words that will help you problem-solve. Words such as "always," "all," "never," "mostly," "primarily," and so forth play significant roles. In all types of questions, distractors with terms such as "always" or "never" most often are incorrect. Adjectives and adverbs can completely change the meaning of questions—pay close attention to them. The knowledge and application of grammar often are key to dissecting questions.

Multiple-Choice Questions

Read the question and the choices carefully to become familiar with the data provided. Remember, in multiple-choice questions there is one correct answer and there are four distractors, or incorrect answers. (Distractors are plausible and possibly correct, or they would not be called distractors.) They are generally correct for part of the question but not for the entire question. Dissecting the question into parts helps eliminate distractors.

Many students think that they must always start at option A and make a decision before they move to B, thus forcing decisions they are not ready to make. Your first decisions should be made on those choices you feel the most confident about.

Compare the choices with each part of the question. To be wrong, a choice needs to be incorrect for only part of the question. To be correct, it must be totally correct. If you believe a choice is partially incorrect, tentatively eliminate that choice. Make notes next to the choices regarding tentative decisions. One method is to place a minus sign next to the choices you are certain are incorrect and a plus sign next to those that potentially are correct. Finally, place a zero next to any choice you do not understand or need to come back to for further inspection. Do not feel that you must make final decisions until you have examined all choices carefully.

When you have eliminated as many choices as you can, decide which of those that remain has the highest probability of being correct. Above all, be honest with yourself. If you do not know the answer, eliminate as many choices as possible and choose reasonably.

Multiple True-False Questions

Multiple true-false questions are not as difficult as some students make them. These are the questions for which you must select:
A if only I is correct.
B if only III is correct.
C if I and II are correct.
D if II and III are correct.
E if all (I, II, and III) are correct.

Remember that the name for this type of question is multiple true-false, and then use this concept. Become familiar with each choice, and make notes. Then concentrate on the one choice you feel is definitely incorrect. If you can find one incorrect alternative, you can eliminate three choices immediately and be down to a 50-50 probability of guessing the correct answer. If choice A is incorrect, so are C and E; if choice B is incorrect, so are choices D and E. Therefore, you are down to a 50-50 probability of guessing the correct answer.

After eliminating the choices you are sure are incorrect, concentrate on the choice that will make your final decision. For instance, if you discard choice I, you have eliminated alternatives A, C, and E. This leaves B (III) and D (II and III). Concentrate on choice II, and decide if it is true or false. (Take the path of least resistance and concentrate on the smallest possible number of items while making a decision.) Obviously, if none of the choices is found to be incorrect, the answer is E (all).

Guessing
Nothing takes the place of a firm knowledge base, but having little information to work with, you may find it necessary to guess at the correct answer. A few simple rules can help increase your guessing accuracy. Always guess consistently if you have no idea what is correct; that is, after eliminating all that you can, make the choice that agrees with your intuition or choose the option closest to the top of the list that has not been eliminated as a potential answer.

When guessing at questions that present with choices in numeric form, you will often find the choices listed in an ascending or descending order. It is generally not wise to guess the first or last alternative, since these are usually extreme values and are most likely incorrect.

Using a Practice Exam to Learn
All too often, students do not take full advantage of practice exams. There is a tendency to complete the exam, score it, look up the correct answer to those questions missed, and then forget the entire thing.

In fact, great educational benefits could be derived if students would spend more time using practice tests as learning tools. As mentioned previously, incorrect choices in test questions are plausible and partially correct, or they would not fulfill their purpose as distractors. This means that it is just as beneficial to look up the incorrect choices as the correct choices to discover specifically why they are incorrect. In this way, it is possible to learn better test-taking skills as the subtlety of question construction is uncovered.

In addition, it is advisable to go back and attempt to restructure each question to see if all the choices can be made correct by modifying the question. By doing this, you will learn four times as much. By all means, look up the right answer and explanation. Then, focus on each of the other choices, and ask yourself under what conditions they might be correct.

Summary
Ideally, examinations are designed to determine how much material students have learned and how that material is used in the successful completion of the examination. Students will be successful if these suggestions are followed:
- Develop a positive attitude, and maintain that attitude.
- Be realistic in determining the amount of material you attempt to master and in the score you hope to attain.
- Read the directions for each type of question and the questions themselves closely, and follow the directions carefully.
- Bring differential reasoning to each question in the examination.
- Guess intelligently and consistently when guessing strategies must be used.
- Use the test as an opportunity to display your knowledge and as a tool for developing prescriptions for further study and learning.

Board examinations are not easy. They may be almost impossible for those who have unrealistic expectations or for those who allow misinformation concerning the exams to produce anxiety out of proportion to the task at hand. Examinations are manageable if they are approached with a positive attitude and with consistent use of all of the information the student has learned.

Michael J. O'Donnell

Introduction to the NAPLEX®

After graduation from an accredited pharmacy program, the prospective pharmacist must demonstrate the competency to practice pharmacy. The standards of competence for the practice of pharmacy are set by each state board of pharmacy. The NAPLEX™ is the principal instrument used by the state board of pharmacy to assess the knowledge and proficiency necessary for a candidate to practice pharmacy. The National Association of Boards of Pharmacy™ (NABP™) develops examinations that enable boards of pharmacy to assess the competence of candidates seeking licensure to practice pharmacy. Each state board of pharmacy may impose additional examinations. The two major examinations developed by NABP are:

- The North American Pharmacist Licensure Examination™ (NAPLEX™)
- Multistate Pharmacy Jurisprudence Examination™ (MPJE™)

Registration information and a description of these computerized examinations may be found on the NABP website: http://www.nabp.org. Before submitting registration materials, the pharmacy candidate should contact the board of pharmacy for additional information regarding procedures, deadline dates, and required documentation.

The NAPLEX™ is a computer-adaptive test that measures a candidate's knowledge and ability by assessing the answers before presenting the next test question. If the answer is correct, the computer will select a more difficult question from the test item pool in an appropriate content area; if the answer is incorrect, an easier question will be selected by the computer. The NAPLEX™ score is based on the difficulty level of the questions answered correctly.

NAPLEX™ consists of 185 multiple-choice test questions. Of these, 150 questions are used to calculate the test score. The remaining 35 items serve as pretest questions and does not affect the NAPLEX™ score. Pretest questions are administered to evaluate the item's difficulty level for possible inclusion as a scored question in future exams. These pretest questions are dispersed throughout the exam and cannot be identified by the candidate.

A majority of the questions on the NAPLEX™ are asked in a scenario-based format (i.e., patient profiles with accompanying test questions). To properly analyze and answer the questions presented, the candidate must refer to the information provided in the patient profile. Some questions appear in a stand-alone format and should be answered solely from the information provided in the question.

All NAPLEX™ questions are based on competency statements that are reviewed and revised periodically. The NAPLEX™ Competency Statements describe the knowledge, judgment, and skills that the candidate is expected to demonstrate as an entry-level pharmacist. A complete description of the NAPLEX™ Competency Statements is published on the NABP website. The NAPLEX™ examines three general areas of competence:

- Management of drug therapy to optimize patient outcomes
- Safe and accurate preparation and dispensing of medications
- Drug information and promotion of public health

The NAPLEX™ *Candidates' Review Guide* may be obtained from a school or college of pharmacy or from the National Association of Boards of Pharmacy.

1
Drug Product Development in the Pharmaceutical Industry

Anton H. Amann
Leon Shargel

I. INTRODUCTION

A. Active pharmaceutical ingredient (API)

1. A **drug substance** is the API or component that produces pharmacological activity.

2. The API may be **produced by** chemical synthesis, recovery from a natural product, enzymatic reaction, recombinant DNA technology, fermentation, or a combination of these processes. Further purification of the API may be needed before it can be used in a drug product.

3. A **new chemical entity (NCE)** is a drug substance with unknown clinical, toxicologic, physical, and chemical properties. In addition, the United States Food and Drug Administration (FDA) considers an NCE as an API that has not been approved for marketing in the United States.

B. Drug product

1. A drug product is the **finished dosage form** (e.g., capsule, tablet, ointment) that contains the API, generally in association with other excipients, or inert substances.

2. Different **approaches** are generally used to produce drug products that contain NCEs, product line extensions, generic drug products, and specialty drug products.

C. Drug products containing new chemical entities. The following phases of product development proceed sequentially.

1. **Preclinical stage.** Animal pharmacology and toxicology data are obtained to determine the safety and efficacy of the drug. An **investigational new drug (IND) application** for human testing is submitted to the FDA. Because little is known about the human and the therapeutic/toxicologic potential, many drug products will not reach the marketplace. No attempt is made to develop a final formulation during the preclinical stage. **Nonclinical** studies are nonhuman studies that may continue at any stage of research to obtain additional information concerning the pharmacology and toxicology of the drug.

2. **Phase I**
   a. Clinical testing takes place after the IND application is submitted.
   b. Healthy volunteers are used in phase I clinical studies to determine drug tolerance and toxicity.
   c. For oral drug administration, a simple hard gelatin capsule formulation containing the API is usually used for the IND studies.
   d. Toxicologic studies including acute, chronic, subchronic, mutagenicity, and other toxicologic studies in various animal species are planned during this phase.

3. **Phase II**
   a. A limited number of patients with the disease or condition for which the drug was developed are treated under close supervision.

    b. Dose–response studies and pharmacokinetics are performed to determine the optimum dosage regimen for treating the disease.

    c. Safety is measured by attempting to determine the **therapeutic index** (ratio of toxic dose to effective dose).

    d. A final drug formulation is developed. This formulation is bioequivalent to the dosage form used in the initial clinical studies.

    e. Chronic toxicity studies are started in two species, which will normally last more than 2 years' duration.

  4. Phase III

    a. Large-scale, **multicenter clinical studies** are performed with the final dosage form developed in phase II. These studies are done to determine the safety and efficacy of the drug product in a large patient population with the disease or condition for which the drug was developed.

    b. Side effects are monitored. In a large population, new toxic effects may occur that were not evident in previous clinical trials.

  5. Submission of a **new drug application (NDA).** An NDA is submitted to the FDA for review and approval after the completion of clinical trials that show to the satisfaction of the medical community that the drug product is effective by all parameters, and is reasonably safe as demonstrated by animal and human studies.

  6. Phase IV

    a. After the NDA is submitted and before approval to market the product is obtained from the FDA, manufacturing **scale-up** activities occur. Scale-up is the increase in the batch size from the clinical batch, the submission batch, or both, up to the full-scale production batch size, using the finished, marketed product.

    b. The **drug formulation** may be modified slightly as a result of data obtained during the manufacturing scale-up and validation process.

  7. Phase V

    a. After the FDA grants market approval of the drug, product development may continue.

    b. The drug product may be improved as a result of equipment, regulatory, supply, or market demands.

    c. Additional clinical studies may be performed in special populations such as the elderly, pediatric, renal-impaired patients, and others to obtain information on the efficacy of the drug in these subjects.

    d. Additional clinical studies may be performed to determine if the drug can be used for a new indication.

D. Product line extensions are dosage forms in which the physical form or strength, but not the use or indication, of the product changes. Product line extension is usually performed during phase III, IV, or V.

E. Generic drug products

  1. After **patent expiration** of the brand drug product, a generic drug product may be marketed. A generic drug product is **therapeutically equivalent to the brand name drug product** and contains the same amount of the drug in the same type of dosage form (e.g., tablets, liquids, injectables).

  2. A generic drug product must be **bioequivalent** (i.e., have the same rate and extent of drug absorption) to the brand drug product. Therefore, a generic drug product is expected to give the same clinical response (see Chapter 7). These studies are normally performed with healthy human volunteers.

  3. The generic drug product may differ from the brand product in **physical appearance** (i.e., size, color, shape) or in the amount and type of excipients only for tablets.

  4. A generic drug product may not differ in both the qualitative and quantitative compositions for liquids, injectables, semisolids, transdermals, inhalation products, and ophthalmic products, unless adequate safety studies have been performed.

  5. Before a drug product is marketed, the manufacturer must submit an **abbreviated new drug application (ANDA)** to the FDA for approval. Because preclinical safety and efficacy studies have already been performed for the NDA-approved brand product, human bioequivalence studies are generally required for the ANDA instead of clinical trials. The chemistry, manufacturing, and controls requirements for the generic drug product are similar to those for the brand name drug product.

F. Specialty drug products are existing products that are developed as a new delivery system or for a new therapeutic indication. The safety and efficacy of the drug product was established in the initial NDA-approved dosage form. For example, the nitroglycerin transdermal delivery system (patch) was developed after experience with nitroglycerin sublingual tablets.

II. PRODUCT DEVELOPMENT. For each drug, various activities and information are required to develop a safe, effective, and stable dosage form.

A. New chemical entities

    1. Preformulation is the characterization of the physical and chemical properties of the active drug substance and dosage form. The therapeutic indication of the drug and the route of administration will dictate the type of drug product or drug delivery system (e.g., immediate release, controlled release, suppository, parenteral, transdermal) that needs to be developed.

        a. Preformulation activities are usually performed during the preclinical stage. However, these activities may continue into phases I and II.

        b. The following information is obtained during preformulation.

            (1) General characteristics, including particle size and shape, crystalline features, polymorphism, density, surface area, hygroscopicity (ability to take up and retain moisture), and powder flow

            (2) Solubility characteristics, including intrinsic dissolution, pH solubility profile, and general solubility characteristics in various solvents

            (3) Chemical characteristics, including surface energy, pH stability profile, pK_a, temperature stability (dry or under various humidity conditions), and excipient interactions

            (4) Analytical methods development, including development of a stability indicating method (measures both the API and degradation products), cleaning methods, and the identification of impurities

    2. Formulation development is a continuing process. Initial drug formulations are developed for early clinical studies. When the submission of an NDA is considered, the manufacturer attempts to develop the final (marketed) dosage form. The dose of the drug and the route of administration are important in determining the modifications needed.

        a. Injectable drug product

            (1) A final injectable drug product is usually developed in the preclinical phase.

            (2) A major concern is the stability of the drug in solution.

            (3) Because few excipients are allowed in injectable products, the formulator must choose a final product early in the development process.

            (4) If the formulation is changed, bioavailability studies are not required for intravenous injections because the product is injected directly into the body.

            (5) Formulation changes may require acute toxicity studies.

        b. Topical drug products for local application include antibacterials, antifungals, corticosteroids, and local anesthetics.

            (1) The final dosage form for a topical drug product is usually developed during phase I because any major formulation changes may require further clinical trials.

            (2) The release of the drug from the matrix is measured in vitro with various diffusion cell models.

            (3) Significant problems encountered with locally acting topical drug products include local irritation and systemic drug absorption.

        c. Topical drug products for systemic drug absorption include drug delivery through the skin (transdermal), mucous membranes (intranasal), and rectal mucosa.

            (1) A prototype formulation is developed for phase I.

            (2) A final topical drug product is developed during phase III after the available technology and desired systemic levels are considered.

        d. Oral drug products

            (1) Prototype dosage forms are often developed during the **preclinical phase** to assure that the drug is optimally available and that the product dissolves in the gastrointestinal tract.

  (2) In the early stages of product development, **hard gelatin** capsule dosage forms are often developed for **phase I** clinical trials. If the drug shows efficacy, the same drug formulation may be used in phase II studies.
  (3) Final product development begins when the drug proceeds during phase II and prior to initiating phase III clinical studies.

  3. Final drug product. Considerations in the development of a final dosage form include:
  a. Color, shape, size, taste, viscosity, sensitivity, skin feel, and physical appearance of the dosage form
  b. Size and shape of the package or container
  c. Production equipment
  d. Production site
  e. Country of origin in which the drug is to be manufactured
  f. Country in which to market the drug

B. Product line extensions generally are defined as drug products containing an NDA-approved drug in a different dosage strength or in a different dosage form (e.g., modified release, oral liquid).

  1. Solid oral product line extensions
  a. The simplest dosage form to develop is a different dosage strength of a drug in a tablet or capsule. Only bioequivalence studies are needed.
  b. A **modified-release** dosage form is more difficult to develop when only an instant-release dosage form exists. Clinical trials are normally required.
  c. Considerations in developing these dosage forms are similar to those for the final drug product (see II A 3).
  d. Marketing has a role in the choice of the dosage form.
  e. Because the original brand drug product information contributes to the body of knowledge about the drug, no preformulation is needed. All other factors considered for the original product are similar. If the relation between *in vitro* dissolution and *in vivo* bioavailability is known, the innovator can progress to a finished dosage form relatively quickly.
  f. Regulatory approval is based on the following:
    (1) Stability information
    (2) Analytical and manufacturing controls
    (3) Bioequivalence studies
    (4) Clinical trials (in the case of modified-release dosage forms)
  g. A new therapeutic indication for a drug requires new **efficacy studies** and a new NDA.

  2. Liquid product line extensions
  a. If the current marketed product is a liquid preparation, then the same factors as for the solid oral dosage forms are considered (see II B 1 a–g).
  b. If the marketed product is a solid oral dosage form and the product line extension is a liquid, product development must proceed with caution because the rate and extent of absorption for liquid and solid dosage forms may not be the same.
  c. Regulatory approval requires:
    (1) Bioequivalence studies
    (2) Stability information
    (3) Analytical and manufacturing controls
    (4) Safety studies (e.g., depending on the drug substance, local irritation)
    (5) Clinical trials, if the rate and extent of drug absorption are drastically altered from the original dosage form

C. Combination products are products comprised of two or more regulated components (i.e., drug/device, biologic/device, drug//biologic, or drug/device/biologic) that are physically, chemically, or otherwise combined or mixed and produced as a single entity.

  1. These may be two or more separate products packaged together in a single package or as a unit and comprised of drug and device products, device and biological products, or biological and drug products.

  2. Examples may include an inhalation steroid (e.g., beclomethasone inhalation aerosol) in which the device component is important for delivery of the steroid.

III. PREAPPROVAL INSPECTIONS (PAIs)

A. The **manufacturing facility** is inspected by the Food and Drug Administration (FDA) after an NDA, abbreviated antibiotic drug application (AADA), or ANDA is submitted, and before the application is approved.

B. A PAI may be initiated if a **major change** is reported in a supplemental application to an NDA, AADA, or ANDA.

C. During the PAI, the FDA investigator:

1. **Performs** a general current good manufacturing practice (cGMP) inspection relating specifically to the drug product intended for the market

2. **Reviews** the development report to verify that the drug product has enough supporting documentation to ensure a validated product and a rationale for the manufacturing directions

3. **Consults** the chemistry, manufacturing, and control (CMC) section of the NDA, AADA, or ANDA and determines the capability of the manufacturer to produce the drug product as described

4. **Verifies** the traceability of the information submitted in the CMC section to the original laboratory notebooks, electronic information, and batch records

5. **Recommends** whether to approve the manufacture of the drug product after the PAI

IV. SCALE-UP AND POSTAPPROVAL CHANGES (SUPAC)

A. Purpose. These guidelines are intended to reduce the number of manufacturing changes that require preapproval by the FDA. The guidelines are published by the FDA on the Internet (http://www.fda.gov/cder/guidance/index.htm).

B. Function. These guidelines provide recommendations to sponsors of NDAs, AADAs, and ANDAs during the following changes in the postapproval period.

1. To make slight changes in the amount of the excipient to aid in the processing of the product during scale-up

2. To change the **site** of manufacture

3. To **scale-up** (increase) or **scale-down** (decrease) the batch size of the formulation

4. To change the manufacturing **process** or **equipment**

C. The FDA must be notified about a proposed change to a drug product through different **regulatory documentation,** depending on the type of change proposed.

1. **Annual report.** Changes that are unlikely to have any detectable effect on formulation quality and performance can be instituted without approval by the FDA, and reported annually. Examples of these changes include:
   a. **Compliance** with an official compendium
   b. **Label description** of the drug product or how it is supplied (not involving dosage strength or dosage form)
   c. Deletion of an **ingredient** that affects only the color of the product
   d. Extension of the expiration date based on full shelf-life data obtained from a protocol approved in the application
   e. **Container** and **closure system** for the drug product (except a change in container size for nonsolid dosage forms) based on equivalency to the approved system under a protocol approved in the application or published in an official compendium
   f. Addition or deletion of an **alternate analytical method**

2. **Changes being effected (CBE) supplement.** Changes that probably would not have any detectable effect, but require some validation efforts, require specific documentation, depending on the change. A supplement is submitted, and the change can be implemented without previous approval by the FDA or, in some cases, FDA has 30 days to review the

change (**CBE-30**). FDA may reject this supplement. Some examples of reasons for submitting a supplement include:

    a. Addition of a **new specification** or test method or changes in methods, facilities, or controls

    b. **Label change** to add or strengthen a contraindication, warning, precaution, or adverse reaction

    c. Use of a **different facility** to manufacture the drug substance and drug product (the manufacturing process in the new facility does not differ materially from that in the former facility, and the new facility has received a satisfactory current good manufacturing practice inspection within the previous 2 years covering that manufacturing process)

3. Preapproval supplement. Changes that could have a significant effect on formulation quality and performance require specific documentation. This supplement must be approved before the proposed change is initiated. Some appropriate examples for preapproval supplement are:

    a. Addition or deletion of an **ingredient**

    b. Relaxation of the limits for a **specification**

    c. Establishment of a new **regulatory analytical method**

    d. Deletion of a **specification** or regulatory analytical method

    e. Change in the method of **manufacture** of the drug product, including changing or relaxing an in-process control

    f. Extension of the **expiration date** of the drug product based on data obtained under a new or revised stability testing protocol that has not been approved in the application

D. When any change to a drug product is proposed, the manufacturer must show that the resultant drug product is **bioequivalent** and **therapeutically equivalent** to the original approved drug product (see Chapter 7).

    1. A **minor change** is a change that has minimal potential to have an adverse effect on the identity, strength, quality, purity, or potency of the product as they may relate to the safety or effectiveness of the product. If the proposed change is considered **minor** by the FDA, bioequivalence may be demonstrated by comparative dissolution profiles for the original and new formulations.

    2. A **major change** is one that has substantial potential to have an adverse effect on the identity, strength, quality, purity, or potency of a product as they may relate to the safety or effectiveness of the product. If the proposed change is considered **major** by the FDA, bioequivalence must be demonstrated by an in vivo bioequivalence study comparing the original and new formulations.

V. GOOD MANUFACTURING PRACTICES (GMPs) are regulations developed by the FDA. GMPs are minimum requirements that the industry must meet when manufacturing, processing, packing, or holding human and veterinary drugs. These regulations, also known as **cGMPs,** establish criteria for personnel, facilities, and manufacturing processes to ensure that the finished drug product has the correct identity, strength, quality, and purity characteristics.

A. Quality control (QC) is the group within the manufacturer that is responsible for establishing process and product specifications.

    1. Specifications are the criteria to which a drug product should conform to be considered acceptable quality for its intended use.

    2. The QC unit **tests** the product and verifies that the specifications are met. QC testing includes the **acceptance** or **rejection** of the incoming raw materials, packaging components, drug products, water system, and environmental conditions (e.g., heating, ventilation, and air-conditioning; air quality; microbial load) that exist during the manufacturing process.

B. Quality assurance (QA) is the group within the manufacturer that determines that the systems and facilities are adequate, and that the **written procedures** are followed to ensure that the finished drug product meets the applicable specifications for quality.

STUDY QUESTIONS

Directions: Each item below contains three suggested answers of which **one or more** is correct. Choose the answer

- **A**   if **I only** is correct
- **B**   if **III only** is correct
- **C**   if **I and II** are correct
- **D**   if **II and III** are correct
- **E**   if **I, II, and III** are correct

1. Healthy human volunteers are used in drug development for

I. phase I testing after the submission of an investigational new drug (IND) application

II. generic drug development for an abbreviated new drug application (ANDA) submission

III. phase III testing just before the submission of a new drug application (NDA)

2. The required information contained in a new drug application (NDA) that is NOT included in the abbreviated new drug application (ANDA) consists of

I. preclinical animal toxicity studies

II. clinical efficacy studies

III. human safety and tolerance studies

3. A product line extension contains the new drug application (NDA) approved drug in a

I. new dosage form

II. new dosage strength

III. new therapeutic indication

Directions: Each of the numbered items or incomplete statements in this section is followed by answers or by completions of the statement. Select the **one** lettered answer or completion that is **best** in each case.

4. The regulations developed by the United States Food and Drug Administration (FDA) for the pharmaceutical industry for meeting the minimum requirements in the manufacturing, processing, packing, or holding of human and veterinary drugs are known as

(A)   good manufacturing practices (GMPs)
(B)   quality assurance
(C)   quality control
(D)   preapproval inspection (PAI)
(E)   scale-up and postapproval changes

5. The unit within the pharmaceutical manufacturer that ensures that the finished dosage form has met all the specifications for its intended use is

(A)   analytical methods unit
(B)   marketing and sales unit
(C)   preapproval inspection unit
(D)   quality assurance unit
(E)   quality control unit

6. Manufacturers may make a change in the formulation after market approval. If the change in the formulation is considered a minor change, the manufacturer needs only to report the change to the FDA in

(A)   annual report
(B)   preapproval supplement
(C)   investigational new drug (IND) submission
(D)   changes being effected supplement—30 days
(E)   no report is required for a minor change

ANSWERS AND EXPLANATIONS

1. The answer is C (I, II) *[I C 2 b, 4 a].*
Phase I testing is the first set of human studies performed during new drug development. Phase I studies establish the tolerance and toxicity of the drug in humans. Clinical studies for generic drug development are most often performed in healthy human volunteers. These studies establish the bioequivalence of the generic drug product against the brand drug product. Phase III testing entails large-scale, multicenter clinical studies performed in patients with the disease or condition to be treated. Phase III studies determine the safety and efficacy of the drug in a large patient population.

2. The answer is E (I, II, and III) *[I C 5, E 5].*
The development of a new drug requires extensive toxicity and efficacy testing in animals and humans. The new drug application (NDA) documents all studies performed on the drug. The abbreviated new drug application (ANDA) is used for generic drug product submissions. The generic drug product is similar to the original brand drug product that has already been marketed. Because the efficacy, safety, and toxicity of this drug product have been studied and documented, further studies of this nature are unnecessary.

3. The answer is C *(I, II) [I D].*
Product line extensions are developed after further studies with the original new drug application (NDA) approved drug product. From these studies, the manufacturer may develop a new dosage form (e.g., controlled-release product) or a new dosage strength. A new therapeutic indication requires an NDA.

4. The answer is A *[V].*
Quality control and quality assurance follow good manufacturing practice (GMP) regulations in ensuring that the finished product meets all applicable specifications for quality. The United States Food and Drug Administration (FDA) may inspect a manufacturing site [preapproval inspection (PAI)] before the drug application is approved. Additionally, the FDA must be notified about any proposed changes to an approved drug product.

5. The answer is E *[V A].*
The quality control unit performs the appropriate tests on the dosage form. Preapproval inspection is performed by the United States Food and Drug Administration (FDA) compliance inspectors who inspect the pharmaceutical manufacturer and review the procedures and records for manufacturing the finished dosage form prior to market approval by the FDA. The analytical development unit develops the analytical methods used in testing the drug product.

6. The answer is A *[IV D].*
All changes in the formulation must be reported to the United States Food and Drug Administration (FDA). A **minor change** is a change that has minimal potential to have an adverse effect on the identity, strength, quality, purity, or potency of the product as they may relate to the safety or effectiveness of the product. Changes that are unlikely to have any detectable effect on formulation quality and performance can be instituted without approval by the FDA, and only need to be reported annually in the annual report.

2
Pharmaceutical Calculations and Statistics
Riccardo L. Boni

I. FUNDAMENTALS OF MEASUREMENT AND CALCULATION

A. Ratio and proportion

1. **Ratio.** The relative magnitude of two like quantities is a ratio, which is expressed as a fraction. Certain basic principles apply to the ratio, as they do to all fractions.
   a. When the two terms of a ratio are multiplied or divided by the same number, the value of the ratio is unchanged.
   $$1/3 \times 2/2 = 2/6 = 1/3$$
   b. Two ratios with the same value are equivalent. Equivalent ratios have equal cross products and equal reciprocals. As an example,
   $$1/3 = 2/6$$
   and
   $$1 \times 6 = 3 \times 2 = 6$$
   If two ratios are equal, then their reciprocals are equal:
   $$\text{if } 1/3 = 2/6, \text{ then } 3/1 = 6/2$$

2. **Proportion.** The expression of the equality of two ratios is a proportion. The product of the extremes is equal to the product of the means for any proportion. Furthermore, the numerator of the one fraction equals the product of its denominator and the other fraction (i.e., one missing term can always be found given the other three terms).
   a. Most pharmaceutical calculations can be performed by use of proportion. Several examples follow.
      (1) If 240 mL of a cough syrup contain 480 mg of dextromethorphan hydrobromide, then what mass of drug is contained in a child's dose (5 mL) of syrup?
      $$\frac{240 \text{ mL}}{5 \text{ mL}} = \frac{480 \text{ mg}}{X \text{ mg}}$$
      $$X = \frac{480 \times 5}{240} = 10 \text{ mg}$$

      (2) If a child's dose (5 mL) of a cough syrup contains 10 mg of dextromethorphan hydrobromide, what mass of drug is contained in 240 mL?
      $$\frac{240 \text{ mL}}{5 \text{ mL}} = \frac{X \text{ mg}}{10 \text{ mg}}$$
      $$X = \frac{240 \times 10}{5} = 480 \text{ mg}$$

      (3) If the amount of dextromethorphan hydrobromide in 240 mL of cough syrup is 480 mg, what would be the volume required for a child's dose of 10 mg?
      $$\frac{X \text{ mL}}{240 \text{ mL}} = \frac{10 \text{ mg}}{480 \text{ mg}}$$
      $$X = \frac{10 \times 240}{480} = 5 \text{ mL}$$

   b. **Mixed ratios.** Some pharmacists use mixed ratios (where dissimilar units are used in the numerator and denominator of each ratio) in their proportion calculations. Such computations generally give correct answers, providing the conditions where mixed ratios cannot be used are known. A later example shows mixed ratios leading to failure in the case of dilution, where inverse proportions are required. For **inverse proportions,** similar units must be used in the numerator and denominator of each ratio. Following is an example of a mixed ratio calculation using the previous example problem.

$$\frac{X \text{ mL}}{10 \text{ mL}} = \frac{240 \text{ mg}}{480 \text{ mg}}$$

$$X = \frac{240 \times 10}{480} = 5 \text{ mL}$$

The **same answer** is obtained in this example whether we use proper ratios, with similar units in numerator and denominator, or mixed ratios. This is not the case when dealing with inverse proportions.

3. **Inverse proportion.** The most common example of the need for inverse proportion for the pharmacist is the case of **dilution.** Whereas in the previous examples of proportion the relationships involved direct proportion, the case of dilution calls for an inverse proportion (i.e., as volume increases, concentration decreases). The necessity of using inverse proportions for dilution problems is shown in this example.

If 120 mL of a 10% stock solution are diluted to 240 mL, what is the final concentration? Using inverse proportion,

$$\frac{120 \text{ mL}}{240 \text{ mL}} = \frac{X\%}{10\%}$$

$$\frac{120 \times 10}{240} = 5\%$$

As expected, the final concentration is one half the original concentration because the volume is doubled. However, if the pharmacist attempts to use direct proportion and neglects to estimate an appropriate answer, the resulting calculation would provide an answer of 20%, which is twice the actual concentration.

$$\frac{120 \text{ mL}}{240 \text{ mL}} = \frac{10\%}{X\%}$$

$$\frac{240 \times 10}{120} = 20\% \text{ (incorrect answer)}$$

Likewise, the pharmacist using mixed ratios fails in this case.

$$\frac{120 \text{ mL}}{10\%} = \frac{240 \text{ mL}}{X\%}$$

and

$$\frac{10 \times 240}{120} = 20\% \text{ (again, an incorrect answer)}$$

B. **Aliquot.** A pharmacist requires the aliquot method of measurement when the **precision** of his measuring device is not great enough for the required measurement. Aliquot calculations can be used for measurement of solids or liquids, allowing the pharmacist to realize the required precision through a process of measuring a multiple of the desired amount followed by dilution and finally selection and measurement of an aliquot part that contains the desired amount of material. This example problem involves weighing by the aliquot method, using a prescription balance.

A prescription balance has a sensitivity requirement of 6 mg. How would you weigh 10 mg of drug with an accuracy of ±5%, using a suitable diluent?

1. First, calculate the least weighable quantity for the balance with a sensitivity requirement of 6 mg, assuming ±5% accuracy is required.

$$\frac{100 \times 6 \text{ mg}}{5} = 120 \text{ mg (least weighable quantity for our balance)}$$

2. Now, it is obvious that an aliquot calculation is required because 10 mg of drug are required, whereas the least weighable quantity is 120 mg in order to achieve the required percentage of error. Using the least weighable quantity method of aliquot measurement, use the smallest quantity weighable on the balance at each step in order to preserve materials.

   a. Weigh 12 x 10 mg = 120 mg of drug.
   b. Dilute the 120 mg of drug (from step **a**) with a suitable diluent to achieve a mixture that will provide 10 mg of drug in each 120 mg aliquot. The amount of diluent to be used can be determined through **proportion.**

$$\frac{120 \text{ mg drug}}{10 \text{ mg drug}} = \frac{X \text{ mg total mixture}}{120 \text{ mg aliquot mixture}}$$

$$X = 1440 \text{ mg total mixture}$$

$$1440 \text{ mg total} - 120 \text{ mg drug} = 1320 \text{ mg diluent}$$

   c. Weigh 120 mg (1/12) of the total mixture, which will contain the required 10 mg of drug.

II. SYSTEMS OF MEASURE.
The pharmacist must be familiar with **three systems** of measure, including the **metric system** and two common systems of measure (the **avoirdupois** and **apothecaries'** systems). The primary system of measure in pharmacy and medicine is the metric system. Most students find it easiest to convert measurements in the common systems to metric units. A table of conversion equivalents is provided and should be memorized by the pharmacist (see Appendix A). The metric system, because of its universal acceptance and broad use, will not be reviewed here.

A. Apothecaries' system of fluid measure. The apothecaries' system of fluid measure is summarized in Appendix A.

B. Apothecaries' system for measuring weight. The apothecaries' system for measuring weight includes units of grains, scruples, drams, ounces, and pounds (see Appendix A).

C. Avoirdupois system of measuring weight. The avoirdupois (AV) system of measuring weight includes the grain, ounce, and pound. The grain is a unit common with the apothecaries' system and allows for easy conversion between the systems. The avoirdupois pound, however, is 16 AV ounces in contrast to the apothecaries' pound, which is 12 apothecaries' ounces (see Appendix A).

D. Conversion equivalents (see Appendix A)

III. REDUCING AND ENLARGING FORMULAS.
The pharmacist is often required to reduce or enlarge a recipe. Problems of this type are solved through proportion, or by multiplication or division by the appropriate factor to obtain the required amount of each ingredient that will give the desired total mass or volume of the formula. Formulas can be provided in amounts or in parts.

A. Formulas that indicate parts. When dealing with formulas that specify parts, parts by weight will require the determination of weights of ingredients, whereas parts by volume warrant the calculation of volumes of ingredients. Always find the total number of parts indicated in the formula, and equate that total with the total mass or volume of the desired formula in order to set up a proportion. Such a proportion will allow calculation of the mass or volume of each ingredient in units common to the total mass or volume.

What quantities should be used to prepare 100 g of camphorated parachlorophenol?

$$R_x \qquad \text{Parachlorophenol} \quad 7 \text{ parts}$$
$$\text{Camphor} \qquad 13 \text{ parts}$$
$$7 \text{ parts} + 13 \text{ parts} = 20 \text{ parts total}$$

$$\frac{7 \text{ parts}}{20 \text{ parts}} = \frac{X \text{ g}}{100 \text{ g}}, \ X = 35 \text{ g of parachlorophenol}$$

$$\frac{13 \text{ parts}}{20 \text{ parts}} = \frac{X \text{ g}}{100 \text{ g}}, \ X = 65 \text{ g of camphor}$$

B. Formulas that indicate quantities

The previous prescription for cold cream provides a 100 g quantity. What mass of each ingredient is required to provide one pound (AV) of cream?

R$_x$	White wax	12.5 g
	Mineral oil	60.0 g
	Lanolin	2.5 g
	Sodium borate	1.0 g
	Rose water	24.0 g

454/100 = 4.54, a factor to use in calculating the quantities of each ingredient.

$$12.5 \text{ g} \times 4.54 = 56.8 \text{ g of white wax}$$
$$60.0 \text{ g} \times 4.54 = 272 \text{ g of mineral oil}$$
$$2.5 \text{ g} \times 4.54 = 11.4 \text{ g of lanolin}$$
$$1.0 \text{ g} \times 4.54 = 4.54 \text{ g of sodium borate}$$
$$24.0 \text{ g} \times 4.54 = 109 \text{ g of rose water}$$

IV. CALCULATING DOSES. Calculation of doses generally can be performed with dimensional analysis. **Problems** encountered in the pharmacy include calculation of the number of doses, quantities in a dose or total mass/volume, amount of active or inactive ingredients, and size of dose. Calculation of **children's doses** is commonly performed by the pharmacist. Dosage is optimally calculated by using the child's body weight or mass and the appropriate dose in mg/kg. Without this data, the following formulas based on an adult dose can be used.

A. Fried's rule for infants:

$$\frac{\text{age (in months)} \times \text{adult dose}}{150} = \text{dose for infant}$$

B. Clark's rule:

$$\frac{\text{weight (in lb)} \times \text{adult dose}}{150 \text{ lb (avg wt of adult)}} = \text{dose for child}$$

C. Child's dosage based on body surface area (BSA):

$$\frac{\text{BSA of child (in m}^2) \times \text{adult dose}}{1.73 \text{ m}^2 \text{ (avg adult BSA)}} = \text{approximate child's dose}$$

V. PERCENTAGE, RATIO STRENGTH, AND OTHER CONCENTRATION EXPRESSIONS

A. Percentage weight-in-volume (w/v)

1. **Definition.** Percentage, indicating parts per hundred, is an important means of expressing concentration in pharmacy practice. Percentage w/v indicates the number of grams of a constituent per 100 mL of solution or liquid formulation. The pharmacist may be required to perform **three types** of calculations: determine the **weight** of active ingredient in a certain volume when given the percentage strength, determine the **percentage w/v** when the weight of substance and volume of liquid formulation are known, and determine the **volume** of liquid mixture when the percentage strength and amount of substance are known.

2. **Tolu balsam syrup.** Tolu balsam tincture contains 20% w/v tolu balsam.

   What is the percentage concentration of tolu balsam in the syrup?

Tolu balsam tincture	50 mL
Magnesium carbonate	10 g
Sucrose	820 g
Purified water, qs ad	1000 mL

   a. First, determine what the amount of tolu balsam is in the 50 mL quantity of tincture used for the syrup. Then, by proportion, calculate the concentration of tolu balsam in the syrup.

$$\text{tolu balsam tincture} = 50 \text{ mL} \times \frac{20 \text{ g}}{100 \text{ mL}} = 10 \text{ g tolu balsam,}$$

$$\frac{10 \text{ g}}{1000 \text{ mL}} = \frac{X \text{ g}}{100 \text{ mL}}, X = 1 \text{ g}/100 \text{ mL} = 1\% \text{ tolu balsam in the syrup}$$

In answering this one question, the first two types of problems listed above have been solved, while exhibiting two methods of solving percentage problems, namely, by **dimensional analysis** and **proportion.**

    b. For an example of the **third type** of percentage w/v problem, determine what volume of syrup could be prepared if we had only 8 g of magnesium carbonate. Use proportion to find the total volume of syrup that can be made using only 8 g of magnesium carbonate. If we have 8 g of magnesium carbonate in 1000 mL of solution, according to the recipe, then 800 mL of solution can be prepared using 8 g of the drug.

$$\frac{10 \text{ g}}{1000 \text{ mL}} = \frac{8 \text{ g}}{X \text{ mL}}, X = 800 \text{ mL}$$

B. Percentage volume-in-volume (v/v). Percentage v/v indicates the number of milliliters of a constituent in 100 mL of liquid formulation. The percentage strength of mixtures of liquids in liquids is indicated by % v/v, which indicates the parts by volume of a substance in 100 parts of the liquid preparation. The **three types** of problems that are encountered involve calculating **percentage strength,** calculating **volume of ingredient,** or calculating **volume of the liquid preparation.** Using the same tolu balsam syrup formula from above, we'll now work a % v/v problem.

What is the percentage strength v/v of the tolu balsam tincture in the syrup preparation? By proportion, we can solve the problem in one step.

$$\frac{50 \text{ mL tolu balsam tincture}}{X \text{ mL tolu balsam tincture}} = \frac{1000 \text{ mL syrup}}{100 \text{ mL syrup}}, X = 5\%$$

C. Percentage weight-in-weight (w/w). Percentage w/w indicates the number of grams of a constituent per 100 g of formulation (solid or liquid). Solution of problems involving percentage w/w is straightforward when the total mass of the mixture is available or if the total mass can be determined from the available data. In calculations similar to those for percentage w/v or v/v, the pharmacist might need to solve several types of problems, including determination of the weight of a constituent, the total weight of a mixture, or the percentage w/w.

    1. How many grams of drug substance should be used to prepare 240 g of a 5% w/w solution?
        a. The first step in any percentage w/w problem is to attempt identification of the total mass of the mixture. In this problem, the total mass is obviously provided (240 g).
        b. The problem can be solved easily through **dimensional analysis.**

$$240 \text{ g mixture} \times \frac{5.0 \text{ g drug}}{100 \text{ g mixture}} = 12 \text{ g}$$

    2. When the total mass of the mixture is unavailable or cannot be determined, an **extra step** is required in the calculations. Because it is usually impossible to know how much volume is displaced by a solid material, the pharmacist is unable to prepare a specified volume of a solution given the percentage w/w.

    How much drug should be added to 30 mL of water to make a 10% w/w solution?
    The volume of water that is displaced by the drug is unknown, so the final volume is unknown. Likewise, even though the mass of solvent is known (30 mL x 1 g/mL = 30 g), it is not known how much drug is needed, so the total mass is unknown. The water represents 100% − 10% = 90% of the total mixture. Then, by proportion, the mass of drug to be used can be identified.

$$\frac{30 \text{ g of mixture (water)}}{X \text{ g of mixture (drug)}} = \frac{90\%}{10\%}, X = 3.33 \text{ g of drug required to make a solution}$$

    The **common error** that many students make in solving problems of this type is to assume that 30 g is the total mass of the mixture. Solving the problem with that assumption gives the following incorrect answer.

$$\frac{X \text{ g drug}}{10 \text{ g drug}} = \frac{30 \text{ g mixture}}{100 \text{ g mixture}}, X = 3 \text{ g of drug (incorrect answer)}$$

D. **Ratio strength.** Solid or liquid formulations that contain low concentrations of active ingredients will often have concentration expressed in **ratio strength.** Ratio strength, as the name implies, is the expression of concentration by means of a ratio. The numerator and denominator of the ratio indicate g or mL of a solid or liquid constituent in the total mass (g) or volume (mL) of a solid or liquid preparation. Because **percentage strength** is essentially a ratio of parts per hundred, conversion between ratio strength and percentage strength is easily accomplished by proportion.

1. **Express 0.1 percent w/v as a ratio strength.**
   a. Ratio strengths are by convention expressed in reduced form, so in setting up our proportion to solve for ratio strength, use the numeral 1 in the numerator of the right-hand ratio as shown below:

   $$\frac{0.1 \text{ g}}{100 \text{ mL}} = \frac{1 \text{ part}}{X \text{ parts}}, X = 1000 \text{ parts, for a ratio strength of } 1{:}1000$$

   b. Likewise, conversion from ratio strength to percentage strength by proportion is easy, as seen in the following example. Keep in mind the definition of percentage strength (parts per hundred) when setting up the proportion.

2. **Express 1:2500 as a percentage strength.**

   $$\frac{1 \text{ part}}{2500 \text{ parts}} = \frac{X \text{ parts}}{100 \text{ parts}}, X = 0.04, \text{ indicating } 0.04\%$$

E. **Other concentration expressions**
   1. **Molarity** (M) is the expression of the number of moles of solute dissolved per liter of solution. It is calculated by dividing the moles of solute by the volume of solution in liters.

   $$M_A = \frac{n_A}{\text{solutions, liters}}$$

   2. **Normality.** A convenient way of dealing with acids, bases, and electrolytes involves the use of equivalents. One equivalent of an acid is the quantity of that acid that supplies or donates one mole of H^+ ions. One equivalent of a base is the quantity that furnishes one mole of OH^- ions. One equivalent of acid reacts with one equivalent of base. Equivalent weight can be calculated for atoms or molecules.

   $$\text{Equivalent weight} = \frac{\text{atomic weight or molecular weight}}{\text{valence}}$$

   The **normality** (N) of a solution is the number of gram-equivalent weights (equivalents) of solute per liter of solution. Normality is analogous to molarity; however, it is defined in terms of equivalents rather than moles.

   $$\text{Normality} = \frac{\text{\# equivalents of solute}}{\text{\# liters of solution}}$$

   3. **Molality** (m) is the moles of solute dissolved per kilogram of solvent. Molality is calculated by dividing the number of moles of solute by the number of kilograms of solvent. Molality offers the advantage over molarity because it is based on solvent weight and avoids problems associated with volume expansion or contraction on the addition of solutes.

   $$m_A = \frac{n_A}{\text{mass}_{\text{solvent, kg}}}$$

   4. **Mole fraction** (X) is the ratio of the number of moles of one component to the total moles of a mixture or solution.

   $$X_A = \frac{n_A}{n_A + n_B + n_C + \ldots}, \text{ where } X_A + X_B + X_C + \ldots = 1$$

VI. **DILUTION AND CONCENTRATION.** If the amount of drug remains constant in a dilution or concentration, then any change in the mass or volume of a mixture is inversely proportional to the concentration.

A. Dilution and concentration problems can be solved by:

1. Inverse proportion (as mentioned earlier)

2. The equation: quantity$_1$ x concentration$_1$ = quantity$_2$ x concentration$_2$

3. Determining the amount of active ingredient present in the initial mixture and, with the assumption that the initial quantity does not change, calculation of the final concentration of the new total mass or volume

4. **Alligation medial**—a method for calculating the average concentration of a mixture of two or more substances

5. **Alligation alternate**—a method for calculation of the number of parts of two or more components of known concentration to be mixed when the final desired concentration is known

B. Dilution of alcohols and acids

1. **Dilution of alcohols.** When alcohol and water are mixed, a contraction of volume occurs. As a result, the final volume of solution cannot be determined accurately. Nor can the volume of water needed to dilute to a certain percentage v/v be identified. Accordingly, percentage w/w is often used for solutions of alcohol.

2. The **percentage strength** of concentrated acids is expressed as percentage w/w. The concentration of diluted acids is expressed as percentage w/v. Determining the volume of concentrated acid to be used in preparing a diluted acid requires the specific gravity of the concentrated acid.

C. Dilution and concentration of liquids and solids. Dilution and concentration problems are often easily solved by identifying the amount of drug involved followed by use of an appropriate proportion.

1. **How many milliliters of a 1:50 stock solution of ephedrine sulfate should be used in compounding the following prescription?**

   R$_x$ Ephedrine sulfate 0.25%
                   Rose water ad 30 mL

   0.25 g/100 mL $\times$ 30 mL = 0.075 g drug required

   $$\frac{50 \text{ mL}}{1 \text{ g}} = \frac{X \text{ mL}}{0.075 \text{ g}}, X = 3.75 \text{ mL of stock solution required for the prescription}$$

2. **How many milliliters of a 15% w/v concentrate of benzalkonium chloride should be used in preparing 300 mL of a stock solution such that 15 mL diluted to 1 L will yield a 1 to 5000 solution?**

   a. First, determine the amount of drug in 1 liter of 1 to 5000 solution.

   $$\frac{5000 \text{ mL}}{1000 \text{ mL}} = \frac{1 \text{ g}}{X \text{ g}}, X = 0.2 \text{ g of benzalkonium chloride in the final solution}$$

   b. Now, because 15 mL of the stock solution is being diluted to 1 L, a stock solution is needed where 15 mL contain 0.2 g of drug. By proportion, the amount of drug required to make 300 mL of the stock solution is found.

   $$\frac{0.2 \text{ g}}{X \text{ g}} = \frac{50 \text{ mL}}{300 \text{ mL}}, \text{ and } X = 4 \text{ g of drug required to make 300 mL of solution}$$

   c. Finally, to determine the amount of 15% concentrate required,

   $$\frac{15 \text{ g}}{4 \text{ g}} = \frac{100 \text{ mL}}{X \text{ mL}}, \text{ and } X = 26.7 \text{ mL of 15\% solution required to obtain necessary drug}$$

3. When the relative amount of components must be determined for preparation of a mixture of a desired concentration, the problem is most easily solved using alligation alternate.

   How many grams of 2.5% hydrocortisone cream should be mixed with 360 g of 0.25% cream to make a 1% hydrocortisone cream?

2.5% — 0.75 parts of 2.5% cream = 1 part   0.75/2.25 = 1/3
            1%
0.25% — 1.5 parts of 0.25% cream = 2 parts   1.5/2.25 = 2/3
            2.25 parts total   = 3 parts

The relative amounts of the 2.5% and 1% creams are 1 to 2, respectively. By proportion, the mass of 2.5% cream to use can be determined. If 2 parts of 0.25% cream is represented by 360 g, then the total mass (3 parts) is represented by what mass?

$$\frac{2 \text{ parts}}{3 \text{ parts}} = \frac{360 \text{ g}}{X \text{ g}}, \; X = 540 \text{ g total}$$

With the total mass known, the amount of 2.5% cream can be identified. If 3 parts represent the total mass of 540 g, then 1 part represents the mass of 2.5% cream (X g = 180 g).

$$\frac{1 \text{ part}}{3 \text{ parts}} = \frac{X \text{ g}}{540 \text{ g}}, \; X = 180 \text{ g of 2.5\% cream}$$

VII. ELECTROLYTE SOLUTIONS. Electrolyte solutions contain species (electrolytes) that dissociate into ions. The **milliequivalent** (mEq) is the unit used to express the concentration of electrolytes in solution. Table 2-1 exhibits some physiologically important ions and their properties.

A. **Milliequivalents.** The milliequivalent is the amount, in milligrams, of a solute equal to 1/1000 of its gram-equivalent weight. Conversion of concentrations in the form of milliequivalent to concentrations in percentage strength, mg/mL or any other terms, begins with calculation of the number of milliequivalents of drug. The following examples exhibit the calculation of milliequivalents and manipulation of data from the table in order to perform the required calculations for preparing electrolyte solutions.

What is the concentration, in percent w/v, of a solution containing 2 mEq of potassium chloride per milliliter?

Calculations involving milliequivalents are easily solved if the practitioner follows a predefined procedure to determine the milliequivalent weight. This involves three steps.
1. Find the molecular weight.

Atomic wt K = 39
Atomic wt Cl = 35.5   39 + 35.5 = 74.5 g = mol wt of KCl

2. Calculate the equivalent weight of KCl.

Eq wt = mol wt/valence = 74.5/1 = 74.5 g

3. Determine the milliequivalent weight, which is 1/1000 of the equivalent weight.

mEq wt = 74.5 g/1000 = 0.0745 g or 74.5 mg

Now that we know the milliequivalent weight, we can calculate by dimensional analysis and proportion the concentration in percentage in a fourth step.

4. 0.0745 g/mEq x 2 mEq = 0.149 g of drug

$$\frac{0.149 \text{ g drug}}{1 \text{ mL}} = \frac{X \text{ g drug}}{100 \text{ mL}}, \; X = 14.9 \text{ g/100 mL} = 14.9\%$$

How many milliequivalents of Na^+ would be contained in a 15-mL volume of the following buffer?

$Na_2HPO_4 \cdot 7H_2O$		180 g
$NaH_2PO_4 \cdot H_2O$		480 g
Purified water	ad	1000 mL

For each salt, the mass (and milliequivalents) must be found in a 15-mL dose.
mol wt $Na_2HPO_4 \cdot 7H_2O$ (disodium hydrogen phosphate) = 268 g
Eq wt = 268/2 = 134 g
1 mEq = 0.134 g or 134 mg

Table 2-1. Valences, Atomic Weights, and Milliequivalent Weights of Selected Ions

Ion	Formula	Valence	Atomic/Formula Weight	Milliequivalent Weight (mg)
Aluminum	Al^{+++}	3	27	9
Ammonium	NH_4^+	1	18	18
Calcium	Ca^{++}	2	40	20
Ferric	Fe^{+++}	3	56	18.7
Ferrous	Fe^{++}	2	56	28
Lithium	Li^+	1	7	7
Magnesium	Mg^{++}	2	24	12
Bicarbonate	HCO_3^-	1	61	61
Carbonate	CO_3^-	1	60	30
Chloride	Cl^-	1	35.5	35.5
Citrate	$C_6H_5O_7^{---}$	3	189	63
Gluconate	$C_6H_{11}O_7^-$	1	195	195
Lactate	$C_3H_5O_3^-$	1	89	89
Phosphate	$H_2PO_4^-$	1	97	97
Sulfate	SO_4^{--}	2	96	48
Potassium	K^+	1	29	39
Sodium	Na^+	1	23	23
Acetate	$C_2H_3O_2^-$	1	59	59

$$\frac{180 \text{ g}}{X \text{ g}} = \frac{1000 \text{ mL}}{15 \text{ mL}}, \; X = 2.7 \text{ g of disodium hydrogen phosphate in each 15 mL}$$

$$2.7 \text{ g} \times \frac{1 \text{ mEq}}{0.134 \text{ g}} = 20.1 \text{ mEq of disodium hydrogen phosphate}$$

mol wt $NaH_2PO_4 \cdot H_2O$ (sodium biphosphate) $= 138$ g
Eq wt $= 138$ g
1 mEq $= 0.138$ g

$$\frac{480 \text{ g}}{X \text{ g}} = \frac{1000 \text{ mL}}{15 \text{ mL}}, \; X = 7.2 \text{ g of sodium biphosphate in each 15 mL}$$

$$7.2 \text{ g} \times \frac{1 \text{ mEq}}{0.138 \text{ g}} = 52.2 \text{ mEq of sodium biphosphate}$$

20.1 mEq + 52.2 mEq = 72.3 mEq of sodium in each 15 mL of solution

B. Milliosmoles (mOsmol). Osmotic pressure is directly proportional to the total number of particles in solution. The milliosmole is the unit of measure for osmotic concentration. For nonelectrolytes, 1 millimole represents 1 milliosmole. However, for electrolytes, the total number of particles in solution is determined by the number of particles produced in solution and influenced by the degree of dissociation. Assuming complete dissociation, 1 millimole of KCl represents 2 milliosmoles of total particles, 1 millimole of $CaCl_2$ represents 3 milliosmoles of total particles, etc. The ideal osmolar concentration can be calculated with the following equation.

$$\text{mOsmol/L} = \frac{\text{wt of substance in g/L}}{\text{molecular weight in g}} \times \text{number of species} \times 1000$$

The pharmacist should recognize the difference between **ideal** osmolar concentration and **actual** osmolarity. As the concentration of solute increases, interaction between dissolved particles increases, resulting in a reduction of the actual osmolar values.

C. Isotonic solutions. An **isotonic** solution is one that has the same osmotic pressure as body fluids. **Isosmotic** fluids are fluids with the same osmotic pressure. Solutions to be administered to patients should be isosmotic with body fluids. A **hypotonic** solution is one with a lower osmotic pressure than body fluids, whereas a **hypertonic** solution will have an osmotic pressure that is greater than body fluids.

1. **Preparation of isotonic solutions.** Colligative properties, including freezing point depression, are representative of the number of particles in solution and considered in preparation of isotonic solutions.

    a. When 1 g mol wt of any nonelectrolyte is dissolved in 1000 g of water, the freezing point of the solution is depressed by 1.86°C. By proportion, the weight of any nonelectrolyte needed to make the solution isotonic with body fluid can be calculated.

    b. Boric acid (H_3BO_3) has a mol wt of 61.8 g. Thus, 61.8 g of H_3BO_3 in 1000 g of water should produce a freezing point of −1.86°C. Therefore, knowing that the freezing point depression of body fluids is −0.52°C,

    $$-1.86°C/-0.52°C = 61.8 \text{ g/X g, and X} = 17.3 \text{ g}$$

    and 17.3 g of H_3BO_3 in 1000 g of water provide a solution that is **isotonic.**

    c. The degree of dissociation of electrolytes must be taken into account in such calculations. For example, NaCl is approximately 80% dissociated in weak solutions, yielding 180 particles in solution for each 100 molecules of NaCl. Therefore,

    $$-1.86°C \times 1.8/-0.52°C = 58.5 \text{ g/X g, and X} = 9.09 \text{ g}$$

    indicating that 9.09 g of NaCl in 1000 g of water (0.9% w/v) should make a solution isotonic. Lacking any information on the degree of dissociation of an electrolyte, the following **dissociation values** (*i*) may be used.

    (1) Substances that dissociate into 2 ions: 1.8
    (2) Substances that dissociate into 3 ions: 2.6
    (3) Substances that dissociate into 4 ions: 3.4
    (4) Substances that dissociate into 5 ions: 4.2

2. **Sodium chloride equivalents.** The pharmacist will often be required to prepare an isotonic solution by adding an appropriate amount of another substance (drug or inert electrolyte or nonelectrolyte). Considering that isotonic fluids contain the equivalent of 0.9% NaCl, the question arises: How much of the added ingredient is required to make the solution isotonic? A **common method** for computing the amount of added ingredient to use for reaching isotonicity involves the use of **sodium chloride equivalents.**

    a. **Definition.** The sodium chloride equivalent represents the amount of NaCl that is equivalent to the amount of particular drug in question. For every substance, there is one quantity that should have a constant tonic effect when dissolved in 1000 g of water. This is 1 g mol wt of the substance divided by its *i*, or dissociation value.

    b. **Examples**

    (1) Considering H_3BO_3, from the last section, 17.3 g of H_3BO_3 are equivalent to 0.52 g of NaCl in tonicity. Therefore, the relative quantity of NaCl that is equivalent to H_3BO_3 in tonicity effects is determined as follows:

    $$\frac{\text{mol wt of NaCl}/i \text{ value}}{\text{mol wt of } H_3BO_3/i \text{ value}} = \frac{58.5/1.8}{61.8/1.0}$$

    Applying this method to atropine sulfate, recall that the mol wt of NaCl and the mol wt of atropine sulfate are 58.5 and 695 g, respectively, and their *i* values are 1.8 and 2.6, respectively. Calculate the mass of NaCl represented by 1 g of atropine sulfate (Table 2-2). 695 × 1.8/58.5 × 2.6 = 1 g/X g, and X = 0.12 g NaCl represented by 1 g of atropine sulfate.

    (2) An example of the practical use of sodium chloride equivalents is seen in the following problem.

    How many grams of boric acid should be used in compounding the following prescription?

R_x	Phenacaine hydrochloride	1%
	Chlorobutanol	0.5%
	Boric acid	q.s.
	Purified water ad	60.0 mL
	Make isoton. sol.	

The prescription calls for 0.3 g of chlorobutanol and 0.6 g of phenacaine. How much boric acid is required to prepare this prescription? The question is best answered in four steps.

(a) Find the mass of sodium chloride represented by all ingredients.

$0.20 \times 0.6 = 0.120$ g of sodium chloride represented by phenacaine hydrochloride
$0.24 \times 0.3 = \underline{0.072}$ g of sodium chloride represented by chlorobutanol
0.192 g of sodium chloride represented by the two active ingredients

(b) Find the mass of sodium chloride required to prepare an equal volume of isotonic solution.

$$\frac{0.9 \text{ g NaCl}}{100 \text{ mL}} = \frac{X \text{ g NaCl}}{60 \text{ mL}}, X = 0.540 \text{ g of sodium chloride in 60 mL of an isotonic sodium chloride solution}$$

(c) Calculate, by subtraction, the amount of NaCl required to make the solution isotonic.

0.540 g NaCl required for isotonicity
$\underline{0.192}$ g NaCl represented by ingredients
0.348 g NaCl required to make isotonic solution

(d) Because the prescription calls for boric acid to be used, one last step is required. 0.348 g $\div 0.52$ (sodium chloride eq. for boric acid) $= 0.669$ g of boric acid to be used.

VIII. STATISTICS

A. Introduction. Statistics can be used to describe and compare data distributions. Such **frequency distributions** are constructed by classifying individual observations into categories corresponding to fixed numeric intervals and plotting the number of observations in each such category (i.e., **interval frequency**) versus the category descriptor (e.g., the interval mean or range). Because of random errors, repeated observations or measurements (of the same value) are not identical. These observations have a **"normal distribution."** Normally, distributed data are described by a **bell-shaped (Gaussian) curve** with a maximum, μ **(population mean)**, corresponding to the central tendency of the population, and a spread characterized by σ (the **population standard deviation**). Statistics derived from a **sample** or subset of a population can be used as estimates of the population parameters.

B. Frequency distribution

1. **Estimates of population mean.** The population mean, μ, is the best estimate of the true value.
   a. **The sample mean.** For a finite number of observations, the arithmetic average or mean, $\overline{X}$, is the best estimate of the true value, μ.

$$\overline{X} = \frac{\sum x_i}{n}$$

   where $\sum x_i$ is the sum of all (n) observations.
   (1) Accuracy is the degree to which a measured value (X or $\overline{X}$) agrees with the "true" value (μ).
   (2) Error (or bias) is the difference between a measured value (X or $\overline{X}$) and the "true" value (μ).

Table 2-2. Sodium Chloride (NaCl) Equivalents

Substance	NaCl Equivalent
Atropine sulfate (H_2O)	0.12
Boric acid	0.52
Chlorobutanol	0.24
Dextrose (anhydrous)	0.18
Ephedrine hydrochloride	0.29
Phenacaine hydrochloride	0.20
Potassium chloride	0.78

b. **Median.** The median is the "midmost" value of a data distribution. When all the values are arranged in increasing (or decreasing) order, the median is the middle value for an **odd** number of observations. For an **even** number of observations, the median is the arithmetic mean of the two middle values. For a **normal distribution, median equals mean.** The median is less affected by "outliers" or by a "skewed" distribution.

c. **Mode.** The mode is the most frequently occurring value (or values) in a frequency distribution. The mode is useful for non-normal distributions, especially those that are **bimodal**.

2. **Estimates of variability.** For an **infinite** number of observations, the **population variance, σ^2,** can be used to describe the variability or "spread" of observations in a data distribution. For a **finite** number of observations, the **sample variance, s^2,** can be used to describe the variability or spread of observations in a data distribution.

a. **Sample variance, s^2,** is estimated by

$$s^2 = \frac{\sum(x_i - \overline{X})^2}{(n-1)}$$

or

$$s^2 = \frac{\sum x_i{}^2 - \frac{(\sum x_i)^2}{n}}{(n-1)}$$

where $\overline{X}$ is the mean and $(n-1)$ is the number of degrees of freedom (df).

b. **Range.** For a very small number of observations, the **range (w)** can be used to describe the variability in the data set:

$$w = \left| X_{largest} - X_{smallest} \right|$$

c. The **standard deviation** (s; SD), one of the most commonly encountered estimates of variability, is equal to the square root of the variance.

$$s = \sqrt{s^2} = \sqrt{\frac{\sum(x_i - \overline{X})^2}{(n-1)}}$$

or

$$s = \sqrt{s^2} = \sqrt{\frac{\sum x_i{}^2 - \frac{(\sum x_i)^2}{n}}{(n-1)}}$$

d. **Precision** (reproducibility) is the degree to which replicate measurements "made in exactly the same way" agree with each other. **Precision** is often expressed as the **relative standard deviation (RSD, %RSD):**

$$\%RSD = \left(\frac{s}{\overline{X}}\right) \times 100$$

3. The **standard deviation of the mean (S_m),** or standard error of the mean (SEM), is an estimate of the **variability** or **error in the mean** obtained from *n* observations. It is often used to establish confidence intervals for describing the mean of a data set or when comparing the means of two data sets.

$$S_m = \frac{s}{\sqrt{n}}$$

STUDY QUESTIONS

Directions: Each of the numbered items or incomplete statements in this section is followed by answers or by completions of the statement. Select the **one** lettered answer or completion that is **best** in each case.

1. If a vitamin solution contains 0.5 mg of fluoride ion in each milliliter, then how many milligrams of fluoride ion would be provided by a dropper that delivers 0.6 mL?

(A) 0.3 mg
(B) 0.1 mg
(C) 1 mg
(D) 0.83 mg

2. How many chloramphenicol capsules, each containing 250 mg, are needed to provide 25 mg per kg per day for 7 days for a person weighing 200 lb?

(A) 90 capsules
(B) 64 capsules
(C) 13 capsules
(D) 25 capsules

3. If 3.17 kg of a drug are used to make 50,000 tablets, how many milligrams will 30 tablets contain?

(A) 1.9 mg
(B) 1900 mg
(C) 0.0019 mg
(D) 3.2 mg

4. A capsule contains 1/8 gr of ephedrine sulfate, 1/4 gr of theophylline, and 1/16 gr of phenobarbital. What is the total mass of the active ingredients in milligrams?

(A) 20 mg
(B) 8 mg
(C) 28 mg
(D) 4 mg

5. If one fluid ounce of a cough syrup contains 10 gr of sodium citrate, how many milligrams are contained in 10 mL?

(A) 650 mg
(B) 65 mg
(C) 217 mg
(D) 20 mg

6. How many capsules, each containing 1/4 gr of phenobarbital, can be manufactured if a bottle containing 2 avoirdupois ounces of phenobarbital is available?

(A) 771 capsules
(B) 350 capsules
(C) 3500 capsules
(D) 1250 capsules

7. Using the formula for calamine lotion, determine the amount of calamine (in grams) necessary to prepare 240 mL of lotion.

Calamine	80 g
Zinc oxide	80 g
Glycerin	20 mL
Bentonite magma	250 mL
Calcium hydroxide topical solution, a sufficient quantity to make 1000 mL	

(A) 19.2 g
(B) 140 g
(C) 100 g
(D) 24 g

8. From the following formula, calculate the amount of white wax required to make 1 lb of cold cream. Determine the mass in grams.

Cetyl esters wax	12.5 parts
White wax	12.0 parts
Mineral oil	56.0 parts
Sodium borate	0.5 parts
Purified water	19.0 parts

(A) 56.75 g
(B) 254.24 g
(C) 54.48 g
(D) 86.26 g

9. How many grams of aspirin should be used to prepare 1.255 kg of the powder?

ASA	6 parts
Phenacetin	3 parts
Caffeine	1 part

(A) 125 g
(B) 750 g
(C) 175 g
(D) 360 g

10. A solution contains 1.25 mg of a drug per milliliter. At what rate should the solution be infused (drops/min) if the drug is to be administered at a rate of 80 mg/hour? (1 mL = 30 drops)

(A) 64 drops/min
(B) 1.06 drops/min
(C) 32 drops/min
(D) 20 drops/min

11. The recommended maintenance dose of aminophylline for children is 1.0 mg/kg/hour by injection. If 10 mL of a 25 mg/mL solution of aminophylline is added to a 100-mL bottle for dextrose, what should be the rate of delivery in mL/hour for a 40-lb child?

(A) 2.30 mL/hour
(B) 8.00 mL/hour
(C) 18.9 mL/hour
(D) 18.2 mL/hour

12. For children, streptomycin is to be administered at a dose of 30 mg/kg of body weight daily in divided doses every 6 to 12 hours. The dry powder is dissolved by adding water for injection, USP in an amount to yield the desired concentration as indicated in the following table (for a 1-gram vial).

Approximate concentration (mg/mL)	Volume (mL)
200	4.2
250	3.2
400	1.8

Reconstituting at the lowest possible concentration, what volume (mL) would be withdrawn to obtain one day's dose for a 50-pound child?

(A) 3.4 mL
(B) 22.73 mL
(C) 2.50 mL
(D) 2.27 mL

13. The atropine sulfate is available only in the form of 1/150 gr tablets. How many atropine sulfate tablets would you use to compound the prescription?

Atropine sulfate	gr 1/200
Codeine phosphate	gr 1/4
Aspirin	gr 5
d.t.d.	#24 caps.
Sig:	cap 1 prn.

(A) 3 tablets
(B) 6 tablets
(C) 12 tablets
(D) 18 tablets

14. In 25.0 mL of a solution for injection, there are 4.00 mg of the drug. If the dose to be administered to a patient is 200 µg, what quantity (in milliliters) of this solution should be used?

(A) 1.25 mL
(B) 125 mL
(C) 12.0 mL
(D) None of the above

15. How many milligrams of papaverine will the patient receive each day?

R_x	Papaverine hydrochloride	1.0 g
	Aqua	30.0 mL
	Syrup tolu qs ad	90.0 mL
	Sig:	One tsp. t.i.d.

(A) 56 mg
(B) 5.6 mg
(C) 166 mg
(D) 2.5 mg

16. Considering the following prescription, how many grams of sodium bromide should be used in filling this prescription?

R_x	Sodium bromide	1.2 g
	Syrup tolu	2.0 mL
	Syrup wild cherry qs ad	5.0 mL
	d.t.d.	#24

(A) 1.2 g
(B) 1200 g
(C) 28.8 g
(D) 220 g

17. How many milliliters of a 7.5% stock solution of $KMnO_4$ should be used to obtain the KMnO needed?

> $KMnO_4$ qs.
> Distilled water ad 1000
> Sig: Two teaspoons diluted to 500 mL yield a
> 1 to 5000 solution

(A) 267 mL
(B) 133 mL
(C) 26.7 mL
(D) 13.3 mL

18. The formula for Ringer's solution follows. How much sodium chloride is needed to make 120 mL?

> R_x Sodium chloride   8.60 g
> Potassium chloride   0.30 g
> Calcium chloride   0.33 g
> Water for injection qs ad 1000 mL

(A) 120 g
(B) 1.03 g
(C) 0.12 g
(D) 103 g

19. How many grams of talc should be added to 1 lb of a powder containing 20 g of zinc undecylenate per 100 g to reduce the concentration of zinc undecylenate to 3%?

(A) 3026.7 g
(B) 2572.7 g
(C) 17 g
(D) 257 g

20. How many milliliters of a 0.9% aqueous solution can be made from 20.0 g of sodium chloride?

(A) 2222 mL
(B) 100 mL
(C) 222 mL
(D) 122 mL

21. The blood of a reckless driver contains 0.1% alcohol. Express the concentration of alcohol in parts per million.

(A) 100 ppm
(B) 1000 ppm
(C) 1 ppm
(D) 250 ppm

22. Syrup is an 85% w/v solution of sucrose in water. It has a density of 1.313 g/mL. How many milliliters of water should be used to make 125 mL of syrup?

(A) 106.25 mL
(B) 164.1 mL
(C) 57.9 mL
(D) 25.0 mL

23. How many grams of benzethonium chloride should be used in preparing 5 gallons of a 0.025% w/v solution?

(A) 189.25 g
(B) 18.9 g
(C) 4.73 g
(D) 35 g

24. How many grams of menthol should be used to prepare this prescription?

> R_x Menthol   0.8%
> Alcohol qs ad   60.0 mL

(A) 0.48 g
(B) 0.8 g
(C) 4.8 g
(D) 1.48 g

25. How many milliliters of a 1 to 1500 solution can be made by dissolving 4.8 g of cetylpyridinium chloride in water?

(A) 7200 mL
(B) 7.2 mL
(C) 48 mL
(D) 4.8 mL

26. The manufacturer specifies that one Domeboro tablet dissolved in a pint of water makes a modified Burow's solution approximately equivalent to a 1 to 40 dilution. How many tablets should be used in preparing a half gallon of a 1 to 10 dilution?

(A) 16 tablets
(B) 189 tablets
(C) 12 tablets
(D) 45 tablets

27. How many milliosmoles of calcium chloride ($CaCl_2 \cdot 2H_2O$ − mol wt = 147) are represented in 147 mL of a 10% w/v calcium chloride solution?

(A) 100 mOsmol
(B) 200 mOsmol
(C) 300 mOsmol
(D) 3 mOsmol

28. How many grams of boric acid should be used in compounding the following prescription?

> Phenacaine HCl 1.0% (NaCl eq. = 0.17)
> Chlorobutanol 0.5%   (NaCl eq. = 0.18)
> Boric acid qs.   (NaCl eq. = 0.52)
> Purified H_2O ad 30 mL
> Make isotonic solution
> Sig: One drop in each eye

(A) 0.37 g
(B) 0.74 g
(C) 0.27 g
(D) 0.47 g

29. A pharmacist prepares 1 gallon of KCl solution by mixing 565 grams of KCl (valence = 1) in an appropriate vehicle. How many milliequivalents of K^+ are in 15 mL of this solution? (Atomic weights: K = 39, Cl = 35.5)

(A) 7.5 mEq
(B) 10 mEq
(C) 20 mEq
(D) 30 mEq
(E) 40 mEq

Questions 30–33

Five ibuprofen tablets were assayed for drug content and the following results obtained by HPLC analysis: 198.2, 199.7, 202.5, 201.3, 196.4 mg.

30. What is the mean ibuprofen content?

(A) 196.9 mg
(B) 200.2 mg
(C) 199.6 mg
(D) 249.5 mg
(E) 202.5 mg

31. What is the standard deviation of ibuprofen content in the analyzed tablets?

(A) 2.17 mg
(B) 3.35 mg
(C) 2.42 mg
(D) 3.00 mg
(E) − 2.17 mg

32. What is the percent relative standard deviation (%RSD) for this ibuprofen tablet analysis?

(A) 1.69%
(B) 1.21%
(C) 8.25%
(D) 3.35%
(E) 1.50%

33. What is the standard deviation of the mean drug content of this sample?

(A) 0.480 mg
(B) 0.605 mg
(C) 1.21 mg
(D) 1.08 mg
(E) 0.825 mg

ANSWERS AND EXPLANATIONS

1. The answer is A *[V E]*.

2. The answer is B *[II]*.

3. The answer is B *[II]*.

4. The answer is C *[1 A 2; III A]*.

5. The answer is C *[I A 2]*.

6. The answer is C *[II]*.

7. The answer is A *[V]*.

8. The answer is C *[V]*.
The formula tells the pharmacist that white wax represents 12 parts out of the total 100 parts in the prescription. What we wish to determine is the mass of white wax required to prepare 454 g (1 lb) of the recipe. This can be easily solved by proportion:

$$\frac{12 \text{ parts W.W.}}{100 \text{ parts total}} = \frac{X}{454 \text{ parts (grams)}}, \; X = 54.48 \text{ g}$$

9. The answer is B *[V]*.

10. The answer is C *[VI]*.

11. The answer is B *[IV]*.

12. The answer is A *[IV]*.

13. The answer is D *[V]*.

14. The answer is A *[VI]*.
Dimensional analysis is often useful for calculating doses. Considering that 4 mg of drug are present in each 25 mL of solution, we can easily calculate the number of mL to be used to give a dose of 0.200 mg (200 μg). Always include units in your calculations.

$$25 \text{ mL/4 mg} \times 0.200 \text{ mg} = 1.25 \text{ mL}$$

15. The answer is C *[V A 1]*.

16. The answer is C *[V A 1]*.

17. The answer is B *[I A]*.
First, determine the mass of drug in the final diluted solution.

$$\frac{1 \text{ part}}{5000 \text{ parts}} = \frac{X \text{ g}}{500 \text{ g}}, \; X = 0.1 \text{ g}$$

Now, if 0.1 g of drug is present in 500 mL of 1 to 5000 solution, two teaspoonfuls (10 mL) of the prescription contain the same amount of drug (0.1 g) before dilution. From this, the amount of drug in 1000 mL (the total volume) of the prescription can be determined:

$$\frac{0.1 \text{ g}}{10 \text{ ml}} = \frac{X \text{ g}}{1000 \text{ mL}}, \; X = 10 \text{ g}$$

Finally, to obtain the correct amount of drug to formulate the prescription (10 g), we are to use a 7.5% stock solution. Recalling the definition of percentage strength w/v:

$$100 \text{ mL/7.5 g} \times 10 \text{ g} = 133.3 \text{ mL or } 133 \text{ mL}$$

18. The answer is B *[IV]*.

19. The answer is B *[V]*.

20. The answer is A *[I A 3]*.
Using dimensional analysis: 20 g × 100 mL/0.9 g = 2222 mL

21. The answer is B *[V A]*.

22. The answer is C *[I A; V A 1]*.
Using the density, the weight of 125 mL of syrup can be calculated:

$$125 \text{ mL} \times 1.313 \text{ g/mL} = 164.125 \text{ g}$$

Using proportion and the sucrose concentration in w/v, the weight of sucrose in 125 mL of syrup can be calculated:

$$\frac{100}{\text{mL}} = \frac{85 \text{ g}}{\text{X g}}, \text{ X} = 106.25 \text{ g}$$

Finally, the weight of water in 125 mL of syrup can be calculated:

$$164.125 \text{ g} - 106.25 \text{ g} = 57.875 \text{ g}$$

which has a volume of 57.9 milliliters.

23. The answer is C *[I; V]*.

24. The answer is A *[I; V]*.

25. The answer is A *[I; V]*.
The problem is easily solved by proportion. The question to be answered is: If 1 g of drug is present in 1500 mL of solution, what volume can be made with 4.8 g of drug?

$$\frac{1 \text{ g}}{4.8 \text{ g}} = \frac{1500 \text{ mL}}{\text{X mL}}, \text{ X} = 7200 \text{ mL (the volume of 1:1500 solution that can be prepared from 4.8 g of drug)}$$

26. The answer is A *[I; V]*.

27. The answer is C *[VII B]*.
Recalling the expression for ideal osmolar concentration:

$$\text{mOsmol/L} = \frac{100 \text{ g/L}}{147 \text{ g/mole}} \times 3 \times 1000 = 2040 \text{ mOsmol/L} \times 0.147 \text{ L} = 300 \text{ mOsmol}$$

28. The answer is A *[VII C]*.

29. The answer is D *[VII A]*.

30. The answer is C *[VIII B 1]*.
The mean is calculated directly from the equation:

$$\overline{X} = \frac{\Sigma x_i}{n} = \frac{998.1}{5} = 199.6 \text{ mg}$$

31. The answer is C *[VIII B 3].*
The standard deviation can be calculated with either of the two most commonly used equations:

x_i	$(x_i - \overline{X})$	$(x_i - \overline{X})^2$
198.2	-1.4	1.96*
199.7	0.1	0.01
202.5	2.9	8.41
201.3	1.7	2.89
196.4	-3.2	10.24
$\sum x_i = 998.1$		$\sum(x_i - \overline{X})^2 = 23.51$

$$s = \sqrt{s^2} = \sqrt{\frac{\sum(x_i - \overline{X})^2}{(n-1)}} = \sqrt{\frac{23.51}{(5-1)}} = 2.42 \text{ mg}$$

or

x_i	x_i^2
198.2	39,283.24*
199.7	39,880.09
202.5	41,006.25
201.3	40,521.69
196.4	38,572.96
$\sum x_i = 998.1$	$\sum x_i^2 = 199,264.23$

$$s = \sqrt{s^2} = \sqrt{\frac{199,264.23 - \frac{(998.1)^2}{5}}{(5-1)}} = 2.42 \text{ mg}$$

*Note: It is important to carry enough significant figures through the calculation in order to minimize roundoff error.

32. The answer is B *[VIII B 4].*

$$\%RSD = \left(\frac{s}{\overline{X}}\right) \times 100 = \left(\frac{2.42}{199.6}\right) \times 100 = 1.21\%$$

33. The answer is D *[VIII C].*

$$s_m = \frac{s}{\sqrt{n}} = \frac{2.42}{\sqrt{5}} = 1.08 \text{ mg}$$

3
Pharmaceutical Principles and Drug Dosage Forms
Lawrence H. Block

I. INTRODUCTION. Pharmaceutical principles are the underlying physicochemical principles that allow a drug to be incorporated into a pharmaceutical **dosage form** (e.g., solution, capsule). These principles apply whether the drug is extemporaneously compounded by the pharmacist or manufactured for commercial distribution as a **drug product.**

   A. The finished **dosage form** contains the active drug ingredient in association with nondrug (usually inert) ingredients **(excipients)** that comprise the **vehicle,** or **formulation matrix.**

   B. The **drug delivery system** concept that has evolved over the last four decades is a more holistic concept. It embraces not only the drug (or prodrug) and its formulation matrix, but also the dynamic interactions among the drug, its formulation matrix, its container, and the physiologic milieux of the patient. These dynamic interactions are the subject of **biopharmaceutics** (see Chapter 4).

II. INTERMOLECULAR FORCES OF ATTRACTION

   A. Introduction. The application of pharmaceutical principles to drug dosage forms is illustrated when drug dosage forms are **categorized** according to their **physical state, degree of heterogeneity,** and **chemical composition.** The usual relevant states of matter are **gases, liquids,** and **solids.** Intermolecular forces of attraction are weakest in gases and strongest in solids. Conversions from one physical state to another can involve simply overcoming intermolecular forces of attraction by adding energy (heat). Chemical composition can have a dramatic effect on physicochemical properties and behavior. For this reason, it is necessary to distinguish between **polymers,** or **macromolecules,** and more conventional (i.e., smaller) molecules, or **micromolecules.**

   B. Intermolecular forces of attraction. Because atoms vary in their electronegativity, electron sharing between different atoms is likely to be unequal. This asymmetric electron distribution causes a shift in the overall electron cloud in the molecule. As a result, the molecule tends to behave as a **dipole** (i.e., as if it had a positive and a negative pole). The dipole associated with each covalent bond has a corresponding **dipole moment** (μ) defined as the product of the distance of charge separation (d) and the charge (q):

$$\mu = q \cdot d$$

The molecular dipole moment may be viewed as the vector sum of the individual bond moments.

   1. Nonpolar molecules that have **perfect symmetry** [e.g., carbon tetrachloride (Figure 3-1)] have dipole moments of zero.

   2. Polar molecules are **asymmetric** and have nonzero dipole moments.

   3. When **dipolar** molecules approach one another close enough "positive to positive" or "negative to negative" so that their electron clouds interpenetrate, **intermolecular repulsive**

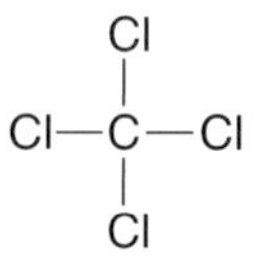

```
        Cl
        |
Cl —— C —— Cl
        |
        Cl
```

Figure 3-1. Carbon tetrachloride molecule.

forces arise. When these dipolar molecules approach one another so that the positive pole of one is close to the negative pole of the other, molecular **attraction** occurs **(dipole–dipole interaction).** When the identically charged poles of the two molecules are closer, **repulsion** occurs.

C. Types of intermolecular forces of attraction include:

1. Nonpolar molecules do not have permanent dipoles. However, the instantaneous electron distribution in a molecule can be asymmetric. The resultant transient dipole moment can induce a dipole in an adjacent molecule. This **induced dipole–induced dipole interaction (London dispersion force),** with a force of approximately 0.5–1 kcal/mol, is sufficient to facilitate order in a molecular array. These relatively weak electrostatic forces are responsible for the liquefaction of nonpolar gases.

2. The transient dipole induced by a permanent dipole, or **dipole–induced dipole interaction (Debye induction force),** is a stronger interaction, with a force of approximately 1–3 kcal/mol.

3. **Permanent dipole interactions (Keesom orientation forces),** with a force of approximately 1–7 kcal/mol, together with Debye and London forces, constitute **van der Waals forces.** Collectively, they are responsible for the more substantive structure and molecular ordering found in liquids.

4. **Hydrogen bonds.** Because they are small and have a large electrostatic field, hydrogen atoms can approach highly electronegative atoms (e.g., fluorine, oxygen, nitrogen, chlorine, sulfur) and interact electrostatically to form a hydrogen bond. Depending on the electronegativity of the second atom and the molecular environment in which hydrogen bonding occurs, hydrogen bond energy varies from approximately 1–8 kcal/mol.

5. **Ion–ion, ion–dipole, and ion-induced dipole forces. Positive–negative ion interactions** in the solid state involve forces of 100–200 kcal/mol. Ionic interactions are reduced considerably in liquid systems in the presence of other electrolytes. **Ion–dipole** interaction, or **dipole induction by an ion,** can also affect molecular aggregation, or ordering, in a system.

III. STATES OF MATTER

A. Gases. Molecules in the gaseous state can be pictured as moving along straight paths, in all directions and at high velocities (e.g., mean velocity for H_2O vapor, 587 m/sec; for O_2, 440 m/sec), until they collide with other molecules. As a result of these random collisions, molecular velocities and paths change, and the molecules continue to collide with other molecules and with the boundaries of the system (e.g., the walls of a container holding the gas). This process, repeated incessantly, is responsible for the **pressure** exhibited within the confines of the system.

1. The interrelation among **volume (V), pressure (P),** and the **absolute temperature (T)** is given by the **ideal gas law,** which is the equation of state for an ideal gas:

$$PV = nRT$$
$$PV = (g/M)RT,$$

where n is the number of moles of gas [equivalent to the number of grams (g) of gas divided by the molecular weight of the gas (M)] and R is the **molar gas constant** (0.08205 L atm/mole deg).

2. Pharmaceutical gases include the **anesthetic gases** (e.g., nitrous oxide, halothane). **Compressed gases** include oxygen (for therapy), nitrogen, and carbon dioxide. **Liquefiable gases,** including certain **halohydrocarbons** and **hydrocarbons,** are used as propellants in **aerosol products (pressurized packaging),** as are compressed gases such as nitrous oxide, nitrogen, and carbon dioxide. Ethylene oxide is a gas used to sterilize or disinfect heat-labile objects.

3. In general, as the temperature of a substance increases, its **heat content,** or **enthalpy,** increases as well.

   a. Substances can undergo a change of state, or phase change, from the solid to the liquid state **(melting)** or from the liquid to the gaseous state **(vaporization).**

b. Volatile liquids (e.g., ether, halothane, methoxyflurane) are used as inhalation anesthetics. Amyl nitrite is a volatile liquid that is inhaled for its vasodilating effect in acute angina.

c. Sublimation occurs when a solid is heated directly to the gaseous, or vapor, state without passing through the liquid state (e.g., camphor, iodine). Ice sublimes at pressures below 3 torr. The process of **freeze-drying,** or **lyophilization,** is a form of vacuum drying in which water is removed by sublimation from the frozen product. It is an especially useful process for drying aqueous solutions or dispersions of heat- or oxygen-sensitive drugs and biologicals (e.g., proteins, peptides).

d. The reverse process (i.e., direct transition from the vapor state to the solid state) is also referred to as sublimation, but the preferred term is **deposition.** Some forms of sulfur and colloidal silicon dioxide are prepared in this way.

4. The intermolecular forces of attraction in gases are virtually nonexistent at room temperature. Gases display little or no ordering.

B. Liquids. The intermolecular forces of attraction in liquids **(van der Waals forces)** are sufficient to impose some ordering, or regular arrangement, among the molecules. **Hydrogen bonding** increases the likelihood of cohesion in liquids and further affects their physicochemical behavior. However, these forces are much weaker than **covalent** or **ionic** forces. Therefore, liquids tend to display short-range rather than long-range order. Hypothetically, although molecules of a liquid would tend to aggregate in localized clusters, no defined structuring would be evident.

1. Surface and interfacial tension

a. Molecules in the bulk phase of a liquid (Figure 3-2A) are surrounded by other molecules of the same kind. Molecules at the surface of a liquid (Figure 3-2B) are not completely surrounded by like molecules. As a result, molecules at or near the surface of a liquid experience a net inward pull from molecules in the interior of the liquid. Because of this net inward intermolecular attraction, the liquid surface tends to spontaneously contract. Thus, liquids tend to assume a spherical shape (i.e., a volume with the minimum surface area). This configuration has the least free energy.

b. Any expansion of the surface increases the free energy of the system. Thus, **surface free energy** can be defined by the work required to increase the surface area A of the liquid by 1 area unit. This value is expressed as the number of milli-Newtons (mN) needed to expand a 1-m^2 surface by 1 unit:

$$\text{work} = \gamma \cdot \Delta A$$

where ΔA is the increase in surface area and γ is the **surface tension,** or **surface free energy,** in mN m^{-1} [equivalent to centimeter-gram-second (CGS) units of dynes cm^{-1}]. Water has a surface tension at 20°C of 72 mN m^{-1}, whereas n-octanol has a surface tension of 27 mN m^{-1}. Thus, more work must be expended to expand the surface of water than to expand the surface of n-octanol (i.e., to proceed from a given volume of bulk liquid to the corresponding volume of small droplets).

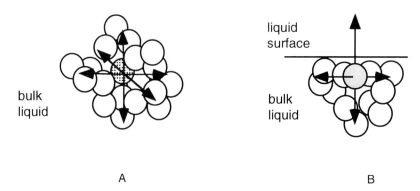

A   B

Figure 3-2. (*A*) Molecules in the bulk phase. (*B*) Molecules at the surface of the liquid.

c. At the **boundary,** or **interface,** between two immiscible liquids that are in contact with one another, the corresponding **interfacial tension** (i.e., free energy, or work required to expand the interfacial area) reflects the extent of the intermolecular forces of attraction and repulsion at the interface. When the interface is between two liquids, substantial molecular interaction occurs across the interface between the two phases. This interaction reduces the imbalance in forces of attraction within each phase. The interfacial tension between n-octanol and water is reduced to 8.5 mN m^{-1} from 72 mN m^{-1} (γ air/water). This reduction indicates, in part, the interfacial interaction between n-octanol and water.

2. The flow of a liquid across a solid surface can be examined in terms of the **velocity,** or rate of movement, of the liquid relative to the surface across which it flows. More insight can be gained by visualizing the flow of liquid as involving the movement of numerous parallel layers of liquid between an upper, movable plate and a lower, fixed plate (Figure 3-3). The application of a constant force (F) to the upper plate causes both this plate and the uppermost layer of liquid in contact with it to move with a velocity $\Delta y/\Delta x$. The interaction between the fixed bottom plate and the liquid layer closest to it prevents the movement of the bottom layer of liquid. The **velocity** (v) of the remaining layers of liquid between the two plates is proportional to their distance from the immovable plate (i.e., $\Delta y/\Delta x$). The **velocity gradient** leads to deformation of the liquid with time. This deformation is the **rate of shear,** dv/dx, or D. **Newton** defined flow in terms of the ratio of the force F applied to a plate of area A [**shear stress (τ)**] divided by the velocity gradient (D) induced by τ:

$$F/A = \eta \frac{dv}{dx}$$

or

$$\tau/D = \eta$$

The proportionality constant η is the coefficient of **viscosity.** It indicates the resistance to flow of adjacent layers of fluid. The reciprocal of η is **fluidity.** Units of viscosity in the CGS system are dynes cm^{-2}s^{-1}, or poise. In the SI system, the units are Newtons m^{-2}s^{-1}, which corresponds to 10 poise. The viscosity of water at 20°C is approximately 0.01 poise, or 1 centipoise (cps), which corresponds to 1 mN m^{-2}s^{-1}.

a. Substances that flow in accordance with the above equation (Newton's law) are known as **Newtonian substances.** Liquids that consist of simple molecules and dilute dispersions tend to be **Newtonian.**

b. Non-Newtonian substances do not obey Newton's equation of flow. These substances tend to exhibit **shear-dependent** or **time-dependent viscosity.** In either case, viscosity is more aptly termed **apparent viscosity** because Newton's law is not strictly obeyed. Heterogeneous liquids and solids are most likely non-Newtonian.

(1) Shear-dependent viscosity involves either an *increase* in apparent viscosity (i.e., **shear thickening, or dilatancy**) or a *decrease* in apparent viscosity (i.e., **shear thinning, or pseudoplasticity**) with an increase in the rate of shear. Shear thickening is displayed by suspensions that have a high solids content of small, deflocculated

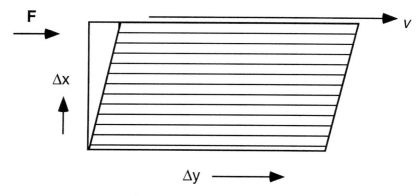

Figure 3-3. Depiction of liquid flow.

particles. Shear thinning is displayed by polymer or macromolecule solutions. **Plastic,** or **Bingham body,** behavior is exemplified by flocculated particles in concentrated suspensions that show no apparent response to low-level stress. Flow begins only after a limiting yield stress **(yield value)** is exceeded.

(2) Time-dependent viscosity

   (a) The yield value of **plastic** systems may be time-dependent (i.e., may depend on the time scale involved in the application of force). **Thixotropic** systems display shear-thinning behavior, but do not immediately recover their higher apparent viscosity when the rate of shear is lowered. In a thixotropic system, structural recovery is relatively slow compared with structural breakdown.

   (b) Thixotropy occurs with heterogeneous systems that involve a three-dimensional structure or network. When such a system is at rest, it appears to have a relatively rigid consistency. Under shear, the structure breaks down and fluidity increases (i.e., **gel–sol** transformation).

   (c) Negative thixotropy, or **antithixotropy,** occurs when the apparent viscosity of the system continues to increase with continued application of shear up to some equilibrium value at a given shear rate. These systems display a **sol–gel** transformation. One explanation for antithixotropic behavior is that continued shear increases the frequency of particle or macromolecule interactions and leads to increased structure in the system.

C. Solids. Intermolecular forces of attraction are stronger in solids than in liquids or gases.

   1. Crystalline solids have the following attributes:
      a. Fixed **molecular order** (i.e., molecules occupy set positions in a specific array)
      b. A distinct melting point
      c. Anisotropicity (i.e., their properties are not the same in all directions), with the exception of cubic crystals

   2. Amorphous solids have these attributes:
      a. Randomly arranged molecules
      b. Nondistinct melting points
      c. Isotropicity (i.e., properties are the same in all directions)

   3. Polymorphism is the condition wherein substances can exist in more than one crystalline form. These **polymorphs** have different molecular arrangements or crystal lattice structures. As a result, the different polymorphs of a drug solid can have different properties. For example, the melting point, solubility, dissolution rate, density, and stability can differ considerably among the polymorphic forms of a drug. Many drugs exhibit polymorphic behavior. One drug class in which the incidence of polymorphism is especially high is **steroids.** Fatty (triglyceride) excipients (e.g., theobroma oil, cocoa butter) are recognized for their polymorphic behavior.

   4. Melting point and heat of fusion. The melting point of a solid is the temperature at which the solid is transformed to a liquid. When 1 g of a solid is heated and melts, the heat absorbed in the process is referred to as the **latent heat of fusion.**

D. Phase diagrams and phase equilibria. A **phase diagram (Figure 3-4)** represents the states of matter (i.e., solid, liquid, and gas) that exist as temperature and pressure are varied. The data arrays separating the phases in the figure delineate the temperatures and pressures at which the phases can coexist. Thus, gas (or vapor) and liquid coexist along "curve" BC, solid and liquid coexist along "curve" AB, and solid and gas (or vapor) coexist along "curve" DB. Depending upon the change in temperature and pressure, **evaporation** or **condensation** occur along "curve" BC, **fusion** or **melting** along "curve" AB, and **sublimation** or **deposition** along "curve" DB. The three "curves" intersect at point B. Only at this unique temperature and pressure, known as the **triple point,** do all three phases exist in equilibrium. (The triple point for water is 0.01°C and $6.04 \cdot 10^{-3}$ atm.) Continuing along "curve" BC, to higher temperatures and pressures, one ultimately reaches point C, known as the **critical point,** above which there is no distinction between the liquid and gas phases. Substances that exist above this critical point are known as **supercritical fluids.** Supercritical fluids such as carbon dioxide (critical point, 30.98°C and 73.8 atm) often exhibit markedly altered physicochemical properties (e.g., density, diffusivity, or solubility characteristics) that render them useful as solvents and processing aids in the production of pharmaceuticals and drug delivery systems.

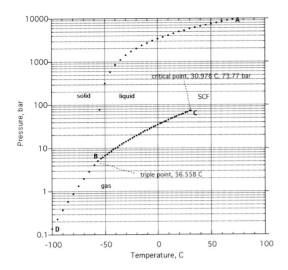

Figure 3-4. Phase diagram for CO_2 showing the variation of the state of matter as pressure and temperature are varied. The solid state exists in the region **ABD**; the liquid state, in the region **ABC**; and the gas state, in the region to the right of curve **CD**. **B** corresponds to the triple point, the pressure and temperature at which all three phases coexist. **C** corresponds to the critical point, the pressure and temperature above which the liquid and gas phases are indistinguishable.

IV. PHYSICOCHEMICAL BEHAVIOR

A. Homogeneous systems

1. A **solution** is a homogeneous system in which a **solute** is molecularly dispersed, or dissolved, in a **solvent.** The solvent is the predominant species. **Saturated solutions** are solutions that, at a given temperature and pressure, contain the maximum amount of solute that can be accommodated by the solvent. If the saturation, or solubility, limit is exceeded, a fraction of the solute can separate from the solution and exist in equilibrium with it.

   a. **Solutes** can be gases, liquids, or solids, and nonelectrolytes or electrolytes.

      (1) **Nonelectrolytes** are substances that **do not form ions** when dissolved in water. Examples are estradiol, glycerin, urea, and sucrose. Their aqueous solutions do not conduct electric current.

      (2) **Electrolytes** are substances that **do form ions** in solution. Examples are sodium chloride, hydrochloric acid, and atropine. As a result, their aqueous solutions conduct electric current. Electrolytes are characterized as **strong** or **weak.** Strong electrolytes (e.g., sodium chloride, hydrochloric acid) are **completely ionized** in water at all concentrations. Weak electrolytes (e.g., aspirin, atropine) are **partially ionized** in water.

   b. The **colligative properties of a solution** are dependent on the total **number of ionic and nonionic solute molecules in the solution.** These properties are dependent on ionization, but **independent of other chemical properties of the solute.**

2. **Colligative properties** include the following:

   a. **Lowering of vapor pressure.** The **partial vapor pressure** of each volatile component in a solution is equal to the product of the mol fraction of the component in the solution and the vapor pressure of the pure component. This is **Raoult's law:**

   $$p_A = p_A{}^0 \cdot x_A$$

   where p_A is the partial vapor pressure above a solution in which the mol fraction of the solute A is x_A and $p_A{}^0$ is the **vapor pressure** of the pure component A. The vapor pressure is the pressure at which an equilibrium is established between the molecules of A in the liquid state and the molecules of A in the gaseous (vapor) state in a closed, evacuated container. The vapor pressure is temperature dependent, but independent of the amount of liquid and vapor. Raoult's law holds for ideal solutions of nonelectrolytes. For a **binary solution** (i.e., a solution of component B in component A)

   $$(p_A{}^0 - p_A)/p_A{}^0 = (1 - x_A) = x_B$$

   The lowering of the vapor pressure of the solution relative to the vapor pressure of the pure solvent is proportional to the number of molecules of solute in the solution. The actual lowering of the vapor pressure by the solute, Δp_A, is given by

   $$\Delta p_A = (p_A{}^0 - p_A) = x_B p_A{}^0$$

b. Elevation of the boiling point. The **boiling point** is the temperature at which the vapor pressure of a liquid equals an external pressure of 760 mm Hg. A solution of a nonvolatile solute has a higher boiling point than a pure solvent because the solute lowers the vapor pressure of the solvent. The amount of elevation of the boiling point (ΔT_b) depends on the concentration of the solute:

$$\Delta T_b = \frac{RT_0^2\, M_1\, m}{1000 \cdot \Delta H_{vap}} = K_b m$$

where K_b is the molal boiling point elevation constant, R is the molar gas constant, T is absolute temperature ($^\circ$K), M_1 is the molecular weight of the solute, m is the molality of the solution, and ΔH_{vap} is the molal enthalpy of vaporization of the solvent.

c. Depression of the freezing point. The **freezing point,** or melting point, of a pure compound is the temperature at which the solid and the liquid phases are in equilibrium under a pressure of 1 atmosphere (atm). The freezing point of a solution is the temperature at which the solid phase of the pure solvent and the liquid phase of the solution are in equilibrium under a pressure of 1 atm. The amount of depression of the freezing point (ΔT_f) depends on the molality of the solution:

$$\Delta T_f = \frac{RT_0^2\, M_1\, m}{1000 \cdot \Delta H_{fusion}} = K_f m$$

where K_f is the molal freezing point constant and ΔH_{fusion} is the molal heat of fusion.

d. Osmotic pressure. Osmosis is the process by which solvent molecules pass through a semipermeable membrane (a barrier through which only solvent molecules may pass) from a region of dilute solution to one of more concentrated solution. Solvent molecules transfer because of the inequality in chemical potential on the two sides of the membrane. Solvent molecules in a concentrated solution have a lower chemical potential than solvent molecules in a more dilute solution.

(1) Osmotic pressure is the **pressure** that must be applied to the solution to prevent the flow of pure solvent into the concentrated solution.

(2) Solvent molecules move from a region where their **escaping tendency is high** to one where their **escaping tendency is low.** The presence of dissolved solute lowers the escaping tendency of the solvent in proportion to the solute concentration.

(3) The **van't Hoff equation** defines the osmotic pressure π as a function of the number of moles of solute n_2 in the solution of volume V:

$$\pi V = n_2\, RT$$

3. Electrolyte solutions and ionic equilibria

a. Acid–base equilibria

(1) According to the **Arrhenius dissociation theory,** an **acid** is a substance that liberates H^+ in aqueous solution. A **base** is a substance that liberates hydroxyl ions (OH^-) in aqueous solution. This definition applies only under aqueous conditions.

(2) The **Lowry-Brønsted theory** is a more powerful concept that applies to aqueous and nonaqueous systems. It is most commonly used for pharmaceutical and biologic systems because these systems are primarily aqueous.

(a) According to this definition, an **acid** is a substance (charged or uncharged) that is capable of donating a proton. A **base** is a substance (charged or uncharged) that is capable of accepting a proton from an acid. The dissociation of an acid (HA) always produces a base (A^-) according to the following formula:

$$HA \leftrightarrow H^+ + A^-$$

(b) HA and A^- are a **conjugate acid–base pair** (an acid and a base that exist in equilibrium and differ in structure by a proton). The proton of an acid does not exist free in solution, but combines with the solvent. In water, this **hydrated proton is a hydronium ion** (H_3O^+).

(c) The relative **strengths** of acids and bases are determined by their ability to donate or accept protons. For example, in water, HCl donates a proton more readily than does acetic acid. Thus, HCl is a stronger acid. Acid strength is also determined by the affinity of the solvent for protons. For example, HCl may dissociate completely in liquid ammonia, but only very slightly in glacial acetic acid. Thus, HCl is a strong acid in liquid ammonia and a weak acid in glacial acetic acid.

(3) The **Lewis theory** extends the acid–base concept to reactions that do not involve protons. It defines an **acid** as a molecule or ion that accepts an electron pair from another atom and a **base** as a substance that donates an electron pair to be shared with another atom.

b. **H^+ concentration** values are very small. Therefore, they are expressed in **exponential notation as pH.** The pH is the logarithm of the reciprocal of the H^+ concentration

$$pH = \log \frac{1}{[H^+]}$$

where $[H^+]$ is the molar concentration of H^+. Because the logarithm of a reciprocal equals the **negative logarithm** of the number, this equation may be rewritten as:

$$pH = -\log[H^+]$$
or
$$[H^+] = 10^{-pH}$$

Thus, the pH value may be defined as the negative logarithm of the $[H^+]$ value. For example, if the H^+ concentration of a solution is 5×10^{-6}, the pH value may be calculated as follows:

$$
\begin{aligned}
pH &= -\log[5 \times 10^{-6}] \\
\log 5 &= 0.699; \log 10^{-6} = -6.0 \\
pH &= -[-6 + 0.699] \\
&= -[-5.301] \\
&= 5.301
\end{aligned}
$$

c. As pH decreases, **H^+ concentration increases exponentially.** When the pH decreases from 6 to 5, the H^+ concentration increases from 10^{-6} to 10^{-5}, or 10 times its original value. When the pH falls from 5 to 4.7, the H^+ concentration increases from 1×10^{-5} to 2×10^{-5}, or double its initial value.

d. **Dissociation constants. Ionization** is the complete separation of the ions in a crystal lattice when the salt is dissolved. **Dissociation** is the separation of ions in solution when the ions are associated by interionic attraction.

(1) For **weak electrolytes,** dissociation is a reversible process. The equilibrium of this process can be expressed by the law of mass action. This law states that the rate of the chemical reaction is proportional to the product of the concentration of the reacting substances, each raised to a power of the number of moles of the substance in solution.

(2) For **weak acids,** dissociation in water is expressed as:

$$HA \leftrightarrow H^+ + A^-$$

The dynamic equilibrium between the simultaneous forward and reverse reactions is indicated by the arrows. By the law of mass action,

$$
\begin{aligned}
\text{rate of forward reaction} &= K_1[HA] \\
\text{rate of reverse reaction} &= K_2[H^+][A^-]
\end{aligned}
$$

At equilibrium, the forward and reverse rates are equal. Therefore,

$$K_1[HA] = K_2[H^+][A^-]$$

Thus, the **equilibrium expression for the dissociation of a weak acid** is written as:

$$K_a = \frac{K_1}{K_2} = \frac{[H^+][A^-]}{[HA]}$$

where K_a represents the acid dissociation constant. For a weak acid, the **acid dissociation constant** is conventionally expressed as **pK_a,** which is $-\log[K_a]$. For example, the K_a of acetic acid at 25°C is 1.75×10^{-5}. The pK_a is calculated as follows:

$$
\begin{aligned}
pK_a &= -\log[1.75 \times 10^{-5}] \\
\log 5 &= 0.243; \log 10^{-5} = -5 \\
pH &= -[0.243 + (-5)] \\
&= -[-4.757] \\
&= 4.76
\end{aligned}
$$

(3) For **weak bases,** dissociation may also be expressed with the K_a expression for the **conjugate acid of the base.** This acid is formed when a proton reacts with the base. For a base that does not contain a hydroxyl group,

$$BH^+ \leftrightarrow H^+ + B$$

The **dissociation constant** for this reaction is expressed as:

$$K_a = \frac{[H^+][B]}{[BH^+]}$$

However, a **base dissociation constant** is traditionally defined for a weak base with this expression:

$$B + H_2O \leftrightarrow OH^- + BH^+$$

$$K_b = \frac{[OH^-][BH^+]}{[B]}$$

where K_b represents the dissociation constant of a weak base. This **dissociation constant** can be expressed as **pK_b,** as follows:

$$pK_b = -\log [K_b]$$

(4) Certain compounds (acids or bases) can accept or donate more than one proton. Consequently, they have **more than one dissociation constant.**

e. **Henderson-Hasselbalch equations** describe the relation between the ionized and unionized species of a weak electrolyte.

(1) For **weak acids,** the Henderson-Hasselbalch equation is obtained from the equilibrium relation described above [IV A 3d (2)]:

$$pH = pK_a + \log \frac{[salt]}{[acid]}$$

(2) Similarly, the Henderson-Hasselbalch equation for **weak bases** is as follows:

$$pH = pK_a + \log \frac{[B]}{[BH^+]}$$

where B is the unionized weak base and BH^+ is the protonated base.

f. The **degree of ionization (α),** the fraction of a weak electrolyte that is ionized in solution, is calculated from the following equation:

$$\alpha = \frac{[I]}{[I] + [U]}$$

where [I] and [U] represent the concentrations of the ionized and unionized species, respectively. The degree of ionization depends solely on the pH of the solution and the pK_a of the weak electrolyte. **When pH = pKa,** the Henderson-Hasselbalch equations are, for a weak acid and a weak base, respectively:

$$pH - pK_a = 0 = \log \frac{[A^-]}{[HA]}$$

$$thus, \frac{[A^-]}{[HA]} = 1$$

$$pH - pK_a = 0 = \log \frac{[B]}{[BH^+]}$$

$$thus, \frac{[B]}{[BH^+]} = 1$$

In effect, when the pH of the solution is numerically equivalent to the pK_a of the weak electrolyte, whether a weak base or a weak acid, [I] = [U] and the degree of ionization $\alpha = 0.5$ (i.e., 50% of the solute is ionized).

g. **Solubility of a weak electrolyte** varies as a function of pH.

(1) For a **weak acid,** the total solubility C_s is given by the expression:

$$C_s = [HA] + [A^-]$$

where [HA] is the intrinsic solubility of the unionized weak acid and is denoted as C_0, whereas [A$^-$] is the concentration of its anion. Because [A$^-$] can be expressed in terms of C_0 and the dissociation constant K_a,

$$C_s = C_0 + \frac{K_a C_0}{[H^+]}$$

Thus, the **solubility of a weak acid increases with increasing pH** (i.e., with an increasing degree of ionization, as the anion is more polar and therefore more water-soluble than the unionized weak acid).

(2) Similarly, for **weak bases,**

$$C_s = C_0 + \frac{C_0 [H^+]}{K_a}$$

Thus, the **solubility decreases with increasing pH** because more of the weak base is in the unprotonated form. This form is less polar and therefore less water-soluble.

h. Buffers and buffer capacity

(1) A **buffer** is a mixture of salt with acid or base that resists changes in pH when small quantities of acid or base are added. A buffer can be a **combination** of a weak acid and its conjugate base (salt) or a combination of a weak base and its conjugate acid (salt). However, buffer solutions are more **commonly prepared** from weak acids and their salts. They are not ordinarily prepared from weak bases and their salts because weak bases are often unstable and volatile.

(a) For a **weak acid and its salt,** the buffer equation below is satisfactory for calculations with a pH of 4–10. It is important in the preparation of buffered pharmaceutical solutions:

$$pH = pK_a + \log \frac{[salt]}{[acid]}$$

(b) For a **weak base and its salt,** the buffer equation is similar, but also depends on the dissociation constant of water (pK_w). The equation becomes:

$$pH = pK_w - pK_b + \log \frac{[base]}{[salt]}$$

(2) **Buffer action** is the resistance to a change in pH.

(3) **Buffer capacity** is the ability of a buffer solution to resist changes in pH. The **smaller the pH change** caused by addition of a given amount of acid or base, the **greater the buffer capacity** of the solution.

(a) Buffer capacity is the number of gram equivalents of an acid or base that changes the pH of 1 L of buffer solution by 1 unit.

(b) Buffer capacity is affected by the concentration of the buffer constituents. A higher concentration provides a greater acid or base reserve. Buffer capacity (β) is related to total concentration (C) as follows:

$$\beta = 2.3\, C\, \frac{K_a [H^+]}{[K_a + (H^+)]^2}$$

where C represents the molar concentrations of the acid and the salt.

(c) Thus, buffer capacity depends on the value of the ratio of the salt to the acid form. It increases as the ratio approaches unity. Maximum buffer capacity occurs when pH = pK_a, and is represented by $\beta = 0.576 \cdot C$.

B. Heterogeneous (disperse) systems

1. Introduction

a. A **suspension** is a two-phase system that is composed of a solid material dispersed in an oily or aqueous liquid. The particle size of the dispersed solid is usually greater than 0.5 μm.

b. An **emulsion** is a heterogeneous system that consists of at least one immiscible liquid that is intimately dispersed in another in the form of droplets. The droplet diameter usually exceeds 0.1 μm. Emulsions are **inherently unstable** because the droplets of the dispersed liquid tend to coalesce to form large droplets until all of the dispersed droplets have coalesced. The third component of the system is an **emulsifying agent.** This agent prevents coalescence and maintains the integrity of the individual droplets.

2. **Dispersion stability.** In an **ideal dispersion,** the dispersed particles do not interact. The particles are uniform in size and undergo no change in position other than the random movement that results from Brownian motion. In contrast, in a **real dispersion,** the particles are not uniformly sized (i.e., they are not **monodisperse**). The particles are subject to particulate aggregation, or clumping, and the dispersion becomes more heterogeneous with time. The **rate of settling (separating, or creaming)** of the dispersed phase in the dispersion medium is a function of the particle size, dispersion phase viscosity, and difference in density between the dispersed phase and the dispersion medium, in accordance with **Stokes' law:**

$$\text{Sedimentation rate} = \frac{d^2 g (\rho_1 - \rho_2)}{18 \, \eta}$$

where d is the particle diameter, g is the acceleration due to gravity, η is the viscosity of the dispersion medium, and $(\rho_1 - \rho_2)$ is the difference between the density of the particles (ρ_1) and the density of the dispersion medium (ρ_2). Although Stokes' law was derived to determine the settling, or sedimentation, of noninteracting spherical particles, it also provides guidance for determining the stabilization of dispersion:
   a. **Particle size** should be as **small** as possible. Smaller particles yield slower sedimentation, or flotation, rates.
   b. **High particulate (dispersed phase) concentrations** increase the rate of particle–particle collisions and interaction. As a result, particle aggregation occurs, and instability increases as the aggregates behave as larger particles. In the case of liquid–liquid dispersions, particle–particle collisions can lead to coalescence (i.e., larger particles) and decrease dispersion stability.
   c. **Avoidance of particle–particle interactions**
      (1) Aggregation can be prevented if the particles have a similar electrical charge. Particles in an aqueous system always have some electrical charge because of **ionization** of chemical groups on the particle surface or **adsorption** of charged molecules or ions at the interface. If the adsorbed species is an **ionic surfactant** (e.g., sodium lauryl sulfate), the charge associated with the surfactant ion (e.g., lauryl sulfate anion) will accumulate at the interface. However, if a relatively non–surface-active electrolyte is adsorbed, the sign of the charge of the adsorbed ion is less readily predicted.
      (2) The **magnitude of the charge** is the difference in electrical potential between the charged surface of the particle and the bulk of the dispersion medium. This magnitude is approximated by the **electrokinetic, or zeta, potential (ζ).** The zeta potential is measured from the fixed, avidly bound layers of ions and solvent molecules on the particle surface. When ζ is high (e.g., ≥ 25 mV), interparticle **repulsive forces** exceed the attractive forces. As a result, the dispersion is **deflocculated** and relatively stable to collision and subsequent aggregation **(flocculation).** When ζ is so low that interparticulate **attractive forces** predominate, loose particle aggregates, or **flocs,** form (i.e., **flocculation** occurs).
   d. **Density** can be manipulated to decrease the rate of dispersion instability. The settling rate decreases as $(\rho_1 - \rho_2)$ approaches zero. However, the density of the dispersion medium usually cannot be altered sufficiently to halt the settling (or flotation) process. In the dispersed phase, the density of solid particles is not readily altered; altering the density of liquid particles would require the addition of a miscible liquid of higher (or lower) density. Altering the composition of suspensions is also problematic because most solid particles are denser than the dispersion medium. Additives of higher (or lower) density might alter the biopharmaceutical characteristics of the formulation (e.g., rate of drug release, residence time at the site of administration or absorption).
   e. The sedimentation, or **flotation, rate** is inversely proportional to the **viscosity.** An **increase** in the **viscosity of the dispersion medium** decreases the rate of settling, or flotation. However, although the rate of destabilization can be slowed by an increase in viscosity, it cannot be halted.

3. **Emulsion stability. Coalescence** occurs in emulsion systems when the liquid particles of the dispersed phase merge to form larger particles. Coalescence is largely prevented by the **interfacial film** of surfactant around the droplets. This film prevents direct contact of the

liquid phase of the droplets. Coalescence of droplets in oil-in-water (o/w) emulsions is also inhibited by the **electrostatic repulsion** of similarly charged particles. **Creaming** is the **reversible** separation of a layer of emulsified particles. Because mixing or shaking may be sufficient to reconstitute the emulsion system, creaming is not necessarily unacceptable. However, **cracking, or irreversible phase separation,** is never acceptable. **Phase inversion,** or emulsion-type reversal, involves the reversion of an emulsion from an o/w to a water-in-oil (w/o) form, or vice versa. Phase inversion can change the consistency or texture of the emulsion or cause further deterioration in its stability.

V. CHEMICAL KINETICS AND DRUG STABILITY

A. Introduction. The **stability** of the **active component** of a drug is a major criterion in the rational design and evaluation of drug dosage forms. Problems with **stability** can determine whether a given formulation is accepted or rejected.

   1. Extensive chemical degradation of the active ingredient can cause **substantial loss** of active ingredient from the dosage form.

   2. Chemical degradation can produce a **toxic product** that has undesirable side effects.

   3. Instability of the drug product can cause **decreased bioavailability.** As a result, the therapeutic efficacy of the dosage form may be substantially reduced.

B. Rates and orders of reactions

   1. The **rate of a reaction,** or degradation rate, is the velocity with which the reaction occurs. This rate is expressed as dC/dt (the change in concentration, or C, within a given time interval, or dt).

   a. Reaction rates depend on certain conditions (e.g., **reactant concentration, temperature, pH, presence of solvents or additives**). Radiation and catalytic agents (e.g., polyvalent cations) also have an effect.

   b. The effective study of reaction rates in the body requires application of **pharmacokinetic principles** (see Chapter 6).

   2. The **order of a reaction** is the way in which the concentration of the drug or reactant in a chemical reaction affects the rate. The rate of a reaction, dC/dt, is proportional to the concentration to the nth power, where n is the order of the reaction. That is,

$$\frac{dC}{dt} \propto C^n$$

The study of reaction orders is a crucial aspect of pharmacokinetics (see Chapter 6). Usually, **pharmaceutical degradation** can be treated as a **zero-order, first-order,** or **higher order reaction.** The first two are summarized below.

   a. In a **zero-order reaction,** the **rate is independent of the concentration of the reactants** (i.e., $dC/dt \propto C^0$) [see Chapter 6]. Other factors, such as absorption of light in certain photochemical reactions, determine the rate.

   (1) A **zero-order reaction** can be expressed as:

$$C = -k_o t + C_o$$

where C is the drug concentration, k_o is the zero-order rate constant in units of concentration/time, t is the time, and C_o is the initial concentration.

   (2) When this equation is plotted with C on the vertical axis (ordinate) against t on the horizontal axis (abscissa), the **slope of the line is equal to** $-k_o$ (Figure 3-5). The negative sign indicates that the slope is decreasing.

   b. In a **first-order reaction,** the **rate depends on the first power of the concentration of a single reactant** (i.e., $dC/dt + C^1$).

   (1) In a first-order reaction, **drug concentration decreases exponentially with time,** in accordance with the equation

$$C = C_o e^{-k_1 t}$$

where C is the concentration of the reacting material, C_o is the initial concentration, k_1 is the first-order rate constant in units of reciprocal time, and t is time. A plot of

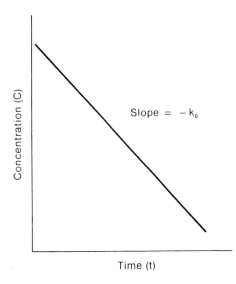

Figure 3-5. Concentration *(C)* versus time *(t)* for a zero-order reaction. The slope of the line equals $-k_0$. The slope of the line is not equal to the rate constant because it includes the minus sign.

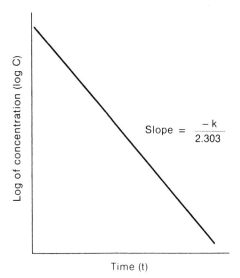

Figure 3-6. Logarithm of concentration *(log C)* versus time *(t)* for a first-order reaction. The slope of the line equals $-k/2.303$.

the logarithm of concentration against time produces a straight line with a slope of $-k/2.303$ (Figure 3-6).

(2) The **half-life** $(t_{1/2})$ of a reaction is the time required for the concentration of a drug to decrease by one-half. For a first-order reaction, half-life is expressed by:

$$t_{1/2} = \frac{0.693}{k_1}$$

(3) The **time required for a drug to degrade** to 90% of its original concentration ($t_{90\%}$) is also important. This time represents a reasonable limit of degradation for the active ingredients. The $t_{90\%}$ can be calculated as:

$$t_{90\%} = \frac{2.303}{k_1} \log\left(\frac{100}{90}\right) = \frac{0.105}{k_1}$$

(a) Because

$$k_1 = \frac{0.693}{t_{1/2}}$$

(b) Then

$$t_{90\%} = \frac{0.105}{0.693/t_{1/2}} = 0.152 \cdot t_{1/2}$$

(4) Both $t_{1/2}$ and $t_{90\%}$ are **concentration-independent.** Thus, for $t_{1/2}$, it takes the same amount of time to reduce the concentration of the drug from 100 mM to 50 mM as it does from 50 mM to 25 mM.

C. **Factors that affect reaction rates.** Factors other than concentration can affect the reaction rate and stability of a drug. These factors include temperature, the presence of a solvent, pH, and the presence of additives.

   1. **Temperature.** An **increase in temperature** causes an increase in reaction rate, as expressed in the equation first suggested by Arrhenius:

   $$k = Ae^{-Ea/RT} \text{ or } \log k = \log A - \left(\frac{Ea}{2.303} \times \frac{1}{RT} \right)$$

   where k is the specific reaction rate constant, A is a constant known as the frequency factor, Ea is the energy of activation, R is the molar gas constant (1.987 cal/degree × mole), and T is the absolute temperature.
      a. The **constants A and Ea** are obtained by determining k at several temperatures and then plotting log k against 1/T. The slope of the resulting line equals $-Ea/(2.303 \cdot R)$. The intercept on the vertical axis equals log A.
      b. The activation energy (Ea) is the amount of energy required to put the molecules in an **activated state.** Molecules must be activated to react. As **temperature increases,** more molecules are activated, and the **reaction rate increases.**

   2. **Presence of solvent.** Many dosage forms require the incorporation of a water-miscible solvent [e.g., low–molecular-weight alcohols, such as the polyethylene glycols (PEGs)] to stabilize the drug.
      a. A change in the solvent system **alters** the transition state and the **activity coefficients** of the reactant molecules. It can also cause simultaneous changes in physicochemical parameters, such as pK_a, surface tension, and viscosity. These changes **indirectly affect the reaction rate.**
      b. In some cases, **additional reaction pathways** are generated. For example, with an increasing concentration of ethanol in an aqueous solution, aspirin degrades by an extra route and forms the ethyl ester of acetylsalicylic acid. However, a **change in solvent can also stabilize the drug.**

   3. **Change in pH.** The magnitude of the rate of a hydrolytic reaction catalyzed by H^+ and OH^- can vary considerably with pH.
      a. H^+ **catalysis** predominates at **lower pH,** whereas OH^- **catalysis** operates at **higher pH.** At **intermediate pH,** the rate may be **pH-independent** or may be catalyzed by **both H^+ and OH^-.** Rate constants in the intermediate pH range are typically less than those at higher or lower pH.
      b. To determine the **effect of pH on degradation kinetics,** decomposition is measured at several H^+ concentrations. The **pH of optimum stability** can be determined by plotting the logarithm of the rate constant (k) as a function of pH (Figure 3-7). The **point of inflection** of the plot is the pH of optimum stability. This value is useful in the development of a stable drug formulation.

   4. **Presence of additives**
      a. **Buffer salts** must be added to many drug solutions to maintain the formulation at optimum pH. These salts **can affect the rate of degradation,** primarily as a result of salt increasing the ionic strength.
         (1) Increasing salt concentrations, particularly from polyelectrolytes (e.g., citrate, phosphate), can **substantially affect the magnitude of pK_a.** In this way, they change the rate constant.
         (2) Buffer salts can also **promote drug degradation** through general acid or base catalysis.

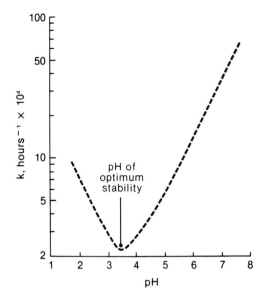

Figure 3-7. Semilogarithmic plot of the rate constant (k) versus *pH*. This plot is used to determine the pH of optimum stability.

    b. The **addition of surfactants** may accelerate or decelerate drug degradation.
       (1) Acceleration of degradation is common and is caused by micellar catalysis.
       (2) Stabilization of a drug through the addition of a surfactant is less common.
    c. Complexing agents can improve drug stability. Aromatic esters (e.g., benzocaine, procaine, tetracaine) **increase in half-life** in the presence of caffeine. This increased stability appears to result from the formation of a less reactive complex between the aromatic ester and caffeine.

D. Modes of pharmaceutical degradation. The decomposition of active ingredients in a dosage form occurs through several pathways (e.g., hydrolysis, oxidation, photolysis) [see Chapter 12 II A].

  1. Hydrolysis is the most common type of degradation because many medicinal compounds are esters, amides, or lactams.
    a. H^+ **and** OH^- are the most common catalysts of hydrolytic degradation in solution.
    b. Esters usually undergo hydrolytic reactions that cause drug instability. Because esters are rapidly degraded in aqueous solution, formulators are reluctant to incorporate drugs that have ester functional groups into liquid dosage forms.

  2. Oxidation is usually mediated through reaction with atmospheric oxygen under ambient conditions (auto-oxidation).
    a. Medicinal compounds that undergo auto-oxidation at room temperature are affected by **oxygen dissolved in the solvent** and in the head space of their packages. These compounds should be packed in an **inert atmosphere** (e.g., nitrogen) to exclude air from their containers.
    b. Most oxidation reactions involve a **free radical mechanism** and a **chain reaction.** Free radicals tend to take electrons from other compounds.
       (1) Antioxidants in the formulation react with the free radicals by providing electrons and easily available hydrogen atoms. In this way, they prevent the propagation of chain reactions.
       (2) Commonly used antioxidants include ascorbic acid, butylated hydroxyanisole (BHA), butylated hydroxytoluene (BHT), propyl gallate, sodium bisulfite, sodium sulfite, and the tocopherols.

  3. Photolysis is the degradation of drug molecules by normal sunlight or room light.
    a. Molecules may absorb the proper wavelength of light and **acquire sufficient energy to undergo reaction.** Usually, photolytic degradation occurs on exposure to light of wavelengths less than 400 nm.
    b. An **amber glass bottle** or an **opaque container** acts as a barrier to this light, thereby preventing or retarding photolysis. For example, sodium nitroprusside in aqueous solution

has a shelf life of only 4 hours if exposed to normal room light. When protected from light, the solution is stable for at least 1 year.

E. Determination of shelf life. The shelf life of a drug preparation is the amount of time that the product can be stored before it becomes unfit for use, through either chemical decomposition or physical deterioration.

1. **Storage temperature** affects shelf life. It is generally understood to be ambient temperature unless special storage conditions are specified.

2. **In general, a preparation is considered fit for use if it varies from the nominal concentration or dose by no more than 10%,** provided that the decomposition products are not more toxic or harmful than the original material.

3. **Shelf-life testing** aids in determining the standard shelf life of a formulation.
   a. Samples are stored at approximately 3–5°C and at room temperature (20–25°C). The samples are then analyzed at various intervals to determine the **rate of decomposition.** Shelf life is calculated from this rate.
   b. Because storage time at these temperatures can result in an extended testing time, **accelerated testing** is conducted as well, with a range of higher temperatures. The **rate constants** obtained from these samples are used to predict shelf life at ambient or refrigeration temperatures. **Temperature-accelerated stability testing** is not useful if temperature changes are accompanied by changes in the reaction mechanism or by physical changes in the system (e.g., change from the solid to the liquid phase).
   c. **Stability at room temperature** can be predicted from accelerated testing data by the Arrhenius equation:

$$\log\left(\frac{k_{T_2}}{k_{T_1}}\right) = \frac{Ea(T_2 - T_1)}{2.303 \cdot R \cdot T_2 \cdot T_1}$$

   where k_{T_2} and k_{T_1} are the rate constants at the absolute temperatures T_2 and T_1, respectively; R is the molar gas constant; and Ea is the energy of activation.
   d. Alternatively, an expression of concentration can be plotted as a linear function of time. Rate constants (k) for degradation at several temperatures are obtained. The logarithm of the rate constant ($\log k$) is plotted against the reciprocal of absolute temperature ($1/T$) to obtain, by extrapolation, the rate constant for degradation at room temperature (Figure 3-8).

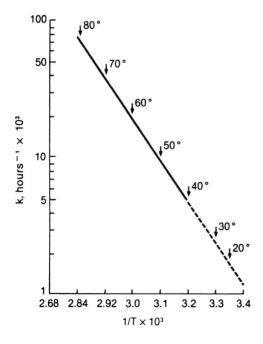

Figure 3-8. Semilogarithmic plot of the rate constant *(k)* versus the reciprocal of absolute temperature *(1/T)*, showing the temperature dependency of degradation

e. The **length of time that the drug will maintain its required potency** can also be predicted by calculation of the t$_{90\%}$ [see V B 2 b (3)]. This method applies to chemical reactions with activation energies of 10–30 kcal/mol, the magnitude of the activation energy for many pharmaceutical degradations that occur in solution.

VI. DRUG DOSAGE FORMS AND DELIVERY SYSTEMS

A. Oral solutions. The *United States Pharmacopeia* (USP) 26/National Formulary (NF) 21 categorizes **oral solutions** as "liquid preparations, intended for oral administration, that contain one or more substances with or without flavoring, sweetening, or coloring agents dissolved in water or cosolvent-water mixtures." Oral solutions can contain certain polyols (e.g., sorbitol, glycerin) to inhibit crystallization and to modify solubility, taste, mouth feel, and other vehicle properties. They can be "formulated for direct oral administration to the patient or they may be dispensed in a more concentrated form that must be diluted prior to administration. . . ." **Drugs in solution** are more homogeneous and easier to swallow than drugs in solid form. For drugs that have a slow dissolution rate, onset of action and bioavailability are also improved. However, drugs in solution are bulkier dosage forms, degrade more rapidly, and are more likely to interact with constituents than those in solid form.

1. **Water** is the **most commonly used vehicle** for drug solutions. The **USP** recognizes six types of water for the preparation of dosage forms:
   a. Purified water USP is water obtained by distillation, ion exchange, reverse osmosis, or other suitable treatment. It cannot contain more than 10 parts per million (ppm) of total solid and should have a pH between 5 and 7. Purified water is used in prescriptions and finished manufactured products except parenteral and ophthalmic products.
   b. Water for injection USP is water obtained by distillation or by reverse osmosis. It conforms to the standards of purified water, but is also free of pyrogen. Water for injection is used as a solvent for the preparation of parenteral solutions.
   c. Sterile water for injection USP is water for injection that is sterilized and packaged in single-dose containers of type I and II glass. These containers do not exceed a capacity of 1 L. The limitations for total solids depend on the size of the container.
   d. Bacteriostatic water for injection USP is sterile water for injection that contains one or more suitable antimicrobial agents. It is also packaged in single- or multiple-dose containers of type I or II glass. These containers do not exceed the capacity of 30 mL.
   e. Sterile water for inhalation USP is water that is purified by distillation or by reverse osmosis (i.e., water for injection) and rendered sterile. It contains no antimicrobial agents, except where used in humidifiers or similar devices. This type of water should not be used for parenteral administration or for other sterile dosage forms.
   f. Sterile water for irrigation USP is water for injection that is sterilized and suitably packaged. It contains no antimicrobial agents or other added substance.

2. **Oral drug solutions** include **syrups** and **elixirs** as well as other less widely prescribed classic **(galenical)** formulations, such as **aromatic waters, tinctures, fluidextracts,** and **spirits.**
   a. Syrups are traditionally peroral solutions that contain high concentrations of sucrose or other sugars. Through common usage, the term syrup has also come to include any other liquid dosage form prepared in a sweet, viscous vehicle, including peroral suspensions.
      (1) Syrup NF (simple syrup) is a concentrated or nearly saturated aqueous solution of sugar (85% w/v).
      (2) Syrups have a **low solvent capacity for water-soluble drugs** because the hydrogen bonding between sucrose and water is very strong. For this reason, it can be difficult or impossible to dissolve a drug in a syrup. Often, the drug is best dissolved in a small quantity of water, and the flavoring syrup is added.
      (3) The **sucrose concentration** of syrup plays a crucial role in the control of microbial growth. Dilute sucrose solutions are excellent media for microorganisms. As the concentration of sucrose approaches saturation, the syrup becomes self-preserving (i.e., requires no additional preservative). However, a saturated solution is undesirable because temperature fluctuations may cause crystallization. **Syrup NF** is a self-preserved solution with a minimal tendency to undergo crystallization.
   b. Elixirs are traditionally peroral solutions that contain alcohol as a cosolvent. Many peroral solutions are not described as elixirs, but contain alcohol.

(1) To be considered an elixir, the solution **must contain alcohol.** Traditionally, the alcohol content of elixirs has varied from 5%–40%. Most elixirs become turbid when moderately diluted by aqueous liquids. Elixirs are not the preferred vehicle for salts because alcohol accentuates saline taste. Salts also have limited solubility in alcohol. Therefore, the alcoholic content of salt-containing elixirs must be low.

(2) **Aromatic elixir NF,** prepared in part from syrup, contains approximately 22% alcohol. The limited usefulness of this elixir as a solvent for drugs was offset by the development of **iso-alcoholic elixir.** It is a combination of **low-alcoholic elixir,** an elixir with low alcoholic content (8%–10% alcohol), and **high-alcoholic elixir,** an elixir with high alcoholic content (73%–78% alcohol). Mixing appropriate volumes of the two elixirs provides an alcoholic content sufficient to dissolve the drugs.

B. Miscellaneous solutions

1. **Aromatic waters** are clear, **saturated aqueous solutions of volatile oils** or other aromatic or volatile substances. Aromatic waters may be used as pleasantly flavored vehicles for a water-soluble drug or as an aqueous phase in an emulsion or suspension. If a large amount of water-soluble drug is added to an aromatic water, then an insoluble layer may form at the top. This **"salting out"** is a competitive process. The molecules of water-soluble drugs have more attraction for the solvent molecules of water than the "oil" molecules. The associated water molecules are pulled away from the "oil" molecules, which are no longer held in solution. Aromatic waters should be stored in tight, light-resistant bottles to reduce volatilization and degradation from sunlight. Aromatic waters are usually prepared by any of the following methods:

   a. **Distillation** is a universal method, but it is not practical or economical for most products. It is the only method, however, for preparing strong rose water and orange flower water.

   b. With the **solution method,** the volatile, or aromatic, substance is admixed with water, with or without the use of a dispersant (e.g., talc).

2. **Spirits,** or **essences,** are alcoholic or hydroalcoholic solutions of volatile substances, that contain 50%–90% alcohol. This **high alcoholic content** maintains the water-insoluble volatile oils in solution. If water is added to a spirit, the oils separate. Some spirits are **medicinal** (e.g., aromatic ammonia spirit). Many spirits (e.g., compound orange spirit, compound cardamom spirit) are used as flavoring agents. Spirits should be stored in tight containers to reduce loss by evaporation.

3. **Tinctures** are alcoholic or hydroalcoholic solutions of chemicals or soluble constituents of vegetable drugs. Although tinctures vary in drug concentration (≤50%), those prepared from potent drugs are usually 10% in strength (i.e., 100 mL of the tincture has the activity of 10 g of the drug). Tinctures are usually considered stable. The alcohol content of the official tinctures varies from 17%–21% with opium tincture USP and from 74%–80% with compound benzoin tincture USP. Most tinctures are prepared by an **extraction process** of maceration or percolation. The selection of a **solvent,** or menstruum, is based on the solubility of the active and inert constituents of the crude drugs. Aging can cause precipitation of the inactive constituents of tinctures. Glycerin may be added to the hydroalcoholic solvent to increase the solubility of the active constituent and reduce precipitation on storage. Tinctures must be tightly stoppered and kept from excessive temperatures. Because many of their constituents undergo a photochemical change when exposed to light, tinctures must be stored in light-resistant containers.

4. **Fluidextracts** are liquid extracts of vegetable drugs that contain alcohol as a solvent, preservative, or both. Fluidextracts are prepared by percolation so that each milliliter contains the therapeutic constituents of 1 g of the standard drug. Because of their high drug content, fluidextracts are sometimes referred to as "100% tinctures." Fluidextracts of potent drugs are usually 10 times as concentrated, or potent, as the corresponding tincture. For example, the usual dose of tincture belladonna is 0.6 mL; the equivalent dose of the more potent fluidextract is 0.06 mL. Many fluidextracts are considered too potent for self-administration by patients, so they are almost never prescribed. In addition, many fluidextracts are simply too bitter. Today, most fluidextracts are modified by either flavoring or sweetening agents.

5. **Nasal, ophthalmic, otic,** and **parenteral solutions** are classified separately because of their specific use and method of preparation.

6. **Mouthwashes** are solutions that are used to cleanse the mouth or treat diseases of the oral mucous membrane. They often contain alcohol or glycerin to aid in dissolving the volatile ingredients. Mouthwashes are more often used cosmetically than therapeutically.

7. **Astringents** are locally applied solutions that precipitate protein. They reduce cell permeability without causing injury. Astringents cause **constriction,** with wrinkling and blanching of the skin. Because astringents **reduce secretions,** they can be used as antiperspirants.
   a. **Aluminum acetate** and **aluminum subacetate solutions** are used as wet dressings in contact dermatitis. The precipitation is minimized by the addition of boric acid.
   b. **Calcium hydroxide solution** is a mild stringent that is used in lotions as a reactant and an alkalizer.

8. **Antibacterial topical solutions** (e.g., benzalkonium chloride, strong iodine, povidone–iodine) kill bacteria when applied to the skin or mucous membrane in the proper strength and under appropriate conditions.

C. **Suspensions**

1. **Lotions, magmas** (i.e., suspensions of finely divided material in a small amount of water), and **mixtures** are all suspensions that have had official formulas for some time (e.g., calamine lotion USP, kaolin mixture with pectin NF). Official formulas are given in the USP/NF.
   a. A **complete formula** and a **detailed method of preparation** are available for some official suspensions. For others, only the **concentration** for the active ingredients is given, and the manufacturer has considerable latitude in the formulation.
   b. Some drugs are packaged in a **dry form** to circumvent the instability of aqueous dispersions. Water is added at the time of dispensing to reconstitute the suspension.

2. **Purposes of suspension**
   a. **Sustaining effect.** For a sustained release preparation, a suspension necessitates drug dissolution prior to absorption.
   b. **Stability.** Drug degradation in suspension or solid dosage forms occurs much more slowly than degradation in solution form.
   c. **Taste.** A drug with an unpleasant taste can be converted into an insoluble form and then prepared as a suspension.
   d. **Basic solubility.** When suitable solvents are not available, the suspension provides an alternative. For example, only water can be used as a solvent for ophthalmic preparations because of the possibility of corneal damage. Ophthalmic suspensions provide an alternative to ophthalmic solutions.

3. **Suspending agents** include hydrophilic colloids, clays, and a few other agents. Some are also used as **emulsifying agents** (see VI D 3).
   a. **Hydrophilic colloids** (i.e., **hydrocolloids**) increase the viscosity of water by binding water molecules, thus limiting their mobility, or fluidity. Viscosity is proportional to the concentration of the hydrocolloid. These agents **support the growth of microorganisms** and require a preservative. They are mostly **anionic,** with the exception of methyl cellulose (neutral) and chitosan (cationic). Thus, the anionic hydrocolloids are incompatible with quaternary antibacterial agents and other positively charged drugs. Chitosan is incompatible with negatively charged drugs and excipients. Most hydrocolloids are **insoluble in alcoholic solutions.**
      (1) **Acacia** is usually used as a 35% dispersion in water (mucilage). Its viscosity is greatest between pH 5 and 9. Acacia is susceptible to microbial decomposition.
      (2) **Tragacanth** is usually used as a 6% dispersion in water (mucilage). It has an advantage over acacia in that less is needed. Also, tragacanth does not contain the oxidase that is present in acacia. This oxidase catalyzes the decomposition of organic chemicals. The viscosity of tragacanth is greatest at pH 5.
      (3) **Methyl cellulose** is a polymer that is nonionic and stable to heat and light. It is available in several viscosity grades. Because it is soluble in cold water, but not in hot water, dispersions are prepared by adding methyl cellulose to boiling water and then cooling the preparation until the material dissolves.
      (4) **Carboxymethylcellulose** is an anionic material that is soluble in water. Prolonged exposure to heat causes loss of viscosity.

b. Clays (e.g., bentonite, Veegum®) are silicates that are anionic in aqueous dispersions. They are strongly hydrated and exhibit **thixotropy** (the property of forming a gel-like structure on standing and becoming fluid on agitation).

    (1) The official form of **bentonite** is the 5% magma.

    (2) Veegum® is hydrated to a greater degree than bentonite. Thus, it is more viscous at the same concentration.

c. Other agents include agar, chondrus (carrageenan), gelatin, pectin, and gelatinized starch. Their use is limited by their susceptibility to bacterial attack, their incompatibilities, and their cost. Xanthan gum is used in many modern suspension formulations because of its cosolvent compatibility, its stability, and its solution's high viscosity relative to concentration.

4. Preparation

a. Solids are wetted initially to separate individual particles and coat them with a layer of dispersion medium. Wetting is accomplished by **levigation** (i.e., addition of a suitable nonsolvent, or **levigating agent,** to the solid material, followed by blending to form a paste), using a glass mortar and pestle or an ointment slab. A **surfactant** can also be used.

b. Suspending agents are then added as dry powder along with the active ingredient. For best results, the suspending agent is added in the form of its **aqueous dispersion.**

    (1) The aqueous dispersion is added to the solid (or the levigated solid) by **geometric dilution.**

    (2) The preparation is brought to the desired volume by stirring in the appropriate vehicle.

D. Emulsions

1. Purposes of emulsions

a. Increased drug solubility. Many drugs have limited aqueous solubility, but have maximum solubility in the oil phase of an emulsion. Drug partitioning from the oil phase to the water phase can maintain or enhance activity.

b. Increased drug stability. Many drugs are more stable when incorporated into an emulsion rather than an aqueous solution.

c. Prolonged drug action. Incorporation of a drug into an emulsion can prolong bioavailability, as with certain intramuscular injection preparations.

d. Improved taste. Drugs with an unpleasant taste are more palatable and thus more conveniently administered in emulsion form.

e. Improved appearance. Oily materials intended for topical application are more appealing in an emulsified form.

2. Phases of emulsions. Most emulsions are considered **two-phase systems.**

a. The **liquid droplet** is known as the **dispersed, internal,** or **discontinuous phase.** The other liquid is known as the **dispersion medium, external phase,** or **continuous phase.**

b. In pharmaceutical applications, one phase is usually an **aqueous solution.** The other phase is usually **lipid** or **oily.** The lipids range from vegetable or hydrocarbon oils to semisolid hydrocarbons and waxes. Emulsions are usually described in terms of water and oil. Oil is the lipid, or nonaqueous, phase, regardless of its composition.

    (1) If water is the **internal phase,** the emulsion is classified as **w/o.**

    (2) If water is the **external phase,** the emulsion is classified as **o/w.**

c. The **type of emulsion** formed is primarily determined by the **relative phase volumes** and the **emulsifying agent** used.

    (1) For an ideal emulsion, the maximum concentration of internal phase is 74% (i.e., theoretically, an o/w emulsion can be prepared containing ≤74% oil).

    (2) The choice of an emulsifying agent is more important than the relative phase volumes in determining the final emulsion type. Most agents preferentially form one type of emulsion or the other if the phase volume permits.

3. Emulsifying agents. Any compound that lowers the interfacial tension and forms a film at the interface can potentially function as an emulsifying agent. The effectiveness of the emulsifying agent depends on its chemical structure, concentration, solubility, pH, physical properties, and electrostatic effect. **True emulsifying agents** (primary agents) can form and stabilize emulsions by themselves. **Stabilizers** (auxiliary agents) do not form acceptable emulsions when used alone, but assist primary agents in stabilizing the product (e.g., increase viscosity). Emulsifying agents are either **natural** or **synthetic.**

a. Natural emulsifying agents:
   (1) Acacia forms a good, stable emulsion of low viscosity. It tends to cream easily, is acidic, and is stable at a pH range of 2–10. Like other gums, it is negatively charged, dehydrates easily, and usually requires a preservative. It is incompatible with Peruvian balsam, bismuth salts, and carbonates.
   (2) Tragacanth forms a stable emulsion that is coarser than acacia emulsion. It is anionic and difficult to hydrate, and is used mainly for its effects on viscosity. Less than 1/10 of the amount used for acacia is needed.
   (3) Agar is an anionic gum that is primarily used to increase viscosity. Its stability is affected by heating, dehydration, and destruction of charge. It is also susceptible to microbial degradation.
   (4) Pectin is a quasi-emulsifier that is used in the same proportion as tragacanth.
   (5) Gelatin provides good emulsion stabilization in a concentration of 0.5%–1.0%. It may be anionic or cationic, depending on its isoelectric point. Type A gelatin (+), prepared from an acid-treated precursor, is used in acidic media. Type B gelatin (−), prepared from an alkali-treated precursor, is used in basic media.
   (6) Methyl cellulose is nonionic and induces viscosity. It is used as a primary emulsifier with mineral oil and cod liver oil, and yields an o/w emulsion. It is usually used in 2% concentration.
   (7) Carboxymethylcellulose is anionic and is usually used to increase viscosity. It tolerates alcohol up to 40%, forms a basic solution, and precipitates in the presence of free acids.
b. Synthetic emulsifying agents are anionic, cationic, or nonionic. Although these surfactants are amphiphilic molecules, their lipophilic and hydrophilic regions are seldom inverse equals of each other: some surfactant molecules tend to be predominantly lipophilic whereas others are predominantly hydrophilic. This imbalance is reflected in the HLB or hydrophilic-lipophilic balance (HLB) scale: the larger the HLB value, the more hydrophilic the molecule. Table 3-1 lists HLB values for surfactants and their corresponding utility.
   (1) Anionic synthetic agents include **sulfuric acid esters** (e.g., sodium lauryl sulfate), **sulfonic acid derivatives** (e.g., dioctyl sodium sulfosuccinate), and **soaps.** Soaps are for external use. They have a high pH and are therefore sensitive to the addition of acids and electrolytes.
      (a) Alkali soaps are hydrophilic and form an o/w emulsion.
      (b) Metallic soaps are water-insoluble and form a w/o emulsion.
      (c) Monovalent soaps form an o/w emulsion.
      (d) Polyvalent soaps form a w/o emulsion.
   (2) Cationic synthetic agents (e.g., benzalkonium chloride) are used as surface-active agents in 1% concentration. They are incompatible with soaps.
   (3) Nonionic synthetic agents are resistant to the addition of acids and electrolytes (Table 3-1).
      (a) The **sorbitan esters** known as **Spans** are hydrophobic in nature and form w/o emulsions. They have low hydrophilic–lipophilic balance values (1–9) [Table 3-2].
      (b) The **polysorbates** known as **Tweens** are hydrophilic and tend to form o/w emulsions. They may form complexes with phenolic compounds. They have high hydrophilic–lipophilic balance values (11–20).

Table 3-1. Hydrophilic–Lipophilic Balance (HLB)

HLB Value Range	Surfactant Application
0–3	Antifoaming agents
4–6	Water-in-oil emulsifying agents
7–9	Wetting agents
8–18	Oil-in-water emulsifying agents
13–15	Detergents
10–18	Solubilizing agents

Table 3-2. Commonly Used Surfactants and Their Hydrophilic–Lipophilic Balance (HLB) Values

Agent	HLB Value
Sorbitan trioleate (Span 85, Arlacel 85)	1.8
Sorbitan tristearate (Span 65)	2.1
Propylene glycol monostearate (pure)	3.4
Sorbitan sesquioleate (Arlacel C)	3.7
Sorbitan monooleate (Span 80y)	4.3
Sorbitan monostearate (Arlacel 60)	4.7
Sorbitan monopalmitate (Span 40, Arlacel 40)	6.7
Sorbitan monolaurate (Span 20, Arlacel 20)	8.6
Glyceryl monostearate (Aldo 28, Tegin)	5.5
Gelatin	9.8
Triethanolamine oleate (Trolamine)	12.0
Polyoxyethylene alkyl phenol (Igepal CA-630)	12.8
Tragacanth	13.2
Polyoxyethylene sorbitan monolaurate (Tween 21)	13.3
Polyoxyethylene castor oil (Atlas G-1794)	13.3
Polyoxyethylene sorbitan monooleate (Tween 80)	15.0
Polyoxyethylene sorbitan monopalmitate (Tween 40)	15.6
Polyoxyethylene sorbitan monolaurate (Tween 20)	16.7
Polyoxyethylene lauryl ether (Brij 35)	16.9
Sodium oleate	18
Sodium lauryl sulfate	40

4. **Preparation.** Various methods are used to prepare emulsions, depending upon the type of emulsifying agent.
   a. Classical, acacia-stabilized emulsions are prepared by one of the following four methods:
      (1) **Wet gum (English) method.** A primary emulsion of fixed oil, water, and acacia (in a 4:2:1 ratio) is prepared as follows:
         (a) Two parts of water are added all at once to one part of acacia. The mixture is triturated until a smooth mucilage is formed.
         (b) Oil is added in small increments (1–5 mL) with continuous trituration until the primary emulsion is formed.
         (c) The mixture (an o/w emulsion) is triturated for another 5 minutes.
         (d) The o/w mixture can then be brought to volume with water and mixed to achieve homogeneity.
      (2) **Dry gum (continental) method.** A primary emulsion of the fixed oil, water, and acacia (in a 4:2:1 ratio) is prepared as follows:
         (a) Oil is added to the acacia, and the mixture is triturated until the powder is distributed uniformly throughout the oil. Water is added all at once, followed by rapid trituration to form the primary emulsion.
         (b) Any remaining water and other ingredients are added to finish the product.
            (i) **Electrolytes in high concentration** tend to crack an emulsion. They should be added last and in as dilute a form as possible.
            (ii) **Alcoholic solutions** tend to dehydrate and precipitate hydrocolloids. They should be added in as dilute a concentration as possible.
      (3) **Bottle method** (a variation of the dry gum method used for volatile oils). Oil is added to the acacia in a bottle. The ratio of oil, water, and acacia should be 3:2:1 or 2:1:1. The low viscosity of the volatile oil requires a higher proportion of acacia.
      (4) **Nascent soap method.** A soap is formed by mixing relatively equal volumes of an oil and an aqueous solution that contains a sufficient amount of alkali. The soap acts as an emulsifying agent.
         (a) This method is used to form an o/w or a w/o emulsion, depending on the soap formed. For example, olive oil, which contains oleic acid, is mixed with lime water during the preparation of calamine lotion to calcium oleate, an emulsifying agent.

(b) A 50:50 ratio of oil to water ensures sufficient emulsion, provided that the oil contains an adequate amount of free fatty acid. Olive oil usually does. Cotton-seed oil, peanut oil, and some other vegetable oils do not.

(c) The addition of an acid destroys the emulsifying soap and causes the emulsion to separate.

b. Emulsions stabilized by synthetic emulsifying agents are readily prepared by a two-phase procedure:

(1) Oil-miscible ingredients and water-miscible ingredients are separately admixed, using heat if necessary to ensure liquefaction and ease of mixing of each phase.

—High melting point oil-miscible ingredients (e.g., waxes) are melted before lower melting point ingredients (e.g., oils) are added.

(2) The two phases are heated to about 70–80° and then combined with stirring until the resultant emulsion has cooled.

—In general, heat-labile or volatile ingredients should not be incorporated in the separate phases but in the resultant emulsion after it has cooled to about 40°C. or less.

(3) Further mechanical processing of the emulsion by a hand homogenizer, immersion blender, or other equipment may be warranted to improve the homogeneity and stability of the product.

5. Incorporation of medicinal agents. Medicinal agents can be incorporated into an emulsion either during or after its formation.

a. Addition of a drug during emulsion formation. It is best to incorporate a drug into a vehicle during emulsion formation, when it can be incorporated in molecular form. Soluble drugs should be dissolved in the appropriate phase (e.g., drugs that are soluble in the external phase of the emulsion should be added as a solution to the primary emulsion).

b. Addition of a drug to a preformed emulsion can present some difficulty, depending on the type of emulsion and the nature of the emulsifier (Table 3-3).

(1) Addition of oleaginous materials to a w/o emulsion presents no problem because of the miscibility of the additive with the external phase. However, **addition of oleaginous materials to an o/w emulsion** can be difficult after emulsion formation.

(a) Occasionally, a small amount of oily material is added if excess emulsifier was used in the original formation.

(b) A small amount of an oil-soluble drug can be added if it is dissolved in a very small quantity of oil with geometric dilution techniques.

(2) Addition of water or an aqueous material to a w/o emulsion is extremely difficult, unless enough emulsifier has been incorporated into the emulsion. However, **addition of aqueous materials to an o/w emulsion** usually presents no problems if the added material does not interact with the emulsifying agent. Potential interactions should be expected with cationic compounds and salts of weak bases.

Table 3-3. Selected Commercial Emulsion Bases: Emulsion Type and Emulsifier Used

Commercial Base	Emulsion Type	Emulsifier Type
Allercreme Skin Lotion	o/w	Triethanolamine stearate
Almay Emulsion Base	o/w	Fatty acid glycol esters
Cetaphil	o/w	Sodium lauryl sulfate
Dermovan	o/w	Fatty acid amides
Eucerin	w/o	Wool wax alcohol
HEB Base	o/w	Sodium lauryl sulfate
Keri Lotion	o/w	Nonionic emulsifiers
Lubriderm	o/w	Triethanolamine stearate
Neobase	o/w	Polyhydric alcohol esters
Neutragena Lotion	o/w	Triethanolamine lactate
Nivea Cream	w/o	Wool wax alcohols
pHorsix	o/w	Polyoxyethylene emulsifiers
Polysorb Hydrate	w/o	Sodium sesquioleate
Velvachol	o/w	Sodium lauryl sulfate

w/o = water-in-oil

o/w = oil-in-water

(3) Addition of small quantities of alcoholic solutions to an o/w emulsion is possible if the solute is compatible or dispersible in the aqueous phase of the emulsion. If acacia or another gum is used as the emulsifying agent, the alcoholic solution should be diluted with water before it is added. Table 3-3 lists some commercial emulsion bases and their general composition.

(4) Addition of crystalline drugs to a w/o emulsion occurs more easily if the drugs are dissolved or dispersed in a small quantity of oil before they are added.

E. Ointments

1. **Introduction. Ointments** are **semisolid preparations intended for external use.** They are easily spread. Modifying the formulation controls their plastic viscosity. Ointments are typically used as:
   a. **Emollients** to make the skin more pliable
   b. **Protective barriers** to prevent harmful substances from coming in contact with the skin
   c. **Vehicles** in which to incorporate medication

2. **Ointment bases**
   a. **Oleaginous bases** are anhydrous and insoluble in water. They cannot absorb or contain water and are not washable in water.
      (1) **Petrolatum** is a good base for oil-insoluble ingredients. It forms an occlusive film on the skin, absorbs less than 5% water under normal conditions, and does not become rancid. Wax can be incorporated to stiffen the base.
      (2) **Synthetic esters** are used as constituents of oleaginous bases. These esters include glyceryl monostearate, isopropyl myristate, isopropyl palmitate, butyl stearate, and butyl palmitate. Long-chain alcohols (e.g., cetyl alcohol, stearyl alcohol, PEG) can also be used.
      (3) **Lanolin derivatives** are often used in topical and cosmetic preparations. Examples are lanolin oil and hydrogenated lanolin.
   b. **Absorption bases** are anhydrous and water-insoluble. Therefore, they are not washable in water, although they can absorb water. These bases permit water-soluble medicaments to be included through prior solution and uptake as the internal phase.
      (1) **Wool fat** (anhydrous lanolin) contains a high percentage of cholesterol as well as esters and alcohol that contain fatty acids. It absorbs twice its weight in water and melts between 36°C and 42°C.
      (2) **Hydrophilic petrolatum** is a white petrolatum combined with 8% beeswax, 3% stearyl alcohol, and 3% cholesterol. These components are added to a w/o emulsifier. Prepared forms include Aquaphor, which uses wool alcohol to render white petrolatum emulsifiable. Aquaphor is superior in its ability to absorb water.
   c. **Emulsion bases** may be w/o emulsions, which are water-insoluble and are not washable in water. These emulsions can absorb water because of their aqueous internal phase. Emulsion bases may also be o/w emulsions, which are water-insoluble, but washable in water. They can absorb water in their aqueous external phase.
      (1) **Hydrous wool fat** (lanolin) is a w/o emulsion that contains approximately 25% water. It acts as an emollient and occlusive film on the skin, effectively preventing epidermal water loss.
      (2) **Cold cream** is a w/o emulsion that is prepared by melting white wax, spermaceti, and expressed almond oil together, adding a hot aqueous solution of sodium borate, and stirring until the mixture is cool.
         (a) The use of mineral oil rather than almond oil makes a more stable cold cream. However, cold cream prepared with almond oil makes a better emollient base.
         (b) This ointment should be freshly prepared.
      (3) **Hydrophilic ointment** is an o/w emulsion that uses sodium lauryl sulfate as an emulsifying agent. It absorbs approximately 30%–50% w/w without losing its consistency. It is readily miscible with water and is removed from the skin easily.
      (4) **Vanishing cream** is an o/w emulsion that contains a large percentage of water as well as humectant (e.g., glycerin, propylene glycol) that retards moisture loss. An excess of stearic acid in the formula helps to form a thin film when the water evaporates.
      (5) **Other emulsion bases** include Dermovan, a hypoallergenic, greaseless emulsion base, and Unibase, a nongreasy emulsion base that absorbs approximately 30% of its weight in water and has a pH close to that of the skin.

d. Water-soluble bases may be anhydrous or may contain some water. They are washable in water and absorb water to the point of solubility.

  (1) PEG ointment is a blend of water-soluble polyethylene glycols that form a semisolid base. This base can solubilize water-soluble drugs and some water-insoluble drugs. It is compatible with a wide range of drugs.

    (a) This base contains 40% PEG 3350 and 60% PEG 400. It is prepared by the fusion method (see VI E 3 b).

    (b) Only a small amount of liquid (<5%) can be incorporated without loss of viscosity. This base can be made stiffer by increasing the amount of PEG 3350 to 60%.

    (c) If 6% to 25% of an aqueous solution is to be incorporated, 5 g of the 40 g of PEG 3350 can be replaced with an equal amount of stearyl alcohol.

  (2) Propylene glycol and **propylene glycol–ethanol** form a clear gel when mixed with 2% hydroxypropyl cellulose. This base is a popular dermatologic vehicle.

3. Incorporation of medicinal agents. Medicinal substances may be incorporated into an ointment base by **levigation** or by the **fusion method.** Insoluble substances should be reduced to the finest possible form and levigated before incorporation with a small amount of compatible levigating agent or with the base itself.

  a. Levigation. The substance is incorporated into the ointment by levigation on an ointment slab.

  (1) A stainless steel spatula with a long, broad, flexible blade should be used. If the substance may interact with a metal spatula (e.g., when incorporating iodine and mercuric salts), then a hard rubber spatula can be used.

  (2) Insoluble substances should be powdered finely in a mortar and mixed with an equal quantity of base until a smooth, grit-free mixture is obtained. The rest of the base is added in increments.

  (3) Levigation of powders into a small portion of base is facilitated by the use of a melted base or a small quantity of compatible levigation aid (e.g., mineral oil, glycerin).

  (4) Water-soluble salts are incorporated by dissolving them in the smallest possible amount of water and incorporating the aqueous solution directly into a compatible base.

    (a) Usually, organic solvents (e.g., ether, chloroform, alcohol) are not used to dissolve the drug because the drug may crystallize as the solvent evaporates.

    (b) Solvents are used as levigating aids only if the solid will become a fine powder after the solvent evaporates.

  b. Fusion method. This method is used when the base contains solids that have higher melting points (e.g., waxes, cetyl alcohol, glyceryl monostearate). This method is also useful for solid medicaments, which are readily soluble in the melted base.

  (1) The oil phase should be melted separately, starting with materials that have the highest melting point. All other oil-soluble ingredients are added in decreasing order of melting point.

  (2) The ingredients in the water phase are combined and heated separately to a temperature that is equal to or several degrees above that of the melted oil phase.

  (3) The two phases are combined. If a w/o system is desired, then the hot aqueous phase is incorporated into the hot oil phase with agitation. If an o/w system is preferred, then the hot oil phase is incorporated into the hot aqueous phase.

  (4) Volatile materials (e.g., menthol, camphor, iodine, alcohol, perfumes) are added after the melted mixture cools to 40°C or less.

F. Suppositories

1. Introduction. A suppository is a **solid or semisolid mass intended to be inserted into a body orifice** (i.e., rectum, vagina, urethra). After it is inserted, a suppository either melts at body temperature or dissolves (or disperses) into the aqueous secretions of the body cavity.

  a. Suppositories are often used for local effects (e.g., relief of hemorrhoids or infection).

  b. When used rectally, suppositories can provide systemic medication. The absorption of a drug from a suppository through the rectal mucosa into the circulation involves two steps:

  (1) The drug is released from a vehicle and diffuses through the mucosa.

  (2) The drug is transported through the veins or lymph vessels into systemic fluids or tissues. The first-pass effect is avoided because the rectal veins "bypass the liver."

  c. Rectal suppositories are useful when oral administration is inappropriate, as with infants, debilitated or comatose patients, and patients who have nausea, vomiting, or gastrointestinal disturbances. Some drugs can cause disturbances of the gastrointestinal tract.

2. Types of suppositories

a. Rectal suppositories are usually cylindrical and tapered to a point, forming a bullet-like shape. As the rectum contracts, a suppository of this shape moves inward rather than outward. Suppositories for adults weigh approximately 2 g. Suppositories for infants and children are smaller.

b. Vaginal suppositories are oval and typically weigh approximately 5 g. Drugs administered by this route are intended to have a local effect, but systemic absorption can occur. Antiseptics, contraceptive agents, and drugs used to treat trichomonal, monilial, or bacterial infections are often formulated as vaginal suppositories.

c. Urethral suppositories are typically long and tapered. They are approximately 60 mm long and 4–5 mm in diameter. They are administered for a local effect and are most often used for anti-infective agents. Alprostadil, or prostaglandin E1 (PGE1), when used to treat erectile dysfunction, is available for urethral insertion in the form of a micropellet, or microsuppository, that is only 3–6 mm long and 1.4 mm in diameter.

3. Suppository bases

a. Criteria for satisfactory suppository bases. Suppository bases should:

(1) Remain firm at room temperature to allow insertion. The suppository should not soften below 30°C to avoid melting during storage.

(2) Have a narrow, or sharp, melting range

(3) Yield a clear melt just below body temperature or dissolve rapidly in the cavity fluid

(4) Be inert and compatible with a variety of drugs

(5) Be nonirritating and nonsensitizing

(6) Have wetting and emulsifying properties

(7) Have an acid value of less than 0.2, a saponification value of 200–245, and an iodine value of less than 7 if the base is fatty

b. Selecting a suppository base. Lipid–water solubility must be considered because of its relation to the drug-release rate.

(1) If an oil-soluble drug is incorporated into an oily base, then the rate of absorption is somewhat less than that achieved with a water-soluble base. The lipid-soluble drug tends to remain dissolved in the oily pool from the suppository. It is less likely to escape into the mucous secretions from which it is ultimately absorbed.

(2) Conversely, a water-soluble drug tends to pass more rapidly from the oil phase to the aqueous phase. Therefore, if rapid onset of action is desired, the water-soluble drug should be incorporated into the oily base.

c. Bases that melt include **cocoa butter,** other **combinations of fats and waxes, Witepsol bases,** and **Wecobee bases** (Table 3-4).

(1) Cocoa butter (theobroma oil) is the most widely used suppository base. It is firm and solid up to a temperature of 32°C, at which point it begins to soften. At 34–35°C, it melts to produce a thin, bland, oily liquid.

(a) Cocoa butter is a good base for a **rectal suppository,** but it is less than ideal for a vaginal or urethral suppository.

Table 3-4. Composition, Melting Range, and Congealing Range of Selected Bases That Melt

Base	Composition	Melting Range (°C)	Congealing Range (°C)
Cocoa butter	Mixed triglycerides of oleic, palmitic, and stearic acids	34–35	28 or less
Cotmar	Partially hydrogenated cottonseed oil	34–75	. . .
Dehydag	Hydrogenated fatty alcohols and esters		
Base I		33–36	32–33
Base II		37–39	36–37
Base III		9 ranges	9 ranges
Wecobee R	Glycerides of saturated fatty acids C_{12}–C_{18}	33–35	31–32
Wecobee SS	Triglycerides derived from coconut oil	40–43	33–35
Witepsol	Triglycerides of saturated fatty acids		
H-12	C_{12}–C_{18}, with varied portions of the	32–33	29–32
H-15	corresponding partial glycerides	33–35	32–34
H-85		42–44	36–38

(b) A mixture of triglycerides, cocoa butter exhibits polymorphism. Depending on the fusion temperature, it can crystallize into any one of four crystal forms.

(c) **Major limitations of cocoa butter.** Because of the following limitations, many combinations of fats and waxes are used as substitutes (see Table 3-4):

(i) An inability to absorb aqueous solutions. The addition of nonionic surfactants to the base ameliorates this problem to some extent. However, the resultant suppositories have poor stability and may turn rancid rapidly.

(ii) The lowering of the melting point produced by certain drugs (e.g., chloral hydrate)

(2) **Witepsol** bases contain natural saturated fatty acid chains between C_{12} and C_{18}. Lauric acid is the major component. All 12 bases of this series are colorless and almost odorless. The drug-release characteristics of Witepsol H15 are similar to those of cocoa butter.

(a) Unlike cocoa butter, Witepsol bases do not exhibit polymorphism when heated and cooled.

(b) The interval between softening and melting temperature is very small. Because Witepsol bases solidify rapidly in the mold, lubrication of the mold is not necessary.

(3) **Wecobee** bases are derived from coconut oil. Their action is similar to that of Witepsol bases. Incorporation of glyceryl monostearate and propylene glycol monostearate makes these bases emulsifiable.

d. **Bases that dissolve** include **PEG** polymers with a molecular weight of 400–6000.

(1) At room temperature, PEG 400 is a liquid, PEG 1000 is a semisolid, PEG 1500 and 1600 are fairly firm semisolids, and PEG 3350 and 6000 are firm, wax-like solids.

(2) These bases are water-soluble, but the dissolution process is very slow. In the rectum and vagina, where the amount of fluid is very small, they dissolve very slowly, but they soften and spread.

(3) PEGs complex with several drugs and affect drug release and absorption.

(4) Mixtures of PEG polymers in varying proportions provide a base of different properties (Table 3-5).

4. **Preparation.** Suppositories are prepared by the following three methods:

a. **Hand-rolling** involves molding the suppository with the fingers after a plastic mass is formed.

(1) A finely powdered drug is mixed with the grated base in a mortar and pestle, using levigation and geometric dilution techniques. A small quantity of fixed oil may be added to facilitate preparation.

(2) The uniformly mixed semiplastic mass is kneaded further, rolled into a cylinder, and divided into the requisite number of suppositories. Each small cylinder is rolled by hand until a suppository shape is fashioned.

b. **Compression** is generally used when cocoa butter is used as a base.

(1) A uniform mixture of drug and base is prepared as for the hand-rolling method.

(2) The mixture is placed into a suppository compression device. Pressure is applied, and the mixture is forced into lubricated compression mold cavities. The mold is then cooled and the suppositories ejected.

Table 3-5. Mixtures of Polyethylene Glycol (PEG) Bases Providing Satisfactory Room Temperature Stability and Dissolution Characteristics

Base	Comments	Components	Proportion (%)
1	Provides a good general-purpose, water-soluble suppository base	PEG 6000	50
		PEG 1540	30
		PEG 400	20
2	Provides a good general-purpose base that is slightly softer than base 1 and dissolves more rapidly	PEG 4000	60
		PEG 1500	30
		PEG 400	10
3	Has a higher melting point than the other bases, which is usually sufficient to compensate for the melting-point lowering effect of such drugs as chloral hydrate and camphor	PEG 6000	30
		PEG 1540	70

Table 3-6. Cocoa Butter Density Factors of Drugs Commonly Used in Suppositories

Drug	Cocoa Butter Density Factor	Drug	Cocoa Butter Density Factor
Aloin	1.3	Dimenhydrinate	1.3
Aminophylline	1.1	Diphenhydramine hydrochloride	1.3
Aminopyrine	1.3	Gallic acid	2.0
Aspirin	1.1	Morphine hydrochloride	1.6
Barbital sodium	1.2	Pentobarbital	1.2
Belladonna extract	1.3	Phenobarbital sodium	1.2
Bismuth subgallate	2.7	Salicylic acid	1.3
Chloral hydrate	1.3	Secobarbital sodium	1.2
Codeine phosphate	1.1	Tannic acid	1.6
Digitalis leaf	1.6		

(3) This procedure generally produces a 2-g suppository. However, a large volume of the active ingredients can affect the amount of cocoa butter required for an individual formula.

(a) The amount of cocoa butter needed is determined by calculating the total amount of active ingredient to be used, dividing this number by the cocoa butter density factor (Table 3-6), and subtracting the resulting number from the total amount of cocoa butter required for the desired number of suppositories.

(b) For example, suppose 12 suppositories, each containing 300 mg aspirin, are required. Each mold cavity has a 2-g capacity. For 13 suppositories (calculated to provide one extra), 3.9 g aspirin (13×0.3 g = 3.9 g) is required. This number is divided by the density factor of aspirin (1.1) [see Table 3-6]. Thus, 3.9 g of aspirin replaces 3.55 g of cocoa butter. The total amount of cocoa butter needed for 13 suppositories of 2 g each equals 26 g. The amount of cocoa butter required is 26 g − 3.55 g, or 22.45 g.

c. The **fusion method** is the principal way that suppositories are made commercially. This method is used primarily for suppositories that contain cocoa butter, PEG, and glycerin–gelatin bases. Molds made of aluminum, brass, or nickel–copper alloys are used and can make 6–50 suppositories at one time.

(1) The **capacity of the molds** is determined by melting a sufficient quantity of base over a steam bath, pouring it into the molds, and allowing it to congeal. The "blank" suppositories are trimmed, removed, and weighed. Once the weight is known, the drug-containing suppositories are prepared.

(a) To prepare suppositories, the drug is reduced to a fine powder. A small amount of grated cocoa butter is liquefied in a suitable container placed in a water bath at 33°C or less.

(b) The finely powdered drug is mixed with melted cocoa butter with continuous stirring.

(c) The remainder of the grated cocoa butter is added with stirring. The temperature is maintained at or below 33°C. The liquid should appear creamy rather than clear.

(d) The mold is very lightly lubricated with mineral oil, and the creamy melt is poured into the mold at room temperature. The melt is poured continuously to avoid layering.

(e) After the suppositories congeal, they are placed in a refrigerator to harden. After 30 minutes, they are removed from the refrigerator, trimmed, and unmolded.

(2) The fusion process should be used carefully with **thermolabile drugs** and **insoluble powders.**

(a) Insoluble powders in the melt may settle or float during pouring, depending on their density. They may also collect at one end of the suppository before the melt congeals, and cause a nonuniform drug distribution.

(b) Hard crystalline materials (e.g., iodine, merbromin) can be incorporated by dissolving the crystals in a minimum volume of suitable solvent before they are incorporated into the base.

(c) Vegetable extracts can be incorporated by moistening with a few drops of alcohol and levigating with a small amount of melted cocoa butter.

G. Powders

1. **Introduction.** A pharmaceutical powder is a mixture of finely divided drugs or chemicals in dry form. The powder may be used internally or externally.
   a. **Advantages** of powders
      (1) Flexibility of compounding
      (2) Good chemical stability
      (3) Rapid dispersion of ingredients because of the small particle size
   b. **Disadvantages** of powders
      (1) Time-consuming preparation
      (2) Inaccuracy of dose
      (3) Unsuitability for many unpleasant-tasting, hygroscopic, and deliquescent drugs
   c. **Milling** is the mechanical process of reducing the particle size of solids (**comminution**) before mixing with other components, further processing, or incorporation into a final product (Tables 3-7 and 3-8). The particle size of a powder is related to the proportion of the powder that can pass through the opening of standard sieves of varying dimensions in a specified amount of time. **Micromeritics** is the study of particles.
      (1) **Advantages** of milling
         (a) Milling increases the surface area, which may increase the dissolution rate as well as bioavailability (e.g., griseofulvin).
         (b) Milling increases extraction, or leaching, from animal glands (e.g., liver, pancreas) and from crude vegetable extracts.
         (c) Milling facilitates drying of wet masses by increasing the surface area and reducing the distance that moisture must travel to reach the outer surface. Micronization and subsequent drying, in turn, increase stability as occluded solvent is removed.
         (d) Milling improves mixing, or blending, of several solid ingredients if they are reduced to approximately the same size. It also minimizes segregation and provides greater dose uniformity.
         (e) Milling permits uniform distribution of coloring agents in artificially colored solid pharmaceuticals.
         (f) Milling improves the function of lubricants used to coat the surface of the granulation or powder in compressed tablets and capsules.
         (g) Milling improves the texture, appearance, and physical stability of ointments, creams, and pastes.
      (2) **Disadvantages** of milling
         (a) Milling can change the polymorphic form of the active ingredient, rendering it less active.

Table 3-7. *United States Pharmacopeia* (USP) Standards for Powders of Animal and Vegetable Drugs

Type of Powder	Sieve Size All Particles Pass Through	Sieve Size Percentage of Particles Pass Through
Very coarse (#8)	#20 sieve	20% through a #60 sieve
Coarse (#20)	#20 sieve	40% through a #60 sieve
Moderately coarse (#40)	#40 sieve	40% through a #80 sieve
Fine (#60)	#60 sieve	40% through a #100 sieve
Very fine (#80)	#80 sieve	No limit

Table 3-8. *United States Pharmacopeia* (USP) Standards for Powders of Chemicals

Type of Powder	Sieve Size All Particles Pass Through	Sieve Size Percentage of Particles Pass Through
Coarse (#20)	#20 sieve	60% through a #40 sieve
Moderately coarse (#40)	#40 sieve	60% through a #60 sieve
Fine (#80)	#80 sieve	No limit
Very fine (#120)	#120 sieve	No limit

(b) Milling can degrade the drug as a result of heat buildup, oxidation, or adsorption of unwanted moisture because of increased surface area.

(c) Milling decreases the bulk density of the active compound and excipients, causing flow problems and segregation.

(d) Milling decreases the particle size of the raw materials, and may create problems with static charge that may cause particle aggregation and decrease the dissolution rate.

(e) Milling increases surface area, which may promote air adsorption and inhibit wettability.

(3) Comminution techniques. On a large scale, various mills and pulverizers (e.g., rotary cutter, hammer, roller, fluid energy mill) are used during manufacturing. On a small scale, the pharmacist usually uses one of the following comminution techniques:

(a) Trituration. The substance is reduced to small particles by rubbing it in a mortar with a pestle. Trituration also describes the process by which fine powders are intimately mixed in a mortar.

(b) Pulverization by intervention. Substances are reduced and subdivided with an additional material (i.e., solvent) that is easily removed after pulverization. This technique is often used with gummy substances that reagglomerate or resist grinding. For example, camphor is readily reduced after a small amount of alcohol or other volatile solvent is added. The solvent is then permitted to evaporate.

(c) Levigation. The particle size of the substance is reduced by adding a suitable nonsolvent (levigating agent) to form a paste. The paste is then rubbed in a mortar and pestle or using an ointment slab and spatula. This method is often used to prevent a gritty feel when solids are incorporated into dermatologic or ophthalmic ointments and suspensions. Mineral oil is a common levigating agent.

2. Mixing powders. Powders are mixed, or blended, by the following five methods:

a. Spatulation. A spatula is used to blend small amounts of powders on a sheet of paper or a pill tile.

(1) This method is not suitable for large quantities of powders or for powders that contain potent substances because homogeneous blending may not occur.

(2) This method is particularly useful for solid substances that liquefy or form **eutectic mixtures** (i.e., mixtures that melt at a lower temperature than any of their ingredients) when in close, prolonged contact with one another because very little compression or compaction results.

(a) These substances include phenol, camphor, menthol, thymol, aspirin, phenylsalicylate, phenacetin, and similar chemicals.

(b) To diminish contact, powders prepared from these substances are commonly mixed with an inert diluent (e.g., light magnesium oxide or magnesium carbonate, kaolin, starch, bentonite).

(c) Silicic acid (approximately 20%) prevents eutexia with aspirin, phenylsalicylate, and other troublesome compounds.

b. Trituration is used both to comminute and to mix powders.

(1) If comminution is desired, a porcelain or ceramic mortar with a rough inner surface is preferred to a glass mortar with a smooth working surface.

(2) A glass mortar is preferable for chemicals that stain a porcelain or ceramic surface as well as for simple admixture of substances without special need for comminution. A glass mortar cleans more readily after use.

c. Geometric dilution is used when potent substances must be mixed with a large amount of diluent.

(1) The potent drug and an approximately equal volume of diluent are placed in a mortar and thoroughly mixed by trituration.

(2) A second portion of diluent, equal in volume to the powder mixture in the mortar, is added, and trituration is repeated. The process is continued, with equal volumes of diluent added to the powder mixture in the mortar until all of the diluent is incorporated.

d. Sifting. Powders are mixed by passing them through sifters similar to those used to sift flour. This process results in a light, fluffy product. Usually, it is not acceptable for incorporating potent drugs into a diluent base.

e. Tumbling is the process of mixing powders in a large container rotated by a motorized process. These blenders are widely used in industry, as are large-volume powder mixers that use motorized blades to blend the powder in a large mixing vessel.

3. **Use and packaging of powders.** Depending on their intended use, powders are packaged and dispensed by pharmacists as bulk powders or divided powders.
    a. **Bulk powders** are dispensed by the pharmacist in bulk containers. A **perforated,** or **sifter, can** is used for external dusting, and an **aerosol container** is used for spraying onto skin. A **wide-mouthed glass** permits easy removal of a spoonful of powder.
        (1) Powders commonly dispensed in bulk form
            (a) **Antacid and laxative powders** are used by mixing the directed amount of powder (usually approximately 1 teaspoonful) in a portion of liquid, which the patient then drinks.
            (b) **Douche powders** are dissolved in warm water and applied vaginally.
            (c) **Medicated and nonmedicated powders for external use** are usually dispensed in a sifter for convenient application to the skin.
            (d) **Dentifrices,** or **dental cleansing powders,** are used for oral hygiene.
            (e) Powders for the **ear, nose, throat, tooth sockets,** or **vagina** are administered with an insufflator, or powder blower.
        (2) **Nonpotent substances** are usually dispensed in bulk powder form. Those intended for external use should be clearly labeled.
        (3) **Hygroscopic, deliquescent,** or **volatile** powders should be packed in glass jars rather than pasteboard containers. Amber or green glass should be used if needed to prevent decomposition of light-sensitive components. All powders should be stored in tightly closed containers.
    b. **Divided powders** are dispensed in individual doses, usually in folded **papers** (i.e., chartulae). They may also be dispensed in metal foil, small heat-sealed or resealable **plastic bags,** or other containers.
        (1) After the ingredients are weighed, comminuted, and mixed, the powders must be accurately **divided** into the prescribed number of doses.
        (2) Depending on the potency of the drug substance, the pharmacist decides whether to **weigh** each portion separately before packaging or to approximate portions by the **block-and-divide method.**
        (3) **Powder papers** can be of any convenient size that fits the required dose. Four basic types are used:
            (a) **Vegetable parchment** is a thin, semiopaque, moisture-resistant paper.
            (b) **White bond** is an opaque paper that has no moisture-resistant properties.
            (c) **Glassine** is a glazed, transparent, moisture-resistant paper.
            (d) **Waxed paper** is a transparent waterproof paper.
        (4) Hygroscopic and volatile drugs are best protected with waxed paper that is double-wrapped and covered with a bond paper to improve the appearance. Parchment and glassine papers are of limited use for these drugs.

4. **Special problems.** Volatile substances, eutectic mixtures, liquids, and hygroscopic or deliquescent substances present problems when they are mixed into powders that require special treatment.
    a. **Volatile substances** (e.g., camphor, menthol, essential oils) can be lost by volatilization after they are incorporated into powders. This process is prevented or retarded by the use of heat-sealed plastic bags or by double-wrapping with waxed or glassine paper inside white bond paper.
    b. **Liquids** are incorporated into divided powders in small amounts.
        (1) Magnesium carbonate, starch, or lactose can be added to increase the absorbability of the powders by increasing the surface area.
        (2) When the liquid is a solvent for a nonvolatile heat-stable compound, it is evaporated gently in a water bath. Some fluidextracts and tinctures are treated in this way.
    c. **Hygroscopic and deliquescent substances** that become moist because of an affinity for moisture in the air can be prepared as divided powders by adding inert diluents. Double-wrapping is desirable for further protection.
    d. **Eutectic mixtures**

H. Capsules

1. **Introduction.** Capsules are solid dosage forms in which one or more medicinal or inert substances (as powder, compact, beads, or granulation) are enclosed within a small gelatin shell. Gelatin capsules may be hard or soft. Most capsules are intended to be swallowed whole, but occasionally, the contents are removed from the gelatin shell and used as a premeasured dose.

2. Hard gelatin capsules

a. Preparation of filled hard capsules includes preparing the formulation, selecting the appropriate capsule, filling the capsule shells, and cleaning and polishing the filled capsules.

(1) Empty hard capsule shells are manufactured from a mixture of gelatin, colorants, and sometimes an opacifying agent (e.g., titanium dioxide). The USP also permits the addition of 0.15% sulfur dioxide to prevent decomposition of gelatin during manufacture.

(2) Gelatin USP is obtained by partial hydrolysis of collagen obtained from the skin, white connective tissue, and bones of animals. Types A and B are obtained by acid and alkali processing, respectively.

(3) Capsule shells are cast by dipping cold metallic molds or pins into gelatin solutions that are maintained at a uniform temperature and an exact degree of fluidity.

(a) Variation in the viscosity of the gelatin solution increases or decreases the thickness of the capsule wall.

(b) After the pins are withdrawn from the gelatin solution, they are rotated while being dried in kilns. A strong blast of filtered air with controlled humidity is forced through the kilns. Each capsule is then mechanically stripped, trimmed, and joined.

b. Storage. Hard capsules should be stored in tightly closed glass containers and protected from dust and extremes of humidity and temperature.

(1) These capsules contain 12%–16% water, varying with storage conditions. When humidity is low, the capsules become brittle. When humidity is high, the capsules become flaccid and shapeless.

(2) Storage at high temperatures also affects the quality of hard gelatin capsules.

c. Sizes. Hard capsules are available in a variety of sizes.

(1) Empty capsules are **numbered** from 000, which is the largest size that can be swallowed, to 5, the smallest size. The approximate capacity of capsules ranges from 600 to 30 mg for capsules from 000 to 5, respectively. The capacity varies because of varying densities of powdered drug materials and the degree of pressure used to fill the capsules.

(2) Large capsules are available for **veterinary medicine.**

(3) Selecting capsules. Capsule size should be chosen carefully. A properly filled capsule should have its body filled with the drug mixture and its cap fully extended down the body. The cap is meant to enclose the powder, not to retain additional powder. Typically, hard gelatin capsules are used to encapsulate between 65 mg and 1 g of powdered material, including the drug and any diluents needed.

(a) If the drug dose is inadequate to fill the capsule, a diluent (e.g., lactose) is added.

(b) If the amount of drug needed for a usual dose is too large to place in a single capsule, two or more capsules may be required.

(c) Lubricants such as magnesium stearate (frequently, 1%) are added to facilitate the flow of the powder when an automatic capsule-filling machine is used.

(d) Wetting agents (e.g., sodium lauryl sulfate) may be added to capsule formulations to enhance drug dissolution.

d. Filling capsules. Whether on a large or a small production scale, the cap is first separated from the body of the capsule before filling the capsule body with the formulation and then reattaching the cap. Automated and semi-automated capsule filling equipment fill the capsule bodies with the formulation by gravity fill, tamping, or a screw-feed (i.e., auger) mechanism. Extemporaneously compounded capsules are usually filled by the punch method.

(1) The powder is placed on paper and flattened with a spatula so that the layer of powder is no more than approximately one-third the length of the capsule. The paper is held in the left hand. The body of the capsule is held in the right hand and repeatedly pressed into the powder until the capsule is filled. The cap is replaced and the capsule weighed.

(2) Granular material that does not lend itself well to the punch method can be poured into each capsule from the powder paper on which it was weighed.

(3) Crystalline materials, especially those that consist of a mass of filament-like crystals (e.g., quinine salts) will not fit into a capsule easily unless they are powdered.

(4) After they are filled, capsules must be cleaned and polished.

   (a) On a **small scale,** capsules are cleaned individually or in small numbers by rubbing them on a clean gauze or cloth.
   (b) On a **large scale,** many capsule-filling machines have a cleaning vacuum that removes any extraneous material as the capsules leave the machine.

3. **Soft gelatin capsules**
   a. **Preparation**
      (1) Soft gelatin capsules are prepared from gelatin shells. Glycerin or a polyhydric alcohol (e.g., sorbitol) is added to these shells to make them elastic or plastic-like.
      (2) These shells contain preservatives (e.g., methyl and propyl parabens, sorbic acid) to prevent the growth of fungi.
   b. **Uses.** Soft gelatin shells are oblong, elliptical, or spherical. They are used to contain liquids, suspensions, pastes, dry powders, or pellets.
      (1) Drugs that are commercially prepared in soft capsules include demeclocycline hydrochloride (Declomycin, Lederle), chloral hydrate, digoxin (Lanoxicaps, GlaxoSmithKline), vitamin A, and vitamin E.
      (2) Soft gelatin capsules are usually prepared by the plate process or by the rotary or reciprocating die process.

4. **Uniformity and disintegration**
   a. The **uniformity** of dosage forms can be demonstrated by either weight variation or content uniformity methods. The official compendia should be consulted for details of these procedures.
   b. **Disintegration** tests are not usually required for capsules unless they have been treated to resist solution in gastric fluid (enteric-coated). In this case, they must meet the requirements for disintegration of enteric-coated tablets.

I. Tablets

1. **Introduction**
   a. The **oral route** is the most important method for administering drugs for systemic effect. Oral drugs can be given as solids or liquids.
      (1) Advantages of solid dosage forms
         (a) Accurate dosage
         (b) Easy shipping and handling
         (c) Less shelf space needed per dose than for liquid
         (d) No preservation requirements
         (e) No taste-masking problem
         (f) Generally more stable than liquids, with longer expiration dates
      (2) Advantages of liquid dosage forms
         (a) For some drugs (e.g., adsorbents, antacids), greater effectiveness than solid form
         (b) Useful for patients who have trouble swallowing solid dosage forms
   b. **Tablets** are the **most commonly used solid dosage forms.**
      (1) Advantages
         (a) Precision and low content variability of the unit dose
         (b) Low manufacturing cost
         (c) Easy to package and ship
         (d) Simple to identify
         (e) Easy to swallow
         (f) Appropriate for special-release forms
         (g) Best suited to large-scale production
         (h) Most stable of all oral dosage forms
         (i) Essentially tamperproof
      (2) Disadvantages
         (a) Some drugs resist compression into tablets.
         (b) Some drugs (i.e., those with poor wetting, slow dissolution properties, intermediate to large doses, optimum absorption high in the gastrointestinal tract, or any combination of these features) may be difficult to formulate to provide adequate bioavailability.
         (c) Some drugs (e.g., those with an objectionable taste or odor, those sensitive to oxygen or atmospheric moisture) require encapsulation or entrapment before compression. These drugs are more appropriate in capsule form.

2. Tablet design and formulation

a. Characteristics of ideal tablets

(1) Free of defects (e.g., chips, cracks, discoloration, contamination)
(2) Strong enough to withstand the mechanical stresses of production
(3) Chemically and physically stable over time
(4) Capable of releasing medicinal agents in a predictable and reproducible manner

b. Tablet excipients.
Tablets are manufactured by **wet granulation, dry granulation, or direct compression.** Regardless of the method of manufacture, tablets for oral ingestion usually contain excipients, which are components added to the active ingredients that have special functions (Table 3-9).

(1) **Diluents** are fillers designed to make up the required bulk of the tablet when the drug dosage amount is inadequate. Diluents may also improve cohesion, permit direct compression, or promote flow.

(a) **Common diluents** include kaolin, lactose, mannitol, starch, microcrystalline cellulose, powdered sugar, and calcium phosphate.

(b) **Selection of the diluent** is based on the experience of the manufacturer as well as on the cost of the diluent and its compatibility with the other tablet ingredients. For example, calcium salts cannot be used as fillers for tetracycline products because calcium interferes with the absorption of tetracycline from the gastrointestinal tract.

(2) **Binders and adhesives** are added in either dry or liquid form to promote granulation or to promote cohesive compacts during direct compression.

(a) **Common binding agents** include a 10%–20% aqueous preparation of cornstarch; a 25%–50% solution of glucose; molasses; various natural gums (e.g., acacia); cellulose derivatives (e.g., methylcellulose, carboxymethylcellulose, microcrystalline cellulose); gelatins; and povidone. The natural gums are variable in composition and are usually contaminated with bacteria.

Table 3-9. Some Common Tablet Excipients

Diluents	Disintegrants
Calcium phosphate dihydrate NF (dibasic)	Alginates
Calcium sulfate dihydrate NF	Cellulose
Cellulose NF (microcrystalline)	Cellulose derivatives
Cellulose derivatives	Clays
Dextrose	PVP (cross-linked)
Lactose USP	Starch
Lactose USP (anhydrous)	Starch derivatives
Lactose USP (spray-dried)	
Mannitol USP	**Lubricants**
Starches (directly compressible)	PEGs
Starches (hydrolyzed)	Stearic acid
Sorbitol	Stearic acid salts
Sucrose USP (powder)	Stearic acid derivatives
Sucrose-based materials	Surfactants
	Talc
	Waxes
Binders and adhesives	
Acacia	**Glidants**
Cellulose derivatives	Cornstarch
Gelatin	Silica derivatives
Glucose	Talc
PVP	
Sodium alginate and alginate derivatives	**Colors, flavors, and sweeteners**
Sorbitol	FD&C and D&C dyes and lakes
Starch (paste)	Flavors are available in two forms:
Starch (pregelatinized)	spray-dried and oils
Tragacanth	Artificial sweeteners
	Natural sweeteners

D&C = drugs and cosmetics; FD&C = food, drugs, and cosmetics; NF = National Formulary; PEG = polyethylene glycol; PVP = polyvinylpyrrolidone, more commonly called povidone.

   (b) If the drug substance is adversely affected by an aqueous binder, a **nonaqueous binder** can be used, or the binder can be added dry. The binding action is usually more effective when the binder is mixed in liquid form.

   (c) The **amount** of binder or adhesive used depends on the experience of the manufacturer as well as on the other tablet ingredients. Overwetting usually produces granules that are too hard to allow proper tableting. Underwetting usually produces tablets that are too soft and tend to crumble.

  (3) Disintegrants are added to tablet formulations to facilitate disintegration when the tablet contacts water in the gastrointestinal tract. Disintegrants function by drawing water into the tablet, swelling, and causing the tablet to burst.

   (a) Tablet disintegration may be critical to the subsequent dissolution of the drug and to satisfactory drug bioavailability.

   (b) Common disintegrants include cornstarch and potato starch; starch derivatives (e.g., sodium starch glycolate); cellulose derivatives (e.g., sodium carboxymethylcellulose, croscarmellose sodium); clays (e.g., Veegum, bentonite); and cation exchange resins.

   (c) The total **amount of disintegrant** is not always added to the drug–diluent mixture. A portion can be added, with the lubricant, to the prepared granulation of the drug. This approach causes double disintegration of the tablet. The portion of disintegrant that is added last causes the tablet to break into small pieces, or chunks. The portion that is added first breaks the pieces of tablet into fine particles.

  (4) Lubricants, antiadherents, and glidants have overlapping function.

   (a) Lubricants reduce the friction that occurs between the walls of the tablet and the walls of the die cavity when the tablet is ejected. Talc, magnesium stearate, and calcium stearate are commonly used.

   (b) Antiadherents reduce sticking, or adhesion, of the tablet granulation or powder to the faces of the punches or the die walls.

   (c) Glidants promote the flow of the tablet granulation or powder by reducing friction among particles.

  (5) Colors and dyes disguise off-color drugs, provide product identification, and produce a more aesthetically appealing product. **Food, drug,** and **cosmetic dyes** are applied as solutions. **Lakes** are dyes that have been absorbed on a hydrous oxide. Lakes are typically used as dry powders.

  (6) Flavoring agents are usually limited to chewable tablets or tablets that are intended to dissolve in the mouth.

   (a) Water-soluble flavors usually have poor stability. For this reason, flavor oils or dry powders are typically used.

   (b) Flavor oils may be added to tablet granulations in solvents, dispersed on clays and other adsorbents, or emulsified in aqueous granulating agents. Usually, the maximum amount of oil that can be added to a granulation without affecting its tablet characteristics is 0.5%–0.75%.

  (7) Artificial sweeteners, like flavors, are typically used only with chewable tablets or tablets that are intended to dissolve in the mouth.

   (a) Some **sweetness** may come from the diluent (e.g., mannitol, lactose). Other agents (e.g., saccharin, aspartame) may also be added.

   (b) Saccharin has an unpleasant aftertaste.

   (c) Aspartame is not stable in the presence of moisture and heat.

  (8) Adsorbents (e.g., magnesium oxide, magnesium carbonate, bentonite, silicon dioxide) hold quantities of fluid in an apparently dry state.

 3. Tablet types and classes. Tablets are classified according to their route of administration, drug delivery system, and form and method of manufacture (Table 3-10).

  a. Tablets for oral ingestion are designed to be swallowed intact, with the exception of chewable tablets. Tablets may be coated for a number of reasons: to mask the taste, color, or odor of the drug; to control drug release; to protect the drug from the acid environment of the stomach; to incorporate another drug and provide sequential release or avoid incompatibility; or to improve appearance.

   (1) Compressed tablets are formed by compression and have no special coating. They are made from powdered, crystalline, or granular materials, alone or in combination with excipients such as binders, disintegrants, diluents, and colorants.

   (2) Multiple compressed tablets are layered or compression-coated.

Table 3-10. Tablet Types and Classes

Tablets for oral ingestion	Tablets used in the oral cavity
Compressed tablets	Buccal tablets
Multiple compressed tablets	Sublingual tablets
Layered tablets	Troches, lozenges, and dental cones
Compression-coated tablets	**Tablets used to prepare solutions**
Repeat-action tablets	Effervescent tablets
Delayed-action and enteric-coated tablets	Dispensing tablets
Sugar-coated and chocolate-coated tablets	Hypodermic tablets
Film-coated tablets	Tablet triturates
Air suspension-coated tablets	
Chewable tablets	

    (a) Layered tablets are prepared by compressing a tablet granulation around a previously compressed granulation. The operation is repeated to produce multiple layers.

    (b) Compression-coated, or dry-coated, tablets are prepared by feeding previously compressed tablets into a special tableting machine. This machine compresses an outer shell around the tablets. This process applies a thinner, more uniform coating than sugar-coating, and it can be used safely with drugs that are sensitive to moisture. This process can be used to separate incompatible materials, to produce repeat-action or prolonged-action products, or to produce tablets with a multilayered appearance.

  (3) Repeat-action tablets are layered or compression-coated tablets in which the outer layer or shell rapidly disintegrates in the stomach (e.g., Repetabs, Schering; Extentabs, Wyeth). The components of the inner layer or inner tablet are insoluble in gastric media, but soluble in intestinal media.

  (4) Delayed-action and **enteric-coated tablets** delay the release of a drug from a dosage form. This delay is intended to prevent destruction of the drug by gastric juices, to prevent irritation of the stomach lining by the drug, or to promote absorption, which is better in the intestine than in the stomach.

    (a) Enteric-coated tablets are coated and remain intact in the stomach, but yield their ingredients in the intestines (e.g., Ecotrin, SmithKline Beecham). Enteric-coated tablets are a form of delayed-action tablet. However, not all delayed-action tablets are enteric or are intended to produce an enteric effect.

    (b) Agents used to coat these tablets include fats, fatty acids, waxes, shellac, and cellulose acetate phthalate.

  (5) Sugar-coated and **chocolate-coated tablets** are compressed tablets that are coated for various reasons. The coating may be added to protect the drug from air and humidity, to provide a barrier to a drug's objectionable taste or smell, or to improve the appearance of the tablet.

    (a) Tablets may be coated with a colored or an uncolored sugar. The process includes **seal coating** (waterproofing), **subcoating, syrup coating** (for smoothing and coloring), and **polishing.** These steps take place in a series of mechanically operated coating pans.

    (b) Disadvantages of sugar-coated tablets include the time and expertise required for the process and the increase in tablet size and weight. Sugar-coated tablets may be 50% larger and heavier than the original tablets.

    (c) Chocolate-coated tablets are rare today.

  (6) Film-coated tablets are compressed tablets that are coated with a thin layer of a water-insoluble or water-soluble polymer (e.g., hydroxypropyl methylcellulose, ethylcellulose, povidone, PEG).

    (a) The film is usually colored, and it is more durable, less bulky, and less time-consuming to apply than sugar-coating. Although the film typically increases tablet weight by only 2%–3%, it increases formulation efficiency, resistance to chipping, and output.

      (b) Film-coating solutions usually contain a film former, an alloying substance, a plasticizer, a surfactant, opacifiers, sweeteners, flavors, colors, glossants, and a volatile solvent.

      (c) The volatile solvents used in these solutions are expensive and potentially toxic when released into the atmosphere. Specifically formulated **aqueous dispersion**s of polymers (e.g., ethylcellulose) are now available as alternatives to organic solvent–based coating solutions.

   (7) **Air suspension–coated tablets** are fed into a vertical cylinder and supported by a column of air that enters from the bottom of the cylinder. As the coating solution enters the system, it is rapidly applied to the suspended, rotating solids **(Wurster process).** Rounding coats can be applied in less than 1 hour when blasts of warm air are released in the chamber.

   (8) **Chewable tablets** disintegrate smoothly and rapidly when chewed or allowed to dissolve in the mouth. These tablets contain specially colored and flavored mannitol and yield a creamy base.

      (a) Chewable tablets are especially useful in formulations for children.

      (b) They are commonly used for multivitamin tablets and are used for some antacids and antibiotics.

 b. **Tablets used in the oral cavity** are allowed to dissolve in the mouth.

   (1) **Buccal** and **sublingual tablets** allow absorption through the oral mucosa after they dissolve in the buccal pouch (buccal tablets) or below the tongue (sublingual tablets). These forms are useful for drugs that are destroyed by gastric juice or poorly absorbed from the intestinal tract. Examples include sublingual nitroglycerin tablets, which dissolve very promptly to give rapid drug effects, and buccal progesterone tablets, which dissolve slowly.

   (2) **Troches, lozenges,** and **dental cones** dissolve slowly in the mouth and provide primarily local effects.

 c. **Tablets used to prepare solutions** are dissolved in water before administration.

   (1) **Effervescent tablets** are prepared by compressing granular effervescent salts or other materials (e.g., citric acid, tartaric acid, sodium bicarbonate) that release carbon dioxide gas when they come into contact with water. Commercial alkalinizing analgesic tablets are often made to effervesce to encourage rapid dissolution and absorption (e.g., Alka-Seltzer, Bayer).

   (2) **Other tablets** used to prepare solutions include dispensing tablets, hypodermic tablets, and tablet triturates.

4. **Processing problems**

 a. **Capping** is the partial or complete separation of the top or bottom crown from the main body of the tablet. **Lamination** is separation of a tablet into two or more distinct layers. These problems are usually caused by entrapment of air during processing.

 b. **Picking** is removal of the surface material of a tablet by a punch. **Sticking** is adhesion of tablet material to a die wall. These problems are caused by excessive moisture or the inclusion of substances with low melting temperatures in the formulation.

 c. **Mottling** is unequal color distribution, with light or dark areas standing out on an otherwise uniform surface. This problem occurs when a drug has a different color than the tablet excipients or when a drug has colored degradation products. Colorants solve the problem but can create other problems.

5. **Tablet evaluation and control**

 a. The **general appearance** of tablets is an important factor in consumer acceptance. It also allows monitoring of lot-to-lot uniformity, tablet-to-tablet uniformity, and elements of the manufacturing process. The appearance of the tablet includes visual identity and overall appearance. The **appearance** of the tablet is **controlled** by measurement of attributes such as size, shape, color, odor, taste, surface, texture, physical flaws, consistency, and legibility of markings.

 b. **Hardness** and **resistance** to friability are necessary for tablets to withstand the mechanical shocks of manufacture, packaging, and shipping, and to ensure consumer acceptance. Hardness involves both tablet disintegration and drug dissolution. Certain tablets that are intended to dissolve slowly are made hard. Other tablets that are intended to dissolve rapidly are made soft. Friability is the tendency of the tablet to crumble.

   (1) **Tablet hardness testers** measure the degree of force required to break a tablet.

(2) Friabilators determine friability by allowing the tablet to roll and fall within a rotating tumbling apparatus. The tablets are weighed before and after a specified number of rotations, and the weight loss is determined.

    (a) Resistance to weight loss indicates the ability of the tablet to withstand abrasion during handling, packaging, and shipping. Compressed tablets that lose less than 0.5%–1% of their weight are usually considered acceptable.

    (b) Some chewable tablets and most effervescent tablets are **highly friable** and require special unit packaging.

c. Tablets are routinely **weighed** to ensure that they contain the proper amount of drug.

    (1) The USP defines a **weight variation standard** to which tablets must conform.

    (2) These standards apply to tablets that contain 50 mg or more of drug substance when the drug substance is 50% or more (by weight) of the dosage form unit.

d. Content uniformity is evaluated to ensure that each tablet contains the desired amount of drug substance, with little variation among contents within a batch. The USP defines content uniformity tests for tablets that contain 50 mg or less of drug substance.

e. Disintegration is evaluated to ensure that the drug substance is fully available for dissolution and absorption from the gastrointestinal tract.

    (1) All USP tablets must pass an **official disintegration test** that is conducted in vitro with special equipment.

        (a) Disintegration times for **uncoated USP tablets** are as low as 2 minutes (nitroglycerin) to 5 minutes (aspirin). Most have a maximum disintegration time of less than 30 minutes.

        (b) Buccal tablets must disintegrate within 4 hours.

        (c) Enteric-coated tablets must show no evidence of disintegration after 1 hour in simulated gastric fluid. In simulated intestinal fluid, they should disintegrate in 2 hours plus the time specified.

    (2) Dissolution requirements in the USP have replaced earlier disintegration requirements for many drugs.

f. Dissolution characteristics are tested to determine drug absorption and physiologic availability.

    (1) The USP gives **standards for tablet dissolution.**

    (2) An increased emphasis on testing tablet dissolution and determining drug bioavailability has increased the use of sophisticated testing systems.

J. Aerosol products

1. Introduction. Aerosol products, or aerosols, are pressurized dosage forms. They are designed to deliver drug systemically or topically with the aid of a liquefied or propelled gas **(propellant).** Aerosol products consist of a **pressurizable container** (tin-plated steel, aluminum, glass, or plastic); a **valve** that allows the pressurized product to be expelled from the container, either continuously or intermittently, when the **actuator** is pressed; and a **dip tube** that conveys the formulation from the bottom of the container to the valve assembly. Aerosols are prepared by special methods (cold filling, pressure filling) because of the gaseous components.

2. Systemic or pulmonary drug delivery is provided by aerosol drug delivery systems, or **metered dose inhalers (MDIs).** These devices allow a drug to be inhaled as a fine mist of drug or drug-containing particles. **MDIs** use special metering valves to regulate the amount of formulation and drug that is dispensed with each dose (i.e., each actuation of the container). Aerosol products are used for topical drug delivery. The formulations range from solutions to dispersions. Metering valves may also be used with topical aerosol products to regulate the amount of drug applied per application.

3. Propellants used in aerosol products

    a. Compressed gases include carbon dioxide, nitrogen, and nitrous oxide. Aerosol products that contain compressed gas tend to lose pressure over time as the product is dispensed. The drop in pressure reflects the expansion of the head space in the container (i.e., increase in the volume that the gas can occupy) as formulation is withdrawn for use. For this reason, higher initial pressures are typically used with compressed gas–based systems than with liquefiable gas–based formulations.

    b. Liquefiable gases include **saturated hydrocarbons** (n-butane, isobutane, propane); chlorofluorocarbons (CFCs), including tetrafluorodichloroethane (propellant 114), dichlorodifluoromethane (propellant 12), and trichlorofluoromethane (propellant 11);

dimethyl ether; and **hydrofluorocarbons,** such as 1,1,1,2-fluoroethane (propellant 134a) and 1,1-difluoroethane (propellant 152a). The negative impact of older CFCs on atmospheric ozone and the potential for global warming led to the worldwide reduction in CFC production under the Montreal Protocol. This plan called for a general ban on CFC production in industrialized countries by January 1996. As a result, the use of CFCs in pharmaceutical products is being phased out. Temporary exemptions for CFCs in MDIs will eventually lapse as stable, safe, and effective alternative formulations are developed with more acceptable propellants (e.g., **hydrofluorocarbons**).

4. **Advantages** of aerosol products include the convenience of push-button dispensing of medication and the stability afforded by a closed, pressurized container that minimizes the likelihood of tampering and protects the contents from light, moisture, air (oxygen), and microbial contamination. Aerosol formulations and packaging components (valves, actuators) permit a wide range of products to be dispensed as sprays, foams, or semisolids.

5. The principal **disadvantage** of aerosol products is environmental (e.g., disposal of pressurized packages, venting of propellants to the atmosphere).

K. Controlled-release dosage forms

1. **Introduction.** Controlled-release dosage forms are also known as delayed-release, sustained-action, prolonged-action, sustained-release, prolonged-release, timed-release, slow-release, extended-action, and extended-release forms. They are designed to **release drug substance slowly** to provide prolonged action in the body.

2. **Advantages** of controlled-release forms
   a. Fewer problems with patient compliance
   b. Use of less total drug
   c. Fewer local or systemic side effects
   d. Minimal drug accumulation with long-term dosage
   e. Fewer problems with potentiation or loss of drug activity with long-term use
   f. Improved treatment efficiency
   g. More rapid control of the patient's condition
   h. Less fluctuation in drug level
   i. Improved bioavailability for some drugs
   j. Improved ability to provide special effects (e.g., morning relief of arthritis by bedtime dosing)
   k. Reduced cost

3. **Sustained-release forms** can be grouped according to their pharmaceutical mechanism.
   a. **Coated beads or granules** (e.g., Spansules, GlaxoSmithKline; Sequels, Wyeth) produce a blood level profile similar to that obtained with multiple dosing.
      (1) A solution of the drug substance in a nonaqueous solvent (e.g., alcohol) is coated onto small, inert beads, or granules, made of a combination of sugar and starch. When the drug dose is large, the starting granules may be composed of the drug itself.
      (2) Some of the granules are left uncoated to provide immediate release of the drug.
      (3) Coats of a lipid material (e.g., beeswax) or a cellulosic material (e.g., ethylcellulose) are applied to the remaining granules. Some granules receive few coats, and some receive many. The various coating thicknesses produce a sustained-release effect.
   b. **Microencapsulation** is a process by which solids, liquids, or gases are encased in microscopic capsules. Thin coatings of a "wall" material are formed around the substance to be encapsulated.
      (1) **Coacervation** is the most common method of microencapsulation. It occurs when a hydrophilic substance is added to a colloidal drug dispersion and causes layering and the formation of microcapsules.
      (2) **Film-forming substances** that are used as the coating material include a variety of natural and synthetic polymers. These materials include shellacs, waxes, gelatin, starches, cellulose acetate phthalate, and ethylcellulose. After the coating material dissolves, all of the drug inside the microcapsule is immediately available for dissolution and absorption. The thickness of the wall can vary from 1–200 mm, depending on the amount of coating material used (3%–30% of total weight).
   c. **Matrix tablets** use insoluble plastics (e.g., polyethylene, polyvinyl acetate, polymethacrylate); hydrophilic polymers (e.g., methylcellulose, hydroxypropyl methylcellu-

lose); or fatty compounds (e.g., various waxes, glyceryl tristearate). Examples include Gradumet (Abbott) and Dospan (Aventis).

   (1) The most common method of preparation is **mixing of the drug with the matrix material** followed by **compression of the material into tablets.**

   (2) The primary dose, or the portion of the drug to be released immediately, is placed on the tablet as a layer, or coat. The rest of the dose is released slowly from the matrix.

d. Osmotic systems include the **Oros system (Alza),** which is an oral osmotic pump composed of a core tablet and a semipermeable coating that has a small hole (0.4 mm in diameter) for drug exit. The hole is produced by a laser beam. Examples include Glucotrol XL (glipizide extended-release tablets, Pfizer) and Procardia XL (nifedipine extended-release tablets, Pfizer).

   (1) This system requires only osmotic pressure to be effective. It is essentially independent of pH changes in the environment.

   (2) The drug-release rate can be changed by changing the tablet surface area, the nature of the membrane, or the diameter of the drug-release aperture.

e. Ion-exchange resins can be complexed with drugs by passage of a cationic drug solution through a column that contains the resin. The drug is complexed to the resin by replacement of hydrogen atoms. Examples include Ionamin capsules (Celltech; resin complexes of phentermine), and the Pennkinetic system (Celltech), which incorporates a polymer barrier coating and bead technology in addition to the ion-exchange mechanism.

   (1) After the components are complexed, the **resin–drug complex** is washed and tableted, encapsulated, or suspended in an aqueous vehicle.

   (2) Release of drug from the complex depends on the ionic environment within the gastrointestinal tract and on the properties of the resin. Usually, release is greater in the highly acidic stomach than in the less acidic small intestine.

f. Complex formation is used for certain drug substances that combine chemically with other agents. For example, hydroxypropyl-β-cyclodextrin forms a chemical complex that can be only slowly soluble from body fluids, depending on the pH of the environment. Tannic acid (i.e., tannates) complexes with the amino groups of weak bases dissolve at a slow rate in the gastrointestinal tract, thereby providing for a prolonged release of drug. Examples of the latter include brompheniramine tannate (Brovex, Athlon) and chlorpheniramine/phenylephrine tannates (Rynatan, Wallace).

STUDY QUESTIONS

Directions: Each of the numbered items or incomplete statements in this section is followed by answers or by completions of the statement. Select the **one** lettered answer or completion that is **best** in each case.

1. Which substance is classified as a weak electrolyte?

(A) Glucose
(B) Urea
(C) Ephedrine
(D) Sodium chloride
(E) Sucrose

2. The pH value is calculated mathematically as the

(A) log of the hydroxyl ion (OH^-) concentration
(B) negative log of the OH^- concentration
(C) log of the hydrogen ion (H^+) concentration
(D) negative log of the H^+ concentration
(E) ratio of H^+/OH^- concentration

3. Which property is classified as colligative?

(A) Solubility of a solute
(B) Osmotic pressure
(C) Hydrogen ion (H^+) concentration
(D) Dissociation of a solute
(E) Miscibility of the liquids

4. The colligative properties of a solution are related to the

(A) pH of the solution
(B) number of ions in the solution
(C) total number of solute particles in the solution
(D) number of unionized molecules in the solution
(E) pK_a of the solution

5. The pH of a buffer system can be calculated with the

(A) Noyes-Whitney equation
(B) Henderson-Hasselbalch equation
(C) Michaelis-Menten equation
(D) Young equation
(E) Stokes equation

6. Which mechanism is most often responsible for chemical degradation?

(A) Racemization
(B) Photolysis
(C) Hydrolysis
(D) Decarboxylation
(E) Oxidation

7. Which equation is used to predict the stability of a drug product at room temperature from experiments at accelerated temperatures?

(A) The Stokes equation
(B) The Young equation
(C) The Arrhenius equation
(D) The Michaelis-Menten equation
(E) The Hixson-Crowell equation

8. Based on the relation between the degree of ionization and the solubility of a weak acid, the drug aspirin (pK_a 3.49) will be most soluble at

(A) pH 1.0
(B) pH 2.0
(C) pH 3.0
(D) pH 4.0
(E) pH 6.0

9. Which solution is used as an astringent?

(A) Strong iodine solution USP
(B) Aluminum acetate topical solution USP
(C) Acetic acid NF
(D) Aromatic ammonia spirit USP
(E) Benzalkonium chloride solution NF

10. The particle size of the dispersed solid in a suspension is usually greater than

(A) 0.5 mm
(B) 0.4 mm
(C) 0.3 mm
(D) 0.2 mm
(E) 0.1 mm

11. In the extemporaneous preparation of a suspension, levigation is used to

(A) reduce the zeta potential
(B) avoid bacterial growth
(C) reduce particle size
(D) enhance viscosity
(E) reduce viscosity

12. Which compound is a natural emulsifying agent?

(A) Acacia
(B) Lactose
(C) Polysorbate 20
(D) Polysorbate 80
(E) Sorbitan monopalmitate

13. Vanishing cream is an ointment that may be classified as

(A) a water-soluble base
(B) an oleaginous base
(C) an absorption base
(D) an emulsion base
(E) an oleic base

14. Rectal suppositories intended for adult use usually weigh approximately

(A) 1 g
(B) 2 g
(C) 3 g
(D) 4 g
(E) 5 g

15. In the fusion method of making cocoa butter suppositories, which substance is most likely to be used to lubricate the mold?

(A) Mineral oil
(B) Propylene glycol
(C) Cetyl alcohol
(D) Stearic acid
(E) Magnesium silicate

16. A very fine powdered chemical is defined as one that

(A) completely passes through a #80 sieve
(B) completely passes through a #120 sieve
(C) completely passes through a #20 sieve
(D) passes through a #60 sieve and not more than 40% through a #100 sieve
(E) passes through a #40 sieve and not more than 60% through a #60 sieve

17. Which technique is typically used to mill camphor?

(A) Trituration
(B) Levigation
(C) Pulverization by intervention
(D) Geometric dilution
(E) Attrition

18. The dispensing pharmacist usually blends potent powders with a large amount of diluent by

(A) spatulation
(B) sifting
(C) trituration
(D) geometric dilution
(E) levigation

19. Which type of paper best protects a divided hygroscopic powder?

(A) Waxed paper
(B) Glassine
(C) White bond
(D) Blue bond
(E) Vegetable parchment

20. Which capsule size has the smallest capacity?

(A) 5
(B) 4
(C) 1
(D) 0
(E) 000

21. The shells of soft gelatin capsules may be made elastic or plastic-like by the addition of

(A) sorbitol
(B) povidone
(C) polyethylene glycol (PEG)
(D) lactose
(E) hydroxypropyl methylcellulose

22. The *United States Pharmacopeia* (USP) content uniformity test for tablets is used to ensure which quality?

(A) Bioequivalency
(B) Dissolution
(C) Potency
(D) Purity
(E) Toxicity

23. All of the following statements about chemical degradation are true EXCEPT

(A) as temperature increases, degradation decreases
(B) most drugs degrade by a first-order process
(C) chemical degradation may produce a toxic product
(D) chemical degradation may result in a loss of active ingredients
(E) chemical degradation may affect the therapeutic activity of a drug

24. All of the following statements concerning zero-order degradation are true EXCEPT

(A) its rate is independent of the concentration
(B) a plot of concentration versus time yields a straight line on rectilinear paper
(C) its half-life is a changing parameter
(D) its concentration remains unchanged with respect to time
(E) the slope of a plot of concentration versus time yields a rate constant

25. All of the following statements about first-order degradation are true EXCEPT

(A) its rate is dependent on the concentration
(B) its half-life is a changing parameter
(C) a plot of the logarithm of concentration versus time yields a straight line
(D) its $t_{90\%}$ is independent of the concentration
(E) a plot of the logarithm of concentration versus time allows the rate constant to be determined

26. A satisfactory suppository base must meet all of the following criteria EXCEPT

(A) it should have a narrow melting range
(B) it should be nonirritating and nonsensitizing
(C) it should dissolve or disintegrate rapidly in the body cavity
(D) it should melt below 30°C
(E) it should be inert

27. Cocoa butter (theobroma oil) exhibits all of the following properties EXCEPT

(A) it melts at temperatures between 33°C and 35°C
(B) it is a mixture of glycerides
(C) it is a polymorph
(D) it is useful in formulating rectal suppositories
(E) it is soluble in water

28. *United States Pharmacopeia* (USP) tests to ensure the quality of drug products in tablet form include all of the following EXCEPT

(A) disintegration
(B) dissolution
(C) hardness and friability
(D) content uniformity
(E) weight variation

Directions: Each question below contains three suggested answers of which **one or more** is correct. Choose the answer.

    A   if **I only** is correct
    B   if **III only** is correct
    C   if **I and II** are correct
    D   if **II and III** are correct
    E   if **I, II, and III** are correct

29. Forms of water that are suitable for use in parenteral preparations include

  I. purified water USP
  II. water for injection USP
  III. sterile water for injection USP

30. The particles in an ideal suspension should satisfy which of the following criteria?

  I. Their size should be uniform
  II. They should be stationary or move randomly
  III. They should remain discrete

31. The sedimentation of particles in a suspension can be minimized by

  I. adding sodium benzoate
  II. increasing the viscosity of the suspension
  III. reducing the particle size of the active ingredient

32. Ingredients that may be used as suspending agents include

  I. methylcellulose
  II. acacia
  III. talc

33. Mechanisms that are thought to provide stable emulsifications include the

  I. formation of interfacial film
  II. lowering of interfacial tension
  III. presence of charge on the ions

34. Nonionic surface-active agents used as synthetic emulsifiers include

  I. tragacanth
  II. sodium lauryl sulfate
  III. sorbitan esters (Spans)

35. Advantages of systemic drug administration by rectal suppositories include

  I. avoidance of first-pass effects
  II. suitability when the oral route is not feasible
  III. predictable drug release and absorption

36. True statements about the milling of powders include

  I. a fine particle size is essential if the lubricant is to function properly
  II. an increased surface area may enhance the dissolution rate
  III. milling may cause degradation of thermolabile drugs

37. Substances used to insulate powder components that liquefy when mixed include

  I. Talc
  II. Kaolin
  III. Light magnesium oxide

38. A ceramic mortar may be preferable to a glass mortar when

  I. a volatile oil is added to a powder mixture
  II. colored substances (dyes) are mixed into a powder
  III. comminution is desired in addition to mixing

39. Divided powders may be dispensed in

  I. individual-dose packets
  II. a bulk container
  III. a perforated, sifter-type container

40. True statements about the function of excipients used in tablet formulations include

  I. binders promote granulation during the wet granulation process
  II. glidants help to promote the flow of the tablet granulation during manufacture
  III. lubricants help the patient to swallow the tablets

41. Which manufacturing variables would be likely to affect the dissolution of a prednisone tablet in the body?

  I. The amount and type of binder added
  II. The amount and type of disintegrant added
  III. The force of compression used during tableting

42. Agents that may be used to coat enteric-coated tablets include

  I. hydroxypropyl methylcellulose
  II. carboxymethylcellulose
  III. cellulose acetate phthalate

Directions: Each group of items in this section consists of lettered options followed by a set of numbered items. For each item, select the **one** lettered option that is most closely associated with it. Each lettered option may be selected once, more than once, or not at all.

Questions 43–46

For each tablet processing problem listed below, select the most likely reason for the condition.

(A) Excessive moisture in the granulation
(B) Entrapment of air
(C) Tablet friability
(D) Degraded drug
(E) Tablet hardness

43. Picking

44. Mottling

45. Capping

46. Sticking

Questions 47–49

For each description of a comminution procedure below, select the process that it best describes.

(A) Trituration
(B) Spatulation
(C) Levigation
(D) Pulverization by intervention
(E) Tumbling

47. Rubbing or grinding a substance in a mortar that has a rough inner surface

48. Reducing and subdividing a substance by adding an easily removed solvent

49. Adding a suitable agent to form a paste and then rubbing or grinding the paste in a mortar

Questions 50–53

Match the drug product below with the type of controlled-release dosage form that it represents.

(A) Matrix formulations
(B) Ion-exchange resin complex
(C) Drug complexes
(D) Osmotic system
(E) Coated beads or granules

50. Ionamin capsules

51. Thorazine Spansule capsules

52. Rynatan pediatric suspension

53. Procardia XL

ANSWERS AND EXPLANATIONS

1. The answer is C *[IV A 1 a, 3 d]*.
Glucose, urea, and sucrose are nonelectrolytes. Sodium chloride is a strong electrolyte. Electrolytes are substances that form ions when dissolved in water. Thus, they can conduct an electric current through the solution. Ions are particles that bear electrical charges: cations are positively charged, and anions are negatively charged. Strong electrolytes are completely ionized in water at all concentrations. Weak electrolytes (e.g., ephedrine) are only partially ionized at most concentrations. Because nonelectrolytes do not form ions when in solution, they are nonconductors.

2. The answer is D *[IV A 3 b]*.
The pH is a measure of the acidity, or hydrogen ion concentration, of an aqueous solution. The pH is the logarithm of the reciprocal of the hydrogen ion (H^+) concentration expressed in moles per liter. Because the logarithm of a reciprocal equals the negative logarithm of the number, the pH is the negative logarithm of the H^+ concentration. A pH of 7.0 indicates neutrality. As the pH decreases, the acidity increases. The pH of arterial blood is 7.35–7.45; of urine, 4.8–7.5; of gastric juice, approximately 1.4; and of cerebrospinal fluid, 7.35–7.40. The concept of pH was introduced by Sörensen in the early 1900s. Alkalinity is the negative logarithm of $[OH^-]$ and is inversely related to acidity.

3. The answer is B *[IV A 2 d]*.
Osmotic pressure is an example of a colligative property. The osmotic pressure is the magnitude of pressure needed to stop osmosis across a semipermeable membrane between a solution and a pure solvent. The colligative properties of a solution depend on the total number of dissociated and undissociated solute particles. These properties are independent of the size of the solute. Other colligative properties of solutes are reduction in the vapor pressure of the solution, elevation of its boiling point, and depression of its freezing point.

4. The answer is C *[IV A 1 b]*.
The colligative properties of a solution are related to the total number of solute particles that it contains. Examples of colligative properties are the osmotic pressure, lowering of the vapor pressure, elevation of the boiling point, and depression of the freezing, or melting, point.

5. The answer is B *[IV A 3 e]*.
The Henderson-Hasselbalch equation for a weak acid and its salt is as follows:

$$pH = pK_a + \log \frac{[salt]}{[acid]}$$

where pK_a is the negative log of the dissociation constant of a weak acid and [salt]/[acid] is the ratio of the molar concentration of salt and acid used to prepare a buffer.

6. The answer is C *[V D 1]*.
Although all of the mechanisms listed can be responsible, the chemical degradation of medicinal compounds, particularly esters in liquid formulations, is usually caused by hydrolysis. For this reason, drugs that have ester functional groups are formulated in dry form whenever possible. Oxidation is another common mode of degradation and is minimized by including antioxidants (e.g., ascorbic acid) in drug formulations. Photolysis is reduced by packaging susceptible products in amber or opaque containers. Decarboxylation, which is the removal of COOH groups, affects compounds that include carboxylic acid. Racemization neutralizes the effects of an optically active compound by converting half of its molecules into their mirror-image configuration. As a result, the dextrorotatory and levorotatory forms cancel each other out. This type of degradation affects only drugs that are characterized by optical isomerism.

7. The answer is C *[V E 3 d]*.
Testing of a drug formulation to determine its shelf life can be accelerated by applying the Arrhenius equation to data obtained at higher temperatures. The method involves determining the rate constant (k) values for the degradation of a drug at various elevated temperatures. The log of k is plotted against the reciprocal of the absolute temperature, and the k value for degradation at room temperature is obtained by extrapolation.

8. The answer is E *[IV A 3 d]*.
The solubility of a weak acid varies as a function of pH. Because pH and pK_a (the dissociation constant) are related, solubility is also related to the degree of ionization. Aspirin is a weak acid that is completely ionized at a pH that is 2 units greater than its pK_a. Therefore, it is most soluble at pH 6.0.

9. The answer is B *[VI B 7]*.
Aluminum acetate and aluminum subacetate solutions are astringents that are used as antiperspirants and as wet dressings for contact dermatitis. Strong iodine solution and benzalkonium chloride are topical antibacterial solutions. Acetic acid is added to products as an acidifier. Aromatic ammonia spirit is a respiratory stimulant.

10. The answer is A *[IV B 1 a]*.
A suspension is a two-phase system that consists of a finely powdered solid dispersed in a liquid vehicle. The particle size of the suspended solid should be as small as possible to minimize sedimentation, but it is usually greater than 0.5 μm.

11. The answer is C *[VI E 3 a]*.
Levigation is the process of blending and grinding a substance to separate the particles, reduce their size, and form a paste. Levigation is performed by adding a small amount of suitable levigating agent (e.g., glycerin) to the solid and blending the mixture with a mortar and pestle.

12. The answer is A *[VI D 3]*.
Acacia, or gum arabic, is the exudate obtained from the stems and branches of various species of *Acacia,* a woody plant native to Africa. Acacia is a natural emulsifying agent that provides a stable emulsion of low viscosity. Emulsions are droplets of one or more immiscible liquids dispersed in another liquid. Emulsions are inherently unstable: the droplets tend to coalesce into larger and larger drops. The purpose of an emulsifying agent is to keep the droplets dispersed and prevent them from coalescing. Polysorbate 20, polysorbate 80, and sorbitan monopalmitate are also emulsifiers, but are synthetic, not natural, substances.

13. The answer is D *[VI E 1]*.
Ointments are typically used as emollients to soften the skin, as protective barriers, or as vehicles for medication. A variety of ointment bases are available. Vanishing cream, an emulsion type of ointment base, is an oil-in-water emulsion that contains a high percentage of water. Stearic acid is used to create a thin film on the skin when the water evaporates.

14. The answer is B *[VI F 2 a, b]*.
By convention, a rectal suppository for an adult weighs approximately 2 g. Suppositories for infants and children are smaller. Vaginal suppositories typically weigh approximately 5 g. Rectal suppositories are usually shaped like an elongated bullet (cylindrical and tapered at one end). Vaginal suppositories are usually ovoid.

15. The answer is A *[VI F 4 c]*.
In the fusion method of making suppositories, molds made of aluminum, brass, or nickel–copper alloys are used. Finely powdered drug mixed with melted cocoa butter is poured into a mold that is lubricated very lightly with mineral oil.

16. The answer is B *[VI G; Table 3-8]*.
The *United States Pharmacopeia* (USP) defines a very fine chemical powder as one that completely passes through a standard #120 sieve, which has 125-μm openings. The USP classification for powdered vegetable and animal drugs differs from that for powdered chemicals. To be classified as very fine, powdered vegetable and animal drugs must pass completely through a #80 sieve, which has 180-μm openings.

17. The answer is C *[VI G 1 c (3) (b)]*.
Pulverization by intervention is the milling technique that is used for drug substances that are gummy and tend to reagglomerate or resist grinding (e.g., camphor, iodine). In this sense, intervention is the addition of a small amount of material that aids milling and can be removed easily after pulverization is complete. For example, camphor can be reduced readily if a small amount of volatile solvent (e.g., alcohol) is added. The solvent is then allowed to evaporate.

18. The answer is D *[VI G 2 b, c]*.
The pharmacist uses geometric dilution to mix potent substances with a large amount of diluent. The potent drug and an equal amount of diluent are first mixed in a mortar by trituration. A volume of diluent equal to the mixture in the mortar is added, and the mix is again triturated. The procedure is repeated, and each time, diluent equal in volume to the mixture then in the mortar is added, until all of the diluent is incorporated.

19. The answer is A *[VI G 3 b (4)]*.
Hygroscopic and volatile drugs are best protected by waxed paper, which is waterproof. The packet may be double-wrapped with a bond paper to improve the appearance of the completed powder.

20. The answer is A *[VI H 2 c (1)]*.
Hard capsules are numbered from 000 (largest) to 5 (smallest). Their approximate capacity ranges from 600 to 30 mg; however, the capacity of the capsule depends on the density of the contents.

21. The answer is A *[VI H 3 a, b]*.
The shells of soft gelatin capsules are plasticized by the addition of a polyhydric alcohol (polyol), such as glycerin or sorbitol. An antifungal preservative can also be added. Both hard and soft gelatin capsules can be filled with a powder or another dry substance. Soft gelatin capsules are also useful dosage forms for fluids or semisolids.

22. The answer is C *[VI H 4 a]*.
A different uniformity test is a test of potency. To ensure that each tablet or capsule contains the intended amount of drug substance, the *United States Pharmacopeia* (USP) provides two tests: weight variation and content uniformity. The content uniformity test can be used for any dosage unit, but is required for coated tablets, for tablets in which the active ingredient comprises less than 50% of the tablet, for suspensions in single-unit containers or in soft capsules, and for many solids that contain added substances. The weight variation test can be used for liquid-filled soft capsules, for any dosage form unit that contains at least 50 mg of a single drug if the drug comprises at least 50% of the bulk, for solids that do not contain added substances, and for freeze-dried solutions.

23. The answer is A *[V B]*.
The reaction velocity, or degradation rate, of a pharmaceutical product is affected by several factors, including temperature, solvents, and light. The degradation rate increases two to three times with each 10° increase in temperature. The effect of temperature on reaction rate is given by the Arrhenius equation:

$$k = Ae^{-Ea/RT}$$

where k is the reaction rate constant, A is the frequency factor, Ea is the energy of activation, R is the gas constant, and T is the absolute temperature.

24. The answer is D *[V B 2 a]*.
In zero-order degradation, the concentration of a drug decreases over time. However, the change of concentration with respect to time is unchanged. In the equation:

$$-\frac{dC}{dt} = k$$

the fact that dC/dt is negative signifies that the concentration is decreasing. However, the velocity of the concentration change is constant.

25. The answer is B *[V B 2 b (2)]*.
The half-life ($t_{1/2}$) is the time required for the concentration of a drug to decrease by one-half. For a first-order degradation:

$$t_{1/2} = \frac{0.693}{k}$$

Because both k and 0.693 are constants, $t_{1/2}$ is a constant.

26. The answer is D *[VI F 3]*.
A satisfactory suppository base should remain firm at room temperature. Preferably, it should not melt below 30°C to avoid premature softening during storage and insertion. It should also be inert, nonsensitizing, nonirritating, and compatible with a variety of drugs. Moreover, it should melt just below body

temperature and should dissolve or disintegrate rapidly in the fluid of the body cavity into which it is inserted.

27. The answer is E *[VI F 3 c (1)]*.
Cocoa butter is a fat that is obtained from the seed of *Theobroma cacao*. Chemically, it is a mixture of stearin, palmitin, and other glycerides that are insoluble in water and freely soluble in ether and chloroform. Depending on the fusion temperature, cocoa butter can crystallize into any one of four crystal forms. Cocoa butter is a good base for rectal suppositories, although it is less than ideal for vaginal or urethral suppositories.

28. The answer is C *[VI I 5]*.
To satisfy the *United States Pharmacopeia* (USP) standards, tablets are required to pass one of two tests. A weight variation test is used if the active ingredient comprises the bulk of the tablet. A content uniformity test is used if the tablet is coated or if the active ingredient comprises less than 50% of the bulk of the tablet. Many tablets for oral administration are required to meet a disintegration test. Disintegration times are specified in the individual monographs. A dissolution test may be required instead if the active component of the tablet has limited water solubility. Hardness and friability would affect the disintegration and dissolution rates, but hardness and friability tests are in-house quality control tests, not official USP tests.

29. The answer is D (II, III) *[VI A 1]*.
Water for injection USP is water that has been purified by distillation or by reverse osmosis. This water is used to prepare parenteral solutions that are subject to final sterilization. For parenteral solutions that are prepared aseptically and not subsequently sterilized, sterile water for injection USP is used. Sterile water for injection USP is water for injection USP that has been sterilized and suitably packaged. This water meets the USP requirements for sterility. Bacteriostatic water for injection USP is sterile water for injection USP that contains one or more antimicrobial agents. It can be used in parenteral solutions if the antimicrobial additives are compatible with the other ingredients in the solution, but it cannot be used in newborns. Purified water USP is not used in parenteral preparations.

30. The answer is E (all) *[VI C]*.
An ideal suspension would have particles of uniform size, minimal sedimentation, and no interaction between particles. Although these ideal criteria are rarely met, they can be approximated by keeping the particle size as small as possible, the densities of the solid and the dispersion medium as similar as possible, and the dispersion medium as viscous as possible.

31. The answer is D (II, III) *[IV B 2]*.
As Stokes' law indicates, the sedimentation rate of a suspension is slowed by reducing its density, reducing the size of the suspended particles, or increasing its viscosity by incorporating a thickening agent. Sodium benzoate is an antifungal agent and would not reduce the sedimentation rate of a suspension.

32. The answer is C (I, II) *[VI C 3]*.
Acacia and methylcellulose are common suspending agents. Acacia is a natural product, and methylcellulose is a synthetic polymer. By increasing the viscosity of the liquid, these agents enable particles to remain suspended for a longer period.

33. The answer is E (all) *[VI D 3]*.
Emulsifying agents provide a mechanical barrier to coalescence. They also reduce the natural tendency of the droplets in the internal phase (oil or water) of the emulsion to coalesce. Three mechanisms appear to be involved. Some emulsifiers promote stability by forming strong, pliable interfacial films around the droplets. Emulsifying agents also reduce interfacial tension. Finally, ions (from the emulsifier) in the interfacial film can lead to charge repulsion that causes droplets to repel one another, thereby preventing coalescence.

34. The answer is B (III) *[VI D 3]*.
All of the substances listed are emulsifying agents, but only sorbitan esters are nonionic synthetic agents. Tragacanth, like acacia, is a natural emulsifying agent. Sodium lauryl sulfate is an anionic surfactant. Sorbitan esters (known colloquially as Spans because of their trade names) are hydrophobic and form water-in-oil emulsions. The polysorbates (known colloquially as Tweens) are also nonionic, synthetic sorbitan derivatives. However, they are hydrophilic and therefore form oil-in-water emulsions. Sodium lauryl sulfate, as an alkali soap, is also hydrophilic and thus forms oil-in-water emulsions.

35. The answer is C (I, II) *[VI F 1–2].*
Rectal suppositories are useful for delivering systemic medication under certain circumstances. Absorption of a drug from a rectal suppository involves release of the drug from the suppository vehicle, diffusion through the rectal mucosa, and transport to the circulation through the rectal veins. The rectal veins bypass the liver, so this route avoids rapid hepatic degradation of certain drugs (first-pass effect). The rectal route is also useful when a drug cannot be given orally (e.g., because of vomiting). However, the extent of drug release and absorption is variable. It depends on the properties of the drug, the suppository base, and the environment in the rectum.

36. The answer is E (all) *[VI G 1 c].*
Milling is the process of mechanically reducing the particle size of solids before they are formulated into a final product. To work effectively, a lubricant must coat the surface of the granulation or powder. Hence, fine particle size is essential. Decreasing the particle size increases the surface area and can enhance the dissolution rate. Thermolabile drugs may undergo degradation because of the buildup of heat during milling.

37. The answer is D (II, III) *[VI G 2 a (2)].*
Some solid substances (e.g., aspirin, phenylsalicylate, phenacetin, thymol, camphor) liquefy or form eutectic mixtures when in close, prolonged contact with one another. These substances are best insulated by the addition of light magnesium oxide or magnesium carbonate. Other inert diluents that can be used are kaolin, starch, and bentonite.

38. The answer is B (III) *[VI G 2 b].*
When powders are mixed, if comminution is especially important, a porcelain or ceramic mortar that has a rough inner surface is preferred over the smooth working surface of a glass mortar. Because a glass mortar cleans more easily after use, it is preferred for chemicals that may stain a porcelain or ceramic mortar as well as for simple mixing of substances that do not require comminution.

39. The answer is A (I) *[VI G 3 a, b].*
Powders for oral use can be dispensed by the pharmacist in bulk form or divided into premeasured doses (divided powders). Divided powders are traditionally dispensed in folded paper packets (chartulae) made of parchment, bond paper, glassine, or waxed paper. However, individual doses can be packaged in metal foil or small plastic bags if the powder needs greater protection from humidity or evaporation.

40. The answer is C (I, II) *[VI I 2 b].*
Tablets for oral ingestion usually contain excipients that are added to the formulation for their special functions. Binders and adhesives are added to promote granulation or compaction. Diluents are fillers that are added to make up the required tablet bulk. They can also aid in the manufacturing process. Disintegrants aid in tablet disintegration in gastrointestinal fluids. Lubricants, antiadherents, and glidants aid in reducing friction or adhesion between particles or between tablet and die. For example, lubricants are used in the manufacture of tablets to reduce friction when the tablet is ejected from the die cavity. Lubricants are usually hydrophobic substances that can affect the dissolution rate of the active ingredient.

41. The answer is E (all) *[VI I 2 b (3)].*
Disintegrants are added to tablet formulations to facilitate disintegration in gastrointestinal fluids. Disintegration of the tablet in the body is critical to its dissolution and subsequent absorption and bioavailability. The binder and the compression force used during tablet manufacturing affect the hardness of the tablet as well as tablet disintegration and drug dissolution.

42. The answer is B (III) *[VI I 3 a (4)].*
An enteric-coated tablet has a coating that remains intact in the stomach, but dissolves in the intestines to yield the tablet ingredients there. Enteric coatings include various fats, fatty acids, waxes, and shellacs. Cellulose acetate phthalate remains intact in the stomach because it dissolves only when the pH exceeds 6. Other enteric-coating materials include povidone (polyvinylpyrrolidone), polyvinyl acetate phthalate, and hydroxypropyl methylcellulose phthalate.

43–46. The answers are: 43-A, 44-D, 45-B, 46-A *[VI I 4].*
Sticking is adhesion of tablet material to a die wall. It may be caused by excessive moisture or by the use of ingredients that have low melting temperatures. Mottling is uneven color distribution. It is most often caused by poor mixing of the tablet granulation, but may also occur when a degraded drug pro-

duces a colored metabolite. Capping is separation of the top or bottom crown of a tablet from the main body. Capping implies that compressed powder is not cohesive. Reasons for capping include excessive force of compression, use of insufficient binder, worn tablet tooling equipment, and entrapment of air during processing. Picking is adherence of tablet surface material to a punch. It can be caused by a granulation that is too damp, by a scratched punch, by static charges on the powder, and particularly by the use of a punch tip that is engraved or embossed.

47–49. The answers are: 47-A, 48-D, 49-C *[VI G 1 c, 2].*
Comminution is the process of reducing the particle size of a powder to increase its fineness. Several comminution techniques are suitable for small-scale use in a pharmacy. Trituration is used both to comminute and to mix dry powders. If comminution is desired, the substance is rubbed in a mortar that has a rough inner surface. Pulverization by intervention is often used for substances that tend to agglomerate or resist grinding. A small amount of easily removed (e.g., volatile) solvent is added. After the substance is pulverized, the solvent is allowed to evaporate or is otherwise removed. Levigation is often used to prepare pastes or ointments. The powder is reduced by adding a suitable nonsolvent (levigating agent) to form a paste and then either rubbing the paste in a mortar with a pestle or rubbing it on an ointment slab with a spatula. Spatulation and tumbling are techniques that are used to mix or blend powders, not to reduce them. Spatulation is blending small amounts of powders by stirring them with a spatula on a sheet of paper or a pill tile. Tumbling is blending large amounts of powder in a large rotating container.

50–53. The answers are: 50-B, 51-E, 52-C, 53-D *[VI I 3 a (3), (4)].*
Controlled-release dosage forms are designed to release a drug slowly for prolonged action in the body. A variety of pharmaceutical mechanisms are used to provide the controlled release. Ion-exchange resins may be complexed to drugs by passing a cationic drug solution through a column that contains the resin. The drug is complexed to the resin by replacement of hydrogen atoms. Release of drug from the complex depends on the ionic environment within the gastrointestinal tract and on the properties of the resin. Coated beads (e.g., Thorazine Spansule capsules) or granules produce blood levels similar to those obtained with multiple dosing. The various coating thicknesses produce a sustained-release effect.

Matrix devices may use insoluble plastics, hydrophilic polymers, or fatty compounds. These components are mixed with the drug and compressed into a tablet. The primary dose, or the portion of the drug to be released immediately, is placed on the tablet as a layer or coat. The remainder of the dose is released slowly from the matrix. Relatively insoluble tannate-amine complexes provide for a prolonged gastrointestinal absorption phase and sustained systemic concentrations of the weak bases. Osmotic systems employ osmotic pressure to control the release of the active ingredient from the formulation. Osmotic tablet formulations provide a semipermeable membrane as a coating that surrounds the osmotically active core. The coating allows water to diffuse into the core but does not allow drug to diffuse out. As water flows into the tablet, the drug dissolves. The laser-drilled hole in the coating allows the drug solution within the tablet to flow to the outside at a rate that is equivalent to the rate of water flow into the tablet. The osmotic pressure gradient, and a zero-order drug-release rate, will be maintained as long as excess osmotically active solute (e.g., electrolyte) remains in the tablet core.

4

Biopharmaceutics and Drug Delivery Systems

Lawrence H. Block

I. INTRODUCTION

A. Biopharmaceutics is the study of the relation of the physical and chemical properties of a drug to its bioavailability, pharmacokinetics, and pharmacodynamic and toxicologic effects.

1. A **drug product** is the finished dosage form (e.g., tablet, capsule, solution) that contains the active drug ingredient in association with nondrug (usually inactive) ingredients **(excipients)** that make up the **vehicle, or formulation matrix.**

2. The phrase *drug delivery system* is often used interchangeably with the terms *drug product* or *dosage form.* However, a **drug delivery system** is a more comprehensive concept that includes the drug formulation and the dynamic interactions among the drug, its formulation matrix, its container, and the patient.

3. **Bioavailability** is a measurement of the rate and extent (amount) of systemic absorption of the therapeutically active drug.

B. Pharmacokinetics is the study of the time course of drug movement in the body during absorption, distribution, and elimination (excretion and biotransformation).

C. Pharmacodynamics is the study of the relation of the drug concentration or amount at the site of action (receptor) and its pharmacologic response as a function of time.

II. DRUG TRANSPORT AND ABSORPTION

A. Transport of drug molecules *across* cell membranes. Drug absorption requires the drug to be transported across various cell membranes. Drug molecules may enter the bloodstream and be transported to the tissues and organs of the body. Drug molecules may cross additional membranes to enter cells. Drug molecules may also cross an intracellular membrane, such as the nuclear membrane or endoplasmic reticulum, to reach the site of action. **Figure 4-1** is a representation of some of the key transport processes involved in drug absorption.

1. General principles
   a. A **cell membrane** is a semipermeable structure composed primarily of lipids and proteins.
   b. Drugs may be transported by **passive diffusion, partitioning, carrier-mediated transport, paracellular transport,** or **vesicular transport.**
   c. Usually, **proteins, drugs bound to proteins,** and **macromolecules** do not cross cell membranes easily.
   d. **Nonpolar lipid-soluble drugs** traverse cell membranes more easily than **ionic** or **polar water-soluble drugs.**
   e. **Low-molecular-weight drugs** diffuse across a cell membrane more easily than **high-molecular-weight drugs.**

2. **Passive diffusion and partitioning**
   a. *Within* **the cytoplasm** or in **interstitial fluid,** most drugs undergo transport by simple **diffusion.**
   b. **Fick's law of diffusion. Simple passive diffusion** involves the transfer of drugs from an area of high concentration (C_1) to an area of lower concentration (C_2) according to Fick's law of diffusion:

$$\frac{dQ}{dt} = \frac{DA}{h}(C_1 - C_2),$$

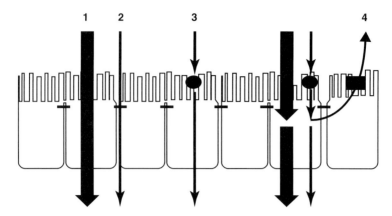

Figure 4-1. Diagram of the key drug transport processes in intestinal epithelial cells. (1) Transcellular passive (diffusion and partitioning); (2) paracellular transport (diffusion and convection); (3) carrier-mediated transport; and (4) P-glycoprotein-mediated efflux. [after D. J. Brayden, Pharm News 4 (1):11–15 (1997)]

where dQ/dt is the rate of drug diffusion, D is the diffusion coefficient for the drug, A is the surface area of the plane across which transfer occurs, h is the thickness of the region through which diffusion occurs, and $(C_1 - C_2)$ is the difference between the drug concentration in area 1 and area 2, respectively.

   c. Passive drug transport *across* cell membranes involves the successive **partitioning** of a solute between aqueous and lipid phases as well as **diffusion** within the respective phases. Modifying Fick's law of diffusion to accommodate the partitioning of drug gives the following:

$$\frac{dQ}{dt} = \frac{DAK}{h}(C_1 - C_2)$$

The rate of drug diffusion, dQ/dt, now reflects its direct dependence on K, the oil:water partition coefficient of the drug, as well as on A and $(C_1 - C_2)$.

   d. Ionization of a weak electrolyte is affected by the pH of the medium in which the drug is dissolved as well as by the pK_a of the drug. The nonionized species is more lipid soluble than the ionized species, and it partitions more readily across cell membranes.

3. Carrier-mediated transport

   a. Active transport of the drug across a membrane is a carrier-mediated process that has the following characteristics:

   (1) The drug moves against a concentration gradient.

   (2) The process requires energy.

   (3) The carrier may be selective for certain types of drugs that resemble natural substrates, or metabolites that are normally actively transported.

   (4) The carrier system may be saturated at a high drug concentration.

   (5) The process may be competitive (i.e., drugs with similar structures may compete for the same carrier).

   b. Facilitated diffusion is also a carrier-mediated transport system. However, facilitated diffusion occurs with (i.e., in the direction of) a concentration gradient and does not require energy.

4. Paracellular transport. Drug transport across tight (narrow) junctions between cells or transendothelial channels of cells is known as **paracellular transport.** It involves both diffusion and the **convective** (bulk) flow of water and accompanying water-soluble drug molecules through the paracellular channels.

5. Vesicular transport is the process of engulfing particles or dissolved materials by a cell. Vesicular transport is the only transport mechanism that does not require a drug to be in an aqueous solution to be absorbed. **Pinocytosis** and **phagocytosis** are forms of vesicular transport.

   a. Pinocytosis is the engulfment of small solute or fluid volumes.

    b. Phagocytosis is the engulfment of larger particles, or macromolecules, generally by macrophages.

    c. Endocytosis and **exocytosis** are the movement of macromolecules into and out of the cell, respectively.

6. Other transport mechanisms: transporter proteins. Various **transporter proteins** (e.g., **P-glycoprotein**) are embedded in the lipid bilayer of cell membranes in tandem in α-helical transmembrane regions or domains. These proteins are adenosine triphosphate (ATP; energy)-dependent "pumps," which can facilitate the efflux of drug molecules from the cell. Because these transmembrane efflux pumps are often found in conjunction with metabolizing enzymes such as **cytochrome P450 3A4,** their net effect is to substantially reduce intracellular drug concentrations. Thus, they determine, to a large extent, the pharmacokinetic disposition and circulating plasma concentrations of drugs (e.g., cyclosporin, nifedipine, digoxin) that are substrates for these proteins.

B. Routes of drug administration

  1. Parenteral administration

    a. Intravenous bolus injection. The drug is injected directly into the bloodstream, distributes throughout the body, and acts rapidly. Any side effects, including an intense pharmacologic response, anaphylaxis, or overt toxicity, also occur rapidly.

    b. Intra-arterial injection. The drug is injected into a specific artery to achieve a high drug concentration in a specific tissue before drug distribution occurs throughout the body. Intra-arterial injection is used for diagnostic agents and occasionally for chemotherapy.

    c. Intravenous infusion. The drug is given intravenously at a constant input rate. Constant-rate intravenous infusion maintains a relatively constant plasma drug concentration once the infusion rate is approximately equal to the drug's elimination rate from the body (i.e., once steady state is reached).

    d. Intramuscular injection. The drug is injected deep into a skeletal muscle. The rate of absorption depends on the vascularity of the muscle site, the lipid solubility of the drug, and the formulation matrix.

    e. Subcutaneous injection. The drug is injected beneath the skin. Because the subcutaneous region is less vascular than muscle tissues, drug absorption is less rapid. The factors that affect absorption from intramuscular depots also affect subcutaneous absorption.

    f. Miscellaneous parenteral routes

      (1) Intra-articular injection. The drug is injected into a joint.

      (2) Intradermal (intracutaneous) injection. The drug is injected into the dermis (i.e., the vascular region of the skin below the epidermis).

      (3) Intrathecal injection. The drug is injected into the spinal fluid.

  2. Enteral administration

    a. Buccal and sublingual administration. A tablet or lozenge is placed under the tongue **(sublingual)** or in contact with the mucosal **(buccal)** surface of the cheek. This type of administration allows a nonpolar, lipid-soluble drug to be absorbed across the epithelial lining of the mouth. After buccal or sublingual administration, the drug is absorbed directly into the systemic circulation, bypassing the liver and any first-pass effects.

    b. Peroral (oral) drug administration. The drug is administered orally, is swallowed, and undergoes absorption from the gastrointestinal tract through the mesenteric circulation to the hepatic portal vein into the liver and then to the systemic circulation. The peroral route is the most common route of administration.

      (1) The peroral route is the most convenient and the safest route.

      (2) Disadvantages of this route include the following:

        (a) The drug may not be absorbed from the gastrointestinal tract consistently or completely.

        (b) The drug may be digested by gastrointestinal enzymes or decomposed by the acid pH of the stomach.

        (c) The drug may irritate mucosal epithelial cells or complex with the contents of the gastrointestinal tract.

        (d) Some drugs may be incompletely absorbed because of first-pass effects or presystemic elimination (e.g., the drug is metabolized by the liver before systemic absorption occurs).

        (e) The absorption rate may be erratic because of delayed gastric emptying or changes in intestinal motility.

    (3) Most drugs are **xenobiotics** or **exogenous** molecules and, consequently, are absorbed from the gastrointestinal tract by **passive diffusion** and **partitioning. Carrier-mediated transport, paracellular transport,** and **vesicular transport** play smaller, but critical, roles, particularly for endogenous molecules.

    (4) Drug molecules are absorbed throughout the gastrointestinal tract, but the **duodenal region,** which has a very large surface area because of the villi and microvilli, is the primary absorption site. The large blood supply provided by the mesenteric vessels allows the drug to be absorbed more efficiently (see II A 2).

    (5) Altered gastric emptying affects arrival of the drug in the duodenum for systemic absorption. **Gastric emptying time** is affected by food content, emotional state, and drugs that alter gastrointestinal tract motility (e.g., anticholinergics, narcotic analgesics, prokinetic agents).

    (6) Normal intestinal motility from **peristalsis** brings the drug in contact with the intestinal epithelial cells. A sufficient period of contact (residence time) is needed to permit drug absorption across the cell membranes from the mucosal to the serosal surface.

    (7) Some drugs, such as **cimetidine** and **acetaminophen,** when given in an immediate-release peroral dosage form to fasted subjects, produce a systemic drug concentration time with two peaks. This **double-peak phenomenon** is attributed to variability in stomach emptying, variable intestinal motility, and enterohepatic cycling.

  c. Rectal administration. The drug in solution (enema) or suppository form is placed in the rectum. Drug diffusion from the solution or release from the suppository leads to absorption across the mucosal surface of the rectum. Drug absorbed in the lower two-thirds of the rectum enters the systemic circulation directly, bypassing the liver and any first-pass effects.

3. Respiratory tract administration
  a. Intranasal administration. The drug contained in a solution or suspension is administered to the nasal mucosa, either as a spray or as drops. The medication may be used for local (e.g., nasal decongestants, intranasal steroids) or systemic effects.

  b. Pulmonary inhalation. The drug, as liquid or solid particles, is inhaled perorally (with a nebulizer or a metered-dose aerosol) into the pulmonary tree. In general, **particles larger than 60 μm** are primarily deposited in the **trachea. Particles larger than 20 μm** do not reach the bronchioles, and **particles smaller than 0.6 μm** are not deposited and are **exhaled.** Particles between **2 and 6 μm** can reach the **alveolar ducts,** although only particles of **1 to 2 μm are retained in the alveoli.**

4. Transdermal and topical administration
  a. Transdermal (percutaneous) drug absorption is the placement of the drug (in a lotion, ointment, cream, paste, or patch) on the skin surface for systemic absorption. An occlusive dressing or film improves systemic drug absorption from the skin. Small lipid-soluble molecules, such as nitroglycerin, nicotine, scopolamine, clonidine, fentanyl, and steroids (e.g., 17-β-estradiol, testosterone), are readily absorbed from the skin.

  b. Drugs (e.g., antibacterials, local anesthetic agents) are applied **topically** to the skin for a local effect.

5. Miscellaneous routes of drug administration include **ophthalmic, otic, urethral,** and **vaginal** administration. These routes of administration are generally used for local therapeutic activity. However, some systemic drug absorption may occur.

C. Local drug activity versus **systemic drug absorption.** The route of administration, absorption site, and bioavailability of the drug from the dosage form are major factors in the design of a drug product.

  1. Drugs intended for **local activity,** such as topical antibiotics, anti-infectives, antifungal agents, and local anesthetics are formulated in dosage forms that minimize systemic absorption. The concentration of these drugs at the application site affects their activity.

  2. When **systemic absorption** is desired, the bioavailability of the drug from the dosage form at the absorption site must be considered (e.g., a drug given intravenously is 100% bioavailable because all of the drug is placed directly into the systemic circulation). The amount, or dose, of drug in the dosage form is based on the extent of drug absorption and the desired systemic drug concentration. The type of dosage form (e.g., immediate release, controlled release) affects the rate of drug absorption.

III. BIOPHARMACEUTIC PRINCIPLES

A. Physicochemical properties

1. **Drug dissolution.** For most drugs with limited water solubility, the rate at which the solid drug enters into solution (i.e., the rate of dissolution) is often the rate-limiting step in bioavailability. The **Noyes-Whitney** equation describes the diffusion-controlled rate of drug dissolution (dm/dt; i.e., the change in the amount of drug in solution with respect to time):

$$\frac{dm}{dt} = \frac{DA}{\delta}(C_s - C_b),$$

   where D is the diffusion coefficient of the solute, A is the surface area of the solid undergoing dissolution, δ is the thickness of the diffusion layer, C_s is the concentration of the solvate at saturation, and C_b is the concentration of the drug in the bulk solution phase.

2. **Drug solubility** in a saturated solution (see Chapter 3 VI) is a static (equilibrium) property. The dissolution rate of a drug is a dynamic property related to the rate of absorption.

3. **Particle size** and **surface area** are inversely related. As solid drug particle size decreases, particle surface area increases.
   a. As described by the Noyes-Whitney equation, the dissolution rate is directly proportional to the surface area. An increase in surface area allows for more contact between the solid drug particles and the solvent, resulting in a faster dissolution rate (see III A 1).
   b. With certain **hydrophobic drugs,** excessive particle size reduction does not always increase the dissolution rate. Small particles tend to reaggregate into larger particles to reduce the high surface free energy produced by particle size reduction.
   c. To prevent the formation of aggregates, small drug particles are molecularly dispersed in polyethylene glycol (PEG), polyvinylpyrrolidone (PVP; povidone), dextrose, or other agents. For example, a molecular dispersion of griseofulvin in a water-soluble carrier such as PEG 4000 (e.g., Gris–PEG) enhances dissolution and bioavailability.

4. **Partition coefficient and extent of ionization**
   a. The **partition coefficient** of a drug is the ratio of the solubility of the drug, at equilibrium, in a nonaqueous solvent (e.g., *n*-octanol) to that in an aqueous solvent (e.g., water; pH 7.4 buffer solution). Hydrophilic drugs with higher water solubility have a faster dissolution rate than hydrophobic or lipophilic drugs, which have poor water solubility.
   b. **Extent of ionization.** Drugs that are weak electrolytes (acids or bases) exist in both an ionized form and a nonionized form. The extent of ionization depends on the pK_a of the weak electrolyte and the pH of the solution. The ionized form is more polar, and therefore more water soluble, than the nonionized form. The **Henderson–Hasselbalch equation** describes the relation between the ionized and nonionized forms of a drug as a function of pH and pK_a. When the pH of the medium equals the pK_a of the drug, 50% of the drug in solution is nonionized and 50% is ionized, as shown in the following equations.
      (1) **For weak acids:**

$$pH = pK_a + \log\left(\frac{[salt]}{[nonionized\ acid]}\right)$$

      (2) **For weak bases:**

$$pH = pK_a + \log\left(\frac{[nonionized\ base]}{[salt]}\right)$$

5. **Salt formation**
   a. The choice of salt form for a drug depends on the desired physical, chemical, or pharmacologic properties. Certain salts are designed to provide slower dissolution, slower bioavailability, and longer duration of action. Other salts are selected for greater stability, less local irritation at the absorption site, or less systemic toxicity.
      (1) Some soluble salt forms are less stable than the nonionized form. For example, sodium aspirin is less stable than aspirin in the acid form.
      (2) A solid dosage form containing buffering agents may be formulated with the free acid form of the drug (e.g., buffered aspirin).

       (a) The buffering agent forms an alkaline medium in the gastrointestinal tract, and the drug dissolves in situ.

       (b) The dissolved salt form of the drug diffuses into the bulk fluid of the gastrointestinal tract, forms a fine precipitate that redissolves rapidly, and becomes available for absorption.

  b. Effervescent granules or **tablets** containing the acid drug in addition to sodium bicarbonate, tartaric acid, citric acid, or other ingredients are added to water just before oral administration. The excess sodium bicarbonate forms an alkaline solution in which the drug dissolves. Carbon dioxide is also formed by the decomposition of carbonic acid.

  c. For weakly acidic drugs, potassium and sodium salts are more soluble than divalent cation salts (e.g., calcium, magnesium) or trivalent cation salts (e.g., aluminum).

  d. For weak bases, common water-soluble salts include the hydrochloride, sulfate, citrate, and gluconate salts. The estolate, napsylate, and stearate salts are less water soluble.

6. Polymorphism is the ability of a drug to exist in more than one crystalline form.

  a. Different polymorphs have different physical properties, including melting point and dissolution rate.

  b. Amorphous, or **noncrystalline, forms** of a drug have faster dissolution rates than crystalline forms.

7. Chirality is the ability of a drug to exist as **optically active stereoisomers** or **enantiomers.** Individual enantiomers may not have the same pharmacokinetic and pharmacodynamic activity. Because most chiral drugs are used as racemic mixtures, the results of studies with such mixtures may be misleading because the drug is assumed to behave as a single entity. For example, ibuprofen exists as the *R*- and *S*-enantiomers; only the *S*-enantiomer is pharmacologically active. When the racemic mixture of ibuprofen is taken orally, the *R*-enantiomer undergoes presystemic inversion in the gut to the *S*-enantiomer. Because the rate and extent of inversion are site specific and formulation dependent, ibuprofen activity may vary considerably.

8. Hydrates. Drugs may exist in a **hydrated,** or **solvated, form** or as an **anhydrous molecule.** Dissolution rates differ for hydrated and anhydrous forms. For example, the anhydrous form of ampicillin dissolves faster and is more rapidly absorbed than the hydrated form.

9. Complex formation. A **complex** is a species formed by the reversible or irreversible association of two or more interacting molecules or ions. **Chelates** are complexes that typically involve a ring-like structure formed by the interaction between a partial ring of atoms and a metal. Many biologically important molecules (e.g., hemoglobin, insulin, cyanocobalamin) are chelates. Drugs such as tetracycline form chelates with divalent (e.g., Ca^{++}, Mg^{++}) and trivalent (e.g., Al^{+++}, Bi^{+++}) metal ions. Many drugs adsorb strongly on charcoal or clay (e.g., kaolin, bentonite) particles by forming complexes. Drug complexes with proteins, such as albumin or α_1-acid glycoprotein, often occur.

  a. Complex formation usually alters the physical and chemical characteristics of the drug. For example:

    (1) The chelate of tetracycline with calcium is less water soluble and is poorly absorbed.

    (2) Theophylline complexed with ethylenediamine to form aminophylline is more water soluble and is used for parenteral and rectal administration.

    (3) Cyclodextrins are used to form complexes with many drugs to increase their water solubility.

  b. Large drug complexes, such as drug–protein complexes, do not cross cell membranes easily. These complexes must dissociate to free the drug for absorption at the absorption site, or to permit transport across cell membranes or glomerular filtration before the drug is excreted into the urine.

B. Drug product and delivery system formulation

  1. General considerations

    a. Design of the appropriate dosage form or **delivery system** depends on the:

      (1) Physical and chemical properties of the drug

      (2) Dose of the drug

      (3) Route of administration

      (4) Type of drug delivery system desired

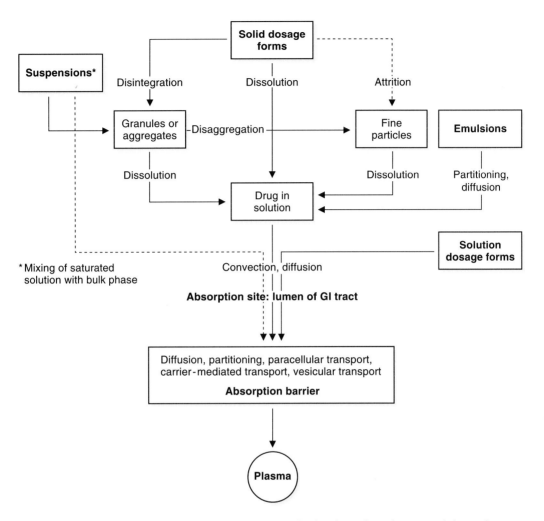

Figure 4-2. Schematic representation of the processes involved in drug release from peroral dosage forms.

    (5) Desired therapeutic effect
    (6) Physiologic release of the drug from the delivery system
    (7) Bioavailability of the drug at the absorption site
    (8) Pharmacokinetics and pharmacodynamics of the drug
  b. Bioavailability. The more complicated the formulation of the finished drug product (e.g., controlled-release tablet, enteric-coated tablet, transdermal patch), the greater the potential for a bioavailability problem. For example, the **release** of a drug from a peroral dosage form and its subsequent bioavailability depend on a succession of rate processes (Figure 4-2). These processes may include:
    (1) Attrition, disintegration, or **disaggregation** of the drug product
    (2) Dissolution of the drug in an aqueous environment
    (3) Convection and **diffusion** of the drug molecules to the absorbing surface
    (4) Absorption of the drug across cell membranes into the systemic circulation
  c. The **rate-limiting step** in the bioavailability of a drug from a drug product is the slowest step in a series of kinetic processes.
    (1) For most conventional solid drug products (e.g., capsules, tablets), the dissolution rate is the slowest, or rate-limiting, step for bioavailability.
    (2) For a controlled- or sustained-release drug product, the release of the drug from the delivery system is the rate-limiting step.

2. **Solutions** are homogeneous mixtures of one or more solutes dispersed molecularly in a dissolving medium (solvent).
   a. Compared with other oral and peroral drug formulations, a drug dissolved in an aqueous solution is in the most bioavailable and consistent form. Because the drug is already in solution, no dissolution step is necessary before systemic absorption occurs. Peroral drug solutions are often used as the reference preparation for solid peroral formulations.
   b. A drug dissolved in a hydroalcoholic solution (e.g., elixir) also has good bioavailability. Alcohol aids drug solubility. However, when the drug is diluted by gastrointestinal tract fluid and other gut contents (e.g., food), it may form a finely divided precipitate in the lumen of the gastrointestinal tract. Because of the extensive dispersion and large surface area of such finely divided precipitates, redissolution and subsequent absorption occur rapidly.
   c. A viscous drug solution (e.g., syrup) may interfere with dilution and mixing with gastrointestinal tract contents. The solution decreases the gastric emptying rate and the rate of transfer of drug solution to the duodenal region, where absorption is most efficient.

3. **Suspensions** are dispersions of finely divided solid particles of a drug in a liquid medium in which the drug is not readily soluble. The liquid medium of a suspension comprises a saturated solution of the drug in equilibrium with the solid drug.
   a. The bioavailability of the drug from suspensions may be similar to that of a solution because the finely divided particles are dispersed and provide a large surface area for rapid dissolution. On the other hand, a slow dissolution rate decreases the absorption rate.
   b. **Suspending agents** are often hydrophilic colloids (e.g., cellulose derivatives, acacia, xanthan gum) added to suspensions to increase viscosity, inhibit agglomeration, and decrease the rate at which particles settle. Highly viscous suspensions may prolong gastric emptying time, slow drug dissolution, and decrease the absorption rate.

4. **Capsules** are solid dosage forms with hard or soft gelatin shells that contain drugs, usually admixed with excipients. **Coating** the capsule shell or the drug particles within the capsule can affect bioavailability.
   a. **Hard gelatin capsules** are usually filled with a powder blend that contains the drug. Typically, the powder blend is simpler and less compacted than the blend in a compressed tablet. After ingestion, the gelatin softens, swells, and begins to dissolve in the gastrointestinal tract. Encapsulated drugs are released rapidly and dispersed easily, and bioavailability is good. Hard gelatin capsules are the preferred dosage form for early clinical trials of new drugs.
   b. **Soft gelatin capsules** may contain a nonaqueous solution, a powder, or a drug suspension. The vehicle may be water miscible (e.g., PEG). The cardiac glycoside digoxin, dispersed in a water-miscible vehicle (Lanoxicaps), has better bioavailability than a compressed tablet formulation (Lanoxin). However, a soft gelatin capsule that contains the drug dissolved in a **hydrophobic** vehicle (e.g., vegetable oil) may have poorer bioavailability than a compressed tablet formulation of the drug.
   c. **Aging** and **storage conditions** can affect the moisture content of the gelatin component of the capsule shell and the bioavailability of the drug.
      (1) At low moisture levels, the capsule shell becomes brittle and is easily ruptured.
      (2) At high moisture levels, the capsule shell becomes moist, soft, and distorted. Moisture may be transferred to the capsule contents, particularly if the contents are hygroscopic.

5. **Compressed tablets** are solid dosage forms in which high pressure is used to compress a powder blend or granulation that contains the drug and other ingredients, or excipients, into a solid mass.
   a. **Excipients,** including diluents (fillers), binders, disintegrants, lubricants, glidants, surfactants, dye, and flavoring agents, have the following properties.
      (1) They permit the efficient manufacture of compressed tablets.
      (2) They affect the physical and chemical characteristics of the drug.
      (3) They affect bioavailability. The higher the ratio of excipient to active drug, the greater the likelihood that the excipients affect bioavailability.
   b. **Examples**
      (1) **Disintegrants** (e.g., starch, croscarmellose, sodium starch glycolate) vary in action, depending on their concentration, the method by which the disintegrant is mixed with the powder formulation or granulation, and the degree of tablet compaction. Although tablet disintegration is usually not a problem because it often occurs more

rapidly than drug dissolution, it is necessary for dissolution in immediate-release formulations. Inability to disintegrate may interfere with bioavailability.

   (2) Lubricants are usually hydrophobic, water-insoluble substances such as stearic acid, magnesium stearate, hydrogenated vegetable oil, and talc. They may reduce wetting of the surface of the solid drug particles, slowing the dissolution and bioavailability rates of the drug. Water-soluble lubricants, such as L-leucine, do not interfere with dissolution or bioavailability.

   (3) Glidants (e.g., colloidal silicon dioxide) improve the flow properties of a dry powder blend before it is compressed. Rather than posing a potential problem with bioavailability, glidants may reduce tablet-to-tablet variability and improve product efficacy.

   (4) Surfactants enhance drug dissolution rates and bioavailability by reducing interfacial tension at the boundary between solid drug and liquid and improving the wettability (contact) of solid drug particles by the solvent.

  c. Coated compressed tablets have a sugar coat, a film coat, or an enteric coat with the following properties:

   (1) It protects the drug from moisture, light, and air.

   (2) It masks the taste or odor of the drug.

   (3) It improves the appearance of the tablet.

   (4) It may affect the release rate of the drug.

  d. In addition, **enteric coatings** minimize contact between the drug and the gastric region by resisting dissolution or attrition and preventing contact between the underlying drug and the gastric contents or gastric mucosa. Some enteric coatings minimize gastric contact because they are insoluble at acidic pHs. Other coatings resist attrition and remain whole long enough for the tablet to leave the gastric area. By resisting dissolution or attrition, enteric coatings may decrease bioavailability. Enteric coatings are used to:

   (1) Minimize irritation of the gastric mucosa by the drug

   (2) Prevent inactivation or degradation of the drug in the stomach

   (3) Delay release of the drug until the tablet reaches the small intestine, where conditions for absorption may be optimal

6. Modified-release dosage forms are drug products that alter the rate or timing of drug release. Because modified-release dosage forms are more complex than conventional immediate-release dosage forms, more stringent quality control and bioavailability tests are required. **Dose dumping,** or the abrupt, uncontrolled release of a large amount of drug, is a problem.

  a. Extended-release dosage forms include **controlled-release, sustained-action,** and **long-acting drug delivery systems.** These delivery systems allow at least a twofold reduction in dosing frequency compared with conventional immediate-release formulations.

   (1) The extended, slow release of controlled-release drug products produces a relatively flat, sustained plasma drug concentration that avoids toxicity (from high drug concentrations) or lack of efficacy (from low drug concentrations).

   (2) Extended-release dosage forms provide an immediate (initial) release of the drug, followed by a slower sustained release.

  b. Delayed-release dosage forms release active drug at a time other than immediately after administration at a desired site in the gastrointestinal tract. For example, an enteric-coated drug product does not allow for dissolution in the acid pH environment of the stomach, but rather, in the less acidic pH environment of the small intestine.

7. Transdermal drug delivery systems, or patches, are controlled-release devices that contain the drug for systemic absorption after topical application to the skin surface. Transdermal drug delivery systems are available for a number of drugs (nitroglycerin, nicotine, scopolamine, clonidine, fentanyl, 17-β-estradiol, and testosterone). Although the formulation matrices of these delivery systems differ somewhat, they all differ from conventional topical formulations in the following ways:

  a. They have an impermeable **occlusive backing film** that prevents insensible water loss from the skin beneath the patch. This film causes increased hydration and skin temperature under the patch and enhanced permeation of the skin by the drug.

  b. The formulation matrix of the patch maintains the drug concentration gradient within the device after application so that drug delivery to the interface between the patch and skin is sustained. As a result, drug partitioning and diffusion into the skin persist, and systemic absorption is maintained throughout the dosing interval.

    c. Transdermal drug delivery systems are kept in place on the skin surface by an **adhesive layer,** ensuring drug contact with the skin and continued drug delivery.

8. Targeted (site-specific) drug delivery systems are drug carrier systems that place the drug at or near the receptor site. Examples include macromolecular drug carriers (protein drug carriers), particulate drug delivery systems (e.g., liposomes, nanoparticles), and monoclonal antibodies. With targeted drug delivery, the drug may be delivered:
    a. To the capillary bed of the active site
    b. To a special type of cell (e.g., tumor cells), but not to normal cells
    c. To a specific organ or tissue by complexing with a carrier that recognizes the target

9. Inserts, implants, and devices are used to control drug delivery for localized or systemic drug effects. The drug is impregnated into a biodegradable or nonbiodegradable material and is released slowly. The inserts, implants, and devices are inserted into a variety of cavities (e.g., vagina, buccal cavity, skin). For example, the L-norgestrel implant (Norplant) is inserted beneath the skin of the upper arm. It provides contraceptive protection for nearly 5 years.

STUDY QUESTIONS

Directions: Each of the numbered items or incomplete statements in this section is followed by answers or by completions of the statement. Select the **one** lettered answer or completion that is **best** in each case.

1. Which statement best describes bioavailability?

(A) Relation between the physical and chemical properties of a drug and its systemic absorption

(B) Measurement of the rate and amount of therapeutically active drug that reaches the systemic circulation

(C) Movement of drug into body tissues over time

(D) Dissolution of the drug in the gastrointestinal tract

(E) Amount of drug destroyed by the liver before systemic absorption from the gastrointestinal tract occurs

2. The route of drug administration that gives the most rapid onset of the pharmacologic effect is

(A) intramuscular injection

(B) intravenous injection

(C) intradermal injection

(D) peroral administration

(E) subcutaneous injection

3. The route of drug administration that provides complete (100%) bioavailability is

(A) intramuscular injection

(B) intravenous injection

(C) intradermal injection

(D) peroral administration

(E) subcutaneous injection

4. After peroral administration, drugs generally are absorbed best from the

(A) buccal cavity

(B) stomach

(C) duodenum

(D) ileum

(E) rectum

5. The characteristics of an active transport process include all of the following EXCEPT

(A) active transport moves drug molecules against a concentration gradient

(B) active transport follows Fick's law of diffusion

(C) active transport is a carrier-mediated transport system

(D) active transport requires energy

(E) active transport of drug molecules may be saturated at high drug concentrations

6. The passage of drug molecules from a region of high drug concentration to a region of low drug concentration is known as

(A) active transport

(B) bioavailability

(C) biopharmaceutics

(D) simple diffusion

(E) pinocytosis

7. What equation describes the rate of drug dissolution from a tablet?

(A) Fick's law

(B) Henderson–Hasselbalch equation

(C) Law of mass action

(D) Michaelis–Menten equation

(E) Noyes-Whitney equation

8. Which condition usually increases the rate of drug dissolution from a tablet?

(A) Increase in the particle size of the drug

(B) Decrease in the surface area of the drug

(C) Use of the free acid or free base form of the drug

(D) Use of the ionized, or salt, form of the drug

(E) Use of sugar coating around the tablet

9. Dose dumping is a problem in the formulation of

(A)   compressed tablets
(B)   modified-release drug products
(C)   hard gelatin capsules
(D)   soft gelatin capsules
(E)   suppositories

10. The rate-limiting step in the bioavailability of a lipid-soluble drug formulated as an immediate-release compressed tablet is the rate of

(A)   disintegration of the tablet and release of the drug
(B)   dissolution of the drug
(C)   transport of the drug molecules across the intestinal mucosal cells
(D)   blood flow to the gastrointestinal tract
(E)   biotransformation, or metabolism, of the drug by the liver before systemic absorption occurs

11. The extent of ionization of a weak electrolyte drug is dependent on the

(A)   pH of the media and pK_a of the drug
(B)   oil:water partition coefficient of the drug
(C)   particle size and surface area of the drug
(D)   Noyes-Whitney equation for the drug
(E)   polymorphic form of the drug

12. The rate of drug bioavailability is most rapid when the drug is formulated as a

(A)   controlled-release product
(B)   hard gelatin capsule
(C)   compressed tablet
(D)   solution
(E)   suspension

13. The amount of drug that a transdermal patch (i.e., transdermal drug delivery system) delivers within a 24-hour period depends on the

(A)   patch composition that includes an occlusive backing and an adhesive film in contact with the skin
(B)   affinity of the drug for the formulation matrix relative to its affinity for the stratum corneum
(C)   rate of drug partitioning and/or diffusion through the patch to the skin surface
(D)   surface area of the patch
(E)   all of the above

ANSWERS AND EXPLANATIONS

1. The answer is B *[I A 3]*.
Bioavailability is the measurement of the rate and extent (amount) of therapeutically active drug that reaches the systemic circulation. The relation of the physical and chemical properties of a drug to its systemic absorption (i.e., bioavailability) is known as its biopharmaceutics. The movement of a drug into body tissues is an aspect of pharmacokinetics, which is the study of drug movement in the body over time. The dissolution of a drug in the gastrointestinal tract is a physicochemical process that affects bioavailability. Significant destruction of a drug by the liver before it is systemically absorbed (known as the first-pass effect because it occurs during the first passage of the drug through the liver) decreases bioavailability.

2. The answer is B *[II B 1 a]*.
When the active form of the drug is given intravenously, it enters the systemic circulation directly. The drug is delivered rapidly to all tissues, including the drug receptor sites. For all other routes of drug administration except intra-arterial injection, the drug must be systemically absorbed before it is distributed to the drug receptor sites. For this reason, the onset of pharmacologic effects is slower. If the drug is a prodrug that must be converted to an active drug, oral administration, not intravenous injection, may not provide the most rapid onset of activity if conversion to the active form takes place in the gastrointestinal tract or liver.

3. The answer is B *[II C 2]*.
When a drug is given by intravenous injection, the entire dose enters the systemic circulation. With other routes of administration, the drug may be lost before it reaches the systemic circulation. For example, with first-pass effects, a portion of an orally administered drug is eliminated, usually through degradation by liver enzymes, before the drug reaches its receptor sites.

4. The answer is C *[II B 2 b (4)]*.
Drugs given orally are well absorbed from the duodenum. The duodenum has a large surface area because of the presence of villi and microvilli. In addition, because the duodenum is well perfused by the mesenteric blood vessels, a concentration gradient is maintained between the lumen of the duodenum and the blood.

5. The answer is B *[II A 2–3]*.
Fick's law of diffusion describes passive diffusion of drug molecules moving from a high concentration to a low concentration. This process is not saturable and does not require energy.

6. The answer is D *[II A 2]*.
The transport of a drug across a cell membrane by passive diffusion follows Fick's law of diffusion: the drug moves with a concentration gradient (i.e., from an area of high concentration to an area of low concentration). In contrast, drugs that are actively transported move against a concentration gradient.

7. The answer is E *[III A 1]*.
The Noyes-Whitney equation describes the rate at which a solid drug dissolves. Fick's law is similar to the Noyes-Whitney equation in that both equations describe drug movement caused by a concentration gradient. Fick's law generally refers to passive diffusion, or passive transport, of drugs. The law of mass action describes the rate of a chemical reaction, the Michaelis–Menten equation involves enzyme kinetics, and the Henderson–Hasselbalch equation gives the pH of a buffer solution.

8. The answer is D *[III A 1–3]*.
The ionized, or salt, form of a drug has a charge and is generally more water soluble and, therefore, dissolves more rapidly than the nonionized (free acid or free base) form of the drug. The dissolution rate is directly proportional to the surface area and inversely proportional to the particle size. An increase in the particle size or a decrease in the surface area slows the dissolution rate.

9. The answer is B *[III B 6]*.
A modified-release, or controlled-release, drug product contains two or more conventional doses of the drug. An abrupt release of the drug, known as dose dumping, may cause intoxication.

10. The answer is B *[III B 1 c].*
For lipid-soluble drugs, the rate of dissolution is the slowest (i.e., rate-limiting) step in drug absorption and thus in bioavailability. The disintegration rate of an immediate-release or conventional compressed tablet is usually more rapid than the rate of drug dissolution. Because the cell membrane is a lipoprotein structure, transport of a lipid-soluble drug across the cell membrane is usually rapid.

11. The answer is A *[III A 4 b].*
The extent of ionization of a weak electrolyte is described by the Henderson–Hasselbalch equation, which relates the pH of the solvent to the pK_a of the drug.

12. The answer is D *[III B 2 a].*
Because a drug in solution is already dissolved, no dissolution is needed before absorption. Consequently, compared with other drug formulations, a drug in solution has a high rate of bioavailability. A drug in aqueous solution has the highest bioavailability rate and is often used as the reference preparation for other formulations. Drugs in hydroalcoholic solution (e.g., elixirs) also have good bioavailability. The rate of drug bioavailability from a hard gelatin capsule, compressed tablet, or suspension may be equal to that of a solution if an optimal formulation is manufactured and the drug is inherently rapidly absorbed.

13. The answer is E *[III B 7].*
Drug delivery from a transdermal drug delivery system depends on all of the factors cited, i.e., on the presence of an occlusive backing (to maintain skin hydration and elevate skin temperature slightly) and an adhesive film to maintain contact of the formulation matrix with the skin to enable drug transfer from the patch into the skin. If the drug's affinity for the formulation matrix is greater than its affinity for the stratum corneum, the drug's escaping tendency from the patch will be reduced, minimizing the gradient for drug transfer into the skin. The microviscosity of the formulation matrix, the presence of a membrane between the drug reservoir in the patch and the skin surface, and interaction of the drug with the formulation matrix affect the rate and extent of diffusion and/or partitioning of the drug through the patch to the skin surface. Finally, the extent of drug delivery from the patch is directly proportional to the surface area of the patch in contact with the skin surface.

5

Extemporaneous Prescription Compounding

Loyd V. Allen, Jr.

I. INTRODUCTION

A. Definitions

1. Compounding vs Manufacturing

2. It is important, but difficult, to distinguish between compounding and manufacturing.

3. **Compounding** has been defined by the National Association of Boards of Pharmacy as "the preparation, mixing, assembling, packaging, or labeling of a drug or device (i) as the result of a practitioner's prescription drug order or initiative based on the pharmacist/patient/prescriber relationship in the course of professional practice or (ii) for the purpose of, as an incident to research, teaching, or chemical analysis and not for sale or dispensing. Compounding also includes the preparation of drugs and devices in anticipation of prescription drug orders based on routine, regularly observed patterns."

4. **Manufacturing** has been defined as "the production, preparation, propagation, conversion or processing of a drug or device, either directly or indirectly, by extraction from substances of natural origin or independently by means of chemical or biological synthesis, and includes any packaging or repackaging of the substance(s) or labeling or relabeling of its container, and the promotion and marketing of such drugs or devices. Manufacturing also includes the preparation and promotion of commercially available products from bulk compound for resale by pharmacies, practitioners, or other persons."

5. The purpose of pharmaceutical compounding is to prepare an individualized drug treatment for a patient based on an order from a duly licensed prescriber. The fundamental difference between compounding and manufacturing is the existence of a pharmacist/prescriber/patient relationship that controls the preparation of the drug product. Compounded drugs are not for resale, but rather, are personal and responsive to the patient's immediate needs. They are produced and administered by the patient's health-care professionals, which allows for the monitoring of patient outcomes. On the other hand, drug manufacturers produce batches consisting of tens or hundreds of thousands of dosage units, such as tablets or capsules, for resale utilizing many personnel and large-scale manufacturing equipment. These products are distributed through the normal channels of interstate commerce to individuals unknown to the company. Manufacturers are not required to, and do not, provide oversight of individual patients.

B. Regulation

1. **Current Good Manufacturing Practices** (cGMP) are the standards of practice used in the pharmaceutical industry and are regulated by the Food and Drug Administration (FDA). Community pharmacists must comply with state board of pharmacy regulations and guidelines to ensure a quality product, which includes using proper materials, weighing equipment, documented techniques, and dispensing and storage instructions.

2. **Legal considerations**
   a. Extemporaneous compounding by the pharmacist or a prescription order from a licensed practitioner, as with the dispensing of any other prescription, is controlled by the state boards of pharmacy.
   b. The legal risk (liability) of compounding is no greater than the risk of filling a prescription for a manufactured product because the pharmacist must ensure that the correct drug, dose, and directions are provided. The pharmacist is also responsible for preparing a quality pharmaceutical product, providing proper instructions regarding its storage, and advising the patient of any adverse effects.

3. **Food and Drug Administration.** The FDA has developed a list of products that should not be extemporaneously compounded. This list was developed primarily from commercial products that have been removed from the market due to safety and/or efficacy concerns. This is a lengthy list and must be read very carefully because in some cases, only certain dosage forms of a specific drug are included on the list and others are not. The list is too extensive to include here but can be viewed at: http://www.fda.gov/cder/pharmcomp/pcwd.txt.

C. **Stability and quality control of compounded preparations**

1. **Beyond-use dates.** The assignment of a beyond-use date is one of the most difficult tasks required of a compounding pharmacist. Chapters <795> and <797> of the *United States Pharmacopeia* (USP) provide guidelines for this task. Chapter <795> involves nonsterile products, and Chapter <797> involves sterile products. Current USP criteria for nonaqueous liquids and solid formulations (where a manufactured drug product is the source of active ingredients) is a beyond-use date not later than 25% of the time remaining until the product's expiration date or 6 months, whichever is earlier. Where a USP or *National Formulary* (NF) substance is the source of active ingredient, the beyond-use date is not later than 6 months. For water-containing formulations (prepared from ingredients in solid form), the beyond-use date is not later than 14 days when stored at cold temperatures. For all other formulations, the beyond-use date is not later than the intended duration of therapy or 30 days, whichever is earlier. These beyond-use dates may be exceeded when there is supporting valid scientific stability information that is directly applicable to the specific preparation.

2. **Quality control.** Quality control is becoming one of the fastest growing aspects of pharmacy compounding. Pharmacists are becoming more involved in the final testing of compounded preparations, or are sending them to contract laboratories for testing. For example, the following quality control tests can be considered for the respective compounded dosage forms:
   a. **Ointments/creams/gels:** Theoretical weight compared to actual weight, pH, specific gravity, active drug assay, physical observations (color, clarity, texture–surface, texture–spatula spread, appearance, feel), and rheological properties.
   b. **Hard gelatin capsules:** Weight overall, average weight, individual weight variation, dissolution of capsule shell, disintegration of capsule contents, active drug assay, physical appearance (color, uniformity, extent of fill, locked), and physical stability (discoloration, changes in appearance).
   c. **Special hard gelatin capsules:** Weight overall, average weight, individual weight variation, dissolution of capsule shell, disintegration of capsule contents, active drug assay, physical appearance (color, uniformity of appearance, uniformity of extent of fill, closures), and physical stability (discoloration or other changes).
   d. **Suppositories, troches, lollipops, and sticks:** Weight, specific gravity, active drug assay, physical observations (color, clarity, texture of surface, appearance, feel), melting test, dissolution test, physical stability.
   e. **Oral and topical liquids:** Weight/volume, pH, specific gravity, active drug assay, globule size range, rheological properties/pourability, physical observations (color, clarity), and physical stability (discoloration, foreign materials, gas formation, mold growth).
   f. **Parenteral preparations:** Weight/volume, pH, specific gravity, osmolality, assay, physical observations, (color, clarity), particulate matter, sterility, and pyrogenicity.

II. REQUIREMENTS FOR COMPOUNDING

A. **Sources for chemicals and drugs.** Pharmacists must obtain small quantities of the appropriate chemicals or drugs from wholesalers or chemical supply houses. These suppliers then may act as consultants to the pharmacists by ensuring them of their product's purity and quality.

B. **Equipment.** The correct equipment is important when compounding. Many state boards of pharmacy have a required minimum list of equipment for compounding prescriptions. Suggested equipment, which varies according to the amount of material needed and the type of compounded prescription (e.g., parenteral), includes:
   1. Class A prescription balance and/or electronic balance
   2. Hot plate

3. Magnetic stirrers
4. Electric mixer
5. Special containers for packaging (e.g., applicator tip bottles, insufflators)
6. Graduated cylinders from 10 mL to 1000 mL
7. Glass, Wedgwood, and porcelain mortars and pestles of various sizes
8. Funnels of various sizes
9. Spatulas of various sizes, including several plastic spatulas
10. Weighing and filter papers
11. Stirring rods (glass)
12. Ointment/pill tile
13. Capsule filling machine
14. Ointment filling machine
15. Autoclave
16. Laminar flow clean bench
17. Special suppository molds
18. Record-keeping system (compounding log book)
19. Glass beakers from 50 mL to 1000 mL

C. **Location of compounding area.** Many pharmacies actively involved in compounding have dedicated a separate area in the pharmacy to this process. The ideal location is away from heavy foot traffic and is near a sink where there is enough space to work and store all chemicals and equipment. For compounding of sterile products, a laminar air-flow hood (minimal) and a clean room are current practice, or isolation barrier technology equipment.

D. **Sources of Information**

1. Library at a college of pharmacy

2. References
   a. Allen Jr LV. *The Art, Science and Technology of Pharmaceutical Compounding,* 2nd ed. Washington, DC: American Pharmaceutical Association; 2002.
   b. Gennaro AR, ed. *Remington: The Science and Practice of Pharmacy.* 20th ed. Easton, PA: Mack Publishing Co; 2000.
   c. Budavari S, ed. *Merck Index.* 12th ed. Whitehouse Station, NJ: Merck & Co; 1996.
   d. *United States Pharmacopeia* (USP) 25; *National Formulary* (NF) 20. United States Pharmacopeial Convention.
   e. Ansel HC, Allen Jr LV, Popovich NG. *Pharmaceutical Dosage Forms and Drug Delivery Systems.* Media, PA: Williams & Wilkins; 1999.

3. Journals
   a. International Journal of Pharmaceutical Compounding
   b. U.S. Pharmacist
   c. Pharmacy Times
   d. Lippincott's Hospital Pharmacy
   e. Journal of the American Society of Health-System Pharmacists

4. Manufacturers' drug product information inserts; compounding specialty suppliers

III. COMPOUNDING OF SOLUTIONS

A. **Definition.** USP 25 defines **solutions** as liquid preparations that contain one or more chemical substances dissolved (i.e., molecularly dispersed) in a suitable solvent or mixture of mutually miscible solvents. Although the uniformity of the dosage in a solution can be assumed, the stability, pH, solubility of the drug or chemicals, taste (for oral solutions), and packaging need to be considered.

B. **Types of solutions**

1. **Sterile parenteral and ophthalmic solutions** require special consideration for their preparation (see XI).

2. **Nonsterile solutions** include oral, topical, and otic solutions.

C. Preparation of solutions. Solutions are the easiest of the dosage forms to compound extemporaneously, as long as a few general rules are followed.

1. Each drug or chemical is dissolved in the solvent in which it is most soluble. Thus, the solubility characteristics of each drug or chemical must be known.

2. If an alcoholic solution of a poorly water-soluble drug is used, the aqueous solution is added to the alcoholic solution to maintain as high an alcohol concentration as possible.

3. The salt form of the drug, and not the free-acid or base form, which both have poor solubility, is used.

4. Flavoring or sweetening agents are prepared ahead of time.

5. When adding a salt to a syrup, dissolve the salt in a few milliliters of water first; then add the syrup to volume.

6. The proper vehicle (e.g., syrup, elixir aromatic water, purified water) must be selected.

D. Examples

1. Example 1
   a. Medication order
      Phenobarbital 1 g
      Belladonna Tr 5 mL
      Preserved flavored syrup q.s. 120 mL
   b. Compounding procedure. Sodium phenobarbital (equivalent to 1 g of phenobarbital) is dissolved in the preserved, flavored syrup. The solution is then slowly added, in individual portions, to the tincture contained in a beaker and is stirred continuously.

2. Example 2
   a. Medication order
      Potassium chloride 500 mg/10 mL
      Preserved flavored oral vehicle q.s. 60 mL
   b. Compounding procedure. Potassium chloride (3 g) is dissolved in the smallest amount of purified water possible. A sufficient amount of preserved, flavored oral vehicle is added to bring the final volume up to 60 mL.

3. Example 3
   a. Medication order
      Salicylic acid 2%
      Lactic acid 6 mL
      Flexible collodion ad 30 mL
   b. Compounding procedure. Pharmacists must use caution when preparing this prescription because flexible collodion is extremely flammable. A 1-oz applicator tip bottle is calibrated, using ethanol, which is poured out and allowed to evaporate, resulting in a dry bottle. Salicylic acid (0.6 g) is added directly into the bottle, to which is added the 6 mL of lactic acid. The bottle is agitated or a glass stirring rod is used to dissolve the salicylic acid. Flexible collodion is added up to the calibrated 30-mL mark on the applicator tip bottle.

4. Example 4
   a. Medication order
      Iodine 2%
      Sodium iodide 2.4%
      Alcohol q.s. 30 mL
   b. Compounding procedure. Iodine (0.6 g) and sodium iodide (0.72 g) are dissolved in the alcohol, and the final solution is placed in an amber bottle. A **rubber or plastic spatula** is used because **iodine is corrosive.**

IV. COMPOUNDING OF SUSPENSIONS

A. Definition. Suspensions are defined by the USP 25 as liquid preparations that consist of solid particles dispersed throughout a liquid phase in which the particles are not soluble.

B. General characteristics

    1. Some suspensions should contain an antimicrobial agent as a preservative.

    2. Particles settle in suspensions even when a suspending agent is added; thus, suspensions must be well shaken before use to ensure the distribution of particles for a uniform dose.

    3. Tight containers are necessary to ensure the stability of the final product.

    4. Principles to keep in mind when compounding include the following:
        a. Insoluble powders should be small and uniform in size to decrease settling.
        b. The suspension should be viscous.
        c. Topical suspensions should have a smooth, impalpable texture.
        d. Oral suspensions should have a pleasant odor and taste.

C. Formation of suspensions. Suspensions are easy to compound; however, physical stability after compounding the final product is problematic. The following steps may minimize stability problems.

    1. The particle size of all powders used in the formulation must be reduced.

    2. A thickening (suspending) agent may be used to increase viscosity. Common thickening agents include bentonite, Veegum, methylcellulose, and tragacanth.

    3. A levigating agent may aid in the initial dispersion of insoluble particles. Common levigating agents include glycerin, propylene glycol, alcohol, syrups, and water.

    4. Flavoring agents and preservatives should be selected and added if the product is intended for oral use. Common preservatives include methylparabens, propylparabens, benzoic acid, and sodium benzoate. Flavoring agents may be any flavored syrup or flavor concentrate (Table 5-1).

    5. The source of the active ingredients (e.g., bulk powders versus tablets or capsules) must be considered.

D. Preparation of suspensions

    1. The insoluble powders are triturated to a fine powder.

    2. A small portion of liquid is used as a levigating agent, and the powders are triturated until a smooth paste is formed. The levigating agent is added slowly and mixed deliberately.

    3. The vehicle containing the suspending agent is added in divided portions. A high-speed mixer greatly increases the dispersion.

Table 5-1. Selected Flavor Applications

Drug Category	Preferred Flavors
Antibiotics	Cherry, maple, pineapple, orange, raspberry, banana-pineapple, banana-vanilla, butterscotch-maple, coconut custard, strawberry, vanilla, lemon custard, cherry custard, fruit-cinnamon
Antihistamines	Apricot, black currant, cherry, cinnamon, custard, grape, honey, lime, loganberry, peach-orange, peach-rum, raspberry, root beer, wild cherry
Barbiturates	Banana-pineapple, banana-vanilla, black currant, cinnamon-peppermint, grenadine-strawberry, lime, orange, peach-orange, root beer
Decongestants and expectorants	Anise, apricot, black currant, butterscotch, cherry, coconut custard, custard mint-strawberry, grenadine-peach, strawberry, lemon, coriander, orange-peach, pineapple, raspberry, strawberry, tangerine
Electrolyte solutions	Cherry, grape, lemon-lime, raspberry, wild cherry syrup, black currant, grenadine-strawberry, lime, port wine, sherry wine, root beer, wild strawberry

4. The product is brought to the required volume using the vehicle.

5. The final mixture is transferred to a "tight" bottle for dispensing to the patient.

6. All suspensions are dispensed with a "shake well" label.

7. Suspensions are not filtered.

8. The water-soluble ingredients, including flavoring agents, are mixed in the vehicle before mixing with the insoluble ingredients.

E. Examples

1. **Example 1**
   a. **Medication order**
      Propranolol HCl 4 mg/mL
      Disp 30 mL
      Sig: 1 mL p.o. t.i.d.
   b. **Calculations.** Propranolol HCl, 4 mg/mL X 30 mL = 120 mg. Propranolol HCl is available as a powder or in immediate-release and extended-release (long-acting) dosage forms. Only the powder or the immediate-release tablets are used for compounding prescriptions; therefore, some combination of propranolol HCl tablets, which yields 120 mg active drug (e.g., 3 X 40 mg tablets), may be used.
   c. **Compounding procedure.** The propranolol tablets are reduced to a fine powder in a mortar. The powder or the comminuted tablets are levigated to a smooth paste, using a 2% methylcellulose solution. To this mixture, about 10 mL of a suitable flavoring agent is added. The mixture is transferred to a calibrated container and brought to the final volume with purified water. A "shake well" label is attached to the prescription container.

2. **Example 2**
   a. **Medication order**
      Zinc oxide 10
      Ppt sulfur 10
      Bentonite 3.6
      Purified water ad 90 mL
      Sig: Apply t.i.d.
   b. **Compounding procedure.** The powders are reduced to a fine uniform mixture in a mortar. The powders are mixed to form a smooth paste using water and transferred to a calibrated bottle. The final volume is attained with purified water. A "shake well" label is attached to the prescription container.

3. **Example 3**
   a. **Medication order**
      Rifampin suspension 20 mg/mL
      Disp 120 mL
      Sig: u.d.
   b. **Calculations.** Rifampin, 20 mg/mL X 120 mL = 2400 mg. Rifampin is available in 150-mg and 300-mg capsules. Hence, 8 capsules containing 300 mg of rifampin in each capsule or 16 capsules containing 150 mg of rifampin per capsule are needed.
   c. **Compounding procedure.** The contents of the appropriate number of rifampin capsules are emptied into a mortar and comminuted with a pestle. This powder is levigated with a small amount of 1% methylcellulose solution. Twenty milliliters of simple syrup are added and mixed. The mixture is brought to the final volume with simple syrup. "Shake well" and "refrigerate" labels are attached to the prescription container.

V. EMULSIONS

A. Definition. Emulsions are **two-phase systems** in which one liquid is dispersed throughout another liquid in the form of small droplets (see Chapter 3 VI D).

B. General characteristics. Emulsions can be used **externally** as lotions and creams or **internally** to mask the taste of medications.

1. The two liquids in an emulsion are immiscible and require the use of an **emulsifying agent.**

2. Emulsions are classified as either **oil-in-water (o/w)** or **water-in-oil (w/o).**

3. Emulsions are **unstable,** and the following steps must be taken to prevent the two phases of an emulsion from separating into two layers after preparation.

    a. The correct **proportions** of oil and water should be used during preparation. The internal phase should represent about 40%–60% of the total volume.

    b. An emulsifying **agent** is needed for emulsion formation.

    c. A **hand homogenizer,** which reduces the size of globules of the internal phase, may be used.

    d. **Preservatives** should be added if the preparation is intended to last longer than a few days. Generally, a combination of methylparaben (0.2%) and propylparaben (0.02%) may be used.

    e. A **"shake well" label** should be placed on the final product.

    f. The product should be **protected** from light and extreme temperature. Both freezing and heat may have an effect on stability.

C. Emulsifying agents

1. **Gums,** such as acacia or tragacanth, are used to form o/w emulsions. These emulsifying agents are for general use, especially for emulsions intended for internal administration (Table 5-2).

    a. One gram of acacia powder is used for every 4 mL of fixed oil or 1 g to 2 mL for a volatile oil.

    b. If using tragacanth in place of acacia, 0.1 g of tragacanth is used for every 1 g of acacia.

2. **Methylcellulose and carboxymethylcellulose** are used for o/w emulsions. The concentrations of these agents vary, depending on the grade that is used. Methylcellulose is available in several viscosity grades, ranging from 15 to 4000 and designated by a centipoise number, which is a unit of viscosity.

3. **Soaps** can be used to prepare o/w or w/o emulsions for external preparations.

4. **Nonionic emulsifying agents** can be used for o/w and w/o emulsions.

D. Formation and preparation of emulsions. The procedure for preparing an emulsion depends on the desired emulsifying agent in the formulation.

1. A **mortar** and **pestle** are frequently all the equipment that is needed.

    a. A mortar with a **rough surface** (e.g., Wedgwood) should be used. This rough surface allows maximal dispersion of globules to produce a fine particle size.

    b. A **rapid motion** is essential when triturating an emulsion using a mortar and pestle.

    c. The mortar should be able to hold at least three times the **quantity** being made. Trituration seldom requires more than 5 minutes to create the emulsion.

2. **Electric mixers** and hand homogenizers are useful for producing emulsions after the coarse emulsion is formed in the mortar.

3. The **order** of mixing of ingredients in an emulsion depends on the type of emulsion being prepared (i.e., o/w or w/o) as well as the emulsifying agent chosen. Methods used for compounding include the following:

    a. **Dry gum** (continental) method is used for forming emulsions using natural emulsifying agents and requires a specific order of mixing.

    b. **Wet gum** (English) method is used for forming emulsions using natural emulsifying agents and requires a specific order of mixing.

    c. **Bottle method** is used for forming emulsions using natural emulsifying agents and requires a specific order of mixing.

    d. **Beaker method** is used to prepare emulsions using synthetic emulsifying agents and produces a satisfactory product regardless of the order of mixing.

4. **Preservatives.** If the emulsion is kept for an extended period of time, refrigeration is usually sufficient. The product should not be frozen. If a preservative is used, it must be soluble in the water phase to be effective.

5. **Flavoring agents.** If the addition of a flavor is needed to mask the taste of the oil phase, the flavor should be added to the external phase before emulsification (Table 5-3).

Table 5-2. Agents Used in Prescription Compounding

Ointments

Oleaginous or hydrocarbon bases
    Anhydrous
    Nonhydrophilic
    Insoluble in water
    Not water removable (occlusive)
    Good vehicles for antibiotics
  Examples
    Petrolatum

Absorption, or hydrophilic, bases
    Anhydrous
    Hydrophilic
    Insoluble in water
    Not water removable (occlusive)
  Examples
    Hydrophilic petrolatum
    Lanolin USP (anhydrous)

Hydrous emulsion bases (w/o)
    Hydrous
    Hydrophilic
    Insoluble in water
    Not water removable (occlusive)
  Examples
    Cold cream
    Hydrous lanolin

Emulsion bases (o/w)
    Hydrous
    Hydrophilic
    Insoluble in water
    Water removable
    Can absorb 30%–50% of weight
  Examples
    Hydrophilic ointment USP
    Acid mantle cream

Water soluble
    Anhydrous or hydrous
    Soluble in water
    Water removable
    Hydrophilic
  Example
    Polyethylene glycol ointment

Suspending Agents

Acacia 10%
Bentonite 6%
Carboxymethylcellulose 1%–3%
Methylcellulose 1%–7%

Sodium alginate 1%–2%
Tragacanth 1%–3%
Veegum 6%

Preservatives

Methylparaben 0.02%–0.2%

Propylparaben 0.01%–0.04%

Emulsifying Agents

Hydrophilic colloids
  Acacia
  Tragacanth
  Pectin   Favor o/w
  Carboxymethylcellulose
  Methylcellulose
Proteins
  Gelatin
  Egg whites   Favor o/w
Inorganic gels and magmas
  Milk of magnesia
  Bentonite   Favor o/w

Surfactants, nonionic
  Concentrations used (1%–30%)
  Tweens (e.g., polysorbate 80)
  Spans

Soaps
  Triethanolamine
  Stearic acid
Others
  Sodium lauryl sulfate
  Dioctyl sodium sulfosuccinate
  Cetyl pyridinium chloride

o/w = oil-in-water; w/o = water-in-oil.

Table 5-3. Flavor Selection Guide

Taste	Masking Flavor
Salt	Butterscotch, maple
Bitter	Wild cherry, walnut, chocolate mint, licorice
Sweet	Fruit, berry, vanilla
Acid	Citrus

E. Examples

1. Example 1

a. Medication order

Mineral oil 18 mL
Acacia q.s.
Distilled water q.s. ad 90.0 mL
Sig: 1 tbsp q.d.

b. Compounding procedure. With the dry gum method, an initial emulsion (primary emulsion) is formed, using 4 parts (18 mL) of oil, 2 parts (9 mL) of water, and 1 part (4.5 g) of powdered acacia. The mineral oil is triturated with the acacia in a Wedgwood mortar. The 9 mL of water are added all at once and, with rapid trituration, form the primary emulsion, which is triturated for about 5 minutes. The remaining water is incorporated in small amounts with trituration. The emulsion is transferred to a 90-mL prescription bottle, and a "shake well" label is attached to the container.

2. Example 2

a. Medication order

Zinc oxide 8 g
Calamine 8 g
Olive oil 30 mL
Lime water 30 mL

b. Compounding procedure. The olive oil is placed in a suitably sized beaker. Using an electric mixer, the zinc oxide, the calamine, and the lime water are added in that order. This yields a w/o emulsion. This procedure is known as the nascent soap method. The olive oil reacts with the calcium hydroxide solution (lime water) and forms a soap. For this reaction to occur, fresh lime water (calcium hydroxide solution) is required.

3. Example 3

a. Medication order

Mineral oil 50 mL
Water q.s. 100 mL
Sig: 2.5 mL p.o. h.s.

b. Compounding procedure. Using a combination of nonionic emulsifying agents, such as Span 40 and Tween 40, the correct hydrophilic–lipophilic balance (HLB) is obtained. Next, the mineral oil is warmed in a water bath to about 60°C, and the Span 40 is dissolved in the heated mineral oil. The water is warmed to about 65°C, and the Tween 40 is dissolved in the heated water. This mixture is added to the mineral oil and dissolved Span 40 and stirred until cooled. An "external use only" label is added to the container.

VI. POWDERED DOSAGE FORMS

A. Definition. Powders are intimate mixtures of dry, finely divided drugs and/or chemicals that may be intended for internal (oral powders) or external (topical powders) use. The major types are powder papers, bulk powders, and insufflations.

B. General characteristics

1. Powder dosage forms are used when **drug stability** or **solubility** is a concern. These dosage forms may also be used when the powders are too bulky to make into capsules and when the patient has difficulty swallowing a capsule.

2. Some **disadvantages** to powders include unpleasant-tasting medications and, occasionally, the rapid deterioration of powders.

3. **Blending** of powders may be accomplished by using trituration in a mortar, stirring with a spatula, and sifting. Geometric dilution should be used if needed. When heavy powders are mixed with lighter ones, the heavier powder should be placed on top of the lighter one and then blended. When mixing two or more powders, each powder should be pulverized separately to about the same particle size before blending together.

   a. The mortar and pestle method is preferred when **pulverization** and a thorough mixing of ingredients are desired (geometric dilution). A Wedgwood mortar is preferable, but glass or porcelain may also be used.

   b. Light powders are mixed best by using the **sifting method.** The sifting is repeated three to four times to ensure thorough mixing of the powders.

C. Preparation of powder dosage forms

1. **Bulk powders,** which may be used internally or topically, include dusting powders, douche powders, laxatives, antacids, and insufflation powders.

2. After a bulk powder has been pulverized and blended, it should be dispensed in an appropriate container.

   a. **Hygroscopic** or **effervescent** salts should always be placed in a tight, wide-mouthed jar.

   b. **Dusting** powders should be placed in a container with a sifter top.

3. **Eutectic mixtures** of powders can cause problems because they may liquefy. One remedy is to add an inert powder, such as magnesium oxide, to separate the eutectic materials.

4. **Powder papers** are also called divided powders.

   a. The entire powder is initially blended. Each dose is then individually weighed.

   b. The dosage should be weighed, then transferred onto a powder paper and folded. This technique requires practice. Hygroscopic, deliquescent, and effervescent powders require the use of glassine paper as an inside lining. Plastic bags or envelopes with snap-and-seal closures offer a convenient alternative to powder papers.

   c. The folded papers are dispensed in a powder box or other suitable container; however, these containers are not child-resistant.

D. Examples

1. **Example 1**

   a. **Medication order**

      Camphor 100 mg
      Menthol 200 mg
      Zinc oxide 800 mg
      Talc 1900 mg
      M foot powder
      Sig: Apply to feet b.i.d.

   b. **Compounding procedure.** The camphor and menthol are triturated together in a glass mortar, where a liquid eutectic is formed. The zinc oxide and talc are blended and mixed with the eutectic, using geometric dilution. This mixing results in a dry powder, which is passed through a wire mesh sieve. The final product is dispensed in a container with a sifter top.

2. **Example 2**

   a. **Medication order**

      Psyllium mucilloid 2 g
      Citric acid 0.3 g
      Sodium bicarbonate 0.25 g
      M. Ft d.t.d. charts v
      Sig: Empty the contents of one chart into a glass of water and take h.s.

   b. **Calculations.** Calculate for one extra powder paper:

      Psyllium mucilloid 2 g X 6 doses = 12 g
      Citric acid 0.3 g X 6 doses = 1.8 g

Sodium bicarbonate 0.25 g X 6 doses = 1.5 g
Total weight = 15.3 g
15.3 g/6 doses = 2.55 g/dose

    c. **Compounding procedure.** The ingredients are first pulverized and weighed. The citric acid and sodium bicarbonate are mixed together first; the psyllium mucilloid is then added, using geometric dilution. Each dose (2.55 g) of the resultant mixture is weighed and placed into a powder paper. This preparation is an effervescent powder. When dissolved in water, the citric acid and sodium bicarbonate react to form carbonic acid, which yields carbon dioxide, making the solution more palatable.

VII. CAPSULES

A. Definition. Capsules are solid dosage forms in which the drug is enclosed within either a hard or soft soluble container or shell. The shells are usually made from a suitable gelatin. Hard gelatin capsules may be manually filled for extemporaneous compounding.

B. Capsule sizes

  1. A list of capsule sizes and the approximate amount of powder that may be contained in the capsule appear on the side of the capsule box (Table 5-4).

  2. Capsule sizes for oral administration in humans range from no. 5, the smallest, to no. 000, the largest.

  3. No. 0 is usually the largest oral size suitable for patients.

  4. Capsules for veterinarians are available in nos. 10, 11, and 12, containing approximately 30, 15, and 7.5 g, respectively.

C. Preparation of hard and soft capsules

  1. As with the bulk powders, all ingredients are triturated and blended, using geometric dilution.

  2. The correct size capsule must be determined by trying different capsule sizes, weighing them, and then choosing the appropriate size.

  3. Before filling capsules with the medication, the body and cap of the capsule are separated. Filling is accomplished by using the "punch" method.
    a. The powder formulation is compressed with a spatula on a pill tile or paper sheet with a uniform depth of approximately half the length of the capsule body.
    b. The empty capsule body is repeatedly pressed into the powder until full.
    c. The capsule is then weighed to ensure an accurate dose. An empty tare capsule of the same size is placed on the pan containing the weights.
    d. For a large number of capsules, capsule-filling machines can be used for small-scale use to save time.

  4. The capsule is wiped clean of any powder or oil and dispensed in a suitable prescription vial.

Table 5-4. Approximate Amount of Powder
Contained in Capsules

Capsule Size	Range of Powder Capacity (mg)
No. 5	60–130
No. 4	95–260
No. 3	130–390
No. 2	195–520
No. 1	225–650
No. 0	325–910
No. 00	390–1300
No. 000	650–2000

D. Examples

1. Example 1

a. Medication order

    Rifampin 100 mg
    dtd #50
    Sig: 1 cap p.o. q.d.

b. Calculations. Calculate for at least one extra capsule.

    51 caps X 100 mg/cap = 5100 mg rifampin
    5100 mg rifampin ÷ 300 mg/cap = 17 caps

c. Compounding procedure. Seventeen rifampin capsules, each containing 300 mg rifampin, are used. The content of each capsule is emptied, and the powder is weighed. The **equivalent** powder equal to 100 mg rifampin is placed in a capsule and sufficient lactose added to fill the capsule. The capsule contents weigh 200 mg. The **equivalent** weight is subtracted to obtain the amount of lactose required per capsule. This is multiplied by 51 capsules. Enough lactose is added to make a total of 10.2 g of powder. The powders are combined, using geometric dilution, and 50 capsules can be punched out. Each capsule should weigh 10.2 g/51 caps or 200 mg.

2. Example 2

a. Medication order. This order is for veterinary use only.

    Castor oil 8 mL
    Disp 12 caps
    Sig: 2 caps p.o. h.s.

b. Calculations. No calculations are necessary.

c. Compounding procedure. A no. 11 veterinary capsule is used. Using a calibrated dropper or a pipette, 8 mL of the oil are carefully added to the inside of each capsule body. Next, the lower inside portion of the cap is moistened, using a glass rod or brush. The cap and body are joined together, using a twisting motion, to form a tight seal. The capsules are placed on a piece of filter paper and checked for signs of leakage. The capsules are dispensed in the appropriate size and type of prescription vial.

VIII. MOLDED TABLETS (TABLET TRITURATES)

A. Definition. Tablet triturates are small, usually cylindrical molded or compressed tablets. They are made of powders created by moistening the powder mixture with alcohol and water. They are used for compounding potent drugs in small doses.

B. Formulation and preparation of tablet triturates

1. Tablet triturates are made in special molds consisting of a pegboard and a corresponding perforated plate.

2. In addition to the mold, a diluent, usually a mixture of lactose and sucrose (80/20), and a moistening agent, usually a mixture of ethyl alcohol and water (60/40), are required.

3. The diluent is triturated with the active ingredients.

4. A paste is then made, using the alcohol and water mixture.

5. This paste is spread into the mold; the tablets are punched out and remain on the pegs until dry.

C. Example

1. Medication order

    Atropine sulfate 0.4 mg
    Disp #500 TT
    Sig. u.d.

2. Calculations. For 500 TT: 500 X 0.4 mg = 200 mg atropine sulfate

3. Compounding procedure. The mold prepares 70-mg tablets. The 200 mg of atropine sulfate, 6.8 g of sucrose, and 28 g of lactose are weighed and mixed by geometric dilution. The powder is wet with a mixture of 40% purified water and 60% ethyl alcohol (95%). The paste

that is formed is spread onto the tablet triturate mold; the tablets are then punched out of the mold and allowed to dry on the pegs. This procedure is repeated until the required number of tablet triturates has been prepared.

IX. OINTMENTS, CREAMS, PASTES, AND GELS

A. Definitions

1. **Ointments, creams, and pastes** are semisolid dosage forms intended for topical application to the skin or mucous membranes. **Ointments** are characterized as being oleaginous in nature; **creams** are generally o/w or w/o emulsions, and **pastes** are characterized by their high content of solids (about 25%).

2. **Gels** (sometimes called jellies) are semisolid systems consisting of suspensions made up of either small inorganic particles or large organic molecules interpenetrated by a liquid.

B. General characteristics. These dosage forms are semisolid preparations generally applied externally. Semisolid dosage forms may contain active drugs intended to:

1. Act solely on the surface of the skin to produce a local effect (e.g., antifungal agent)

2. Release the medication, which, in turn, penetrates into the skin (e.g., cortisol cream)

3. Release medication for systemic absorption through the skin (e.g., nitroglycerin)

C. Types of ointment bases

1. Hydrophobic bases feel greasy and contain mixtures of fats, oils, and waxes. Hydrophobic bases cannot be washed off using water.

2. Hydrophilic bases are usually emulsion bases. The o/w-type emulsion bases can be easily washed off with water, but the w/o type is slightly more difficult to remove.

D. Preparation of ointments, creams, pastes, and gels

1. Mixing can be done in a mortar or on an ointment slab/tile.

2. Liquids are incorporated by gradually adding them to an absorption-type base and mixing.

3. Insoluble powders are reduced to a fine powder and then added to the base, using geometric dilution.

4. Water-soluble substances are dissolved with water and then incorporated into the base.

5. The final product should be smooth (impalpable) and free of any abrasive particles.

E. Examples

1. **Example 1**
   a. Medication order
   > Sulfur
   > Salicylic acid aa 600 mg
   > White petrolatum ad 30 g
   > Sig: Apply t.i.d.

   b. Compounding procedure. The particle sizes of the sulfur and salicylic acid are reduced separately in a Wedgwood mortar and then blended together. Using a pill tile, the powder mixture is levigated with the base. Using geometric dilution, the base and powders are blended to the final weight. An ointment jar or plastic tube is used for dispensing, and an "external use only" label is placed on the container.

2. **Example 2**
   a. Medication order
   > Methylparaben 0.25 g
   > Propylparaben 0.15 g
   > Sodium lauryl sulfate 10 g
   > Propylene glycol 120 g
   > Stearyl alcohol 250 g

White petrolatum 250 g
Purified water 370 g
Disp 60 g
Sig: Apply u.d.

   b. Compounding procedure. The stearyl alcohol and the white petrolatum are melted on a steam bath and heated to about 75°C. The other ingredients, previously dissolved in purified water at about 78°C, are added. The mixture is stirred until it congeals. An ointment jar is used for dispensing, and an "external use only" label is placed on the jar.

3. Example 3
   a. Medication order

Scopolamine hydrobromide 250 mg
Soy lecithin 12 g
Isopropyl palmitate 12 g
Pluronic F-127 20% gel q.s. 100 mL
Sig: Apply 0.1 mL t.i.d.

   b. Compounding procedure. Mix the soy lecithin with the isopropyl palmitate. Dissolve the scopolamine hydrobromide in about 3 mL of purified water and add to about 70 mL of the Pluronic F-127 gel. Add the soy lecithin–isopropyl palmitate mixture, and mix well. Add sufficient Pluronic F-127 gel to volume, and mix well. Package and label.

X. SUPPOSITORIES

A. General characteristics

1. Suppositories are **solid bodies** of various weights and shapes, adapted for introduction into the rectal, vaginal, or urethral orifices of the human body. They are used to deliver drugs for their local or systemic effects.

2. Suppositories differ in **size** and **shape** and include:
   a. Rectal
   b. Vaginal
   c. Urethral

B. Common suppository bases

1. Cocoa butter (theobroma oil), which melts at body temperature, is a fat-soluble mixture of triglycerides that is most often used for rectal suppositories. Witepsol is a synthetic triglyceride. Fatty acid bases include Fattibase.

2. Polyethylene glycol (PEG, Carbowax) derivatives are water-soluble bases suitable for vaginal and rectal suppositories. Polybase is an example.

3. Glycerinated gelatin is a water-miscible base often used in vaginal and rectal suppositories.

C. Suppository molds

1. Suppository molds can be made of rubber, plastic, brass, stainless steel, or other suitable material.

2. The formulation and volume of the base depend on the size of the mold used, less the displacement caused by the active ingredient.

D. Methods of preparing and dispensing suppositories

1. Molded suppositories are prepared by first melting the base and then incorporating the medications uniformly into the base. This mixture is then poured into the suppository mold (fusion method).

2. Hand-rolled suppositories require a special technique. With proper technique, it is possible to make a product equal in quality to the molded suppositories.

3. Containers for the suppositories are determined by the method and base used in preparation. Hand-rolled and molded suppositories should be dispensed in special boxes that prevent the suppositories from coming in contact with each other.

4. **Storage conditions.** If appropriate, a "refrigerate" label should appear on the container. Regardless of the base or medication used in the formulation, the patient should be instructed to store the suppositories in a cool dry place.

E. **Examples**

1. **Example 1**
   a. **Medication order**
      Naproxen suppository 500 mg
      Disp #12
      Sig: Insert u.d. into rectum
   b. **Calculations.** Each standard adult suppository should weigh 2 g, but it depends on the mold used.
      2 g (total weight) − 0.540 g (weight of each 500-mg tablet) naproxen per suppository
      = 1.46 g cocoa butter per suppository X 13 suppositories
      = 18.98 g cocoa butter
   c. **Compounding procedure.** The 13 naproxen 500-mg tablets are triturated to a fine powder, using a Wedgwood mortar. The 18.98 g cocoa butter base is melted in a beaker, using a water bath. The temperature of the water bath should not exceed 36°C. The powder is then added and stirred until mixed. The mixture is poured into an appropriate rectal suppository mold (about 2 g per suppository) and placed into a refrigerator until the suppositories congeal. Any excess is scraped from the top of the mold, and a suppository box is used for dispensing. A "refrigerate" label is placed on the box.

2. **Example 2**
   a. **Medication order**
      Progesterone 50 mg
      Disp #14
      Sig: 1 per vagina once daily on days 14–28 of cycle
   b. **Calculations.** Total weight of each vaginal suppository is 1.9 g.
      50 mg progesterone/suppository X 15 = 750 mg progesterone
      1.9 g (total weight) − 0.050 g progesterone
      = 1.85 g PEG X 15 suppositories
      = 27.75 g PEG total
   c. **Compounding procedure.** The PEG is melted to 55–57°C, and 750 mg progesterone is added. This mixture is poured into a vaginal suppository mold, allowed to cool, cleaned, and dispensed.

XI. PARENTERAL PRODUCTS

A. **General requirements.** The extemporaneous compounding of sterile products is no longer confined only to the hospital environment; it now is done by community pharmacists engaged in home care practice. Minimum requirements include:

1. Proper equipment and supplies

2. Proper facilities, including a laminar-flow clean bench and a clean room or isolation barrier technology equipment

3. Proper documentation of all products made

4. Quality control, including batch sterility testing

5. Proper storage both at the facility and in transport to the patient's home

6. Proper labeling of the prescription product

7. Knowledge of product's stability and incompatibilities

8. Knowledge of all ancillary equipment involved in production or delivery of the medications

B. **Preparation of parenteral products**

1. Preparation of sterile products requires special skills and training. Preparing parenteral products or providing this service without proper training should not be attempted.

2. These products must be prepared in a clean environment, using aseptic technique (i.e., working under controlled conditions to minimize contamination).

3. Dry powders of parenteral drugs for reconstitution are used for drug products that are unstable as solutions. It is important to know the correct diluents that can be used to yield a solution.

4. Solutions of drugs for parenteral administration may also be further diluted before administration. If further dilution is required, then the pharmacist must know the stability and compatibility of the drug in the diluent.

C. Reconstitution of a dry powder from a vial

1. Work takes place in a clean-air environment, observing aseptic technique.

2. The manufacturer's instructions should be checked to determine the required volume of diluent.

3. The appropriate needle size and syringe are chosen, keeping in mind that the capacity of the syringe should be slightly larger than the volume required for reconstitution.

4. Using the correct diluent, the surface of the container is cleaned, using an alcohol prep pad, after which the alcohol is permitted to evaporate.

5. The syringe is filled with the diluent to the proper volume.

6. The surface of the vial containing the sterile powder is cleaned, using an alcohol prep pad, after which it is permitted to dry. The diluent is injected into the vial containing the dry powder.

7. The vial is gently shaken or rolled, and the powder is allowed to dissolve.

8. After the powder has dissolved, the vial is inverted and the desired volume is withdrawn.

9. The vehicle is prepared by swabbing the medication port of the bag or bottle with an alcohol prep pad.

10. The solution in the syringe is injected into the vehicle. If a plastic container is used, care must be taken not to puncture the side walls of the container with the tip of the needle.

11. The container should be shaken or kneaded or rotated to assure thorough mixing of the contents.

12. The contents of the container should be checked for particulate matter.

13. A sterile seal or cap is applied over the port of the container.

14. All needles and syringes should be properly discarded.

15. The bag is labeled.

D. Removing the fluid contents from an ampule

1. The ampule is held upright to open it, and the top is tapped to remove any solution trapped in this area.

2. The neck of the ampule is swabbed with an alcohol swab.

3. The ampule is grasped on each side of the neck with the thumb and index finger of each hand and quickly snapped open.

4. A 5-μm filter needle is attached to a syringe of the appropriate size.

5. The ampule is tilted, and the needle is inserted.

6. The needle is positioned near the neck of the ampule, and the solution is withdrawn from the ampule.

7. If the solution is for an intravenous push (bolus injection), the filter needle is removed from the syringe and replaced with a cap.

8. If the solution is for an intravenous infusion, then the filter needle is removed and replaced with a new needle of the appropriate size. The drug is injected into the appropriate vehicle.

9. All materials should be discarded properly, and the final product should be labeled.

E. Removing drug solution from a vial

1. The tab around the rubber closure on the vial is removed, and this surface is swabbed with an alcohol prep pad.

2. An equivalent amount of sterile air is injected into the vial to prevent a negative vacuum from being created and to allow the drug to be removed.

3. Using the appropriate needle size and syringe, the needle is inserted into the rubber closure with the bevel at a 45° angle.

4. The plunger is pushed down, and air is released into the vial; when the plunger is pulled back, the solution is withdrawn.

5. The solution is then injected into the appropriate vehicle.

F. Examples

1. **Example 1**
   a. **Medication order**
      Progesterone 5 g
      Benzyl alcohol 10 mL
      Sesame oil q.s. 100 mL
   b. **Compounding procedure.** Dissolve the progesterone in the benzyl alcohol. Add sufficient sesame oil to make 100 mL. Sterilize by filtration through a sterile 0.2-μm filter or by dry heat (170°C for 1.5 hours). Package in sterile vials and label.

2. **Example 2**
   a. **Medication order**
      Fentanyl (as the citrate) 2 mg
      Bupivacaine hydrochloride 125 mg
      0.9% Sodium chloride injection q.s. 100 mL
   b. **Compounding procedure.** Using commercially available injections, accurately measure the volume of each and fill into a sterile ambulatory pump reservoir. An air bubble can be injected and used to thoroughly mix the solution. Remove the air from the reservoir, and tightly seal/close the outlet. Label.

3. **Example 3**
   a. **Medication order**
      Morphine sulfate 5 g
      Citric acid 100 mg
      Sodium chloride 180 mg
      Methylparaben 150 mg
      Sterile water for injection q.s. 100 mL
   b. **Compounding procedure.** Dissolve the methylparaben in about 90 mL of sterile water for injection. A small amount of heat may be required. Cool the solution to room temperature; then add the morphine sulfate, citric acid, and sodium chloride. Add sufficient sterile water for injection to volume and mix well. Package in sterile vials or reservoirs and label.

STUDY QUESTIONS

Directions: Each of the numbered items or incomplete statements in this section is followed by answers or by completions of the statement. Select the **one** lettered answer or completion that is **best** in each case.

Questions 1-3

The following medication order is given to the pharmacist by the physician.

Olive oil 60.0 mL
Vitamin A 60,000 units
Water 120.0 mL
Sig: 15 mL t.i.d.

1. The final dosage form of this prescription will be

(A) a solution
(B) an elixir
(C) an emulsion
(D) a suspension
(E) a lotion

2. When preparing this prescription, the pharmacist needs to add

(A) Tween 80
(B) acacia
(C) glycerin
(D) alcohol
(E) propylene glycol

3. Which of the following caution labels should the pharmacist affix to the container when dispensing this product?

(A) Do not refrigerate
(B) Shake well
(C) For external use only
(D) No preservatives added

Directions: Each item below contains three suggested answers of which **one or more** is correct. Choose the answer

A   if **I only** is correct
B   if **III only** is correct
C   if **I and II** are correct
D   if **II and III** are correct
E   if **I, II, and III** are correct

4. Correct statements about the prescription below include which of the following?

Morphine 1 mg/mL
Flavored vehicle q.s. ad 120 mL
Sig: 5–20 mg p.o. q 3–4 hours prn pain

I. The amount of morphine needed is 240 mg
II. Powdered morphine alkaloid should be used when compounding this prescription
III. The final dosage form of this prescription is a solution

5. When preparing the following prescription

Podophyllum 5%
Salicylic acid 10%
Acetone 20%
Flexible collodion ad 30 mL
Sig: Apply q h.s.

the pharmacist should:

I. triturate 1.5 g of podophyllum with the 8 mL of acetone
II. add 3 g of salicylic acid to the collodion with trituration
III. affix an "external use only" label to the container

6. Correct statements about the prescription below include which of the following?

> Sulfur 6 g
> Purified water
> Camphor water aa q.s. ad 60

 I. Precipitated sulfur can be used to prepare this prescription
 II. The sulfur can be triturated with glycerin before mixing with other ingredients
 III. A "shake well" label should be affixed to the bottle

7. Correct statements about the prescription below include which of the following?

> Starch 10%
> Menthol 1%
> Camphor 2%
> Calamine q.s. ad 120

 I. The powders should be blended together in a mortar, using geometric dilution
 II. The prescription should be prepared by dissolving the camphor in a sufficient amount of 90% alcohol
 III. A eutectic mixture should be avoided

8. When preparing the following prescription:

> Salicylic acid 3 g
> Sulfur ppt 7 g
> Lanolin 10 g
> White petrolatum 10 g

the pharmacist should:

 I. reduce the particle size of the powders, using a mortar and pestle, or using the pill tile with a spatula
 II. place on an ointment tile and levigate the ingredients, using geometric dilution
 III. package the ointment in an ointment jar or tube

9. An equal volume of air is injected when removing drug solutions from

 I. vials
 II. ampules
 III. syringes

ANSWERS AND EXPLANATIONS

1–3. The answers are: 1-C [*V B 1*], **2-B** [*V B 2, C 1*], **3-B** [*V B 3*].
Because olive oil and water are two immiscible liquids, their incorporation requires a two-phase system in which one liquid is dispersed throughout another liquid in the form of small droplets. To accomplish this, an emulsifying agent is necessary. Acacia is the most suitable emulsifying agent when forming an oil-in-water emulsion that is intended for internal use.

Emulsions are physically unstable, and they must be protected against the effects of microbial contamination and physical separation. Shaking before use redistributes the two layers of emulsion. Because light, air, and microorganisms also affect the stability of an emulsion, preservatives can be added.

4. The answer is B (III) [*III A, C 3*].
The concentration of morphine needed for the prescription described in the question is 1 mg/mL, and because 120 mL is the final volume, 120 mg of morphine is needed to compound this prescription. Morphine alkaloid has poor solubility; therefore, one of the salt forms should be used. Because morphine is dissolved in the vehicle, resulting in a liquid preparation, the final dosage form is a solution.

5. The answer is B (III) [*III C 1, 5, D 3*].
Calculating for the amount of each ingredient of the prescription in the question requires 1.5 g of podophyllum, 3 g of salicylic acid, and 6 mL of acetone. The correct procedure would be to triturate the podophyllum with the acetone, then add the triturated salicylic acid to a calibrated bottle containing the podophyllum and acetone. Flexible collodion is then added up to the 30-mL calibration. An "external use only" label should be affixed to the container.

6. The answer is E (all) [*IV B 2, C 5, D 1, 2*].
While precipitated sulfur can be used to prepare the prescription described in the question, it is difficult to triturate; therefore, it must first be levigated with a suitable levigating agent (e.g., glycerin). All suspensions, due to their instability, require shaking before use to redistribute the insoluble ingredients.

7. The answer is A (I) [*VI C 3, D 1*].
The proper procedure for compounding the prescription described in the question is to first form a liquid eutectic. This is done by triturating the menthol and camphor together in a mortar. This eutectic is then blended with the powdered starch and calamine, using geometric dilution.

8. The answer is E (all) [*IX D 1-3, E 1*].
The proper procedure for preparing the prescription given in the question is to reduce the particle size of each powder and mix them together, using geometric dilution. This ensures the proper blending of the powders. Next, this powdered mixture is incorporated, geometrically, with the petrolatum. Then, the lanolin is added geometrically.

9. The answer is A (I) [*XI E 2*].
An equal volume of air must be injected when removing a drug solution from a vial. This is done to prevent the formation of a vacuum within the vial. This problem does not occur with ampules and syringes containing drug solutions; therefore, it is unnecessary to inject any air when removing them.

6
Basic Pharmacokinetics
Leon Shargel

I. PHARMACOKINETICS

A. Introduction

1. **Rates and orders of reactions.** The **rate** of a chemical reaction or process is the velocity with which it occurs. The **order** of a reaction is the way in which the concentration of a drug or reactant in a chemical reaction affects the rate.

   a. **Zero-order reaction.** The drug concentration changes with respect to time at a constant rate, according to the following equation:

$$\frac{dC}{dt} = -k_0$$

   where C is the drug concentration and k_0 is the **zero-order rate constant** expressed in units of concentration per time (e.g., milligrams per milliliter per hour). Integration of this equation yields the linear (straight-line) equation:

$$C = -k_0 t + C_0$$

   where k_0 is the slope of the line **(see Chapter 3, Figure 3-4)** and C_0 is the y intercept, or drug concentration, when time (t) equals zero. The negative sign indicates that the slope is decreasing.

   b. **First-order reaction.** The drug concentration changes with respect to time equal the product of the rate constant and the concentration of drug remaining, according to the following equation:

$$\frac{dC}{dt} = -kC$$

   where k is the first-order rate constant, expressed in units of reciprocal time, or $time^{-1}$ (e.g., 1/hr or hr^{-1}).

   (1) Integration of this equation yields the following mathematically equivalent equations:

$$C = C_0 e^{-kt}$$
$$\ln C = -kt + \ln C_0$$

$$\log C = -\frac{kt}{2.3} + \log C_0$$

   (2) A graph of the equation in **Chapter 3, Figure 3-6,** shows the linear relation of the log of the concentration versus time. In **Figure 3-6,** the slope of the line is equal to $-k/2.3$, and the y intercept is C_0. The values for C are plotted on logarithmic coordinates, and the values for t are shown on linear coordinates.

   (3) The **half-life ($t_{1/2}$)** of a reaction is the time required for the concentration of a drug to decrease by one-half. For a first-order reaction, the half-life is a constant and is related to the first-order rate constant, according to the following equation:

$$t_{1/2} = \frac{0.693}{k}$$

2. **Models and compartments**

   a. A **model** is a mathematic description of a biologic system and is used to express quantitative relationships.

   b. A **compartment** is a group of tissues with similar blood flow and drug affinity. A compartment is not a real physiologic or anatomic region.

3. Drug distribution
  a. Drugs distribute rapidly to tissues with high blood flow and more slowly to tissues with low blood flow.
  b. Drugs rapidly cross capillary membranes into tissues because of **passive diffusion** and **hydrostatic pressure. Drug permeability** across capillary membranes varies.
   (1) Drugs easily cross the capillaries of the glomerulus of the kidney and the sinusoids of the liver.
   (2) The capillaries of the brain are surrounded by glial cells that create a **blood–brain barrier** that acts as a thick lipid membrane. Polar and ionic hydrophilic drugs cross this barrier slowly.
  c. Drugs may accumulate in tissues as a result of their physicochemical characteristics or special affinity of the tissue for the drug.
   (1) Lipid-soluble drugs may accumulate in adipose (fat) tissue because of partitioning of the drug.
   (2) Tetracycline may accumulate in bone because complexes are formed with calcium.
  d. Plasma protein binding of drugs affects drug distribution.
   (1) A drug bound to a protein forms a complex that is too large to cross cell membranes.
   (2) Albumin is the major plasma protein involved in drug protein binding. α_1-**Glycoprotein,** also found in plasma, is important for the binding of such basic drugs as propranolol.
   (3) Potent drugs, such as phenytoin, that are highly bound (more than 90%) to plasma proteins may be displaced by other highly bound drugs. The displacement of the bound drug results in more free (nonbound) drug, which rapidly reaches the drug receptors and causes a more intense pharmacologic response.

B. One-compartment model

  1. Intravenous bolus injection. The entire drug dose enters the body rapidly, and the rate of absorption is neglected in calculations **(Figure 6-1).** The entire body acts as a single compartment, and the drug rapidly equilibrates with all of the tissues in the body.
  a. Drug elimination is a first-order kinetic process, according to the equations in **I A 1 b.**

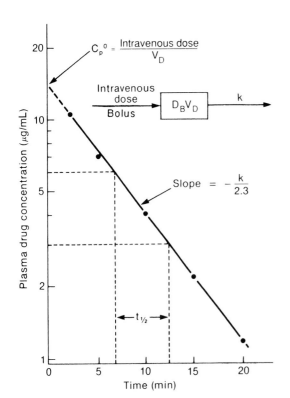

Figure 6-1. Generalized pharmacokinetic model for a drug administered by rapid intravenous bolus injection. C_p^0 = extrapolated drug concentration; V_D = apparent volume of distribution; D_B = amount of drug in the body; k = elimination rate constant; $t_{1/2}$ = elimination half-life. (Adapted with permission from Gibaldi M, Perrier D: *Pharmacokinetics,* 2nd ed. New York, Marcel Dekker, 1982, p. 4.)

(1) The first-order elimination rate constant (k or k_{el}) is the sum of the rate constants for removal of drug from the body, including the rate constants for renal excretion and metabolism **(biotransformation)** as described by the following equation:

$$k = k_e + k_m$$

where k_e is the rate constant for renal excretion and k_m is the rate constant for metabolism. This equation assumes that all rates are first-order processes.

(2) The **elimination half-life ($t_{1/2}$)** is given by the following equation:

$$t_{1/2} = \frac{0.693}{k}$$

b. Apparent volume of distribution (V_D) is the hypothetical volume of body fluid in which the drug is dissolved. This value is not a true anatomic or physical volume.

(1) V_D is needed to estimate the amount of drug in the body relative to the concentration of drug in the plasma, as shown in the following:

$$V_D \times C_p = D_B$$

where V_D is the apparent volume of distribution, C_p is the plasma drug concentration, and D_B is the amount of drug in the body.

(2) To calculate the V_D after an intravenous bolus injection, the equation is rearranged to give:

$$V_D = \frac{D_B{}^0}{C_p{}^0}$$

where $D_B{}^0$ is the dose (D_o) of drug given by intravenous bolus and $C_p{}^0$ is the extrapolated drug concentration at zero time on the y axis, after the drug equilibrates **(Figure 6-1)**.

(3) According to the equation, V_D is increased and $C_p{}^0$ is decreased when the drug is distributed more extravascularly into the tissues. When more drug is contained in the vascular space or plasma, $C_p{}^0$ is increased and V_D is decreased.

2. Single oral dose. If the drug is given in an oral dosage form (e.g., tablet, capsule), the drug is rapidly absorbed by first-order kinetics. Elimination of the drug also follows the principles of first-order kinetics **(Figure 6-2)**.

a. The following equation describes the pharmacokinetics of **first-order absorption and elimination:**

$$C_p = \frac{FD_o k_A}{V_D(k_A - k)}\,(e^{-kt} - e^{-kt})$$

where k_A is the first-order absorption rate constant and F is the fraction of drug bioavailable. Changes in F, D_o, V_D, k_A, and k affect the plasma drug concentration.

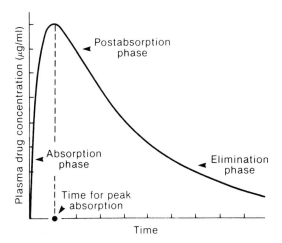

Plasma drug concentration (μg/ml)

Postabsorption phase

Absorption phase

Time for peak absorption

Elimination phase

Time

Figure 6-2. Generalized plot for a one-compartment model showing first-order drug absorption and first-order drug elimination. (Adapted with permission from Shargel L, Yu ABC: *Applied Biopharmaceutics and Pharmacokinetics,* 4th ed. McGraw-Hill, New York, 1999, p. 224.)

b. The time for maximum, or **peak, drug absorption** is given by the following equations:

$$t_{max} = \frac{2.3 \log (k_A/k)}{k_A - k}$$

t_{max} depends only on the rate constants k_A and k, not on F, D_0, or V_D.

c. After t_{max} is obtained, the peak drug concentration (C_{max}) is calculated, using the equation in I B 2 a and substituting t_{max} for t.

d. The area under the curve (AUC) may be determined by integration of $\int_0^t C_p \, dt$, using the trapezoidal rule, or by the following equation:

$$\int_0^t C_p dt = [AUC]_0^t \int_0^\infty C_p dt = \frac{FD_0}{V_D k}$$

where changes in F, D_0, k, and V_D affect the AUC. Minor changes in k_A do not affect the AUC.

e. To obtain $[AUC]_0{}^{00}$, obtain the [AUC] from 0 to t by the trapezoidal rule and add on the extrapolated section of AUC, which is the last measurable drug concentration at time t divided by the slope of the terminal elimination curve, as shown in the following equation:

$$[AUC] = [AUC] + C_p t/k$$

f. Lag time occurs at the beginning of systemic drug absorption. For some individuals, systemic drug absorption is delayed after oral drug administration because of delayed stomach emptying or other factors.

3. Intravenous infusion

a. Intravenous infusion is an example of zero-order absorption and first-order elimination **(Figure 6-3).**

b. A few oral controlled-release drug products release the drug by zero-order kinetics and have **zero-order systemic absorption.**

c. The plasma drug concentration at any time after the start of an intravenous infusion is given by the following equation:

$$C_p = \frac{R}{V_D k} (1 - e^{-kt})$$

where R is the zero-order rate of infusion given in units as milligrams per hour or milligrams per minute.

d. If the intravenous infusion is discontinued, the plasma drug concentration declines by a first-order process. The elimination half-life, or elimination rate constant, k, may be obtained from the declining plasma drug concentration versus time curve.

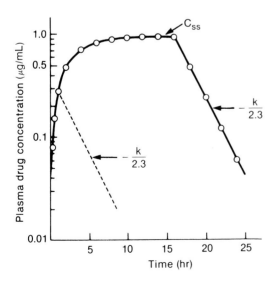

Figure 6-3. Generalized semilogarithmic plot for a drug showing zero-order absorption and first-order elimination. C_{ss} = steady-state concentration; k = elimination rate constant. (Adapted with permission from Gibaldi M, Perrier D: *Pharmacokinetics*, 2nd ed. New York, Marcel Dekker, 1982, p. 30.)

    e. As the drug is infused, the plasma drug concentration increases to a plateau, or **steady-state concentration (C_{ss}).**

        (1) Under steady-state conditions, the fraction of drug absorbed equals the fraction of drug eliminated from the body.

        (2) The plasma concentration at steady state (C_{ss}) is given by the following equation:

$$C_{ss} = \frac{R}{V_D k}$$

        (3) The rate of drug infusion (R) may be calculated from a rearrangement of the equation if the desired C_{ss}, the V_D, and the k are known. These values can often be obtained from the drug literature. To calculate the rate of infusion, the following equation is used:

$$R = C_{ss} V_D k$$

        where C_{ss} is the desired (target) plasma drug concentration. The product, $V_D k$, is also equal to total body clearance, Cl_T.

    f. A **loading dose (D_L)** is given as an initial intravenous bolus dose to produce the C_{ss} as rapidly as possible. The intravenous infusion is started at the same time as the D_L.

        (1) The time to reach C_{ss} depends on the elimination half-life of the drug. Reaching 90%, 95% or 99% of the C_{ss} without a D_L takes 3.32, 4.32, or 6.65 half-lives, respectively. Thus, for a drug with an elimination $t_{1/2}$ of 8 hr, it will take 3.32 × 8 hr or 26.56 hr to reach 90% of C_{ss} if no loading dose is given.

        (2) The D_L is the amount of drug that, when dissolved in the apparent V_D, produces the desired C_{ss}. Thus, D_L is calculated by the following equation:

$$D_L = C_{ss} V_D \text{ and } D_L = R/k$$

    g. An intravenous infusion provides a relatively constant plasma drug concentration and is particularly useful for drugs that have a narrow therapeutic range. The IV infusion keeps the plasma drug concentration between the minimum toxic concentration (MTC) and the minimum effective concentration (MEC).

4. Intermittent intravenous infusions

    a. Intermittent intravenous infusions are infusions in which the drug is infused for short periods to prevent accumulation and toxicity.

    b. Intermittent intravenous infusions are used for a few drugs, such as the aminoglycosides. For example, gentamicin may be given as a 1-hour infusion every 12 hours. In this case, steady-state drug concentrations are not achieved.

    c. The peak drug concentration in the plasma for a drug given by intermittent intravenous infusion may be calculated by the following equation:

$$Cp_n = \frac{R(1 - e^{-kt})(1 - e^{-nk\tau})}{Cl(1 - e^{-k\tau})}$$

    where Cp_n is the peak drug concentration, R is the rate of drug infusion, Cl is total body clearance, k is the dosage interval, n is the number of infusions, and t is the time for the infusion.

5. Multiple doses. Many drugs are given intermittently in a multiple-dose regimen for continuous or prolonged therapeutic activity. This regimen is often used to treat chronic disease.

    a. If drug doses are given frequently before the previous dose is completely eliminated, then plasma drug concentrations accumulate and increase to a steady-state level.

    b. At **steady state,** plasma drug concentration fluctuates between a maximum (C^{∞}_{max}) and a minimum (C^{∞}_{min}) value **(Figure 6-4).**

    c. When a multiple-dose regimen is calculated, the **superposition principle** assumes that previous drug doses have no effect on subsequent doses. Thus, the predicted plasma drug concentration is the total plasma drug concentration obtained by adding the residual drug concentrations found after each previous dose.

    d. When a multiple-dose regimen is designed, only the **dosing rate** (D_0/τ) can be adjusted easily.

        (1) The dosing rate is based on the **size of the dose** (D_0) and the **interval (τ) between doses,** or the **frequency of dosing.**

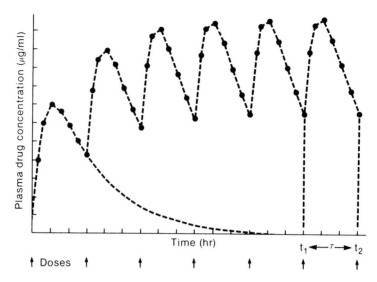

Figure 6-4. Generalized plot showing plasma drug concentration levels after administration of multiple doses and levels of accumulation when equal doses are given at equal time intervals. τ = time interval between doses (t), or the frequency of dosing. (Adapted with permission from Shargel L, Yu ABC: *Applied Biopharmaceutics and Pharmacokinetics,* 4th ed. McGraw-Hill, New York, 1999, p. 420.)

   (2) The dosing rate is given by the following equation:

$$\text{Dosing rate} = D_0/\tau$$

   (3) As long as the dosing rate is the same, the expected **average drug concentration at steady state (C^{∞}_{av})** is the same **(Figure 6-4).**
   (a) For example, if a 600-mg dose is given every 12 hours, the dosing rate is 600 mg/12 hr, or 50 mg/hr.
   (b) A dose of 300 mg every 6 hours or 200 mg every 4 hours also gives the same dosing rate (50 mg/hr), with the same expected C^{∞}_{av}. However, the C^{∞}_{max} and C^{∞}_{min} values will be different.
   (c) For a larger dose given over a longer interval (e.g., 600 mg every 12 hours), the C^{∞}_{max} is higher and the C^{∞}_{min} lower compared with a smaller dose given more frequently (e.g., 200 mg every 4 hours).
   e. Certain antibiotics are given by **multiple rapid intravenous bolus injections.**
   (1) The peak, or **maximum, serum drug concentration** at steady state may be estimated by the following equation:

$$C^{\infty}_{max} = \frac{D_0/V_D}{1 - e^{-k\tau}}$$

   (2) The **minimum serum drug concentration** (C^{∞}_{min}) at steady state is the drug concentration after the drug declines one dosage interval. Thus, C^{∞}_{min} is determined by the following equation:

$$C^{\infty}_{min} = C^{\infty}_{max}\, e^{-kt}$$

   (3) The **average drug concentration** (C^{∞}_{av}) at steady state is estimated with the equation used for multiple oral doses:

$$C^{\infty}_{av} = \frac{FD_o}{kV_D\tau}$$

   For intravenous bolus injections, F = 1.
   f. Orally administered drugs given in **immediate-release dosage forms** (e.g., solutions, conventional tablets, capsules) by multiple oral doses are usually rapidly absorbed and slowly eliminated ($k_A \geq k$). C^{∞}_{max} and C^{∞}_{min} for these drugs are approximated by the equations shown in I B 5 e (1) (2).

(1) For more exact calculations of C^{∞}_{min} and C^{∞}_{max} after multiple oral doses, the following equations are used:

$$C^{\infty}_{max} = \frac{FD_o}{V_D} \frac{1}{1 - e^{-k\tau}} \text{ and}$$

$$C^{\infty}_{min} = \frac{FD_o k_A}{V_D(k_A - k)} \frac{1}{1 - e^{-k\tau}} e^{-kt}$$

(2) The calculation of C^{∞}_{av} is the same as for multiple intravenous bolus injections, using the equation shown in I B 5 e (3).

(3) The term $1/(1 - e^{-k\tau})$ is known as the **accumulation rate.**

(4) The fraction of drug remaining in the body (f) after a dosage interval is given by the following equation:

$$f = e^{-k\tau}$$

g. Loading dose. An initial loading dose **(D_L)** is given to obtain a therapeutic steady-state drug level quickly.

(1) For multiple oral doses, D_L is calculated by:

$$D_L = D_M \frac{1}{1 - e^{-k\tau}}$$

where D_M is the maintenance dose.

(2) If D_M is given at a dosage interval equal to the elimination half-life of the drug, then D_L equals twice the maintenance dose.

C. Multicompartment models

1. Drugs that exhibit multicompartment pharmacokinetics distribute into different tissue groups at different rates. Tissues with high blood flow equilibrate with a drug more rapidly than tissues with low blood flow. Drug concentration in various tissues depends on the physical and chemical characteristics of the drug and the nature of the tissue. For example, highly lipid-soluble drugs accumulate slowly in fat (lipid) tissue.

2. Two-compartment model (intravenous bolus injection)

a. After an intravenous bolus injection, the drug distributes and equilibrates rapidly into highly perfused tissues **(central compartment)** and more slowly into peripheral tissues **(tissue compartment)**

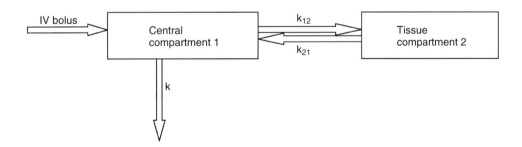

b. The initial rapid decline in plasma drug concentration is known as the **distribution phase.** The slower rate of decline in drug concentration after complete equilibration is achieved is known as the **elimination phase (Figure 6-5).**

c. The **plasma drug concentration** at any time is the sum of two first-order processes, as given in the following equation:

$$C_p = Ae^{-at} + Be^{-bt}$$

where a and b are hybrid first-order rate constants and A and B are y intercepts.

(1) The **hybrid first-order rate constant b** is obtained from the slope of the elimination phase of the curve **(see Figure 6-5)** and represents the first-order elimination of drug from the body after the drug equilibrates with all tissues.

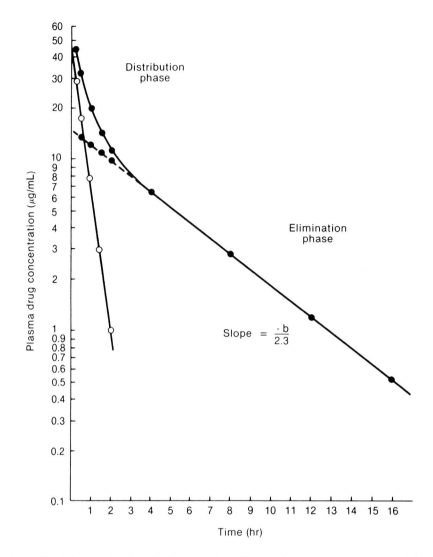

Figure 6-5. Generalized plot showing drug distribution and equilibration for a two-compartment model (intravenous bolus injection). The distribution phase is the initial rapid decline in plasma drug concentration. The elimination phase is the slower rate of decline after complete equilibration of the drug is achieved. (Adapted with permission from Shargel L, Yu ABC: *Applied Biopharmaceutics and Pharmacokinetics,* 4th ed. McGraw-Hill, New York, 1999, p. 73.)

  (2) The **hybrid first-order rate constant a** is obtained from the slope of the residual line of the distribution phase after the elimination phase is subtracted.
 d. The **apparent volume of distribution** depends on the type of pharmacokinetic calculation. Volumes of distribution include the volume of the central compartment (V_p), the volume of distribution at steady state (V_{ss}), and the volume of the tissue compartment (V_t).

3. Two-compartment model (oral drug administration)
 a. A drug with a rapid distribution phase may not show two-compartment characteristics after oral administration. As the drug is absorbed, it equilibrates with the tissues so that the elimination half-life of the elimination portion of the curve equals 0.693/b.
 b. Two-compartment characteristics are seen if the drug is absorbed rapidly and the distribution phase is slower.

4. Models with additional compartments

    a. The addition of each new compartment to the model requires an additional first-order plot.

    b. The addition of a third compartment suggests that the drug slowly equilibrates into a deep tissue space. If the drug is given at frequent intervals, the drug begins to accumulate into the third compartment.

    c. The terminal linear phase generally represents the elimination of the drug from the body after equilibration occurs. The rate constant from the elimination phase is used to calculate dosage regimens.

    d. Adequate pharmacokinetic description of multicompartment models is often difficult and depends on proper plasma sampling and determination of drug concentrations.

5. Elimination rate constants

    a. The elimination rate constant, k, represents drug elimination from the central compartment.

    b. The terminal elimination rate constant (b or λ in the two-compartment model) represents drug elimination after drug distribution is mostly completed.

D. Nonlinear pharmacokinetics are also known as capacity-limited, dose-dependent, or saturation pharmacokinetics. Nonlinear pharmacokinetics do not follow first-order kinetics as the dose increases **(Figure 6-6).** Nonlinear pharmacokinetics may result from the saturation of an enzyme- or carrier-mediated system.

1. Characteristics of nonlinear pharmacokinetics include:

    a. The AUC is not proportional to the dose.

    b. The amount of drug excreted in the urine is not proportional to the dose.

    c. The elimination half-life may increase at high doses.

    d. The ratio of metabolites formed changes with increased dose.

2. Michaelis-Menten kinetics describe the velocity of enzyme reactions. Michaelis-Menten kinetics are used to describe nonlinear pharmacokinetics.

    a. The **Michaelis-Menten equation** describes the rate of change (velocity) of plasma drug concentration after an intravenous bolus injection, as follows:

$$-\frac{dC_p}{dt} = \frac{V_{max}\, C_p}{k_M + C_p}$$

where V_{max} is the maximum velocity of the reaction, C_p is the substrate or plasma drug concentration, and k_M is the rate constant equal to the C_p at 0.5 V_{max}.

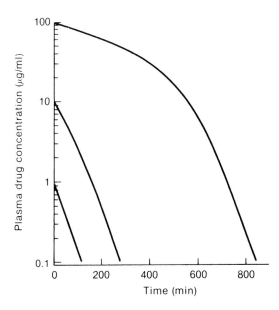

Figure 6-6. Generalized plot showing plasma drug concentration versus time for a drug with Michaelis-Menten (nonlinear) elimination kinetics. For this one-compartment model (intravenous injection), the doses are 1 mg, 10 mg, and 100 mg, and the apparent in vivo rate constant (kM) is 10 mg. The maximum velocity of the reaction (V_{max}) is 0.2 mg/min. (Adapted with permission from Gibaldi M, Perrier D: *Pharmacokinetics,* 2nd ed. New York, Marcel Dekker, 1982, p. 271.)

b. At low C_p values, where $k_M >> C_p$, this equation reduces to a first-order rate equation because both k_M and V_{max} are constants.

$$-\frac{dC_p}{dt} = \frac{V_{max}\,C_p}{k_M} = k'Cp$$

c. At high C_p values, where $C_p >> k_M$, the Michaelis-Menten equation is a zero-order rate equation, as follows:

$$-\frac{dC_p}{dt} = V_{max}$$

3. Drugs that follow nonlinear pharmacokinetics may show zero-order elimination rates at high drug concentrations, a mix of zero- and first-order elimination rates at intermediate drug concentrations, and first-order elimination rates at low drug concentrations (see Figure 6-6).

E. Clearance is a measurement of drug elimination from the body. Units for clearance are volume/time (e.g., liters/hour).

1. Total body clearance (Cl_T) is the drug elimination rate divided by the plasma drug concentration. According to the concept of clearance, the body contains an apparent volume of distribution in which the drug is dissolved. A constant portion of this volume is cleared, or removed, from the body per unit time.

a. The following equations express the measurement of total body clearance:

$$Cl_T = \frac{\text{drug elimination}}{\text{plasma drug concentration}} = \frac{dDe/dt}{C_p},$$

$$Cl_T = V_D k, \text{ and}$$

$$Cl_T = \frac{FD_\infty}{AUC}$$

b. For drugs that follow first-order (linear) pharmacokinetics, total body clearance is the sum of all the clearances in the body, as shown in the following equation:

$$Cl_T = Cl_R + Cl_{NR}$$

where Cl_R is renal clearance and Cl_{NR} is nonrenal clearance. Nonrenal clearance, Cl_{NR}, is often equated with hepatic clearance, Cl_H.

c. The relation between Cl_T and $t_{1/2}$ is obtained by substituting $0.693/t_{1/2}$ for k in the equation in I E 1 a to obtain the following expression:

$$t_{1/2} = \frac{0.693\,V_D}{Cl_T}$$

V_D and Cl_T are considered independent variables, and $t_{1/2}$ is considered a dependent variable.

d. As clearance decreases (e.g., in renal disease), $t_{1/2}$ increases. Changes in V_D also cause proportional changes in $t_{1/2}$.

2. Renal drug excretion is the major route of drug elimination for polar drugs, water-soluble drugs, drugs with low molecular weight (mol wt less than 500), or drugs that are biotransformed slowly. The relation between the drug excretion rate and the plasma drug concentration is shown in **Figure 6-7.** Drugs are excreted through the kidney into the urine by glomerular filtration, tubular reabsorption, and active tubular secretion.

a. Glomerular filtration is a passive process by which small molecules and drugs are filtered through the glomerulus of the nephron.

(1) Drugs bound to plasma proteins are too large to be filtered at the glomerulus.

(2) Drugs such as **creatinine and inulin** are not actively secreted or reabsorbed. They are used to measure the **glomerular filtration rate (GFR).**

b. Tubular reabsorption is a passive process that follows Fick's law of diffusion.

(1) Lipid-soluble drugs are reabsorbed from the lumen of the nephron back into the systemic circulation.

(2) For weak electrolyte drugs, urine pH affects the ratio of nonionized and ionized drug.

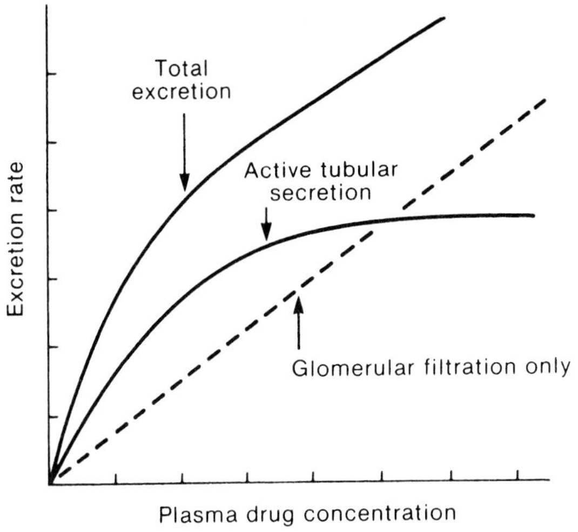

Figure 6-7. Generalized plot showing the excretion rate versus plasma drug concentration for a drug with active tubular secretion and for a drug secreted by glomerular filtration only. (Adapted with permission from Shargel L, Yu ABC: *Applied Biopharmaceutics and Pharmacokinetics,* 4th ed. McGraw-Hill, New York, 1999, p. 343.)

   (a) If the drug exists primarily in the nonionized or lipid-soluble form, then it is reabsorbed more easily from the lumen of the nephron.
   (b) If the drug exists primarily in the ionized or water-soluble form, then it is excreted more easily in the urine.
   (c) Depending on the pK_a of the drug, alteration of urine pH alters the ratio of ionized to nonionized drug and affects the rate of drug excretion. For example, alkalinization of the urine by the administration of sodium bicarbonate increases the excretion of salicylates (weak acids) into the urine.
   (3) An increase in urine flow caused by simultaneous administration of a diuretic decreases the time for drug reabsorption. Consequently, more drug is excreted if given with a diuretic.
 c. Active tubular secretion is a carrier-mediated active transport system that requires energy.
   (1) Two active tubular secretion pathways exist in the kidney: one system for weak acids and one system for weak bases.
   (2) The active tubular secretion system shows competition effects. For example, **probenecid** (a weak acid) competes for the same system as penicillin, decreasing the rate of penicillin excretion, resulting in a longer penicillin $t_{1/2}$.
   (3) The renal clearance of drugs that are actively secreted, such as **p-aminohippurate (PAH),** is used to measure **effective renal blood flow (ERBF).**
 3. Renal clearance is the volume of drug contained in the plasma that is removed by the kidney per unit time. **Units for renal clearance** are expressed in volume per time (e.g., millimeters per minute or liters per hour).
 a. Renal clearance may be measured by dividing the rate of drug excretion by the plasma drug concentration, as shown in the following equation:

$$Cl_R = \frac{\text{Rate of drug excretion}}{C_p} = \frac{dD_U/dt}{C_p}$$

 b. Measurement of renal clearance may also be expressed by the following equation:

$$Cl_R = k_e V_D$$

where k_e is the first-order renal excretion rate constant and

$$Cl_R = \frac{D^\infty_U}{AUC}$$

where D^∞_U is the total amount of parent (unchanged) drug excreted in the urine.
 c. Renal clearance is measured without regard to the physiologic mechanism of renal drug excretion. The probable mechanism for renal clearance is obtained with a **clearance ratio,** which relates drug clearance to inulin clearance (a measure of GFR).

(1) If the clearance ratio is less than 1.0, the mechanism for drug clearance may result from filtration plus reabsorption.

(2) If the ratio is 1.0, the mechanism may be filtration only.

(3) If the ratio is more than 1.0, the mechanism may be filtration plus active tubular secretion.

4. **Hepatic clearance** is the volume of plasma containing drug that is cleared by the liver per unit time.

   a. **Measurement of hepatic clearance.** Hepatic clearance is usually measured indirectly, as the difference between total body clearance and renal clearance, as shown in the following equation:

   $$Cl_H = Cl_T - Cl_R$$

   where Cl_H is the hepatic clearance. Hepatic clearance is generally considered to be equivalent to Cl_{NR}, or nonrenal drug clearance. Hepatic clearance can also be calculated as the **product of the liver blood flow (Q)** and the **extraction ratio (ER),** as shown in the following equation:

   $$Cl_H = QER$$

   (1) The **extraction ratio** is the fraction of drug that is irreversibly removed by an organ or tissue as the plasma-containing drug perfuses that tissue.

   (2) The extraction ratio is obtained by measuring the plasma drug concentration entering the liver and the plasma drug concentration exiting the liver:

   $$ER = \frac{C_a - C_v}{C_a}$$

   where C_a is the arterial plasma drug concentration entering the liver and C_v is the venous plasma drug concentration exiting the liver.

   (3) Values for the ER range from 0 to 1. For example, if the ER is 0.9, then 90% of the incoming drug is removed as the plasma perfuses the liver. If the ER is 0, then no drug is removed by the liver.

   b. **Blood flow, intrinsic clearance,** and **protein binding** affect hepatic clearance.

   (1) **Blood flow** to the liver is approximately 1.5 L/min and may be altered by exercise, food, disease, or drugs.

   (a) Blood enters the liver through the hepatic portal vein and hepatic artery and leaves through the hepatic vein.

   (b) After oral drug administration, the drug is absorbed from the gastrointestinal tract into the mesenteric vessels and proceeds to the hepatic portal vein, liver, and systemic circulation.

   (2) **Intrinsic clearance, Cl_{int}** describes the ability of the liver to remove the drug independently of blood flow.

   (a) Intrinsic drug clearance primarily occurs because of the inherent ability of the **biotransformation enzymes** (mixed-function oxidases) to metabolize the drug as it enters the liver.

   (b) Normally, basal level mixed-function oxidase enzymes biotransform drugs. Levels of these enzymes may be increased by various drugs (e.g., phenobarbital) and environmental agents (e.g., tobacco smoke). These enzymes may be inhibited by other drugs and environmental agents (e.g., cimetidine, acute lead poisoning).

   (3) **Protein binding.** Drugs that are bound to protein are not easily cleared by the liver or kidney because only the free, or nonplasma protein-bound, drug crosses the cell membrane into the tissue.

   (a) **The free drug** is available to drug-metabolizing enzymes for biotransformation.

   (b) A sudden increase in free-drug plasma concentration results in more available drug at pharmacologic receptors, producing a more intense effect in the organs (e.g., kidney, liver) involved in drug removal.

   (c) **Blood flow (Q), intrinsic clearance (Cl_{int}),** and **free-plasma drug concentration (f)** are related to hepatic clearance as shown in the following equation:

   $$Cl_H = Q \frac{fCl_{int}}{Q + Cl_{int}}$$

(1) The hepatic clearance of drugs that have high extraction ratios and high Cl_{int} values (e.g., propranolol) is most affected by changes in blood flow and inhibitors of the drug metabolism enzymes.

(2) The hepatic clearance of drugs that have low extraction ratios and low Cl_{int} values (e.g., theophylline) is most affected by changes in Cl_{int} and is affected only slightly by changes in hepatic blood flow.

(3) Only drugs that are highly plasma protein-bound (i.e., more than 95%) and have a low intrinsic clearance (e.g., phenytoin) are affected by a sudden shift in protein binding. This shift causes an increase in free-drug plasma concentration.

c. Biliary drug excretion, an active transport process, is also included in hepatic clearance. Separate active secretion systems exist for weak acids and weak bases.

(1) Drugs that are excreted in bile are usually high–molecular-weight compounds (i.e., mol wt more than 500) or polar drugs, such as reserpine, digoxin, and various glucuronide conjugates.

(2) Drugs may be recycled by the **enterohepatic circulation.**

(a) Some drugs are absorbed from the gastrointestinal tract through the mesenteric and hepatic portal veins, proceeding to the liver. The liver may secrete some of the drug (unchanged or as a glucuronide metabolite) into the bile.

(b) The bile and drug are stored in the gallbladder and will empty into the gastrointestinal tract through the bile duct and then may be reabsorbed.

(c) If the drug is a **glucuronide metabolite,** bacteria in the gastrointestinal tract may hydrolyze the glucuronide moiety, allowing the released drug to be reabsorbed.

d. First-pass effects (presystemic elimination) occur with drugs given orally. A portion of the drug is eliminated before systemic absorption occurs.

(1) First-pass effects generally result from rapid drug biotransformation by liver enzymes. Other mechanisms include metabolism of the drug by gastrointestinal mucosal cells, intestinal flora, or biliary secretion.

(2) First-pass effects are usually observed by measuring the **absolute bioavailability** (F) of the drug (see Chapter 7). If F is less than 1, then some of the drug was eliminated before systemic drug absorption occurred.

(3) Drugs that have a **high hepatic extraction ratio,** such as propranolol and morphine, show first-pass effects.

(4) To obtain better systemic absorption of a drug that demonstrates high first-pass effects, then either

(a) The drug dose could be increased (e.g., propranolol, penicillin).

(b) The drug could be given by an alternate route of administration (e.g., nitroglycerin sublinqual, insulin subcutaneous, estradiol transdermal).

(c) The dosage form could be modified as a delayed-release drug product (e.g., enteric-coated aspirin, mesalamine) so that the drug may be absorbed more distally in the GI tract.

F. Noncompartment methods. Some pharmacokinetic parameters for absorption, distribution, and elimination may be estimated with noncompartment methods. These methods usually require comparison of the areas under the curve.

1. Mean residence time

a. Mean residence time (MRT) is the average time for the drug molecules to reside in the body. MRT is also known as the mean transit time or mean sojourn time.

b. The MRT depends on the route of administration and assumes that the drug is eliminated from the central compartment.

c. The MRT is the total residence time for all molecules in the body divided by the total number of molecules in the body, as shown in the following equation:

$$MRT = \frac{\text{Total residence time for all drug molecules in the body}}{\text{Total number of drug molecules}}$$

d. MRT after IV bolus injection

(1) The MRT after a bolus intravenous injection is calculated by the following equation:

$$MRT_{IV} = \frac{AUMC}{AUC_{o-\infty}}$$

where AUMC is the area under the first moment versus time curve from t = 0 to t = infinity and $AUC_{0-\infty}$ is the area under the plasma drug concentration versus time curve from t = 0 to t = infinity. $AUC_{0-\infty}$ is also known as the zero moment curve.

(2) The MRT_{IV} is related to the elimination half-life by the following expression:

$$MRT_{IV} = 1/k$$

(3) During MRT_{IV}, 62.3% of the intravenous bolus dose is eliminated.

(4) The MRT for a drug given by a noninstantaneous input is longer than the MRT_{IV}.

2. **Mean absorption time (MAT)** is the difference between MRT and MRT_{IV} after an extravascular route is used.

$$MAT = MRT_{po} - MRT_{IV}$$

When first-order absorption occurs, MAT = 1/ka.

3. **Clearance** is the volume of plasma cleared of drug per unit time and may be calculated without consideration of the compartment model.

$$Cl = \frac{FD_o}{AUC_{0-\infty}}$$

After an IV dose, F = 1

4. **Steady-state volume of distribution (Vss)**
   a. The steady-state volume of distribution is the amount of drug in the body at steady state and the average steady-state drug concentration.
   b. After an intravenous bolus injection, V_{ss} is calculated by the following equation:

$$V_{ss} = \frac{Dose_{IV}\,(AUMC)}{(AUC)^2}$$

II. CLINICAL PHARMACOKINETICS is the application of pharmacokinetic principles for the rational design of an individualized dosage regimen. The two main objectives are **maintenance of an optimum drug concentration at the receptor site** to produce the desired therapeutic response for a specific period and **minimization of any adverse or toxic effects** of the drug.

III. TOXICOKINETICS is the application of pharmacokinetic principles to the design, conduct, and interpretation of drug safety evaluation studies.

A. Toxicokinetics is also used to validate dose-related exposure in animals. Toxicokinetic studies are performed in animals during preclinical drug development to aid in prediction of human drug toxicity. Toxicokinetic (nonclinical) studies may continue after the drug has been tested in humans.

B. **Clinical toxicology** is the study of adverse effects of drugs and toxic substances (poisons) in the human body. The pharmacokinetics of a drug in an overmedicated (intoxicated) patient may be very different from the pharmacokinetics of the same drug given in therapeutic doses. For example, a very high toxic dose may show nonlinear pharmacokinetics due to saturation kinetics compared to the drug given at lower therapeutic doses in which the drug levels follow linear pharmacokinetics.

IV. POPULATION PHARMACOKINETICS is the study of sources and correlates of variability in drug concentrations among individuals who are the target patient population. Population pharmacokinetics is most often applied to the clinical patient who is receiving relevant doses of a drug of interest. Both pharmacokinetic and nonpharmacokinetic data may be considered, including gender, age, weight, creatine clearance, and concomitant disease.

STUDY QUESTIONS

Directions: Each of the numbered items or incomplete statements in this section is followed by answers or by completions of the statement. Select the **one** lettered answer or completion that is **best** in each case.

1. Creatinine clearance is used as a measurement of

(A) renal excretion rate
(B) glomerular filtration rate (GFR)
(C) active renal secretion
(D) passive renal absorption
(E) drug metabolism rate

Questions 2–5

A new cephalosporin antibiotic was given at a dose of 5 mg/kg by a single intravenous bolus injection to a 58-year-old man who weighed 75 kg. The antibiotic follows the pharmacokinetics of a one-compartment model and has an elimination half-life of 2 hours. The apparent volume of distribution is 0.28 L/kg, and the drug is 35% bound to plasma proteins.

2. What is the initial plasma drug concentration (C_p^0) in this patient?

(A) 0.24 mg/L
(B) 1.80 mg/L
(C) 17.9 mg/L
(D) 56.0 mg/L

3. What is the predicted plasma drug concentration (C_p) at 8 hours after the dose?

(A) 0.73 mg/L
(B) 1.11 mg/L
(C) 2.64 mg/L
(D) 4.02 mg/L
(E) 15.10 mg/L

4. How much drug remains in the patient's body (D_B) 8 hours after the dose?

(A) 15.3 mg
(B) 23.3 mg
(C) 84.4 mg
(D) 100.0 mg
(E) 112.0 mg

5. How long after the dose is exactly 75% of the drug eliminated from the patient's body?

(A) 2 hours
(B) 4 hours
(C) 6 hours
(D) 8 hours
(E) 10 hours

Questions 6–11

A 35-year-old man who weighs 70 kg and has normal renal function needs an intravenous infusion of the antibiotic carbenicillin. The desired steady-state plasma drug concentration is 15 mg/dl. The physician wants the antibiotic to be infused into the patient for 10 hours. Carbenicillin has an elimination half-life ($t_{1/2}$) of 1 hour and an apparent volume distribution (V_D) of 9 L in this patient.

6. Assuming that no loading dose was given, what rate of intravenous infusion is recommended for this patient?

(A) 93.6 mg/hr
(B) 135.0 mg/hr
(C) 468.0 mg/hr
(D) 936.0 mg/hr
(E) 1350.0 mg/hr

7. Assuming that no loading intravenous dose was given, how long after the initiation of the intravenous infusion would the plasma drug concentration reach 95% of the theoretic steady-state drug concentration?

(A) 1.0 hour
(B) 3.3 hours
(C) 4.3 hours
(D) 6.6 hours
(E) 10.0 hours

8. What is the recommended loading dose?

(A) 93.6 mg
(B) 135.0 mg
(C) 468.0 mg
(D) 936.0 mg
(E) 1350.0 mg

9. To infuse the antibiotic as a solution containing 10 g drug in 500 mL 5% dextrose, how many milliliters per hour of the solution would be infused into the patient?

(A) 10.0 mL/hr
(B) 46.8 mL/hr
(C) 100.0 mL/hr
(D) 936.0 mL/hr
(E) 1141.0 mL/hr

10. What is the total body clearance rate for carbenicillin in this patient?

(A) 100 mL/hr
(B) 936 mL/hr
(C) 4862 mL/hr
(D) 6237 mL/hr
(E) 9000 mL/hr

11. If the patient's renal clearance for carbenicillin is 86 mL/min, what is the hepatic clearance for carbenicillin?

(A) 108 mL/hr
(B) 1077 mL/hr
(C) 3840 mL/hr
(D) 5160 mL/hr
(E) 6844 mL/hr

12. The earliest evidence that a drug is stored in tissue is

(A) an increase in plasma protein binding
(B) a large apparent volume of distribution (V_D)
(C) a decrease in the rate of formation of metabolites by the liver
(D) an increase in the number of side effects produced by the drug
(E) a decrease in the amount of free drug excreted in the urine

13. The intensity of the pharmacologic action of a drug is most dependent on the

(A) concentration of the drug at the receptor site
(B) elimination half-life ($t_{1/2}$) of the drug
(C) onset time of the drug after oral administration
(D) minimum toxic concentration (MTC) of the drug in plasma
(E) minimum effective concentration (MEC) of the drug in the body

14. Drugs that show nonlinear pharmacokinetics have which property?

(A) A constant ratio of drug metabolites is formed as the administered dose increases
(B) The elimination half-life ($t_{1/2}$) increases as the administered dose increases
(C) The area under the plasma drug concentration versus time curve (AUC) increases in direct proportion to an increase in the administered dose
(D) Both low and high doses follow first-order elimination kinetics
(E) The steady-state drug concentration increases in direct proportion to the dosing rate

15. The loading dose (D_L) of a drug is usually based on the

(A) total body clearance (Cl_T) of the drug
(B) percentage of drug bound to plasma proteins
(C) fraction of drug excreted unchanged in the urine
(D) apparent volume of distribution (V_D) and desired drug concentration in plasma
(E) area under the plasma drug concentration versus time curve (AUC)

16. The renal clearance of inulin is used as a measurement of

(A) effective renal blood flow
(B) rate of renal drug excretion
(C) intrinsic enzyme activity
(D) active renal secretion
(E) glomerular filtration rate (GFR)

17. All of the following statements about plasma protein binding of a drug are true EXCEPT

(A) displacement of a drug from plasma protein binding sites results in a transient increased volume of distribution (V_D)
(B) displacement of a drug from plasma protein binding sites makes more free drug available for glomerular filtration
(C) displacement of a potent drug that is normally more than 95% bound may cause toxicity
(D) albumin is the major protein involved in protein binding of drugs
(E) drugs that are highly bound to plasma proteins generally have a greater V_D compared with drugs that are highly bound to tissue proteins

18. The onset time for a drug given orally is the time for the

(A) drug to reach the peak plasma drug concentration
(B) drug to reach the minimum effective concentration (MEC)
(C) drug to reach the minimum toxic concentration (MTC)
(D) drug to begin to be eliminated from the body
(E) drug to begin to be absorbed from the small intestine

19. The initial distribution of a drug into tissue is determined chiefly by the

(A) rate of blood flow to tissue
(B) glomerular filtration rate (GFR)
(C) stomach emptying time
(D) affinity of the drug for tissue
(E) plasma protein binding of the drug

20. Which tissue has the greatest capacity to biotransform drugs?

(A) Brain
(B) Kidney
(C) Liver
(D) Lung
(E) Skin

21. The principle of superposition in designing multiple-dose regimens assumes that

(A) each dose affects the next subsequent dose, causing nonlinear elimination
(B) each dose of drug is eliminated by zero-order elimination
(C) steady-state plasma drug concentrations are reached at approximately 10 half-lives
(D) early doses of drug do not affect subsequent doses
(E) the fraction of drug absorbed is equal to the fraction of drug eliminated

Questions 22–24

A new cardiac glycoside is developed for oral and intravenous administration. The drug has an elimination half-life ($t_{1/2}$) of 24 hours and an apparent volume of distribution (V_D) of 3 L/kg. The effective drug concentration is 1.5 ng/mL. Toxic effects of the drug are observed at drug concentrations greater than 4 ng/mL. The drug is bound to plasma proteins at approximately 25%. The drug is 75% bioavailable after an oral dose.

22. What is the oral maintenance dose, if given once a day, for a 68-year-old man who weighs 65 kg and has congestive heart failure (CHF) and normal renal function?

(A) 0.125 mg
(B) 0.180 mg
(C) 0.203 mg
(D) 0.270 mg
(E) 0.333 mg

24. If the drug is available in tablets of 0.125 mg and 0.250 mg, what is the patient's plasma drug concentration if he has a dosage regimen of 0.125 mg every 12 hours?

(A) 1.39 ng/mL
(B) 1.85 ng/mL
(C) 2.78 ng/mL
(D) 3.18 ng/mL
(E) 6.94 ng/mL

23. What is the loading dose (D_L) for this patient?

(A) 0.270 mg
(B) 0.293 mg
(C) 0.450 mg
(D) 0.498 mg
(E) 0.540 mg

Directions: The question below contains three suggested answers of which **one or more** is correct. Choose the answer

A   if **I only** is correct
B   if **III only** is correct
C   if **I and II** are correct
D   if **II and III** are correct
E   if **I, II, and III** are correct

25. Which equation is true for a zero-order reaction rate of a drug?

I. $\dfrac{dA}{dt} = -k$

II. $t_{1/2} = \dfrac{0.693}{k}$

III. $A = A_o e^{-kt}$

ANSWERS AND EXPLANATIONS

1. The answer is B *[I E 2 a].*
A substance that is used to measure the glomerular filtration rate (GFR) must be filtered, but not reabsorbed or actively secreted. Although inulin clearance gives an accurate measurement of GFR, creatinine clearance is generally used because no exogenous drug must be given. However, creatinine formation depends on muscle mass and muscle metabolism, which may change with age and various disease conditions.

2–5. The answers are: 2-C *[I B 1 b (2)],* **3-B** *[I C 2 c],* **4-B** *[I B 1 b (1)],* **5-B** *[I B 5 f (4)].*
Substituting the data for this patient in the equation for the initial plasma drug concentration (C_p^0) gives:

$$C_p^0 = \frac{D_o}{V_D} = \frac{5 \text{ mg/kg}}{0.28 \text{ kg}} = 17.9 \text{ mg/L}$$

To obtain the patient's plasma drug concentration (C_p) 8 hours after the dose, the following calculation is performed:

$$C_p = C_p^0 \, e^{-kt}$$

$$k = \frac{0.693}{t_{1/2}} = \frac{0.693}{2} = 0.347 \text{ hr}^{-1}$$

$$C_p = 17.9 \, e^{-(0.347)(8)}$$

$$C_p = (17.9)(0.0623) = 1.11 \text{ mg/L}$$

The amount of drug in the patient's body at 8 hours is calculated as follows:

$$D_B = C_p V_D = (1.11)(0.28)(75) = 23.3 \text{ mg}$$

For any first-order elimination process, 50% of the initial amount of drug is eliminated at the end of the first half-life, and 50% of the remaining drug (i.e., 75% of the original amount) is eliminated at the end of the second half-life. Because the drug in the current case has an elimination half-life ($t_{1/2}$) of 2 hours, 75% of the dose is eliminated in two half-lives, or 4 hours.

6–11. The answers are: 6-D *[I B 3 d (3)],* **7-C** *[I B 3 b],* **8-E** *[I B 5 f (5) (a)],* **9-B** *[I B 3 d (3)],* **10-D** *[I B 3 d (3)],* **11-B** *[I E 4 a].*
The equation for the plasma concentration at steady state (C_{ss}) provides the formula for calculating the rate of an intravenous infusion (R). The equation is:

$$C_{ss} = \frac{R}{kV_D}$$

where k is the first-order elimination rate constant and V_D is the apparent volume of distribution. Rearranging the equation and substituting the data for this patient give the following calculations:

$$R = C_{ss}kV_D = \frac{15 \text{ mg}}{100 \text{ mL}} \times \frac{0.693}{1 \text{ hr}} \times 9000 \text{ mL}$$

$$R = 936 \text{ mg/hr}$$

The time it takes for an infused drug to reach the C_{ss} depends on the elimination half-life of the drug. The time required to reach 95% of the C_{ss} is equal to 4.3 times the half-life, whereas the time required to reach 99% of the C_{ss} is equal to 6.6 times the half-life. Because the half-life in the current case is 1 hour, the time to reach 95% of the C_{ss} is 4.3 × 1 hour, or 4.3 hours.
The loading dose (D_L) is calculated as follows:

$$D_L = C_{ss}V_D = \frac{15 \text{ mg}}{100 \text{ ml}} \times 9000 \text{ mL} = 1350 \text{ mg}$$

The answer to question 6 shows that the infusion rate should be 936 mg/hr. Therefore, if a drug solution containing 10 g in 500 mL is used, the required infusion rate is:

$$\frac{936 \text{ mg}}{1 \text{ hr}} \times \frac{500 \text{ mL}}{10{,}000 \text{ mg}} = 46.8 \text{ mL/hr}$$

The patient's total body clearance (Cl_T) is calculated as follows:

$$Cl_T = kV_D,$$

$$Cl_T = \frac{0.693}{1} \times 9000 \text{ mL} = 6237 \text{ mL/hr}$$

The hepatic clearance (Cl_H) is the difference between total clearance (Cl_T) and renal clearance (Cl_R):

$$Cl_H = Cl_T - Cl_R$$
$$Cl_H = 6237 - (86 \text{ mL/min} \times 60 \text{ min/hr}) = 1077 \text{ mL/hr}$$

12. The answer is B *[I B 1 b (1)]*.
A large apparent volume of distribution (V_D) is an early sign that a drug is not concentrated in the plasma, but is distributed widely in tissue. An increase in plasma protein binding suggests that the drug is located in the plasma rather than in tissue. A decrease in hepatic metabolism, an increase in side effects, or a decrease in urinary excretion of free drug is caused by a decrease in drug elimination.

13. The answer is A *[I A 3 d (3)]*.
As more drug is concentrated at the receptor site, more receptors interact with the drug to produce a pharmacologic effect. The intensity of the response increases until it reaches a maximum. When all of the available receptors are occupied by drug molecules, additional drug does not produce a more intense response.

14. The answer is B *[I D]*.
Nonlinear pharmacokinetics is a term used to indicate that first-order elimination of a drug does not occur at all drug concentrations. With some drugs, such as phenytoin, as the plasma drug concentration increases, the elimination pathway for metabolism of the drug becomes saturated and the half-life increases. The area under the plasma drug concentration versus time curve (AUC) of the drug is not proportional to the dose; neither is the rate of metabolite formation. The metabolic rate is related to the effects of the drug.

15. The answer is D *[I B 3 f (2)]*.
A loading dose (D_L) of a drug is given to obtain a therapeutic plasma drug level as rapidly as possible. The D_L is calculated on the basis of the apparent volume of distribution (V_D) and the desired plasma level of the drug.

16. The answer is E *[I E 3 c]*.
Inulin is neither reabsorbed nor actively secreted. Therefore, it is excreted by glomerular filtration only. The inulin clearance rate is used as a standard measure of the glomerular filtration rate (GFR), a test that is useful both clinically and in the development of new drugs.

17. The answer is E *[I A 3 d]*.
Drugs that are highly bound to plasma proteins diffuse poorly into tissue and have a low apparent volume of distribution (V_D).

18. The answer is B *[I B 3 f]*.
The onset time is the time from the administration of the drug to the time when absorbed drug reaches the minimum effective concentration (MEC). The MEC is the drug concentration in the plasma that is proportional, but not necessarily equal, to the minimum drug concentration at the receptor site that elicits a pharmacologic response.

19. The answer is A *[I A 3 a]*.
The initial distribution of a drug is chiefly determined by blood flow, whereas the affinity of the drug for tissue determines whether the drug concentrates at that site. The glomerular filtration rate (GFR) affects the renal clearance of a drug, not its initial distribution. The gastric emptying time and degree of plasma protein binding affect drug distribution, but are less important than the rate of blood flow to tissue.

20. The answer is C *[I E 4 b (2)]*.
The kidney, lung, skin, and intestine all have some capacity to biotransform, or metabolize, drugs, but the brain has little capacity for drug metabolism. The liver has the highest capacity for drug metabolism.

21. The answer is D *[I B 5 c]*.
The superposition principle, which underlies the design of multiple-dose regimens, assumes that earlier drug doses do not affect subsequent doses. If the elimination rate constant or total body clearance of the drug changes during multiple dosing, then the superposition principle is no longer valid. Changes in the total body clearance (Cl_T) may be caused by enzyme induction, enzyme inhibition, or saturation of an elimination pathway. Any of these changes would cause nonlinear pharmacokinetics.

22–24. The answers are: 22-D *[I B 5 g (1)]*, **23-E** *[I B 5 f (5) (a)]*, **24-A** *[I B 1 b (1)]*.
The oral maintenance dose (D_o) should maintain the patient's average drug concentration (C^∞_{av}) at the effective drug concentration. The bioavailability of the drug (F), the apparent volume of distribution (V_D), the frequency of dosing (t), and the excretion rate constant (k) must be considered in calculating the dose. The equation used is:

$$C^\infty_{av} = \frac{FD_o}{kV_D\tau}$$

For this drug, F = 0.75, k = 0.693/24 hr, V_D = 3 L/kg × 65 kg, τ = 25 hours, and C^∞_{av} = 1.5 ng/mL, or 1.5 µg/L. Therefore, by substitution, D_o = 270 µg, or 0.270 mg. When the maintenance dose is given at a dosage frequency equal to the half-life, then the loading dose is equal to twice the maintenance dose, in this case 540 µg, or 0.540 mg. To determine the plasma drug concentration for a dosage regimen of 0.125 mg every 12 hours, the C^∞_{av} formula is used. This time, F = 0.75, D_o = 0.125, k = 0.693/24 hr, V_D = 3 L/kg × 65 kg, and τ = 12 hours. Therefore, C^∞_{av} = 1.39 ng/mL. For cardiac glycosides, the peak (C_{max}) and trough (C_{min}) concentrations are calculated, and plasma drug concentrations are monitored after dosing. The loading dose (D_L) may be given in small increments over a specified period, according to the dosage regimen suggested by the manufacturer.

25. The answer is A (I) *[I A 1 a]*.
The first equation in the question describes a zero-order reaction (dA/dt) in which the reaction rate increases or decreases at a constant rate (k). A zero-order reaction produces a graph of a straight line with the equation of A = −kt + A_o when A is plotted against time (t). The other equations in the question represent first-order reactions.

7
Bioavailability and Bioequivalence

Leon Shargel

I. DEFINITIONS

A. Bioavailability is a measurement of the rate and extent (amount) to which the active ingredient or active moiety becomes available at the site of action. Bioavailability is also considered as a measure of the rate and extent of therapeutically active drug that is systemically absorbed. For drug products that are not intended to be absorbed into the bloodstream, bioavailability may be assessed by measurements intended to reflect the rate and extent to which the active ingredient or active moiety becomes available at the site of action.

B. Bioequivalent drug products. A generic drug product is considered bioequivalent to the **Reference Listed Drug Product (RLD—generally the brand name)** if both products are pharmaceutical equivalents and the generic drug product's rate and extent of systemic drug absorption (bioavailability) do not show a statistically significant difference when administered in the same dose of the active ingredient, in the same chemical form, in a similar dosage form, by the same route of administration, and under the same experimental conditions.

C. Generic drug product

1. The generic drug product requires an **Abbreviated New Drug Application** (ANDA) for approval by the United States Food and Drug Administration (FDA) and may be marketed after patent expiration of the Reference drug product.

2. The generic drug product must be a **therapeutic equivalent** to the Reference drug product but may differ in certain characteristics, including shape, scoring configuration, packaging, and excipients (such as colors, flavors, preservatives, expiration date, and minor aspects of labeling).

D. Pharmaceutical equivalents are drug products that contain the same therapeutically active drug ingredient(s); same salt, ester, or chemical form; are of the same dosage form; and are identical in strength, concentration and route of administration. Pharmaceutical equivalents may differ in characteristics such as shape, scoring configuration, release mechanisms, packaging, and excipients (including colors, flavoring, and preservatives).

E. The **Reference drug product** is usually the currently marketed, brand-name product with a full **New Drug Application** (NDA) approved by the FDA. The reference listed drug (RLD) is the reference drug product identified by FDA (see "orange book" www.fda.gov/cder/ob/default.htm).

F. Therapeutic equivalent drug products are pharmaceutical equivalents that can be expected to have the same clinical effect and safety profile when administered to patients under the same conditions specified in the labeling. Therapeutic equivalent drug products have the following criteria:

1. The products are safe and effective.

2. The products are pharmaceutical equivalents that contain the same active drug ingredient in the same dosage form, given by the same route of administration; meet compendial or other applicable standards of strength, quality, purity, and identity; and meet an acceptable *in vitro* standard.

3. The drug products are bioequivalent in that they do not present a known potential problem and are shown to meet an appropriate bioequivalence standard.

4. The drug products are adequately labeled.

5. The drug products are manufactured in compliance with current Good Manufacturing Practice regulations.

G. Pharmaceutical alternatives are drug products that contain the same therapeutic moiety but are different salts, esters, or complexes (e.g., tetracycline hydrochloride versus tetracycline phosphate) or are different dosage forms (e.g., tablet versus capsule; immediate-release dosage form versus controlled-release dosage form) or strengths.

II. BIOAVAILABILITY AND BIOEQUIVALENCE may be determined directly using pharmacokinetic studies (e.g., plasma drug concentration versus time profiles, urinary drug excretion studies), measurements of an acute pharmacodynamic effect, comparative clinical studies, or *in vitro* studies. The choice of study used is based on the site of action of the drug and the ability of the study design to compare drug delivered to that site by the two products.

A. Acute pharmacodynamic effects, such as changes in heart rate, blood pressure, electrocardiogram (ECG), clotting time, or forced expiratory volume in 1 second (FEV_1) can be used to measure bioavailability when no assay for plasma drug concentration is available or when the plasma drug concentration does not relate to the pharmacological response (e.g., a bronchodilator such as albuterol given by inhalation). Quantitation of the pharmacological effect versus time profile can be used as a measure of bioavailability and/or bioequivalence (Figure 7-1).

1. **Onset time.** As the drug is systemically absorbed, the drug concentration at the receptor rises to a **minimum effective concentration** (MEC) and a pharmacological response is initiated. The time from drug administration to the MEC is known as the onset time.

2. **Intensity.** The intensity of the pharmacological effect is proportional to the number of receptors occupied by the drug up to a *maximum* pharmacological effect. The maximum pharmacological effect may occur before, after, or at peak drug absorption.

3. **Duration of action.** As long as the drug concentration remains above the MEC, pharmacological activity is observed. The duration of action is the time for which the drug concentration remains above the MEC.

4. **Therapeutic window.** As the drug concentration increases, other receptors may combine with the drug to exert a toxic or adverse response. This drug concentration is the ***minimum toxic concentration*** (MTC). The drug concentration range between the MEC and MTC is the therapeutic window.

B. Plasma drug concentration. The plasma drug concentration versus time curve is most often used to measure the systemic bioavailability of a drug from a drug product (Figure 7-2).

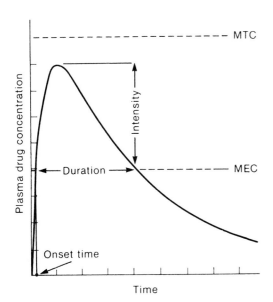

Figure 7-1. Generalized plasma drug concentration versus time curve after oral drug administration. MEC = minimum effective concentration; MTC = minimum toxic concentration. (Adapted with permission from Shargel L, Yu ABC: *Applied Biopharmaceutics and Pharmacokinetics,* 4th ed. New York, McGraw-Hill, 1999, p. 33).

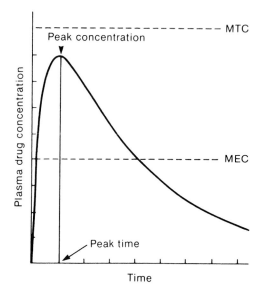

Figure 7-2. Generalized plasma drug concentration versus time curve, showing peak time and peak concentration. MEC = minimum effective concentration; MTC = minimum toxic concentration. (Adapted with permission from Shargel L, Yu ABC: *Applied Biopharmaceutics and Pharmacokinetics,* 4th ed. New York, McGraw-Hill, 1999, p. 33).

1. **Time for peak plasma drug concentration** (T_{max}) relates to the rate constants for systemic drug absorption and elimination. If two oral drug products contain the same amount of active drug but different excipients, the dosage form that yields the faster rate of drug absorption has the shorter T_{max} because the elimination rate constant for the drug from both dosage forms is the same.

2. **Peak plasma drug concentration** (C_{max}). The plasma drug concentration at T_{max} relates to the intensity of the pharmacological response. Ideally, C_{max} should be within the therapeutic window.

3. **Area under the plasma drug concentration versus time curve** (AUC) relates to the amount or extent of drug absorption. The amount of systemic drug absorption is directly related to the AUC. The AUC is usually calculated by the **trapezoidal rule** and is expressed in units of concentration multiplied by time (e.g., mg $\times$ hr/ml).

C. **Urinary drug excretion.** Measurement of urinary drug excretion can determine bioavailability from a drug product. This method is most accurate if the active therapeutic moiety is excreted unchanged in significant quantity in the urine (Figure 7-3).

1. **The cumulative amount of active drug excreted in the urine** (D_U^∞) is directly related to the extent of systemic drug absorption.

2. **The rate of drug excretion in the urine** (dD_U/dt) is directly related to the rate of systemic drug absorption.

3. **The time for the drug to be completely excreted** (t^∞) corresponds to the total time for the drug to be systemically absorbed and completely excreted after administration.

D. **Comparative clinical trials** to a drug can be used to measure bioavailability quantitatively. Clinical studies are highly variable and less precise than other methods because of individual differences in drug pharmacodynamics and subjective measurements.

E. ***In vitro* measurements of bioequivalence.** Bioequivalence may sometimes be demonstrated using an *in vitro* bioequivalence standard, especially when such an *in vitro* test has been correlated with human *in vivo* bioavailability data. For example, the rate of drug dissolution *in vitro* for certain drug products correlates with drug bioavailability *in vivo*. If the dissolution test *in vitro* is considered statistically adequate to predict drug bioavailability, then, in some cases, dissolution may be used in place of an *in vivo* bioavailability study.

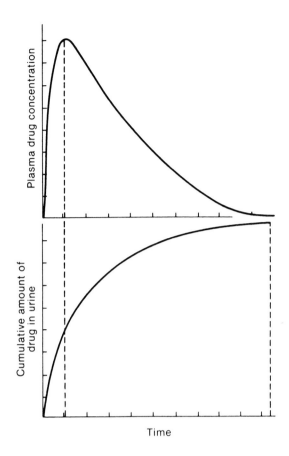

Figure 7-3. These corresponding plots show the relationship of the plasma drug concentration versus time curve to the cumulative amount of drug in the urine versus time curve. (Adapted with permission from Shargel L, Yu ABC: *Applied Biopharmaceutics and Pharmacokinetics,* 4th ed. New York, McGraw-Hill, 1999, p. 255).

III. RELATIVE AND ABSOLUTE BIOAVAILABILITY

A. Relative bioavailability is the systemic availability of the drug from a dosage form as compared to a Reference standard given by the same route of administration. Relative bioavailability is calculated as the ratio of the AUC for the dosage form to the AUC for the Reference dosage form given in the same dose. A relative bioavailability of 1 (or 100%) implies that drug bioavailability from both dosage forms is the same but does not indicate the completeness of systemic drug absorption. The determination of relative bioavailability is very important in generic drug studies (e.g., bioequivalence studies).

B. Absolute bioavailability (F) is the fraction of drug systemically absorbed from the dosage form. F is calculated as the ratio of the AUC for the dosage form given orally to the AUC obtained after intravenous (IV) drug administration (adjusted for dose). A parenteral drug solution given by IV administration is considered to have 100% systemic absorption (i.e., F = 1). An F value of 0.80 (or 80%) indicates that only 80% of the drug was systemically available from the oral dosage form.

IV. BIOEQUIVALENCE STUDIES FOR SOLID ORAL DRUG PRODUCTS

A. Design of bioequivalence studies

1. For many drug products, the Division of Bioequivalence, Office of Generic Drugs (FDA) provides guidance for the performance of *in vitro* dissolution and *in vivo* bioequivalence studies. These guidances are available on the Internet at http://www.fda.gov/cder/guidances.

2. **Fasting study.** Bioequivalence studies are usually evaluated by a single-dose, two-period, two-treatment, two-sequence, open-label, randomized crossover design, comparing equal doses of the Test (generic) and Reference (brand) products in fasted, adult, healthy subjects.
   a. Both men and women may be used in the study.
   b. Blood sampling is performed just before the dose (zero time) and at appropriate intervals after the dose to obtain an adequate description of the plasma drug concentration versus time profile.

3. **Food intervention study.** If the bioavailability of the active drug ingredient is known to be affected by food, the generic drug manufacturer must include a single-dose, randomized, crossover, food effects study comparing equal doses of the Test product and Reference products given immediately after a standard high-fat–content breakfast.

4. **Other study designs.** Crossover studies may not be practical in drugs with a long half-life in the body, and a parallel study design may be used instead. Alternate study methods, such as *in vitro* studies or equivalence studies with clinical or pharmacodynamic end points, are used for drug products where plasma concentrations are not useful to determine delivery of the drug substance to the site of activity (such as inhalers, nasal sprays, and topical products applied to the skin).

5. **Waiver of an *in vivo* bioequivalence study**
   a. A comparative *in vitro* dissolution (drug release) study between the Test and Reference products may be used in lieu of an *in vivo* bioequivalence study for some immediate-release (conventional) oral drug products.
   b. No bioequivalence study is required for certain drug products given as a solution such as oral, parenteral, ophthalmic, or other solutions because bioequivalence is self-evident.

B. **Pharmacokinetic evaluation of the data**
   Pharmacokinetic analysis includes calculation for each subject of the AUC to the last quantifiable concentration (AUC_{0-t}) and to infinity ($AUC_{0-\infty}$), T_{max}, and C_{max}. Additionally, the elimination rate constant (k), the elimination half-life ($t_{1/2}$), and other parameters may be estimated.

C. **Statistical evaluation of the data**

1. The statistical methodology for analyzing bioequivalence studies is called the two one-sided test procedure. Two situations are tested with this statistical methodology.
   a. The first of the two one-sided tests determines whether a generic product (Test), when substituted for a brand-name product (Reference) is significantly less bioavailable.
   b. The second of the two one-sided tests determines whether a brand-name product when substituted for a generic product is significantly less bioavailable.
   c. Based on the opinions of FDA medical experts, a difference of greater than 20% for each of the above tests was determined to be significant and, therefore, undesirable for all drug products.

2. An analysis of variance (ANOVA) should be performed on the log transformed AUC and C_{max} values obtained from each subject. The confidence interval for both pharmacokinetic parameters, AUC and C_{max}, must be entirely within the 80% to 125% boundaries cited above. Because the mean of the study data lies in the center of the 90% confidence interval, the mean of the data is usually close to 100% (a test/reference ratio of 1) (Table 7-1).

Table 7-1. Bioavailability Comparison of a Generic (Test) and Brand (Reference) Drug Product

Parameter	Units	Test	Ratio Reference	(%) T/R	90% Confidence Limits
AUC_{0-t}	μg hr/mL	1466	1494	98.1	93.0–102.5
$AUC_{0-\infty}$	μg hr/mL	1592	1606	99.1	94.5–104.1
C_{max}	μg mL	11.6	12.5	92.8	88.5–98.6
T_{max}	hr	1.87	2.10	89.1	

The results were obtained from a two-way crossover, single-dose, fasting study in 24 healthy adult volunteers. Mean values are reported. No statistical differences were observed between AUC and C_{max} values for the Test and Reference products.

3. Different statistical criteria are sometimes used when bioequivalence is demonstrated through comparative clinical trials, pharmacodynamic studies, or comparative *in vitro* methodology.

4. The bioequivalence methodology and criteria described above simultaneously control for both differences in the average response between Test and Reference as well as the precision with which the average response in the population is estimated. This precision depends on the within-subject (normal volunteer or patient) variability in the pharmacokinetic parameters (AUC and C_{max}) of the two products and on the number of subjects in the study. The width of the 90% confidence interval is a reflection in part of the within-subject variability of the test and reference products in the bioequivalence study.

V. BIOEQUIVALENCE ISSUES

A. Problems in determining bioequivalence include lack of an adequate study design; inability to accurately measure the drug analytes, including metabolites and enantiomers (chiral drugs); and lack of systemic drug absorption (Table 7-2.)

B. Bioequivalence studies for which objective blood drug concentrations cannot be obtained require either a pharmacodynamic study, clinical trial, or an *in vitro* study that has been correlated with human *in vivo* bioavailability data.

    1. Pharmacodynamic measurements are more difficult to obtain and the data tend to be variable, requiring a larger number of subjects compared to the bioequivalence studies for systemically absorbed drugs.

        a. A bioequivalence study using pharmacodynamic measurements tries to obtain a pharmacodynamic effect versus time profile for the drug in each subject.

        b. The area under the effect versus time profile, peak effect, and time for peak effect are obtained for the Test and Reference products and are then statistically analyzed.

    2. Comparative clinical trials are difficult to run, do not have easily quantifiable observations, and are quite costly.

    3. *In vitro* studies may require the development of a reliable surrogate marker that may be correlated with human *in vivo* bioavailability data. For example, the penetration of drug into layers of skin with respect to time (*dermatopharmacokinetics*) has been suggested as a method for measuring the bioequivalence of topical drug products intended for local activity.

Table 7- 2. Problem Issues in the Determination of Bioequivalence

Problem Issues	Example
Drugs with highly variable bioavailability*	Propranolol, verapamil
Drugs with active metabolites	Selegilene
Chiral drugs	Ibuprofen, albuterol
Drugs with nonlinear pharmacokinetics	Phenytoin
Orally administered drugs that are not systemically absorbed	Cholestyramine resin, sulcralfate
Drugs with long elimination half-lives	Probucol
Variable dosage forms	Dyazide, conjugated estrogens
Nonoral drug delivery	
Topical drugs	Steroids, antifungals
Transdermal delivery systems	Estrogen patch
Drugs given by inhalation aerosols	Bronchodilators, steroids
Intranasal drugs	Intranasal steroids
Biotechnology derived drugs	Erythropoietin, interferon
Bioavailable drugs that should not reach peak drug levels	Potassium supplements, hormone replacement therapy
Target population used in the bioequivalence studies	Pediatric patients; renal disease

*These drugs have high intra-subject variability.

VI. DRUG PRODUCTION SELECTION

A. Generic drug substitution

1. **Generic drug substitution** is the process of dispensing a generic drug product in place of the prescribed drug product (e.g., generic product for brand-name product, generic product for another generic product, brand-name product for generic product). The substituted product must be a therapeutic equivalent to the prescribed product.

2. Generic drug products that are classified as therapeutic equivalents by the FDA are expected to produce the same clinical effect and safety profile as the prescribed drug.

3. **Prescribability** refers to the measurement of average bioequivalence in which the comparison of population means of the Test and Reference products falls within acceptable statistical criteria. Prescribability is the current basis for FDA approval of therapeutic equivalent generic drug products.

4. **Switchability** refers to the measurement of individual bioequivalence, which requires knowledge of individual variability (intra-subject variability) and subject-by-formulation effects. Switchability assures that the substituted generic drug product produces the same response in the individual patient.

B. Therapeutic substitution

1. Therapeutic substitution is the process of dispensing a therapeutic alternative in place of the prescribed drug product. For example, amoxicillin is dispensed for ampicillin.

2. The substituted drug product is usually in the same therapeutic class (e.g., calcium channel blocker) and is expected to have a similar clinical profile.

C. Formulary issues

1. A **formulary** is a list of drugs. A **positive** formulary lists all the drugs that may be substituted, whereas a **negative** formulary lists drugs for which the pharmacist may not substitute. A **restrictive** formulary lists only those drugs that may be reimbursed without justification by the prescriber; for drugs not listed in the restrictive formulary, the prescriber must justify the need for the nonlisted drug.

2. Many states have legal requirements that address the issue of drug product selection. States may provide information and guidance in drug product selection through positive, negative, or restrictive formularies.

Table 7-3. Therapeutic Equivalence Evaluation Codes

A Codes	Drug products that are considered to be therapeutically equivalent to other pharmaceutically equivalent products
AA	Products in conventional dosage forms not presenting bioequivalence problems
AB	Products meeting bioequivalence requirements
AN	Solutions and powders for aerosolization
AO	Injectable oil solutions
AP	Injectable aqueous solutions
AT	Topical products
B Codes	Drug products that the FDA does not at this time consider to be therapeutically equivalent to other pharmaceutically equivalent products
BC	Extended-release tablets, extended-release capsules, and extended-release injectables
BD	Active ingredients and dosage forms with documented bioequivalence problems
BE	Delayed-release oral dosage forms
BN	Products in aerosol-nebulizer drug delivery systems
BP	Active ingredients and dosage forms with potential bioequivalence problems
BR	Suppositories or enemas for systemic use
BS	Products with drug standard deficiencies
BT	Topical products with bioequivalence issues
BX	Insufficient data

3. The FDA annually publishes *Approved Drug Products with Therapeutic Equivalence Evaluations* (the "Orange Book"). This publication is also reproduced in the *United States Pharmacopeia*/DI Vol III Approved Drug Products and Legal Requirements, published annually by the U.S.P. Convention. The "Orange Book" may also be found at http://www.fda.gov/cder/ob/default.htm.
   a. The "Orange Book" provides therapeutic evaluation codes for drug products (Table 7-3).
      (1) "A" rated drug products are drug products that contain active ingredients and dosage forms that are *not* regarded as presenting either actual or potential bioequivalence problems or drug quality standards issues. However, all oral dosage forms must meet an appropriate *in vitro* bioequivalence standard that is acceptable to the FDA in order to be approved as therapeutically equivalent and may be interchanged.
      (2) "B" rated drug products are drug products for which actual or potential bioequivalence problems have not been resolved by adequate evidence of bioequivalence. These products often have specific dosage form problems rather than a problem with the active ingredients (e.g., two different nicotine patches). "B" rated drug products are *not* considered therapeutically equivalent to other pharmaceutically equivalent products and are *not* interchangeable.
      (3) Certain products present special situations that deserve a more complete explanation than can be provided by the two-codes used in the "Orange Book." These drugs have particular problems with standards of identity, analytical methodology, or bioequivalence that are considered individually. For these drugs, consult the "Orange Book."
   b. For some drug products, bioequivalence has not been established or no generic product is currently available.

4. Various hospitals, institutions, insurance plans, health maintenance organizations (HMOs), and other third-party plans may have a formulary that provides guidance for drug product substitution.

STUDY QUESTIONS

Directions: Each of the numbered items or incomplete statements in this section is followed by answers or by completions of the statement. Select the **one** lettered answer or completion that is **best** in each case.

1. The parameters used to describe bioavailability are

(A) C_{max}, AUC_{0-t}, and $AUC_{0-\infty}$
(B) C_{max}, AUC_{0-t}, $AUC_{0-\infty}$, and T_{max}
(C) C_{max}, AUC_{0-t}, $AUC_{0-\infty}$, and $t_{1/2}$
(D) C_{max} and AUC_{0-t}
(E) C_{max}, AUC_{0-t}, $AUC_{0-\infty}$, T_{max}, and $t_{1/2}$

2. To determine the absolute bioavailability of a drug given as an oral extended-release tablet, the bioavailability of the drug must be compared to the bioavailability of the drug from

(A) an immediate-release oral tablet containing the same amount of active ingredient
(B) an oral solution of the drug in the same dose
(C) a parenteral solution of the drug given by IV bolus or IV infusion
(D) a Reference (brand) extended-release tablet that is a pharmaceutical equivalent
(E) an immediate-release hard gelatin capsule containing the same amount of active drug and lactose

3. A single-dose, four-way crossover, fasting, comparative bioavailability study was performed in 24 healthy, adult male subjects. Plasma drug concentrations were obtained for each subject, and the following results were obtained:

Table 7Q-3

Drug Product	Dose (mg)	C_{max} ($\mu g/ml$)	T_{max} (hr)	$AUC_{0-\infty}$ ($\mu g\ hr/ml$)
IV bolus injection	100			1714
Oral solution	200	21.3	1.2	3143
Generic tablet	200	17.0	2.1	2822
Reference tablet	200	16.5	1.9	2715

The relative bioavailability of the drug from the generic tablet compared to the Reference tablet is

(A) 82.3%
(B) 69.8%
(C) 91.7%
(D) 96.2%
(E) 103.9%

Directions: Each question below contains three suggested answers of which **one or more** is correct. Choose the answer

A   if **I only** is correct
B   if **III only** is correct
C   if **I and II** are correct
D   if **II and III** are correct
E   if **I, II, and III** are correct

4. For two drug products, generic (Test) and brand (Reference), to be considered bioequivalent

I. there should be no statistical difference between the extent of bioavailability of the drug from the Test product compared to the Reference product
II. the 90% confidence intervals about the ratio of the means of the C_{max} and AUC values for the Test product/Reference product must be within 80%–125% of the Reference product
III. there should be no statistical differences between the mean C_{max} and AUC values for the Test product compared to the Reference product

5. For which of the following products is measuring plasma drug concentrations not appropriate to estimate bioequivalence?

I. Metered-dose inhaler containing a bronchodilator
II. Antifungal agent for the treatment of a vaginal infection
III. Enteric-coated tablet containing a nonsteroidal anti-inflammatory agent

ANSWERS AND EXPLANATIONS

1. The answer is B *[II B].*
AUC relates to the extent of drug absorption. C_{max} and T_{max} relate to the rate of drug absorption. The elimination $t_{1/2}$ of the drug is usually independent of the route of drug administration and is not used as a measure of bioavailability.

2. The answer is C *[II B].*
After an IV bolus injection or IV infusion, all the dose is absorbed into the body. The ratio of the AUC of the drug given orally to the AUC of the drug given by IV injection is used to obtain the absolute bioavailability (F) of the drug.

3. The answer is E *[III A].*
The relative bioavailability is determined from the ratio of the AUC of the generic (Test) product to the AUC of the Reference standard. Thus, the relative bioavailability can exceed 100%, whereas the absolute bioavailability cannot exceed 100%.

4. The answer is E *[IV C].*
Although T_{max} is an indication of rate of drug absorption, T_{max} is a discrete measurement and usually too variable to use for statistical comparisons in bioequivalence studies. Statistical comparisons use AUC and C_{max} values from Test and Reference drug products as the basis of bioequivalence.

5. The answer is C *[IV A].*
Although some systemic absorption may be demonstrated after administering a metered dose inhaler containing a bronchodilator or a vaginal antifungal agent, bioequivalence can only be determined using a clinical response measurement.

8
Functional Group Chemistry and Biochemistry
Marc W. Harrold

I. FUNCTIONAL GROUP CHEMISTRY

A. Introduction. Drug molecules can be viewed as a collection of functional groups (i.e., groups of atoms present within the drug that confer specific chemical and physical properties [Figure 8-1]). Functional groups determine such characteristics as ionization, solubility in aqueous and lipid environments (aka polarity), reactivity, chemical stability, and in vivo metabolic stability. Additionally, these functional groups are **capable of forming specific bonds** (primarily noncovalent) with their receptors and are thus extremely important in drug activity and potency.

1. Functional groups that impart **hydrophilicity** are likely to increase the drug's water solubility, while functional groups that impart **lipophilicity** (hydrophobicity) are likely to increase the drug's tendency to cross cellular membranes through passive diffusion. See Chapter 12 VIII B 1 for a further discussion of water and lipid solubility.
    a. Acidic and basic functional groups allow for **drug ionization** and, in most cases, impart enhanced water solubility to the molecule. One notable exception to this is seen in **amphoteric drugs** (i.e., those compounds possessing both acidic and basic functional groups). As exemplified by ampicillin in Figure 8-2, amphoteric compounds can form **zwitterions,** or **internal salts.** Since the zwitterion form of ampicillin has a net overall charge of zero, it has difficulty dissolving in aqueous environments such as the gastrointestinal (GI) tract.
    b. Neutral functional groups (i.e., those that are incapable of ionization) can enhance either water or lipid solubility depending on their ability to form **hydrogen bonds with water.** Hydrogen bonding is the primary mechanism for increasing the water solubility of nonelectrolytes (i.e., compounds that do not possess acidic, basic, or quaternary ammonium functional groups).

2. Functional group **reactivity** affects **drug shelf life, stability,** and **storage.** There are a number of functional groups that will degrade, primarily through air oxidation and hydrolysis, under **normal environmental conditions.** Two examples of this latter concern are seen with aspirin and nitroglycerin. Both compounds are subject to rapid hydrolysis if exposed to moist environments.

3. Functional groups also affect **in vivo stability** and the duration of drug action. The susceptibility of a given drug to metabolic biotransformation depends in part upon the functional groups that are present (see Chapter 17 II, III).
    a. Drugs that contain a large number or percentage of hydrophilic functional groups are often eliminated from the body unchanged or with minimal metabolism.
    b. Drugs that contain a large number or percentage of lipophilic functional groups often require extensive metabolism.

B. Acidic functional groups

1. **Types.** Shown in Figure 8-3 are examples of the six most common acidic functional groups. In general, carboxylic acids tend to be more acidic than any of the other five functional groups. The tetrazole ring provides the best charge delocalization since resonance allows the charge to be equally shared among all five atoms in the ring.

2. **Common attributes**
    a. Acidic functional groups impart **hydrophilicity** to a drug molecule due to their potential for ionization.

Alkyl chain
OH
O
Carboxylic acid
CH3
CH3
Alkyl group
H3C
Aromatic ring

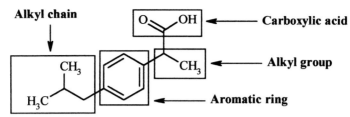

Figure 8-1. Ibuprofen, a nonsteroidal anti-inflammatory agent, is comprised of an ionizable, hydrophilic carboxylic acid and three hydrophobic functional groups: an isobutyl alkyl chain, an ethyl alkyl group, and an aromatic ring.

Ampicillin

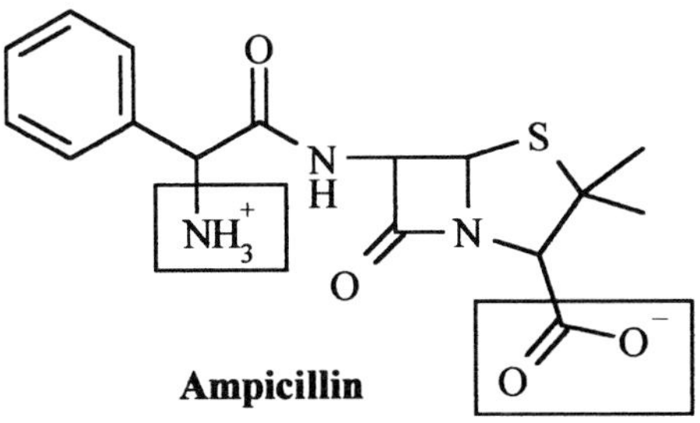

Figure 8-2. Ampicillin is an amphoteric compound. It contains an acidic carboxylic acid and a basic amine and exists in vivo as a zwitterion. The proton from the carboxylic acid binds to the basic amine, producing a molecule with an overall net charge equal to zero.

b. Acidic functional groups can form **ionic, ion–dipole, and hydrogen bonds** with receptors, enzymes, transport proteins, and other macromolecules.
c. Acidic functional groups can form **salts when combined with bases.**

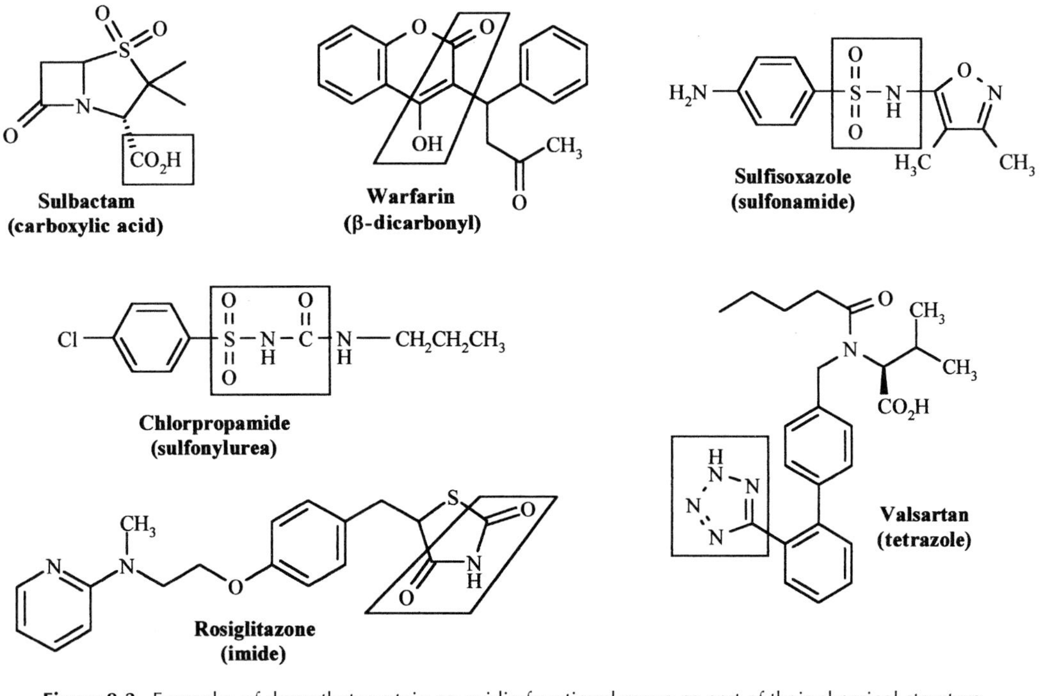

Sulbactam
(carboxylic acid)
Warfarin
(β-dicarbonyl)
Sulfisoxazole
(sulfonamide)
Chlorpropamide
(sulfonylurea)
Valsartan
(tetrazole)
Rosiglitazone
(imide)

Figure 8-3. Examples of drugs that contain an acidic functional group as part of their chemical structure.

    d. Carboxylic acids are often **esterified** for the purposes of prodrug formation (see Chapter 17, section VI for additional information). They can also undergo acid- or enzyme-catalyzed **decarboxylation** reactions.

    e. Metabolism. Acidic functional groups can undergo **conjugation** with glucuronic acid, glycine, and glutamine.

C. Basic functional groups

1. Types

    a. Aliphatic and alicyclic amines are the most common basic functional groups. As shown in Figure 8-4, these amines can be **primary, secondary, or tertiary,** depending on the number of substituents attached to the nitrogen.

    b. Aromatic amines, such as that seen in procainamide (Figure 8-4), are much less basic and for all intents and purposes can be considered neutral.

    c. Aromatic, heterocyclic nitrogens vary in their basicity, but in general are much less basic than aliphatic and alicyclic amines (Figure 8-5).

    d. Additional basic functional groups include **imines, hydrazines, amidines, and guanidines** (Figure 8-6). Imines tend to be less basic than aliphatic and alicyclic amines, whereas guanidines tend to be much more basic. The basicity of the other two functional groups lies somewhere in between.

2. Common attributes

    a. Basic functional groups impart **hydrophilicity** to a drug molecule due to their potential for ionization and their ability to form hydrogen bonds.

    b. Basic functional groups can form **ionic, ion–dipole, and hydrogen bonds** with receptors, enzymes, transport proteins, and other macromolecules.

    c. Basic functional groups can form **salts when combined with acids.**

    d. Metabolism. Common metabolic pathways for primary amines are **oxidative deamination, acetylation, and N-oxidation.** Common pathways for secondary and tertiary amines are **acetylation** (secondary amines only), **oxidative N-dealkylation, and N-oxidation.** Aromatic amines can be **acetylated,** while aromatic heterocyclic nitrogens can undergo **N-oxidation or N-dealkylation.** Imine, hydrazine, amidine, and guanidine groups can undergo similar reactions as those listed for primary, secondary, and tertiary amines. Additionally, amines can be **glucuronidated, sulfated,** and **methylated** by **phase II conjugation** reactions.

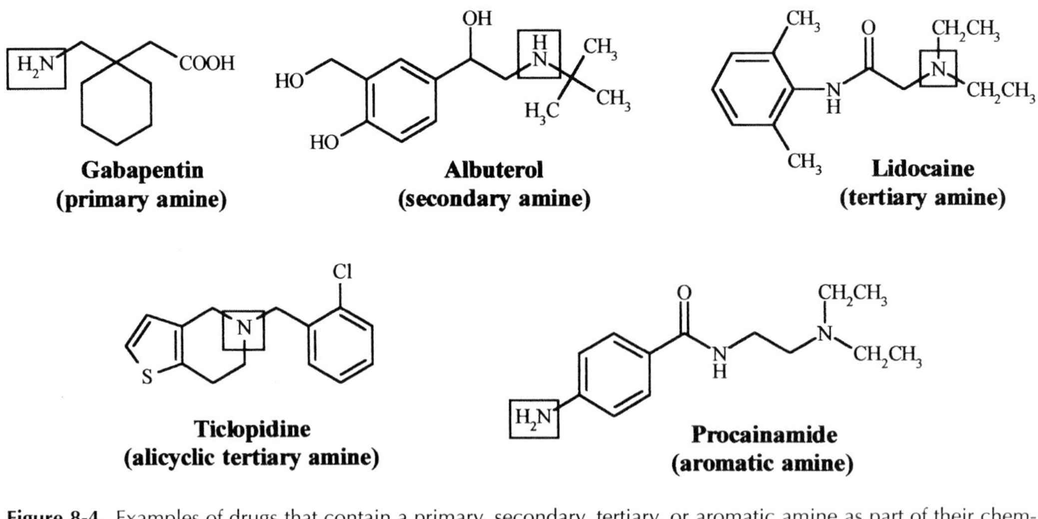

Figure 8-4. Examples of drugs that contain a primary, secondary, tertiary, or aromatic amine as part of their chemical structure. Whenever an amine is part of a nonaromatic ring (e.g., ticlopidine), it is referred to as an alicyclic amine. Whenever an amine amino is part of a side chain or is attached to a nonaromatic ring, it is referred to as an aliphatic or alkyl amine. Whenever an amine is directly attached to an aromatic ring (e.g., procainamide), it is referred to as an aromatic amine.

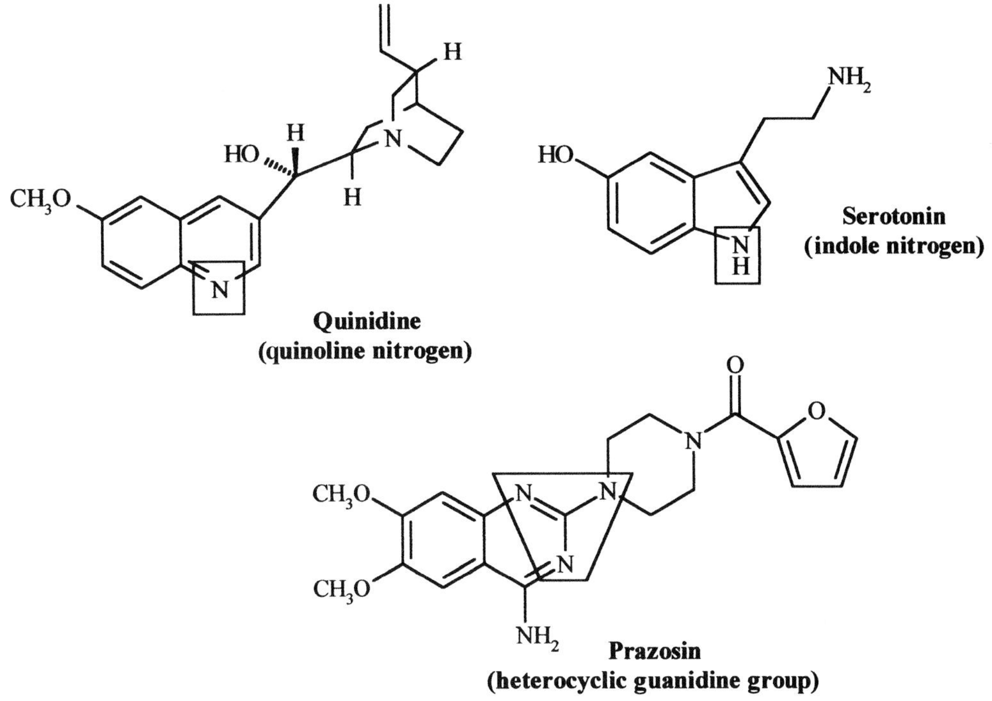

Figure 8-5. Examples of drugs that contain aromatic, heterocyclic nitrogens as part of their chemical structure.

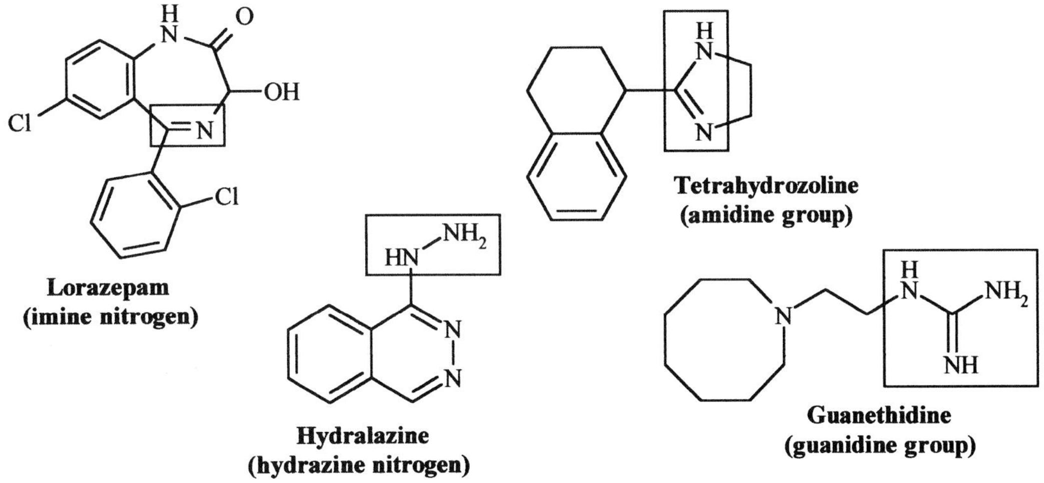

Figure 8-6. Examples of drugs that contain a basic imine, hydrazine, amidine, or guanidine functional group as part of their chemical structure.

D. Additional hydrophilic functional groups

1. Similar to amines, **hydroxyl groups (or alcohols)** may be classified as **primary, secondary, or tertiary,** depending on the number of substituents attached to their respective carbons. A good example of this is seen with the glucocorticoid fludrocortisone (Figure 8-7).

   a. Hydroxyl groups can form **ion–dipole and hydrogen bonds** with receptors, enzymes, transport proteins, and other macromolecules.

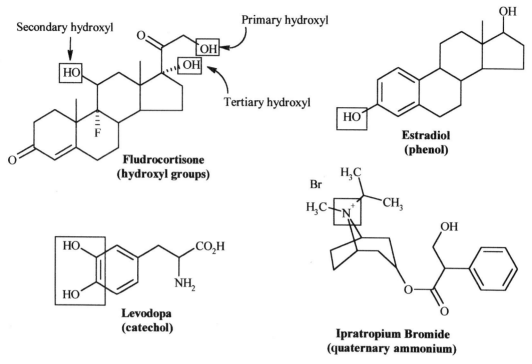

Figure 8-7. Examples of drugs that contain a hydroxyl group, phenol, catechol, or quaternary ammonium functional group as part of their chemical structure. Fludrocortisone contains a primary, secondary, and tertiary hydroxyl group. This designation is similar to that used for amines and depends on the number of substituents attached to the respective carbons. As illustrated with levodopa, a catechol is simply two phenol groups that are *ortho* to one another.

      b. Hydroxyl groups **enhance water solubility** due to their ability to form hydrogen bonds with water.

      c. Hydroxyl groups are often **esterified** in order to produce prodrugs. See Chapter 17 VI for additional information on prodrugs.

      d. Metabolism. Primary hydroxyl groups are initially **oxidized to aldehydes** and then to **carboxylic acids.** Secondary hydroxyl groups are **oxidized to ketones,** while tertiary hydroxyl groups are not usually oxidized. Hydroxyl groups may also undergo **phase II glucuronide or sulfate conjugation.**

2. Phenols, as exemplified by estradiol (Figure 8-7), are hydroxyl groups that are directly attached to an aromatic ring.

      a. Due to resonance stabilization of the aromatic ring, phenols can be ionized in basic environments; however, most phenols are **primarily unionized** at physiological pH and as such should be treated as **neutral,** nonionizable functional groups.

      b. Similar to alcohols, phenols primarily form **ion–dipole and hydrogen bonds.** They can also **enhance water solubility** and be esterified to form prodrugs (see Chapter 17 VI).

      c. Drug molecules containing phenols or **catechols** (see **levodopa** in Figure 8-7) are susceptible to **air oxidation** and to **oxidation on contact with ferric ions.**

      d. Metabolism. Phenols undergo **sulfation, glucuronidation, aromatic hydroxylation,** and *O*-methylation.

3. Quaternary ammonium salts, as exemplified by ipratropium bromide (Figure 8-7), are neither acidic nor basic but contain a **permanent positive charge.**

      a. These salts **enhance water solubility;** however, due to the permanence of the positive charge, compounds containing this functional group often have **difficulty passing through lipid membranes.**

      b. Similar to amines, quaternary ammonium salts can participate in **ionic** and **io–dipole bonds.**

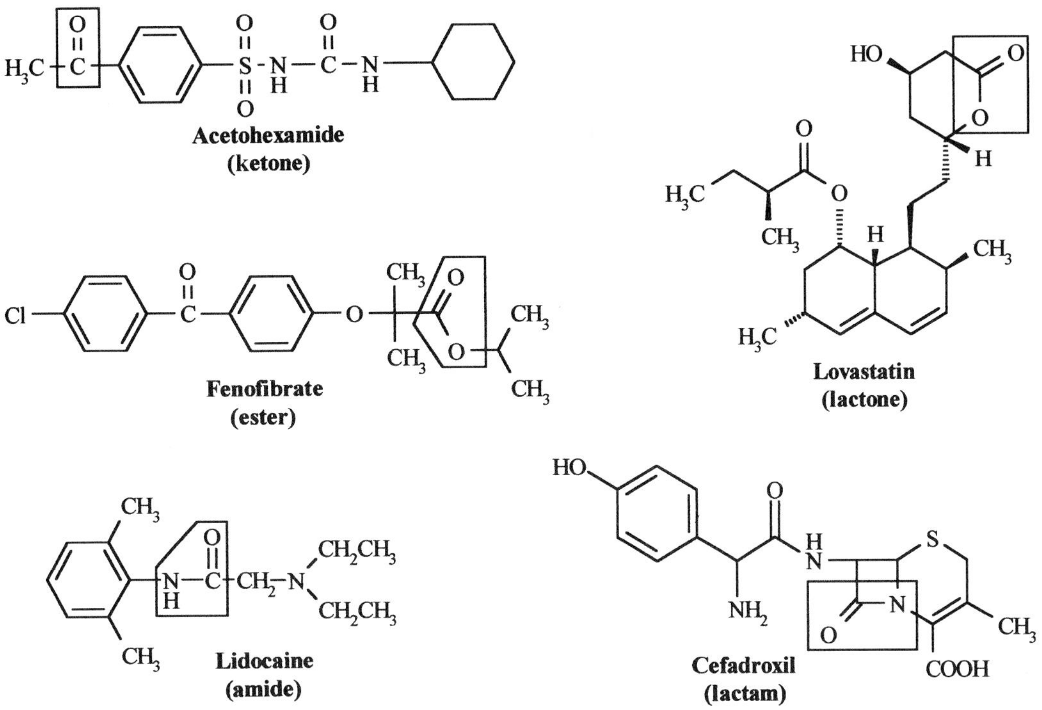

Figure 8-8. Examples of drugs that contain a ketone, ester, amide, lactone, or lactam as part of their chemical structure.

    c. Quaternary ammonium salts are generally not metabolized; however, **N-dealkylation** could occur in some cases.

E. Functional groups with intermediate polarity

    1. Ketones are less prevalent than alcohols and phenols in the structures of drug molecules. One example is seen in the oral hypoglycemic agent, acetohexamide, shown in Figure 8-8.
        a. Ketones are primarily lipid soluble; however, they are able to form **hydrogen bonds** with alcohols and certain amines. They can also form **ion–dipole** bonds.
        b. Metabolism. Ketones are very stable. Their primary route of metabolism is **reduction to an alcohol.**

    2. Compounds containing **esters, amides** and their respective cyclic forms, **lactones, and lactams** can be seen in Figure 8-8.
        a. These functional groups are capable of forming **hydrogen bonds** with receptors, enzymes, transport proteins, other macromolecules, and water. Similar to ketones, esters and lactones can function as **hydrogen-bond acceptors,** while amides and lactams can function as either **hydrogen-bond donors or acceptors.**
        b. Metabolism. Enzymatic **hydrolysis** is the primary route of metabolism for these functional groups. Esters and lactones are hydrolyzed to alcohols and carboxylic acids, while amides and lactams are hydrolyzed to amines and carboxylic acids. Esters and lactones are more susceptible to hydrolysis than are amides and lactams. Additionally, some lactams may undergo **N-dealkylation** prior to or in place of hydrolytic cleavage.

F. Lipophilic functional groups

    1. Alkyl groups are **saturated hydrocarbon chains, links, and rings** that can vary in size from single-carbon **methyl** and **methylene** groups to large chains. Similar to the designations previously given for amines, the designation **alicyclic** refers to alkyl groups that are part of a nonaromatic ring, while the designation **aliphatic** refers to those that are part of a side chain or that function to connect, or bridge, other functional groups. Examples of alkyl groups are illustrated in Figure 8-9.

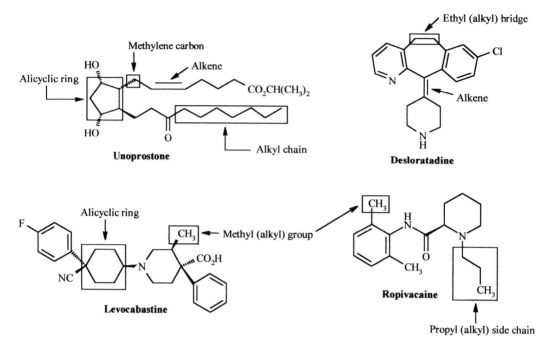

Figure 8-9. Examples of drugs that contain alkyl groups and alkenes as part of their chemical structure. For the sake of clarity, only certain functional groups have been highlighted.

> **a.** Alkyl groups can participate in **van der Waals interactions** (i.e., induced dipole–induced dipole bonds) and **hydrophobic bonding.**
> **b. Metabolism.** Oxidation is the major route of metabolism. Alkyl side chains are usually oxidized at either the **terminal (ω)** or **penultimate (ω-1)** carbon atoms.

2. **Alkenes,** also known as **olefins,** are **unsaturated** analogs of alkyl groups (see Figure 8-9).
    a. The binding ability of alkenes is similar to that of saturated alkyl groups.
    b. Metabolism. Alkenes are somewhat more reactive than alkyl groups and are subject to metabolic **hydration, epoxidation, peroxidation,** and **reduction.**

3. Most **aromatic hydrocarbons** are analogs of either **benzene** or **naphthalene** (see Figure 8-10 for examples). When attached to a drug molecule, benzene is referred to as a **phenyl group.**
    a. Similar to alkyl groups and alkenes, aromatic hydrocarbons can participate in **van der Waals interactions** and **hydrophobic bonding.** Additionally, aromatic rings can participate in **charge-transfer interactions.** Electron-rich aromatic rings (i.e., those with electron-donating groups) can form dipole-like interactions with electron-poor aromatic rings (i.e., those with electron-withdrawing groups).
    b. Metabolism. Oxidation is the primary route of metabolism for aromatic hydrocarbons, with **hydroxylation, epoxidation,** and **diol formation** comprising the three most common pathways.

4. **Ether** functional groups contain an oxygen atom bound on both sides by either alkyl or aromatic carbons. They can be present as either a terminal functional group, such as the **methoxy group** of naproxen, or as part of a central chain/backbone, such as that seen in gemfibrozil (Figure 8-10).
    a. The contribution of ethers to drug binding is minimal; however, these functional groups can participate in **dipole–induced dipole interactions** and can serve as **hydrogen-bond acceptors.**
    b. Metabolism. Methyl and ethyl ethers can undergo *O*-**dealkylation,** while those larger do not generally undergo metabolism. While ethers used as organic solvents (e.g., diethylether) can form **peroxides and may explode,** this property is generally not present in drug molecules.

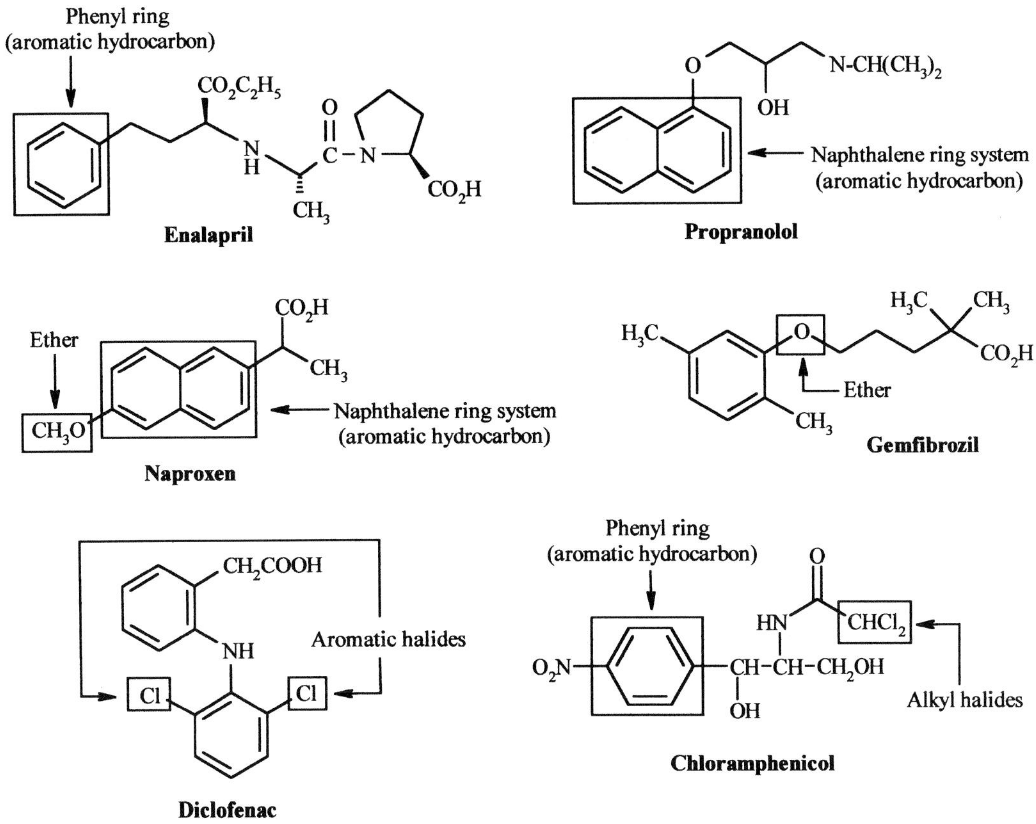

Figure 8-10. Examples of drugs that contain an aromatic hydrocarbon, ether, and/or alkyl or aromatic halide as part of their chemical structure. For the sake of clarity, only certain functional groups have been highlighted.

5. **Alkyl and aromatic halides** are **electron-withdrawing** functional groups. They are often used to "lock" a drug molecule in a desired conformation and/or to decrease aromatic oxidation of the drug. Fluorine is the smallest halogen, with its size very similar to that of hydrogen. Chlorine is the second smallest, followed by bromine and iodine, respectively. See Figure 8-10 for specific examples.

   a. With the exception of fluorine, which can serve as a hydrogen-bond acceptor, halides do not directly participate in the binding of drugs to their receptors or other macromolecules.

   b. **Metabolism.** Aromatic halides are not normally metabolized. Alkyl halides can undergo **oxidative dehalogenation** to form aldehydes.

II. BIOCHEMISTRY

A. **Introduction.** Biochemistry is the study of chemical principles that support life processes. It influences drug metabolism, therapeutic effectiveness, and biotransformation. Biochemically significant molecules include amino acids, carbohydrates, lipids, pyrimidines, purines, and biopolymers—proteins and enzymes, which are built from amino acids; polysaccharides, which are built from carbohydrates; and nucleic acids, which are built from pyrimidines and purines.

B. **Amino acids** are the monomeric units of proteins and enzymes and have the following general formula:

$$R-\underset{\underset{NH_2}{|}}{CH}-COOH$$

1. With the exception of glycine, naturally occurring amino acids are L, α-amino acids. Proteins are made up of the 20 different amino acids, which differ in the side chain (R) attached to the α-carbon. The 20 different side chains vary in size, shape, charge, hydrogen-bonding capacity, and chemical reactivity. A protein can be hydrolyzed into its component α-amino acids by acids, bases, or enzymes.
   a. Amino acids with **acidic side chains** include aspartic acid and glutamic acid.
   b. Amino acids with **basic side chains** include arginine, lysine, and histamine.
   c. Amino acids with **polar, nonionic side chains** include glycine, serine, cysteine, threonine, tyrosine, asparagine, and glutamine.
   d. Amino acids with **nonpolar, hydrophobic side chains** include alanine, valine, leucine, isoleucine, phenylalanine, methionine, proline, and tryptophan.

2. Amino acids have a **zwitterion structure,** which accounts for their high melting point and low water solubility. Amino acids in solution have the following general formula:

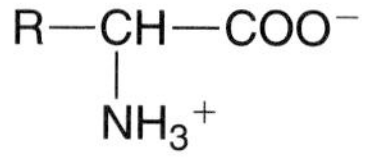

$$R-\underset{\underset{NH_3^+}{|}}{CH}-COO^-$$

3. **Ionization** of amino acids to the zwitterion form or other forms depends on pH (Figure 8-11).

C. **Carbohydrates.** These are polyhydroxy aldehydes or ketones. Three major classes of carbohydrates exist.

1. **Monosaccharides** (simple sugars), such as glucose or fructose, consist of a single polyhydroxy aldehyde or ketone unit.
   a. **Aldehydic** monosaccharides are reducing sugars.
   b. Monosaccharides can be linked together by **glycosidic bonds,** which are hydrolyzed by acids but not by bases.

2. **Oligosaccharides,** such as sucrose, maltose, and lactose, consist of short chains of monosaccharides joined covalently.
   a. **Sucrose** cannot be absorbed by the intestine until it is converted by sucrase into its components, glucose and fructose.
   b. **Maltose** is hydrolyzed by maltase into two molecules of glucose.
   c. **Lactose** (or milk sugar) cannot be absorbed by the intestine until it is converted by lactase into its components, galactose and glucose.

3. **Polysaccharides,** such as **cellulose** and **glycogen,** consist of long chains of monosaccharides.

D. **Pyrimidines and purines.** These are bases that, when bonded with ribose, form nucleosides, which when subsequently bonded to phosphoric acid form nucleotides—the structural building blocks of nucleic acids.

1. **Pyrimidine bases** include:
   a. **Cytosine** (C), found in deoxyribonucleic acid (DNA) and ribonucleic acid (RNA)
   b. **Uracil** (U), found in RNA only
   c. **Thymine** (T), found in DNA only

2. **Purine bases** include:
   a. **Adenine** (A), found in DNA and RNA
   b. **Guanine** (G), found in DNA and RNA

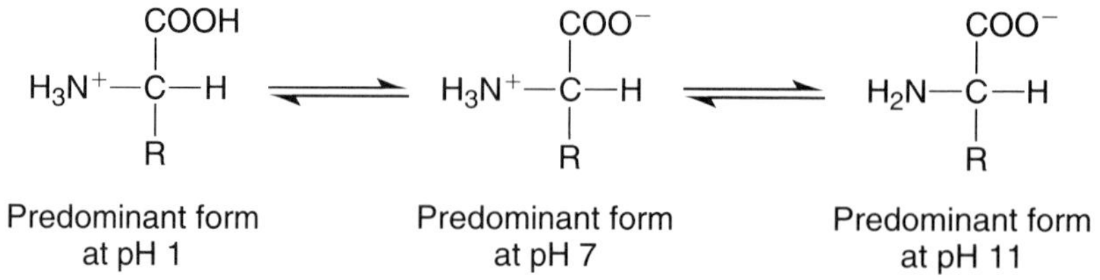

Figure 8-11. Amino acid ionization in solution. The carboxyl and amino groups are either in ionized or unionized form depending on the pH of the solution.

3. Pyrimidines and purines exhibit **tautomerism** (a form of stereoisomerism) and can exist in either **keto** (lactam) or **enol** (lactim) forms.

E. Biopolymers

1. Proteins are polymers of amino acids that are linked together by **peptide bonds** (i.e., links between carbonyl carbons and amino nitrogens [Figure 8-12]). Proteins have four structural levels.

   a. Primary structure refers to the sequence of amino acids and location of disulfide bonds in the protein.

   b. Secondary structure refers to the spatial arrangement of sequenced amino acids (for example, α–conformation [helical coil] or β-conformation [pleated sheet]).

   c. Tertiary structure refers to the three-dimensional structure of a single protein.

   d. Quaternary structure refers to the arrangement of individual subunit chains into complex molecules.

2. Enzymes are proteins capable of acting as catalysts for biologic reactions. They may be simple or complex and may require cofactors or coenzymes for biologic activity.

   a. An enzyme enhances the rate of a specific chemical reaction by lowering the **activation energy** of the reaction. It does not change the reaction's equilibrium point, and it is not used up or permanently changed by the reaction.

   b. A cofactor may be an **inorganic component** (usually a metal ion) or a **nonprotein organic molecule.** A cofactor may be biologically inactive without an apoenzyme (the protein portion of a complex enzyme). A cofactor firmly bound to the apoenzyme is called a **prosthetic group.** An organic cofactor that is not firmly bound but is actively involved during catalysis is called a **coenzyme.**

   c. A complete, catalytically active enzyme system is referred to as a **holoenzyme.**

   d. Enzymes fall into six major classes.

   (1) Oxidoreductases (e.g., dehydrogenases, oxidases, peroxidases) are important in the oxidative metabolism of drugs.

   (2) Transferases catalyze the transfer of groups, such as phosphate and amino groups.

   (3) Hydrolases (e.g., proteolytic enzymes, amylases, esterases) hydrolyze their substrates.

   (4) Lyases (e.g., decarboxylases, deaminases) catalyze the removal of functional groups by means other than hydrolysis.

   (5) Ligases (e.g., DNA ligase, which binds nucleotides together during DNA synthesis) catalyze the coupling of two molecules.

   (6) Isomerases catalyze various isomerizations, such as the change from D to L forms or the change from cisisomers to transisomers.

3. Polysaccharides (also called glycans) are long-chain polymers of carbohydrates and may be linear or branched. They are classified as homopolysaccharides or heteropolysaccharides.

   a. Homopolysaccharides (e.g., starch, glycogen, cellulose) contain only one type of monomeric unit.

   (1) Starch (a reserve food material of plants) is composed of two glucose polymers—amylose (linear and water soluble) and amylopectin (highly branched and water insoluble). It yields mainly maltose (a glucose disaccharide) after enzymatic hydrolysis with salivary or pancreatic amylase; only glucose after complete hydrolysis by strong acids.

   (2) Glycogen, like amylopectin, is a highly branched, compact chain of D-glucose. The main storage polysaccharide of animal cells, it is found mostly in liver and muscle and can be hydrolyzed by salivary or pancreatic amylase into maltose and D-glucose.

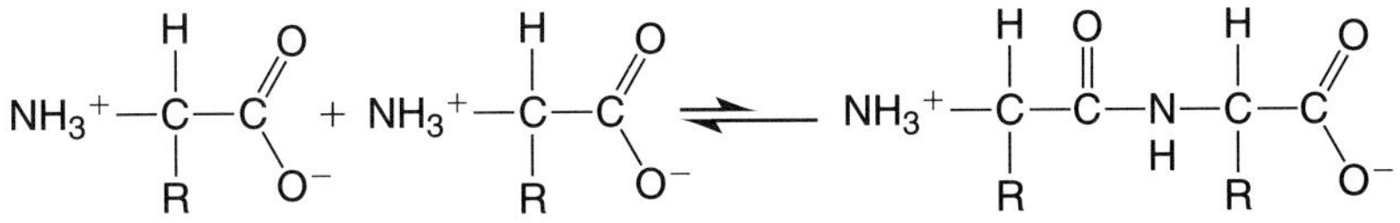

Figure 8-12. Peptide bond formation occurs as a result of the condensation of the carboxyl group of one amino acid with the amino group of another. Water is eliminated during this process.

(3) **Cellulose** (a water-insoluble structural polysaccharide found in plant cell walls) is a linear, unbranched chain of D-glucose. It cannot be digested by humans because the human intestinal tract secretes no enzyme capable of hydrolyzing it.

b. Heteropolysaccharides (e.g., heparin, hyaluronic acid) contain two or more types of monomeric units.

(1) **Heparin** (an acid mucopolysaccharide) consists of sulfate derivatives of *N*-acetyl-D-glucosamine and D-iduronate. It can be isolated from lung tissue and is used medically to prevent blood clot formation.

(2) **Hyaluronic acid,** a component of bacterial cell walls as well as of the vitreous humor and synovial fluid, consists of alternating units of *N*-acetyl-D-glucosamine and *N*-acetyl-muramic acid.

4. **Nucleic acids** are linear polymers of nucleotides—pyrimidine and purine bases linked to ribose or deoxyribose sugars (nucleosides) and bound to phosphate groups. The backbone of the nucleic acid consists of alternating phosphate and pentose units with a purine or pyrimidine base attached to each.

a. Nucleic acids are closely associated with **cellular cations** and such basic proteins as **histones** and **protamines.**

b. The two main types of nucleic acids are **DNA** and **RNA**. RNA exists in three forms.

(1) **Ribosomal** RNA (rRNA) functions as a framework to bind both messenger and transfer RNA. It is comprised of numerous subunits with the 40S and 60S being the most well known. Ribosomal RNA is also thought to have other functions; however, these have not been fully elucidated.

(2) **Messenger** RNA (mRNA) serves as the template for protein synthesis and specifies a polypeptide's amino acid sequence.

(3) **Transfer** RNA (tRNA) carries activated amino acids to the ribosomes, where the amino acids are incorporated into the growing polypeptide chain.

c. In both DNA and RNA, the successive nucleotides are joined by **phosphodiester bonds** between the 5'-hydroxy group of one nucleotide's pentose and the 3'-hydroxy group of the next nucleotide's pentose.

d. DNA differs from RNA in that it **lacks a hydroxyl group** at the pentose's C_2' position, and it contains T rather than U.

e. DNA structure consists of two α-helical DNA strands coiled around the same axis to form a double helix. The strands are antiparallel—the 5', 3'-internucleotide phosphodiester links run in opposite directions.

(1) **Hydrogen bonding** between specific base pairs A–T and cytosine (C)–G holds the two DNA strands together. The strands are complementary (the base sequence of one strand determines the base sequence of the other).

(2) The **hydrophobic bases** are on the inside of the helix; the hydrophilic deoxyribose–phosphate backbone is on the outside.

III. BIOCHEMICAL METABOLISM

A. **Overview.** Biochemical metabolism is the review of pathways that lead to the synthesis or breakdown of compounds important to the life of an organism.

1. **Control of metabolism.** Metabolism is controlled by substrate concentration, enzymes (constitutive or induced), allosteric (regulatory) enzymes, hormones, and compartmentation.

2. **Catabolism** is the sum of degradation reactions that usually release energy for useful work (e.g., mechanical, osmotic, biosynthetic).

3. **Anabolism** is the sum of biosynthetic (build-up) reactions that consume energy to form new biochemical compounds (metabolites).

4. **Amphibolic pathways** are those that may be used for both catabolic as well as anabolic purposes. **Krebs cycle** breaks down metabolites primarily to release 90% of the total energy of an organism. It also draws off metabolites to form compounds such as amino acids (e.g., aspartic, glutamic, alanine). Hemoglobin has its heme moiety formed from succinyl coenzyme A (succinyl CoA) and glycine followed by a complex set of reactions.

B. Bioenergetics

1. **Substrate level phosphorylation** entails the formation of one unit of adenosine triphosphate (ATP) per unit of metabolite transformed (e.g., succinyl CoA to succinate, phosphoenolpyruvate to pyruvate). These reactions do not need oxygen.

2. **Oxidative phosphorylation** entails the formation of one-and-a-half or two-and-a-half units of ATP per unit of metabolite transformed by oxidoreductase enzymes (e.g., dehydrogenases); these enzymes use flavin A dinucleotide (FAD) formed from the vitamin riboflavin, or nicotinamide A dinucleotide (NAD^+) from the vitamin nicotinamide as cofactors. The reactions are coupled to the electron transport system, and the energy released is used to form ATP in the mitochondria.

C. Carbohydrate metabolism

1. **Catabolism.** This process releases stored energy from carbohydrates.
   a. **Glycogenolysis** is the breakdown of glycogen into glucose phosphate in the liver and skeletal muscle. It is controlled by the hormones glucagon and epinephrine.
   b. **Glycolysis** is the breakdown of sugar phosphates (e.g., glucose, fructose, glycerol) into pyruvate (aerobically) or lactate (anaerobically).

2. **Anabolism.** This process consumes energy to build up complex molecules from simpler molecules.
   a. **Glycogenesis** is the formation of glycogen in the liver and muscles from glucose consumed in the diet; its synthesis is controlled by the pancreatic hormone insulin.
   b. **Gluconeogenesis** is the formation of glucose from noncarbohydrate sources, such as lactate, alanine, pyruvate, and Krebs cycle metabolites; fatty acids cannot form glucose.

D. Krebs cycle. This pathway is also known as the citric acid cycle, serves both breakdown and synthetic purposes, and occurs in the mitochondrial compartment.

1. **Catabolism.** This pathway converts pyruvate (glycolysis), acetyl CoA (fatty acid degradation), and amino acids to carbon dioxide and water with a release of energy. The cycle is strictly oxygen-dependent (aerobic). Mature red blood cells lack mitochondria; hence, there is no Krebs cycle activity.

2. **Anabolism.** This pathway forms amino acids such as aspartate and glutamate from cycle intermediates; also, the porphyrin ring of heme (e.g., hemoglobin, myoglobin, cytochromes) is formed from a cycle intermediate.

3. **Anaplerotic reactions.** Because metabolites are used to make amino acids or heme (e.g., succinyl CoA), the metabolite must be replaced by intermediates from other sources (e.g., glutamate from the breakdown of protein forms α-ketoglutarate).

4. **Electron transport.** The electron transport system accepts electrons and hydrogen from the oxidation of Krebs cycle metabolites and couples the energy released to synthesize ATP in the mitochondria.

E. Lipid metabolism

1. **Catabolism. Triglycerides** (triacylglycerols) stored in fat cells (adipocytes) are hydrolyzed by hormone-sensitive lipases into three fatty acids and glycerol.
   a. **Fatty acids** are broken down by beta oxidation to acetyl CoA (two carbon units), which enter the Krebs cycle to complete the oxidation to carbon dioxide and water with release of considerable energy. Too rapid breakdown of fatty acids leads to ketone bodies (ketogenesis) as in diabetes mellitus.
   b. **Glycerol** enters glycolysis and is oxidized to pyruvate and, via the Krebs cycle, to carbon dioxide and water.
   c. **Steroids** may be converted to other compounds such as bile acids, vitamin D, or steroidal hormones (e.g., cortisone, estrogens, androgens); they are not broken down completely.

2. **Anabolism. Biosynthesis** forms fatty acids, steroids, and other terpene-related metabolites.
   a. **Fatty acids** are formed in the cytoplasm, and unsaturation occurs in the mitochondria or endoplasmic reticulum. Humans cannot make linoleic acid; thus, it is important that it be included in the diet (essential fatty acid).

b. Terpene compounds are derived from acetyl CoA via mevalonate and include:
   (1) Cholesterol and other steroids
   (2) Fat-soluble vitamins (i.e., A, D, E, K)
   (3) Bile acids
c. Sphingolipids contain sphingenine formed from palmitoyl CoA and serine. Sphingenine forms a ceramide backbone when joined to fatty acids. The addition of sugars, sialic acid, or choline phosphate forms compounds such as cerebrosides, gangliosides, or sphingomyelin found in nerve tissues and membranes.
d. Phosphatidyl compounds, such as phosphatidyl choline (lecithin), phosphatidyl serine, or ethanolamine, are also important parts of membranes.

F. Nitrogen metabolism. Nitrogen metabolism involves amino acid metabolism and nucleic acid metabolism (see Chapter 9 for a discussion of the nucleic acid role in cell activity).

1. **Catabolism**
   a. Amino acids. The amino group is removed by a transaminase enzyme. The carbon skeleton is broken down to acetyl CoA (ketogenic amino acids) or to citric acid cycle intermediates (glycogenic amino acids) and oxidized to carbon dioxide and water for energy. Glycogenic amino acids form glucose as needed via gluconeogenesis; some amino acids are both ketogenic and glycogenic (e.g., tyrosine).
   b. Purines are salvaged (90%), and the remaining 10% are degraded in a sequence that includes xanthine oxidase forming uric acid in humans.
   c. Pyrimidines are catabolized to β-alanine, ammonia, and carbon dioxide.

2. **Anabolism**
   a. Amino acids are formed from the citric acid cycle intermediates (see III D 2); others must be eaten daily in dietary proteins. The latter are called essential amino acids (phenylalanine, valine, tryptophan [PVT]; threonine, isoleucine, methionine [TIM]; histidine, arginine in infants, lysine, leucine [HALL]).
   b. Purines are formed by complex reactions using carbamoyl phosphate, aspartate, glutamine, glycine, carbon dioxide, and formyl tetrahydrofolate.
   c. Pyrimidines are formed from aspartate and carbamoyl phosphate in a multistep process.

G. Nitrogen excretion. Excess nitrogen must be eliminated because it is toxic. Humans primarily excrete urea but also excrete uric acid.

1. **Urea synthesis.** The **Krebs-Henseleit pathway** is used to form urea principally in the liver. The ammonia is removed from amino acids by amino acid transferases (transaminases) that use pyridoxal phosphate (vitamin B_6) as a coenzyme. **Glutamine** is formed from glutamate (an intermediate) and ammonia; glutamine and carbon dioxide form carbamoyl phosphate, which enters the urea cycle and after several steps forms urea.

2. **Uric acid synthesis.** Although most purines are salvaged, humans excrete the remaining purines as uric acid.

STUDY QUESTIONS

Directions: Each of the numbered items or incomplete statements in this section is followed by answers or by completions of the statement. Select the **one** lettered answer or completion that is **best** in each case.

1. Which of the following functional groups can react with hydrochloric acid to form a salt?

(A) Tertiary amines
(B) Carboxylic acids
(C) Amides
(D) Ethers
(E) Secondary alcohols

2. The compound shown contains all of the following functional groups EXCEPT:

(A) a phenol
(B) a substituted phenyl ring
(C) an ester
(D) an alicyclic nitrogen
(E) a ketone

3. Which of the following functional groups is most susceptible to hydrolysis?

(A) R—CO—R
(B) R—COOR
(C) R—O—R
(D) R—NH—CH$_3$
(E) R—COOH

4. Monomer units of proteins are known as

(A) monosaccharides
(B) prosthetic groups
(C) amino acids
(D) purines
(E) nucleosides

5. Which of the following formulas represents the zwitterion form of an amino acid?

(A) H_2N—CH—COO$^-$
       |
       R

(B) $H_3\overset{+}{N}$—CH—COOH
         |
         R

(C) H_2N—CH—COOH
       |
       R

(D) $H_3\overset{+}{N}$—CH—COO$^-$
         |
         R

(E) H_2N—CH—CONH—CH—COOH
       | |
       R   R

6. Glucose is a carbohydrate that cannot be hydrolyzed into a simpler substance. It is best described as

(A) a sugar
(B) a monosaccharide
(C) a disaccharide
(D) a polysaccharide
(E) an oligosaccharide

7. All of the following carbohydrates are considered to be polysaccharides EXCEPT

(A) heparin
(B) starch
(C) glycogen
(D) maltose
(E) cellulose

8. Which of the following compounds are considered the building blocks of nucleic acids?

(A) Nucleotides
(B) Nucleosides
(C) Monosaccharides
(D) Purines
(E) Amino acids

9. Which of the following terms best describes a cofactor that is firmly bound to an apoenzyme?

(A) Holoenzyme
(B) Prosthetic group
(C) Coenzyme
(D) Transferase
(E) Heteropolysaccharide

10. Enzymes that uncouple peptide linkages are best classified as

(A) hydrolases
(B) ligases
(C) oxidoreductases
(D) transferases
(E) isomerases

11. The sugar that is inherent in the nucleic acids RNA and DNA is

(A) glucose
(B) sucrose
(C) ribose
(D) digitoxose
(E) maltose

Directions: Each item below contains three suggested answers of which **one or more** is correct. Choose the answer

A	if **I only** is correct
B	if **III only** is correct
C	if **I and II** are correct
D	if **II and III** are correct
E	if **I, II, and III** are correct

12. Which of the following functional groups can form a hydrogen bond?

I. An aromatic amine
II. A tertiary hydroxyl
III. An aromatic hydrocarbon

13. Which of the following functional groups commonly undergoes conjugation with glucuronic acid?

I. A carboxylic acid
II. A primary amine
III. A phenol

Questions 14–16

The following questions refer to the drug molecule shown below.

14. The functional groups that enhance this compound's ability to cross cell membranes include:

I. the phenyl rings
II. the central alkyl chain
III. the secondary and tertiary hydroxyls

15. Based upon the functional groups present, this drug would be expected to be able to form:

I. van der Waals interactions
II. ionic bonds
III. hydrogen bonds

16. Possible metabolic pathways for this drug include:

I. reduction of the carboxylic acid
II. hydrolytic cleavage
III. aromatic oxidation

ANSWERS AND EXPLANATIONS

1. The answer is A *[I C 2 c]*.
Substances that react with acids to form salts must be bases. Only organic compounds that contain the nitrogen-containing amine group are bases. While amides contain nitrogen, the adjacent carbonyl group decreases the basicity; therefore, they are essentially neutral.

2. The answer is C *[Figures 8-4, 8-7, 8-8, 8-10]*.
As shown in Figure 8-8, esters have a carbonyl atom directly bonded to an oxygen atom. This structural feature is not present in this compound. However, the compound does have three substituted phenyl rings, two phenols, a tertiary alicyclic nitrogen, a ketone, and an ether.

3. The answer is B *[I E 2 b]*.
Hydrolysis is a double decomposition reaction in which water is one of the reactants. Esters, particularly simple esters, commonly undergo hydrolysis. Certain types of ethers such as glycosides also undergo hydrolysis, but they usually require strongly alkaline conditions or a catalyst such as an enzyme. Ketones, amines, or carboxylic acids do not undergo hydrolysis.

4. The answer is C *[II B 1, II E 1]*.
Proteins are large molecules with molecular weights ranging from 5000 to more than 1 million daltons. All proteins are composed of chains of amino acids and can be hydrolyzed to yield a mixture of their respective amino acids. There are 20 α-amino acids, which are commonly found in proteins. All the naturally occurring amino acids in proteins are L-enantiomers, with the exception of glycine. All have at least one amino group and one carboxyl group. The amino acids are linked together through the amino group of one amino acid and the carboxyl group of another amino acid with the splitting out of a water molecule to form an amide linkage, which in a protein is referred to as a peptide.

Monosaccharides are simple, nonhydrolyzable sugars. Purines and pyrimidines are organic bases, while a prosthetic group is a cofactor that is firmly bound to an apoenzyme.

5. The answer is D *[I A 1 a, II B 2, 3, II E 1, Figures 8-2, 8-11, 8-12]*.
A zwitterion is a single species containing both negative and positive charges. It sometimes is referred to as an internal salt. Amino acids have an amino group and a carboxyl group in the same molecule. The amino group, which is basic, attracts the proton from the carboxyl group and becomes positively charged, while the carboxyl group becomes negatively charged when it donates its proton to the amino group. Amino acids exist as zwitterions at near neutral pH such as occurs within a cell or in the bloodstream.

6. The answer is B *[II C 1]*.
While glucose is a sugar, it is more specifically a simple sugar that cannot be hydrolyzed into more simple sugars—thus, it is classified as a monosaccharide. Sugars may be simple, such as glucose, or complex, such as sucrose, and are classified as disaccharides or oligosaccharides, respectively. Polysaccharides consist of long chains of monosaccharides such as cellulose and glycogen.

7. The answer is D *[II C 2 b, 3, E 3 a, b]*.
Polysaccharides are long-chain polymers of sugars. As the prefix "poly" indicates, there are many sugar units in the molecule. Maltose is composed of two molecules of glucose and is classified as a disaccharide or an oligosaccharide.

8. The answer is A *[II D, E 4]*.
Nucleic acids are linear polymers of nucleotides that consist of three different molecules that are covalently linked to form one unit: (1) an organic base of either a purine or a pyrimidine; (2) a 5-carbon sugar (e.g., pentose); and (3) a phosphoric acid group. A nucleoside consists of the organic base and the pentose. A monosaccharide is a simple nonhydrolyzable carbohydrate, which may be considered a building block of polysaccharides. Purines are heterocyclic bases. Adenine and guanine are the two purines found in deoxyribonucleic acid (DNA) and ribonucleic acid (RNA). Amino acids are the building blocks of protein.

9. The answer is B *[II E 2 b–d]*.
Complex, or conjugated, enzymes contain a nonprotein group called a cofactor, which is required for biologic activity. In many cases, the cofactor is quite firmly bound to the protein. In others, the binding occurs only during the reaction that the enzyme catalyzes. Cofactors that are firmly bound to the

protein are known as prosthetic groups, whereas those that are actively bound to the protein only during catalysis are referred to as coenzymes.

A holoenzyme is a complete, catalytically active enzyme system. A transferase is an enzyme that catalyzes the transfer of groups from one substance to another, such as catechol-*O*-methyl transferase (COMT). A heteropolysaccharide is a polysaccharide that contains two or more different monomeric units, such as heparin.

10. The answer is A *[II E 2 d].*
A peptide linkage is an amide functional group formed from the loss of a molecule of water from two amino acids. Uncoupling this linkage is the reverse of this reaction, a hydrolysis reaction. A hydrolase is an enzyme that catalyzes hydrolysis reactions. More specific terms for an enzyme that catalyzes the hydrolysis of proteins are amidase or peptidase. A ligase catalyzes the coupling of two molecules. An oxidoreductase catalyzes oxidation reactions. A transferase catalyzes the transfer of groups from one substance to another. An isomerase catalyzes the interconversion of one isomer to another.

11. The answer is C *[II E 4].*
Nucleic acids are biopolymers consisting of long chains of nucleotides. Nucleotides contain a pentose monosaccharide as one of their three constituents. RNA contains, as the name suggests, the monosaccharide ribose, whereas DNA contains deoxyribose. The only difference between these two sugars is the absence of oxygen in the 2 position of the ribose ring. Glucose, also known as dextrose, is a hexose. Digitoxose is a deoxyhexose present in the digitalis glycosides. Sucrose and maltose are disaccharides.

12. The answer is C (I, II) *[I C 2 b, D 1 a, F 3 a].*
Hydrogen bonds are a specialized type of dipole bond in which a hydrogen atom serves as a bridge between two electronegative atoms. Hydrogen-bond donors include hydroxyl groups, phenols, amines, and amides. Hydrogen-bond acceptors include hydroxyl groups, phenols, unionized nitrogen atoms, ketones, and ethers. Hydrocarbons, regardless if they are aliphatic, alicyclic, or aromatic, are not capable of forming hydrogen bonds.

13. The answer is E (I, II, and III) *[I B 2 e, C 2 d, D 2 d].*
Glucuronide conjugation is the most common phase II metabolic pathway for two reasons: (1) The body has a readily available supply of glucuronic acid, and (2) there are a large number of functional groups that can react with this compound. Included among these functional groups are carboxylic acids, primary, secondary and tertiary amines, and phenols.

14–16. The answers are: 14-C (I, II) *[I A 1, D 1 b, F 1, 3],* **15-E (I, II, and III)** *[I B 2 b, C 2 b, D 1 a, F 1 a, 3 a],* **16-B (III)** *[I B 2 e, E 2 b, F 3 b].*
Lipophilic functional groups increase a drug's ability to cross cell membranes. The three aromatic phenyl rings, as well as the aliphatic butyl chain connecting the central phenyl ring to the nitrogen of the piperadine ring, are all lipophilic (i.e., hydrophobic) and contribute to the drug's passage through cell membranes. The hydroxyl groups, as well as the acidic carboxylic acid and the basic alicyclic amine, are all hydrophilic and enhance the overall water solubility of the compound.

The phenyl rings, as well as the central alkyl chain and the methyl groups, are capable of forming van der Waals interactions with aromatic and aliphatic hydrocarbon regions on receptor molecules. The carboxylic acid and the basic nitrogen are capable of forming both ionic and hydrogen bonds, while the hydroxyl groups are also capable of forming hydrogen bonds.

Of the metabolic pathways listed, aromatic oxidation is the only plausible choice. The two unsubstituted phenyl rings are very susceptible to hydroxylation, epoxidation, and/or diol formation. Carboxylic acids are not normally reduced, but rather conjugated with either glucuronic acid, glycine or glutamine. Esters, amides and their cyclic derivatives, lactones and lactams, are the primary functional groups that undergo hydrolysis. None of these functional groups are present in the compound shown.

9
Microbiology
Carolyn Dabirsiaghi

I. SCOPE OF MICROBIOLOGY

Microbiology is the study of organisms from three domains, as well as acellular entities that are not considered to be living in the biological sense.

A. Domains of living organisms

1. **Archaea** includes prokaryotes with cell walls that are biochemically different from bacteria and that inhabit extreme environments of heat, cold, pH, or salts.

2. **Eukarya** contains some microorganisms, for example, fungi (yeasts and molds), protozoa, and algae, along with macroscopic organisms like mushrooms, plants, and animals. **Dimorphic fungi** are those that can exist in either the unicellular (yeast) or filamentous (mold) phase depending on the incubation temperature (e.g., *Histoplasma* and *Blastomyces*).

   a. **Fungi** are classified into phyla based on the type of reproductive structures observed or the lack of observable sexual reproductive structures.
      (1) **Ascomycota** (ascus) (e.g., *Candida* & *Histoplasma*)
      (2) **Basidiomycota** (basidium) (e.g., *Cryptococcus*)
      (3) **Zygomycota** (zygote) (e.g., *Rhizopus*)
      (4) **Deuteromycota** (asexual, also called Fungi Imperfecti) (e.g., *Coccidioides*)

   b. **Protozoa,** unicellular, non-photosynthetic eukaryotes characterized by mode of motility include:
      (1) **Mastigophora** (flagellates) (e.g., *Giardia*)
      (2) **Sarcodina** (amoebae) (e.g., *Entamoeba*)
      (3) **Ciliophora** (ciliates) (e.g., *Balantidium*)
      (4) **Sporozoa** (non-motile) (e.g., *Plasmodium*)

3. **Bacteria** contains a wide variety of prokaryotes including gram-positive and gram-negative bacteria. The sections that follow (II–VII) characterize bacteria in more detail.

B. Non–living, but medically significant entities are:

1. **Viruses,** which are classified by:
   a. **Capsid structure,** which is the protein coating around the nucleic acid,
   b. **Type and strandedness of nucleic acid,** which could be either deoxyribonucleic acid (DNA) or ribonucleic acid (RNA), either single or double stranded,
   c. Presence or absence of a **lipid-envelope** surrounding the protein capsid, and
   d. Presence of **enzymes,** which may either be incorporated into the lipid envelope or found near the nucleic acid.

2. **Prions,** thought to be **infectious proteins,** are implicated in some spongiform encephalopathies (e.g., mad cow disease, *nv*Creutzfeldt-Jakob disease, and kuru).

II. TAXONOMY AND NOMENCLATURE OF BACTERIA

A. **Taxonomy** is classification or ordering into groups based on degree of relatedness. Bacteria are **prokaryotes** that belong to the Bacteria domain and the Eubacteria kingdom and are grouped and named primarily by morphology, biochemical and metabolic differences, and immunologic and genetic relationships. Bacteria are named using the **Linnaean** or **binomial** system as a genus and species (e.g., *Homo sapiens* is the genus and species for humans).

B. **Morphology** is classification of bacteria by shape and structure.

1. **Cultural morphology** is based on the size, shape, and texture of colonies that are grown in an **axenic,** or pure, culture. Each colony originates from a **colony-forming unit (CFU),** consisting of a single cell or group of adherent cells.

2. **Microscopic morphology** describes bacteria on the basis of the size, shape, and arrangement of the cells.

C. **Stains.** Because of their small size and relative transparency, bacteria must be stained to be visible with the light microscope. Staining is also used as a classification system. The major types of staining reactions are:

1. **Simple** stain: a single dye (e.g., Gentian violet, safranin) that colors the cells.

2. **Gram** stain: a differential staining procedure that divides bacterial cells into either gram-positive (purple) or gram-negative (pink).

3. **Acid–fast** stain: a vigorous procedure that stains cells that have an outer layer of a waxy–lipid (acid–fast) but not those that lack this layer material (non–acid–fast).

4. **Spore** stain: heat is used to facilitate the dye entering the spore.

5. **Capsule** stain: two dyes are used to stain the cell and the background, allowing visualization of the unstained capsular material.

D. **Bacterial cell shape and arrangement**

1. **Cocci** are spherical and exist in chains (streptococci), pairs or diplococci *(Streptococcus pneumoniae, Neisseria gonorrhoeae),* clusters (staphylococci), and packets of four or eight (sarcinae).

2. **Bacilli** are cylindrical and rod–shaped organisms (pseudomonads, *Escherichia*).

3. **Coccobacilli** are a combination of small rods or flattened cocci *(Brucella).*

4. **Spirochetes** are helical like a corkscrew *(Treponema pallidum).*

5. **Fusobacteria** have tapered ends and are slightly curved (i.e., fusiform) *(Fusobacterium mortiferum).*

6. **Filamentous** organisms are branching *(Actinomyces bovis).*

7. **Vibrios** are comma shaped *(Vibrio cholerae).*

8. **Pleomorphic** organisms exist in varied forms *(Haemophilus, Legionella, Corynebacteria).*

E. **Other parameters** used for classification

1. The **presence** or **absence** of:
   a. **Spores**
   b. **Capsules** or **slime layers**

2. **Motility** and the type of **flagella**
   a. **Monotrichous:** a single flagellum at either pole
   b. **Lophotrichous:** a tuft of flagella at either or both poles
   c. **Amphitrichous:** a flagellum at both poles
   d. **Peritrichous:** flagella distributed evenly over the entire cell
   e. **Axial filaments:** periplasmic flagella wrapped around spirochetes
   f. **Gliding motility:** as demonstrated by slime molds

III. STRUCTURE OF THE PROKARYOTIC CELL

A. **Overview.** Prokaryotic cells (bacteria) are **small** and **simple** in design. They have the following characteristics:

1. **Less complex inside,** but more complex outside

2. Lack a true nucleus, a nuclear membrane, and intracytoplasmic membranous organelles (e.g., plastids, endoplasmic reticulum, vacuoles)

3. Cytoplasm is immobile (e.g., no cytoplasmic streaming, pseudopodia, endocytosis or exocytosis seen)

4. Multiply asexually by **binary fission** rather than by mitosis or meiosis

5. **Protein synthesis** is mediated by 70s rather than by 80s ribosomes.

6. Bacterial genetic information is arranged on a single supercoiled circular strand of DNA, the **nucleoid.**

B. External structures

1. **Capsule and slime layer**
   a. The **capsule** is an expressed, adherent, large polymer surface coat that differs in composition between genera and usually is polysaccharide in nature; however, the capsule of *Bacillus* is polypeptide. The capsule has several functions:
      (1) Increases the **virulence** (degree of organism pathogenicity) of a microorganism
      (2) Prevents **phagocytosis** of the organism by macrophages and neutrophils
      (3) Aids in **adherence** of the organism to host cells
   b. If the polysaccharide is nonadherent, it is called a **slime layer.**
   c. **Transformation** from smooth to rough colonies on media is indicative of **capsule loss.** Concurrently, there is a loss of virulence. This capsular material is immunogenic, thereby inducing the production of **antibodies,** which act as opsonins to enhance phagocytosis (**opsonization**).

2. **Flagella** are proteinaceous, helically coiled organs of locomotion that extend outward from the cytoplasm through the cell wall into the environment. Flagella rotate either clockwise or counter-clockwise, allowing a series of runs and tumbles in response to chemicals in the environment. The direction of movement is controlled by a complex mechanism involving chemoreceptors and an intracellular cascade of methylation and phosphorylation reactions, causing bacteria to move toward nutrient chemoattractants and away from repellants.
   a. **Structure**
      (1) Flagella are composed of **flagellin,** a protein that is antigenically distinct from other flagella and cell antigens and is termed **H antigen.**
      (2) **Three parts** comprise flagella:
         (a) **Basal body**
            (i) Attaches the flagella to the cell envelope (cytoplasmic membrane and cell wall)
            (ii) The number of rings that make up the basal body differ in gram-positive (two) and gram-negative (four) organisms**.**
         (b) **Hook**
         (c) **Filament**
   b. **Periplasmic flagella,** also called **axial filaments,** occur in spirochetes and are embedded into the cell wall's outer membrane. Because they cause a corkscrew type of motion on contraction, these organisms are not hindered by viscosity of media.

3. **Pili (fimbriae)** are proteinaceous, hair-like extensions that are shorter than flagella, composed of regularly arranged protein subunits called **pilin** or **fimbrilin.** They are more common in gram-negative organisms, but can be found in gram-positive organisms. There are two morphological and functional varieties:
   a. **Common** (attachment) pili
      (1) Appear in greater numbers than sex pili
      (2) Have adhesive properties, which are important in the formation of biofilms
      (3) Are lectins that are responsible for trophism, the ability of the organism to bind to specific receptors on host cells
   b. **Sex** (conjugative or F) pili
      (1) Are longer than common pili
      (2) Form in groups of less than 10
      (3) Are involved in the transport of DNA between donor and recipient cells

C. The cell wall, periplasmic space, and cytoplasmic membrane

1. The **cell wall** is rigid; while it provides the general shape of the cell, its function is to protect the cell from osmotic shock. If the cell wall is destroyed, the bacterial cells are very susceptible to alterations in the tonicity of the environment. The wall is composed of a basic **peptidoglycan** or **murein layer.** This layer is composed of repeating disaccharide units, with a four-amino–acid side chain that is covalently linked to amino acids from neighboring

disaccharide units, forming a stable cross-linked structure. This complex structure is a polymer of **N–acetylglucosamine** and **N–acetylmuramic acid.** Most bacteria are designated as either gram-positive or gram-negative, based on fundamental differences in the components of the cell wall. Due to the uniqueness and the importance of the cell wall to bacterial viability, it is the target of many antibiotic agents.

a. **Gram-positive organisms** have a thick cell wall, which is 90% peptidoglycan, with extensive cross-linking that is approximately 40 layers thick and forms a sacculus in parallel layers or layered network around the cytoplasmic membrane. Within the cell wall, a variety of elements serve to stabilize the cell wall, maintain its association with the cytoplasmic membrane, and act as receptors and antigenic determinants.

   (1) **Proteins**

   (2) **Polysaccharides**

   (3) **Teichoic acids** (glycerol or ribitol phosphodiesters)

      (a) **Membrane-associated teichoic acids** (lipoteichoic acid) are covalently linked to glycolipids of the cytoplasmic membrane.

      (b) **Wall-associated teichoic acids** are covalently linked to the glycan chain of peptidoglycan.

b. **Gram-negative organisms** have cell walls that are multilayered with a thin peptidoglycan layer that has no teichoic acids. External to this is the **outer membrane,** a complex cell wall layer, linked to the peptidoglycan layer by the **lipoprotein** layer. The outer membrane acts as a hydrophobic diffusion barrier and consists of:

   (1) **Phospholipid,** a bilayer similar to the cytoplasmic membrane with protein channels called **porins** for nutrient transport

   (2) The **lipopolysaccharide (LPS)** component projects from the cell surface and is both toxic and antigenic **(O antigen).** In the gram-negative organism, the LPS **blocks diffusion** of low-molecular-weight substances into the cell, so antibiotics and chemicals that attack the cell wall (e.g., lysozyme, penicillin) cannot pass through easily. LPS, also known as gram-negative **endotoxin,** is toxic to humans and is composed of three parts:

      (a) **Lipid A:** toxic portion that can either slough off intact cells or be released into circulation upon lysis of the cell, causing nonspecific inflammation including diarrhea, fever, and septic shock

      (b) **Core polysaccharide:** similar within genera

      (c) **O-specific side chain:** species specific

   (3) **Protein**

2. The **periplasmic space,** an area between the cell wall and the cytoplasmic membrane, contains a gel of several types of molecules (e.g., hydrolytic enzymes, periplasmic-binding proteins) that process molecules before they enter the cytoplasm. It also contains proteins that act as chemoreceptors for chemotaxis, others that act as carriers of nutrient (similar to carriers in the cytoplasmic membrane), and antibiotic inactivating enzymes.

3. The **cytoplasmic membrane** is a phospholipid bilayer matrix of a fatty-acid core (hydrophobic) and glycerol phosphate backbone (hydrophilic). With the presence of proteins embedded in the matrix, these membranes are actively and passively engaged in several **cellular functions.**

a. **Transportation** of nutrients through:

   (1) Passive diffusion

   (2) Facilitated diffusion

   (3) Active transport (this method is the only one that actively uses energy because molecules are moving into the cell against a concentration gradient)

b. The site of **respiration proteins** used for:

   (1) **Electron transport** and energy formation

   (2) **Enzymes** involved in the assembly of the cell wall components

   (3) **Secretion of exotoxins** and other substances for the breakdown of macromolecules

D. **Internal structures**

1. **Storage granules** have inclusion bodies of metachromatic granules used for food or energy storage (e.g., polyphosphate complexes, carbohydrate).

2. **Ribosomes** are cellular units that synthesize protein by the translation of messenger RNA (mRNA)–base sequences into amino-acid protein sequences. These ribosomes, unlike

those in eukaryotic cells, are 70s units and are not associated with membranes, such as mitochondria or rough endoplasmic reticulum.

3. The **nuclear region** of bacteria is a condensed area (a nucleoid) containing the bacterial DNA or genome that lacks a nuclear membrane and consists of a long, double-stranded, supercoiled, circular DNA molecule.

4. Some organisms contain **plasmids,** circular double-stranded pieces of DNA that are found outside of the bacterial chromosome. These structures are autonomous (not controlled by the bacterial chromosome), contain information for heavy metal and antibiotic resistance, are conjunctive, and carry genetic elements called **transposons.**

IV. MICROBIAL PHYSIOLOGY

A. Nutritional types

1. **Autotrophs** use carbon dioxide as their sole or main carbon source.
   a. **Photoautotrophs** use light as an energy source.
   b. **Chemoautotrophs** oxidize organic or inorganic compounds to produce energy.

2. **Heterotrophs** use organic compounds as their main carbon source.
   a. **Photoheterotrophs** use light as an energy source.
   b. **Chemoheterotrophs** oxidize organic and inorganic compounds to produce energy.

3. **Prototrophs** are parent cells that have no special nutritional requirements. They require the same nutrients as the major number of the natural members of the species.

4. **Auxotrophs** are mutated so that they cannot synthesize the same essential nutrients (usually amino acids) as their parent cell.

5. **Subsets**
   a. **Holophytic:** organisms whose nutrients must be in a soluble, diffusible form
   b. **Holozoic:** organisms that need complex nutrients, often solid materials that are ingested and then broken down
   c. **Saprophytic:** organisms whose nutrients are obtained from dead or decaying organic matter
   d. **Parasitic:** organisms whose nutrients are obtained from and at the expense of a living organism (human pathogens)

B. Nutritional requirements.
Bacteria use a wide variety of nutrients to obtain energy and to construct new cellular components. There are six elements that are used as the main components of carbohydrates, lipids, proteins, and nucleic acids. These are carbon, oxygen, hydrogen, nitrogen, phosphorus, and sulfur. There are several minor and trace elements as well as cations that play various roles in the microorganisms.

C. Temperature relations

1. **Psychrophile:** an organism that grows well at 0°C, has optimal growth at 15°C or less, and a maximum growth temperature of 20°C

2. **Mesophile:** an organism with optimal growth at 20°C–45°C, minimum growth temperatures between 15°C and 20°C, and maximum at approximately 45°C

3. **Thermophile:** an organism that can grow at 55°C or greater, with a minimum growth temperature of approximately 45°C

D. Oxygen requirements.
How organisms use oxygen can be a major factor in their classification.

1. **Aerobes** have the ability to grow in the presence of atmospheric oxygen.
   a. **Obligate** aerobes are completely dependent on oxygen for growth. Oxygen serves as terminal electron acceptor in aerobic respiration.
   b. **Facultative** aerobes have the ability to grow with or without molecular oxygen.

2. **Anaerobes** have the ability to grow without oxygen.
   a. **Obligate** anaerobes do not tolerate oxygen at all and die in its presence. Many strains lack catalase and superoxide dismutase that protect cells from the destructive oxidizing

capabilities of hydrogen peroxide and superoxide ions, which are normally produced under aerobic conditions.

   b. Facultative anaerobes do not require oxygen but grow better in its presence.

  3. Microaerophiles require oxygen levels below normal.

E. Bacterial growth curve. Bacterial growth is defined as an increase in the number of cells present. Because bacteria reproduce by **binary fission,** growth can be plotted as the log of the cell number versus time to produce a curve with four distinct phases.

  1. Lag phase is a transition period when the bacteria are replicating DNA and enzymes needed for the new environment are induced. The cells are increasing in size but not in number. During this phase of growth, the cells are most permeable.

  2. Logarithmic (log) phase division occurs at constant and maximal rate, and the number of cells increases in a geometric progression. The generation time, which varies among species, usually is 15–20 minutes (*Escherichia*), but may be hours (*Mycobacterium*). Because the cell wall is being synthesized so rapidly, bacterial cells are most susceptible to cell wall inhibitors during this phase.

  3. Stationary phase is when the growth rate tapers off and growth and death rates are nearly equal. A fairly constant population of viable cells results. During this phase, cellular metabolites are polluting the environment.

  4. Death phase describes when the concentration of viable cells decreases at a geometric rate because of the accumulation of toxic wastes and autolytic enzymes.

V. METABOLISM AND ENERGY PRODUCTION. Microorganisms derive energy from nutrients by a series of chemical reactions, in which the energy stored in chemical bonds is transferred to newly formed chemical bonds to provide energy storage in a useful form, such as adenosine triphosphate (ATP).

A. ATP generation

  1. Substrate-level phosphorylation releases energy through direct transfer of high-energy phosphate groups from an intermediate metabolic compound to adenosine diphosphate (ADP). No molecular oxygen or other inorganic final electron acceptor is required.

  2. Oxidative phosphorylation removes electrons from organic compounds and passes these electrons through a series of electron acceptors along an electron transport chain, with molecular oxygen or some other inorganic compound as the final acceptor.

B. Fermentation refers to energy-producing oxidative sequences, in which organic compounds serve as both electron donors and acceptors. This process occurs in the absence of external electron acceptors.

  1. Glycolysis is the first step in fermentation and respiration and causes the oxidation of glucose to pyruvic acid with a yield of two moles of ATP. There are different pathways for pyruvic acid production in microorganisms:
  a. The **Embden–Meyerhof (glycolytic) pathway** is the major pathway.
  b. The **Entner–Doudoroff pathway** is an alternate.
  c. The **hexose monophosphate shunt** used with the glycolytic pathway is an alternative.

  2. Secondary fermentation process. Many bacteria use pyruvate to oxidize **reduced nicotinamide adenine dinucleotide (NADH)** produced in glycolysis to produce a variety of final products.
  a. Lactic acid fermentation: the simplest process, in which pyruvate is converted to lactate *(Lactobacillus, Streptococcus)*
  b. Alcohol fermentation: pyruvate is converted to ethanol and carbon dioxide *(Saccharomyces)*
  c. Mixed acid fermentation: a combination of lactic, formic, and acetic acids is produced with ethanol, hydrogen, and carbon dioxide *(Escherichia coli)*
  d. Butanediol fermentation: pyruvate is converted to acetoin, which is reduced to 2,3-butanediol *(Enterobacter)*

e. Butyric acid fermentation: produces butanol, isopropanol, and acetone *(Clostridium)*
f. Propionic acid fermentation: pyruvate is converted to oxaloacetate with the addition of carbon dioxide, then to propionic acid *(Propionibacterium)*

C. **Respiration** refers to energy-producing oxidative sequences, in which inorganic compounds act as the last electron acceptor in a series of reactions. This process includes **glycolysis, tricarboxylic acid (TCA) cycle,** and the **electron transport system,** which yields ATP when coupled with oxidative phosphorylation.

1. **Aerobic respiration:** Oxygen serves as the final electron acceptor.
   a. Pyruvate is converted to **acetyl coenzyme A** and carbon dioxide and water through the **TCA cycle.**
   b. The **electron transport system** plays a role in the transport of electrons along a series of carriers found in the cytoplasmic membrane, each with successively higher oxidation potentials. Major components of the electron transport system include:
      (1) Cytochromes
      (2) Flavoproteins
      (3) Ubiquinones

2. **Anaerobic respiration:** An inorganic electron acceptor other than oxygen (e.g., nitrate, sulfate, carbonate) serves as the final electron acceptor.

VI. GENETICS

A. **Definition and terms.** Genetics is the study of what genes are, how they carry information, and how they are replicated and passed on.

1. **Chromosomes** are bodies that have the DNA that contain genetic information. Bacteria have only one chromosome—a single, continuous (closed), double-stranded, circular piece of DNA.
   a. **Duplication** occurs by semiconservative replication, in which the two strands of the helix separate **(origin)** and at this point **(two replication forks)** new strands are synthesized, bidirectionally, with the originals serving as templates.
   b. **Structure.** The cell membrane is attached to the chromosome, and as the cell grows, it separates the daughter chromosomes. Therefore, each daughter cell has one original and one new strand.

2. **Genes** are DNA segments that are processed in two steps to produce various proteins. A normal bacterial cell is **haploid.**

B. **Regulation and expression of genetic information**

1. **DNA** has many **functions.**
   a. It is **duplicated** for transfer to progeny during cell division.
   b. It is **transcribed** into RNA that can be translated into a protein.
   c. It contains **control signals** that ultimately control the synthesis of protein.
   d. It can be **mutated** to alter specific characteristics that are encoded by genes.
   e. It can be duplicated and transferred to **other bacterial cells** in processes other than cell division (e.g., conjugal transfer).

2. **DNA replication, transcription,** and **translation** affect cellular growth and development.
   a. Bacterial **replication** involves accurate duplication of chromosomal DNA, which enables the formation of two identical daughter cells.
   b. **Transcription** of information from DNA to RNA is the first of two steps needed to produce necessary proteins. One gene can be transcribed into many copies of RNA. Simplistically, RNA polymerase locates the beginning of the gene (promotor), and this area undergoes localized unwinding to allow RNA polymerase to **transcribe** RNA (called **mRNA**) from the DNA template. The RNA is not processed, as in eukaryotes. There are no introns and exons, no capping of the 5′ end, and no polyadenine tails added to the 3′ end.
   c. **Translation** is the processing of genetic information to synthesize proteins. Before transcription is completed, a ribosome will attach to the 5′ end of the message. The 70s bacterial **ribosome** is composed of two subunits, 30s and 50s. The ribosome **translates** the message into protein by reading the **triplet codon** (three nucleotides) as a specific

amino acid. This amino acid is carried to the site by **transfer RNA (tRNA)** and pairs with the codon by an **anticodon.** Amino acids are joined, and the ribosome moves to the next codon. This continues until the complete protein is synthesized.

3. **Regulation.** The products of cellular growth must be produced in correct proportions for the cell to live and function. The two most common mechanisms of metabolic and genetic regulation are as follows:
   a. **Feedback inhibition** of enzyme activity (metabolic regulation) inhibits the synthesis of the cell growth product. The product binds with an allosteric site on the enzyme, thereby inactivating the active site.
   b. **Repression** of enzyme activity (genetic regulation) inhibits the synthesis of the enzyme at the transcriptional level.

C. **Other methods of DNA transfer.** Microorganisms can change their genetic constitution by the transfer of genetic material from a donor chromosome to a recipient chromosome (recombination). Recombinations occur between homologous segments (those that have similar nucleotide sequences). There are three general mechanisms.

1. **Transformation** involves the recipient cell taking up cell-free, fragmented (i.e., naked) DNA and recombining genetic elements.
   a. This process is **primitive** and naturally occurs within only a few genera.
   b. Requirements include competent recipient cells (exhibiting DNA receptors) or a **"leaky" bacterial cell wall** so that DNA can be introduced into the cell.
   c. It is generally associated with **recombinant DNA technology** or **cloning,** a technique to amplify a specific gene in preparation for analysis. However, in this process, the bacterial cell walls are made "leaky" by chemical treatment.
      (1) Cloning involves splicing a gene into a plasmid DNA **(vector).** All vectors share several common characteristics:
         (a) Typically small, well-characterized molecules of DNA
         (b) Contain at least one replicon and can be replicated within the host even when they contain foreign DNA
         (c) Code for a phenotypic trait that can be used to detect the presence of foreign DNA, which often can be used to distinguish parental from recombinant vectors
      (2) **Selectable markers** are used to find cells that contain these vectors.
      (3) **Plasmids** cannot maintain stability unless they are beneficial to the host, so the plasmid should contain a gene essential for cellular survival—either an enzyme required in a metabolic pathway or a gene that resists certain antibiotics (see III D 4).

2. **Conjugation** is an important means of gene transfer, particularly among gram-negative organisms. This process involves two mating types [the donor **(F⁺)** and recipient **(F⁻)** cells] and the extrachromosomal piece known as the sex or fertility factor **(F factor).** The F factor (e.g., F plasmid or episome) is not under the control of the chromosome and can replicate autonomously. Plasmid-mediated exchange of genetic information can only occur through the expression of transfer genes. These genes encoded on the plasmid result in the transfer of a single strand of DNA through the sex pilus into the recipient cell. The F factor has several genes that code for formation and aid in donor attachment of sex pili. During this process, a copy is made, a single strand is transferred, and the recipient becomes F⁺. Along with the F plasmids, there can be R plasmids, which encode for resistance to certain antibiotics or heavy metals. When an F plasmid integrates into the cellular chromosome, the bacterial strain is said to be a **high-frequency recombination (Hfr)** strain. During the conjugal transfer involving an Hfr strain, and dependent on the length of time, the whole bacterial chromosome may be transferred. Antibiotic resistance genes are often parts of **transposons** (see III D 4), which are responsible for additions, deletions, and inversions of large (4–80 kb) sequences. When different transposons "jump" into transferable plasmids, contagious resistance to multiple antibiotics can occur.

3. **Transduction** is the transfer of genetic material by **bacteriophage** (viruses that infect bacteria). These viruses can be classified into two different groups:
   a. **Lytic phages** enter the cell, replicate, and package their DNA and then lyse the cell to release mature infective virions.
   b. **Lysogenic (temperate) phages** can alternate between two pathways:
      (1) By the lytic pathway
      (2) By integrating into the host DNA and remaining dormant

    (a) The viral DNA does not replicate but is integrated into the host genome and is known as **prophage.**

    (b) The prophage suppresses the lytic state by synthesizing a protein known as a repressor, which protects the cell from further infection by a virus.

    (c) Some prophages can change the cell's phenotype **(phage** or **lysogenic conversion),** which allows the organism to elaborate materials (exotoxins or virulence factors) that are detrimental to the human host. Lysogenic conversion thereby increases the virulence or the symptoms of a specific pathogen [e.g., *Corynebacterium diphtheriae* (diph-toxin), *Streptococcus pyogenes* (erythrogenic toxin in scarlet fever), *Clostridium tetani* (tetanus toxin)].

VII. EXAMPLES OF UNIQUE BACTERIA

A. *Chlamydia* are obligate intracellular parasites that:

    1. Lack the ability to generate ATP; hence, they must obtain it from the host cell.

    2. Have a **two-phase life cycle.**

        a. The infectious form, or **elementary body,** is a dense, nonreplicating cell that is resistant to drying in the environment.

        b. The **reticulate body** forms from engulfed elementary body and undergoes binary fission. After multiple divisions, the reticulate bodies become the dense, elementary bodies, which are released from the host cell [e.g., *Chlamydia trachomatis,* which causes blindness and sexually transmitted dieases (STDs)].

B. *Rickettsia,* which are obligate intracellular parasites transmitted by arthropods, appear to have the ability to generate ATP, but instead **utilize the host cell products, including ATP, amino acids, NAD, and coenzyme A** (e.g., *Rickettsia rickettsii,* which causes Rocky Mountain spotted fever).

C. *Mycoplasma* are the smallest bacteria and they are unique in that:

    1. They **lack a cell wall.**

    2. The plasma membrane contains **sterols** for added strength (e.g., *Mycoplasma pneumonia,* which causes an atypical or walking pneumonia).

STUDY QUESTIONS

Directions: Each of the numbered items or incomplete statements in this section is followed by answers or by completions of the statement. Select the **one** lettered answer or completion that is **best** in each case.

1. Cell envelopes of both gram-positive and gram-negative bacteria are composed of complex macromolecules. Which of the following statements describes both types of cell envelopes?

(A) They contain significant amounts of teichoic acid.
(B) They contain all the common amino acids.
(C) Their antigenic specificity is determined by the polysaccharide O antigen.
(D) They form a diffusion barrier to large macromolecules.

2. Which of the following descriptions best characterizes sex pili? They

(A) enable DNA transport between bacteria during conjugation.
(B) play a role in the adhesion of bacteria to their target cells.
(C) are numerous on the bacterial cell surface.
(D) are found only on gram-positive organisms.

3. The mode of gene transfer in which naked DNA is taken up is called

(A) transformation
(B) transduction
(C) conjugation
(D) cell fusion

4. Bacteria that make either a fermentative or respiratory set of enzymes are known as

(A) obligate anaerobes
(B) obligate aerobes
(C) microaerophiles
(D) facultative organisms

5. Which of the following statements describes plasmids? They

(A) are single-stranded DNA molecules.
(B) carry optional genes.
(C) carry genes essential for growth.
(D) are always found in linear form.

6. All of the following statements describe the nuclear body EXCEPT that it

(A) is referred to as nucleoid.
(B) is free of ribosomes.
(C) is composed of ribosomes.
(D) lacks a nuclear membrane.

7. Bacteria that grow at temperatures as high as 55°C are known as

(A) psychrophiles
(B) thermophiles
(C) mesophiles
(D) auxotrophs

8. Which of the following organisms can use only molecular oxygen as the final acceptor?

(A) Obligate anaerobes
(B) Facultative anaerobes
(C) Obligate aerobes
(D) Strict anaerobes

9. Viruses are classified by all of the following EXCEPT

(A) structure of capsid
(B) type of nucleic acid
(C) oxygen requirements
(D) presence of lipid envelope

10. Protozoa are classified by

(A) shape
(B) cell wall type
(C) sexual reproductive structures
(D) mode of motility

Directions: Each question below contains four suggested answers, of which **one or more** is correct. Choose the answer

A	if **I, II, and III** are correct
B	if **I** and **III** are correct
C	if **II and IV** are correct
D	if **IV only** is correct

11. Gram-negative and gram-positive cell walls share which of the following characteristics?

I. Peptide cross-links between polysaccharides
II. Hydrolysis by lysozyme
III. Rigid polysaccharide framework
IV. A wide variety of complex lipids

12. A declining growth rate occurs during which of the following phases of bacterial cell growth?

I. Lag phase
II. Exponential phase
III. Stationary phase
IV. Death phase

13. The peptidoglycan backbone of a bacterial cell contains

I. tetrapeptide chains
II. *N*-acetylmuramic acid
III. teichoic acid
IV. *N*-acetylglucosamine

14. Entities that are acellular do not fit the classical definition of living things. They are

I. bacteria
II. viruses
III. fungi
IV. prions

15. Dimorphic fungi have

I. a yeast phase
II. a sexual phase
III. a mold phase
IV. basidium

ANSWERS AND EXPLANATIONS

1. The answer is D *[III C 1].*
The envelope is composed of the cytoplasmic membrane and the cell wall. The membrane is a diffusion barrier for large macromolecules; the cell wall of gram-positive bacteria is a thick layer of peptidoglycan with a large amount of teichoic acids (surface antigens). The gram-negative bacteria have only a small amount of peptidoglycan, no teichoic acid, and an outer membrane composed of lipoprotein and lipopolysaccharide, of which the polysaccharide comprises the O antigen.

2. The answer is A *[III B 3 b].*
Sex pili are found only on gram-negative organisms and in very small numbers (less than 10). They act as fragile transport tubes for DNA exchange. Common pili are adhesions.

3. The answer is A *[VI C 1].*
Of the three methods of DNA transfer, only transformation takes up DNA without an intermediary.

4. The answer is D *[III D 4, IV A1].*
Facultative organisms can grow without air and make either a fermentative or a respiratory set of enzymes, depending on the conditions.

5. The answer is B *[III C 4, V C 1].*
The chromosome carries all of the genes essential for growth, whereas plasmids are extrachromosomal, double-stranded, circular pieces of DNA that carry optional genes that add extra properties.

6. The answer is C *[III D 2, 3].*
Ribosomes are found in the cytoplasm, not in the nucleoid (a long, circular, double-stranded DNA without a nuclear membrane).

7. The answer is B *[IV C 1–3].*
Thermophiles grow at 55°C and are found in hot springs and compost piles. Mesophiles grow at approximately 37°C, psychrophiles grow at 15°C and lower, and auxotrophs are mutant organisms.

8. The answer is C *[IV D 1–2].*
Obligate aerobes require oxygen and lack an alternative fermentative pathway. Obligate anaerobes are strict anaerobes that cannot live in the presence of oxygen. Facultative anaerobes can use oxygen as the final acceptor or to provide an alternate fermentative pathway.

9. The answer is C *[I B 1].*
Viruses are classified by the structure of the capsid, the type and strandedness of the nucleic acid, the presence of a lipid envelope, and the presence of enzymes. Viruses do not generate their own energy, hence there is no need for oxygen. Viruses utilize the energy in the host cell.

10. The answer is D *[I A 2 b].*
Protozoa are unicellular, nonphotosynthetic eukaryotes that are classified by their mode of motility or lack of motility. The types of motility include flagella, cilia, and amoeboid movement.

11. The answer is B (I, III) *[III C 1].*
Peptidoglycan is the basic layer of the cell wall in both gram-positive and gram-negative organisms. It provides a rigid framework that is susceptible to the action of lysozyme. Gram-positive cells are deficient in lipids; however, gram-negative cells are rich in complex lipids (e.g., lipopolysaccharide). Both types of cell walls have cross-links between polysaccharides.

12. The answer is D (IV) *[IV E 1–4].*
During the lag phase, the cells prepare for growth, so there is no actual growth. Growth is maximal during the exponential phase and levels out during the stationary phase with no net increase in cell number. There is a decline in organism number during the death phase because there are more organisms dying than being produced.

13. The answer is C (II, IV) *[III C 1].*
The cell wall of both gram-positive and gram-negative organisms is composed of repeating disaccharide units. These units contain N-acetylglucosamine and N-acetylmuramic acid, to which tetrapeptide chains are cross-linked. Only gram-positive organisms have teichoic acid.

14. The answer is C (II, IV) *[I B 1–2].*
Viruses are basically proteins and nucleic acids, while prions are proteins, neither of which are cells. Bacteria are prokaryotic cells, and fungi are eukaryotic cells.

15. The answer is B (I, III) *[I A 2 a 1–4].*
Dimorphic fungi like *Blastomyces, Coccidioides,* and *Histoplasma* can be grown in either a yeast (unicellular) or mold (filamentous) phase, depending on the temperature of incubation. Fungi are placed in phyla based on the type of sexual reproduction observed: either ascus, basidium, or zygote. Fungi imperfecti consist of species without observable sexual reproductive structures.

10
Immunology
Gail Goodman-Snitkoff

I. THE PHYSIOLOGY OF THE IMMUNE SYSTEM

A. Immunogens, antigens, and haptens

1. **Immunogens** are chemical compounds that cause a specific immune response.

2. **Antigens** are chemical compounds that bind to products of an immune response. When the antigens are recognized by antibody or activated cells, they can be eliminated by a specific immune response.

3. **Immunogen–antigens.** Compounds associated with or secreted by parasitic bacteria, protozoa, fungi, and viruses, and of molecular weight (mol wt) greater than 5000 daltons may act as both immunogens and antigens.
   a. Molecular complexity is as important as molecular weight in determining the status of a compound as an immunogen. For a molecule to be immunogenic, it must contain protein or peptide. Therefore, proteins, glycoproteins, lipoproteins, and nucleoproteins are the most potent immunogen–antigens.
   b. Drugs of sufficient molecular weight (e.g., insulin) can act as immunogen–antigens. The cells of another individual and the cells of one's own body (see III) can act as immunogen–antigens. Immunogen–antigens can be contacted environmentally (e.g., pollens).

4. **Haptens** are low–molecular-weight compounds that act as immunogens after chemically complexing to a larger molecule or cell surface. After they stimulate the immune system in this complex, these compounds can act as antigens in the uncomplexed or complexed state.
   a. Haptens may be present in the environment (e.g., pentadecyl catechol of poison ivy).
   b. Several types of drugs act as haptens (e.g., penicillin).

5. **Tolerogens** are chemical compounds that elicit specific nonresponsiveness. This specific nonresponsiveness may be caused by the ability of the compound to be broken down by the body or by the route of administration of the compound (e.g., oral administration often causes specific nonresponsiveness).

6. In this chapter, the term antigen is used for compounds and cells that are both immunogens and antigens.

B. Cells of the immune system

1. **B lymphocytes and T lymphocytes** are the primary cells of specific immune responses. All B and T lymphocytes are antigen-specific because they have specific antigen receptors as part of their plasma membranes. In this chapter, the terms B cell and T cell are used instead of B lymphocyte and T lymphocyte.

2. **Antigen receptors of B cells** are antibody molecules.
   a. B cells have thousands of identical antibodies in their membranes that allow them to bind chemically to a small group of chemically related antigens. This group defines the antigen specificity of each B cell. Different B cells have different antigen specificities, but each B cell has only one specificity. B cells that recognize specific antigens divide to form new B cells **(memory B cells)** and **plasma cells (antibody-forming cells),** which secrete free, soluble (humoral) antibody molecules into extracellular fluids (Figure 10-1).
   b. Virgin B cells have never responded to an antigen since their release into the circulation from bone marrow. Their membrane antibodies are of the immunoglobulin M and D (IgM, IgD) classes (see I D).
   c. Memory B cells are derived by cell division from another B cell that has responded to an antigen. Their membrane antibodies are of immunoglobulin classes A, E, or G (IgA, IgE, IgG; see I D).

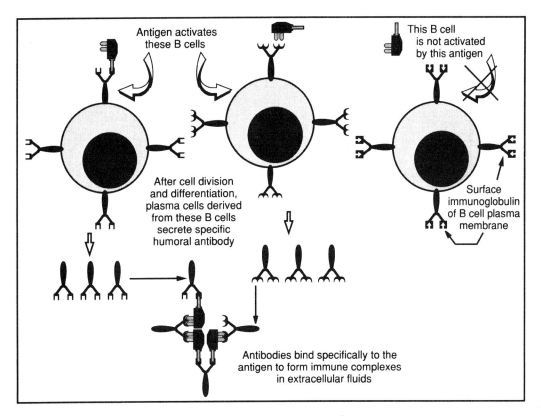

Figure 10-1. B cells: antigen specificity and activation.

3. **Antigen receptors of T cells** have two membrane proteins (α and β or γ and δ) that define the antigen specificity of each T cell and several other integral membrane proteins known as **CD3 complex.** Therefore, T cells are **CD3+.** Each T cell has thousands of identical antigen receptors in its membrane. Different T cells of different antigen specificities differ in the conformation of their antigen receptors.

   a. **Major histocompatibility complex (MHC) proteins.** The antigen receptors of T cells do not recognize antigens alone. Rather, they normally recognize **peptide epitopes** (fragments of antigen) that are chemically combined with MHC proteins on the surface of other body cells (Figure 10-2). MHC proteins are divided into **two major classes:**

     (1) **Class I proteins,** which are present on the surfaces of almost all body cells.

     (2) **Class II proteins,** which are present only on the surfaces of special **antigen-presenting cells (APCs).**

   b. **Thymus gland.** T cells do not enter the circulation directly from bone marrow, but first enter the thymus gland to mature. Most developing T cells die in the thymus. The cells that die either do not recognize normal self-antigens or produce a response against normal self-antigens.

     (1) T cells that are released from the thymus into the circulation are **virgin T cells.**

     (2) T cells that originate through cell division from the responses of other T cells are **memory T cells.**

   c. **Glycoproteins.** Most T cells can be classified by the presence of a membrane glycoprotein known as **CD4,** the **helper,** or **T_H cell,** or the presence of **CD8,** the **cytotoxic T lymphocyte (CTL)** or **T_c cell.**

     (1) **T_H cells** can be divided into two functional groups, **T_H1** and **T_H2.** These cells have different functions in the immune response. These cells regulate immune responses through the production of lymphokines, which are small proteins that act on other cells in an autocrine, paracrine, or endocrine manner.

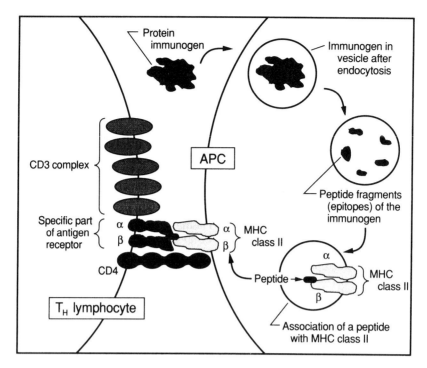

Figure 10-2. Helper T-cell antigen recognition.

        (a) T_H1 cells activate other cells, including some T_H cells, T_c cells, and macrophages. In addition, they can decrease antibody (Ab) production by inhibiting the formation of T_H2 cells.

        (b) T_H2 cells activate B cells to divide and produce Ab. They can also inhibit the formation of T_H1 cells.

    (2) T_c cells are able to kill cells that are infected by viruses. They do this through direct binding with the infected cell, or through the release of cytotoxins.

    (3) T_r cells have recently been described. Most of these cells are CD4+, although there is a CD8+ subset as well. All of these cells suppress immune responses through the secretion of IL-10 and TGF-β; in addition, cells designated CD4+CD25+ are also able to inhibit through direct contact.

    (4) Lymphokines are part of a larger network of regulatory **cytokines.** This network includes secretions of other cell types in addition to those of lymphocytes. Table 10-1 lists the sources and actions of important cytokines that regulate the immune system and inflammation.

4. Natural killer (NK) cells are large, granular lymphocytes without a specific T- or B-cell antigen receptor. Their cytotoxicity is similar to that of CTL cells. NK cells recognize and destroy tumors.

5. APCs are essential for most immune responses and are found in the sites at which these responses originate.

    a. The best understood APCs are the macrophages and **dendritic cells of the lymph nodes, spleen,** and **other lymphoid tissue.** Most immune responses within these organs begin when these cells present epitopes bound to their surface MHC class II molecules to T_H cells (see Figure 10-2) and secrete cytokines as accessory signals.

    b. Any cell in the body can act as an APC for immune responses involving CTL cells. Nucleated cells can present fragments of antigens bound to their surface MHC class I molecules to T_c (CD8) lymphocytes.

    c. Both T and B cells continually circulate from the blood through the lymph nodes, spleen, and other secondary lymphoid tissue and then back into the blood. If there is

Table 10-1. Major Cytokines and Their Actions

Cytokine	Sources of Secretion*	Major Actions
IL-1	Macrophages, antigen-presenting cells, others	T- and B-cell activation, pyrogenic, proinflammatory
TNF-α, TNF-β	Macrophages, T_H1, T_c	Similar to IL-1, but including cytotoxicity
IL-2	T_H0, T_H1	T-, B-, and natural killer (NK)-cell activation
IFN-γ	T_H1 cells	Induction of major histocompatibility complex (MHC), activation of macrophages and NK cells, formation of memory B cells, antiviral
IFN-α, IFN-β	Leukocytes, fibroblasts	Induction of MHC, antiviral and growth inhibition
IL-3	Macrophages, T_H cells	Proliferation of multilineage marrow stem cells
IL-4	T_H2 cells	B-cell activation and memory B-cell formation, increased mast cell precursors, activation of mast cells
IL-5	T_H2 cells	Memory B-cell formation, eosinophil production
IL-6	T_H2 cell, other types	Plasma cell maturation, others similar to IL-1
IL-7	Bone marrow stroma	Lymphocyte maturation
IL-8	T_H1 cells, macrophages, endothelial cells	Neutrophil activation
IL-9	T_H1 cells	Proliferation and differentiation of bone marrow cells and thymocytes
IL-10	Macrophages, T_H2 cells CD8$^+$ T cells, B cells	Increased humoral (antibody), decreased cell-mediated immunity, mast cell growth
IL-11	Bone marrow stroma	Proliferation and differentiation of bone marrow cells and thrombocytes
IL-12	Macrophages, B cells	Promotion of cell-mediated immunity, activation of TC and NK cells, suppression of humoral immunity
IL-13	T_H cells	IL-4–like effects on B cells, inhibition of production of inflammatory cytokines by monocytes
IL-14	T_H cells	Important for the generation of B memory cells
IL-15	Endothelial cells, epithelial monocytes, muscle cells	IL-2–like effects
GM-CSF	T_H1 cells, macrophages	Marrow proliferation of myeloid precursors
G-CSF	Fibroblasts, endothelial cells	Proliferation and survival of neutrophil precursors
M-CSF	Fibroblasts, endothelial cells	Survival of monocyte–macrophages

GM-CSF = granulocyte macrophage colony-stimulating factor; IFN = interferon; IL = interleukin; TNF = tumor necrosis factor.
*Not all sources are listed.

antigen present in the secondary lymphoid tissue, which binds specifically to the receptor on the T or B cell, then an immune response can begin.

6. **Neutrophils, macrophages, eosinophils, basophils, platelets,** and **mast cells** assist in eliminating antigens from the body. Their functions may be phagocytic, proinflammatory, cytotoxic, regulatory, or a combination of these.

C. Humoral immunity: primary and memory responses that produce antibodies

1. **Overview.** In most humoral immune responses, antigens are recognized by antigen-specific B cells and T_H cells (non–antigen-specific B and T_H cells do not respond). Initially, B and T_H^2 cells divide to increase their cell numbers. Responding B cells produce both **memory B cells** and **plasma cells,** aided by cytokines secreted by T_H^2 cells. **T-independent responses** to certain bacterial polysaccharide antigens do not require T_H cells. During T-independent responses, B cells respond alone and produce plasma cells that secrete IgM antibodies, but no memory B cells are produced.

2. **Primary immune response.** The first time a specific antigen is encountered, only **virgin B cells** and **virgin T_H cells** are present to respond to the antigen. Initially, these cells produce plasma cells that secrete IgM antibody. Later in the immune response, plasma cells producing

other classes of antibody develop. The primary immune response is detected in the serum after 4 days and peaks in 7–11 days. In a primary immune response, IgM is produced first and is followed by IgG. Memory B and T_H^2 cells are also produced. Memory B cells can also be activated to produce the other classes of antibody in subsequent immune responses.

3. **Memory immune responses.** The second or subsequent encounter with the same antigen or a closely related antigen produces responses by memory B cells and memory T_H^2 cells. These responses are more rapid because memory cells require less antigen for stimulation and are of greater magnitude because there are more antigen-specific B and T cells to respond. Most antibody produced is IgG, with smaller amounts of IgA and IgE. Significant amounts of antibodies are produced as rapidly as 2–3 days after the reencounter with antigen, and the absolute amount of antibody (measured in milligrams per deciliter of serum) is greater than in primary immune responses. The duration of memory varies among antigens and probably among individuals. Some, but not all, memory is lifelong.

4. **Major roles of antibodies**
   a. The first function of an antibody is to act as an **antigen receptor** for B cells so that the B cells can recognize and respond to antigens.
   b. The second function of an antibody is to aid in the **elimination of antigen.** Elimination occurs through nonspecific functions, such as phagocytosis or complement activation. The mechanism of elimination depends on the class of antibody involved.
   c. The third function of an antibody is **neutralization of toxins.** Neutralization occurs when an antibody binds to the toxin and prevents it from reaching the target organ.

D. **Immunoglobulins: antigen-binding and class-specific functions.** The terms antibody and immunoglobulin are used interchangeably.

1. **Structure.** The standard immunoglobulin unit has four polypeptide chains: two identical light polypeptide chains and two identical heavy polypeptide chains. The structure is represented as H_2L_2. Each chain can be divided into a **C-terminal constant** region and an **N-terminal variable region** of amino acids (Figure 10-3). The N-terminal variable region formed from the H and L variable domains is responsible for antigen binding by the immunoglobulin. The C-terminal constant regions of the H chain determine the class of the immunoglobulin.

2. **Class.** There are five general heavy-chain, constant-region amino acid sequences. These determine the **five general classes of immunoglobulins: IgM, IgG, IgE, IgA,** and **IgD.** Within some classes, variants of the heavy-chain sequence yield subclasses: IgM1, IgM2, IgG1-4, IgA1, and IgA2. The class of an immunoglobulin defines its nonspecific antigen elimination or inflammatory function. These functions are activated only after antigen-antibody complexes are formed, not by unbound antibodies.
   a. **IgM** is the first immunoglobulin secreted during primary immune responses. It plays a minor role in memory responses. It does not leave the blood in significant amounts because of its pentameric structure and large size (mol wt 900,000 daltons). It accounts for approximately 20% of the adult serum immunoglobulin. IgM is the most potent **activator of the complement system** (see I E 2). Its serum half-life is 9–11 days.
   b. **IgG** is the predominant immunoglobulin secreted at the end of the primary immune responses and during memory responses. It can diffuse from blood into other extracellular fluids, particularly in inflamed microvasculature, and it crosses the placenta to enter the fetal circulation. It accounts for approximately 70% of adult serum immunoglobulin. It **opsonizes antigens** for **phagocytosis and activates the complement system.** Its serum half-life is 25–35 days.
   c. **IgE** is secreted during memory responses and may also be secreted late during a primary response. It normally accounts for less than 1% of serum immunoglobulin. It **binds to IgE receptors located on the cell surfaces of blood basophils and on connective tissue mast cells** to trigger the secretion of inflammatory mediators from these cells in the presence of specific antigens. IgE mediates allergic reactions. Its serum half-life is 2–3 days, but its mast cell-bound half-life is several months to years.
   d. **IgA** is secreted during memory responses and may also be secreted late during a primary response. It accounts for 10% of serum immunoglobulin. It is **secreted across mucosal surfaces into gastrointestinal, respiratory, lachrymal, mammary, and genitourinary secretions, where it protects mucosa from colonization** by bacteria and other microorganisms. Its serum half-life is approximately 5 days.

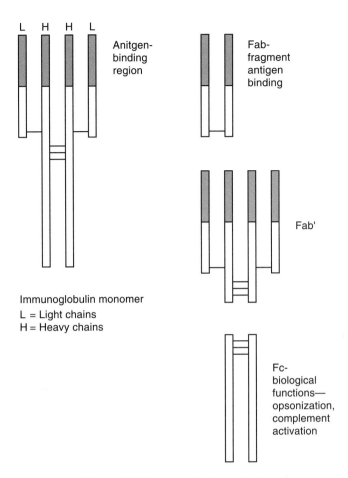

Figure 10-3. Immunoglobulin molecule.

    e. IgD accounts for less than 1% of serum immunoglobulin and has no known function as a secreted immunoglobulin.

3. Specificity. The specificity of each immunoglobulin for antigen binding resides in the two identical antigen-binding sites, each formed by the combination of the variable regions of heavy and light chains. Secreted IgM antibodies have 10 identical antigen-binding sites through the combination of five H_2L_2 units with a joining polypeptide chain to form a pentamer. Likewise, secreted IgA typically exists as a dimer with four binding sites.

4. Quantitation of immunoglobulin: antigen binding and cross-reactivity. 10^8 to 10^{11} unique immunoglobulins with different antigen-binding specificities are formed by the immune system.

    a. Each immunoglobulin specificity can bind to several different, but close structurally related, antigens. This ability illustrates the phenomenon of cross-reactivity of a single antibody for multiple antigens. Each immunoglobulin–antigen interaction is quantitated by its **association constant (K_a).**

    b. Cross-reactivity may also occur through the sharing of some, but not all, antigens by two strains of bacteria, viruses, or other microorganisms.

    c. Because each microorganism has several antigens, each elicits the production of multiple antibodies with unique specificities by the immune system. This response is known as a **polyclonal response** and results in a combination of antibodies known as a **polyclonal antiserum** and defines the serotype of the immunizing organism.

5. Fragments of immunoglobulin for clinical use. Immunoglobulins can be enzymatically cleaved into fragments [e.g., **Fab** and **F(ab')$_2$** (antigen-binding fragments), **Fc** (crystallizable fragment), **Fv** (variable region fragment)]. Fab and F(ab')$_2$ fragments are clinically useful because they retain antigen specificity, but not class-specific (e.g., inflammatory) functions, and are readily excreted renally. Conversely, this characteristic limits their effectiveness in certain situations.

E. Antigen elimination and acute inflammatory mechanisms of humoral immunity

1. **Opsonization** is the preparation of any extracellular antigen for phagocytosis through binding of antibody. Neutrophils and macrophages have a variety of receptors for the constant region of IgG antibodies, which bind antigen–antibody complexes. When the antigen is soluble, the immune complexes must be sufficiently large to induce this reaction. This binding triggers phagocytosis of the antigen–antibody complex and activates the metabolism of the phagocyte, shifting it toward the production of bactericidal oxygen radicals (e.g., superoxide anion, hydrogen peroxide).

2. **Complement** is a group of approximately 20 serum proteins that, when activated, form a proteolytic cascade similar to the clotting and fibrinolytic sequence. Within this complex of proteins, there are some that inhibit complement activation. Complement is responsible for increasing the inflammatory response, phagocytosis of antigen, lysis of cells (usually pathogens), and clearance of immune complexes.

   a. In the **classic activation pathway,** immune complexes of IgM or IgG antibodies bind subunits of complement component 1 (C1) and trigger an initial series of proteolytic cleavages.

   b. In the **alternative activation pathway,** the cell walls of certain microorganisms (e.g., gram-negative bacteria) are able to bind C3b and other complement proteins that initiate a different sequence of proteolytic cleavages, leading to the same end point as the classic activation pathway.

   c. In the **mannose-binding pathway,** mannose-binding protein (MBP) is produced by the liver during the acute-phase response. MBP binds to mannose on the surface of bacteria and in conjunction with associated serum-proteases triggers proteolytic cleavages identical to those seen in the classic pathway of complement.

   d. Certain complement proteins provide opsonization in addition to that provided by IgG in immune complexes.

   e. **Proinflammatory fragments** of certain complement proteins act both by **direct activity on the microvasculature,** promoting arteriole dilation and increased vascular permeability, and by triggering the release of histamine and other proinflammatory mediators from mast cells and basophils.

   f. A complex of complement proteins known as **the membrane attack complex (MAC)** can insert into any lipid bilayer membrane, forming a large channel through which ions and water diffuse. Many bacteria, enveloped viruses, and some human or mammalian cells are subject to this osmotic lysis.

3. **Circulating basophils and connective tissue mast cells** are mainly proinflammatory cells that rapidly initiate acute inflammation. Triggers of secretion include mechanical and thermal trauma and immunologic triggers, complement and IgE.

   a. **IgE antibodies,** regardless of antigen specificity, equilibrate between serum and binding noncovalently to high-affinity IgE receptors on mast cell and basophil surfaces. This activity arms the mast cells and basophils, but the triggering of secretion requires that antigen bind to and cross-link antigen-specific IgE molecules already affixed to their receptors.

   b. Mast cells and basophils, when triggered, immediately secrete the contents of their storage granules, including histamine, proteases, and chemotactic proteins for neutrophils and eosinophils. In addition, activation of phospholipase A$_2$ releases arachidonic acid from membrane phospholipids and results in the synthesis of various leukotrienes, prostaglandins, and thromboxanes. The primary effects of these mediators are:

      (1) Vascular dilation

      (2) Increased vascular permeability

      (3) Contraction of respiratory and gastrointestinal smooth muscle

      (4) Neutrophil and eosinophil chemotaxis

4. **Antibody-dependent cell-mediated cytotoxicity** is mediated by cells with cytotoxic potential as well as receptors for IgG. These cells, NK cells, macrophages, and some T$_c$ cells, bind to and lyse target cells coated with IgG.

5. Acute inflammation causes increased ease of movement of crucial components of the blood into the tissues, including phagocytes, particularly neutrophils, IgG antibodies, complement, clotting proteins, and kinins. The adaptive result is the isolation and removal of invading microorganisms and necrotic tissues, followed by tissue repair and regeneration.

F. Cell-mediated immune responses **(cell-mediated immunity)** are those in which **antibody is not involved in the elimination of antigen.**

1. **Nonviral intracellular parasites** of macrophages, such as *Mycobacteria, Listeria,* and certain protozoa, are primarily eliminated by T-cell–macrophage immunity. CD4$^+$ T$_H$1 cells recognize infected macrophages and secrete lymphokines, particularly interferon-γ (IFN-γ). These lymphokines activate macrophages to produce more bactericidal oxygen radicals (e.g., superoxide anion, hydrogen peroxide) and to also increase the secretory function of the macrophages and inhibit phagocytosis, enabling the macrophages to kill the parasites in the **extracellular** environment.

2. **Viruses** must be eliminated from both extracellular sites and infected cells.
   a. **Antibodies** opsonize virus particles in blood and tissue fluids for phagocytosis, but antibodies are generally ineffective against infected cells.
   b. **CTL cells** recognize infected cells and directly kill them in an antigen-specific manner, secreting lymphokines, such as tumor-necrosis factor-β (TNF-β). Often, the cells are killed before infectious virus particles are assembled. When killed cells release infectious viral particles, they may be opsonized by an antibody. Cell-mediated immunity and humoral immunity must function in concert to provide optimal antiviral defenses.
   c. **NK cells** are believed to kill infected (and tumor) cells in a non–antigen-specific manner.
   d. **IFN-γ,** secreted by CTL, NK, and T$_H$1 cells, and **IFN-α** and **IFN-β,** secreted by macrophages and other cells, provide additional antiviral immunity by binding to receptors on other cells and inducing synthesis of kinases and endonucleases (i.e., antiviral proteins) that inhibit viral and cellular growth. Interferons also upregulate MHC proteins, which make infected cells more visible to CTL cells.

3. **Tumors** are modified host cells and must be eliminated by the immune system, usually by cell-mediated immunity.
   a. **NK cells** are primarily responsible for killing tumor cells. They may act by recognizing changes in cell-surface proteins or by **antibody-dependent cell-mediated cytotoxicity.**
   b. **CTL cells** recognize tumor cells in an antigen-specific manner and kill them by secreting lymphokines, such as TNF-β, and by inducing apoptosis through the binding of FAS and FAS-ligand.
   c. **Macrophages** also kill tumor cells in a nonspecific manner through the release of TNF-α.

4. **Graft rejection** (see V)

II. HYPERSENSITIVITY REACTIONS are **exaggerated, inappropriate, or prolonged immune responses that cause damage to otherwise normal tissue** (Figure 10-4). Four types of hypersensitivity reactions are recognized, primarily on the basis of the mechanisms of pathogenesis. Many different diseases are included within each type. **Allergens** are broadly defined as antigens or haptens that induce hypersensitivity reactions.

A. IgE-mediated type I hypersensitivity reaction (immediate hypersensitivity)

1. A type I hypersensitivity reaction is caused by **inappropriate production and hypersecretion of IgE** to specific allergens, plus auxiliary factors such as increased mucosal permeability to allergens (e.g., SO$_2$, NO$_2$, diesel fumes). The **tendency to hypersecrete IgE is inheritable;** a child's probability of being a hypersecretor is 50% with one hypersecretor parent and 75% with two hypersecretor parents. These individuals are considered to be atopic.
   a. IgE is produced locally following nonsystemic exposure to an antigen.
      (1) In normosecretors (1–10 μg/dl), arming of local mast cells occurs (see I B 6).
      (2) In hypersecretors (typically 100 μg–1 mg/dl), IgE spillover occurs, arming basophils and nonlocal mast cells and causing increased occupancy of mast cell and basophil IgE receptors by IgE.
   b. Because there is a lag period for IgE synthesis and cell arming, a type I reaction usually does not occur on the first (or first seasonal) exposure to a specific allergen.

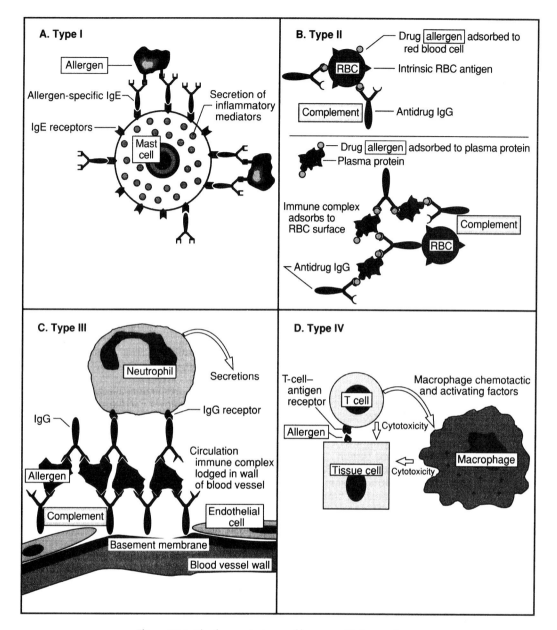

Figure 10-4. The four main types of hypersensitivity reactions.

2. **Common allergens**
    a. **Respiratory allergens** include pollens of various plants (e.g., ragweed, grasses, trees), fungi, animal fur, carpet mites, and other shed allergens.
    b. **Gastrointestinal allergens** include dairy products, shellfish, soybeans, and peanuts.
    c. **Skin and mouth allergens** include topically applied drugs (e.g., procaine).
    d. **Intravenous allergens** include insect venoms and drugs that act as cell or plasma protein-bound haptens (e.g., penicillin, cephalosporins, vaccines). These drugs may cause type II or III hypersensitivity reactions in people who do not hypersecrete IgE in response to these drugs.

3. **Activation of mast cell and basophil secretion** by an allergen requires two or more receptor-bound IgE molecules to be cross-linked by a specific allergen. Hapten-sized drugs that provoke

this reaction both sensitize the immune system and trigger mast cells when the drug is bound to a larger molecule (e.g., a protein). Activation leads to a transient increase in the cyclic adenosine monophosphate (cAMP) level, followed by an increase in the level of cyclic guanosine monophosphate (cGMP) relative to cAMP. This is followed by phospholipase C producing second messengers which lead to a rapid increase in cytoplasmic calcium ions (Ca^{++}). With the increase in cytoplasmic Ca^{++}, there is immediate fusion of vesicles containing inflammatory mediators with the cell membrane and release of these mediators into the extracellular milieu. In addition, phospholipase A2 is activated, and this further activates the local inflammatory response. Prolonged increases in cAMP levels inhibit mast cell activation. Additionally, an increase in cytoplasmic calcium ion (cytoplasmic Ca^{++}) occurs, probably as a result of the second messengers produced by phospholipase C. Immediate secretion of stored inflammatory mediators and activation of phospholipase A_2 follow activation of the mast cell.

4. **Effects of mediators secreted from mast cells and basophils**
   a. Vasodilation and increased capillary permeability are caused by histamine; the leukotrienes C4, D4, and E4; and prostaglandin D_2 (PGD_2) secreted by mast cells.
   b. Gastrointestinal and respiratory smooth muscle constriction is caused primarily by the leukotrienes C4, D4, and E4; PGD_2; and platelet-activating factor secreted by mast cells and other leukocytes.
   c. Eosinophil and neutrophil infiltration is caused by chemotactic factors secreted by mast cells.

5. **Local symptoms of pathogenesis** include inflammation of the upper (rhinitis) and lower respiratory tract (asthma), gastrointestinal tract, and skin.
   a. Common clinical symptoms include urticaria, pruritus (itching), nasal congestion, bronchoconstriction, mucus and lachrymal hypersecretion, laryngeal edema, vomiting, and diarrhea.
   b. Symptoms may be confined to the portal of allergen entry (e.g., respiratory allergen: respiratory symptoms) or may be more widespread as a result of allergen spillover into the circulation (e.g., food allergen: gastrointestinal, skin, respiratory symptoms).
   c. **Atopic dermatitis** typically includes severe pruritic dermatitis, rhinitis or asthma, food allergies, and changes in the cell-mediated immune system.
   d. The local introduction of allergen sometimes leads to anaphylaxis.
   e. Approximately 50% of patients with asthma hypersecrete IgE. This tendency is probably contributory, but ancillary, to the underlying bronchial hyperreactivity present in these patients (see Chapter 48).

6. **Systemic anaphylactic manifestations of pathogenesis.** In sensitized individuals, intravenous injection of an allergen (e.g., bee venom) or absorption across the mucous membranes (e.g., peanuts) can cause systemic edemic and hypovolemic shock, with cardiac arrhythmia, asphyxiation as a result of bronchoconstriction and mucous hypersecretion, and urticaria. Death usually occurs because of asphyxiation. While other sensitized individuals may have only mild local symptoms upon encountering the allergen, these results demonstrate differing host responses to identical proteins.

7. **Time course.** Immediate hypersensitivity reactions have two phases. The **early reaction,** resulting from mediator secretion by mast cells, begins within 1–2 minutes after allergen contact and peaks within 1–2 hours. The **late-phase reaction** begins 3–12 hours after contact with the allergen and lasts for several hours. The late-phase reactions are initiated by products of the early phase, but the late-phase reaction is characterized by increased numbers of eosinophils and is maintained by the products of these cells.

8. **Diagnosis.** In scratch tests, a variety of allergens are injected intradermally to screen for the presence of a wheal and flare (i.e., edema and erythema) response in the skin. **Radioallergenosorbent (RAST)** and **radioimmunosorbent (RIST) assays** use radiolabeled reagents to detect serum IgE concentrations. The results of these assays do not always agree with each other or with clinical manifestations of type I hypersensitivity.

9. **Prophylaxis**
   a. Identifying and avoiding allergens is the most important form of prophylaxis.
   b. **Hyposensitization (desensitization)** is performed by injecting weekly, increasing doses of allergen intramuscularly to elicit an allergen-specific IgG response and decrease the allergen-specific IgE. Once desensitization has been achieved, monthly injections are used to maintain the IgG levels. IgG is able to bind to the allergen and inhibit its binding to the mast-cell bound IgE.

10. Therapy

a. Competitive H_1 antagonists of histamine are useful in local forms, but do not completely reverse the inflammation, because histamine is not the only inflammatory mediator in the reaction. Competitive H_1 antagonists have little effect on anaphylaxis.

b. Epinephrine reverses anaphylaxis through its α-agonist and β-agonist effects. Patients with systemic allergies are given epinephrine self-administration kits. β_2-agonists (e.g., albuterol) are able to promote bronchodilation, and α_1-agonists (e.g., phenylpropanolamine) decrease nasal congestion.

c. Cromolyn sodium (cromoglycate) is a locally administered inhibitor of mast cell degranulation. **Glucocorticoids** are able to block the late phase of the reaction, but are less effective during the early phase. **Anti-leukotriene therapies** are also able to block the late phase of the reaction.

d. Topical steroids inhibit inflammation and immune responses. Topical application via spray or inhaler limits the side effects seen when glucocorticoids are administered systemically. In addition to using topical steroids alone, they are also combined with long-acting β_2-agonists as therapy for asthma.

B. Non–IgE-mediated type I hypersensitivity reactions. These reactions are probably due to several poorly understood causes and are sometimes called **anaphylactoid reactions.** The following factors may contribute to and exacerbate non–IgE-mediated type I reactions.

1. Respiratory β_2-receptor unresponsiveness, which leads to a diminished bronchodilatory effect of the sympathetic nervous system.

2. Hyperreactivity of mast cells through H_2-receptor unresponsiveness. This decreases the negative feedback of histamine on the activation of mast cells.

C. Type II hypersensitivity reactions

1. Pathogenesis. Antibody-mediated cytotoxicity occurs through the production of IgM or IgG. These antibodies are able to bind to specific allergens located on cell surfaces.

a. These allergens may be intrinsic to the cell (i.e., natural cell-surface components) or extrinsic compounds (i.e., drugs) adsorbed to the cell surface.

b. Cytotoxicity may result from activation of complement, phagocytosis of the IgG opsonized cell, or both.

c. A third cytotoxic mechanism, known as antibody-dependent, cell-mediated cytotoxicity, involves the direct killing of antibody-coated cells by macrophages, eosinophils, or NK cells.

d. Type II reactions may exhibit anaphylactic signs and symptoms if enough complement is activated; however, they usually do not progress to this stage.

2. Common allergens. Type II allergens are diverse. It is the pathogenic mechanism that is common to all the reactions.

a. Foreign blood surface antigens may act as allergens to produce **transfusion mismatches** or **Rh disease.**

b. Drug allergens (or drug metabolite allergens) acting as haptens are the **leading cause of hemolytic anemia.**

(1) These allergens may directly adsorb to cell surfaces and be specifically bound by antibodies (e.g., penicillins, cephalosporins, quinidine).

(2) Alternately, they may form serum-phase immune complexes, which adsorb nonspecifically to blood cell surfaces. This makes the cell susceptible to lysis due to the "innocent bystander" effect (e.g., rifampin, sulfonamides, chlorpromazine).

c. Self-antigens are the allergen in certain autoimmune diseases (e.g. Hashimoto's thyroiditis, myasthenia gravis, autoimmune hemolytic anemia; see III) Autoimmune hemolytic anemia is sometimes associated with administration of α-methyldopa, which induces autoantibodies against the red blood cell surface.

d. Hyperacute rejection of transplanted tissue (see V)

3. Chemical mediators. Complement proteins produce cytotoxicity and inflammation, which stimulate **macrophages and granulocytes** to secrete cytokines and enzymes, which in turn enhance inflammation.

4. Clinical symptoms depend on the type of antigen/allergen involved (see II C 2). Hemolytic anemia and thrombocytopenia are the major clinical signs of type II hypersensitivity reactions. In hyperacute graft rejection, the transplanted tissue does not successfully perfuse because of antibody-mediated cytotoxicity to the transplanted vasculature.

5. **Time course**
   a. In the first sensitization to a drug allergen, the blood cell lysis and inflammation begin 7–10 days after initiation of drug therapy. The second exposure to the drug causes symptoms within 3 days.
   b. **Transfusion mismatch.** Hemolysis begins 1–2 hours after transfusion. Peak effects occur after approximately 12 hours.
   c. **Rh disease** does not occur in the first RhD+ pregnancy of an RhD− mother. Maternal IgG is produced in the second and subsequent pregnancies following transplacental maternal sensitization to the RhD+ fetal red blood cells. This sensitization usually takes place in the third trimester. Maternal anti-RhD IgG crosses the placenta, binds to the fetal red blood cells, and activates the fetal complement system prenatally, which leads to perinatal hemolytic anemia.

6. **Prophylaxis and therapy.** In drug-induced hypersensitivity reactions, withdrawing the drug usually reverses the lysis. Preventing recontact is the best prophylaxis. In Rh disease, anti-RhD is administered during pregnancy and within 72 hours postpartum for each Rh+ pregnancy. The simplest explanation for the efficacy of anti-RhD is that this passive immunization (see V I B) binds to fetal red blood cells in the maternal circulation and prevents sensitization of the maternal immune system.

D. **Type III hypersensitivity reactions** involve the persistence of immune complexes in the circulation or at local tissue sites when they are not removed following production of specific antibodies and antigen–antibody complexes. The subtypes of type III hypersensitivity reactions have diverse causes, and only the pathogenic mechanism is common to them all.

1. **Pathogenesis.** Immune complexes activate complement, cause inflammation, and induce positive chemotaxis in neutrophils. Persistence of immune complexes may be caused by:
   a. A **high concentration of antigen or antibody,** which leads to a disparity in the molar ratio of antigen to antibody.
   b. **Chronic formation of immune complexes** in the circulation as a result of **persistence of antigen.**
   c. Other factors, which cause insoluble immune complexes to form and precipitate intravascularly or on basement membranes.

2. **Common allergens**
   a. **Self-antigens in most non–organ-specific** (rheumatologic) **autoimmune disorders** (e.g., systemic lupus erythematosus, rheumatoid arthritis).
   b. **Bacterial or protozoan antigens in persistent or chronic infections** and in the initial stages of viremia for certain viral infections [e.g., prodrome of hepatitis B virus (HBV) infection].
   c. **Drugs** (e.g., penicillin, sulfonamides, thiouracil).
   d. **Antisera** from another species (e.g., horse), can cause serum sickness when used for passive immunization.
   e. **Fungal and bacterial spores** in the local respiratory form of the reaction.

3. **Chemical mediators. Complement proteins** cause inflammation and **stimulate mast cell and basophil secretions,** which enhance inflammation. The increased vascular permeability allows immune complexes to leave the circulation and attach to basement membranes, which underlay the endothelial lining of blood vessels. The kidney glomerulus and certain small arteries are particularly susceptible. Complement and mast cell proteins attract neutrophils; these cells can phagocytize immune complexes and release enzymes that damage local tissue, thus intensifying inflammation. In addition, platelet aggregation and microthrombus formation may occur.

4. **Clinical symptoms** depend on the severity and systemic or local nature of immune complex deposition and persistence.
   a. The first symptoms of systemic reactions are lymphadenopathy, splenomegaly, fever, and rash. These are common in drug-induced and viremia-induced type III hypersensitivity reactions.
   b. More serious symptoms include vasculitis and glomerulonephritis, both of which may become necrotizing. These symptoms often occur with systemic lupus erythematosus (SLE). Arthralgia and arthritis occur in both systemic and local reactions.

    c. The most common types of local type III hypersensitivity reactions are pneumonitis to inhaled fungi and bacteria to which the patient is occupationally exposed (e.g., moldy hay in **farmer's lung**) and reactions to spores borne in aerosol microdroplets from dirty ultrasonic humidifiers (e.g., **humidifier lung**). The etiology of these diseases is not completely understood, but both IgE and IgG are involved. IgE causes the initial inflammation and trapping of antigen, and IgG is responsible for the long-term effects. Symptoms include:
      (1) Nasal congestion and bronchoconstriction
      (2) Joint pain and inflammation of rheumatoid arthritis caused by joint-localized immune complexes involving rheumatoid factor and neutrophil phagocytosis (see Chapter 49)

5. Time course
    a. Systemic. In patients with no prior exposure to the allergen, the symptoms appear in 1–2 weeks (possibly longer) after exposure. In patients with preexisting antibodies, symptoms appear within several hours to 1 day after exposure. Severe symptoms, such as glomerulonephritis, usually require 2 or more weeks to appear.
    b. Local. In patients with preexisting antibodies, hypersensitivity pneumonitis symptoms appear 6–8 hours after exposure to the antigen.

6. Prophylaxis and therapy. In drug-induced reactions, **withdrawing the drug** usually reverses the reaction. Treatment includes antihistamines or corticosteroids. Transient infectious forms resolve spontaneously as immune complexes are removed by phagocytes.

E. Type IV hypersensitivity reactions

1. Pathogenesis. Type IV reactions include prolonged inappropriate and appropriate immune responses mediated by antigen-specific T_H1 cells in concert with activated macrophages. The T_H1 cells infiltrate tissues in which the antigen is presented and recruit and activate macrophages. The release of enzymes and cytokines by these cells results in inflammation and disruption of tissue structure in the absence of antibody.
    a. Reactions to infections involve a T_H1 response against specific intracellular bacterial and protozoan parasites (e.g., *Mycobacteria*). When the response is prolonged and ineffective, granuloma formation will occur.
    b. Contact dermatitis is an inappropriate skin reaction to haptens (e.g., pentadecyl catechols of poison ivy), which bind to epidermal cell surfaces and elicit a T_H1 cell response.
    c. Tuberculin reaction is observed in the dermis and is an appropriate reaction to mycobacterial antigens. This reaction indicates a state of active T_H1 immunity (due to an active infection) or T-cell memory to the organism. (In patients who had a positive tuberculin reaction, a subsequent negative reaction would indicate immunologic anergy or unresponsiveness).

2. Common allergens
    a. Infectious allergens include *Mycobacterium tuberculosis, M. leprae, Listeria monocytogenes,* trypanosomes, and viruses.
    b. Hapten allergens, such as pentadecyl catechols from poison ivy, poison oak, chromates, nickel ions (leached from watch backs and other jewelry), acrylates, hair dyes that contain p-phenylene diamine, para-aminobenzoic acid, and certain antibiotic ointments (e.g., topical neomycin), may induce **contact dermatitis.**
    c. Antigens that induce a tuberculin reaction include purified protein derivative (PPD), tuberculin (Mantoux reaction), Candida, mumps, and other antigens from microorganisms.

3. Chemical mediators are important in type IV reactions. These mediators are cytokines produced by activated T_H1 cells. These cytokines attract and activate macrophages to the site(s) where the pathogen/allergen is located. In turn, the activated macrophages secrete cytokines, which are responsible for inflammation and cytotoxicity (TNF).

4. Clinical symptoms depend on the subtype of reaction.
    a. Granulomas are local aggregations of T cells, macrophages, and giant epithelioid cells (derived from fusion of activated macrophages). They occur at sites of chronic infection and serve to restrict the spread of the infection.
    b. In contact sensitivity, cellular infiltration of the epidermis by T cells and macrophages produces microvesicle formation with spongiosis.
    c. Tuberculin tests cause erythema and induration as a result of cellular infiltration of the dermis, but no epidermal spongiosis is observed.

5. **Time course**
   a. Granulomas form at various times after the onset of a chronic immune response, but generally require a minimum of 2 weeks.
   b. Contact sensitivity may not occur with the first transient exposure. However, in a sensitized individual, skin inflammation will appear 12–24 hours after contact with the antigen and peaks between 24 and 48 hours after exposure.
   c. Tuberculin reactions follow the same time course as contact sensitivity. This reaction is often called **delayed cutaneous hypersensitivity,** or delayed-type hypersensitivity.

6. **Prophylaxis and therapy.** Treatment of granulomas depends on the organism involved. Proper treatment to resolve the infection will also aid in resolving the chronic immune response. For contact sensitivity, it is important to identify the antigen/allergen involved. Removal and avoidance of the allergen is important for prophylaxis. For treatment, topical corticosteroids suppress T-cell and macrophage function. In severe cases, oral corticosteroid therapy may be required.

III. **AUTOIMMUNITY** is a tissue-damaging immune response directed specifically and inappropriately against one or more self-antigens.

A. The **etiology** of autoreactive immune responses is not generally known and probably involves several deregulations in the control networks that normally prevent development of autoimmune disease. These deregulations may include aberrant regulation of T_H and T_c cells, cross-reactivity with antigens from microorganisms, loss of self-tolerance or failure to develop tolerance, and aberrant presentation of self-antigen on specific HLA molecules.

B. **Epidemiology**

1. **Familial clustering** is evident for many, if not most, autoimmune reactions representing a complex inherited predisposition toward autoimmunity. In most cases, this predisposition is associated with specific MHC types (e.g., rheumatoid arthritis with the MHC class II molecule HLA-DR4).

2. These reactions are more common in women. The female-to-male ratio in myasthenia gravis is approximately 2:1 and in SLE is approximately 10:1. In contrast, Sjögren's disease and Goodpasture's syndrome are more common in men than in women.

C. **Pathogenesis**

1. **Overview.** In a specific autoimmune disorder, the primary pathogenic mechanism may be humoral (mediated by antibodies with or without a contribution by complement), T-cell mediated, or involve both humoral and cell-mediated components. These diseases are commonly associated with exacerbation and remission of the disease.

2. **Environmental factors** are thought to contribute to pathogenesis. However, specific associations have been found in only a few cases; these include *Streptococcus* group A pharyngitis and rheumatic fever, exposure to organic solvents and Goodpasture's syndrome, ultraviolet irradiation, and SLE. It is likely that environmental factors act in concert with genetic predisposition to induce disease.

3. **Organ-specific and systemic (non–organ-specific) disorders**
   a. **Organ-specific disorders** (e.g., antithyroid autoimmunity) are limited to and directed specifically against self-antigen in a single organ. Lesions and clinical symptoms are limited primarily to that organ. Cellular damage may be mediated through antibody-mediated and complement-mediated cytotoxicity (type II hypersensitivity) and/or through cell-mediated cytotoxicity (type IV hypersensitivity).
   b. **Systemic disorders** (e.g., SLE)
      (1) These disorders are also known as connective tissue, collagen vascular, or rheumatologic disorders. Autoantibodies are formed against antigens found in most or all tissues, especially those located in the nuclei of cells and containing DNA, RNA, or nuclear-associated proteins (**antinuclear antibodies**). Pathologic changes occur systematically, primarily in the connective tissue and are at least partially caused by type III hypersensitivity reactions. Symptoms may be seen in the blood vessels, kidney glomerula, skin, joints, and serous membranes.

(2) Non–organ-specific disorders are sometimes difficult to distinguish from one another because of the similarities in autoantigens and pathogenesis. For example, most patients with SLE have circulating antinuclear antibodies; however, these also occur in 50%–65% of patients with Sjögren's syndrome and rheumatoid arthritis, as well as in a small percentage of clinically normal individuals. By contrast, rheumatoid factor (anti-IgG) is seen in 75%–90% of patients with rheumatoid arthritis or Sjögren's syndrome, and also in 35% of patients with SLE. The synovitis of rheumatoid arthritis is often a clinical finding in SLE, and the vasculitis of SLE is found in rheumatoid arthritis (Chapter 49).

D. Organ-specific autoimmunities

1. **Rheumatic fever** is not technically an autoimmune response because antibodies are produced against group A streptococci and cross-react with cardiac muscle fibers that are damaged by complement. Increased risk is related to a strong immune response to streptococcal M antigen.

2. **Antithyroid autoimmunities** (see Chapter 52). Aspects of several subtypes may occur in the same patient. Increased risk is associated with MHC class II types DR3 and DR5.
   a. **Primary autoimmune myxedema.** Antibodies against the thyroid-stimulating hormone (TSH) receptor on thyroid follicle cells act as antagonists to the stimulation of growth of the follicle cells normally provoked by TSH. The result is thyroid atrophy with hypothyroidism.
   b. **Hashimoto's thyroiditis.** Antibodies against thyroid peroxidase on follicle cells cause cytotoxicity and inflammation through the activation of complement. Antibodies against thyroglobulin (colloid) also may be present. Cell-mediated immunity may cause some cytotoxic damage. The resulting hypothyroidism is treated with synthetic thyroid hormone.
   c. **Graves' disease.** Antibodies act as agonists of TSH, binding to the TSH receptor and stimulating hypersecretion of thyroid hormone [thyroid-stimulating immunoglobulins (TSIs)]. The result is hyperthyroidism, which is treated by antithyroid drugs (e.g., propylthiouracil) or thyroid ablation with surgery or radiation.

3. **Myasthenia gravis**
   a. **Pathogenesis.** Antibodies against the nicotinic acetylcholine receptor on skeletal muscle plasma membrane at neuromuscular junctions act as competitive antagonists of **acetylcholine** binding. This activity causes weakness and fatigue in skeletal muscles. In addition to this direct blockage of neuromuscular transmission, down regulation of receptors and complement damage to muscle fibers occur. Many patients have swallowing and respiratory muscle dysfunction that may be caused by penicillamine therapy. Increased risk is associated with MHC class I type B8.
   b. **Therapy.** Anticholinesterase therapy (e.g., neostigmine) increases acetylcholine synaptic concentrations (preservation of endogenous acetylcholine). Immunosuppression with corticosteroids is used in severe cases; plasmapheresis to remove autoreactive antibodies from the blood is also helpful. Thymectomy helps many patients.

4. **Autoimmune pernicious anemia**
   a. **Pathogenesis.** Antibodies against intrinsic factor are secreted into the stomach lumen, where they inhibit the association of intrinsic factor with vitamin B_{12}. Thus, the absorption of vitamin B_{12} is decreased. This condition also can result from antibodies against gastrin receptors on parietal cells of the stomach mucosa that block stimulation of the cells by gastrin and decrease their secretion of intrinsic factor.
   b. **Therapy** is intramuscular injection of cyanocobalamin or oral administration of concentrated intrinsic factor preparations.

5. **Goodpasture's syndrome**
   a. **Pathogenesis.** Antibodies against **glomerular capillary basement membrane (GBM)** activate complement- and neutrophil-mediated damage. This activation leads to glomerulonephritis, with rapid deterioration of renal function. These antibodies cross-react with pulmonary capillary basement membrane, producing pulmonary hemorrhage. Increased risk is associated with MHC class II type DR2.
   b. **Therapy.** Immunosuppressive therapy includes corticosteroids, with plasmapheresis to remove autoreactive antibodies.

6. **Autoimmune hemolytic anemia (red blood cell), thrombocytopenia (platelet), neutropenia (neutrophil), and lymphopenia (lymphocyte)**
   a. **Pathogenesis.** Antibodies against membrane antigens of one or more of the indicated cell types may activate complement and opsonize the cells for rapid splenic phagocytosis. It may also occur as part of the spectrum of autoimmunity in non–organ-specific disorders, particularly SLE. These autoimmune varieties must be distinguished from those precipitated by responses to external antigens (e.g., drugs) but the clinical effects are similar.
   b. **Therapy.** These disorders are often acute and self-limiting, but therapy is required when they are chronic. In adults, treatment begins with corticosteroids. Additional options are cyclophosphamide, chlorambucil, and intravenous immune globulin (IVIG).

7. **Insulin-dependent diabetes mellitus (IDDM)** (see Chapter 51). Progressive and ultimately complete destruction of pancreatic B-islet cells occurs in diabetes. Although they are predictively useful, antibodies against insulin and surface cytoplasmic antigens of the B-islet cell are present before clinical onset. The main cytotoxic mechanisms appear to be mediated by T cells and macrophages. This view is supported by the beneficial effects of cyclosporine therapy in patients with early-stage IDDM at levels that have little effect on antibody production. Increased risk is associated with MHC class II types DR3 and DR4.

8. **Multiple sclerosis (MS)**
   a. **Pathogenesis.** T cells and macrophages, which are thought to be cytocidal for oligodendrocytes, infiltrate the central nervous system (CNS) and **attack the basic protein of myelin** as an autoantigen. The immunologic component may be secondary to other, unknown initiating agents. **CNS demyelination with sclerotic plaques** leads to spasticity. Increased risk is associated with MHC class II type DR2. Guillain-Barré syndrome is a related condition that involves peripheral nervous system (PNS) demyelination that, unlike MS, can be acute.
   b. **Therapy.** Spasticity is treated with **baclofen** with variable effectiveness. The peripheral skeletal muscle relaxant **dantrolene** is effective in some patients. **Adrenocorticotropic hormone (ACTH),** rather than corticosteroids, is the favored immunosuppressive therapy. Recombinant IFN-β 1b (Betaseron) IFNβ-1a and glatiramer acetate are approved by the United State Food and Drug Administration (FDA) as a treatment for MS.

E. **Non–organ-specific autoimmunities.** The similarities and differences in this class of disorders are shown by a comparison of Sjögren's syndrome and SLE. Rheumatoid arthritis is discussed in Chapter 48.

1. **Sjögren's syndrome**
   a. **Diagnosis** is usually based on lymphocytic infiltration and the presence of autoantibodies against salivary gland antigens and exocrine glands of the eyes, gastrointestinal and respiratory systems, and vagina. Hypergammaglobulinemia (50%) as a result of hyperactive B cells, antinuclear antibodies (50%–65%), and rheumatoid factors (anti-IgG; 75%–90%) are present in the indicated percentages of patients.
   b. **Pathogenesis.** Primary symptoms include **inhibition of exocrine gland secretion,** with dryness of the eyes, mouth, and gastrointestinal, respiratory, and vaginal mucous membranes; and pain and edema in the salivary glands. Patients with hypergammaglobulinemia often have type III hypersensitivity reactions (e.g., vasculitis with CNS involvement and kidney disease; see II D).
   c. **Therapy.** Mild cases are treated with **artificial tears** and frequent drinking of water. For more serious cases (e.g., vasculitis), treatment is similar to that for SLE (**systemic corticosteroids**).

2. **SLE**
   a. **Diagnosis** is complicated and depends on the presence of four or more of 11 criteria. The most useful criterion is a high concentration of antinuclear antibodies directed against double-stranded DNA and the Smith (Sm) nuclear antigen, both of which are considered specific for SLE. Other diagnostic criteria include the presence of the lupus erythematosus cell (a neutrophil that has phagocytosed nuclei), a discoid erythematous facial rash, photosensitivity, oral ulcers, arthritis, persistent proteinuria, and anticardiolipin, antierythrocyte, or antileukocyte antibodies.
   b. **Pathogenesis** is that of **type III hypersensitivity.** Patients have **hyperactivity of B cells** of unknown origin. This hyperreactivity causes hypergammaglobulinemia, with circulating

immune complexes of DNA and other nuclear antigens that precipitate onto vascular basement membranes and activate complement.

(1) Mild arthritis, fever, rash, and fatigue occur.

(2) Progressive necrotizing vasculitis with CNS involvement and glomerulonephritis are the most serious consequences, occurring in approximately 50% of patients.

(3) Hypertension may develop secondary to kidney disease.

(4) Hemolytic anemia and thrombocytopenia are common.

(5) Behavioral changes occur in approximately 25% of patients.

(6) Several drugs (e.g., **procainamide, hydralazine, quinidine, methyldopa, isoniazid, phenytoin, chlorpromazine)** provoke a lupus-like syndrome that usually resolves when the drug is withdrawn. The basis for this syndrome is not understood. No renal disorder occurs in drug-induced SLE.

c. **Therapy.** Mild disease (e.g., low fever, arthritis) is managed with nonsteroidal anti-inflammatory drugs (NSAIDs). Therapy for patients with severe symptoms is usually oral methylprednisolone. Cyclophosphamide may also be used, and plasmapheresis to remove circulating immune complexes may be helpful.

F. **Prospects for more specific immunologic therapies.** Current therapies involve approaches that suppress all immune responses; however, current clinical trials seek to suppress only lymphocytes that are activated; for example:

1. **Feeding autoantigens** to patients to induce immunologic suppression

2. **Vaccination with autoreactive T cells** to induce immunologic suppression

3. Administration of **anti-T$_H$** monoclonal antibodies (particularly anti-CD4) to eliminate autoreactive T cells

4. Administration of **conjugates of interleukin-2 (IL-2) and toxins** from plants or bacteria to eliminate autoreactive T cells without generalized T-cell suppression

IV. **IMMUNODEFICIENCY** is either primary or secondary. **Primary immunodeficiencies** are either **hereditary** or **congenital,** and at least one element basic to the immune system does not function properly or is absent. **Secondary immunodeficiencies** are the **result of another systemic** disorder or are **iatrogenic in patients given immunosuppressive therapy.** They usually develop in patients who previously showed normal immune function. The expected clinical outcome of an immunodeficiency is governed by the specific portion of the immune system that is affected (e.g., B and T cells, phagocytic cells, and complement).

A. **Primary immunodeficiencies** are, with one exception, rare. Examples are:

1. **X-linked agammaglobulinemia** (hypogammaglobulinemia) is an inherited deficiency in antibody production (humoral immunity) in which T-cell function is relatively normal, but B cells do not fully mature. Serum immunoglobulin levels are low. Because this disorder is linked to the X chromosome, it occurs primarily in men.

a. **Pathogenesis** occurs 6–9 months after birth and is representative of situations in which antibody function is deficient, but T-cell function is intact, such as recurrent infections with extracellular pyogenic bacteria (e.g., streptococci, pneumococci, *Haemophilus*). Immunity to fungi and most viruses is generally functional.

b. **Clinical symptoms** include pneumonia, sinusitis, otitis, meningitis, and septicemia.

c. **Therapy** is **passive immunization with intravenous human immune globulin** (IVIG; see VI B 1 c).

2. **Common variable immunodeficiency** is an acquired deficiency of B-cell maturation to plasma cells. It can occur at any age and in either sex. Symptoms and treatment are similar to those for X-linked agammaglobulinemia; the pathogenesis and etiology vary significantly.

3. **Selective IgA deficiency** is the most common primary immunodeficiency, affecting approximately 0.5% of the United States population. It appears to be inherited. The low secretory IgA (sIgA) concentration predisposes patients to extracellular bacterial infections of the mucosal surfaces, leading to respiratory, urogenital, and gastrointestinal infections. Some affected individuals are asymptomatic for unknown reasons. Certain autoimmunities may be more prevalent. There is no specific immunologic therapy.

4. **DiGeorge syndrome** results from developmental failure of the thymus and parathyroid glands, accompanied by cardiovascular and other developmental anomalies. Patients have a decrease in total T-cell numbers, but relatively normal immunoglobulin levels.
   a. **Pathogenesis** in severe cases (i.e., little functional thymic tissue) is representative of conditions involving T-cell deficiency, such as recurrent infections of the skin, lung, genitourinary tract, and blood with opportunistic pathogens, particularly viruses (e.g., herpes viruses), fungi (e.g., *Candida*), and protozoa (e.g., *Pneumocystis carinii*); increased incidence of certain cancers; graft-versus-host disease (GVH; see V C) after transfusion of whole blood; and death in infancy or early childhood.
   b. **Therapy** for severe T-cell deficiencies is bone marrow transplantation, although thymus grafts may be attempted in DiGeorge syndrome (see V C).

5. **Nezelof syndrome** is probably inherited and causes lymphopenia and thymic abnormalities, but normal or elevated serum immunoglobulin levels. Gram-negative sepsis may occur in addition to the opportunistic infections associated with T-cell deficiency.

6. **Severe combined immunodeficiency disorders (SCIDs)** are a heterogeneous group of inherited disorders with deficiencies in T cells, B cells (variable), and serum immunoglobulin. Infections with opportunistic organisms occur in the first few months postnatally, and survival for longer than 1 year is rare without successful bone marrow transplantation. One form involves the inherited deficiency of the enzyme adenosine deaminase (ADA). Human trials with gene replacement therapy are under way.

7. **Chronic granulomatous disease (CGD)** is a defect in the ability of phagocytes to kill bacteria. The disease is caused by a genetic defect in the production of oxygen radicals that are important for intra- and extracellular killing of bacteria. The defect can occur in any of the four proteins important for producing oxygen radicals, but the most common defect is X-linked. CGD is characterized by chronic infection with organisms such as *Staphylococcus aureus* and is usually fatal.

8. **Leukocyte adhesion deficiency (LAD)** is associated with a defect in the phagocytic cells. These cells lack intercellular adhesion molecules, the proteins necessary for binding to the endothelial cells of the blood vessels and other cell membranes. This defect leads to an inability to exit the blood and enter the tissues. In addition, the phagocytes have a decreased ability to bind to activated components of complement on a bacterial surface, leading to a decrease in phagocytosis. Patients have severe bacterial infections, especially in the mouth and gastrointestinal tract.

9. **Chédiak–Higashi syndrome** is a deficiency in the fusion of lysosomes with phagocytic vesicles. The cause is unknown, but this syndrome leads to bacterial survival in the phagocyte, with an increase in bacterial infections.

10. **Defects in complement** may be due to defects in the activation pathways, membrane attack complex, or regulatory proteins. Defects in the activation pathways and in the membrane attack complex, are associated with increased infections due to pyogenic bacteria and with increased rates of immune complex diseases such as systemic lupus erythematosus. Defects in regulation can be observed as angioneurotic edema and nocturnal hemoglobinuria.

B. **Secondary immunodeficiencies** involve decreased immunologic responsiveness.

1. **Cytotoxic drugs** prevent the division of responding lymphocytes, suppress the production of blood cells in bone marrow, and may directly kill cells. Patients who receive chemotherapy and exhibit a significant loss of neutrophils may be treated with filgrastim, or recombinant G-CSF (Neupogen), to restore the white blood cell count to normal levels. Treatment to increase neutrophil levels in these patients results in decreased morbidity rates as a result of bacterial infection. Corticosteroids broadly suppress immune system cells, including decreased division, cytokine secretion, and chemotaxis, or emigration from the blood into tissues.

2. **Leukemias, lymphomas, and myelomas** are associated with decreased immune responsiveness, at least some of which results from destruction of the architecture of lymphoid organs (e.g., spleen, lymph nodes). Malignancy-related immunodeficiency also occurs in other cancers.

3. **Protein calorie malnutrition** significantly decreases immune competence, particularly in children.

4. **Aging** is associated with decreased immunologic competence.

5. **Acute infections** produce a transient immunodeficiency.

6. **Acquired immune deficiency syndrome (AIDS)** is a secondary immunodeficiency that is usually persistent and is an indirect consequence of infection by **human immunodeficiency virus-1 (HIV-1)** or **HIV-2.**
   a. **Pathogenesis.** The viral envelope glycoprotein 120 (gp120) has a strong affinity for CD4 (see I B 3 c), allowing the virus to directly infect T_H cells. In addition, these proteins use a chemokine receptor CCR5 to gain entry to macrophages and dendritic cells. Because it is a retrovirus, viral entry and uncoating release the viral RNA genome and the associated reverse transcriptase enzyme, which synthesizes a double-stranded DNA copy of the genome (provirus). The proviral copy is integrated into the genome of the infected cell, and the virus enters a period of latency, during which it is essentially hidden from the immune system.
      (1) During **initial infection,** an acute illness that lasts an average of 3 weeks and resembles mononucleosis occurs in some individuals; others have no symptoms.
      (2) **Seroconversion** (i.e., the appearance of antiviral antibodies) occurs 3 weeks to 6 months after the initial exposure to HIV-1. A period of **asymptomatic infection** typically follows seroconversion.
      (3) Infected T_H cells are killed when **viral genes are reactivated from latency** and viruses bud from the cell. In addition, infected T cells may fuse to form syncytia. This fusion may hasten the spread of virus to uninfected T cells and contribute to cell killing. A **progressive depletion of T_H** cells occurs (normal count, 800–1000/mm³). However, even before an obvious loss of CD4⁺ T cells occurs, there is evidence of a defect in CD4⁺ T-cell function. The functional defect is a failure of these cells to respond to antigens to which they were previously sensitized (e.g., tetanus toxoid). The defect in responsiveness may be a function of the CD4⁺ T cells, the APCs, or both.
      (4) Macrophages may produce new virus without being killed and may spread the virus to uninfected T cells and other cell types. CD4⁺ cell lines that are susceptible to HIV infection include neurons, liver, and fibroblasts. In direct cell-to-cell transfer of the virus, minimal exposure to the extracellular immune system (e.g., antibody) may occur.
      (5) **APCs** are also affected by the infection. There is a loss of follicular dendritic cells and interdigitating cells in the lymphoid tissue. This loss leads to decreased antigen presentation to the CD4⁺ T cells. In addition, the cytokines produced by the APCs may produce CD4⁺ T cells that increase B-cell activation, but do not produce the appropriate cytokines for T-cell proliferation. This activity changes the T_H-cell ratios.
   b. **Clinical symptoms**
      (1) **Persistent generalized lymphadenopathy** (extrainguinal) is an indicator of impending progression to full disease. Unexplained fever, night sweats, diarrhea, and other symptoms known as **AIDS-related complex (ARC)** may occur.
      (2) Progression to full-blown AIDS may occur 8 years or longer after the initial infection. Depletion of the T_H-cell level to less than 200/mm³ and oral candidiasis suggest imminent disease. Because CD8⁺ T cells are not significantly affected, the ratio of circulating CD4⁺ to CD8⁺ cells is inverted. In addition, the number of virgin T_H cells relative to memory T_H cells increases. T_H cells are lost, and memory T_H cells are lost in relatively larger numbers. There is also a shift in the type of T_H cell help being generated.
      (3) A diagnosis of AIDS involves the occurrence of **opportunistic infections** or **neoplasms as a result of the progressive immunodeficiency** caused by severe depletion of T_H-cell (CD4) function. Also included in this diagnosis are the HIV wasting syndrome and encephalopathy.
         (a) Opportunistic infections are the major consequence of AIDS, particularly by *P. carinii* (as many as 80% of patients), *Candida albicans, Mycobacterium avium-intracellulare,* herpes simplex virus (HSV), cytomegalovirus (CMV), and others. Tuberculosis occurs as a reactivation of a latent infection in carriers. Cumulatively, **these opportunistic infections are the primary cause of death.**
         (b) **Kaposi's sarcoma,** an otherwise rare cancer, occurs in fewer than one-half of patients with AIDS. Non-Hodgkin's lymphoma is also more common than in the general population.

(4) HIV-associated dementia complex (HADC) affects more than one-half of patients with AIDS. In HADC, macrophages infiltrate the brain and are the most productively infected cell in comparison with neurons or glia. Some patients show demyelination.

(5) Other immune system abnormalities include polyclonal B-cell activation and hypergammaglobulinemia with a concomitant decreased ability to mount humoral immune responses to specific antigens. Chemotaxis, cytokine secretion, and cytotoxic ability of monocyte–macrophages are all diminished. These problems are consequences of impaired T-cell regulation.

c. Therapy
(1) Current therapy includes prophylactic use of antibiotics and antifungal agents. Optimal anti-HIV therapy is combination therapy with three antiretroviral drugs. At present, there are three classes of antiretroviral drugs approved by the FDA. These are nucleoside reverse transcriptase inhibitors (NRTIs) (i.e., zidovudine-AZT, lamivudine, stavudine, zalcitabine-ddC, didansosine-ddI, and abacavir), non-nucleoside reverse transcriptase inhibitors (NNRTIs) (e.g., neviapine, delavirdine, efavirenz), and protease inhibitors (e.g., saquinavir, indinavir, ritonavir, nelfinavir). IFN-α is recommended for the treatment of Kaposi's sarcoma. Other drugs and immunomodulators are currently under development and testing.

(2) An effective active vaccine is necessary to limit the spread of HIV infection. Because of viral antigenic variation, cell-to-cell transmission, and the uncertain role of antibodies in protection, the process of vaccine development is difficult. A live, attenuated vaccine (see VI C 2) is considered too great a risk. Trials of subunit vaccines are under way.

V. GRAFT REJECTION

A. Overview. Individual differences in the molecular structures of cells and tissues occur, except in identical twins, because of the genetic variation inherent in humans. Because of these molecular differences, transplanted tissues or organs (i.e., grafts) are likely to be antigenically different from the recipient and therefore may stimulate an immune response.

1. Although MHC class I and II glycoproteins play an essential role in all T-cell immune responses (see I B 3 a), these molecules are particularly antigenic and variant in structure among different humans (polymorphic).

2. Each person's set of MHC glycoproteins is called his **human leukocyte antigen (HLA), or histocompatibility, type.** Class I glycoproteins are known as HLA-A, -B, and -C antigens. Class II glycoproteins are known as HLA-DR, -DP, and -DQ antigens. Each person receives one set of genes (a haplotype) encoding these protein antigens from each parent.

3. Identical twins have the same histocompatibility type. In others, the probability is approximately 25% (0.25) that two siblings with the same parents are HLA-identical, or matched, and approximately 50% that they are one-half HLA-matched, or haploidentical. Parents and children are almost always haploidentical. Some transplanted tissues are rejected because of HLA incompatibility. In other cases, the reason for rejection is unknown. HLA matching is not always a factor in rejection.

B. Common solid-organ transplants are kidney, heart, liver, heart–lung, and pancreas. Organs are obtained from cadavers or living donors. The probability of an exact HLA match in a cadaver graft is approximately 1 in 10 million.

1. HLA matching
a. The primary problem with organ donation is rejection of the transplanted organ by the host's immune response, a host-versus-graft response. Donation of an organ by an HLA-matched sibling is the best way to avoid this problem.
b. Although HLA-DR and HLA-B matching decreases the rejection reaction in renal and cardiac grafts, rejection does occur in HLA-matched situations. HLA matching is not important in liver transplantation.

2. Types of rejection of organ grafts
a. Hyperacute rejection is mediated by preexisting antibody in the recipient, usually against ABO mismatches. Complement is activated, clotting occurs, and the vasculature

of the transplanted organ is occluded. Rejection occurs within 2 days after transplantation. An ABO-mismatched graft is rarely attempted. Rejection is essentially untreatable.

   b. Acute rejection is most likely a T-cell–macrophage–mediated attack on the graft based on HLA and other tissue antigen mismatches. T cells and macrophages infiltrate the graft and, in 10–14 days, cause cellular necrosis and inflammation perivascularly. The entire graft begins to necrose if untreated.

   c. Chronic rejection occurs several months to several years after transplantation. It causes fibrosis and occlusion of small arteries and arterioles in the kidneys and atherosclerosis in the heart. It may be controlled by immunologic injury, through antibody or cells, and includes the release of inflammatory cytokines by macrophages. Despite the high success rate of MHC-matched, pharmacologically treated grafts in the first year after transplantation (85%–90% kidney grafts), the rejection rate after 5 years is nearly 50%. This form of rejection is resistant to therapy.

C. Bone marrow transplantation is sometimes attempted in patients with immunodeficiency diseases, aplastic anemias, some leukemias, and certain genetic diseases. The graft contains a high proportion of donor lymphocytes that respond to the host HLA and other antigens. This response causes GVH disease.

   1. Graft T-cell recognition of the host is important in GVH disease, as shown by the decreased incidence of GVH disease after procedures that purge mature T cells from the donor marrow.

   2. Clinical symptoms of GVH disease are seen in the skin (e.g., rash, desquamation), gastrointestinal tract (e.g., pain, vomiting, intestinal bleeding), and liver (e.g., necrosis indicated by increased serum bilirubin levels). Death commonly occurs.

   3. HLA matching is important in bone marrow transplantation, but the failure rate, even of matched grafts, as a result of GVH disease is high.

   4. Because the recipient of the marrow (host) is immunosuppressed due to primary immunodeficiency, or by drugs or radiation, the host-versus-graft response is less important.

D. Prophylaxis and treatment of graft rejection

   1. Immunosuppression of the graft recipient
      a. Corticosteroids (e.g., methylprednisolone, prednisone) are administered just before transplantation and rapidly tapered because of their side effects. Corticosteroids are used in combination with azathioprine, cyclosporine, or **antilymphocyte globulins/ antithymocyte globulins (ALG/ATG).**
      b. Azathioprine is given before transplantation. Maintenance doses are given afterward.
      c. Methotrexate is used primarily for bone marrow transplantation in combination with ALG/ATG. It is administered either a few days before or at the time of transplantation.

   2. Specific suppression of T cells
      a. Cyclosporine binds to an intracellular protein known as cyclophilin and blocks the transcription of cytokine genes in a T cell that has recognized antigens. In this way, it inhibits T_H-cell secretion of IL-2 and IFN-γ and prevents complete T-cell activation. It is administered prophylactically because it is more effective if it is present when rejection begins. Cyclosporine is commonly combined with other agents. The major side effect is nephrotoxicity.
      b. Tacrolimus (FK-506) is an immunosuppressive agent that inhibits T_H-cell function in the same way as cyclosporine. Both drugs function through the same pathway and are not used together.
      c. Rampamycin inhibits T_H-cell response to IL-2 and prevents T_H-cell activation. It works through a different pathway than either cyclosporine or tacrolimus and is especially effective in combination with the other drugs.
      d. ALG and **ATG** are antisera derived from animals. They contain a variety of antibody specificities against T-cell antigens. They are used both prophylactically and therapeutically in bone marrow and organ transplantation.
      e. Muromonab-CD3 (OKT3) is a mouse monoclonal antibody specific for the CD3 antigen, which is present on all peripheral T cells. OKT3 is used therapeutically to halt and reverse acute rejection as soon as it is diagnosed.

(1) Its main action is the opsonization of T cells for enhanced phagocytosis. It is administered daily for 10–14 days. Only one course is typically used because it causes an immune response against the foreign mouse antibody.

(2) Acute side effects are common, probably because of nonspecific T-cell activation that causes the release of cytokines. Side effects include high fever, chills, blood pressure changes, vomiting, diarrhea, and respiratory distress. OKT3 is contraindicated in patients who have fluid overload because it may cause fatal pulmonary edema.

(3) OKT3 may also be used in vitro to purge donor bone marrow of T cells to reduce the risk of GVH disease.

3. Investigational agents that are being tested to prevent or reverse graft rejection include anti–T-cell immunotoxins (see VII C 1); conjugates of IL-2 and a toxin; and other monoclonals that prevent T cells from adhering to foreign graft cells. These agents are administered to the graft recipient. In addition, monoclonal antibodies are used to mask HLA antigens on the graft tissue before it is transplanted into the recipient.

VI. VACCINATION

A. Overview

1. Passive vaccination is the intramuscular or intravenous injection of antibody preparations to enhance a patient's immune competence. Protection depends on the serum half-life of the injected antibody and is limited to several weeks to several months for each administration of human sera.

2. Active vaccination is the intramuscular, subcutaneous, or oral introduction of one or more antigens designed to stimulate the immune system to produce a specific immune response. This response generates antibody, activated T cells, and specific memory. Protection through memory varies with the vaccine, but immunity is long-lasting.

B. Passive vaccination (Table 10-2)

1. Preparations. Doses of intramuscular preparations are sometimes given in units per kilogram and sometimes in milliliters per kilogram. The dose varies with the vaccine and patient population. Intravenous preparations are commonly used in high doses.

a. Standard human serum immune globulin for intramuscular vaccination (IGIM) is a polyclonal antiserum prepared from pooled plasma of donors. It contains 165 mg/ml human immunoglobulin, predominantly the four subclasses of IgG. Side effects are rare, minimal, and usually confined to minor inflammation and pain at the site of injection. This preparation is unsuitable for intravenous injection because antibody aggregates form and may activate complement and platelets.

b. Special IGIMs are individual sera prepared from plasma lots of subjects actively immunized against or recovering from specific diseases. Each serum is enriched for antibodies of the desired specificity [e.g., tetanus immune globulin (TIG) contains more antibodies against tetanus toxin than would be found in IGIM].

c. IVIGs are prepared from pooled human serum and modified to minimize antibody aggregation. Chills, nausea, and abdominal pain occur in approximately 10% of patients. Side effects are diminished by reducing the rate of intravenous infusion. Premedication with corticosteroids is recommended, and intravenous epinephrine is used if anaphylaxis occurs.

d. Animal antisera. Equine (horse) antisera are used in certain situations (see Table 10-2). Mouse monoclonal antibody (muromonab-CD3) is used in acute renal rejection (see V D 2 e). The half-lives of animal antibodies are shorter in humans.

2. Rationales for passive vaccination

a. Prophylaxis of infectious disease. Antibodies are given prophylactically to prevent clinical symptoms of a viral or bacterial infectious process, particularly in a patient without previous exposure and therefore without immunologic memory. The vaccine protects the recipient during the incubation period for infection. For example:

(1) *Clostridium tetani* infection has an incubation period of approximately 5 days before significant quantities of tetanus toxin are produced. A primary immune response of 7–10 days is too slow. Passive vaccination with TIG binds the toxin and prevents disease.

Table 10-2. Passive Vaccines

Illness	Vaccine	Rationale
Intramuscular		
Hepatitis B (HBV)	Hepatitis B immune globulin (HBIG)	Prophylaxis
Hepatitis A (HAV)	Immune globulin IM (IGIM)	Prophylaxis
Non-A, non-B hepatitis	IGIM	Prophylaxis, therapy
Measles	IGIM	Prophylaxis, therapy
Rabies	Rabies immune globulin (RIG)	Prophylaxis
Rubella	IGIM	Fetal prophylaxis in exposed mother
Varicella	Varicella zoster immune globulin (VZIG)	Prophylaxis and therapy in immuno-compromised individual
Tetanus	Tetanus immune globulin (TIG)	Prophylaxis
Hypogammaglobulinemia	IGIM	Therapy for antibody deficiency
Rh disease	Rh_o (D) immune globulin (RhoGAM)	Prophylaxis during pregnancy and after delivery of Rh^+ fetus by Rh^- mother
Botulism	Botulism antiserum (equine)	Prophylaxis, therapy
Snakebite	Polyvalent antivenin (equine)	Prophylaxis, therapy
Black widow bite	Black widow antivenin (equine)	Prophylaxis, therapy
Intravenous*		
Hypogammaglobulinemia	Intravenous immune globulin (IVIG)	Therapy for antibody deficiency
Idiopathic thrombocytopenic purpura (ITP)	IVIG	Therapy
Chronic lymphocytic leukemia	IVIG	Therapy for antibody deficiency
Cytomegalovirus (CMV) infection	CMV IVIG	Therapy in renal transplant patients
Acute renal rejection	Muromonab-CD3 (murine)	Reversal of acute rejection

*United States Food and Drug Administration (FDA)–approved uses; many others currently in trials result from vaccine preparation in cells of nonhuman origin. The valence of a vaccine indicates the number of strains of organism included (e.g., trivalent polio vaccine includes three strains of poliovirus).

    (2) Hepatitis B immune globulin (HBIG) is administered to exposed individuals as soon as possible after exposure to prevent viral infection.

  b. Prophylaxis or therapy prevents or attenuates the effects of infection in special populations. Examples are the use of **varicella zoster immune globulin (VZIG)** in immuno-compromised patients and the use of IGIM in pregnant women who are exposed to rubella and have not been actively vaccinated.

  c. Treatment of antibody deficiency. Persons who are deficient in antibody production, either because of primary immunodeficiency (see IV) or as a result of chronic lymphocytic leukemia, receive IVIG or IGIM every 2–4 weeks to maintain humoral immunity. IVIG is preferred.

  d. Other situations. IVIG is used for idiopathic (autoimmune) thrombocytopenia purpura. Intramuscular Rh_o(D) immune globulin (RhoGAM) is used prophylactically for Rh disease (see II C 5 c). Muromonab-CD3 (see V D 2 e) is used for acute renal graft rejection.

C. Active vaccination (Table 10-3) is used for prophylaxis.

  1. Overview

    a. Contents. Active vaccines contain one or more antigens or whole pathogenic organisms, but may also contain preservatives, low doses of antibiotics, and other compounds that do not affect the immune response.

    b. Administration. Active vaccines are administered subcutaneously, intramuscularly, or intradermally. Some are introduced adsorbed to aluminum hydroxide or aluminum phosphate adjuvants. An adjuvant increases the antigenicity of the vaccine. A few vaccines are administered orally or intranasally.

c. **Seroconversion.** For most active vaccines, the success of the series of vaccinations is indicated by seroconversion of the patient. Seroconversion indicates that a person who previously did not have specific serum antibodies (i.e., seronegative) now has these antibodies (i.e., seropositive). Seroconversion does not indicate established immunity for certain vaccines [e.g., bacillus Calmette-Guérin (BCG) vaccine for tuberculosis].

d. **A schedule of active vaccination** is recommended for infants and children (see Table 10-3). The first vaccination is given after the infant is 6 weeks old because responses are normally inadequate in newborns and because maternal antibodies remain in the newborn circulation; some vaccines (e.g., HBV), however, may be given immediately after birth. Some vaccines are intended for use primarily in noninfant populations.

e. Most vaccines require **a series of vaccinations;** others are effective with a single vaccination. For those that require a series, intervals between vaccinations greater than those recommended do not generally diminish protection. The duration of memory varies with each vaccine, and **booster vaccinations** are often necessary.

f. **Side effects** include inflammation at the site of vaccination, malaise, mild fever, chills, headache, myalgia, and arthralgia. More severe side effects include febrile illness, somnolence, seizures, or anaphylactic hypersensitivity to vaccine antigens or accessory components (e.g., antibiotic, chicken protein). Severe reactions contraindicate continuation of a series. A person with severe febrile illness should not be actively vaccinated until the illness resolves.

2. **Types of active vaccines**

   a. **Live, attenuated vaccines** consist of whole organisms (usually viruses). These organisms multiply after vaccination, but are attenuated to reduce their pathogenicity.

      (1) A small dose produces a strong immune response because the antigen concentration increases when the organism multiplies. Some vaccines elicit lifelong immunity in two doses [e.g., measles, mumps, rubella (MMR) vaccine]. Because of their relative genetic instability, viruses can revert to virulence and cause the disease against which the patient is vaccinated [e.g., oral polio vaccine (OPV)].

      (2) Live, attenuated viral vaccines are not recommended for pregnant women or those intending to become pregnant within 3 months of vaccination. Live, attenuated viral or bacterial vaccines are not given to immunocompromised individuals.

   b. **Killed, inactivated vaccines** may contain whole killed cells (e.g., phenol-killed *Bordetella pertussis)* or any antigenic fraction isolated from the organism. They are usually given adsorbed to adjuvant.

      (1) Isolated antigens may require inactivation before they are used in a vaccine [e.g., formaldehyde-modified toxin of *Clostridium tetani,* known as **tetanus toxoid (Td)** after modification]. Inactivation eliminates pathogenicity, but preserves some antigenicity.

      (2) Because no live organisms are present, reversion to pathogenicity is not a problem. However, doses of cells or antigens must be higher than in live, attenuated vaccines, and hypersensitivity reactions to vaccine components are more common. Minimum effective doses are usually measured in numbers of cells or micrograms of antigen.

      (3) Vaccines in which the antigenic fragment is a polysaccharide (e.g., *Haemophilus* b) are usually poor at eliciting immune responses and memory, probably because they do not evoke T-cell activation. These vaccines have been improved by conjugating the polysaccharide to another antigenic compound (e.g., Td). These are known as **conjugate vaccines.**

   c. **Subunit vaccines.** Proteins and glycoproteins of an organism are produced by recombinant DNA technology in bacteria, yeast, or mammalian cells, and are used as the antigens for vaccination. Two vaccines containing proteins produced by recombinant genetic technologies are approved by the FDA for use in humans. These are the HBV vaccine and the Lyme disease vaccine (the Lyme disease vaccine is not currently available).

   d. **Experimental vaccines** include other subunit vaccines; peptides produced by chemical, cell-free synthesis; recombinant DNA viruses containing genes for the antigens of multiple organisms; and anti-idiotype antibodies used for active vaccination.

3. **Specific vaccines** in common use and recommended administration schedules are listed in Table 10-3.

Table 10-3. Commonly Administered Unites States Food and Drug Administration (FDA)–Approved Active Vaccines

Vaccine	Target Population*	Number of Vaccinations	Schedule	Notes
Live, attenuated viral				
Oral polio (OPV; trivalent)	Infants, children, health-and day-care workers	4	2, 4, 15–18 months; 1 at school entry	Approximately 1 in 2.6 million risk of vaccine-induced paralysis; no longer recommended because of risks, substitute killed vaccine
Measles, mumps, rubella (MMR)	Infants, children	2	15 months (<12 months if high risk); 1 at school entry	Generally affords lifelong immunity
Rubella	Adolescent girls not previously vaccinated	1	Postpuberty	Protects future fetus from congenital rubella injury
Varicella	Children, other at-risk individuals	1 (if 13 years or older, 2)	1 between 12–18 months or 2–3 years; after 13 years of age, 2–4 weeks apart	Duration of immunity or effect on development of shingles is unknown
Bacterial				
BCG tuberculosis	Persons exposed to sputum-positive tuberculosis patients	Varies	Depends on success of initial vaccination	Unpredictable effectiveness; induces cell-mediated immunity
Killed, inactivated viral, or viral subunit				
Influenza (tri- or polyvalent)	Geriatric patients, health-care workers, those at risk for complications of flu	1/year	Annually for maximal protection	Variant strains may appear each year; vaccine must be updated annually
Hepatitis B (HBV)	All	3	Between 1–2 months, 2–3 months, after 6 months	Recombinant, subunit
Inactivated polio (IPV; trivalent)	Immunodeficient children and families; as booster in health- and day-care workers	4	2, 4, 15–18 months; 1 at school entry	No sIgA; thus, reduced protection; no paralysis risk
Rabies (HDCV)	Animal-care workers	4 or 5+ with boosters	7 days apart; boosters as required to maintain immunoglobulin (Ig)	Two doses to exposed, already immune individual

Bacterial subunit

Vaccine	Target population*	Doses	Schedule	Comments
Diphtheria, tetanus, pertussis (DTP)	Infants, children	4 with boosters	2, 4, 15–18 months; 1 at school entry	Tetanus toxoid (Td) booster every 10 years or on exposure through a wound
Tetanus and diphtheria toxoids (Td)	Children 7 years or older, adults with no vaccination	3 with boosters	Second dose in 4–8 weeks; third dose 6 months later	Td booster every 10 years or on exposure through a wound if more than 10 years or vaccine history unavailable
Haemophilus b (Hib)	Infants, children, HIV-infected adults	Depends on formulation	Depends on formulation	Polysaccharide capsule is poor antigen; conjugate vaccines enhance potency
Pneumococcus (polyvalent)	At-risk adults or children 2 years or older (e.g., immunocompromised patients, geriatric patients)	1 or 1/year	As necessary in at-risk patients; not given during active infection; 1/year in geriatric patients	Poor response to polysaccharide antigen in children younger than 2 years of age
Meningococcus (quadrivalent A, C, Y, W-135)	College freshmen living in dormitories; high-risk adults or children 2 years or older, including individuals with terminal complement component deficiencies or anatomic or functional asplenia	1 subcutaneously	As necessary in at-risk individuals at 3–5-year intervals	Polysaccharide vaccine gives poor response in children younger than 2 years; does not protect against serotype B, which accounts for 46% of cases

BCG = bacille Calmette-Guérin; HBsAg = hepatitis B surface antigen; HDCV = human diploid cell vaccines; HIV = human immunodeficiency virus; sIgA = secretory immunoglobulin A.

*Entire target population is not listed in all cases.

†Five doses to already exposed individuals.

D. Simultaneous administration of active and passive vaccines. Sometimes active and passive vaccines against a pathogenic organism are administered simultaneously to maximize post-exposure prophylaxis. The immune globulin offers immediate protection, and the active vaccine stimulates an immune response. These vaccines are given at separate sites to prevent antibody (passive) and antigen (active) from reacting and inactivating one another.

1. Infants with **HBV** who are born to mothers who have the hepatitis B surface antigen (HBsAg) are significantly protected from becoming chronic carriers by this combined prophylaxis.

2. **Rabies.** Postexposure prophylaxis typically includes the combined use of active and passive vaccines because of the lethal nature of the unchecked infection. The exception is patients with a previous active vaccination who have sufficient existing serum antibody concentration.

3. **Tetanus.** Combined prophylaxis is sometimes used, depending on the type of wound and the patient's history of active vaccination. Recommended guidelines are as follows:
   a. **A tetanus-prone wound** is one that produces anaerobic conditions (e.g., deep puncture) or one in which exposure to *Clostridium* or its spores is probable (e.g., contaminated with animal feces). If the patient's history of active vaccination is uncertain or includes fewer than three doses, both TIG and Td are administered. The patient returns to complete the toxoid series.
      (1) If the wound is tetanus-prone but the patient received a full series of active vaccination, no treatment is necessary if the last Td dose was received within the last 5 years.
      (2) If the last dose was received more than 10 years ago, Td, but not TIG, is given to boost memory immunity and antibody production.
   b. For a **clean, minor wound,** if the patient's history of active vaccination is uncertain or includes fewer than three doses, Td is administered.
      (1) If the patient received a full series of active vaccinations, no treatment is necessary if the last Td dose was received within 10 years.
      (2) If the last dose was received more than 10 years ago, Td, but not TIG, is given to boost memory immunity and antibody production.

VII. PROSPECTS FOR IMMUNOMODULATION

A. Fab antidigoxin antibody preparations obtained from sheep are approved for the reversal of toxicity associated with toxic digoxin serum levels. The antibody binds digoxin and prevents it from binding to its normal receptor site. The Fab–digoxin complex is excreted renally.

B. Monoclonal antibodies are generally produced through the in vitro fusion of a cancerous plasma cell (myeloma) with an activated mouse B cell. The resulting **hybridoma** secretes murine (mouse) antibodies of a single defined specificity and has the immortality characteristic of the myeloma. Techniques for the production of human monoclonal antibodies and a variety of hybrid mouse–human monoclonal antibodies are not as well refined as the hybridoma technology.

1. **Monoclonal antibodies** [e.g., whole antibodies or Fab or F(ab')$_2$ fragments] are routinely used for in vitro diagnostic tests (e.g., blood group and tissue typing for HLA); screening for cancer-related antigens [e.g., carcinoembryonic antigen (CEA)]; urine testing for drugs and metabolites; and testing for HIV infection. In these and many other diagnostic applications, monoclonal antibodies are often conjugated to enzymes, radioisotopes, or fluorescent dyes.

2. **Muromonab-CD3** is used to treat acute graft rejection. Several other monoclonal antibodies are being tested (see V D 2 e).

3. In clinical trials, **monoclonal antibodies against T cells** show improvement in certain autoimmune disorders.

4. **Monoclonal antibodies against neoplastic cells** show some success, and are useful in treating certain leukemias and lymphomas, as well as breast and colon cancers.

C. Monoclonal antibodies are conjugated to enzymes, drugs, prodrugs, radioisotopes, or plant and bacterial toxins to provide specific delivery of the conjugated agent to one or more focused in vivo sites of action. Several problems are associated with the use of these agents.

1. **Immunotoxins** are usually produced by the conjugation of a monoclonal antibody to a biologic polypeptide toxin (e.g., diphtheria toxin) that is modified to reduce nonspecific toxicity.

2. Although they are being tested for graft rejection and autoimmunity, immunotoxins are primarily used as antineoplastic agents. Clinical trials show moderate success in treating leukemia and lymphoma, with lower success rates against tumors such as breast carcinoma.

3. **Monoclonal antibodies conjugated to radioisotopes** (e.g., ^{90}Y) cause remissions in patients with Hodgkin's disease and acute T-cell leukemia.

4. **Monoclonal antibodies conjugated to enzymes** that activate a prodrug to the active drug at a specific tissue site (e.g., neoplastic cell surface) are in the early stages of human trials.

D. **Immunostimulation** has been attempted with a variety of compounds, ranging from cytokines (see Table 10-1) to bacterial products.

1. IFN-α has many subtypes. Two are currently FDA-approved. Because it inhibits cell growth, it is used to treat hairy cell leukemia, Kaposi's sarcoma in patients with AIDS, and genital warts. At low doses, interferons stimulate immune cellular function (e.g., T cells, NK cells, macrophages), but at high doses, they are immunosuppressive. The use of IFN-α against other cancers produces variable results.

2. IFN-γ provides greater immunostimulation in the intact immune system, but its effects depend on dose and timing. The combined use of IFN-α and IFN-γ yields better results. The most common side effects of interferon therapy are influenza-like symptoms. IFN-γ is approved for use as a macrophage-activating factor in chronic granulomatous disease.

3. Several protocols using **IL-2** show promising results, with apparently complete remissions in some patients with melanoma. With this technique, known as adoptive immunotherapy, a patient's peripheral blood lymphocytes, or tumor-infiltrating lymphocytes, are removed. They are cultured with IL-2 and reinfused with additional IL-2. These IL-2–responsive cells are likely T cells and NK cells. Severe capillary leakage syndrome, occasionally leading to death, is a problematic side effect.

4. **Hormones of the thymus** that induce T-cell maturation and other functions are used to increase certain cell-mediated immune functions, with variable results.

5. Sulfur-containing compounds, such as **levamisole** (a phenylimidothiazole anthelmintic) and diethyldithiocarbamate **(Imuthiol),** have immunostimulatory activity. Their effect is greater on cell-mediated immunity than on humoral immunity. Levamisole is approved as an oral agent for use in colon cancer in combination with fluorouracil.

6. **Inosine pranobex** is licensed for use in many countries as an immunostimulant. It induces T-cell differentiation and augments cell-mediated immune functions, with minimal toxicity.

7. As a component of mycobacterial cell walls, **muramyl dipeptide (MDP)** stimulates macrophage activation and may be used as an adjuvant, given with antigen (see I), or given alone as an immunostimulant.

STUDY QUESTIONS

Directions: Each of the numbered items or incomplete statements in this section is followed by answers or by completions of the statement. Select the **one** lettered answer or completion that is **best** in each case.

1. A man has symptoms of a viral infection of about 4 days' duration. To confirm the diagnosis, the physician draws a blood sample and requests the antibody titer (level) for the suspected agent. The first blood sample shows a low titer of antibody. A week later, another blood sample is drawn, and the titer against the virus is much higher. This situation is an example of

(A) an inflammatory response to the viral infection
(B) a primary immune response to the viral infection
(C) a secondary immune response to the viral infection
(D) a cellular response to the viral infection

2. Which class of antibody has the longest serum half-life and opsonizes antigens for phagocytosis through two different pathways?

(A) Immunoglobulin G (IgG)
(B) Immunoglobulin M (IgM)
(C) Immunoglobulin A (IgA)
(D) Immunoglobulin E (IgE)

3. Urticaria that appears rapidly after the ingestion of food usually indicates which type of hypersensitivity reaction?

(A) Type I
(B) Type II
(C) Type III
(D) Type IV

4. In which autoimmune disorder is the mechanism of pathogenesis classified as type II hypersensitivity?

(A) Systemic lupus erythematosus (SLE)
(B) Insulin-dependent diabetes mellitus (IDDM)
(C) Graves' disease
(D) Hashimoto's thyroiditis

5. A patient receives long-term, high-dose therapy with a sulfonamide. After approximately 3 weeks of therapy, the patient has a low-grade fever, rash, and muscle and joint pain. Which type of hypersensitivity accounts for these symptoms?

(A) Type I
(B) Type II
(C) Type III
(D) Type IV

6. In which type IV hypersensitivity reaction is the tissue-damaging disorder considered an inappropriate response by the immune system?

(A) Poison ivy dermatitis
(B) Chronic tuberculosis
(C) Acute graft rejection
(D) Tuberculin test

7. Which agent is commonly used to treat multiple sclerosis (MS)?

(A) Neostigmine
(B) Cyanocobalamin
(C) IFNβ-1b
(D) Propylthiouracil

8. The therapeutic role of muromonab-CD3 in acute renal graft rejection is probably based on

(A) activation of T-cell function and secretion of cytokines
(B) destruction of T cells by complement
(C) opsonization of T cells for phagocytosis
(D) selective inhibition of T_H-cell function

9. Which is a current clinical application of intravenous human immune globulin (IVIG)?

(A) Prophylaxis after hepatitis B virus (HBV) exposure
(B) Treatment of humoral immunodeficiency
(C) Prophylactic infant immunization for polio
(D) Prophylaxis for Rh disease by infant immunization

10. Which cytokine is approved for the treatment of certain forms of cancer?

(A) Interleukin-2 (IL-2)
(B) Interferon-α (IFN-α)
(C) Interferon-δ (IFN-δ)
(D) Imuthiol

Questions 11 and 12

A 6-year-old child has a deep puncture wound. The parent is unsure of the child's history of vaccination.

11. If no other information is available, what should the physician recommend?

(A) No vaccination
(B) Tetanus immune globulin (TIG)
(C) Tetanus toxoid (Td)
(D) Both TIG and Td at separate sites

12. If the child received a full series of diphtheria, pertussis, tetanus (DPT) vaccinations, the last at entry into school, what should the physician recommend?

(A) No vaccination
(B) Tetanus immune globulin (TIG)
(C) Tetanus toxoid (Td)
(D) Both TIG and Td at separate sites

13. Persistent infections by opportunistic pathogens, such as *Candida albicans* and *Pneumocystis carinii,* could indicate all of the following EXCEPT

(A) inherited T-cell immunodeficiency
(B) humoral immunodeficiency
(C) AIDS
(D) combined immunodeficiency

14. Which statement about human immunodeficiency virus (HIV) infection is NOT correct?

(A) Individuals who become infected with human immunodeficiency virus-1 (HIV-1) always show overt symptoms shortly after infection.
(B) Seroconversion to positive status for anti-HIV-1 antibodies is the primary criterion for diagnosis of a viral carrier.
(C) The incubation period for the pathogenesis of acquired immune deficiency syndrome (AIDS) is believed to be 8 years or longer after the initial infection with HIV.
(D) CD4$^+$ T cells and macrophages may be able to spread HIV to uninfected CD4$^+$ cells without releasing any extracellular virus particles.

Directions: Each question below contains three suggested answers of which **one or more** is correct. Choose the answer

A	if **I only** is correct
B	if **III only** is correct
C	if **I and II** are correct
D	if **II and III** are correct
E	if **I, II, and III** are correct

15. Which statement about the currently approved sheep Fab fragment used to counteract digoxin overdose is true?

I. It is obtained by the immunization of sheep with a digoxin–protein conjugate and subsequent proteolytic cleavage of the collected antibody.
II. It specifically binds digoxin, preventing its activity.
III. It has a serum half-life of approximately 3 weeks.

16. CD4$^+$T cells specifically recognize antigens in which form?

I. Bound to major histocompatibility (MHC) class I molecules on the surface of any body cell
II. In free, soluble form in extracellular fluids
III. Bound to MHC class II molecules on the surface of special antigen-presenting cells (APCs)

17. Which is a normal outcome of the activation of the complement system by either the classic or alternative pathway?

I. Acute inflammation
II. Opsonization of immune complexes
III. Cytolytic action

18. In antiviral immunity, what directly recognizes and kills viral-infected cells?

 I. Cytotoxic T cells (CTLs)
 II. Antiviral antibodies
 III. Interferons

19. A patient is treated with penicillin and produces antibodies against the drug. They are still mostly present. An emergency situation requires administration of an intravenous dose of penicillin. If the patient has a type I penicillin hypersensitivity reaction, which pathologic consequence would be expected, and within what time course of clinical onset?

 I. Hemolytic anemia, with an onset of 1–2 hours after the intravenous dose
 II. Anaphylaxis, with an onset of a few minutes after the intravenous dose
 III. Cutaneous urticaria and pruritus, with an onset of a few minutes after the intravenous dose

20. Which situation occurs in all type IV hypersensitivity reactions?

 I. Infiltration of the affected tissue by mononuclear cells
 II. A delay of 12 hours or longer in the onset of clinical symptoms after allergen contact
 III. Significant beneficial effect of the administration of H_1-antagonists

21. Which immunologic finding is NOT unique to systemic lupus erythematosus (SLE)?

 I. Hypergammaglobulinemia
 II. The presence of circulating antinuclear antibodies
 III. The presence of circulating rheumatoid factors

22. An organ donor who is human leukocyte antigen (HLA)-matched with the recipient of a graft is sought. Which individual is at least somewhat likely to provide a total HLA match?

 I. A sibling of the graft recipient
 II. A parent of the graft recipient
 III. A cadaver

23. Graft-versus-host (GVH) disease is associated primarily with which type of transplantation?

 I. Kidney
 II. Heart
 III. Bone marrow

24. The prophylactic use of cyclosporine in graft rejection is probably based on its ability to

 I. inhibit synthesis of antibodies, thereby preventing hyperacute rejection
 II. inhibit activation of T cells, thereby preventing acute rejection
 III. block transcription of the interleukin-2 (IL-2) gene and synthesis or secretion of IL-2

25. Which is a valid comparison of live, attenuated and killed, inactivated active vaccines?

 I. Replication of the organisms in a live, attenuated vaccine increases the stimulation of the immune system, and a lower dose is often required
 II. Attenuated vaccines often require multiple doses
 III. A killed, inactivated vaccine probably produces lifelong immunity in one or two doses

26. Which active vaccine is recommended for health-care workers, but is not routinely given to infants?

 I. Measles, mumps, rubella (MMR) vaccine
 II. Influenza polyvalent
 III. Tetanus toxoid (Td)

27. Which statement about pneumococcus and meningococcus vaccines is true?

 I. They are composed of purified polysaccharides.
 II. They are recommended for children less than 2 years of age.
 III. The vaccines protect against all serotypes of disease causing pneumococcus or meningococcus.

ANSWERS AND EXPLANATIONS

1. The answer is B *[1 C 2, 3].*
A primary immune response to an infection is characterized by the initial production of IgM, beginning about 4 days after antigen is encountered. A switch to a different immunoglobulin isotype (i.e., IgG, IgE, or IgA) occurs before the peak of antibody production is reached. The peak primary immune response occurs 10–14 days after the antigen is encountered, and the serum contains both IgM and IgG.

2. The answer is A *[I D 2 b, E].*
Immunoglobulin G (IgG) has a serum half-life of 25–35 days, longer than that of any other class, although mast cell–bound immunoglobulin E (IgE) has the longest half-life. In general, immune complexes containing IgG are opsonized for phagocytosis through binding to the IgG receptors on neutrophils and macrophages, and additionally through the activation of complement. Immunoglobulin M (IgM) also opsonizes, but only through the activation of complement.

3. The answer is A *[II A 5 a, b].*
Food allergies are usually type I reactions. In a patient with preexisting hypersecreted immunoglobulin E (IgE) specific to a food allergen and bound to mast cells, the allergic response usually occurs shortly after ingestion. Mast cell secretions lead to vomiting. Systemic spillover of allergen into the circulation may lead to milder effects in other tissues (e.g., urticaria).

4. The answer is D *[II C 2 c; III D 2 b].*
Antithyroid peroxidase antibodies produce complement-mediated cytotoxicity to thyroid follicle cells (a type II pathogenic mechanism). In systemic lupus erythematosus (SLE), persistent circulating immune complexes are responsible for much of the pathogenesis (type III); in Graves' disease, an antibody acting as a thyroid-stimulating hormone (TSH) agonist hyperstimulates the thyroid; in insulin-dependent diabetes mellitus (IDDM), T-cell cytotoxicity to beta islet cells is probably responsible for the major pathogenesis (type IV).

5. The answer is C *[II D 2 c, 4 a, b, 5 a].*
One of the most common causes of type III hypersensitivity is the response to drugs. This type of reaction is often seen after long-term, high-dose therapy. The treatment of choice is to discontinue treatment and substitute an unrelated drug.

6. The answer is A *[II E 1].*
Poison ivy contains a hapten, pentadecyl catechol, which is not known to be toxic. Therefore, its capacity to elicit an immune response is inappropriate because it serves no useful function. In chronic tuberculosis, the immune response is attempting, although unsuccessfully, to eliminate the mycobacterial pathogen. Acute graft rejection is also appropriate, but unfortunate, because it is a response against foreign tissue. A tuberculin test is an appropriate manifestation of the existence of active immunity or memory to Mycobacterium.

7. The answer is C *[III D 8 b].*
Treatment with IFNβ-1b lowers the frequency of attacks by 33% to 50% at 2 years in MS patients. Neostigmine is used as an anticholinergic agent in myasthenia gravis. Cyanocobalamin is administered in autoimmune pernicious anemia to replace nonabsorbed vitamin B_{12}. Propylthiouracil is used as an antithyroid in Graves' disease.

8. The answer is C *[V D 2 e].*
Muromonab-CD3 is a mouse anti-CD3 monoclonal antibody that binds to all T cells because CD3 is a constant part of the antigen receptor of each T cell. The binding of muromonab-CD3 opsonizes the T cells for phagocytosis. Therefore, the total number of T cells is reduced. Mouse antibodies are inefficient at activating human complement. Some T-cell activation with cytokine secretion occurs, but it is an undesirable side effect of muromonab-CD3 administration.

9. The answer is B *[VI B 1 c; Table 10-2].*
Intravenous human immune globulins (IVIGs) are used to replace antibody in immunodeficient individuals. Hepatitis B immune globulin (HBIG) is administered intramuscularly. Anti-Rh antibody is also administered intramuscularly to the mother immediately postpartum (sometimes during pregnancy), but not to the infant. Prophylactic infant immunization for polio is provided through active, not passive, vaccination.

10. The answer is B *[VII D].*
Interferon-α (IFN-α) is approved for use in patients with hairy cell leukemia and patients with acquired immune deficiency syndrome (AIDS) and Kaposi's sarcoma. Some of its beneficial effects probably

derive from its ability to inhibit growth. The other cytokines are in various stages of clinical trials as antineoplastic therapies, although interferon-g (IFN-α) is approved for use in patients with chronic granulomatous disease. Imuthiol is not a cytokine, but a synthetic drug.

11 and 12. The answers are: 11-D, 12-A *[VI D 3 a; Table 10-3].*
A patient with an uncertain history of vaccination and a tetanus-prone wound requires both active and passive vaccination. The tetanus immune globulin (TIG) provides immediate protection if the individual does not have memory. The tetanus toxoid (Td) begins the series that leads to the establishment of memory. A tetanus-prone wound in an individual with a full series of active vaccinations requires no treatment if the last vaccination in the series was administered less than 5 years earlier. These recommendations are general guidelines.

13. The answer is B *[IV A, B 6].*
Opportunistic infections by fungi, viruses, and parasites other than extracellular pyogenic bacteria suggest a deficiency of T-cell function. Inherited T-cell immunodeficiency and acquired immune deficiency syndrome (AIDS) are inherited and acquired T-cell deficiencies, respectively. Combined immunodeficiency includes both humoral and T-cell deficiency. Only humoral immunodeficiency is a primarily humoral deficiency in which the expected signs are recurrent infections by extracellular pyogenic bacteria.

14. The answer is A *[IV B 6 a (1)].*
It is not known what percentage of individuals shows overt symptoms after initial infection. Those who do, however, generally show mononucleosis-like symptoms for approximately 3 weeks. Some individuals display no overt symptoms.

15. The answer is C (I, II) *[I A 4, D 2, 5; VII A].*
Digoxin is a hapten, a molecule that is too small to stimulate responses (be an immunogen) in its free form, but can be recognized by antibodies. To obtain sheep antidigoxin antibodies, the sheep is immunized with digoxin that has been coupled to a larger molecule, in this case, a protein. The antibodies obtained from the sheep are cleaved with proteolytic enzymes to yield the Fab fragment. This fragment is specific to and can bind digoxin, blocking its biologic activity. Animal antibodies have a shorter serum half-life when injected into humans, and all Fab fragments, even human, have a short half-life compared with complete antibody molecules. Only complete human immunoglobulin G (IgG) has a half-life of approximately 1 month.

16. The answer is B (III) *[I B 3, 5].*
CD4$^+$, or helper, T cells have receptors that recognize fragments (epitopes) of immunizing antigens (immunogens) only when the fragments are bound to an MHC class II molecule on the surface of antigen-presenting cells (APCs). As a result, T cells cannot be activated inappropriately by soluble antigens. CD8$^+$T cells recognize fragments bound to MHC class I molecules.

17. The answer is E (all) *[I E 2].*
When complement is activated, different proteins of the complement sequence have functions that lead to all three actions. Acute inflammation allows greater movement of plasma proteins and phagocytes from blood to tissue. Opsonization of immune complexes enhances their phagocytosis. Cytolysis of microorganisms often results in their killing.

18. The answer is A (I) *[I F 2].*
Antiviral antibodies are probably most important in extracellular immunity to viruses, binding virus particles for opsonization and preventing additional infection of cells. Interferons are secreted from viral-infected and other cells (e.g., macrophages, T cells) and, after binding to receptors, induce the appearance of antiviral proteins in other cells. Cytotoxic T cells (CTLs) recognize viral-infected cells and cause direct cytotoxicity.

19. The answer is D (II, III) *[II A 2 d, 6, 7, C 1 b, 5].*
If the patient produced antibodies that are still present and the hypersensitivity reaction is type I, these antibodies are hypersecreted immunoglobulin E (IgE), mostly bound to mast cell and basophil IgE receptors. Their half-life is several months. Intravenous introduction of penicillin causes rapid activation of and secretion by blood basophils. Symptoms of type I hypersensitivity occur within minutes. These symptoms may be severe (anaphylaxis) or less severe (cutaneous, gastrointestinal, or respiratory), depending on the individual. Hemolytic anemia is an expected result of a type II hypersensitivity reaction to penicillin, based on the presence of immunoglobulin M (IgM) or immunoglobulin G (IgG) antibodies in the serum. The onset is delayed by a few hours in a patient with preexisting antibodies.

20. The answer is C (I, II) *[II E 3–6].*
Type IV hypersensitivity reactions are delayed after the introduction of allergen because allergen-specific T cells become activated and attract other cells, such as macrophages, to the site of allergen introduction (e.g., the epidermis of the skin in contact sensitivity, the lungs in tuberculosis). These sites are infiltrated by mononuclear cells. Inflammation is primarily caused by tissue disruption and necrosis as well as by secretion of cytokines by the infiltrating cells. Although histamine secretion can also occur from local mast cells, H1 antagonists of histamine usually do not have significant effects because T-cell and macrophage activation, migration, and secretion are not greatly affected by these drugs.

21. The answer is E (all) *[III C 3 b, E 1, 2].*
All three findings are common to more than one non–organ-specific autoimmune disorder, but occur in different percentages of patients with specific disorders. For example, antinuclear antibodies are probably present in all patients with systemic lupus erythematosus (SLE), but are found in only a fraction of patients with rheumatoid arthritis and Sjögren's syndrome. Rheumatoid factors are more common in rheumatoid arthritis than in SLE or Sjögren's syndrome, and hypergammaglobulinemia is more prevalent in SLE than in Sjögren's syndrome.

22. The answer is A (I) *[V A 3, B].*
Parents and children are rarely human leukocyte antigen (HLA)-matched, but are usually half-matched. An HLA match from a cadaver-derived organ is unlikely. The probability that two siblings are HLA-matched is 25%; the probability that they are half-matched is 50%.

23. The answer is B (III) *[V B 2, C 1].*
In bone marrow transplantation, marrow containing competent lymphocytes is transplanted to a generally immunosuppressed host. The greatest problem is an immune response by the graft against human leukocyte antigens (HLA) and other tissue antigens of the host. In renal and cardiac transplantation, the greatest problem is rejection of the foreign organ by the immune system of the host [host-versus-graft (HVG) disease].

24. The answer is D (II, III) *[V B 2, D 2 a].*
Cell-mediated immune mechanisms are thought to be more important in acute graft rejection, and the inhibition of T-cell activation appears to be the key element in immunosuppression. Responding T cells require signaling from interleukin-2 (IL-2) to reach full activation and progress to cell division. IL-2 is produced by activated T cells and can act autocrinely. Cyclosporine blocks transcription of the IL-2 gene during T-cell activation, inhibits the synthesis of IL-2, and prevents full T-cell activation and division. Its effects are limited to activated T cells. Because it has no direct effect on antibody synthesis, it is not useful in the hyperacute rejection phenomena that are based on antibody-mediated mechanisms. Hyperacute rejection is essentially untreatable because it depends on the presence of antibodies in the graft recipient.

25. The answer is A (I) *[VI C 2 a, b].*
Live, attenuated vaccines introduce organisms that are competent to replicate. This replication stimulates the immune response. For this and probably other reasons, a live, attenuated vaccine (but not a killed, inactivated vaccine) probably provides lifelong immunity in one or two doses.

26. The answer is D (II, III) *[VI C 1 d; Table 10-3].*
The measles, mumps, rubella (MMR) vaccine is administered to infants within or shortly after the first year. A second dose is recommended at school entry. Influenza active vaccine is targeted toward specific adult populations. Health-care workers are included in this target population, as are infants and children at risk; however, the vaccine is not routinely administered to infants. Tetanus toxoid (Td) is not routinely administered to infants, who instead receive diphtheria, tetanus, pertussis (DTP). Td is used primarily for initial vaccinations in adults who were not previously vaccinated and for 10-year booster vaccinations in all individuals, including health-care workers.

27. The answer is A (I) *[VI C 2; Table 10-3].*
The pneumococcal and meningococcal vaccines are multivalent and contain purified polysaccharide from a number of different serotypes. However, these vaccines do not contain polysaccharide from all the relevant infectious agents. Purified polysaccharides do not stimulate immune responses in children less than 2 years of age. For polysaccharide vaccines to be effective in young children, the polysaccharide must be conjugated to a protein as in the HIB vaccine.

11
Biotechnologic Products

Godwin W. Fong
Charles Lee

I. INTRODUCTION. Advances in biotechnology have made many formerly unstable or difficult-to-produce biologic products available for therapeutic use. Some life-threatening diseases are now treated with biotechnology products.

   A. Interferon is an example of a drug that was genetically engineered to inhibit certain types of cancer cells and some viruses.

   B. Cellular hormones known as **interleukins,** lymphotoxins, and tumor necrosis factor are now used to treat cancer and immune deficiency diseases.

   C. Monoclonal antibodies (MABs) can deliver toxins specifically to cancer cells and destroy them. MABs are also used with radioisotopes to diagnose and visualize cancer cells.

   D. Many biopharmaceutical products derived from the body tissues (through cell lines) are now produced on a large scale. Modified natural products also may be further improved.

   E. A synthetic analogue of thyrotropin-releasing hormone prevents paralysis after spinal cord injuries in animal studies.

   F. Superoxide dismutase may be useful in preventing damage to tissues that are deprived of oxygen.

   G. New biotechnologic treatments have been developed for emphysema, congestive heart failure, ulcers, atherosclerosis, and an increasing number of medical conditions. **Table 11-1** lists the biotechnology products that are approved for human use.

II. BASIC TERMINOLOGY

   A. An **antigen** is a substance that stimulates the production of antibodies.

   B. An **antibody** is an immunoglobulin produced by the body in response to stimulation from an antigen.

   C. Antisense DNA is a complementary strand of DNA that is specifically synthesized to attach to the sense DNA and prevent genetic transcription. The sense DNA that carries the information that affects the disease process is usually elucidated before an antisense drug is designed.

   D. Colony-stimulating factors (CSFs) are a class of glycoprotein hormones. CSFs regulate the differentiation and formation of blood cells from precursor cells.

   E. Cytokines are a group of special proteins (nonantibodies) released by cells to trigger action in other cells.

   F. Deoxyribonucleic acid (DNA) is the molecule that contains the genetic instructions of a cell. DNA consists of deoxyribose, phosphate, and repeating bases as building blocks. The four bases are adenine, guanine, thymine, and cytosine.

   G. DNA ligase is an enzyme that seals single-stranded nicks between nucleotides in double-stranded DNA. DNA ligase enables DNA fragments from different sources to be joined.

   H. DNA polymerase is an enzyme that catalyzes the synthesis of DNA. It uses a single strand of DNA as the template and uses nucleotides as the substrates.

Table 11-1. Approved Recombinant Therapeutics and Vaccines

Drug (Trade Name)	Indication	Company (Year introduced)
Human insulin (Humulin)	Diabetes	Eli Lilly/Genentech (1982)
Somatrem for injection (Protropin)	Human growth hormone deficiency in children	Genentech (1985)
Interferon-alpha-2a (Roferon-A)	Hairy cell leukemia	Hoffmann-La Roche (1986)
Interferon-alpha-2b (Intron A)	Hairy cell leukemia	Schering-Plough/Biogen (1986)
	Extension of therapy for chronic hepatitis C from 6 months to 18–24 months	(1997)
	Follicular lymphoma in conjunction with chemotherapy	(1997)
Hepatitis B vaccine recombinant (Recombivax HB)	Prevention of hepatitis B	Merck; Chiron (1986)
Muromonab-CD3 (Ortho-clone OKT3)	Reversal of acute kidney transplant rejection	Ortho Biotech (1986)
Somatropin for injection (Humatrope)	Human growth hormone deficiency in children	Eli Lilly (1987)
Alteplase (Activase)	Acute myocardial infarction	Genentech (1987)
	Acute pulmonary embolism	(1990)
	Restoration of function to central venous access devices (as assessed by the ability to withdraw blood)	(2001)
Interferon-alpha-2a (Roferon-A)	Acquired immune deficiency syndrome (AIDS)-related Kaposi's sarcoma	Hoffmann-La Roche (1988)
Interferon-alpha-2b (Intron A)	AIDS-related Kaposi's sarcoma, genital warts	Schering-Plough; Biogen (1988)
	Hepatitis C	(1991)
Interferon-n3 (Alferon N injection)	Genital warts	Interferon Sciences (1989)
Hepatitis B vaccine (Engerix-B)	Hepatitis B prevention	SmithKline Beecham; Biogen (1989)
	Chronic hepatitis C infection	(1998)
Erythropoietin (Epogen)	Anemia associated with chronic renal failure	Amgen; Johnson & Johnson; Kirin (1989)
Erythropoietin (Procrit)	Anemia associated with AIDS or zidovudine administration	Amgen; Ortho Biotech (1990)
	Anemia associated with chronic renal failure	(1990)
	Chemotherapy-associated anemia in patients with nonmyloid malignancy	(1993)
	Anemia associated with cancer and chemotherapy	(1993)
PEG-adenosine (ADAGEN®)	ADA-deficient severe combined immunodeficiency	Enzon; Eastman Kodak (1990)
Interferon-gamma-1b (Actimmune)	Management of chronic granulomatous disease	Genentech (1990)
	Delaying time to disease progression in patients with severe, malignant osteopetrosis	InterMune Pharmaceuticals (2000)

(Continued on next page)

Table 11-1. Continued.

Drug (Trade Name)	Indication	Company (Year introduced)
Cytomegalovirus (CMV) immune globulin (CytoGam)	Prevention of CMV in kidney transplant recipients	Medimmune (1990)
Filgrastim; granulocyte colony-stimulating factor (G-CSF)	Chemotherapy-induced neutropenia Acute myeloid leukemia	Amgen (1991) (1998)
Glucocerebrosidase (Ceredase)	Type I Gaucher's disease*	Genzyme (1991)
Glucocerebrosidase (Cerezyme)	Type I Gaucher's disease*	Genzyme (1994)
Sargramostim [granulocyte–macrophage colony-stimulating factor (GM-CSF)] (Prokine)	Autologous bone marrow transplantation	Hoechst-Roussel; Immunex (1991)
Sargramostim (GM-CSF) (Leukine)	Neutrophil recovery after bone marrow transplantation	Immunex; Hoechst-Roussel (1991)
Antihemophilic factor (Mononine)	Hemophilia B	Armour (1992)
Antihemophilic factor (Recombinate)	Hemophilia A	Genetics Institute; Baxter Healthcare (1992)
Interleukin-2 (Proleukin)	Renal cell carcinoma Metastatic melanoma	Chiron (1992) (1998)
Indium-111–labeled antibody (OncoScint CR103)	Detection, staging, and follow-up of colorectal cancer	Cytogen; Knoll (1992)
Indium-111–labeled antibody (OncoScint OV103)	Detection, staging, and follow-up of ovarian cancer	(1992)
Interferon-beta-1b (Betaseron)	Relapsing/remitting multiple sclerosis	Chiron; Berlex (1993)
DNase-alfa (Pulmozyme)	Cystic fibrosis	Genentech (1993)
Factor VIII (Kogenate)	Hemophilia A	Genentech; Miles (1993)
Filgrastim (G-CSF) (Neupogen)	Bone marrow transplant	Amgen (1994)
PEG-L-asparaginase (Oncaspar)	Refractory childhood acute lymphoblastic leukemia	Enzon (1994)
Human growth hormone (Nutropin)	Short stature caused by human growth hormone deficiency	Genentech (1994)
Abciximab (ReoPro)	Antiplatelet prevention of blood clots	Centocor (1994)
	Treatment of a broader range of patients undergoing percutaneous coronary intervention; revised dosage and patient management to reduce bleeding	
	Unstable angina that does not respond to conventional medical therapy when percutaneous coronary intervention is planned within 24 hours	
Live varicella virus vaccine (Varivax)	Active immunization of persons 12 months of age and older	Merck (1995)
Respiratory syncytial virus (RSV) immune globulin (RespiGam)	Prevention of serious lower respiratory tract infection in children younger than 24 months old	Massachusetts Public Health Biologic Labs (1996)

Table 11-1. Continued.

Drug (Trade Name)	Indication	Company (Year introduced)
Inactivated hepatitis A vaccine (Vaqta)	Immunization against hepatitis A in children older than 6 years of age	Merck (1996)
Interferon-beta-1a (Avonex)	Multiple sclerosis	Biogen (1996)
Human antihemophilic factor	Hemophilia A	Centeon (1996)
Haemophilus b conjugate (meningococcal protein conjugate) and hepatitis B (recombinant vaccine) (Comvax)	Immunization of persons 6 weeks to 15 months of age born of hepatitis B surface antigen–negative mothers	Merck (1996)
Cryoprecipitated antihemophilic factor A	Control of bleeding associated with Factor VIII deficiency	Blood Bank of the Redwoods (1996)
Reteplase (Retavase)	Acute myocardial infarction in adults	Boehringer Mannheim (1996)
Diphtheria and tetanus toxoids and acellular pertussis (DTaP) vaccine (Infanrix)	Primary and booster immunization of infants and children except as a fifth dose in children who previously received four doses of DTaP	SmithKline Beecham (1997)
Recombinant coagulation Factor IX (BeneFix)	Control and prevention of hemorrhagic episodes in patients with hemophilia B, including perioperative management of patients with hemophilia B who are undergoing surgery	Genetics Institute (1997)
Autologous cultured chondrocytes (Carticel SM Service)	Repair of clinically significant, symptomatic, cartilaginous defects of the femoral condyle (medial, lateral, or trochlear) caused by acute or repetitive trauma	Genzyme Tissue Repair (1997)
Interferon-alfacon-1 (Infergen)	Treatment of chronic hepatitis C virus (HCV) infection in patients 18 years of age or older who have compensated liver disease and anti-HCV serum antibodies or HCV RNA	Amgen (1997)
	Subsequent treatment of HCV-infected patients who tolerated an initial course of interferon therapy	(1997)
Rabies vaccine (RabAvert)	Pre-exposure and postexposure immunization of children and adults	Chiron (1997)
Oprelvekin (Neumega)	Prevention of severe thrombocytopenia and reduction of the need for platelet transfusions after myelosuppressive chemotherapy in patients with nonmyeloid malignancies who are at high risk for severe thrombocytopenia	Genetics Institute (1997)
Rituximab (Rituxan)	Treatment of patients with relapsed or refractory low-grade or follicular B-cell non-Hodgkin's lymphoma	Genentech (1997)
Daclizumab (Zenapax)	Prophylaxis of acute organ rejection in patients receiving renal transplants; part of an immunosuppressive regimen that includes cyclosporine and corticosteroids	Hoffman-La Roche (1997)

(Continued on next page)

Table 11-1. Continued.

Drug (Trade Name)	Indication	Company (Year introduced)
Becaplermin (Regranex)	Lower-extremity diabetic neuropathic ulcers that extend into the subcutaneous tissue or beyond, and have an adequate blood supply	OMJ Pharmaceuticals (1997)
Human T-lymphotropic virus (HTLV) I/II (Vironostika HTLV-I & II MicroElisa System)	Detection of antibodies to HTLV I/II in human serum or plasma	Organon Teknika (1998)
Fibrin sealant (Tisseel VH kit)	Adjunct to hemostasis in surgeries that involve cardiopulmonary bypass; treatment of splenic injuries caused by blunt or penetrating trauma to the abdomen, when control of bleeding by conventional surgical techniques, including suture, ligature, and cautery, is ineffective or impractical; closure of colostomies	Osterreichisches Institut fur Haemoderivate (1998)
Pooled plasma, solvent detergent treated (VIPLAS/SD)	Documented deficiencies of coagulation factors for which there are no concentrate preparations available, including congenital single-factor deficiencies of Factors I, V, VII, XI, and XIII, and acquired multiple coagulation factor deficiencies; reversals of warfarin effect; thrombotic thrombocytopenic purpura	V.I. Technologies (1998)
Basiliximab (Simulect)	Prophylaxis of acute organ rejection in patients undergoing renal transplantation; part of an immunosuppressive regimen that includes cyclosporine and corticosteroids	Novartis (1998)
	Use in renal transplantation in combination with triple immunosuppressive therapy; use in pediatric renal transplantation; and use of an IV bolus injection	(2001)
Palivizumab (Synagis)	Prophylaxis of serious lower respiratory tract disease caused by RSV in pediatric patients at high risk of RSV disease	Medimmune (1998)
Sacrosidase (Sucraid)	Congenital sucrose isomaltase deficiency	Orphan Medical (1998)
Eptifibatide (Integrilin)	Acute coronary syndrome; treatment of patients undergoing percutaneous coronary intervention	COR Therapeutics (1998)
Diphtheria and tetanus toxoids and acellular pertussis vaccine adsorbed (Certiva)	Active immunization of persons 6 weeks to 7 years of age (before the seventh birthday)	North American Vaccine (1998)
Infliximab (Remicade)	Treatment of moderately to severely active Crohn's disease to reduce the signs and symptoms in patients who have an inadequate response to conventional therapies; treatment of patients with fistulizing Crohn's disease to reduce the number of draining enterocutaneous fistulas	Centocor (1998)

Table 11-1. Continued.

Drug (Trade Name)	Indication	Company (Year introduced)
Rotavirus vaccine, live, oral, tetravalent (RotaShield)	Primary immunization of infants at 2, 4, and 6 months of age	Wyeth-Ayerst Laboratories (1998)
Trastuzumab (Herceptin)	Metastatic breast cancer in patients whose tumors overexpress the HER2 protein and who have received one or more chemotherapy regimens for metastatic disease	Genentech (1998)
	Median survival	(2001)
(Etanercept) Enbrel	Reduction in signs and symptoms of moderately to severely active rheumatoid arthritis in patients who have had an inadequate response to one or more disease-modifying antirheumatic drugs	Immunex (1998)
	Reducing the signs and symptoms and delaying structural damage in patients with moderately to severely active rheumatoid arthritis, including those who have not previously failed treatment with a disease-modifying antirheumatic drug (DMARD)	(2000)
	Reducing signs and symptoms of active arthritis in patients with psoriatic arthritis	(2002)
Recombinant OspA (LYMErix)	Active immunization against Lyme disease in people 15–70 years old	SmithKline Beecham (1998)
Vitravene (Fomivirsen)	Local treatment of CMV retinitis in patients with AIDS who are intolerant of or have a contraindication to other treatments for CMV retinitis or who were insufficiently responsive to previous treatments	Isis Pharmaceuticals; Ciba Vision (1998)
Antithymocyte globulin (Thymoglobulin)	Acute rejection in renal transplant patients	Pasteur-Mérieux Serums et Vaccines—France (1998)
Denileukin diftitox (Ontak)	Treatment of patients with persistent or recurrent cutaneous T-cell lymphoma whose malignant cells express the CD25 component of the interleukin-2 receptor	Seragen (1999)
Hepatitis B immune globulin (Nabi-HB)	Treatment of acute exposure to hepatitis B surface antigen (HBsAg), perinatal exposure of infants born to HBsAg-positive mothers, sexual exposure to HBsAg-positive persons, and household exposure of infants to persons with acute hepatitis B virus infection	Nabi (1999)
Recombinant coagulation factor VIIa (NovoSeven)	Treatment of bleeding episodes in hemophilia A or B with inhibitors to Factor VIII or Factor IX	Novo Nordisk A/S—Denmark (1999)
Interferon-alpha-n1, lymphoblastoid (Wellferon)	Chronic HCV infection in patients 18 years of age or older who do not have decompensated liver disease	GlaxoWellcome (1999)

(Continued on next page)

Table 11-1. Continued.

Drug (Trade Name)	Indication	Company (Year introduced)
Antihemophilic factor/ von Willebrand factor complex (Humate-P)	Used in adult patients for treatment and prevention of bleeding hemophilia A (classic hemophilia); in adult and pediatric patients for treatment of spontaneous and trauma-induced bleeding episodes in severe von Willebrand disease and in mild and moderate von Willebrand disease where use of desmopressin is known or suspected to be inadequate	Centeon Pharma—Germany (1999)
Hetastarch (Hextend)	Plasma volume expander for treatment of hypovolemia during surgery	BioTime (1999)
Pneumococcal 7-valent conjugate vaccine (diphtheria CRM197 protein) (Prevnar)	Immunization of infants 2, 4, 6, and 12–15 months of age to prevent invasive pneumococcal disease	Lederle Laboratories Division American Cyanamid (2000)
	Immunization of infants and toddlers against otitis media caused by vaccine serotypes	(2002)
Antihemophilic factor (recombinant) (ReFacto)	Control and prevention of hemorrhagic episodes and for short-term routine and surgical prophylaxis in patients with hemophilia A	Genetics Institute (2000)
BCG, live (PACIS)	Treatment of carcinoma-in-situ (CIS) in the absence of associated invasive cancer of the bladder	BioChem Pharma-Canada (2000)
Tenecteplase (TNKase)	Reduction of mortality associated with acute myocardial infarction (AMI)	Genentech (2000)
Crotalidae polyvalent immune Fab (ovine) (CroFab)	Treatment of minimal and moderate North American Crotalidae envenomation	Protherics (2000)
Botulinum toxin type B (MYOBLOC)	Treatment of cervical dystonia to reduce the severity of abnormal head position and neck pain	Elan Pharmaceuticals (2000)
Botulinum toxin type A (BOTOX or BOTOX COSMETIC)	Treatment of cervical dystonia	Allergan (2002)
	Temporary improvement in the appearance of moderate to severe glabellar lines associated with corrugator and/or procerus muscle activity in adult patients ≥65 years of age	
Peginterferon-alpha-2b (PEG-Intron)	Treatment of chronic hepatitis C in patients not previously treated with interferon-alpha who have compensated liver disease and are at least 18 years of age	Schering (2001)
Alemtuzumab (Campath)	Treatment of patients with B-cell chronic lymphocytic leukemia who have been treated with alkylating agents and who have failed fludarabine therapy	Millennium and ILEX Partners (2001)
Hepatitis A inactivated and hepatitis B (recombinant) vaccine (TWINRIX)	Active immunization of persons 18 years of age or older against disease caused by hepatitis A virus and infection by all known subtypes of hepatitis B virus	SmithKline Beecham Biologicals (2001)
Digoxin immune Fab (Ovine) (DigiFab)	Treatment of patients with life-threatening or potentially life-threatening digoxin toxicity or overdose	Protherics (2001)

Table 11-1. Continued.

Drug (Trade Name)	Indication	Company (Year introduced)
Darbepoetin-alpha (Aranesp)	Treatment of anemia associated with chronic renal failure, including patients on dialysis and patients not on dialysis	Amgen (2001)
	Treatment of anemia in patients with nonmyeloid malignancies where anemia is due to the effect of concomitantly administered chemotherapy	(2002)
Hepatitis B immune globulin (Human) (Nabi-HB)	Treatment of acute exposure to HBsAg following acute exposure to blood containing HBsAg, perinatal exposure of infants born to HBsAg-positive mothers, sexual exposure to HBsAg-positive persons, and household exposure of infants to persons with acute hepatitis B virus infection	Nabi (2001)
Anakinra (Kineret)	Reduction in signs and symptoms of moderately to severely active rheumatoid arthritis, in patients 18 years of age or older who have failed one or more DMARD	Amgen (2001)
Drotrecogin-alpha (activated) (Xigris)	Reduction of mortality in adult patients with severe sepsis (sepsis associated with acute organ dysfunction) who have a high risk of dying from sepsis, as measured by a scoring system based on their general health and the severity of their illness (e.g., by APACHE II)	Eli Lilly (2001)
Pegfilgrastim (Neulasta)	To decrease the incidence of infection, as manifested by febrile neutropenia, in patients with nonmyeloid malignancies receiving myelosuppressive anti-cancer drugs associated with a clinically significant incidence of febrile neutropenia	Amgen (2002)
Ibritumomab tiuxetan (Zevalin)	Treatment of patients with relapsed or refractory low-grade, follicular, or transformed B-cell non-Hodgkin's lymphoma, including patients with rituximab (Rituxan) refractory follicular non-Hodgkin's lymphoma; the therapeutic regimen includes rituximab, indium-111 ibritumomab tiuxetan, and yttrium-90 ibritumomab tiuxetan	IDEC Pharmaceuticals (2002)
Interferon-beta-1a (Rebif)	Treatment of patients with relapsing forms of multiple sclerosis to decrease the frequency of clinical exacerbations and delay the accumulation of physical disability	Serono (2002)

(Continued on next page)

Table 11-1. Continued.

Drug (Trade Name)	Indication	Company (Year introduced)
Diphtheria and tetanus toxoids and acellular pertussis vaccine adsorbed (DTaP) (DAPTACEL)	Active immunization of infants and toddlers at 2, 4, 6, and 17–20 months of age against diphtheria, tetanus, and pertussis	Aventis Pasteur—Canada (2002)
Rasburicase (Elitek)	Initial management of plasma uric acid levels in pediatric patients with leukemia, lymphoma, and solid tumor malignancies who are receiving anti-cancer therapy expected to result in tumor lysis and subsequent elevation of plasma uric acid	Sanofi-Synthelabo (2002)
Peginterferon-alpha-2a (PEGASYS)	Treatment of adults with chronic hepatitis C who have compensated liver disease and who have not been previously treated with interferon-alpha	Hoffman-La Roche (2001)
Urokinase (Abbokinase)	For adults for the lysis of acute massive pulmonary emboli, defined as obstruction of blood flow to a lobe or multiple segments, and for the lysis of pulmonary emboli accompanied by unstable hemodynamics (i.e., failure to maintain blood pressure without supportive measures)	Abbott Laboratories (2001)

*Gaucher's disease is an autosomal dominant or recessive disorder. It is caused by an excess of glucocerebroside in the reticuloendothelial cells because of the lack of a metabolic enzyme, cerebrosidase. Proliferation of abnormal cells leads to splenomegaly, hepatomegaly, skeletal lesions, and other symptoms.

Source: *Biotechnology in the U.S. Pharmaceutical Industry.* Research Triangle Park, NC, Institute for Biotechnology Information, 1995; http://www.fda.gov in 2002.

    I. An **enzyme** is a protein that catalyzes a substrate during its conversion to a product.

    J. A **gene** is a segment of DNA that codes for a specific polypeptide.

    K. A **genome** is the genetic information content of a cell.

    L. A **hormone** is an endogenous substance that is secreted by one type of cell and acts on another type of cell.

    M. A **hybridoma** is a hybrid cell produced by the fusion of a myeloma cell and a specific antibody-producing B lymphocyte. A single hybridoma produces a single type of antibody.

    N. **Interferon** is any of a class of glycoproteins produced by animal cells in response to viral infection.

    O. **Interleukin** is a group of proteins synthesized by macrophages and T lymphocytes in response to antigen and other stimulation.

    P. A **lymphokine** is any of a class of soluble proteins produced by some white blood cells. These proteins stimulate other white blood cells as part of the immune response.

    Q. A **plasmid** is a circular piece of duplex DNA that is not part of a chromosome and can replicate independently. Plasmids are used as vectors for the transfer of DNA in recombinant DNA technology.

R. **Ribonucleic acid (RNA)** is a macromolecule that contains information for protein synthesis. The three types of RNA are ribosomal RNA (rRNA), transfer RNA (tRNA), and messenger RNA (mRNA). RNA is also the genetic material of some viruses.

S. **Recombinant DNA (rDNA)** is a hybrid DNA that is formed when pieces of DNA from different sources are joined. The process is also known as gene splicing.

T. **Restriction endonuclease** is an enzyme that cleaves DNA at sequence-specific sites.

U. **Tumor necrosis factor** is a lymphokine produced by macrophages. It can be activated to kill tumor cells.

V. **Reverse transcripts** is an enzyme present in RNA viruses that catalyzes the formation of DNA from the viral RNA.

III. PROTEINS AND PEPTIDES.
Proteins and peptides play essential roles in all aspects of cellular function. Many **endogenous** substances synthesized in the body are essential proteins. Many enzymes that catalyze vital reactions in the body are proteins.

A. **Hemoglobin** is a large protein involved in oxygen transport.

B. **Globulins** are special proteins in the plasma. They are involved in immunogenic response and antibody formation.

C. **Albumin** is a plasma protein that binds to many drugs. It is also used as a carrier for new drugs.

D. Other well-known proteins include insulin and the enzymes involved in digestion.

E. Protein is an important component of **keratin** in hair and **myosin** in muscles.

F. **Albumin (human) 5% USP** is used to reverse hypovolemia in shock patients, burn patients, and those with chronic hypoalbuminemia.

IV. IMMUNOGLOBULIN (IgG)
is an important class of globulin protein involved in immunity and the allergic response. **IgG** is used therapeutically to modulate or replace antibody in various **immunodeficiency** and disease states. Intramuscular and intravenous preparations are available from various manufacturers **(Tables 11-2, 11-3)**. Most of these products must be stored under refrigeration (2–8°C) and have a limited shelf life.

V. RECOMBINANT HUMAN GRANULOCYTE COLONY-STIMULATING FACTOR

A. These factors are **glycoproteins** that regulate the production of many types of blood cells and components in the body. These include **macrophages, eosinophils, neutrophils, basophils, and platelets.** Natural and modified CSFs are used to treat a number of congenital disorders and several forms of cancer.

Table 11-2. Immunoglobulin Applications

Gammaglobulinemia
Hepatitis A prophylaxis
Measles and rubella prophylaxis
Multiple myeloma with specific antibody deficiency
Prophylaxis in infants and children with human immunodeficiency virus (HIV) exposure
Chronic inflammatory demyelinating neuropathy
Acquired hemophilia
Orphan drug for the treatment of juvenile rheumatoid arthritis
Respiratory tract infections
Immune thrombocytopenic purpura
Orphan drug for the treatment of polymyositis and acute myocarditis
Acute exposure to hepatitis B surface antigen
Kawasaki disease in conjunction with high-dose aspirin

Table 11-3. Immunoglobulin Products

Gamimune-N
Gammagard
Polygram
Gammar
Iveegam
Nabi-HB
RespiGam
Sandoglobulin
Polygam
Venoglobulin

B. Lenograstim is a **recombinant human granulocyte CSF** (rHuG-CSF) derived from Chinese hamster ovary cells. It is glycosylated at the same site as natural HuG-CSF (threonine-133) and consists of 174 amino acids.

C. Filgrastim is an *Escherichia coli*–derived glycoprotein. It is not glycosylated, and it differs in structure from natural HuG-CSF. Like natural HuG-CSF and **filgrastim,** lenograstim selectively promotes the proliferation, differentiation, and maturation of blood cell precursors. Dose-related increases in blood neutrophil counts are observed after lenograstim administration. Lenograstim reduces the duration of **neutropenia** and the severity of infection in patients who are receiving **cytotoxic chemotherapy** for **nonmyeloid malignancy.** Colony-forming assays show that lenograstim is approximately three times as potent as filgrastim. These agents were similarly potent in cell proliferation assays. Both natural and recombinant granulocyte CSF products stimulate the release of mature neutrophils from hematopoietic tissue, prolong their survival, and enhance their phagocytic and cytotoxic activity.

D. Other actions of rHuG-CSF include synergism with **interleukin-3** to induce megakaryocyte formation and with granulocyte–macrophage CSF (GM-CSF) to stimulate granulocyte–macrophage colonies.

VI. GLYCOPROTEINS

A. Many special proteins acquire biologic activity as a result of their covalent linking with a polymer of sugar or **carbohydrate.** The covalently linked protein–carbohydrate molecule is a **glycoprotein.** Glycoproteins form natural structural membranes in the cells of unicellular (e.g., bacteria) and multicellular (e.g., humans, animals) organisms.

B. N-acetylglucosamine (NAG) forms the cell membrane in bacteria. It is an example of a carbohydrate chain linked to a protein through a chain of amino acids. Bacterial resistance to penicillin is linked to the integrity of **NAG** in the cell membrane.

C. The extent and site of **glycosylation** of a protein molecule may affect the physicochemical properties, stability, and specificity of a surface receptor in a cell. Glycoproteins on the surface of red blood cells are involved in recognizing the specific blood type.

D. The charge at the site of a glycoprotein molecule may play a role in the orientation and interaction of the receptor. The charge may be modified by **sialic acid, sulfate,** and **phosphate groups.** The protein molecule presents potential sites for **N-glycosylation** and **O-glycosylation.** Change in glycosylation is a powerful tool for use in engineering the preferred configuration and stability when designing recombinant glycoprotein for therapeutic use.

E. Carbohydrates contribute to activities in a number of ways, including recognition of the terminal sialic acids of glycoproteins by various viruses and bacteria, recognition of polylactosamines on **erythrocytes** by autoimmune antibodies, and recognition of sialylated, fucosylated lactosaminoglycans on leukocytes by E-selectin of endothelial cells.

VII. DNA

A. DNA is the genetic material of all organisms except some viruses whose genetic material is in the form of RNA. Most organisms have double-stranded DNA. Some viruses contain single-stranded DNA. This type of virus replicates itself by entering a host cell, where it makes a complementary copy of itself and temporarily forms a double strand.

B. All DNA molecules consist of many covalently linked subunits called nucleotides. The nucleotides consist of deoxyribose, phosphate, and one of the nitrogen-containing bases (adenine, guanine, thymine, or cytosine). DNA encodes information to produce all of the proteins needed by the organism. The DNA sequence may be modified or recombined with new strands. This recombinant technology may be used to correct genetic defects in living organisms.

VIII. ANTISENSE DRUGS

A. Many diseases occur because of genetic defects or errors in the gene involved in producing essential enzymes or proteins. Genetic information resides in **chromosomes** that house helical strands of DNA within the nucleus. The **Human Genome Initiative** was created several years ago to study all human genes. This national effort is now yielding information on many serious diseases that involve congenital defects, cancer, infection, acquired immune deficiency syndrome (AIDS), and other disorders of the immune system.

B. Strategies are now available to moderate many disease processes by altering or blocking the **transcription** of DNA. If the DNA sequence is altered so that the **complementary strand** is transcribed instead of the normal "sense" gene, then the DNA cannot make a copy of the normal RNA that participates in protein synthesis. The aberrant copies of RNA may "pair up" **(hybridize)** with other RNA strands that complement it and thereby block protein synthesis. This technique involves targeting DNA or RNA with **antisense** drugs.

C. Many oligonucleotides are designed to target viral disease and cancer cells. To further stabilize the drug, phosphodiesters are chemically converted to phosphothioates.

D. Antisense drugs against cytomegalovirus (CMV), human immunodeficiency virus (HIV), and other viruses are in various phases of clinical trial. The first antisense drug, Vitravene, was approved by the FDA in 1998. Vitravene is a very potent biotechnology drug that is indicated for the local treatment of CMV retinitis in patients with AIDS who are intolerant of other treatments, who have a contraindication to other treatments, or who were insufficiently responsive to previous treatments. The recommended labeled dosage is an induction dose on days 1 and 15, followed by a monthly intravitreal injection of 330 µg.

E. When the **nucleotide** base sequence of a gene that controls a specific body function is known, the antisense DNA strand can be synthesized. If necessary, the DNA strand can be modified to provide increased stability and potency. These strands can then be introduced into cells, where they attach themselves to the **complementary** sense DNA strands and depress transcription of these genes. This technique was performed successfully in cell culture for the gene that produces human **squamous cell carcinoma** of the **larynx.**

F. If a duplicate copy of a gene is inserted into a chromosome in **reverse orientation** to the normal gene, then the antisense DNA strand of this gene is transcribed. This process yields an antisense mRNA strand that is complementary to the mRNA strand transcribed for the normal gene. The two complementary RNA strands bind to each other, thereby preventing the **translation** of the normal RNA strand that may control protein synthesis.

IX. GENE THERAPY. The first example of human gene therapy started in 1990, when the FDA approved PEG-ADA (Enzon, Piscataway, NJ) for **adenosine deaminase** deficiency. This rare, but serious, genetic disorder weakens the immune system and causes increased susceptibility to infection. Two girls were reinfused with their own genetically altered white blood cells. The altered cells live and function normally, and the two girls were living a relatively normal life after 5 years.

X. MISCELLANEOUS BIOTECHNOLOGIC PRODUCTS

A. **Alteplase** (Activase, Genentech) is a **thrombolytic** agent formerly known as **tissue plasminogen activator.** Intravenous alteplase effectively produces recanalization of occluded coronary arteries after acute **myocardial infarction.** Intravenous alteplase is also effective in the treatment of acute massive **pulmonary embolism.** Adverse effects, including bleeding complications, **reperfusion arrhythmias,** and reinfarction, are the primary concerns with this therapy. Systemic fibrinolysis is less than that seen with streptokinase. The recommended dose to produce **recanalization** after myocardial. infarction is 100 mg in divided doses. The recommended dose to treat pulmonary embolism is 100 mg infused intravenously over 2 hours.

B. **Antithrombin III** (heparin cofactor, human antithrombin III, ATnativ) is designated an orphan product. It is used as replacement therapy to prevent or treat thromboembolic episodes in congenital deficiency states. The amount of intravenous antithrombin III concentrate to be administered is based on antithrombin III levels. In patients who have congenital or acquired **antithrombin III deficiency,** the goal is to maintain levels between 80% and 120% of normal. Once-daily doses of antithrombin III should maintain serum levels above 80% of normal. Levels should be monitored twice daily until they stabilize, then daily thereafter immediately before the next dose is administered.

C. **Interleukin-3** is a **hematopoietic growth factor** used to treat patients with bone marrow failure. Recombinant human interleukin-3 alone improves neutrophil and platelet counts in patients who have **chemotherapy-related bone marrow failure** and myelodysplastic syndromes. However, only minimal improvements in hematopoiesis are seen in patients who have aplastic anemia. Enhanced responses are seen with the sequential combined use of recombinant human interleukin-3 and other hematopoietic growth factors (e.g., GM-CSF). Recombinant human interleukin-3 is given subcutaneously or intravenously. Intravenous doses range from $30–1000 \ \mu g/m^2/day$ infused over 4 hours.

D. **Aldesleukin,** a lymphokine, is a human recombinant interleukin-2 product that is used to treat **metastatic renal cell carcinoma.** The starting dose is 0.037 mg/kg every 8 hours by a 15-minute intravenous infusion. Aldesleukin is absorbed erratically after intramuscular or subcutaneous injection. It follows two-compartment pharmacokinetics, with an alpha half-life of 13 minutes and a beta half-life of 85 minutes. It is eliminated renally. The principal side effects are hypotension and flu-like symptoms. Most adverse effects are dose-related.

E. **Abciximab** (c7E3 Fab, ReoPro) is a chimeric monoclonal antibody Fab fragment that is specific for platelet glycoprotein IIb—IIIa receptors. Abciximab is extremely effective in reducing fatalities (>50%) in subjects who have **unstable angina** after they undergo **angioplasty.** The recommended dosage is an intravenous bolus of 0.25 mg/kg administered 10–60 minutes before the start of angioplasty, followed by a continuous infusion of 10 μg/min for 12 hours. Platelet aggregation is almost completely inhibited 2 hours after the initiation of abciximab therapy. The major complication of abciximab infusion is dose-related bleeding.

F. **Campath-1** is a MAB that targets human lymphocytes and monocytes. It is used for **immunosuppression** in patients who undergo organ transplant. The intravenous dose is 25 mg once or twice daily. Campath-1 is also used to treat refractory **autoimmune disorders,** including rheumatoid arthritis. It is used experimentally to treat vasculitis. Campath-1 antibodies are used to prevent graft-versus-host disease and to treat **lymphoid malignancy** caused by immunosuppression in patients who undergo organ transplant.

G. **Edobacomab** is an immune globulin directed against **gram-negative bacterial endotoxins.** For **septic shock,** single doses of 2–15 mg/kg intravenously every 24 hours are used. The volume of distribution ranges from 4–8 L. The elimination half-life is approximately 10–18 hours. The main side effects are hypersensitivity reactions and antibody production. The drug is also being investigated for the treatment of gram-negative sepsis and septic shock.

H. **Muromonab-CD3** is an immunosuppressive agent with specific targeting. It is effective in reversing **acute renal allograft rejection.** The usual dose is 5 mg/day intravenously for 10–14 days after the initial signs and symptoms of rejection. The volume of distribution is approximately 6.5 L, and the half-life is 18 hours. Side effects include flu-like symptoms that appear to be associated with the release of cytokines. Symptoms may be self-limiting or severe and life-threatening.

I. Nebacumab is an immune globulin directed against gram-negative bacterial endotoxins. The drug is being investigated for the treatment of **gram-negative sepsis** and **septic shock.** Signs and symptoms of septic shock usually resolve during the first 7 days after treatment. Its half-life is 15.9 hours, and the volume of distribution is 48.5 mL/kg.

J. Satumomab pendetide is an MAB conjugate produced from the murine MAB B72.3. It requires radiolabeling to form indium-111 chloride satumomab pendetide. It is used as a **diagnostic imaging agent** in the staging of patients with known **colorectal** and **ovarian carcinoma.** The metabolic fate of this agent is unclear. The antibody conjugate is cleared slowly. It has a terminal half-life of approximately 56 hours. Approximately 10% of an administered dose appears in urine.

K. Zolimomab aritox (Orthozyme-CD5, Xoma/Ortho Biotech) is an immunoconjugate of monoclonal anti-CD5 murine IgG and the ricin A-chain toxin. Its primary use is in the treatment of steroid-resistant graft-versus-host disease after **allogeneic bone marrow transplant** for hematopoietic neoplasms (e.g., acute myelogenous leukemia). Other potential uses include the treatment of **rheumatoid arthritis** and insulin-dependent diabetes mellitus. After therapeutic doses, peak serum levels range from 1–5 μg/mL. The serum half-life is 1.5–4 hours. The dose varies depending on the indications.

L. Betaseron (interferon beta, Berlex Laboratories) is a glycoprotein with antiviral, antiproliferative, and immunomodulatory activity. Many of its effects are similar to those of interferon alfa. Its uses include the treatment of multiple sclerosis, AIDS, malignant melanoma, herpesvirus, and papillomavirus infections. It is also recommended at a dose of 8 million units subcutaneously every other day to reduce exacerbations in patients who have relapsing–remitting multiple sclerosis. It is administered intravenously, intramuscularly, subcutaneously, intrathecally, topically, or intralesionally for a variety of indications. Its biologic activity is evident in the absence of detectable serum levels. Serum concentrations are not consistently detectable after subcutaneous or intramuscular administration. Interferon beta may cross the disrupted blood–brain barrier. The compound does not appear in urine after systemic administration. Adverse effects include flu-like symptoms, bone marrow suppression, neurotoxic effects with high doses, anorexia and other gastrointestinal symptoms, and elevations of liver enzymes and serum creatinine.

STUDY QUESTIONS

1. Which type of cell does not contain double-stranded deoxyribonucleic acid (DNA)?

(A) Human cells
(B) Bacteria cells
(C) Human immunodeficiency virus (HIV) cells
(D) Viruses

2. Which enzyme is used by the human immuno-deficiency virus (HIV) to form deoxyribonucleic acid (DNA) in the host cell?

(A) Restrictive endonuclease
(B) DNA-directed polymerase
(C) Reverse transcriptase
(D) Both A and B
(E) None of the above

3. Gamma immunoglobulin is considered

(A) deoxyribonucleic acid (DNA)
(B) ribonucleic acid (RNA)
(C) a protein
(D) none of the above

4. Glycoprotein is considered a protein linked to

(A) a carbohydrate
(B) a hormone
(C) a lipid
(D) deoxyribonucleic acid (DNA)
(E) none of the above

5. An enzyme that cleaves deoxyribonucleic acid (DNA) at a specific site is called

(A) restrictive endonuclease
(B) restrictive ribonuclease
(C) trypsin
(D) none of the above

6. An example of a cytokine is

(A) interleukin
(B) insulin
(C) gonadotropin
(D) thyroxine
(E) none of the above

7. A common storage condition for most biotech-nology products after reconstitution is

(A) at room temperature
(B) in a cool place
(C) in a warm place
(D) no excessive heat
(E) in a freezer

8. What drug is used to prevent embolism in the lung and during myocardial infarction?

(A) Alteplase
(B) Human growth hormone
(C) Granulocyte–macrophage colony-stimulating factor (GM-CSF)
(D) Epogen (EPO)
(E) None of the above

9. What base is found in deoxyribonucleic acid (DNA)?

(A) Cytosine
(B) Adenine
(C) Guanine
(D) Thymine
(E) All of the above

ANSWERS AND EXPLANATIONS

1. The answer is C *[VII A].*
Human cells contain double-stranded DNA, whereas lower organisms (e.g., bacteria, viruses) do not.

2. The answer is C *[II V].*
Reverse transcriptase is the enzyme that a virus uses to assemble its DNA from RNA. Unlike higher animals, viral particles have genetic material in the RNA and need a host cell for reproduction.

3. The answer is C *[III C].*
Gamma globulin is a subclass of immunoglobulin protein involved in immunity and allergic response. (See p. 217, Table 11-2)

4. The answer is A *[III B].*
Glycoprotein consists of a carbohydrate linked to a protein. (See p. 218, Section VI, Glycoproteins)

5. The answer is A *[II T].*
Restriction endonuclease is an enzyme that specifically cleaves DNA molecules. Ribonuclease will cleave RNA only, and trypsin is a digestive enzyme found in the gastrointestinal tract. (See p. 217, T)

6. The answer is A *[II O].*
Interleukin is a "messenger" substance synthesized by the cell (cytokine) to communicate and trigger cellular response. (See p. 220, Section X C)

7. The answer is B *[II C].*
Most biologic compounds are heat labile and must be stored at low temperature. (See p. 208, Introduction)

8. The answer is A *[X A].*
Alteplase is a thrombolytic agent formerly known as tissue plasminogen activator (tPA). (See p. 209, Table 11-1 and p. 220, Section X A)

9. The answer is E *[IV B 2].*
All DNA molecules consist of nucleotides, which consist of deoxyribose, phosphate, and one of the nitrogen-containing bases, such as adenine, guanine, thymine, or cytosine. (See p. 219, VII DNA)

12
Principles of Pharmacodynamics and Medicinal Chemistry

Marc W. Harrold
Nelson S. Yee

I. INTRODUCTION. Pharmacodynamics is a branch of pharmacology that focuses on the study of the biochemical and physiological effects of drugs and the mechanisms by which they produce such effects. Analysis of drug action provides the basis for rational design of therapeutic agents and also provides insight into the regulation of cellular functions.

II. EFFECTS OF DRUGS

A. Perturbation of normal physiological processes. The actions of drugs are the consequences of the dynamic interactions between drug molecules and cellular components. Such interactions lead to alteration in the functions of these components, called **receptors.** The resulting biochemical and physiological changes form the basis of the cellular response to the drug. Drugs act by modulating the ongoing processes inside the cells.

B. Agonists and antagonists

1. Potentially, any macromolecular component may act as a **drug receptor.**

2. Certain drug receptors normally serve as receptors for endogenous ligands and, thus, are **physiological receptors.** For example, adrenergic receptors are physiological receptors for catecholamines.

3. Drugs whose responses resemble the effects of the endogenous molecules are receptor **agonists.** For example, bethanechol directly stimulates cholinergic receptors, and it is thus an agonist.

4. **Pharmacological antagonists** are drugs that lack **intrinsic activity** and produce effects by **competitively** or **noncompetitively** inhibiting the action of the endogenous molecules at the receptor.
   a. A **competitive antagonist** acts by interfering with binding of the endogenous ligand to the receptor in a reversible manner. For example, propanolol competes with catecholamines for binding with adrenergic β-receptors.
   b. A **noncompetitive antagonist** acts by interacting with the nonligand binding site of the receptor (for example, through covalent modification), such that normal binding of the endogenous ligand to the receptor is irreversibly inhibited. For instance, monoamine oxidase (MAO) inhibitors such as tranylcypromine (Parnate) initially interact with MAO in a reversible manner but then form covalent adducts that irreversibly inhibit MAO.

5. **Partial antagonists** inhibit the endogenous ligand from binding the receptor but possess some intrinsic activity. Nalorphine is a partial antagonist for the opiate receptor.

6. **Physiological antagonism** occurs when the drugs act independently at different receptor sites, often yielding opposing actions. For example, epinephrine and acetylcholine act on the sympathetic and parasympathetic autonomic nervous system, respectively, and their effects are antagonistic to each other.

7. **Neutralizing antagonism** occurs when two drugs bind with each other to form an inactive compound. For example, digoxin-binding antibody used in digoxin overdose acts by sequestering the drug, resulting in the formation of an inactive complex.

III. MECHANISMS OF DRUG ACTION

A. Cell surface receptors

1. Receptors can be **proteins, glycoproteins,** or **nucleic acids.** Receptors can be located at the cell surface, within the cytoplasm, or inside the nucleus.

2. The binding of drugs to receptors is highly specific and can involve a variety of interactions, including hydrophobic interactions and van der Waals forces with ionic, hydrogen, and covalent bonds. The type of interaction and the binding affinity can influence the duration and reversibility of the drug action.

3. The interaction and binding affinity are related to the chemical structure of both the drug and ligand. Chemical modification of the structure of the drug molecule can change the pharmacological and pharmacokinetic properties of drugs.

4. Through structure–activity relationship studies, synthetic drug analogues can be developed to achieve a high selectivity of drug action—a desirable ratio of therapeutic to toxic effect with a better-tolerated side-effect profile.

B. Signal transduction by cell-surface receptors

1. Cell-surface receptors are composed of extracellular domains that bind the ligands (drugs or physiological molecules).

2. The ligand binding serves as a triggering signal that can be propagated in the target cell through intracellular regulatory molecules, known as **second messengers** or **effectors.** For example, isoproterenol binds with the β-adrenergic receptor, which is functionally coupled to adenylate cyclase via the stimulatory G protein G_s. As a result, adenylate cyclase is activated, and the cyclic adenosine monophosphate (cAMP) level increases.

3. Ligand binding of receptors often leads to interaction of the receptors with the cytoplasmic effectors, which in turn become activated. Integration of the multiple signal transducing events along the receptor–effector system might change the cellular phenotype or gene expression, leading to new protein synthesis.

C. Signaling mediated by intracellular receptors. Thyroid hormone, steroid hormones, vitamin D, and the retinoids act through binding cytoplasmic receptors, which translocate into the nucleus. These receptors are soluble, deoxyribonucleic acid (DNA)-binding proteins that regulate the transcription of specific genes.

D. Target cell desensitization and hypersensitization

1. Cells have the ability to **respond** to endogenous regulatory molecules or exogenously added drugs over a wide range of concentrations. However, protective mechanisms are available for maintaining homeostatic control to prevent overstimulation or understimulation of the target cells.

2. Cell **regulation** can occur at different levels along the signal transduction pathway. Regulation can involve changes in the level of the receptors or alterations in the downstream effector molecules.

3. The expression of receptors is normally under homeostatic control through receptor internalization, recycling, and *de novo* synthesis.

4. **Down-regulation and desensitization**
   a. **Down-regulation** of receptors is caused by continuous prolonged exposure of receptors to drugs that disrupt the homeostatic equilibrium and result in altered levels of the receptors. This disruption involves endocytosis of ligand-bound receptors, resulting in sequestration of receptors from the cell surface and possibly accelerated degradation of the receptors, or inactivation of the receptors.
   b. **Desensitization** is the result of down-regulation. The target cells become desensitized, and the effect of subsequent exposure to the same concentration of the drug is reduced. Therefore, an increased concentration of the drug is required to produce an effect of the same magnitude as the initial exposure with a smaller drug concentration.
   c. Repeated doses of bronchodilator such as albuterol inhaler for the treatment of asthma can lead to down-regulation of β-adrenergic receptors in the bronchial cells. The

patient develops tolerance and requires increased dosage of the drug to achieve relief of the initial extent. In this case, the target cells become desensitized only to ligands that bind to those receptors; this is called **homologous desensitization.**

5. **Heterologous desensitization.** Some forms of desensitization involve alteration of components in the signaling pathway, such as a G protein. When cultured fibroblasts are exposed to prostaglandin (PGE_1), which normally activates adenylate cyclase through a G_s protein, the cells lose responsiveness not only to PGE_1 but also to other ligands binding to other receptors that act through the G_s–adenylate cyclase pathway.

6. **Hyperreactivity** or **supersensitivity** to receptor agonists is expected when target cells are subject to long-term exposure to receptor antagonists followed by abrupt cessation of administration of the drug. This can involve receptor **up-regulation** through synthesis of new receptors.

E. **Pharmacological effects not mediated by receptors.** The effects of some drugs do not involve binding with specific receptors because of interaction with molecules or ions, which are not typically defined as receptors.

1. **Colligative** drug effects are characterized by a lack of requirement for highly specific chemical structure.
   a. Volatile general **anesthetic** agents with diverse structures are lipophilic and interact with the lipid bilayer of cell membranes, resulting in depressed excitability.
   b. **Cathartics,** such as magnesium sulfate and sorbitol, act by increasing the osmolarity of intestinal fluids and, thus, changing the distribution of water.

2. Methotrexate, cytarabine, and 5-fluorouracil are examples of **antimetabolites.** Antimetabolites are structural analogues of endogenous molecules and are incorporated into cellular components that interfere with the normal cellular functions.

3. Certain drugs interact with specific ions normally found in body fluids. For example, **antacids** such as aluminum hydroxide, calcium carbonate, and magnesium hydroxide act by neutralizing gastric acid.

IV. RELATIONSHIP BETWEEN DRUG CONCENTRATION AND EFFECT

A. **Dose-response relationship.** In general, the larger the drug dose, the higher the drug concentration at its site of action and the greater the effect of the drug, up to a maximum effect. Higher drug concentrations (or doses) will not produce an effect greater than the maximum effect.

B. **A quantal dose-response curve** describes the relationship between the number of patients exhibiting a defined response (e.g., a 50% increase in peak flow) produced by a specified dose of a drug (e.g., minimum doses of albuterol for 50% increase in peak flow). This relationship often follows a gaussian (bell-shaped) distribution (Figures 12-1 and 12-2).

C. **A graded dose-response curve** describes the relationship between the magnitude of the effect of a drug (e.g., reduction of blood pressure by nifedipine) in an individual and the doses of the drug (Figure 12-3).

1. Generally, as the dose of a drug increases, the effect produced will reach a maximum level.

2. Graded dose-response curves for different drugs allow comparison of their efficacies and potencies.
   a. **Efficacy** of a drug is measured by its maximum effect.
   b. **Potency** of a drug is a relative measure that compares the different doses (molar doses) of different drugs needed to produce the same effect. From a clinical viewpoint, potency is considered in drug selection (e.g., triazolam is preferred for the treatment of insomnia instead of diazepam).
   c. In **selecting** drugs in clinical situations, a drug with greater efficacy might be needed to achieve the therapeutic outcome (e.g., hydromorphone is preferred to acetaminophen for controlling bone pain in a patient with metastatic breast cancer).

D. A **log dose-response curve** describes the relationship between the drug effect and the log of the dose. This curve facilitates comparison of potency and efficacy among different drugs with the same mechanism of action (and thus they have the same slopes) [Figure 12-4].

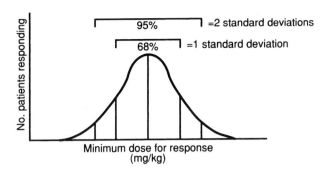

Figure 12-1. Frequency distribution curve, plotting the number of patients showing a quantal response to a drug against the minimum dose needed to produce the response.

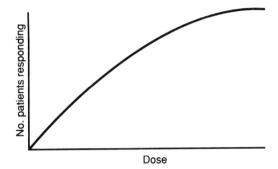

Figure 12-2. Quantal dose-response curve, cumulating the data used in plotting Figure 12-1.

1. The **efficacy** of a drug is determined by the **height** of its log dose-response curve (E_{max}); the higher the curve, the greater the E_{max} and efficacy.

2. The **potency** of two drugs can be compared by determining their ED_{50}. The ED_{50} is the **dose** of each drug producing 50% of the corresponding maximum effect (50% of E_{max}). The smaller the ED_{50}, the greater the potency.

3. A **competitive antagonist** shifts the log dose-response curve to the **right**, and the shift is **parallel.** A greater concentration of the agonist is required to produce the same response than when the competitive antagonist is absent. Even in the presence of the antagonist, the **same E_{max}** can be achieved if enough agonist is added (Figure 12-5).

4. A **noncompetitive antagonist** binds to the same receptor or binds to another site that prevents the agonist from producing a response. The shift of the log dose-response curve is to the **right** and **nonparallel,** resulting in a **lower E_{max}.** The action of the antagonist cannot be overcome even if more agonist is present (Figure 12-6).

V. ENHANCEMENT OF DRUG EFFECTS

A. **Addition** occurs when two different drugs with the same effect are given together, resulting in a drug effect that is equal in magnitude to the sum of the individual effects of the two drugs. For example, trimethoprim and sulfamethoxazole inhibit different steps in the synthesis of folic acid, resulting in the suppression of bacterial growth.

B. **Synergism** occurs when two drugs with the same effect are given together, producing a drug effect that is greater in magnitude than the sum of the individual effects of the two drugs. For example, penicillin and gentamicin are synergistic in their antipseudomonal activities.

C. **Potentiation** occurs when one drug, lacking an effect of its own, increases the effect of another drug that is active. For example, carbidopa is an inactive analogue of dopa. When carbidopa blocks the degradation of dopa and is given with dopa, it prolongs the half-life of dopa and the duration of the anti-Parkinsonian effect.

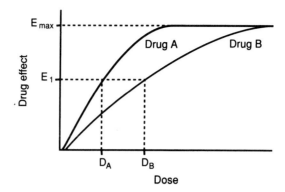

Figure 12-3. Graded dose-response curves for two drugs, A and B. E_{max} = maximum effect; D_A and D_B = amount (dose) of drug A and drug B, respectively, needed to produce the drug effect, E_1.

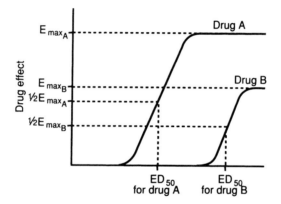

Figure 12-4. Log dose-response curves for two drugs, A and B. E_{max} = maximum effect; ED_{50} = smallest dose showing an effect that is 50% of the E_{max}.

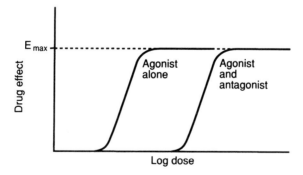

Figure 12-5. Shift in the log dose-response curve that occurs when an agonist is administered in the presence of a competitive antagonist.

VI. SELECTIVITY OF DRUG ACTION

   A. The **therapeutic index** and the **margin of safety** are the relationship (ratio) between the dose of a drug required to produce undesired effects (toxic or lethal) and the dose required to produce the desired effects (therapeutic).

   1. The **therapeutic index** of a drug is a relative measure of the safety and effectiveness in laboratory studies.

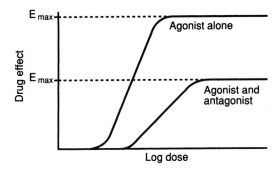

Figure 12-6. Shift in the log dose-response curve and lowering of the maximum effect (E_{max}) that occur when an agonist is given in the presence of a noncompetitive antagonist.

2. The **therapeutic index** is the ratio of the minimum dose that is toxic for 50% of the population (**TD_{50} or median toxic dose**) to the minimum dose that is effective for 50% of the population (**ED_{50} or median effective dose**).

B. In general, the greater the TD_{50} or the smaller the ED_{50}, the greater the therapeutic index, and thus the safer the drug when used at the effective dosage.

C. The **margin of safety** is a more practical term to describe the relative safety and effectiveness of a drug. The margin of safety is the ratio of the minimum toxic dose for 0.1% of the population (**$TD_{0.1}$ or minimal toxic dose**) to the minimum effective dose for 99.9% of the population (**$ED_{99.9}$ or minimal effective dose**).

VII. DRUG SOURCES AND MAJOR CLASSES

A. Natural products are drugs obtained from plant and animal sources.

1. **Alkaloids** are nitrogen-containing compounds obtained primarily from plants through extraction and purification, which possess pharmacological activity. The majority of alkaloids are basic compounds (e.g., **morphine,** from the opium poppy; **atropine,** from the belladonna plant); however, some are neutral amides (e.g., **colchicine,** from the autumn crocus). All alkaloids end in the suffix "-ine"; however, it is important to note that not all drugs that end in "-ine" are alkaloids (e.g., meperidine).

2. **Peptides and polypeptides** are polymers of amino acids, are obtained from either human or animal sources, and are smaller than **proteins.** The amino acid length distinctions between these three classifications are vague and often vary from one source to another. Naturally occurring peptides have little to no oral activity and short half-lives (e.g., **somatostatin,** a 14 amino acid peptide; **glucagon,** a 29 amino acid polypeptide).

3. **Steroids** are chemical derivatives of cyclopentanoperhydrophenanthrene and can be obtained from either human or animal sources (e.g., **estradiol, testosterone, hydrocortisone**).

4. **Hormones** are chemical substances that are formed in one organ or part of the body and carried in the blood to another organ or part. They are principally proteins or steroids and can be obtained either synthetically, through recombinant DNA technology (e.g., **insulin**), or from animal sources (e.g., **thyroid hormones** and **conjugated estrogens**).

5. **Glycosides** are organic substances consisting of a sugar moiety bound to a nonsugar (aglycone) moiety by means of a glycosidic bond (i.e., a bond between the anomeric carbon of the sugar and a hydroxy group on the aglycone). They can be of either plant (e.g., **digitoxin**) or microbial (e.g., **streptomycin, doxorubicin**) origin.

6. **Vitamins** are organic substances that are present in foods and are essential to normal metabolism.
   a. **Water-soluble vitamins** include thiamine (B_1), riboflavin (B_2), niacin (B_3), pyridoxine (B_6), cyanocobalamin (B_{12}), ascorbic acid (C), folic acid, pantothenic acid, and biotin (H).

   b. Lipid-soluble vitamins include retinol (A), ergocalciferol (D), α-tocopherol (E), and phytonadione (K).

7. Polysaccharides are polymers of sugars that can be obtained from either human or animal sources. These compounds can be used either directly (e.g., **heparin**), after partial depolymerization (e.g., **tinzaparin, enoxaparin**), or after structural modification (e.g., **sucralfate**).

8. Antibiotics are chemical substances produced by microorganisms that either suppress or kill other microorganisms (e.g., **penicillin, tetracycline, doxorubicin**).

B. Synthetic products are drugs synthesized from organic compounds.

   1. Synthetic products can have **chemical structures closely resembling those of active natural products** (e.g., **hydroxymorphone,** which resembles morphine; **ampicillin,** which resembles penicillin).

   2. Synthetic products can contain similar spacing of functional groups but lack the general structure of a naturally occurring compound. **Peptidomimetics** are molecules with no peptide bonds, a molecular weight less than 700, and activity similar to the original peptide (e.g., **losartan** is a peptidomimetic and an angiotensin II receptor antagonist).

   3. Synthetic products also can be **completely new products,** obtained by screening synthesized materials for drug activity (e.g., **barbiturates, antibacterial sulfonamides, thiazide diuretics, phenothiazine antipsychotics, benzodiazepine anxiolytics**).

C. Major chemical and pharmacologic classes of drugs (Table 12-1, Figures 12-7, 12-8, 12-9, 12-10, 12-11)

VIII. DRUG ACTION AND PHYSICOCHEMICAL PROPERTIES

A. Drug action results from the interaction of drug molecules with either normal or abnormal physiological processes. Drugs normally interact with receptors, which can be either proteins, enzymes, cell lipids, or pieces of DNA or ribonucleic acid (RNA).

   1. Systemically active drugs must **enter** and **be transported by body fluids.**
      a. The drug must **pass various membrane barriers, escape excessive distribution** into sites of loss, and **penetrate to the active site.**
      b. At the active site, the drug molecules must orient themselves and interact with the receptors to **alter function.**
      c. The drug must be removed from the active site and **metabolized** to a form that is easily **excreted** by the body.

   2. Drug absorption, metabolism, utilization, and excretion all depend on the **drug's physicochemical properties** and the **host's physiological, and biochemical properties.** A drug's physicochemical properties can be altered via the synthesis of chemical analogues, whereas the host's properties usually cannot be altered.

B. Two of the most important **physicochemical properties** of a drug molecule are its polarity and its acid–base nature.

   1. Drug polarity is a relative measure of a drug's lipid and water solubility and is usually expressed in terms of a **partition coefficient.**
      a. The partition coefficient (P) of a drug is defined as the ratio of the solubility of the compound in an organic solvent to the solubility of the same compound in an aqueous environment (i.e., $P = [Drug]_{lipid}/[Drug]_{aqueous}$). The partition coefficient is often expressed as a log value.
      b. Water solubility (or **hydrophilicity**) depends primarily on two factors: ionic character and hydrogen-bonding capabilities. The presence of oxygen- and nitrogen-containing functional groups usually enhances water solubility. Water solubility is required for:
         (1) Dissolution in the gastrointestinal (GI) tract
         (2) Preparation of parenteral solutions (as opposed to suspensions)
         (3) Preparation of ophthalmic solutions
         (4) Adequate urine concentrations (pertains primarily to antibiotics)

Table 12-1. Major Chemical and Pharmacological Classes of Drugs

Classification	Acid/Base Character	Example (See Figures 12-7– 12-11 for structures)
1. **Polyhalogenated Ethers and Hydrocarbons** General anesthetics	Nonelectrolyte	Isoflurane
2. **Barbiturates** Sedative/Hyptonics; Anticonvulsants	Acidic	Phenobarbital
3. **Benzodiazepines** Anxiolytic agents; Sedative/Hypnotics	Basic	Diazepam
4. **Hydantoins** Anticonvulsants	Acidic	Phenytoin
5. **Succinimides** Anticonvulsants	Acidic or nonelectrolyte	Methsuximide
6. **Phenothiazines** Antipsychotics; Antihistamines; Antiemetics	Basic	Chlorpromazine
7. **Thioxanthenes** Antipsychotics	Basic	Thiothixene
8. **Butyrophenones** Antipsychotics	Basic	Haloperidol
9. **Tricyclic Antidepressants** Antidepressant agents	Basic	Imipramine
10. **Selective Serotonin Reuptake Inhibitors** Anxiolytic agents	Basic	Fluoxetine
11. **Benzazepines** Atypical antipsychotics	Basic	Olanzapine
12. **Methyl Xanthines** CNS stimulants; Bronchodilators	Basic (weak)	Theophylline
13. **Opioids** Narcotic analgesics; Antitussives	Basic	Codeine
14. **4-Phenylpiperidines** Narcotic analgesics	Basic	Meperidine
15. **Phenylpropylamines** Narcotic analgesics	Basic	Methadone
16. **Direct-Acting Cholinergics** GI smooth-muscle stimulant; Cataract therapy	Quaternary ammonium salt	Bethanechol
17. **Aminoalkyl Esters** Anticholinergic agents	Basic or quaternary ammonium salt	Dicyclomine
18. **Aminoalkyl Ethers** Anticholinergic agents; Antihistamines (H_1 antagonists)	Basic	Benztropine
19. **Aminoalcohols** Anticholinergic agents	Basic or quaternary ammonium salt	Biperiden
20. **Ethylenediamines** Antihistamines (H_1 antagonists)	Basic	Tripelennamine
21. **Alkylamines (Propylamines)** Antihistamines (H_1 antagonists)	Basic	Chlorpheniramine
22. **Piperazines** Antihistamines (H_1 antagonists); Antivertigo; Antiemetics	Basic	Cyclizine
23. **Mast-Cell Degranulation Inhibitors** Antiallergenics	Basic	Cromolyn sodium
24. **Phenylethylamines** Sympathomimetics (α- and β-adrenergic agonists)	Basic	Albuterol
25. **Adrenergic α$_2$-Agonists** Antihypertensive agents	Basic	Guanabenz
26. **Adrenergic α$_1$-Antagonists** Antihypertensive agents	Basic	Terazosin

(Continued on next page)

Table 12-1. *Continued*

Classification	Acid/Base Character	Example (See Figures 12-7– 12-11 for structures)
27. **Aryloxypropanolamines** β-Adrenergic blockers	Basic	Propranolol
28. **Prostaglandins** Eicosanoids	Acidic	Misoprostol
29. **Salicylates** Nonsteroidal Anti-inflammatory agents (NSAIDs)	Acidic	Aspirin
30. **Fenamates** NSAIDs	Acidic	Mefenamic acid
31. **Pyrazolidinediones** NSAIDs	Acidic	Phenylbutazone
32. **Arylacetic Acids (includes indoleacetic acids, pyrrolacetic acids, and propionic acids)** NSAIDs	Acidic	Tolmetin
33. **Selective COX-II Inhibitors** NSAIDs	Acidic (weak) or nonelectrolyte	Rofecoxib
34. **Triptans** 5-HT$_{1B/1D}$ agonists	Basic	Sumatriptan
35. **Serotonin 5-HT$_3$ Antagonists** Antiemetic agents	Basic	Ondansetron
36. **Coumarins** Oral anticoagulants	Acidic	Warfarin
37. **Sulfated Polysaccharides** Anticoagulants	Acidic	Heparin
38. **Benzothiadiazides (Thiazides)** Diuretics: Saluretics	Acidic	Chlorthiazide
39. **High Ceiling (Loop) Diuretics** Diuretics; Saluretics	Acidic	Furosemide
40. **Organic Nitrates** Antianginal agents	Nonelectrolyte	Isosorbide dinitrate
41. **Dihydropyridines** Antihypertensives; Antianginal agents; Antiarrhythmics	Basic (weak)	Nifedipine
42. **Angiotensin II Receptor Antagonists** Antihypertensive agents	Acidic	Losartan
43. **Angiotensin-Converting Enzyme (ACE) Inhibitors** Antihypertensive agents	Amphoteric	Enalapril
44. **HMG-CoA Reductase Inhibitors** Cholesterol-lowering agents	Acidic	Pravastatin
45. **Bile-Acid Sequestrants** Cholesterol-lowering agents	Basic or quaternary ammonium salt	Cholestyramine
46. **Fibrates** Cholesterol- and triglyceride-lowering agents	Acidic	Gemfibrozil
47. **Steroids** Estrogens; Progestins; Androgens; Adrenocorticoids	Nonelectrolyte	Dexamethasone
48. **Selective Estrogen Receptor Modulators** Estrogen Receptor Agonists and Antagonists	Basic	Raloxifene
49. **5α-Reductase Inhibitors** Antiandrogen	Nonelectrolyte	Finasteride
50. **Androgen Receptor Antagonists** Antiandrogen	Nonelectrolyte	Nilutamide
51. **Sulfonylureas** Oral hypoglycemics	Acidic	Tolbutamide
52. **Meglitinides** Oral hypoglycemics	Acidic	Repaglinide

Table 12-1. *Continued*

Classification	Acid/Base Character	Example (See Figures 12-7–12-11 for structures)
53. **Thiazolidinediones (Glitizones)** Insulin sensitizers; Antidiabetic agents	Amphoteric (acid stronger than base)	Pioglitazone
54. **α-Glucosidase Inhibitors** Antidiabetic agents	Basic	Miglitol
55. **H$_2$-Receptor Antagonists** Antiulcer agents	Basic	Cimetidine
56. **Proton Pump Inhibitors** Antiulcer agents	Basic	Omeprazole
57. **Nitrosoureas** Antineoplastic agents	Nonelectrolyte	Carmustine
58. **β-Chloroethylamines (Nitrogen Mustards)** Antineoplastic agents	Basic	Mechlorethamine
59. **Folate Antimetabolites** Antineoplastic agents; Antibacterial agents; Antifungals	Amphoteric	Methotrexate
60. **Purine Antimetabolites** Antineoplastic agents; Antiviral agents	Basic	6-Mercaptopurine
61. **Pyrimidine Antimetabolites** Antineoplastic agents; Antiviral agents	Basic	Cytarabine
62. **Anthracyclines** Antineoplastic agents	Basic	Doxorubicin
63. **Topoisomerase Inhibitors** Antineoplastic agents	Basic	Topotecan
64. **HIV Protease Inhibitors** Antiretroviral agents	Basic	Saquinavir
65. **Sulfonilamides** Antibacterial agents	Acidic	Sulfamethoxazole
66. **Penicillins** Antibacterial agents	Acidic	Ampicillin
67. **Cephalosporins** Antibacterial agents	Acidic	Cefoxitin
68. **Tetracyclines** Antibacterial agents	Amphoteric	Tetracycline
69. **Aminoglycosides** Antibacterial agents	Basic	Gentimycin
70. **Macrolides** Antibacterial agents	Basic	Erythromycin
71. **4-Quinolones** Antibacterial agents	Amphoteric	Enoxacin
72. **Allylamines** Antifungal agents	Basic	Terbinafine
73. **Polyenes** Antifungal agents	Amphoteric	Amphotericin B
74. **Imidazoles** Antifungal agents	Basic	Oxiconazole

Table 12-1 is not an inclusive list of all drugs or classifications. It is organized according to chemical structure and includes only those classifications that contain multiple compounds with a similar structure. In some instances (e.g., **direct-acting cholinergic agonists** and **H$_2$-receptor antagonists**), drugs are chemically similar, but are usually denoted only by pharmacological classifications. The acid–base character of each class is a general notation, and there are some specific singular agents that fall outside these general notations (i.e., **ampicillin** is amphoteric, whereas the **penicillins,** in general, are acidic molecules).

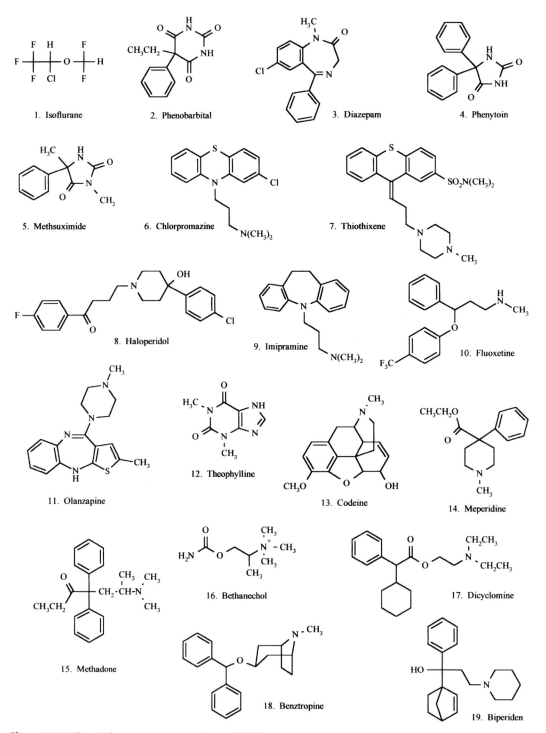

Figure 12-7. Chemical structures representing each of the major chemical classes of drugs listed in Table 12-1 (classifications 1–19).

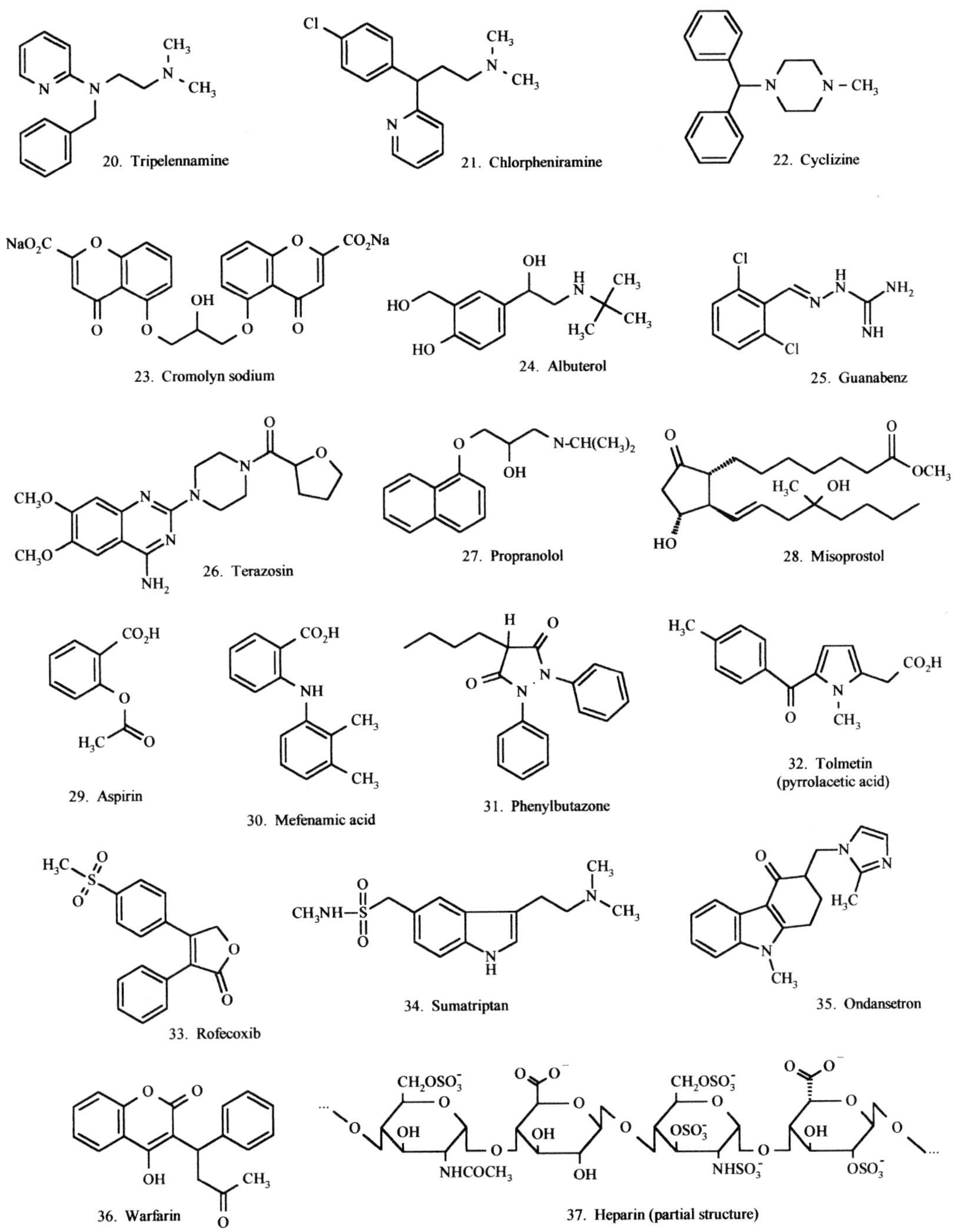

Figure 12-8. Chemical structures representing each of the major chemical classes of drugs listed in Table 12-1 (classifications 20–37).

c. **Lipid solubility (or lipophilicity)** is enhanced by nonionizable hydrocarbon chains and ring systems. Lipid solubility is required for:

(1) Penetration through the lipid bilayer in the GI tract

(2) Penetration through the blood–brain barrier

(3) Preparation of intramuscular (IM) depot injectable formulations

(4) Enhanced pulmonary absorption within the respiratory tract

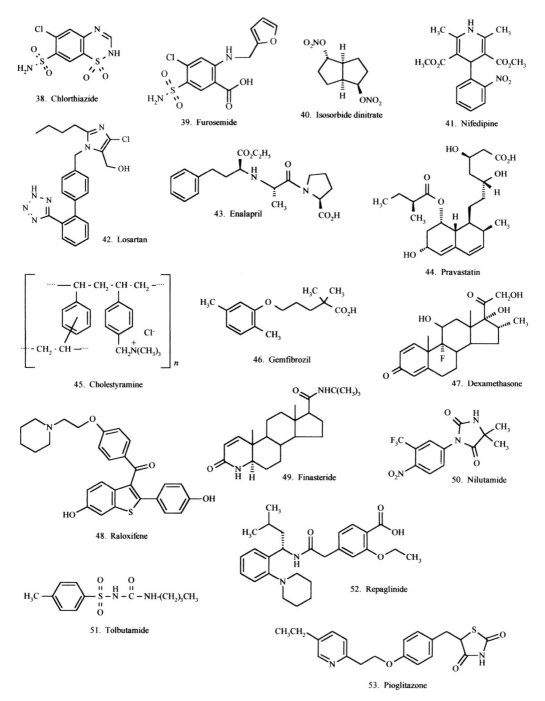

Figure 12-9. Chemical structures representing each of the major chemical classes of drugs listed in Table 12-1 (classifications 38–53).

(5) Enhanced topical potency (seen with many topical glucocorticoids)
(6) Enhanced plasma protein binding

2. Ionization of **acids** and **bases** plays a role with substances that dissociate into ions.
    a. The **ionization constant (K_a)** indicates the relative strength of the acid or base. An acid with a K_a of 1×10^{-3} is stronger (more ionized) than one with a K_a of 1×10^{-5}, whereas a base with a K_a of 1×10^{-7} is weaker (less ionized) than one with a K_a of 1×10^{-9}.

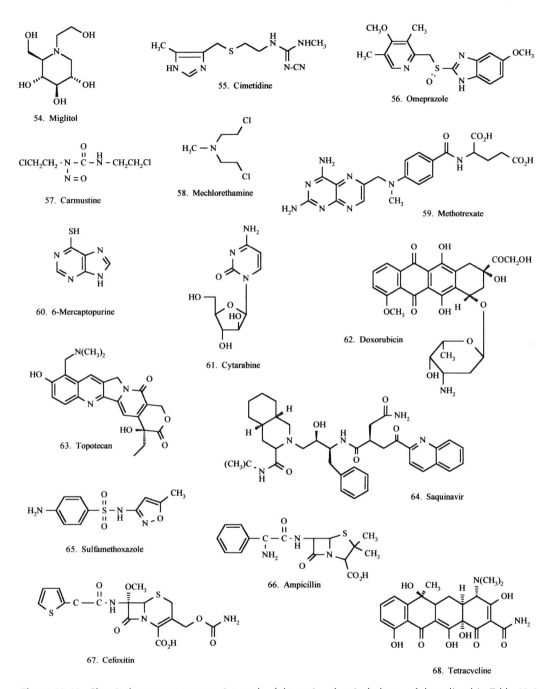

Figure 12-10. Chemical structures representing each of the major chemical classes of drugs listed in Table 12-1 (classifications 54–68).

    b. The **negative log** of the **ionization constant (pK$_a$)** also indicates the relative strength of the acid or base. An acid with a pK$_a$ of 5 (K$_a$ = 1 x 10^{-5}) is weaker (less ionized) than one with a pK$_a$ of 3 (K$_a$ = 1 x 10^{-3}), whereas a base with a pK$_a$ of 9 (K$_a$ = 1 x 10^{-9}) is stronger (more ionized) than one with a pK$_a$ of 7 (K$_a$ = 1 x 10^{-7}).

    c. Strong acids [e.g., **hydrochloric acid** (HCl), sulfuric acid (H$_2$SO$_4$), nitric acid (HNO$_3$), hydrobromic acid (HBr), iodic acid (HIO$_3$), perchloric acid (HClO$_4$)] are completely ionized. Almost all other acids, including organic acids, are weak. **Organic acids** contain one or more of these functional groups:

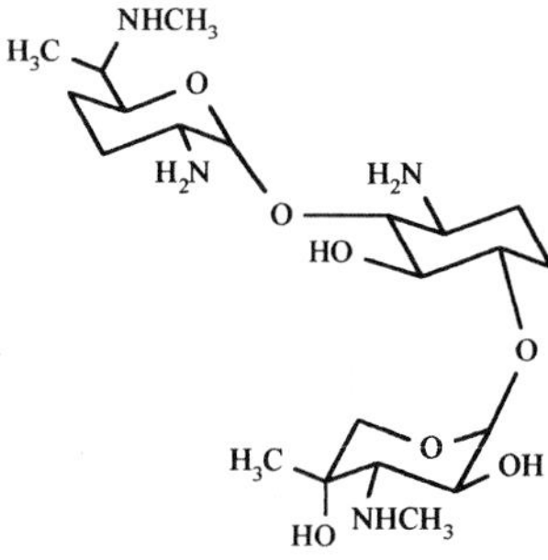

69. Gentimycin

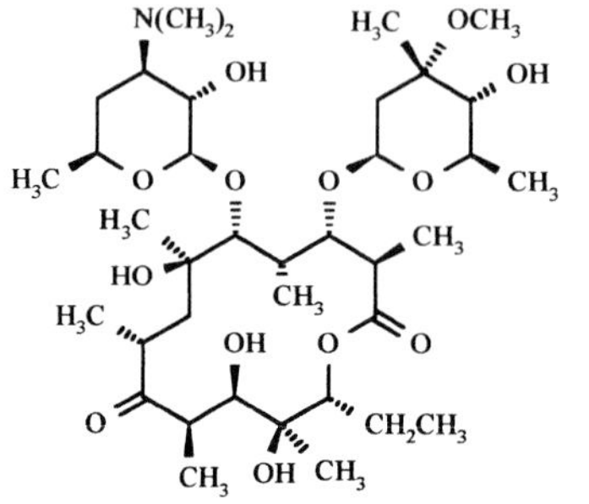

70. Erythromycin

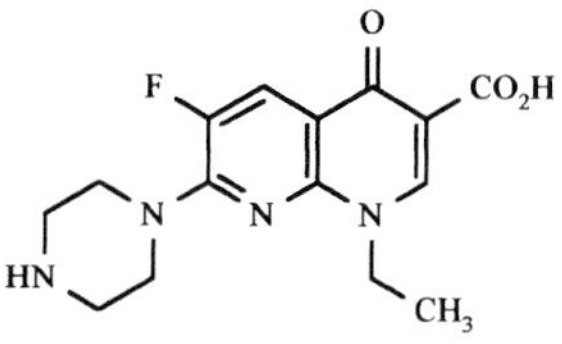

71. Enoxacin

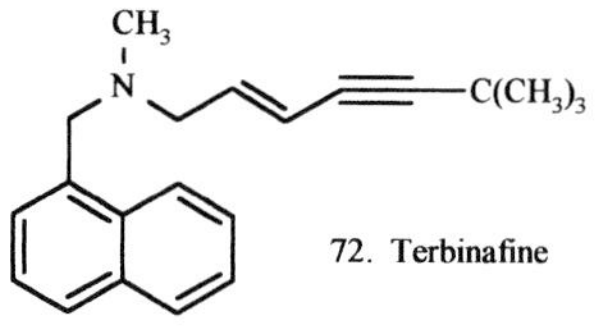

72. Terbinafine

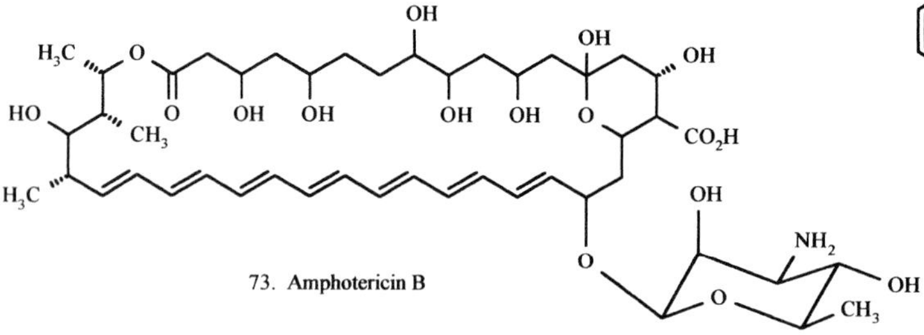

73. Amphotericin B

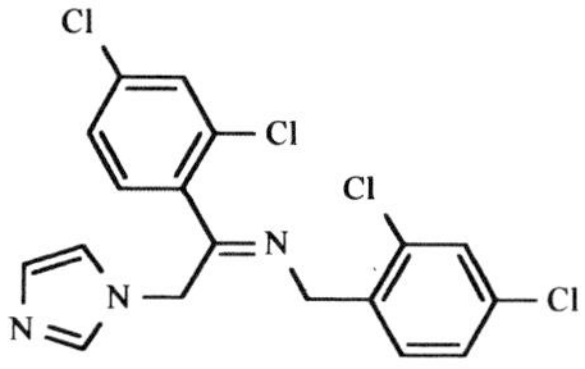

74. Oxiconazole

Figure 12-11. Chemical structures representing each of the major chemical classes of drugs listed in Table 12-1 (classifications 69–74).

- **(1)** Carboxylic acid group (—COOH)
- **(2)** Phenolic group (Ar—OH)
- **(3)** Sulfonic acid group (—SO_3H)
- **(4)** Sulfonamide group (—SO_2NH—R)
- **(5)** Imide group (—CO—NH—CO—)
- **(6)** β-Carbonyl group (—CO—CHR—CO—)
- **(7)** Tetrazole ring (five-member CHN_4 ring; see losartan in Figure 12-9 for example)

d. Strong bases [e.g., sodium hydroxide (NaOH), potassium hydroxide (KOH), magnesium hydroxide [$Mg(OH)_2$], calcium hydroxide [$Ca(OH)_2$], barium hydroxide [$Ba(OH)_2$], and quaternary ammonium hydroxides] are also completely ionized. Almost all other bases, including organic bases, are weak.

- **(1) Organic bases** contain a primary, secondary, or tertiary aliphatic or alicyclic amino group (—NH_2, —NHR, or —NR_2).
- **(2)** Most aromatic or unsaturated heterocyclic nitrogens are so weakly basic that they do not readily form salts with acids. Saturated heterocyclic nitrogens, in contrast, are similar to aliphatic amines.
- **(3)** Additional basic functional groups include imine nitrogens (—N=C—), hydrazine nitrogens (—NH-NH_2), amidine nitrogens (—NH-C=N—), and guanidine nitrogens (four atom functional group, CH_4N_3; see **guanabenz** in Figure 12-8 for example).

e. Weak acids. Ionization of a weak acid (e.g., acetic acid, which has a pK_a of 4.76) takes place as follows:

$$CH_3COOH \rightleftharpoons CH_3COO^- + H^+$$

- **(1)** When a weak acid (such as acetic acid) is placed in an **acid medium,** the equilibrium shifts to the left, suppressing ionization. This decrease in ionization conforms to **Le Chatelier's principle,** which states that when a stress is placed on an equilibrium reaction, the reaction will move in the direction that tends to relieve the stress.
- **(2)** When a weak acid is placed in an **alkaline medium,** ionization increases. The H^+ ions from the acid and the OH^- ions from the alkaline medium combine to form water, shifting the equilibrium to the right.

(3) **Weakly acidic drugs** are less ionized in acid media than in alkaline media. When the pK$_a$ of an acidic drug is greater than the pH of the medium in which it exists, it will be more than 50% in its nonionized (molecular) form and, thus, more likely to cross lipid cellular membranes.

f. **Weak bases.** Ionization of a weak base is the opposite of that for a weak acid.

(1) Weak bases are less ionized in a **basic (alkaline) medium** and more ionized in an **acid medium.**

(2) **Weakly basic** drugs are less ionized in alkaline media than in acid media. When the pK$_a$ of a basic drug is less than the pH of the medium in which it exists, it will be more than 50% in its nonionized (molecular) form and, thus, more likely to cross lipid cellular membranes.

g. **Percent ionization** can be approximated by using the **rule of nines.** If the |pH - pK$_a$| = 1, then a 90 to 10 ratio (note that there is one nine in the ratio) exists. If the |pH - pK$_a$| = 2, the ratio becomes 99 to 1 (two nines in the ratio), and if the |pH - pK$_a$| = 3, the ratio is 99.9 to 0.1 (three nines in the ratio). The predominant form, ionized or unionized, in these ratios can easily be determined [see VIII B 2 e (3), f (2)].

3. A **salt** is the combination of an acid and a base.

a. With a few minor exceptions (mercuric and cadmium halides and lead acetate), **all salts are strong electrolytes.**

b. Because the vast majority of drugs are organic molecules, drug salts can be divided into two classes based upon the chemical nature of the substance forming the salt.

(1) **Inorganic salts** are made by combining drug molecules with inorganic acids and bases, such as hydrochloric acid, sulfuric acid, potassium hydroxide, and sodium hydroxide. The salt form of the drug has increased water solubility in comparison with the parent molecule. Inorganic salts are generally used to increase the aqueous dissolution of a compound.

(2) **Organic salts** are made by combining drug molecules with either **small, hydrophilic** organic compounds (e.g., succinic acid, citric acid) or **lipophilic** organic compounds (e.g., procaine). Water-soluble organic salts are used to increase dissolution and bioavailability, as well as to aid in the preparation of parenteral and ophthalmic formulations (e.g., timolol maleate). Lipid-soluble organic salts are primarily used to make depot injections (e.g., procaine penicillin).

c. **Amphoteric compounds** contain both acidic and basic functional groups and are capable of forming **internal salts,** or zwitterions, which often have dissolution problems.

d. **Dissolution of salts** can alter the pH of an aqueous medium.

(1) Salts of **strong acids** (e.g., HCl, H$_2$SO$_4$) and **basic drugs** (e.g., cimetidine) dissociate in an aqueous medium to yield an **acidic solution.**

(2) Salts of **strong bases** (e.g., NaOH, KOH) and **acidic drugs** (e.g., phenobarbital) dissociate in an aqueous medium to yield a **basic solution.**

(3) Salts of **weak acids** and **weak bases** dissociate in an aqueous medium to yield an **acidic, basic,** or **neutral solution,** depending on the respective ionization constants involved.

(4) Salts of **strong acids** and **strong bases** (e.g., NaCl) do not significantly alter the pH of an aqueous medium.

4. A **neutralization reaction** might occur when an acidic solution of an organic salt (a solution of a salt of a strong acid and a weak base) is mixed with a basic solution (a solution of a salt of a weak acid and a strong base). The nonionized organic acid or the nonionized organic base is likely to **precipitate** in this case. This reaction is the basis for many **drug incompatibilities,** particularly when intravenous solutions are mixed. Neutralization reactions can be avoided by knowing how to predict the approximate pH of the aqueous solutions of common drug salts.

a. Generally, a drug's **salt form** can be recognized when the generic or trade name consists of two separate words, indicating a **cation** and an **anion.**

b. Drugs with **nitrate, sulfate,** or **hydrochloride notations** (e.g., pilocarpine nitrate, morphine sulfate, meperidine hydrochloride) are salts of **strong acids.** Thus, these drugs (e.g., pilocarpine, morphine, meperidine) must be **bases.**

c. Drugs with **sodium** or **potassium cations** (e.g., warfarin sodium, potassium penicillin G) are salts of **strong bases.** Thus, these drugs (e.g., warfarin, penicillin G) must be **acids.**

d. Drugs whose cation name ends with the suffix **"-onium"** or **"-inium"** and whose anion is a chloride, bromide, iodide, nitrate, or sulfate (e.g., benzalkonium chloride, cetylpyridinium chloride), are known as quaternary ammonium salts and form **neutral aqueous solutions.**

IX. STRUCTURAL FEATURES AND PHARMACOLOGIC ACTIVITY. Drugs can be classified as structurally nonspecific or structurally specific.

A. **Structurally nonspecific drugs** are those for which the drug's interaction with the cell membrane depends more on the drug molecule's physical characteristics than on its chemical structure. Usually, the interaction is based on the **cell membrane's lipid nature** and the **drug's lipid attraction.** Most **general anesthetics,** as well as some **hypnotics** and some **bactericidal agents,** act through this mechanism.

B. **Structurally specific drugs** are those for which pharmacological activity is determined by the drug's ability to bind to a **specific endogenous receptor.**

1. **Receptor-site theory** describes the pharmacological activity of such drugs.
   a. The **lock-and-key theory** postulates a completely complementary relationship between the drug molecule and a specific area on the surface of the receptor molecule (i.e., the **active,** or **catalytic, site**). This theory does not account for conformational changes in either drug or receptor molecules and is an oversimplification of a complex process.
   b. The **induced-fit theory** also postulates a complementary relationship between the drug molecule and its active site; however, it provides for **mutual conformational changes** between the drug and its receptor. Conformational changes in the receptor molecule are then translated into biological responses. This theory explains many more phenomena (e.g., **allosteric inhibitors**) than the lock-and-key model.
   c. The **occupational theory of response** further postulates that, for a structurally specific drug, the intensity of the pharmacological effect is directly proportional to the number of receptors occupied by the drug.

2. **Receptor-site binding.** The **ability to bind to a specific receptor,** while not independent of the drug's physical characteristics, is primarily determined by the drug's **chemical structure.**
   a. In such an interaction, the drug's **chemical reactivity** plays an important role, reflected in its **bonding ability** and in the **exactness of its fit** to the receptor.
   b. **Drug interaction** with a specific receptor is analogous to the fitting together of jigsaw puzzle pieces. Only drugs of similar shape (i.e., similar chemical structure) can bind to a specific receptor and initiate a biological response.
   c. Often, only a **critical portion of the drug molecule** (rather than the whole molecule) is involved in receptor-site binding.
      (1) The functional group making up this critical portion is known as a **pharmacophore.**
      (2) Drugs with **similar critical regions** but differences in other parts may have similar qualitative (although not necessarily quantitative) pharmacological activity.
   d. In general, the **better a drug fits** the receptor site, the **higher the affinity** between the drug and the receptor and the **greater** the observed biological response. A drug that binds to a receptor and elicits a biological response is called an **agonist.**
   e. Some drugs, lacking the specific pharmacophore for a receptor, can nonetheless bind to that receptor. Such a drug will have little or no pharmacological effect and also might prevent a molecule having the specific pharmacophore from binding, blocking the expected biological response. A drug that blocks a natural agonist and prevents it from binding to its receptor is called an **antagonist.**

3. The **stereochemistry** of both the receptor-site surface and the drug molecule helps determine the nature and efficiency of the drug-receptor interaction. Stereoisomers can be divided into three main groups: **optical isomers, geometric isomers,** and **conformational isomers.**
   a. **Optical isomers** contain at least one asymmetric, or chiral, carbon atom (i.e., a carbon atom that is covalently bonded to four different substituents). Each asymmetric carbon atom can exist in one of two nonsuperimposable isomeric forms (Figure 12-12).
      (1) **Enantiomers** are optical isomers that are mirror images of one another. Enantiomers have identical physical and chemical properties except that one rotates the plane of

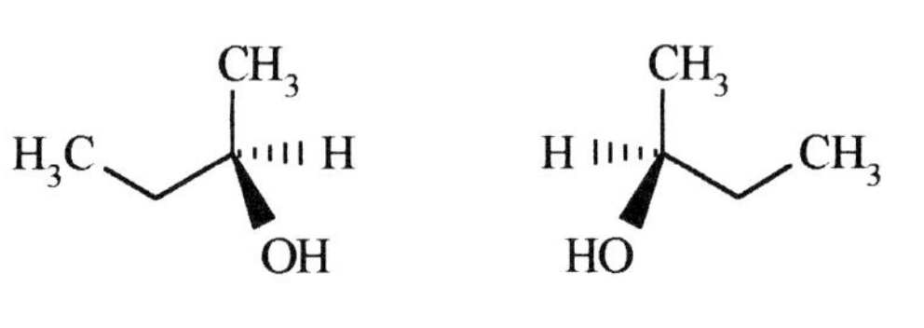

Figure 12-12. The two enantiomers of 2-hydroxybutane. The chiral, or asymmetric, carbon is bonded to four different groups: a methyl group, an ethyl group, a hydroxy group, and a hydrogen. The structures shown are mirror images that cannot be superimposed.

polarized light in a clockwise direction (**dextrorotatory,** designated D or +) and the other in a counterclockwise direction (**levorotatory,** designated L or -).

(2) An equal mixture of D and L enantiomers is called a **racemic mixture** and is optically inactive.

(3) Enantiomers can have large differences in potency, receptor fit, biological activity, transport, and metabolism. These differences result when the drug molecule has an asymmetric interaction with a receptor, a transport protein, or a metabolizing enzyme. For example, **levorphanol** has narcotic, analgesic, and antitussive properties, whereas its mirror image, **dextrorphanol,** has only antitussive activity.

(4) Diastereomers are stereoisomers, which are neither mirror images nor superimposable. A drug must have at least two chiral centers in order to exist in diastereomers. Unlike enantiomers, in which all stereochemical centers are opposite, diastereomers have some stereochemical centers that are identical and some that are opposite. Diastereomers possess different physicochemical properties and, thus, differ in properties, such as solubility, volatility, and melting points.

(5) Epimers are a special type of diastereomers because all epimers are also diastereomers; however, the opposite is not true. Epimers are compounds that are structurally identical in all respects except for the stereochemistry of one chiral center. The process of **epimerization** (in which the stereochemistry of one chiral center is inverted) is important in drug degradation and inactivation (Figure 12-13).

b. Geometric isomers (*cis-trans* isomers) occur as a result of restricted rotation around a chemical bond, owing to double bonds or rigid ring systems in the molecule.

(1) *Cis-trans* isomers are not mirror images and have different physicochemical properties and pharmacologic activity.

(2) Because the functional groups of these isomers are separated by different distances, they generally do not fit the same receptor equally well. If these functional groups are pharmacophores, the isomers will **differ in biological activity.** For example, *cis*-diethylstilbestrol has only 7% of the estrogenic activity of *trans*-diethylstilbestrol (Figure 12-14).

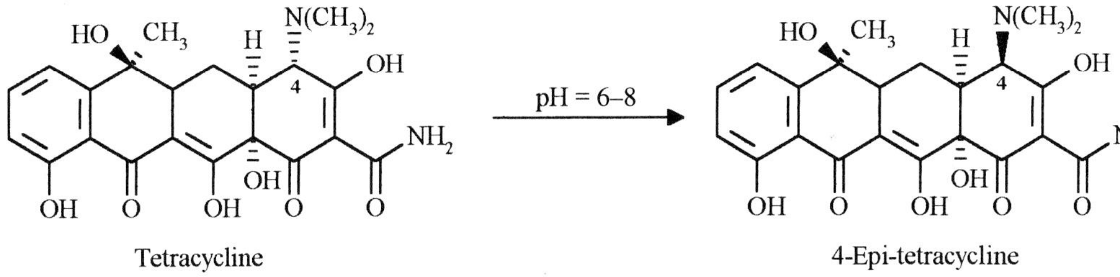

Figure 12-13. Epimerization of tetracycline to 4-epi-tetracycline. The stereochemistry of the 4-dimethylamino group is inverted; however, the stereochemistry of all other chiral centers remains unchanged.

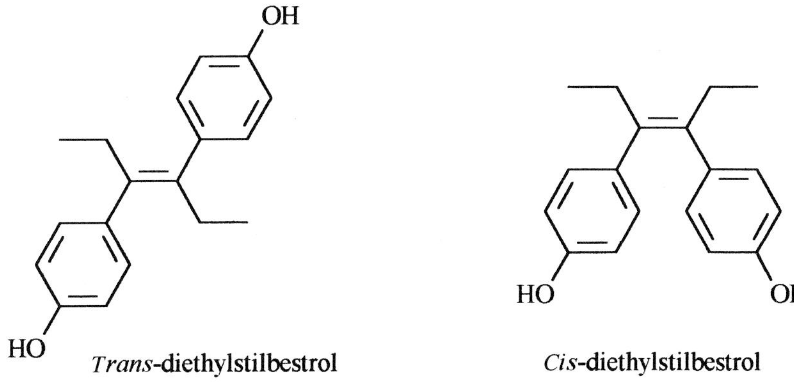

Figure 12-14. The presence of the double bond in diethylstilbestrol allows for the formation of *cis* and *trans* geometric isomers. Only the *trans* isomer has estrogenic activity.

c. **Conformational isomers,** also known as **rotamers** or **conformers,** are nonsuperimposable orientations of a molecule that result from the rotation of atoms around single bonds. Almost every drug can exist in more than one conformation, and this ability allows many drugs to bind to multiple receptors and receptor subtypes. For example, the *trans* conformation of acetylcholine binds to the muscarinic receptor, whereas the *gauche* conformation binds to the nicotinic receptor (Figure 12-15).

d. **Bioisosteres** are molecules containing groups that are spatially and electronically equivalent and, thus, interchangeable without significantly altering the molecules' physicochemical properties. **Isosteric replacement** of functional groups can increase potency, decrease side effects, separate biological activities, and increase the duration of action by altering metabolism. Additionally, **isosteric analogues** may act antagonistically to the parent molecule.

(1) **Procainamide,** an amide, has a longer duration of action than **procaine,** an ester, because of the isosteric replacement of the ester oxygen with a nitrogen atom (Figure 12-16).

(2) **Alloxanthine** is an inhibitor of xanthine oxidase. It is also an isostere of **xanthine,** the normal substrate for the enzyme (see Figure 12-16).

A **B**

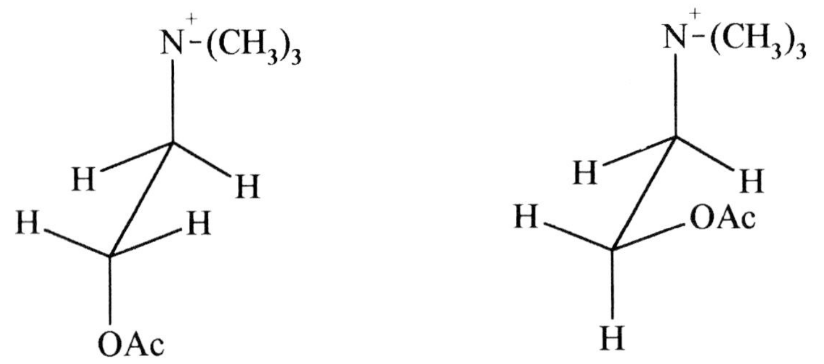

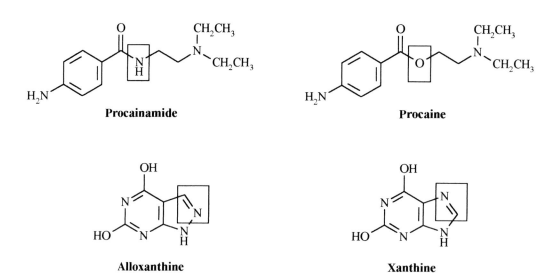

Figure 12-15. The *trans* (A) and *gauche* (B) conformations of acetylcholine occur as the result of rotation around the carbon-carbon single bond.

Procainamide **Procaine**

Alloxanthine **Xanthine**

Figure 12-16. Bioisosteric pairs procainamide/procaine and alloxanthine/xanthine. The isosteric replacements are highlighted.

X. MECHANISMS OF DRUG ACTION

A. Interaction with receptors (see IX B 1–2)

1. **Agonists** interact with specific cellular constituents, known as receptors, and elicit an observable biological response. Agonists have both **affinity** for the receptor and **intrinsic activity.**

2. **Partial agonists** interact with the same receptors as full agonists but are unable to elicit the same maximum response. Partial agonists have lower intrinsic activity than full agonists; however, their affinity for the receptor can be greater than, less than, or equal to that of full agonists.

3. **Antagonists** inhibit the actions of agonists.
   a. **Pharmacological antagonists** bind to the same receptor as the agonist, either at the same site or at an allosteric site. They have affinity for the receptor but lack intrinsic activity. Pharmacological antagonists can be subdivided into reversible, irreversible, competitive, and noncompetitive categories similar to enzyme inhibitors (see X B 2).
   b. **Chemical antagonists** react with one another, resulting in the inactivation of both compounds.
      (1) The anticoagulant **heparin,** an acidic polysaccharide, is chemically antagonized by **protamine,** a basic protein, via an acid–base interaction.
      (2) **Chelating agents** can be used as **antidotes for metal poisoning. Ethylenediamine-tetraacetic acid** (EDTA) chelates calcium and lead; **penicillamine** chelates copper; and **dimercaprol** chelates mercury, gold, antimony, and arsenic.
   c. **Functional (or physical) antagonists** produce antagonistic physiological actions through binding at separate receptors. The adrenergic and cholinergic nervous systems frequently produce this type of antagonism. **Acetylcholine** constricts the pupil by acting on receptors that control the circular muscles of the eye, whereas **norepinephrine** dilates the pupil by acting on receptors that control ocular dilator muscles.

B. Interaction with enzymes

1. **Activation,** or **increased enzyme activity,** can result from induction of enzyme protein synthesis by such drugs as barbiturates, phenytoin and other antiepileptics, rifampin, antihistamines, griseofulvin, and oral contraceptives.
   a. **Allosteric binding.** A drug can enhance enzyme activity by allosteric binding, which triggers a conformational change in the enzyme system and, thus, alters its affinity for substrate binding.
   b. **Coenzymes** play a role in optimizing enzyme activity. Coenzymes include **vitamins** (particularly the **vitamin B complex**) and **cofactors** [mainly metallic ions such as sodium (Na^+), potassium (K^+), magnesium (Mg^{2+}), calcium (Ca^{2+}), zinc (Zn^{2+}), and iron (Fe^{2+})]. Coenzymes activate enzymes by complexation and stereochemical interaction.

2. **Inhibition,** or **decreased enzyme activity,** can result from drugs that interact with the apoenzyme, the coenzyme, or even the whole enzyme complex. The drug might modify or destroy the apoenzyme's protein conformation, react with the coenzyme (thus reducing the enzyme system's capacity to function), or bind with the enzyme complex (rendering it unable to bind with its substrate).
   a. **Reversible inhibition** results from a **noncovalent interaction** between the enzyme and the drug. The drug is free to associate and dissociate with the enzyme, and an equilibrium exists between bound and free drug.
   b. **Irreversible inhibition** results from a stable, **covalent interaction** between the enzyme and the drug. Once bound to the enzyme, the drug is not able to dissociate.
   c. **Competitive inhibition** occurs when there is **mutually exclusive binding** of the substrate and the inhibitor. While it is possible for competitive inhibitors to bind to allosteric sites, these inhibitors are usually structurally similar to the natural substrates and compete with the substrates for common binding sites. Competitive inhibition can be overcome by increasing the concentration of the substrate.
   d. **Noncompetitive inhibition** occurs when a drug binds to an **allosteric site** on the enzyme. This binding induces a conformational change in the enzyme that inhibits enzyme action, even if a substrate is bound to the enzyme. Increasing substrate concentration does not overcome this type of inhibition.

C. Interaction with DNA/RNA formation and function

1. **Inhibition of nucleotide biosynthesis** occurs when folate, purine, and pyrimidine **antimetabolites** interfere with the biosynthesis of purine and pyrimidine building blocks.
   a. **Folic acid analogues** (e.g., methotrexate, trimetrexate) inhibit purine and thymidylate synthesis by inhibiting dihydrofolate reductase.
   b. **Purine analogues** (e.g., 6-mercaptopurine, thioguanine) act as antagonists in the synthesis of purine bases. These analogues do not act as active inhibitors until they are converted to their respective nucleotides.
   c. **Pyrimidine analogues** (e.g., 5-fluorouracil) inhibit the synthesis of thymidylic acid by inhibiting thymidine synthetase. As with purine analogues, pyrimidine analogues are not active until they are converted to their respective nucleotides.

2. **Inhibition of DNA or RNA biosynthesis** occurs when drugs interfere with nucleic acid synthesis. These drugs are used primarily as antineoplastic agents for cancer chemotherapy.
   a. Drugs that interfere with DNA replication and function include intercalating agents (e.g., the **anthracyclines, dactinomycin**), alkylating agents (e.g., **nitrogen mustards, nitrosoureas**), and antimetabolites.
   b. Drugs that can damage and destroy DNA include compounds that produce free radicals (e.g., **bleomycin**, the **anthracyclines**) and compounds that inhibit topoisomerases (e.g., **epipodophyllotoxins, mitoxantrone, irinotecan, topotecan**).
   c. Drugs that interfere with microtubule assembly in the metaphase of **cell mitosis** include the **vinca alkaloids** and **paclitaxel.**

D. Inhibition of protein synthesis

1. **Tetracyclines** interfere with protein synthesis by inhibiting transfer RNA (tRNA) binding to the ribosome and blocking the release of completed peptides from the ribosome.

2. **Chloramphenicol** and **erythromycin** (which compete for the same binding site) bind to the ribosome and inhibit peptidyl transferase, blocking formation of the peptide bond and interrupting formation of the peptide chain.

3. **Aminoglycosides** decrease the fidelity of transcription by binding to the ribosome, which permits formation of an abnormal initiation complex and prohibits addition of amino acids to the peptide chain. Additionally, aminoglycosides cause misreading of the messenger RNA (mRNA) template, so that incorrect amino acids are incorporated into the growing polypeptide chain.

4. **Quinupristin and dalfopristin,** in combination, constrict the exit channel on ribosomal RNA (rRNA). This action prevents newly synthesized polypeptides from being released and in turn inhibits further protein synthesis.

E. Interaction with cell membranes

1. **Digitalis glycosides** inhibit the cell membrane's sodium-potassium pump, inhibiting the influx of K^+ and the outflow of Na^+.

2. **Quinidine** affects the membrane potential of myocardial membranes by prolonging both the polarized and depolarized states.

3. **Local anesthetics** block impulse conduction in nerve cell membranes by interfering with membrane permeability to Na^+ and K^+.

4. **Polyene antifungal drugs** (e.g., amphotericin B, nystatin) affect cell membrane permeability, causing leakage of cellular constituents.

5. **Certain antibiotics** (e.g., polymyxin B, colistin) affect cell membrane permeability through an unknown mechanism.

6. **Acetylcholine** increases membrane permeability to cations.

7. **Omeprazole** and **lansoprazole** inhibit the H^+/K^+ pump (located in parietal cell membranes), thus decreasing the efflux of protons into the stomach.

8. Several **antineoplastic** agents exert their actions by initially binding to **cellular determinants (CDs)** expressed by tumor cells.

    a. Gemtuzumab ozogamicin binds with CD33 expressed by leukemic cells and immature myelomonocytic cells.

    b. Alemtuzumab, a monoclonal antibody, binds to the CD52 antigen expressed on B-lymphocytes, T-lymphocytes, and various other cells.

F. Nonspecific action

  1. Structurally nonspecific drugs form a monomolecular layer over entire areas of certain cells. Because they involve such large surfaces, these drugs are usually given in relatively large doses.

  2. Drugs that act by nonspecific action include the **volatile general anesthetic gases** (e.g., ether, nitrous oxide), some **depressants** (e.g., ethanol, chloral hydrate), and many antiseptic compounds (e.g., phenol, rubbing alcohol).

STUDY QUESTIONS

Directions: Each of the numbered items or incomplete statements in this section is followed by answers or by completions of the statement. Select the **one** lettered answer or completion that is **best** in each case.

1. A 40-year-old man complains of dysuria and urinary urgency and is diagnosed to have uncomplicated gonococcal urethritis. He is given procaine penicillin G intramuscularly. In addition, probenecid is given to prolong the duration of action of penicillin. This type of combined drug effect is known as

(A) synergism
(B) competitive antagonism
(C) addition
(D) potentiation
(E) noncompetitive antagonism

2. A 40-year-old teacher was prescribed lovastatin for the treatment of hypercholesterolemia. She wanted to know the mechanism of the drug before taking it. Her pharmacist explained to her that lovastatin acts by blocking the substrate-binding site of the enzyme HMG-CoA reductase that catalyzes the rate-limiting step in cholesterol biosynthesis. Such drug effect is known as

(A) addition
(B) syngerism
(C) noncompetitive antagonism
(D) potentiation
(E) competitive antagonism

3. A 70-year-old man had prolonged bleeding during an elective knee surgery. Subsequently, the patient admitted to the surgeon that he had been self-administering 81 mg aspirin daily. The consultant pharmacist explained to the patient that, although aspirin has a short plasma half-life, it can irreversibly inhibit platelet function by acetylating the nonsubstrate binding site of the platelet cyclooxygenase, resulting in prolonged effect on platelet aggregation. This drug effect is known as

(A) potentiation
(B) competitive antagonism
(C) synergism
(D) addition
(E) noncompetitive antagonism

4. A 65-year-old woman with intractable pain secondary to bony metastasis of breast cancer had been receiving escalating doses of morphine sulfate intravenously. At 10 a.m., she was found to be unresponsive, her respiratory rate was 4 breaths per minute, and her pupils were pin-pointed. Naloxone, a competitive antagonist of the opiate receptor, was given intravenously and repeated once. She gradually became conscious and began to complain of pain unrelieved by morphine given at the previous dose. This is most likely because

(A) naloxone directly aggravates the pain due to the bony metastasis.
(B) naloxone reduces the E_{max} for morphine.
(C) naloxone reduces the ED_{50} for morphine.
(D) naloxone increases the E_{max} for morphine.
(E) naloxone increases the ED_{50} for morphine.

5. Which of the following statements regarding signal transduction is incorrect?

(A) Thyroxine-bound receptors act on DNA and regulate specific transcription of genes.
(B) Cyclic adenosine monophosphate can act as a second messenger.
(C) The level of drug receptors at the cell surface increases with chronic stimulation by receptor agonists.
(D) Binding of ligand to cell-surface receptors can lead to synthesis of proteins.
(E) Antacids act by interacting with small ions normally found in the gastrointestinal tract.

6. A pharmacist is consulted about selecting a drug that is relatively safe and effective for treating the patient. He searches the literature and obtains the following data that may help guide his decision. The $TD_{0.1}$ and $ED_{99.9}$ for drug A are 20 mg and 0.4 mg, respectively, whereas the $TD_{0.1}$ and $ED_{99.9}$ for drug B are 15 mg and 0.2 mg, respectively. Which of the following statements is true?

(A) Drug A has a higher $TD_{0.1}$ and, thus, should be the drug of choice.
(B) Both drugs have the same margin of safety, so more information is needed.
(C) Drug B has a higher margin of safety and, thus, is preferred to drug A.
(D) Drug A is preferred because it has a greater margin of safety than drug B.
(E) The information obtained is irrelevant.

7. Which of the following statements concerning a drug receptor is true?

(A) It mediates the nonspecific action of volatile anesthetics.
(B) Its expression is induced only by exogenously added drugs.
(C) It can bind endogenous ligand to produce physiological activity.
(D) It mediates the cathartic activity of magnesium citrate.
(E) Down regulation of receptor level can lead to sensitization of the target cell to the receptor agonist.

8. Which of the following statements concerning morphine and hydromorphone is true?

(A) Hydromorphone is a more effective analgesic because it has a smaller ED_{50} than morphine.
(B) Morphine and hydromorphone are equally potent because they have the same E_{max}.
(C) Morphine has a greater ED_{50} and is, thus, a less effective analgesic than hydromorphone.
(D) Hydromorphone is a more potent analgesic because it has a greater E_{max} than morphine.
(E) Hydromorphone has a smaller ED_{50} and, thus, is a more potent analgesic than morphine.

9. A 72-year-old man with hypertension has been taking high-dose propranolol for 20 years. He left home for a week and forgot to bring his medication with him. One day, he was found collapsed on the floor and was brought to the emergency room. His blood pressure was 300/180, heart rate was 180 beats per minute, and retinal hemorrhage was observed. Which of the following best explains this situation?

(A) The β-adrenergic receptors in the cardiac muscles underwent spontaneous mutation and became hyperactive.
(B) Reduction in the chronic antagonism of the β-adrenergic receptor led to down-regulation of the β-adrenergic receptor.
(C) The propranolol that he had previously ingested remained in his body and acted as a receptor agonist.
(D) Long-term administration of propranolol results in desensitization of cardiac muscles to endogenous β-adrenergic stimulation.
(E) Reduction in the chronic level of receptor blockade results in supersensitivity to stimulation with endogenous catecholamines.

10. Which of the following acids has the highest degree of ionization in an aqueous solution?

(A) Aspirin $pK_a = 3.5$
(B) Indomethacin $pK_a = 4.5$
(C) Warfarin $pK_a = 5.1$
(D) Ibuprofen $pK_a = 5.2$
(E) Phenobarbital $pK_a = 7.4$

11. Which of the following salts will most likely yield an aqueous solution with a pH below 7?

(A) Sodium salicylate
(B) Potassium chloride
(C) Magnesium sulfate
(D) Potassium penicillin
(E) Atropine sulfate

12. Which of the following chemical/pharmacological classes of agents is INCORRECTLY matched with its acid/base nature?

(A) Adrenergic α_2-agonists: basic
(B) Prostaglandins: acidic
(C) Organic nitrates: nonelectrolytes
(D) Meglitinides: acidic
(E) 4-Quinolones: basic

13. All of the following medicinal agents are classified as natural products EXCEPT

(A) atropine
(B) diazepam
(C) digitoxin
(D) penicillin
(E) morphine

14. All of the following statements about a structurally specific agonist are true EXCEPT

(A) activity is determined more by its chemical structure than by its physical properties.
(B) the entire molecule is involved in binding to a specific endogenous receptor.
(C) the drug cannot act unless it is first bound to a receptor.
(D) a minor structural change in a pharmacophore can produce a loss in activity.
(E) the higher the affinity between the drug and its receptor, the greater the biological response.

15. The dextro (D) form of β-methacholine (structure shown) is approximately 500 times more active than the levo (L) enantiomer. The observed difference in pharmacological activity between the two isomers is most likely due to differences in

(A) receptor selectivity
(B) dissolution
(C) distribution
(D) interatomic distance between pharmacophore groups
(E) solubility

16. The compound shown below can be classified as a

(A) penicillin
(B) thiazide
(C) coumarin
(D) phenothiazine
(E) hydantoin

17. Which of the following statements concerning the structure shown below is NOT correct? The compound

(A) is an acid.
(B) can be used to treat arthritis.
(C) is a fenamate.
(D) increases prostaglandin production.
(E) is a nonsteroidal anti-inflammatory drug (NSAID).

18. All of the following classes of drugs are used to treat hypertension EXCEPT

(A) aryloxypropanolamines
(B) thiazides
(C) fibrates
(D) dihydropyridines
(E) angiotensin-converting enzyme (ACE) inhibitors

19. Flurazepam has pK_a of 8.2. What percentage of flurazepam will be ionized at a urine pH of 5.2?

(A) 0.1%
(B) 1%
(C) 50%
(D) 99%
(E) 99.9%

Questions 20–24

Directions: Each question below contains three suggested answers, of which **one or more** is correct. Choose the answer

A	if **I only** is correct
B	if **III only** is correct
C	if **I and II** are correct
D	if **II and III** are correct
E	if **I, II, and III** are correct

20. Drugs that act systemically must

I. undergo biotransformation into an active form after reaching their active site.
II. be in a form capable of passage through various membrane barriers.
III. be in or be converted to a form that is readily excreted from the body.

21. Examples of strong electrolytes (i.e., completely dissociated in an aqueous solution) include

I. acetic acid
II. pentobarbital sodium
III. diphenhydramine hydrochloride

22. Precipitation may occur when mixing aqueous solutions of meperidine hydrochloride with which of the following solutions?

I. Sodium bicarbonate injection
II. Atropine sulfate injection
III. Sodium chloride injection

23. Drugs classified as antimetabolites include

I. 5-fluorouracil
II. sulfisoxazole
III. digoxin

24. The excretion of a weakly acidic drug generally is more rapid in alkaline urine than in acidic urine. This process occurs because

I. a weak acid in alkaline media will exist primarily in its ionized form, which cannot be reabsorbed easily.
II. a weak acid in alkaline media will exist in its lipophilic form, which cannot be reabsorbed easily.
III. all drugs are excreted more rapidly in an alkaline urine.

Questions 25–28 refer to the drug meperidine (see structure below).

Questions 25–28

25. Functional groups present in the molecule shown include

I. an ester
II. a tertiary amine
III. a carboxylic acid

26. Meperidine is classified as a

I. weak acid
II. salt
III. weak base

27. Assuming that meperidine is absorbed after oral administration and that a large percentage of the dose is excreted unchanged, the effect of alkalinization of the urine will increase its

I. duration of action
II. rate of excretion
III. ionization in the glomerular filtrate

28. The appropriate chemical classification for meperidine is

I. phenylpropylamines
II. piperazines
III. 4-phenylpiperidines

Directions: The group of items in this section consists of lettered options followed by a set of numbered items. For each item, select the **one lettered** option that is most closely associated with it. Each lettered option may be selected once, more than once, or not at all.

Questions 29–33

For each pair of molecules, select the term that best fits the relationship.

(A) Geometric isomers
(B) Enantiomers
(C) Diastereomers
(D) Bioisosteres
(E) Conformational isomers

29.

30.

31.

32.

33.

ANSWERS AND EXPLANATIONS

1. The answer is D *[V C].*
Probenecid alone is inactive against gonococci. However, it can compete with penicillin for urinary excretion. Thus, probenecid can reduce the elimination rate of penicillin, whose duration of action becomes prolonged. Therefore, probenecid potentiates the activity of penicillin when the two are given together.

2. The answer is E *[II B 4 a, IV D 3].*
Lovastatin reversibly binds to the substrate-binding site of the enzyme HMG-CoA reductase that catalyzes the rate-limiting step in the synthesis of cholesterol, thus lowering the cholesterol level. Therefore, lovastatin inhibits the enzyme by competitive antagonism.

3. The answer is E *[II B 4 b, IV D 4].*
Aspirin can covalently modify the platelet cyclooxygenase through acetylation of the enzyme other than the substrate-binding site, causing irreversible inhibition of platelet aggregation. Therefore, aspirin inhibits platelet function by noncompetitive antagonism of cyclooxygenase.

4. The answer is E *[IV D 3].*
Naloxone is a competitive antagonist of opiate receptor. If one compares the log dose-response curve seen with both morphine and naloxone to that seen with morphine alone, the morphine-naloxone curve would be shifted to the right of the morphine curve. As a result, the ED_{50} for morphine is increased. This means that a larger than previous dose of morphine is required for achieving the same analgesic effect.

5. The answer is C *[III D 4].*
The level of drug receptors at the cell surface usually decreases when the target cells are chronically stimulated by receptor agonists. Down regulation of receptors is a protective mechanism that can prevent the target cells from being over stimulated.

6. The answer is C *[VI C].*
The margin of safety of the two drugs can be helpful in guiding selection of a drug. Margin of safety is the ratio of $TD_{0.1}$ to $ED_{99.9}$. Thus, the margin of safety for drug A is 20 mg / 0.4 mg, or 50, whereas the margin of safety for drug B is 15 mg / 0.2 mg, or 75. Because drug B has a greater margin of safety than drug A, drug B is relatively safe at the dosage given to produce the desired effect.

7. The answer is C *[II B 2, III D 4, III E 1 a, b].*
A drug receptor, such as muscarinic cholinergic receptor that can bind atropine, normally binds endogenous acetylcholine to produce the physiological responses controlled by the parasympathetic autonomic nervous system. Volatile anesthetics act colligatively as solutes in the lipid bilayer of the cell membrane. Drug receptors are endogenously expressed, but their level can be modulated by exogenously added drugs. The cathartic activity of magnesium citrate is a consequence of increase in the osmolarity of the gastrointestinal fluids. Down regulation of receptor level can lead to desensitization, not sensitization, of the target cell to the receptor agonist.

8. The answer is E *[IV D 1, 2].*
The efficacy of a drug is determined by its E_{max}, whereas its potency is measured by the ED_{50}. Hydromorphone has a smaller ED_{50} and, thus, is a more potent analgesic than morphine. Hydromorphone and morphine are both agonists for opiate receptors, and they have the same analgesic efficacy (that is, they have the same E_{max}) if sufficient amounts of both drugs are used.

9. The answer is E *[III D 6].*
Chronic level of blocking the β-adrenergic receptors by propranolol results in up regulation of the receptor level. When the patient ceased taking the drug, the cardiac muscles became supersensitive to stimulation with endogenous catecholamines. This resulted in the hypertensive crisis that caused cerebral hemorrhage and loss of consciousness.

10. The answer is A *[VIII B 2 b].*
The pK_a (the negative log of the acid ionization constant) is indicative of the relative strength of an acidic drug. The lower the pK_a of an acidic drug, the stronger it is as an acid. A strong acid is defined as one that is completely ionized or dissociated in an aqueous solution; therefore, the stronger the acid, the greater the ionization.

11. The answer is E *[VIII B 3 d].*
The solution must contain an acidic substance to have a pH below 7. Atropine sulfate is a salt of a weak base and a strong acid; therefore, its aqueous solution is acidic. Sodium salicylate and potassium penicillin are both salts of strong bases and weak acids; therefore, their aqueous solutions are alkaline. Magnesium sulfate and potassium chloride are salts of strong bases and strong acids; therefore, their aqueous solutions are neutral.

12. The answer is E *[Table 12-1; Figures 12-8, 12-9, and 12-11].*
4-Quinolones are amphoteric compounds. All compounds in this chemical class contain a carboxylic acid as well as a basic nitrogen. Most 4-quinolones contain a basic piperazine ring as well as basic heterocyclic rings; however, some of the older compounds in this class only have the basic heterocyclic rings. All other compounds are correctly matched with their acid/base nature. Please consult the table and figures listed above for confirmation.

13. The answer is B *[VII A, B].*
Diazepam is a benzodiazepine anxiolytic, which, while it is a heterocyclic nitrogen-containing molecule, is not an alkaloid and is prepared synthetically. Natural products refer to those substances biosynthesized in plants or animals. Natural products include alkaloids, such as atropine and morphine; peptides, such as glucagon; steroids, such as estradiol; hormones, such as insulin; glycosides, such as digitoxin; vitamins, such as riboflavin; polysaccharides, such as heparin; and antibiotics, such as penicillin.

14. The answer is B *[IX B].*
The binding of a drug to its receptor usually involves only specific functional groups. These groups comprise what is known as the pharmacophore of the drug molecule. Although the entire drug molecule is present at the receptor site, only a portion of it, the pharmacophore, is required for a biological response.

15. The answer is A *[IX B 3 a; Figure 12-12].*
The term enantiomer and the D and L indicate that the β-methacholine has a chiral center and exhibits optical isomerism. Because the optical isomers have different orientations in space, one orientation will give a better fit than the other and will most likely have greater biological activity than the other. Dissolution, distribution, interatomic distances, and solubility are all related to the physical and chemical properties of the two compounds, which are identical because the compounds are enantiomers.

16. The answer is B *[Table 12-1; Figures 12-7 to 12-10].*
Key structural features of a thiazide, a benzothiadiazine ring with an electron-withdrawing chloride atom and a sulfonyl group on the benzene ring, identify this compound as a thiazide.

17. The answer is D *[Table 12-1, Figure 12-8].*
The carboxylic acid identifies this compound as an acid. Other structural features identify it as a fenamate. Fenamates are NSAIDs (nonsteroidal anti-inflammatory drugs), which can be used for inflammatory disorders (e.g., arthritis, bursitis). The mechanism of action of NSAIDs is inhibition of cyclooxygenase, which results in a decrease in the production of prostaglandins.

18. The answer is C *[Table 12-1].*
Fibrates decrease cholesterol and triglyceride levels. All of the other chemical classes can be used to treat hypertension. Aryloxypropanolamines are β-blockers, thiazides are diuretics, dihydropyridines are calcium channel blockers, and ACE inhibitors decrease the synthesis of angiotensin II, a potent vasoconstrictor.

19. The answer is E *[VIII B 2 f–g; Table 12-1].*
Flurazepam (take note of the suffix, which helps classify the compound) is a benzodiazepine and, thus, a basic compound. Because the pH is less than the pKa, flurazepam is in an acidic environment and, therefore, exists primarily in the ionized form. The percent ionized can be easily calculated by using the rule of nines. The |pH - pKa| is 3, so the ratio is 99.9%:0.01% in favor of the ionized form.

20. The answer is D (II, III) *[VIII A 1, 2].*
Generally, drugs must be lipophilic to pass through lipoprotein membranes and hydrophilic to be excreted by the kidney. Drugs do not have to be converted into an active form at their active site, although most drugs must be in their active form when they reach their active site. Many drugs are active in the

form in which they are administered. Some drugs, usually referred to as prodrugs, are biotransformed into their active form after administration. Theoretically, drugs that reach their active site and then are metabolically activated should be more specific in their action and have fewer side effects. Currently, research efforts are under way to develop site-specific delivery systems and processes.

21. The answer is D (II, III) *[VIII B 2 c, 3 a, 4 a].*
Almost all salts (with very few exceptions) are strong electrolytes, and the terminology pentobarbital sodium and diphenhydramine hydrochloride indicate that both compounds are salts. Acetic acid is a weak acid; therefore, it is a weak electrolyte.

22. The answer is A (I) *[VIII B 3, 4].*
When meperidine hydrochloride solution is mixed with the alkaline solution of sodium bicarbonate, a neutralization reaction occurs with the possible precipitation of the water-insoluble free base meperidine. A neutralization reaction occurs when acidic solutions are mixed with basic solutions, or conversely. No reaction, in terms of acid–base, occurs when solutions are mixed with other acidic or neutral solutions or when basic solutions are mixed with other basic or neutral solutions. There should be no reaction, then, when the meperidine hydrochloride solution, which is acidic, is mixed with the acidic solution of atropine sulfate or the neutral solution of sodium chloride.

23. The answer is C (I, II) *[IX B 3 d; X C 1; X E 1].*
Both sulfisoxazole and 5-fluorouracil compete with and antagonize isosteric normal biological molecules and, therefore, are antimetabolites. Digoxin is a drug that is thought to inhibit Na^+/K^+–ATPase or to affect intracellular influx or use of calcium ion (Ca^{2+}). Because digoxin is steroidal, it is not isosteric with either an enzyme, which is a protein, or an ion; therefore, it is not classified as an antimetabolite.

24. The answer is A (I) *[VIII B 1, 2 e].*
A weakly acidic drug will be more ionized in an alkaline urine; therefore, it will be more polar and, thus, more soluble in the aqueous urine. It would also be less liposoluble, less likely to undergo tubular reabsorption, and thus be more likely to be excreted.

25–28. The answers are: 25-C (I, II), 26-B (III), 27-A (I), 28-B (III) *[VIII B 2, 3; Figure 12-7].*
The molecule contains a basic nitrogen, which is bonded to three carbon atoms (i.e., a tertiary amine), and an ethyl carboxylate, which is an ester group. An ester is the product of the reaction of an alcohol with a carboxylic acid that forms an alkyl carboxylate. There is no free carboxylic acid present. However, if this molecule is subjected to hydrolysis, it forms a carboxylic acid and ethyl alcohol.

Because meperidine contains a tertiary amine, it is classified as a base; because it is an organic base, it is considered weak. The nitrogen is not protonated. It is not ionic and, therefore, is not a salt.

Alkalinization of the urine decreases the ionization of meperidine, making it more liposoluble and, thus, more likely to undergo reabsorption in the kidney tubule. This results in a decreased rate of excretion and an increased duration of action. The six-member, nonaromatic ring is a piperidine ring that is substituted at the 4-position (nitrogen is position 1) with a phenyl ring. The compound does not contain a piperazine ring or a propyl group.

29–33. The answers are: 29-C, 30-B, 31-A, 32-D, 33-E *[IX B 3 a–d].*
The first pair of molecules are isomers that have two asymmetric carbon atoms. They are not superimposable and are not mirror images; therefore, they are known as diastereomers.

The second pair of molecules are isomers that have one asymmetric carbon atom. They are nonsuperimposable mirror images; therefore, they are enantiomers.

The third pair of molecules have different spatial arrangements; however, these molecules do not have an asymmetric center. The presence of the double bond, which restricts the rotation of the groups on each carbon atom involved in the double bond, characterizes this type of isomerism as geometric.

The fourth pair of molecules are neither isomers nor the same compound because one contains three oxygens, whereas the other contains two oxygens and a sulfur. Because oxygen and sulfur are in the same periodic family, they are isosteric and are known as bioisosteres.

The final pair of structures are actually two views of the same compound. Rotation around the side-chain single bonds connecting the ring nitrogen to the tertiary nitrogen produces these two different conformations. Thus, these are conformational isomers.

13
Medicinal Chemistry and Pharmacology: Drugs Affecting the Nervous System

Ashiwel S. Undie

I. INTRODUCTION. Drugs affecting the nervous system modulate neurotransmission in the **central nervous system (CNS),** which consists of the brain and the spinal cord, or in the **peripheral nervous system (PNS),** which includes the **autonomic nervous system (ANS)** and the somatic system that innervates the skeletal muscles. Agents acting in the ANS include adrenergic agonists and antagonists, and cholinergic agonists and antagonists. Drugs affecting the PNS are useful for treating a variety of ailments including blood pressure disturbances, bronchial asthma, cardiac dysfunctions, anaphylactic reactions, nasal congestion, and skeletal muscle spasticity. Drugs affecting the CNS provide anesthesia and sedation, relieve pain and anxiety, suppress movement disorders and epileptic seizures, and treat psychotic and affective disorders. These drugs include general and local anesthetics, anxiolytics and sedative–hypnotics, opioid analgesics, antiparkinsonian agents, antiepileptics, antipsychotics, and antidepressants.

II. GENERAL MECHANISMS OF DRUG ACTION IN THE NERVOUS SYSTEM. Drugs acting in the nervous system achieve their pharmacological effects by modifying the synaptic concentrations or receptor actions of neurotransmitters. Other drugs modulate the intracellular response pathways by which the receptor actions of the transmitters are conveyed to yield the ultimate physiological response. The major neurotransmitters in the nervous system, their primary receptor subtypes, and the predominant effects of receptor stimulation on neurotransmission are shown in Table 13-1. Some general mechanisms by which diverse drugs modulate the activity of the nervous system are summarized in Table 13-2, with examples drawn from the adrenergic and cholinergic components of the PNS. In addition, there are various classes of drugs that modulate neural function by interacting with the pores of ion channels or by binding to allosteric sites on the protein subunits that constitute the channel.

III. ADRENERGIC AGONISTS

A. **Chemistry**

1. **Direct-acting adrenergic agonists** interact directly with adrenergic receptors to elicit a response. These include norepinephrine and epinephrine, which are endogenous or naturally occurring catecholamines. Catecholamines are biosynthesized from tyrosine, an amino acid (Figure 13-1). Examples of other direct-acting adrenergic agonists include naphazoline, terbutaline, and dobutamine (Figure 13-2). The classification of adrenergic agonists and antagonists shown in Table 13-3 should provide a broad perspective on the variety of agents that act on this system to produce their pharmacological and therapeutic effects.

   a. The ethylamine chain common to these agonists is essential to their activity.

   b. N-substituents alter drug activity. Small substituents (e.g., hydrogen, α-methyl group) produce α-receptor activity, as with norepinephrine; larger substituents (e.g., an isopropyl group) produce β-receptor activity, as with isoproterenol.

   c. Removal of the *para* (4) hydroxyl group leaves only α-receptor activity, as with phenylephrine.

   d. The *meta* (3) hydroxyl group is essential for direct α- and β-activity. However, drugs in which the *meta* hydroxyl is replaced by a sulfonamide or a hydroxymethyl group retain activity.

   e. Catecholamines are inactivated by methylation of the *meta* hydroxyl group (catalyzed by catechol O-methyltransferase, COMT) and by oxidative deamination (catalyzed by monoamine oxidase, MAO).

254

Table 13-1. Major Neurotransmitters in the Nervous System and Their Postsynaptic Receptor Effects on Ionic Conductance and Second Messenger (Signaling) Pathways

Neurotransmitter	Primary Receptor Subtypes	Effects of Receptor Stimulation
Acetylcholine	Muscarinic M_1 (and M_3, M_5)	Excitatory ($\uparrow$IP3/DAG)
	Muscarinic M_2 (and M_4)	Inhibitory ($\downarrow$cAMP)
	Nicotinic (N_1 and N_2)	Excitatory ($\uparrow$cation conductance)
Dopamine	D_1 (and D_5)	Excitatory ($\uparrow$cAMP; $\uparrow$IP3/DAG)
	D_2 (and D_3, D_4)	Inhibitory ($\downarrow$cAMP; $\uparrow$K$^+$ conductance)
GABA	GABA$_A$	Inhibitory ($\uparrow$Cl$^-$ ion conductance)
	GABA$_B$	Inhibitory ($\downarrow$Ca^{2+}; $\uparrow$K$^+$ ion conductance)
Glutamate	Ionotropic–NMDA	Excitatory ($\uparrow$Ca^{2+} ion conductance)
	Ionotropic–AMPA/Kainate	Excitatory ($\uparrow$cation conductance)
	Metabotropic	Excitatory ($\uparrow$IP3/DAG; $\downarrow$K$^+$ ion conductance)
Histamine	H_1	Excitatory ($\uparrow$IP3/DAG; $\downarrow$K$^+$ conductance)
	H_2	Excitatory ($\uparrow$cAMP; $\downarrow$K$^+$ conductance)
Norepinephrine	α_1	Excitatory ($\uparrow$IP3/DAG; $\downarrow$K$^+$ conductance)
	α_2	Inhibitory ($\downarrow$cAMP; $\uparrow$K$^+$ conductance)
	β_1	Excitatory ($\uparrow$cAMP; $\downarrow$K$^+$ conductance)
	β_2	Inhibitory in ANS ($\uparrow$cAMP)
Serotonin (5HT)	$5HT_1$	Inhibitory ($\downarrow$cAMP)
	$5HT_2$	Inhibitory ($\downarrow$cAMP; $\uparrow$K$^+$ conductance)
	$5HT_{(3/4/5/6/7)}$	Mixed ($\uparrow$cAMP; ionic conductance)
Opioid peptides	*Mu* (μ)	Inhibitory ($\downarrow$cAMP; $\uparrow$K$^+$ conductance)
	Delta (δ)	Inhibitory ($\downarrow$cAMP; $\uparrow$K$^+$ conductance)
	Kappa (κ)	Inhibitory ($\downarrow$cAMP; $\uparrow$K$^+$ conductance)

Table 13-2. Some General Mechanisms of Drug Action in the Nervous System Exemplified by the Adrenergic and Cholinergic Neurotransmitter Systems

Mechanism	Adrenergic System	Cholinergic System
1. Ganglionic stimulation	Nicotine	
2. Ganglionic blockade	Hexamethonium, trimethaphan	
3. Inhibition of neurotransmitter synthesis	Metyrosine, carbidopa	Hemicholinium
4. Inhibition of neurotransmitter release	Bretylium, guanethidine	Botulinun toxin
5. Facilitation of neurotransmitter release	Amphetamine, tyramine	α-latrotoxin
6. Depletion of vesicular transmitter storage	Reserpine	Vesamicol
7. Blockade of neurotransmitter reuptake	Cocaine, desipramine	See note[a]
8. Inhibition of neurotransmitter metabolism	Clorgyline (inhibits MAO-A)[b] Selegiline (inhibits MAO-B) Tolcapone (inhibits COMT)	Neostigmine and other AChE inhibitors
8. Direct interaction with postsynaptic receptors	Adrenoceptor agonists Adrenoceptor antagonists	Cholinergic agonists Cholinergic antagonists

[a] Reuptake is not a major mechanism for termination of acetylcholine's action; most of the released transmitter is metabolized by acetylcholinesterase (AChE).

[b] MAO-A, MAO-B (monoamine oxidase-A, -B); COMT (catechol-O-methyl transferase).

2. **Indirect-acting adrenergic agonists** are chemically related to the catecholamines, but they do not interact directly with adrenergic receptors. These mostly synthetic compounds induce their pharmacological effects by enhancing the release of the endogenous neurotransmitters. Physiologically, therefore, they have effects similar to the catecholamine neurotransmitters, hence their nickname of sympathomimetic amines. Examples include amphetamine, ephedrine, and tyramine (Figure 13-3).

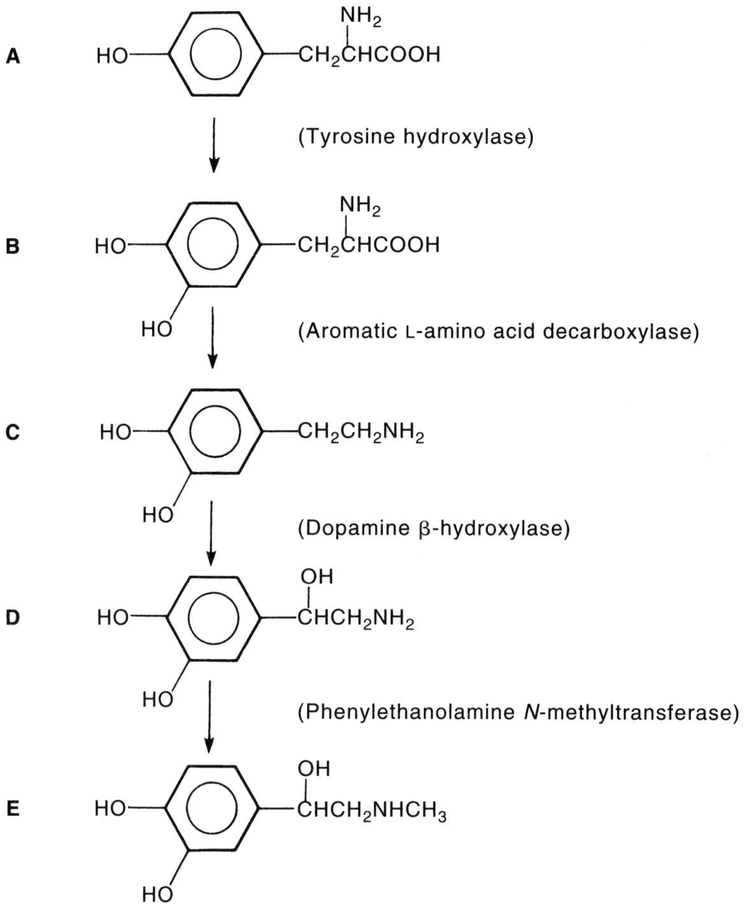

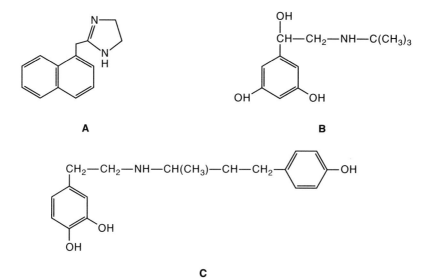

A
HO
NH2
CH2CHCOOH
(Tyrosine hydroxylase)
B
HO
HO
NH2
CH2CHCOOH
(Aromatic L-amino acid decarboxylase)
C
HO
HO
CH2CH2NH2
(Dopamine β-hydroxylase)
D
HO
HO
OH
CHCH2NH2
(Phenylethanolamine N-methyltransferase)
E
HO
HO
OH
CHCH2NHCH3

Figure 13-1. Synthesis of catecholamines from the amino acid tyrosine. In the presence of tyrosine hydroxylase, (*A*) tyrosine is converted to (*B*) dihydroxyphenylalanine (dopa). Further substitutions permit the synthesis of (*C*) dopamine, (*D*) norepinephrine, and (*E*) epinephrine.

N
N
H
A
OH
CH—CH2—NH—C(CH3)3
OH
OH
B
CH2—CH2—NH—CH(CH3)—CH—CH2
OH
OH
OH
C

Figure 13-2. Structural formulas of representative direct-acting sympathomimetic amines. (*A*) Naphazoline, (*B*) terbutaline, (*C*) dobutamine.

Table 13-3. Classification of Adrenoceptor Agonists and Antagonists*

	Class	Adrenoceptor Agonist	Adrenoceptor Antagonist
A.	**Nonselective**		
A.1	Indirect-acting	Tyramine Ephedrine Amphetamine Cocaine	
A.2	Direct-acting	Norepinephrine Epinephrine	Labetalol Carvedilol
B.	**α-Receptor-Selective**		
B.1	Nonselective α	Oxymetazoline Xylometazoline Tetrahydrozoline	Phenoxybenzamine Phentolamine
B.2	Selective α_1	Phenylephrine Methoxamine Metaraminol	Prazosin Terazosin Doxazosin Indoramin
B.3	Selective α_2	Clonidine Guanabenz Guanfacine Rilmenidine Moxonidine α-Methyldopa	Rauwolscine Yohimbine Tolazoline
C.	**β-Receptor-Selective**		
C.1	Nonselective β	Isoproterenol	Propranolol Nadolol Pindolol Carteolol Timolol Sotalol Penbutolol
C.2	Selective β_1	Xamoterol	Acebutolol Atenolol Betaxolol Celiprolol Esmolol Metoprolol
C.3	Selective β_2	Metaproterenol Fenoterol Terbutaline Albuterol (Salbutamol) Ritodrine Salmeterol Formoterol Pirbuterol Bitolterol	Butoxamine
C.4	Selective β_3	BRL 37344	

*To describe the classification of a particular drug, the receptor selectivity class on the left is combined with the receptor activity descriptor on the top of the column; for example, tyramine is an indirect-acting adrenoceptor agonist, and tolazoline is a selective α_2-adrenoceptor antagonist.

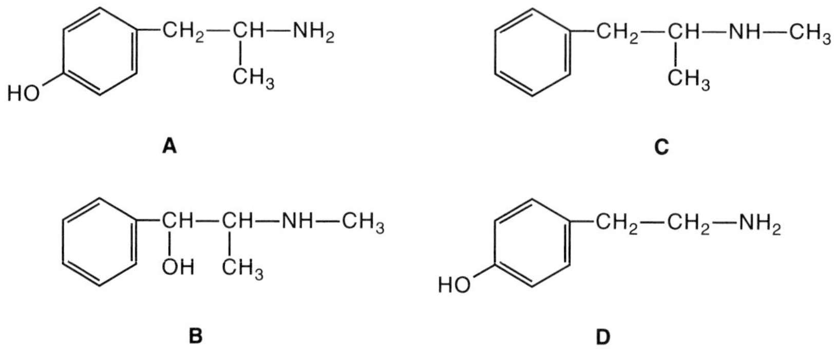

Figure 13-3. Chemical structures of some indirect-acting sympathomimetic amines. (*A*) Hydroxyamphetamine (Paredrine), (*B*) ephedrine or pseudoephedrine (Sudafed), (*C*) methamphetamine (Methedrine), (*D*) tyramine.

    a. Indirect-acting sympathomimetic amines may have one, two, or no hydroxyl groups. The fewer the hydroxyl groups, the higher the lipophilicity, and the greater the absorption and the duration of activity after oral administration. Faster and greater absorption also implies less intestinal destruction of the drug.

    b. Alkyl substitution at the α-carbon (adjacent to the amino group) retards destruction of phenol and phenyl compounds and increases lipophilic character, contributing to prolonged activity.

    c. N-substitution with bulky groups increases direct β-receptor activity, as with the direct-acting agents.

B. Pharmacology

  1. Adrenergic peripheral responses are mediated by both α- and β-adrenoceptors (Table 13-4).

    a. α-Receptors fall into two groups.

      (1) Postjunctional α_1-adrenergic receptors are found in the radial smooth muscle of the iris; in the arteries, arterioles, and veins; in the pilomotor smooth muscle of hair follicles; in the heart; and in the sphincters of the gastrointestinal (GI) tract. Drugs that are **α_1-selective agonists** cause excitatory responses such as vasoconstriction and smooth muscle contraction, and include phenylephrine and methoxamine.

      (2) Prejunctional α_2-adrenergic receptors mediate the inhibition of adrenergic neurotransmitter release. Drugs that are **α_2-selective agonists** also inhibit lipolysis in fat cells and promote platelet aggregation. Examples include clonidine and guanabenz.

    b. β-Receptors fall into three groups.

      (1) Postjunctional β_1-adrenergic receptors are found mainly in the myocardium, where their stimulation increases the force and rate of myocardial contraction. Drugs that are **β_1-selective agonists** include xamoterol and to some extent dobutamine.

      (2) Postjunctional β_2-adrenergic receptors are found in bronchiolar and vascular smooth muscle, where their stimulation causes smooth-muscle dilatation or relaxation. Drugs that are **β_2-selective agonists** include albuterol and terbutaline.

      (3) Postjunctional β_3-adrenergic receptors are expressed on fat cells, and their stimulation causes lipolysis. A number of β_3-agonists such as BRL 37344 are under development as potential antiobesity agents.

  2. Direct-acting adrenergic agonists (e.g., dobutamine, phenylephrine, clonidine, terbutaline) produce their effects primarily by direct stimulation of adrenergic receptors. They may be receptor-selective, as with the drugs listed above, or they may be nonselective. For example, the adrenergic neurotransmitter norepinephrine affects all adrenergic receptors, especially α_1-, α_2-, and β_1-receptors, whereas the adrenal medullary hormone epinephrine affects α_1-, α_2-, β_1-, and β_2-receptors. Isoproterenol affects both β_1- and β_2-receptors but not α-receptors.

  3. Indirect-acting adrenergic agonists work through other primary mechanisms, which ultimately lead to receptor effects. For example, tyramine acts by releasing norepinephrine from storage sites in adrenergic neurons, while cocaine blocks the reuptake of norepinephrine, thereby increasing the duration and activity of the transmitter at the synapse.

Table 13-4. Adrenoceptor-Mediated Responses to Adrenergic Agonists

Organ/Tissue	Receptor Type	Response
Heart	β_1 β_1 β_1	Increases conduction velocity (dromotropic) Increases contraction force (inotropic) Increases contraction rate (chronotropic)
Arterioles	α_1 α_1 α_1 β_2	Constricts cerebral arterioles Constricts cutaneous arterioles Constricts visceral arterioles Dilates skeletal muscle arterioles
Eye	α_1	Contracts iris sphincter muscle, producing mydriasis
Lung	β_2	Relaxes tracheal and bronchial muscles
Intestine	α, β α_1	Decreases peristalsis Contracts sphincters
Urinary bladder	α_1	Contracts trigone and sphincter muscles, inhibiting micturition
Uterus	β_1 α_1 β_2	Relaxes detrusor muscle Excites uterine contractions Inhibits uterine contractions
Adipose tissue	β_3	Causes adipolysis; mobilizes fatty acids

    4. Certain agonists (e.g., ephedrine, metaraminol, mephentermine) produce their effects through both direct and indirect mechanisms.

C. Therapeutic indications

    1. Epinephrine, an α- and β-adrenergic agonist, is indicated to treat bronchospasm and hypersensitivity reactions and is the agent of choice for anaphylactic reactions. It is also used to prolong the activity of local anesthetic solutions and to restore cardiac activity in cardiac arrest. Epinephrine is also used topically in the treatment of glaucoma, presumably decreasing intraocular pressure by enhancing the outflow of aqueous humor and through vasoconstriction-induced decrease in production of aqueous humor. Local application of epinephrine is used to arrest blood flow in epistaxis and gingival surgery.

    2. Phenylephrine, an α_1-selective agonist, is used to provide pressor activity in hypotensive emergencies, to prolong the activity of local anesthetic solutions, and to relieve paroxysmal atrial tachycardia. Phenylephrine or phenylpropanolamine is given systemically for nasal decongestion. Oxymetazoline and xylometazoline, also α_1-agonists, are applied locally to relieve nasal congestion.

    3. Clonidine and related α_2-selective agonists (e.g., methyldopa, guanfacine, guanabenz) are used as antihypertensives based on their inhibition of central sympathetic outflow. Apraclonidine is used topically to decrease intraocular pressure during surgery.

    4. Isoproterenol, a β-adrenergic agonist, is used as a bronchodilator and as a cardiac stimulant in shock and cardiac arrest.

    5. Dobutamine, a relatively β_1-selective agonist, is used to improve myocardial function in congestive heart failure in emergency situations.

    6. Terbutaline and other β_2-selective agonists (e.g., metaproterenol, albuterol, bitolterol, salmeterol) are used as systemic or local bronchodilators in the treatment of bronchospastic conditions such as asthma.

    7. The β_2-selective agonist ritodrine is used exclusively to relax uterine smooth muscle in the treatment of premature labor.

D. Adverse effects. Adrenergic agonists may cause cardiac dysrhythmias, cerebral hemorrhage, pulmonary hypertension and edema, anxiety, headache, and rebound nasal congestion.

IV. ADRENERGIC ANTAGONISTS

A. Chemistry

1. **α-Adrenergic antagonists** (α-blockers) have varied structures and bear little resemblance to the adrenergic agonists. Antagonists include the ergot alkaloids (e.g., ergotamine), the dibenzamines (e.g., phenoxybenzamine), the benzolines (e.g., tolazoline), and the quinazolines (e.g., prazosin) [Figure 13-4].

2. **β-Adrenergic antagonists** (β-blockers) are structurally similar to β-agonists (Figure 13-5). The **catechol ring** can be replaced by a variety of other ring systems without loss of antagonistic activity. The length of the side chain is important, and the side chain hydroxyl as well as a propyl or other bulky substitution on the chain nitrogen are essential for interaction with β-receptors.

B. Pharmacology

1. Adrenergic antagonists inhibit or block adrenergic receptor-mediated responses.

2. **α-Adrenergic antagonists** may be α_1-selective (e.g., prazosin) or nonselective (e.g., phenoxybenzamine). Phenoxybenzamine is an irreversible antagonist because it forms covalent bonds with α-receptors.

3. **β-Adrenergic antagonists** may be β_1-selective (e.g., metoprolol) or nonselective (e.g., propranolol). However, β_1-selective agents may lose their selectivity at higher doses and thus block β_2-receptors as well.

C. Therapeutic indications

1. **Prazosin** and related α_1-selective antagonists (e.g., doxazosin, terazosin, trimazosin, alfuzosin) produce vasodilation and are important antihypertensive agents. They are also useful in the symptomatic treatment of benign prostatic hyperplasia.

2. **Phenoxybenzamine** and **phentolamine** (nonselective α-blockers) can be used to relieve vasospasm in Raynaud's syndrome and for acute hypertensive emergencies resulting from pheochromocytoma or from intake of MAO inhibitors or sympathomimetics. Tolazoline, a similar agent, is used to treat persistent neonatal pulmonary hypertension.

3. **Labetalol,** an agent that possesses both selective α_1-blocking activity and nonselective β-blocking activity, is used in the treatment of hypertension.

4. **Propranolol,** a nonselective β-antagonist, is used for the prophylaxis of angina pectoris, supraventricular and ventricular dysrhythmias, and migraine headache. It is also used as an antihypertensive, a negative inotropic agent in hypertrophic obstructive cardiomyopathy, and a negative chronotropic agent in anxiety and hyperthyroidism.

5. β_1-Selective antagonists (e.g., metoprolol, betaxolol, atenolol, acebutolol) are used in the treatment of hypertension, tachyarrhythmias, and angina.

6. Both β_1-selective (betaxolol) and nonselective (timolol) blockers decrease ciliary body production of aqueous humor and may be used in the topical treatment of glaucoma.

D. Adverse effects

1. **Prazosin** can cause sudden syncope with the first dose, orthostatic hypotension, dizziness, headache, drowsiness, palpitations, fluid retention, and priapism.

2. **Phenoxybenzamine** can cause orthostatic hypotension, tachycardia, inhibition of ejaculation, miosis, and nasal congestion.

3. **Propranolol** can cause bradycardia and congestive heart failure, increased airway resistance, increased serum triglycerides, decreased high-density lipoprotein cholesterol, blood dyscrasias, psoriasis, depression, hallucinations, and transient hearing loss. Sudden withdrawal can be cardiotoxic.

4. **Metoprolol** has adverse effects similar to those of propranolol, except that it is less likely to increase airway resistance given its β_1-selectivity.

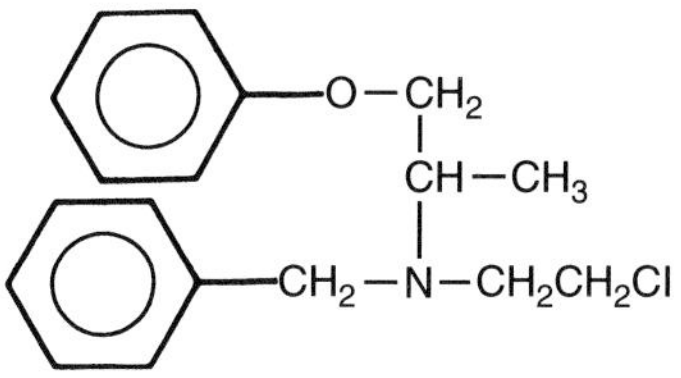

A

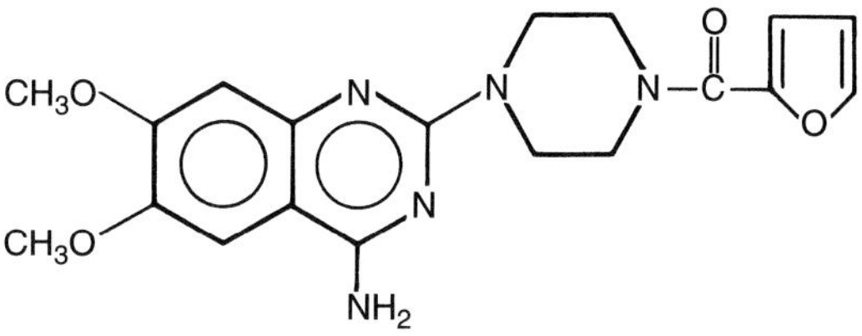

B

Figure 13-4. The structural formulas of (*A*) phenoxybenzamine (Dibenzyline) and (*B*) prazosin (Minipress), representative α-blockers.

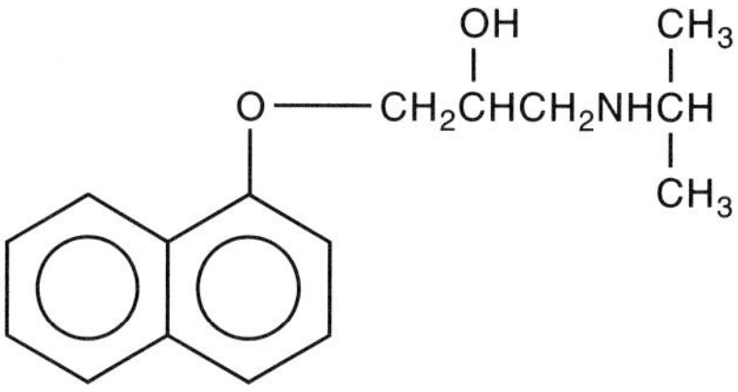

A

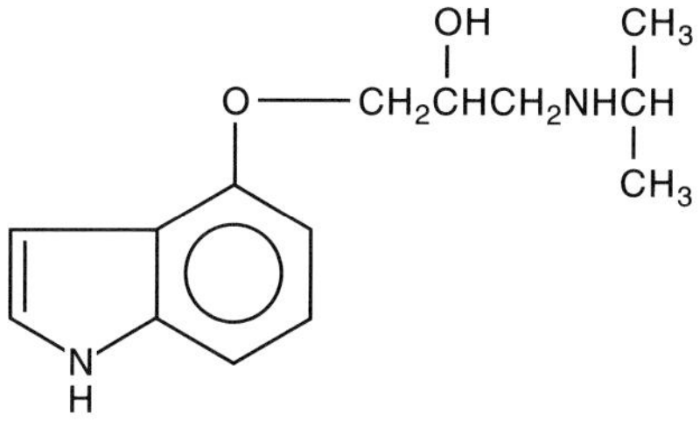

B

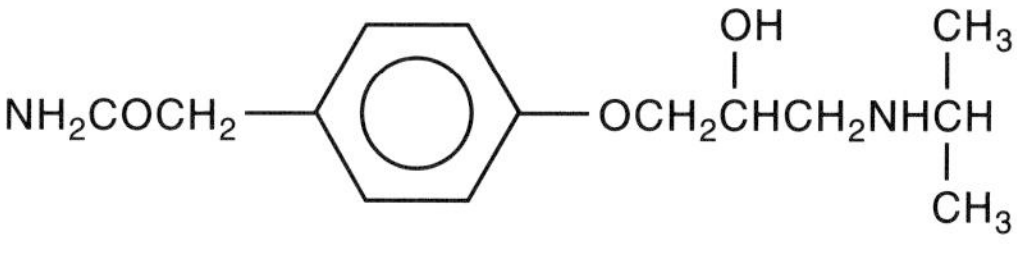

C

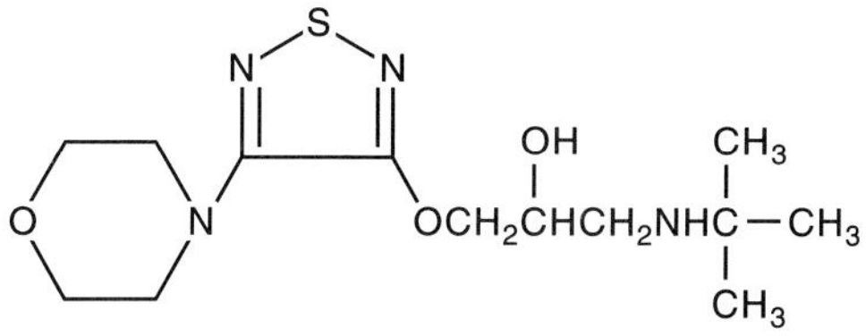

D

Figure 13-5. The structural formulas of (*A*) propranolol (Inderal); (*B*) pindolol (Visken); (*C*) atenolol (Tenormin), and (*D*) timolol (Blocadren), representative β-blockers.

V. CHOLINERGIC AGONISTS

A. Chemistry

1. **Acetylcholine,** the natural endogenous mediator and the most potent cholinergic agonist, is an ester of acetic acid and choline, a quaternary amino alcohol (Figure 13-6). Acetylcholine is unstable and quickly hydrolyzed both in vitro and in vivo. Thus, it is extremely short acting and usually is not a satisfactory therapeutic agent.

2. **Therapeutically useful cholinergic agonists** may be direct acting or indirect acting.
   a. **Direct-acting agonists** may be produced by replacing the acetyl group of acetylcholine with a carbamoyl group or by substituting a methyl group of the β-carbon. These substitutions produce compounds that are more resistant to acetylcholinesterase and thus have longer durations of action. Such stable agonists include methacholine (Provocholine) and bethanechol (Urecholine) [Figure 13-7].
   b. **Indirect-acting agonists** are generally acetylcholinesterase inhibitors and are divided into two major classes.
      (1) **Reversible (short-acting) agents** are principally carbamates (carbamic acid esters), such as physostigmine (Eserine) and neostigmine (Prostigmin) [Figure 13-8].
      (2) **Irreversible (long-acting) agents** are principally organophosphate esters, such as isoflurophate (Floropryl) and echothiophate (Phospholine) [Figure 13-9].

B. Pharmacology

1. **Cholinergic responses** are mediated by both muscarinic and nicotinic receptors (Table 13-5).
   a. **PNS muscarinic receptors** are present at parasympathetic postganglionic neuroeffector sites.
   b. **PNS nicotinic receptors** are present at the ganglia of both the parasympathetic and sympathetic nervous systems and also at the neuromuscular junctions of the somatic nervous system.

2. **Cholinergic agonists act by mimicking the activity of endogenous acetylcholine** at muscarinic and nicotinic receptor sites.
   a. **Direct-acting agonists** interact directly with these receptors.

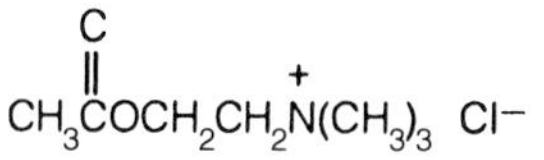

Figure 13-6. The structural formula of acetylcholine.

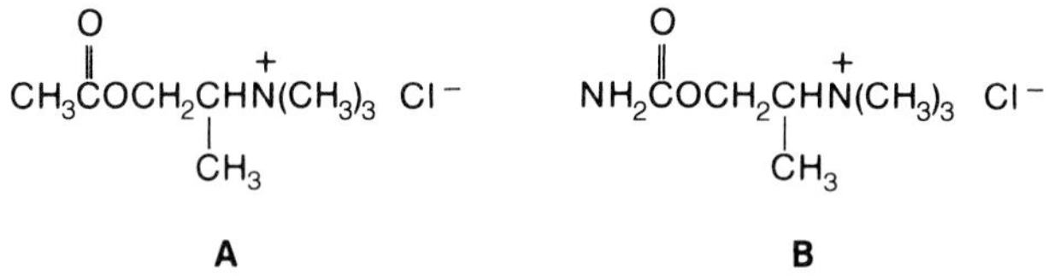

Figure 13-7. Clinically useful direct-acting cholinergic agonists include (*A*) methacholine chloride (Provocholine) and (*B*) bethanechol chloride (Urecholine).

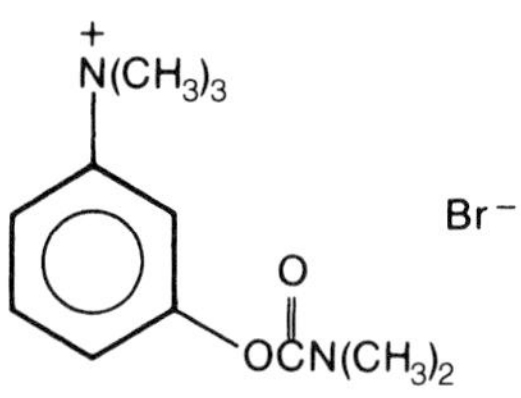

Figure 13-8. The structural formula of neostigmine bromide (Prostigmin), a reversible acetylcholinesterase inhibitor.

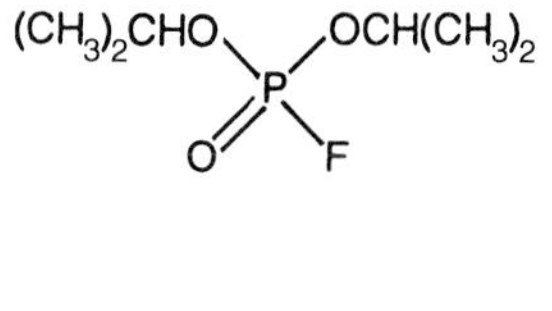

Figure 13-9. The structural formula of isoflurophate (Floropryl), an irreversible acetylcholinesterase inhibitor.

Table 13-5. Cholinoceptor-Mediated Responses to Cholinergic Agonists

Organ	Response
Heart	
Atrioventricular node	Decreased conduction velocity (negative dromotropy)
Atria, ventricles	Decreased contraction force (negative inotropy)
Sinoatrial node	Decreased contraction rate (negative chronotropy)
Eye	
Sphincter muscle	Contraction, producing miosis
Ciliary muscle	Contraction, accommodates for near vision
Lung	
Bronchial muscle	Contraction (bronchoconstriction)
Bronchial glands	Increased secretion
Gastrointestinal tract	
Intestine	Increased motility (peristalsis)
Sphincters	Relaxation of sphincters
Glands	Increased secretions
Urinary bladder	
Detrusor muscle	Contraction
Trigone and sphincter	Relaxation
Glands (sweat, salivary, nasopharyngeal, lacrimal)	Increased glandular secretion

    b. Indirect-acting agonists inhibit or block the activity of cholinesterase enzymes (e.g., acetylcholinesterase, butyrylcholinesterase), which metabolize endogenous acetylcholine to inactive metabolites. Thus, following physiological release of endogenous acetylcholine from nerve terminals, these agents allow the neurotransmitter to accumulate at cholinergic synapses, thereby enhancing cholinergic receptor stimulation. Organophosphate cholinesterase inhibitors, such as certain agricultural insecticides and the so-called nerve gases, can be extremely toxic as they bind to the enzyme to form an irreversible or long-lasting enzyme inhibitor complex.

C. Therapeutic indications

    1. Direct-acting agonists are indicated to:
      a. Initiate micturition in acute nonobstructive urinary retention (e.g., bethanechol)
      b. Produce miosis in the treatment of glaucoma (e.g., pilocarpine)

    2. Indirect-acting agonists are indicated to:
      a. Produce miosis in the treatment of glaucoma (e.g., physostigmine, isoflurophate, echothiophate)
      b. Aid in the differential diagnosis of myasthenia gravis (a disease caused by nicotinic receptor hypofunction at the neuromuscular junction) and hypercholinergic crisis (which produces depolarization blockade of the neuromuscular junction) [e.g., edrophonium]
      c. Treat myasthenia gravis (e.g., ambenonium, neostigmine, pyridostigmine)
      d. Counteract intoxication or adverse effects from compounds with anticholinergic activity (e.g., physostigmine)

D. Adverse effects

    1. Topical adverse effects include congested conjunctivae, myopic accommodation, and transient lenticular opacity.

    2. Systemic adverse effects include headache, syncope, nausea, vomiting, bradycardia, hypotension, bronchospasm, abdominal cramps, diarrhea, epigastric distress, salivation, sweating, lacrimation, flushing, and tremors.

VI. CHOLINERGIC ANTAGONISTS block the actions of acetylcholine at muscarinic or nicotinic cholinoceptors.

A. Chemistry

1. **Atropine,** an alkaloid obtained from the belladonna plant, is the prototypical cholinergic antagonist (anticholinergic agent). A portion of the atropine molecule is structurally similar to acetylcholine (Figure 13-10), permitting the molecule to bind to postganglionic receptors. However, the molecule has no intrinsic activity, and its bulky shape prevents acetylcholine from binding to the receptor.

2. **Synthetic anticholinergic agents** [e.g., dicyclomine (Bentyl), glycopyrrolate (Robinul), propantheline (Pro-Banthine)] are also available. These agents, like atropine, are bulky analogues of acetylcholine (Figure 13-11).

3. An important factor that determines the pharmacological spectrum of anticholinergic agents is the presence of a **quaternary nitrogen** (as in propantheline, glycopyrrolate, and ipratropium), which reduces passage across the blood–brain barrier, or a **tertiary nitrogen** (as in dicyclomine, pirenzepine, tropicamide, and benztropine), which permits a broader volume of distribution.

B. Pharmacology

1. Cholinergic antagonists **competitively inhibit** the activity of endogenous acetylcholine.

2. Antagonists that inhibit muscarinic receptor-mediated responses are called **antimuscarinic agents;** those that inhibit nicotinic receptor-mediated responses at the ganglia are called **ganglionic-blocking agents,** whereas those that inhibit nicotinic receptor-mediated responses at the neuromuscular junction are called **neuromuscular blockers.**

C. Therapeutic indications

1. **Antimuscarinic agents** are indicated to:
   a. Reduce glandular and bronchiolar secretions before anesthesia (e.g., atropine, glycopyrrolate)
   b. Induce sedation (e.g., scopolamine)
   c. Alleviate motion sickness (e.g., scopolamine)
   d. Reduce vagal stimulation of the myocardium (e.g., atropine)
   e. Produce ophthalmic mydriasis and cycloplegia (e.g., homatropine)
   f. Reduce GI smooth-muscle spasms (e.g., propantheline)
   g. Treat bronchospasm associated with chronic obstructive pulmonary disease (e.g., ipratropium)
   h. Control Parkinson's disease and some neuroleptic-induced extrapyramidal disorders (e.g., benztropine, trihexyphenidyl)
   i. Treat intoxication by cholinergic agonists or by acute mushroom poisoning (e.g., atropine)

2. **Ganglionic-blocking agents** are indicated to treat hypertensive crisis (e.g., trimethaphan, mecamylamine). By blocking ganglionic transmission, these agents reduce sympathetic activity, resulting in a hypotensive effect.

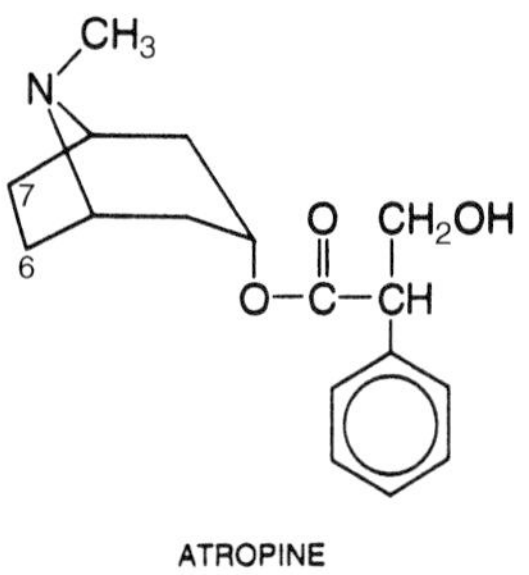

Figure 13-10. Structural formula of atropine, a cholinergic antagonist.

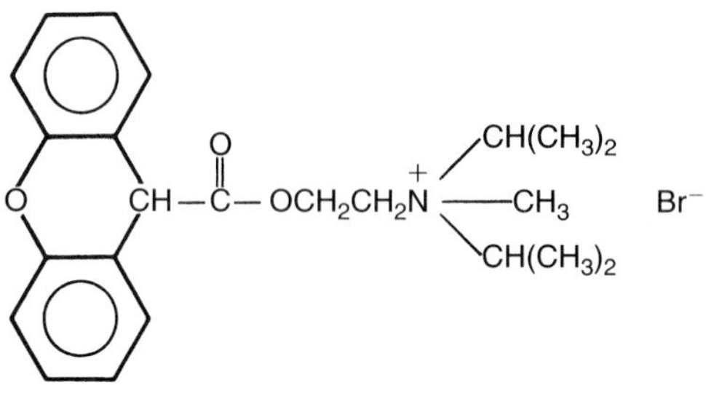

Figure 13-11. Structural formula of propantheline bromide (Pro-Banthine), a synthetic cholinergic antagonist.

D. Adverse effects

1. **Topical adverse effects** include hyperopic accommodation and increased intraocular pressure.

2. **Systemic adverse effects** include headache, nervousness, drowsiness, dizziness, palpitations, tachycardia, dry mouth, mydriasis, blurred vision, nausea, vomiting, constipation, urinary retention, and fever.

VII. NEUROMUSCULAR BLOCKING AGENTS

A. Chemistry

1. **Neuromuscular blocking agents** can be competitive (as with the prototypical curare alkaloids) or depolarizing (as with succinylcholine). They act by blocking the effects of acetylcholine at the nerve–muscle junction of skeletal muscles.

2. The **competitive nondepolarizing agents** include the naturally occurring alkaloids of **curare,** which are bulky and rigid molecules, as well as several synthetic analogues.
   a. The **principal active alkaloid** in curare is tubocurarine (Figure 13-12). A closely related trimethylate derivative is metocurine (Metubine). Their most important structural feature is the presence of a tertiary-quaternary amine in which the distance between the two cations is rigidly fixed at about 14 Å, twice the length of the critical receptor-binding moiety of acetylcholine.
   b. A number of **potent synthetic analogues** have been developed. These include the structurally similar **isoquinolines** atracurium (Tracrium), doxacurium (Nuromax), and mivacurium (Mivacron), as well as the **steroid derivatives** pancuronium (Pavulon), vecuronium (Norcuron), and pipecuronium (Arduan).

3. The **noncompetitive depolarizing agents** include succinylcholine (Anectine) and gallamine (Flaxedil) [Figure 13-13].
   a. Unlike the large, bulky competitive agents, noncompetitive agents are slender aliphatic molecules.
   b. **Succinylcholine** has a short duration of action compared with the other neuromuscular blocking agents. This results from its simple ester functional group, which is rapidly hydrolyzed by plasma and liver pseudocholinesterase (butyrylcholinesterase). Its action may be prolonged, however, in patients with an abnormal genetic variant of pseudocholinesterase, which has only about 20% the activity of normal pseudocholinesterase.

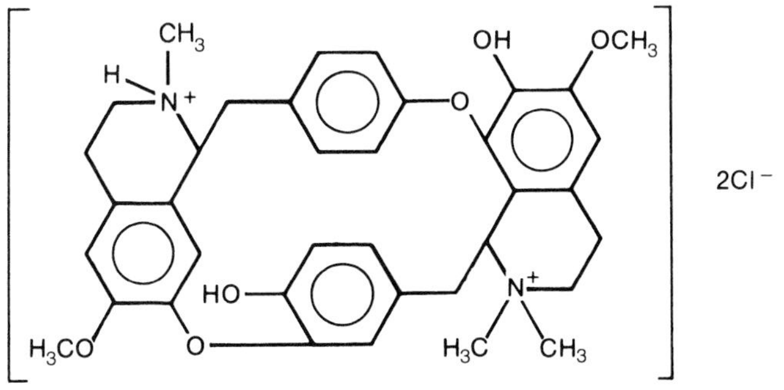

Figure 13-12. Structural formula of tubocurarine chloride (Tubarine), a competitive nondepolarizing agent.

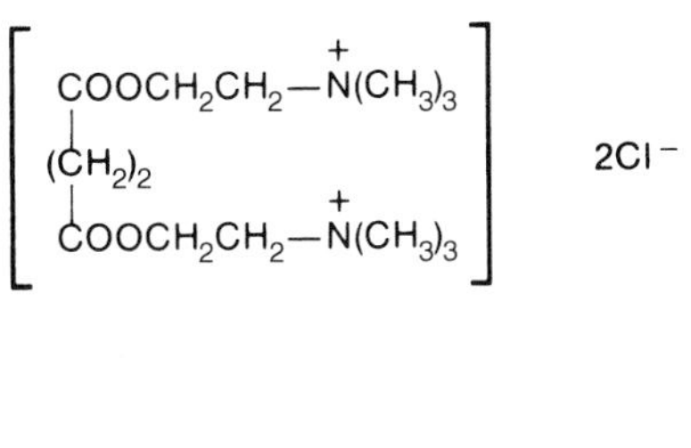

Figure 13-13. Structural formula of succinylcholine chloride, a noncompetitive depolarizing agent.

B. Pharmacology

1. The **competitive nondepolarizing agents** compete with acetylcholine for nicotinic receptors at the neuromuscular junction. These agents decrease the end-plate potential so that the depolarization threshold is not reached. Competitive nondepolarizing agents produce a surmountable blockade of neuromuscular transmission in that administration of cholinesterase inhibitors or prejunctional release of a large quantity of acetylcholine can relieve the blockade.

2. The **noncompetitive depolarizing agents** desensitize the nicotinic receptors at the neuromuscular junction. These agents react with the nicotinic receptors, decreasing receptor sensitivity in a manner similar to that of excess released acetylcholine. They depolarize the excitable membrane for a prolonged period (2–3 minutes); the membrane then becomes unresponsive (desensitized).

C. Therapeutic indications. Neuromuscular blocking agents, which cause only skeletal muscle paralysis (the patient remains conscious and capable of sensation), are used to:

1. Promote skeletal muscle relaxation and facilitate endotracheal intubation, as an adjunct to surgical anesthesia

2. Limit trauma associated with skeletal muscle contraction during electroconvulsive shock therapy

3. Relax the skeletal muscles and facilitate bone placement and manipulations during orthopedic procedures

D. Adverse effects

1. **Competitive nondepolarizing agents** can cause respiratory paralysis, histamine release, bronchospasm, and hypotension (e.g., tubocurarine) or respiratory paralysis, tachycardia, and hypertension (e.g., pancuronium).

2. **Noncompetitive depolarizing agents** (e.g., succinylcholine, gallamine) can cause respiratory paralysis, muscle fasciculation with pain, extraocular muscle contraction with increased intraocular pressure, and increased intragastric pressure. In addition, succinylcholine may cause muscarinic responses such as bradycardia, increased glandular secretions, and cardiac arrest. In combination with the anesthetic halothane, succinylcholine may cause malignant hyperthermia in genetically predisposed individuals.

VIII. GENERAL ANESTHETICS induce a combined state of analgesia, amnesia, loss of consciousness, inhibition of sensory and autonomic reflexes, and skeletal muscle relaxation. Ideal general anesthetics induce anesthesia rapidly and smoothly, and permit rapid recovery of the patient once administration of the agent ceases.

A. Chemistry

1. **Volatile or inhalation anesthetics** are drugs inhaled as gases or vapors. These diverse drugs are relatively simple lipophilic molecules. They include the inorganic agent nitrous oxide (N_2O) and the **nonflammable** halogenated hydrocarbons (e.g., halothane) and ethers (e.g., methoxyflurane, isoflurane, desflurane, sevoflurane).

2. **Nonvolatile or intravenous anesthetics** are administered intravenously or occasionally intramuscularly and come as aqueous solutions, aqueous propylene glycol solutions, or emulsions.
   a. The **water-soluble** and relatively short-acting agents include ultra–short-acting barbiturates (e.g., thiopental, methohexital, thiamylal), cyclohexylamines (e.g., ketamine), benzo-diazepines (e.g., diazepam, midazolam), butyrophenones (e.g., droperidol), and opioid analgesics (e.g., morphine, fentanyl).
   b. The imidazole, etomidate, is prepared as an **aqueous propylene glycol solution,** which is compatible with many preanesthetics.
   c. The dialkylphenol, propofol, is administered as an **emulsion,** which should not be mixed with other therapeutic agents before administration (Figure 13-14).

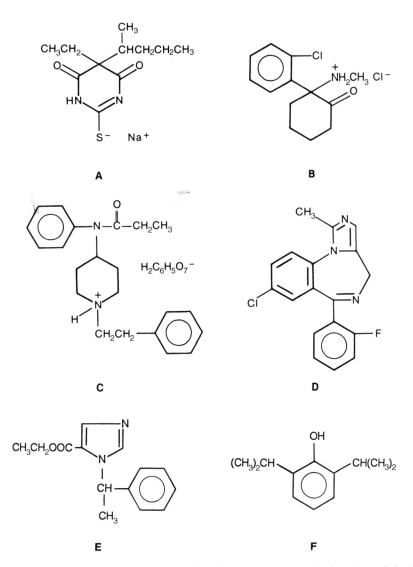

Figure 13-14. Structural formulas of nonvolatile general anesthetics: (*A*) thiopental sodium (Pentothal), (*B*) ketamine hydrochloride (Ketaject), (*C*) fentanyl citrate (Sublimaze), (*D*) midazolam (Versed), (*E*) etomidate (Amidate), and (*F*) propofol (Diprivan).

B. Pharmacology

1. **General anesthetics** depress the CNS, producing a reversible loss of consciousness and loss of all forms of sensation.

2. **Inhalational anesthetics** are absorbed and primarily excreted through the lungs. Frequently, these drugs are supplemented with analgesics, a skeletal muscle relaxant, and an antimuscarinic agent.
   a. Analgesics permit a reduction in the required concentration of inhalational anesthetic.
   b. Skeletal muscle relaxants cause adequate muscle relaxation during surgery.
   c. Antimuscarinic agents decrease bronchiolar secretions.

3. **Nonvolatile anesthetics** are usually administered intravenously (e.g., thiobarbiturates, benzodiazepines), but some agents may also be given intramuscularly (e.g., ketamine).

C. Therapeutic indications

1. **Inhalational anesthetics** are indicated to provide general surgical anesthesia.

2. **Nonvolatile anesthetics** are indicated to induce drowsiness and provide relaxation before the induction of inhalational general anesthesia (e.g., thiopental, diazepam, midazolam).

3. Use of some previously popular volatile anesthetics has been discontinued because of serious toxicity (e.g., chloroform) or because of the flammable and explosive properties of the compounds (e.g., cyclopropane, diethylether).

D. Adverse effects.
General anesthetics depress respiration, circulation, and the CNS. They can also decrease hepatic and kidney function (e.g., methoxyflurane) and cause cardiac dysrhythmias as a result of increased myocardial sensitivity to catecholamines (e.g., halothane).

IX. LOCAL ANESTHETICS

A. Chemistry.
Most local anesthetics are structurally similar to the alkaloid cocaine (Figure 13-15). These drugs consist of a hydrophilic amino group linked through an ester or amide connecting group to a lipophilic aromatic moiety. A few phenols and aromatic alcohols also have local anesthetic activity.

1. **Ester-type agents** are generally short acting due to rapid hydrolysis by plasma esterases. These agents include cocaine, procaine, chloroprocaine, benzocaine, butamben, and tetracaine.

2. **Amide-type agents** are generally longer acting and are metabolized in the liver. Examples of the amide-type local anesthetics include lidocaine, dibucaine, prilocaine, mepivacaine, bupivacaine, and etidocaine.

3. The drug's pK_a influences its chemical state, which in turn determines the anesthetic effectiveness of the compounds. The site of anesthetic action is at the inner surface of the cell membrane. At tissue pH, the drug in the form of a lipophilic, uncharged, secondary or tertiary amine diffuses across connective tissue and cell membranes and enters nerve cells, where it is ionized to a charged ammonium cation. The cationic form of the drug is the active form of the drug that blocks the generation of action potentials at the membrane receptor complex. Also, because of its charged ammonium cation, the ionized molecule poorly penetrates the cell membranes and remains trapped within the cell, thereby enhancing its duration of action.

B. Pharmacology

1. Local anesthetics **reversibly block nerve impulse conduction** and **produce reversible loss of sensation** at their administration site. They do not produce a loss of consciousness.

    a. Small, nonmyelinated nerve fibers, which conduct pain and temperature sensations, are affected first.

    b. Local anesthetics appear to become entrapped within the nerve membrane or to bind to specific membrane sodium ion (Na^+) channels, restricting Na^+ permeability in response to partial depolarization.

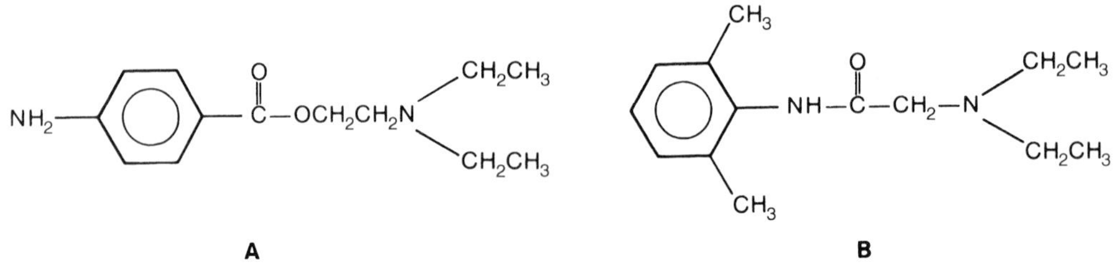

A **B**

Figure 13-15. Structural formulas of local anesthetics structurally similar to cocaine: (*A*) procaine (Novocaine) and (*B*) lidocaine (Xylocaine).

2. Local anesthetic solutions frequently contain the vasoconstrictor **epinephrine,** which reduces vascular blood flow at the administration site. This reduces systemic absorption, and hence prolongs the duration of action and reduces systemic toxicity.

C. **Therapeutic indications.** Local anesthetics are indicated to:

1. Produce regional nerve block for the relief of pain when injected close to the innervating nerve

2. Provide anesthesia for minor operations when infiltrated around the tissue site

3. Provide anesthesia for surgery of the lower limbs and pelvis and for obstetric surgery when injected into the epidural space or the subarachnoid space of the spinal cord

4. Provide anesthesia of the skin and mucous membranes when applied locally. This includes two miscellaneous local anesthetics: **dyclonine,** used primarily in throat lozenges and sprays, and **pramoxine,** used primarily in antihemorrhoidal preparations.

D. **Adverse effects**

1. Ester-type local anesthetics can cause hypersensitivity reactions in susceptible individuals.

2. Systemic absorption of toxic concentrations of local anesthetics can cause seizures; CNS, respiratory, and myocardial depression; and circulatory collapse.

X. **ANTIPSYCHOTICS.** The classic antipsychotic agents are the phenothiazines, thioxanthenes, and butyrophenones. Chemical classes of newer compounds having antipsychotic activity include the dihydroindolones (e.g., molindone), dibenzoxazepines (e.g., loxapine), dibenzodiazepines (e.g., clozapine), diphenylbutylpiperidines (e.g., pimozide), and benzisoxazoles (e.g., risperidone).

A. **Chemistry**

1. **Phenothiazines** (e.g., chlorpromazine, triflupromazine, thioridazine, prochlorperazine, trifluoperazine, fluphenazine) must have a **nitrogen-containing side-chain substituent** on the ring nitrogen for antipsychotic activity (Table 13-6). The ring and side-chain nitrogens must be separated by a three-carbon chain; phenothiazines in which the ring and side-chain nitrogens are separated by a two-carbon chain have only antihistaminic or sedative activity.
   a. The side chains are either aliphatic, piperazine, or piperidine derivatives. Piperazine side chains confer the greatest potency and the highest pharmacological selectivity.
   b. Fluphenazine and long-chain alcohols form stable, **highly lipophilic esters** (e.g., enanthate, decanoate), which possess markedly prolonged activity.

2. **Thioxanthenes** (e.g., chlorprothixene, thiothixene) lack the ring nitrogen of phenothiazines and have a side chain attached by a double bond (Figure 13-16).

3. **Butyrophenones** (e.g., haloperidol) are chemically unrelated to phenothiazines but have similar activity (Figure 13-17).

4. Newer agents derive from diverse chemical classes and include clozapine, olanzapine, loxapine, pimozide, molindone, quetiapine, risperidone, sertindole, and remoxipride.

B. **Pharmacology**

1. These agents have **similar** pharmacodynamic effects in the treatment of psychotic illness. Their antipsychotic action (i.e., improvement of mood and behavior) results primarily from their blockade of dopamine receptors in cortical and limbic areas of the brain, whereas their adverse extrapyramidal effects such as parkinsonian reactions result from antagonism of dopamine receptors in the basal ganglia.

2. Other effects vary among the classes of antipsychotics. These include antiemetic activity and blockade of muscarinic, serotonergic, α_1-adrenergic, and H_1-histaminergic receptors.

3. The atypical antipsychotics (e.g., clozapine) are newer agents that show strong antagonistic properties at serotonin receptors in addition to their blockade of dopamine receptors. Compared to the phenothiazines, butyrophenones, and other classic antipsychotic drugs, the atypical agents are effective in ameliorating a wider range of symptoms, including negative symptoms, and they also are less likely to induce extrapyramidal side effects.

Table 13-6. Antipsychotic Phenothiazines

General Phenothiazine Structure*

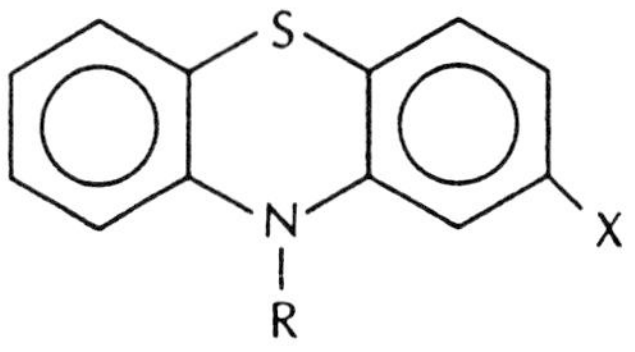

Drug	X-Substituent	R-Substituent*
Chlorpromazine (Thorazine)	—Cl	—(CH$_2$)$_3$—N(CH$_3$)$_2$
Triflupromazine (Vesprin)	—CF$_3$	—(CH$_2$)$_3$—N(CH$_3$)$_2$
Thioridazine (Mellaril)	—SCH$_3$	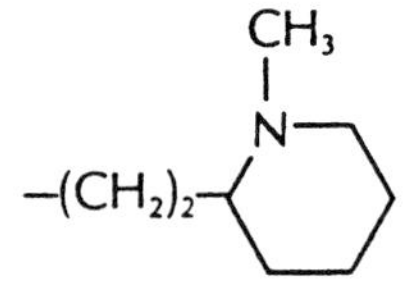 —(CH$_2$)$_2$— (piperidine ring with N—CH$_3$)
Prochlorperazine (Compazine)	—Cl	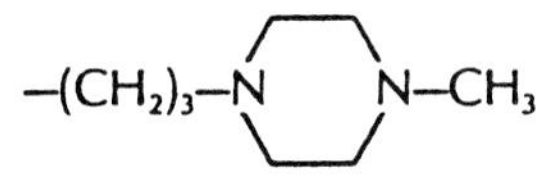 —(CH$_2$)$_3$—N(piperazine)N—CH$_3$
Trifluoperazine (Stelazine)	—CF$_3$	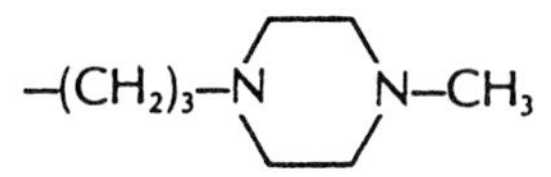 —(CH$_2$)$_3$—N(piperazine)N—CH$_3$
Fluphenazine (Prolixin)	—CF$_3$	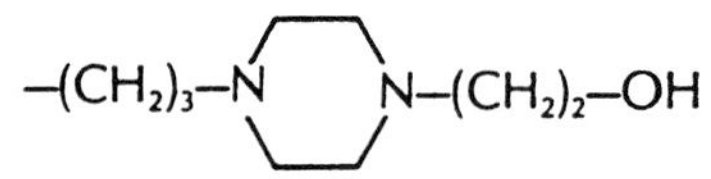 —(CH$_2$)$_3$—N(piperazine)N—(CH$_2$)$_2$—OH

*Antipsychotic phenothiazines have the general structure illustrated in the table. Substituents at positions marked X and R result in different drugs.

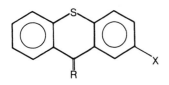

Figure 13-16. Thioxanthenes, similar to phenothiazines, have substituents at X and R positions that alter drug activity. Chlorprothixene (Taractan) has a —Cl substituent at X and CH—(CH$_2$)$_2$—N(CH$_3$)$_2$ at R. Thiothixene (Navane) has a —SO$_2$N(CH$_3$)$_2$ substituent at X and the group:

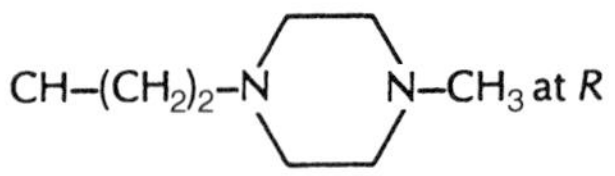

$$CH-(CH_2)_2-N(\text{piperazine})N-CH_3 \text{ at } R$$

C. Therapeutic indications. Antipsychotics are indicated primarily for the treatment of psychosis associated with schizophrenia (e.g., haloperidol, clozapine), paranoia, and Tourette's syndrome (e.g., pimozide).

D. Adverse effects

1. **Centrally mediated adverse effects** include drowsiness; extrapyramidal symptoms such as akathisia, acute dystonia, akinesia, and tardive dyskinesia; alteration of temperature-regulating mechanisms including poikilothermy; increased appetite and weight gain; and al-

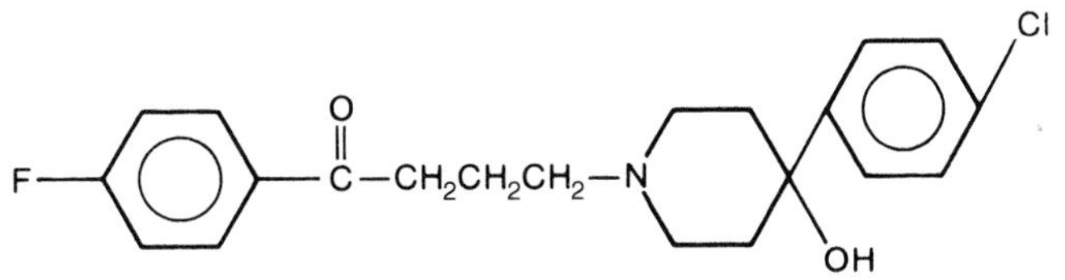

Figure 13-17. Structural formula of haloperidol (Haldol), a butyrophenone antipsychotic.

terations in hypothalamic and endocrine function, such as increased release of corticotropin, gonadotropins, prolactin, growth hormone, and melanocyte-stimulating hormone.

2. **Peripheral adverse effects** include postural hypotension and reflex tachycardia; hepatotoxicity and jaundice; failure of ejaculation; bone marrow depression; photosensitivity; xerostomia; and blurred vision.

XI. **ANTIDEPRESSANT AND ANTIMANIC AGENTS** are classified into four structurally and mechanistically unrelated groups: the monoamine oxidase (MAO) inhibitors, tricyclic antidepressants, atypical antidepressants, and antimanic antidepressants (or mood stabilizers).

A. **Chemistry**
1. **MAO inhibitors** may be weakly potent **hydralazines** [e.g., phenelzine isocarboxazid (Marplan)] or extremely potent **phenylcyclopropylamines** (i.e., ring-closed amphetamine derivatives, such as tranylcypromine) [Figure 13-18].
2. **Tricyclic** antidepressants, which are used commonly, are secondary or tertiary amine derivatives of molecules that have a fused three-ring system.
   a. The principal tricyclic antidepressants are derivatives of dibenzazepine (e.g., imipramine, desipramine, clomipramine, trimipramine) and dibenzocycloheptadiene (e.g., amitriptyline, nortriptyline, protriptyline) [Figures 13-19 and 13-20].
   b. Other closely related tricyclic antidepressants include doxepin, a dibenzoxepine, and amoxapine, a dibenzoxazepine.
   c. A closely related **tetracyclic** agent is maprotiline (Ludiomil).

A

B

Figure 13-18. Structural formulas of (*A*) phenelzine (Nardil), a hydralazine derivative monoamine oxidase (MAO) inhibitor, and (*B*) tranylcypromine (Parnate), a cyclopropylamine derivative MAO inhibitor.

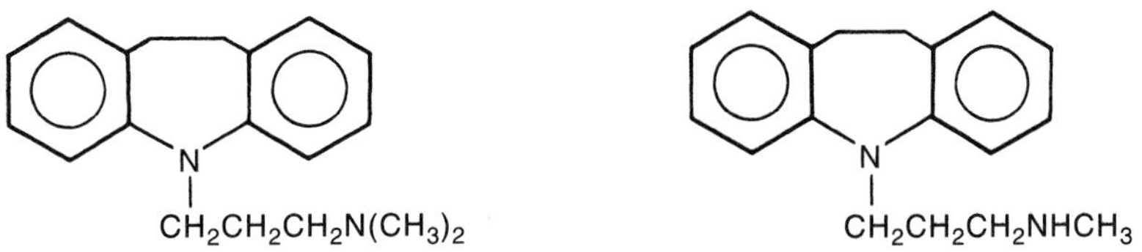

A

B

Figure 13-19. Structural formulas of tricyclic antidepressants derived from dibenzazepine: (*A*) imipramine (Tofranil) and (*B*) desipramine (Norpramin).

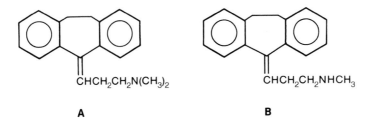

Figure 13-20. Structural formulas of tricyclic antidepressants derived from dibenzocycloheptadiene: (*A*) amitriptyline (Elavil) and (*B*) nortriptyline (Aventyl).

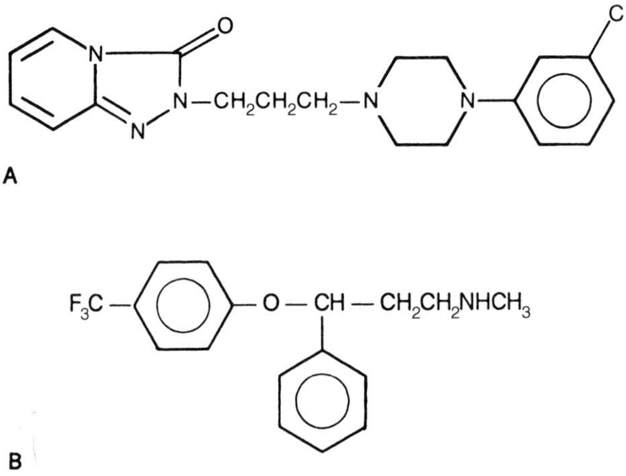

Figure 13-21. Structural formulas of (*A*) trazodone (Desyrel) and (*B*) fluoxetine (Prozac), atypical antidepressants.

3. **Atypical** antidepressants have varied structures ranging from the aminopropiophenone bupropion to the complex heterocyclics trazodone and nefazodone, and the chemically unrelated serotonin reuptake inhibitors fluoxetine, paroxetine, sertraline, fluvoxamine, and venlafaxine (Figure 13-21).

4. **Lithium** is an element that is used in the form of the carbonate salt in the treatment of manic depression or bipolar disease. Other agents in this therapeutic category include the organic compounds **valproic acid** and **carbamazepine.**

B. **Pharmacology**

1. **MAO inhibitors** appear to produce their antidepressant effects by blocking the intraneuronal oxidative deamination of brain biogenic amines (e.g., norepinephrine, serotonin). This action increases the availability of biogenic amines at central aminergic receptors. Other biochemical events (e.g., the down-regulation of central β-adrenergic and serotonergic receptors) that result from chronic inhibition of MAO and reuptake blockade can also explain the therapeutic action of antidepressants. This explanation is suggested by the latency period of MAO inhibitors, which take 2–4 weeks to become effective.

2. **Tricyclic** antidepressants appear to act principally by reducing CNS neuronal reuptake of biogenic amines (e.g., norepinephrine, serotonin). This prolongs the synaptic availability of biogenic amines and hence their action at central aminergic receptors.

3. **Atypical** antidepressants have varying effects on reuptake of biogenic amines. The selective serotonin reuptake inhibitors (SSRIs) selectively inhibit serotonin reuptake into the nerve terminal, thus prolonging the synaptic activity of the amine. Trazodone and other heterocyclics also inhibit amine transmitter reuptake. Bupropion has been approved for clinical use, but its mechanism of action remains unclear.

4. **Lithium** appears to interfere with transmembrane Na$^+$ exchange, alters the release of aminergic neurotransmitters, and blocks inositol metabolism, ultimately leading to depletion of cellular inositol and inhibition of phospholipase C-mediated signal transduction. The relevance of these actions to the mood-stabilizing effects of lithium, however, has not been established.

C. Therapeutic indications

1. **MAO inhibitors** are indicated to treat depression, phobic anxiety, and narcolepsy that has not responded to other treatments. However, their use is limited by their adverse effects (see XI D 1).

2. **Tricyclic and atypical** antidepressants are the agents of choice for endogenous depression. Additionally, imipramine is used to treat enuresis; clomipramine, fluoxetine, and fluvoxamine are used in obsessive-compulsive disorder; and doxepin, for anxiety.

3. **Lithium and valproic acid** are indicated for the treatment of manic-depression (or bipolar disease). The antiepileptic drug, carbamazepine, has also been used as a mood-stabilizer in bipolar illness.

D. Adverse effects

1. **MAO inhibitors** interact with sympathomimetic drugs and with foods that have a high tyramine concentration, such as cheese, wine, and sausage. Hypertensive crises can result. In addition, MAO inhibitors can cause a wide range of adverse effects, including:
   a. CNS effects, such as CNS stimulation, tremors, agitation, overactivity, hyperreflexia, mania, and insomnia followed by weakness, fatigue, and drowsiness
   b. Cardiovascular effects, such as postural hypotension
   c. GI effects, such as nausea, abdominal pain, and constipation
   d. Antimuscarinic effects, such as dry mouth, urinary retention, and constipation

2. **Tricyclic** antidepressants can cause adverse effects, including:
   a. CNS effects, such as drowsiness, dizziness, weakness, fatigue, and confusion
   b. Cardiovascular effects, such as orthostatic hypotension, tachycardia, and interference with atrioventricular conduction
   c. Antimuscarinic effects, such as dry mouth, urinary retention, and constipation
   d. GI effects, such as nausea, vomiting, diarrhea, and anorexia
   e. Bone marrow depression
   f. Mania (in patients with manic-depressive illness)

3. **Atypical** antidepressants can cause adverse effects, including:
   a. CNS effects, such as dizziness, nightmares, confusion, drowsiness, fatigue, headache, insomnia, impaired memory, akathisia, numbness, and tonic-clonic seizures
   b. Cardiovascular effects, such as hypertension, hypotension, tachycardia, chest pain, and syncope
   c. GI effects, such as nausea, vomiting, diarrhea, and constipation
   d. Blurred vision and tinnitus
   e. Antimuscarinic effects, such as urinary retention, dry mouth, and constipation
   f. Bone marrow depression
   g. Sexual dysfunction and menstrual irregularities

4. **Lithium** therapy may be associated with development of fine hand tremors and increased urination; these side effects, however, usually diminish with continued therapy.

XII. ANXIOLYTICS AND SEDATIVE–HYPNOTICS.
Antianxiety and sedative–hypnotic agents in current use comprise the highly effective benzodiazepines (e.g., alprazolam, diazepam, flurazepam) and the atypical azaspirodecanediones (e.g., buspirone) and imidazopyridines (e.g., zolpidem). Diverse classes of agents previously used as anxiolytics and sedative–hypnotics (e.g., barbiturates, meprobamate, and hydroxyzine) are no longer favored because of their liability to produce tolerance, physical dependence, severe withdrawal reactions, and serious toxicity with overdosage.

A. Chemistry

1. **Benzodiazepines** (e.g., alprazolam, chlordiazepoxide, clorazepate, diazepam, halazepam, lorazepam, oxazepam, prazepam) have varying durations of action, which can be correlated with their structures in some cases (Table 13-7).
   a. Agents with a 3-hydroxyl group are easily metabolized by phase II glucuronidation and are short acting (see R3-substituent column in Table 13-7).
   b. Agents lacking a 3-hydroxyl group must undergo considerable phase I metabolism, including 3-hydroxylation. These agents are long acting. Most long-acting agents form the intermediate metabolite desmethyldiazepam, which has a very long half-life. Thus, these agents can have a cumulative action.

Table 13-7. Benzodiazepine Anxiolytics and Sedative–Hypnotics

General Benzodiazepine Structure*

Drug	R_1	R_2	R_3	X (R_2)	Comments
Diazepam (Valium)	$-CH3$	$=O$	$-H$	$-H$	
Chlordiazepoxide (Librium)	$=$ (Ring double bond)	$-NH-CH_3$	$-H$	$-H$	$-O$ (N-oxide) at position 4
Halazepam (Paxipam)	$-CH_2CF_3$	$=O$	$-H$	$-H$	
Clorazepate (Tranxene)	$-H$	$=OH$ ($-OK$)	$-COOH$ ($-COOK$)	$-H$	
Oxazepam (Serax)	$-H$	$=O$	$-OH$	$-H$	
Lorazepam (Ativan)	$-H$	$=O$	$-OH$	$-Cl$	
Alprazolam (Xanax)	R1-C(CH_3)=N-N=R2 (Fused R1-R2 triazolo ring)		$-H$	$-H$	
Flurazepam (Dalmane)	$CH_2CH_2N(C_2H_5)_2$	$=O$	$-H$	$-F$	
Quazepam (Doral)	$-CH_2CF_3$	$=S$	$-H$	F	
Triazolam (Halcion)	R1-C(CH_3)=N-N=R2 (Fused R1-R2 triazolo ring)		$-H$	$-H$	
Temazepam (Restoril)	$-CH_3$	$=O$	$-OH$	H	

*Benzodiazepine anxiolytics and sedative–hypnotics have the general structure illustrated in the table. Substituents at the positions marked R_1, R_2, R_3, R_7, and X (R_2') and the ring nitrogen at the position 2 result in different drugs and clinical properties. Clonazepam, not shown, has an NO_2 substituent at R7 and is used primarily as an anticonvulsant.

   c. Triazolobenzodiazepines (e.g., alprazolam) undergo a different pattern of metabolism and are intermediate in activity.
   d. Agents lacking an amino side chain are not basic enough to form water-soluble salts with acids. For example, intravenous solutions of diazepam contain propylene glycol as a solvent. Precipitation can occur if these solutions are mixed with aqueous solutions.

2. Azaspirodecanediones or azapirones (e.g., buspirone, gepirone, ipsapirone, tiaspirone) are chemically unrelated to the benzodiazepines. Represented by buspirone, these agents have anxiolytic activity resembling that of the benzodiazepines. Unlike the benzodiazepines, buspirone lacks CNS depressant activity and is considered an atypical anxiolytic (Figure 13-22).

3. The **imidazopyridine** zolpidem is a nonbenzodiazepine sedative–hypnotic with actions generally resembling those of the benzodiazepines.

4. Barbiturates are 5,5-disubstituted derivatives of barbituric acid, a saturated triketopyramidine (Table 13-8).
   a. Two side chains in position 5 are essential for sedative–hypnotic activity.
   b. Long-acting agents have a phenyl and an ethyl group in position 5.
   c. Branched side chains, unsaturated side chains, or side chains longer than an ethyl group increase lipophilicity and metabolism rate. Increased lipophilicity leads to a shorter onset of action, a shorter duration of action, and increased potency.
   d. Replacement of the position 2 oxygen with sulfur produces an extremely lipophilic molecule that distributes rapidly into lipid tissues outside the brain.
      (1) These ultra–short-acting barbiturates are not useful as sedative–hypnotics but are effective in facilitating the induction of anesthesia (see XII C 4). The action of these drugs is terminated very quickly.
      (2) The prototype ultra–short-acting barbiturate is thiopental (Pentothal), the 2-thio isostere of pentobarbital.
   e. The barbiturates and many of their metabolites are weak acids, and changes in urinary pH greatly influence their excretion. This is particularly true with overdoses, when a relatively large amount of unchanged drug appears in the glomerular filtrate.
   f. Phenobarbital is one of the most powerful and versatile agents that can induce certain enzyme systems (e.g., the cytochrome P-450 metabolic system). This increases the potential for drug interactions and includes interaction with any drug metabolized by this system. Other barbiturates have less enzyme-inducing effect, except when they are used continuously in higher-than-normal doses.

5. Piperidinediones (e.g., glutethimide, methyprylon) and **aldehydes** (e.g., paraldehyde, chloral hydrate) differ structurally (Figure 13-23) and are used less commonly than the benzodiazepines as sedative–hypnotics.

B. Pharmacology

1. Benzodiazepines appear to produce their calming and hypnotic effects by depressing the limbic system and reticular formation through potentiation of the inhibitory neurotransmitter γ-aminobutyric acid (GABA).
   a. Anxiolytic activity correlates with the drug's binding affinity to a macromolecular complex consisting of $GABA_A$ receptors and chloride channels.
   b. The interaction of benzodiazepines with GABA causes an increase in the frequency of chloride channel opening events, leading to a facilitation of chloride ion conductance, membrane hyperpolarization, and ultimately synaptic inhibition.

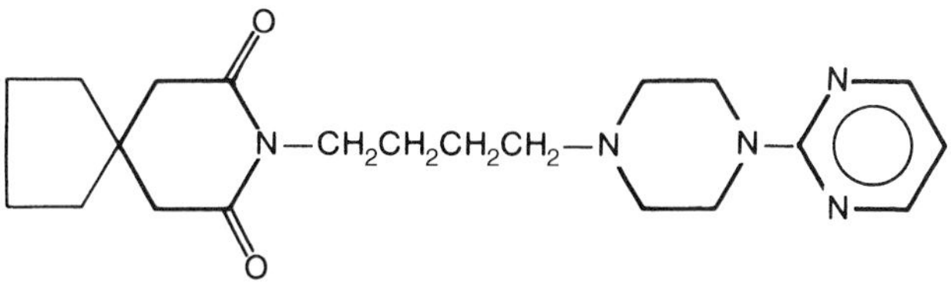

Figure 13-22. Structural formula of buspirone (Buspar), the prototypical azaspirodecanedione anxiolytic.

Table 13-8. Barbiturate Sedative–Hypnotics

General Barbiturate Structure*

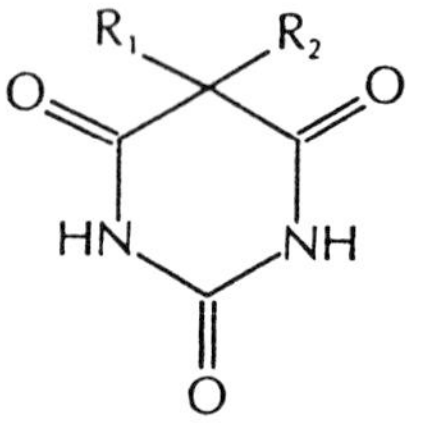

Drug	R_1-Substituent	R_2-Substituent	Duration of Action
Phenobarbital (Luminal)	$-CH_2CH_3$	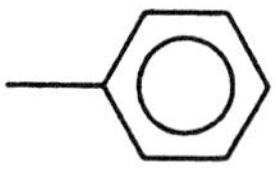 (phenyl)	Long
Amobarbital (Amytal)	$-CH_2CH_3$	$-CH_2CH_2CH(CH_3)_2$	Intermediate
Butabarbital (Butisol)	$-CH_2CH_3$	$-CHCH_2CH_3$ $\quad\lvert$ $\quad CH_3$	Intermediate
Pentobarbital (Nembutal)	$-CH_2CH_3$	$-CHCH_2CH_2CH_3$ $\quad\lvert$ $\quad CH_3$	Short
Secobarbital (Seconal)	$-CH_2CH=CH_2$	$-CHCH_2CH_2CH_3$ $\quad\lvert$ $\quad CH_3$	Short

*Barbiturate sedative–hypnotics have the general structure illustrated in the table. Substituents at R_1 and R_2 positions result in different drugs with different durations of action.

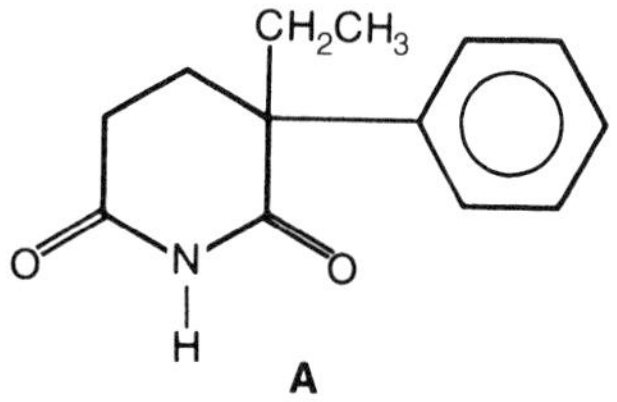

Figure 13-23. Structural formulas of (*A*) glutethimide (Doriden), a piperidine-dione sedative–hypnotic and (*B*) chloral hydrate (Noctec), an aldehyde sedative–hypnotic.

    c. In addition to their anxiolytic properties, most benzodiazepines have other significant CNS actions, including hypnotic, anesthetic, anticonvulsant, and muscle relaxant effects at appropriate doses.

    d. Benzodiazepines increase the depressant effects of alcohol and other CNS depressant drugs.

  2. **Azaspirodecanediones** have multiple biochemical actions, but their principal mechanism of anxiolytic effect is still unknown.

  a. **Buspirone** binds to central dopamine and serotonin receptors rather than to GABA-chloride ionophore receptor complexes. Interactions of azapirones with serotonin receptors may be agonistic when acting at somatodendritic 5-HT1$_A$ autoreceptors or antagonistic when acting at postsynaptic 5-HT1$_A$ receptors.
  b. Buspirone possesses no hypnotic or anticonvulsant properties and does not appear to enhance the depressant effects of alcohol or other CNS depressant drugs.
  c. Buspirone has minimal abuse liability and does not produce rebound anxiety following abrupt discontinuation.

3. **The imidazopyridines** have strong sedative effects with minimal clinical anxiolytic actions.
  a. Zolpidem is as effective as the benzodiazepines in shortening sleep latency and in prolonging total sleep time in patients with insomnia.
  b. Zolpidem is rarely associated with physical dependence, rebound insomnia, or respiratory depression even in overdosage.

4. **Barbiturates** are less selective than benzodiazepines and produce generalized CNS depression.
  a. Barbiturates bind to a site that is distinct from the benzodiazepine binding site on a macromolecular GABA-chloride ionophore receptor complex. Barbiturate binding induces an increase in the duration of channel opening events, and thus mimics or enhances the inhibitory actions of GABA.
  b. Barbiturates have a wide range of dose-dependent pharmacological actions related to CNS depression, including sedation, hypnosis, and anesthesia. They also act as potent respiratory depressants and inducers of hepatic microsomal drug-metabolizing enzyme activity.

5. **Piperidinediones, aldehydes,** and other nonbarbiturate sedative–hypnotics have similar pharmacological actions related to CNS depression.
  a. Chloral hydrate is commonly used to induce sleep in pediatric or geriatric patients. Its low cost is the major factor accounting for its preferred usage in institutional settings.
  b. Chloral hydrate is biotransformed to trichloroethanol, which is responsible for the pharmacological activity of the drug. Chloral hydrate induces hepatic microsomal drug-metabolizing enzyme activity.

C. Therapeutic indications

1. **Benzodiazepines and the azaspirodecanedione buspirone** are indicated to treat anxiety. Buspirone is more effective in patients with generalized anxiety of mild to moderate severity. The antianxiety effects of buspirone may require up to a week to be established.

2. **Benzodiazepines and the imidazopyridine** are indicated to produce drowsiness and promote sleep.

3. **Benzodiazepines** are indicated for use as a preanesthetic medication, as anticonvulsants, and during acute alcohol withdrawal.

4. **Barbiturates** are no longer considered appropriate as anxiolytics or sedative–hypnotics in view of the availability of the safer benzodiazepines. Long-acting barbiturates continue to be widely used as antiepileptics, while the ultra–short-acting barbiturates are used for the induction of general anesthesia and as general anesthetics for short surgical procedures.

5. **Chloral hydrate** is indicated for use as a pediatric or geriatric hypnotic, and also as a preanesthetic agent for minor surgical and dental procedures.

D. Adverse effects

1. Adverse effects associated with **benzodiazepines** include:
  a. CNS effects, such as CNS depression, drowsiness, sedation, ataxia, confusion, and dysarthria
  b. GI effects, such as nausea, vomiting, and diarrhea
  c. Psychiatric effects (rare), such as paradoxical excitement, insomnia, paranoia, and rage reactions
  d. Potential for abuse and dependence

2. Adverse effects of **buspirone** are limited to restlessness, dizziness, headache, nausea, diarrhea, and paresthesias.

3. **Barbiturates** can cause a variety of adverse effects, including:
   a. CNS effects, such as drowsiness, confusion, nystagmus, dysarthria, depressed sympathetic ganglionic transmission, hyperalgesia, impaired judgment, impaired fine motor skills, paradoxical excitement (in geriatric patients), and potentiation of other CNS depressant drugs
   b. Respiratory and cardiovascular effects, such as respiratory depression, bradycardia, and orthostatic hypotension
   c. GI effects, such as nausea, vomiting, constipation, diarrhea, and epigastric distress
   d. Exfoliative dermatitis and Stevens-Johnson syndrome
   e. Headache, fever, hepatotoxicity, and megaloblastic anemia (with the chronic use of phenobarbital)

4. **Trichloroethanol,** the active metabolite of **chloral hydrate,** is metabolized to trichloroacetic acid, which is highly toxic and tends to accumulate with repeated administration of chloral hydrate. Use of chloral hydrate is associated with the following adverse effects.
   a. GI effects, such as GI irritation and upset, nausea, and vomiting
   b. CNS effects, such as CNS depression, disorientation, incoherence, drowsiness, ataxia, headache, and potentiation of other CNS depressants (particularly alcohol)
   c. Leukopenia

XIII. ANTIEPILEPTICS

A. **Chemistry.** Antiepileptics (anticonvulsants) vary widely in structure (Figure 13-24).

1. **Older agents,** which are still widely used, include derivatives of the long-acting barbiturates (e.g., phenobarbital, mephobarbital, metharbital, primidone), hydantoins (e.g., phenytoin, ethotoin), succinimides (e.g., ethosuximide, phensuximide), oxazolidinediones (e.g., trimethadione, dimethadione), and dialkylacetates (e.g., valproic acid).

2. **Newer agents,** which are more structurally diverse, include the iminostilbenes (e.g., carbamazepine), benzodiazepines (e.g., diazepam, clonazepam, clorazepate), GABA-analogue gaba-pentin, phenyltriazine derivative lamotrigine, and dicarbamate felbamate.

B. **Pharmacology**

1. Antiepileptics prevent or reduce excessive discharge and reduce the spread of excitation from CNS seizure foci.

2. The mechanisms of action of antiepileptics appear to be alteration of Na^+ neuronal concentrations by promotion of Na^+ efflux (e.g., hydantoins) and restoration or enhancement of GABA-ergic inhibitory neuronal function (e.g., barbiturates, benzodiazepines, valproic acid).

C. **Therapeutic indications.** These agents are generally categorized by the type of seizure against which they are effective.

1. Drugs that are indicated for the treatment of **tonic-clonic (grand mal) seizures** include phenobarbital, phenytoin, primidone, and carbamazepine.

2. Drugs that are indicated for the treatment of **absence (petit mal) seizures** include phenobarbital, ethosuximide, trimethadione, clonazepam, and valproic acid.

3. Clonazepam is indicated for the treatment of **myoclonic seizures.**

4. Agents that are effective against **partial seizures** include clorazepate, felbamate, gabapentin, and lamotrigine.

5. Phenytoin, phenobarbital, primidone, and carbamazepine are effective against **psychomotor seizures.**

6. Intravenous diazepam, phenytoin, and phenobarbital are indicated for the treatment of **status epilepticus.**

D. **Adverse effects**

1. **Barbiturates** (see XII D 3) and **benzodiazepines** (see XII D 1) used as antiepileptics have the same adverse effects as when used for anxiolytic or sedative–hypnotic purposes. Intravenous use of these agents could cause cardiovascular collapse and respiratory depression.

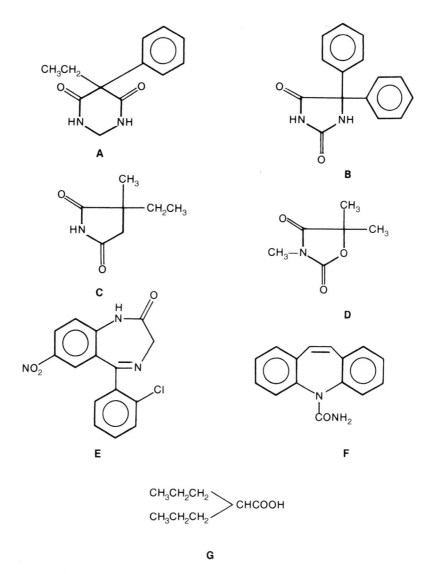

Figure 13-24. Structural formulas of the antiepileptic agents: (*A*) primidone (Mysoline), (*B*) phenytoin (Dilantin), (*C*) ethosuximide (Zarontin), (*D*) trimethadione (Tridione), (*E*) clonazepam (Klonopin), (*F*) carbamazepine (Tegretol), and (*G*) valproic acid (Depakene).

2. Antiepileptic agents generally have the propensity to cause the following side effects:
   a. GI irritation, nausea, and vomiting
   b. CNS sedation, diplopia, nystagmus, ataxia, dizziness, and confusion
   c. Blood dyscrasias, including aplastic anemia and bleeding disorders
   d. Allergic-type reactions, including Stevens-Johnson syndrome
   e. Various organ-system toxicities, including renal and liver failure, pancreatitis, and cardiotoxicity

3. The hydantoins (e.g., phenytoin) can also cause specific **arrhythmias** and **gingival hyperplasia.**

4. Antiepileptics as a class also have the potential to cause various **birth defects,** including cleft palate (e.g., carbamazepine, phenytoin) and neural tube defects (e.g., valproic acid). These effects present a unique problem in treating pregnant women with convulsive disorders. Discontinuation of anticonvulsant therapy can result in a seizure state

that could harm the fetus. However, continued therapy can increase the risk of birth defects and place the mother at risk of bleeding disorders during delivery. Compounding the situation, pregnancy can either increase or decrease seizure incidence of the mother. Risk/benefit evaluation of therapy should be made on individual cases based on the patient's history.

XIV. ANTIPARKINSONIAN AGENTS

A. Chemistry. The principal antiparkinsonian agents are either **dopaminergic agonists** or **cholinergic antagonists.**

1. Some **anticholinergic antiparkinsonian** agents are structurally related to **atropine** (e.g., benztropine, trihexyphenidyl). Other antiparkinsonian anticholinergic agents include procyclidine (Kemadrin), orphenadrine (Norflex), and biperiden (Akineton).

2. The prototypical **dopaminergic** antiparkinsonian agent is the **catecholamine levodopa** (Figure 13-25), a prodrug that must be converted in vivo to dopamine by **dopa decarboxylase.** Direct receptor-acting dopaminergics include **ergot alkaloids** or **ergolines** such as bromocriptine (Parlodel) and pergolide (Permax), and the newer nonergoline dopamine agonists **pramipexole** (Mirapex) and **ropinirole** (Requip).

3. Three agents are available that improve the therapeutic efficacy and safety of levodopa.
   a. Carbidopa, a levodopa analogue that does not cross the blood–brain barrier, is a **decarboxylase inhibitor** that diminishes the decarboxylation and subsequent inactivation of levodopa in **peripheral tissues.** A combination of levodopa and carbidopa (Sinemet) is available for clinical use.
   b. Selegiline (deprenyl), is a **selective monoamine oxidase-B (MAO-B) inhibitor** that inhibits the intracerebral degradation of endogenous or levodopa-derived dopamine.
   c. Tolcapone, a selective inhibitor of COMT, reduces the conversion of levodopa to 3-O-methyldopa, an inactive metabolite that also inhibits levodopa uptake into the brain.

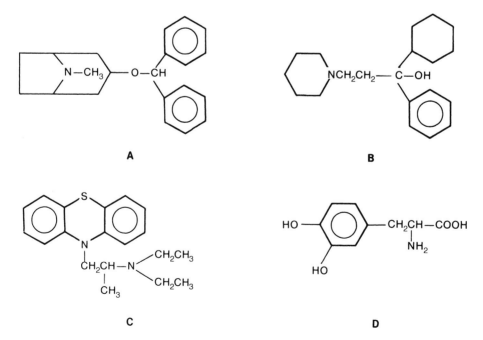

Figure 13-25. Structural formulas of antiparkinsonian agents: (*A*) benztropine (Cogentin), (*B*) trihexyphenidyl (Artane), (*C*) ethopropazine (Parsidol), and (*D*) levodopa (Larodopa).

B. Pharmacology. Antiparkinsonian agents act by restoring the striatal balance of dopaminergic and cholinergic neurotransmission, which is deranged in parkinsonism as a result of degeneration of dopaminergic neurons that supply dopamine to the **striatum (caudate-putamen).**

1. **Levodopa,** which can cross the blood–brain barrier, is the immediate precursor of the striatal neurotransmitter dopamine and is converted to dopamine in the body.

2. **Amantadine,** an antiviral agent, appears to stimulate the release of dopamine from intact striatal dopaminergic terminals.

3. **Bromocriptine, pergolide, pramipexole, and ropinirole,** which are direct dopaminergic receptor agonists, mimic the activity of striatal dopamine.

4. **Selegiline,** an inhibitor of the central MAO-B isoenzyme, blocks the central catabolism of dopamine, increasing its availability in the caudate-putamen.

5. **Anticholinergics,** such as trihexyphenidyl, benztropine, and orphenadrine, block the excitatory cholinergic system, thus reducing the functional imbalance between dopamine and acetylcholine in the striatum.

6. The enzyme inhibitors, **carbidopa and tolcapone,** increase the transport and bioavailability of levodopa in the brain and are thus given as adjunctive treatments with levodopa.

C. Therapeutic indications

1. **Levodopa** is indicated to treat idiopathic, postencephalitic, or arteriosclerotic parkinsonism.

2. **Amantadine** is indicated to treat idiopathic, postencephalitic, or arteriosclerotic parkinsonism, as well as extrapyramidal symptoms induced by antipsychotic drugs (with the exception of tardive dyskinesia).

3. **Bromocriptine** is indicated to treat idiopathic or postencephalitic parkinsonism.

4. **Selegiline, anticholinergics,** and **antihistamines** are indicated for use as adjunctive therapy for all types of parkinsonism, including drug-induced extrapyramidal symptoms (with the exception of tardive dyskinesia).

D. Adverse effects

1. **Levodopa** is associated with these adverse effects:
   a. GI effects, such as GI upset, nausea, vomiting, anorexia, and excessive salivation
   b. Cardiovascular effects, such as orthostatic hypotension, tachycardia, and dysrhythmias
   c. CNS effects, such as headache, dizziness, and insomnia
   d. Abnormal involuntary movements, such as dyskinesia and choreiform or dystonic movements
   e. Psychiatric effects, such as delusions, hallucinations, confusion, psychoses, and depression

2. **Amantadine** is associated with these adverse effects:
   a. CNS effects, such as drowsiness, insomnia, dizziness, slurred speech, and nightmares
   b. Urinary retention and ankle edema
   c. Livedo reticularis (mottling of skin on the extremities)
   d. Psychiatric effects, such as hallucinations and confusion

3. **Bromocriptine** and related ergot alkaloids are associated with these adverse effects:
   a. Nausea
   b. Hypotension
   c. Psychiatric effects, such as confusion and hallucinations
   d. Livedo reticularis
   e. Abnormal involuntary movements, such as dyskinesia and choreiform or dystonic movements

4. **Selegiline** is associated with adverse effects that are similar to those of bromocriptine, including dyskinesias and hallucinations.

5. Anticholinergic antiparkinsonian agents have the same adverse effects as other cholinergic antagonists (see VI D).

XV. OPIOID ANALGESICS and ANTAGONISTS.

Analgesic opioids are opioid receptor agonists that consist of natural opiate alkaloids and their synthetic derivatives.

A. Chemistry. The opiate alkaloids are derived from opium, which is considered the oldest drug on record. **Opium** (the dried exudate of the poppy seed capsule) contains about 25 different alkaloids. Of these, morphine is the most important, both quantitatively and pharmacologically (Figure 13-26).

1. **Morphine's phenolic hydroxyl group** is extremely important for activity; however, analgesic activity appears to depend on a *p*-phenyl-*N*-alkylpiperidine moiety, in which the piperidine ring is in the chair form and is perpendicular to the aromatic ring. The alkyl group is usually methyl. The **morphine molecule** can be altered in a variety of ways; related compounds also can be synthesized from other starting materials.

2. **Natural or synthetic opioids** may be classified into four chemical groups (Figure 13-27):
   a. **Phenanthrenes** (e.g., morphine and hydromorphone, codeine and hydrocodone, nalbuphine and buprenorphine, and nalorphine, naltrexone, and naloxone). Methylation of the phenolic (3)-hydroxyl group with or without modification of the 6-hydroxyl group of morphine yields agents with reduced agonist potency but enhanced oral bioavailability (e.g., codeine, hydrocodone, oxycodone).
   b. **Phenylheptylamines** (e.g., methadone and propoxyphene) are bisphenyl derivatives of heptylamine that have strong (methadone) or moderate (propoxyphene) agonist potency and excellent oral bioavailability.
   c. **Phenylpiperidines** include meperidine, fentanyl, and sufentanil, which are strong agonists that are more effective when given parenterally, and the moderate agonists diphenoxylate and loperamide.
   d. The **morphinan** levorphanol is a strong agonist with high oral bioavailability.

3. **Opioid antagonists** are derived by replacing the methyl group on the nitrogen atom with more bulky substitutions. Thus, nalbuphine and buprenorphine are phenanthrene **mixed agonist–antagonists;** naltrexone and naloxone are phenanthrene **pure antagonists;** and butorphanol and levallorphan are morphinan-derived antagonists (Figure 13-28).

4. Agents having both a free phenolic hydroxyl group and a tertiary amine function (e.g., morphine and nalbuphine) are chemically amphoteric. Amphotericity probably accounts for the erratic absorption of morphine when administered orally.

5. Some newer opioid analgesic agents, such as **tramadol,** are chemically unrelated to the natural, semisynthetic, and synthetic opiate derivatives.

6. Numerous analogues of endogenous opioid peptides have been synthesized and are being used in research.

B. Pharmacology

1. **Opioid analgesics** mimic the actions of endogenous opioid peptides at CNS opioid receptors, raising the pain threshold and increasing pain tolerance. The analgesic actions are mediated primarily through the μ-subtype of opioid receptors.

2. Other actions attributable to stimulation of opioid receptors include induction of euphoria, sedation, cough suppression, and chemoreceptor trigger-zone stimulation leading to nausea and vomiting.

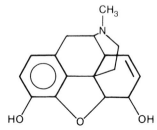

Figure 13-26. Structural formula of morphine.

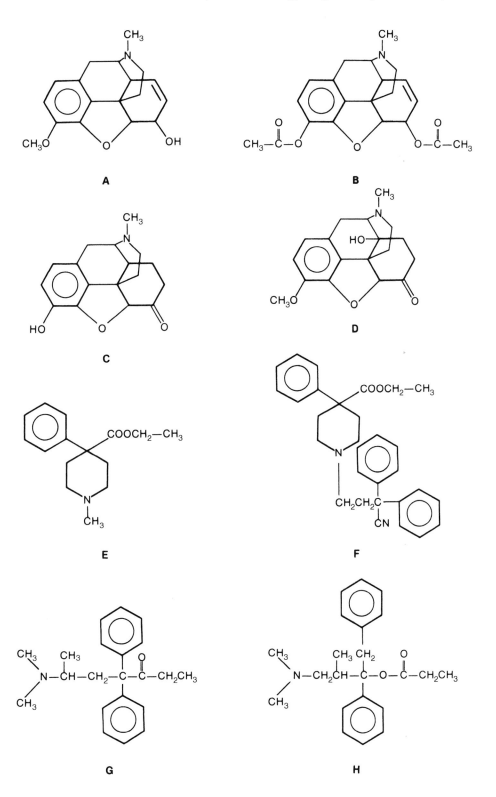

Figure 13-27. Structural formulas of selected opioid agonists, including (*A*) codeine, (*B*) heroin, (*C*) hydromorphone (Dilaudid), and (*D*) oxycodone (Percodan), morphine analogues; (*E*) meperidine (Demerol) and (*F*) diphenoxylate (Lomotil), piperidine analgesics; and (*G*) methadone (Dolophine) and (*H*) propoxyphene (Darvon), methadone analgesics.

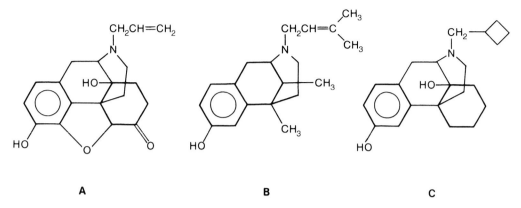

Figure 13-28. Structural formulas of opioid antagonists: (*A*) naloxone (Narcan), (*B*) pentazocine (Talwin), and (*C*) butorphanol (Stadol).

3. **Tramadol** appears to act via a metabolite, which is selective for the μ-opioid receptor and also inhibits reuptake of norepinephrine and serotonin. Its nonopiate character appears to confer no clear benefits over the opiates.

4. **Pure opioid antagonists** such as naloxone block the actions of opioid agonists. **Mixed agonist–antagonists** such as nalbuphine, buprenorphine, butorphanol, and pentazocine block the actions of agonists at some receptor subtypes while directly stimulating other receptor subtypes to produce agonistic effects.

C. Therapeutic indications

1. Opioid analgesics are indicated to relieve **moderate to severe pain,** such as the pain associated with myocardial infarction, cancer, and labor. In the latter use, meperidine is preferred to morphine because meperidine is less likely to induce **neonatal respiratory depression.**

2. Opioids are used also as **preanesthetic medications,** as **analgesic adjuncts during anesthesia,** and occasionally as a primary anesthetic agent.

3. Mild to moderate agonistic opioids are used as **antitussives** (e.g., codeine and dextromethorphan) and as **antidiarrheals** (e.g., diphenoxylate and loperamide).

4. Pure opioid antagonists are used as antidotes to reverse the adverse effects of opioid agonists or opioid agonist–antagonists (e.g., respiratory depression, cardiovascular depression, sedation). Naltrexone is an orally active compound that possesses pure antagonistic activity and is used in the treatment of opioid addiction.

D. Adverse effects

1. **Opioid analgesics** are associated with the following adverse effects:
   a. CNS effects, including CNS depression, miosis, dizziness, sedation, confusion, disorientation, and coma
   b. GI effects, including nausea, vomiting, constipation, biliary spasm, and increased biliary tract pressure
   c. Cardiovascular effects, such as orthostatic hypotension, peripheral circulatory collapse, dysrhythmias, and cardiac arrest
   d. Respiratory depression
   e. Bronchoconstriction
   f. Psychiatric effects, such as euphoria, dysphoria, and hallucinations
   g. Abuse potential and dependence
   h. Precipitation of withdrawal symptoms in opioid-dependent patients (when opioid agonist–antagonists, such as pentazocine or nalbuphine, are used as analgesics)
   i. Classic opioid analgesics can also prompt the release of histamine, causing intense pruritus, vasodilation, and bronchoconstriction, which can be confused with a true allergic reaction.

   j. Tramadol appears to have significantly fewer respiratory depressant effects than the classic opioids. It also does not appear to cause the release of histamine. It has fewer cardiovascular effects with the exception of orthostatic hypotension, which is produced. Tramadol does possess the typical μ–receptor-mediated side effects of constipation, nausea, vomiting, and sedation.

2. Opioid antagonists are associated with the following adverse effects:
   a. Pure opioid antagonists can precipitate a withdrawal syndrome in opioid-dependent patients. Pure antagonists, given in the absence of opioid agonists or agonist–antagonists, produce no clinically significant effects.
   b. In the absence of opioids, mixed agonist–antagonists produce opioid-like effects, such as respiratory depression.

STUDY QUESTIONS

Directions: Each of the numbered items or incomplete statements in this section is followed by answers or by completions of the statement. Select the **one** lettered answer or completion that is **best** in each case.

1. Which of the following drugs would most likely be used in the treatment of bronchospasm that is associated with chronic obstructive pulmonary disease?

(A) Edrophonium
(B) Ipratropium
(C) Ambenonium
(D) Propantheline
(E) Homatropine

2. All of the following adverse effects are manifestations of cholinergic agonists EXCEPT

(A) bradycardia
(B) bronchoconstriction
(C) xerostomia
(D) lacrimation
(E) myopic accommodation

3. Which of the following drugs is considered to be the agent of choice for anaphylactic reactions?

(A) Clonidine
(B) Isoproterenol
(C) Epinephrine
(D) Phenylephrine
(E) Terbutaline

4. Which of the following neuromuscular blocking agents can cause muscarinic responses such as bradycardia and increased glandular secretions?

(A) Tubocurarine
(B) Succinylcholine
(C) Pancuronium
(D) Decamethonium
(E) Gallamine

5. Which of the following agents would NOT be appropriate in the treatment of glaucoma?

(A) Atropine
(B) Pilocarpine
(C) Physostigmine
(D) Timolol
(E) Epinephrine

6. Adverse reactions to atropine include all of the following EXCEPT

(A) photophobia
(B) dry mouth
(C) sedation
(D) diarrhea
(E) tachycardia

7. Which of the following drugs is a volatile substance that is administered by inhalation?

(A) Thiopental
(B) Halothane
(C) Alprazolam
(D) Buspirone
(E) Phenytoin

8. The structure of prochlorperazine is shown below. Which of the following medications, because of its chemical relationship to prochlorperazine, would most likely cause similar side effects?

(A) Fluphenazine
(B) Thioridazine
(C) Alprazolam
(D) Buspirone
(E) Pentobarbital

9. The brief duration of action of an ultra–short-acting barbiturate is due to a

(A) slow rate of metabolism in the liver
(B) low lipid solubility, resulting in a minimal concentration in the brain
(C) high degree of binding to plasma proteins
(D) rapid rate of redistribution from the brain due to its high liposolubility
(E) slow rate of excretion by the kidneys

10. Which of the following mechanisms of action is true and most likely contributes to the treatment of parkinsonism?

(A) The direct-acting dopaminergic agonist amantadine mimics the activity of striatal dopamine.
(B) The antimuscarinic activity of diphenhydramine contributes to the restoration of striatal dopaminergic-cholinergic neurotransmitter balance.
(C) Striatal H_1-receptors are blocked by the antihistaminic trihexyphenidyl.
(D) The ergoline bromocriptine stimulates the release of striatal dopamine from intact terminals.
(E) The ability of dopamine to cross the blood–brain barrier allows it to restore striatal dopaminergic-cholinergic neurotransmitter balance.

11. All of the following adverse effects are associated with the use of levodopa EXCEPT

(A) sialorrhea
(B) orthostatic hypotension
(C) delusions, confusion, and depression
(D) dyskinesia and dystonia
(E) livedo reticularis

12. The activity of which of the following drugs is dependent on a *p*-phenyl-*N*-alkylpiperidine moiety?

(A) Phenobarbital
(B) Chlorpromazine
(C) Diazepam
(D) Imipramine
(E) Meperidine

13. Opioids are used as all of the following agents EXCEPT

(A) antitussives
(B) analgesics
(C) anti-inflammatories
(D) antidiarrheals
(E) preanesthetic medications

14. Which of the following agents would NOT be an alternative to phenobarbital in the treatment of partial seizures?

(A) Trimethadione
(B) Gabapentin
(C) Felbamate
(D) Lamotrigine
(E) None of the above

Directions: Each question below contains three suggested answers, of which **one or more** is correct. Choose the answer

A   if **I only** is correct
B   if **III only** is correct
C   if **I and II** are correct
D   if **II and III** are correct
E   if **I, II, and III** are correct

15. Cholinesterase inhibitors can be used therapeutically

I. as miotic agents in the treatment of glaucoma
II. to increase skeletal muscle tone in the treatment of myasthenia gravis
III. to decrease gastrointestinal (GI) and urinary bladder smooth-muscle tone

16. Antimuscarinic agents are used in the treatment of Parkinson's disease and in the control of some neuroleptic-induced extrapyramidal disorders. These agents include

I. ipratropium
II. benztropine
III. trihexyphenidyl

17. Certain drugs are sometimes incorporated into local anesthetic solutions to prolong their activity and reduce their systemic toxicity. These drugs include

I. dobutamine
II. phenylephrine
III. epinephrine

18. Improper administration of local anesthetics can cause toxic plasma concentrations that may result in

I. seizures and central nervous system (CNS) depression
II. respiratory and myocardial depression
III. circulatory collapse

19. In addition to their anxiolytic properties, benzodiazepines are indicated for use

I. as preanesthetic medications
II. as anticonvulsants
III. during acute withdrawal from alcohol

Directions: Each group of items in this section consists of lettered options followed by a set of numbered items. For each item, select the **one** lettered option that is most closely associated with it. Each lettered option may be selected once, more than once, or not at all.

Questions 20–22

A 58-year-old white male who has a history of essential hypertension and bronchial asthma has recently been diagnosed with prostatic hypertrophy. His medication history includes the following drugs (use to answer the questions below).

(A) Propranolol, for hypertension
(B) Ipratropium, for asthma
(C) Metaproterenol, for asthma
(D) Proscar, for prostatic hypertrophy
(E) Prazosin, for hypertension

20. Which of these agents and uses could worsen the urinary retention he is experiencing as a result of his prostate problems?

21. Which agent and use could worsen or cause an acute asthma attack?

22. Which agent acts selectively at β_2-receptors?

Questions 23–25

A 55-year-old black female has a history of moderate hypertension, glaucoma, and mild osteoarthritis. Her medication history includes

(A) Metoprolol, for hypertension
(B) Pilocarpine gel, for glaucoma
(C) Epinephrine drops, for glaucoma
(D) Isoflurophate, for glaucoma
(E) Timolol, for glaucoma

23. Which of her glaucoma medicines acts via an indirect mechanism?

24. Which two agents could have an additive effect to produce excessive bradycardia?

25. Which two glaucoma agents could lessen the effects of the other?

Questions 26–28

For each statement below, choose the drug that it most closely describes.

(A) Tranylcypromine
(B) Imipramine
(C) Buspirone
(D) Fluoxetine
(E) Phenelzine

26. An anxiolytic drug that does not possess either hypnotic or anticonvulsant properties

27. A prototype tricyclic antidepressant with antimuscarinic properties that make it useful in the treatment of enuresis

28. An antidepressant that inhibits serotonin reuptake and may cause adverse effects such as impaired memory, akathisia, and menstrual irregularities

Questions 29–31

For each of the following structures, select the most appropriate pharmacological category.

(A) General anesthetic
(B) Local anesthetic
(C) Antidepressant
(D) Anxiolytic
(E) Opioid antagonist

29.

$$NH_2 - \text{⬡} - COOCH_2CH_2N(CH_2CH_3)_2$$

30.

31.

Questions 32–33

A 38-year-old man has a history of affective disorders including schizophrenia, depression, obsessive-compulsive disorder, and situational anxiety. His past medications include thiothixene, chlorpromazine, amitriptyline, and diazepam. His current medication profile includes two of the following drugs (use to answer the questions below).

(A) Clozapine
(B) Fluoxetine
(C) Buspirone
(D) Risperidone

32. Which agent is most likely being used to treat his schizophrenic psychosis?

33. Which agent is most likely being used to treat depression and obsessive-compulsive disorder?

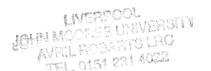

ANSWERS AND EXPLANATIONS

1. The answer is B *[V C 2 b, c; VI C 1 e–g].*
Ipratropium is a newly approved antimuscarinic agent used to treat bronchospasm. Propantheline and homatropine are antimuscarinic agents used as a gastrointestinal (GI) antispasmodic and as a mydriatic, respectively. Edrophonium and ambenonium are indirect-acting cholinergic agonists and, as such, would be expected to induce bronchospasm.

2. The answer is C *[V D].*
Xerostomia, or dry mouth, results from reduced salivary secretions and, therefore, is not a manifestation of cholinergic agonist activity. All of the other effects listed in the question are extensions of therapeutic effects of cholinergic agonists to the point of being adverse effects.

3. The answer is C *[III C 1].*
Of the adrenergic agonists listed in the question, only epinephrine, because of its broad, nonselective α- and β-activity, is an agent of choice for anaphylactic reactions. Epinephrine improves circulatory and respiratory function and counteracts the vascular effects of histamine-related anaphylaxis.

4. The answer is B *[VII D 2].*
Neuromuscular blocking agents interact with nicotinic receptors at the skeletal neuromuscular junction. Succinylcholine is also capable of eliciting autonomic muscarinic responses, such as bradycardia, increased glandular secretions, and cardiac arrest.

5. The answer is A *[V B–D].*
Both direct-acting (e.g., pilocarpine) and indirect-acting (e.g., physostigmine) cholinergics may be used in glaucoma to increase cholinergic activity and facilitate outflow of aqueous humor. Similarly, both β-agonists (e.g., epinephrine) and antagonists (e.g., timolol) may be used respectively to increase outflow and decrease production of aqueous humor. Atropine is contraindicated in glaucoma because its anticholinergic effects can block the outflow of aqueous humor and consequently increase intraocular pressure.

6. The answer is D *[VI D].*
Classic signs and symptoms of muscarinic blockade, as with atropine, include mydriasis, which may cause light sensitivity (photophobia), dry mouth and constipation by decreasing secretory activity and motility in the gastrointestinal (GI) tract, and tachycardia by inhibiting the normal inhibitory cholinergic control of the cardiac system. Diarrhea is one of the common signs of cholinergic agonists (such as salivation, lacrimation or tearing, urination, and diarrhea).

7. The answer is B *[VIII A 1].*
The general anesthetics are divided into two major classes of drugs: those that are gases or volatile liquids, which are administered by inhalation, and those that are nonvolatile salts, which are administered as intravenous solutions. Halothane is a halogenated hydrocarbon, which belongs to the former class. It has the advantage over older volatile anesthetics (e.g., ethyl ether, cyclopropane) of being nonflammable. Thiopental sodium, alprazolam, buspirone, and phenytoin are all nonvolatile substances that are administered orally or parenterally. Thiopental is a general anesthetic and is sometimes referred to as a basal anesthetic because it does not produce significant third-stage surgical anesthesia. Alprazolam and buspirone are anxiolytics, whereas phenytoin is an anticonvulsant.

8. The answer is A *[X A 1; Table 13-6].*
Fluphenazine, like prochlorperazine, is a piperazinyl phenothiazine antipsychotic and would be likely to cause similar side effects. Whereas thioridazine is also a phenothiazine antipsychotic, it is a piperidyl derivative rather than a piperazinyl derivative. Alprazolam, phenytoin, and pentobarbital are not phenothiazines; therefore, structurally, they are not similar to prochlorperazine.

9. The answer is D *[XII A 4 c, d; Figure 13-14].*
Ultra–short-acting barbiturates are characterized by having branched or unsaturated 5,5-side chains and by having a sulfur atom in place of oxygen in the 2 position of the barbituric acid molecule. These modifications of barbituric acid result in an extremely liposoluble molecule that is very soluble in lipid tissues. After administration, an ultra–short-acting barbiturate readily crosses the blood–brain barrier but then is quickly redistributed into extracerebral tissue, resulting in a rapid loss of activity. Whereas these agents do remain in the body for a long time and seem to have slow rates of metabolism and excretion, their long retention time is due more to their slow rate of leaching out of lipid tissue.

10. The answer is B *[XIV B]*.
The H_1-antagonist diphenhydramine possesses antimuscarinic activity, which allows it to be of use in the restoration of striatal dopaminergic-cholinergic neurotransmitter balance. Amantadine appears to stimulate the release of striatal dopamine; it does not mimic the action of dopamine. Trihexyphenidyl is an antimuscarinic, not antihistaminic, agent; it blocks cholinergic, not H_1, receptors. Bromocriptine is a dopaminergic agonist and mimics the activity of striatal dopamine. The neurotransmitter dopamine is not able to cross the blood–brain barrier and is, therefore, not effective as an antiparkinsonian drug.

11. The answer is E *[XIV D 1]*.
Livedo reticularis is a circulatory disorder characterized by large, bluish areas on the extremities. It is an adverse effect associated with the use of amantadine and bromocriptine but not with the use of levodopa.

12. The answer is E *[XV A 1, 2; Figure 13-27, E]*.
The *p*-phenyl-*N*-alkylpiperidine moiety is common to the structurally specific opioid analgesics. Meperidine is an opioid analgesic and is an *N*-methyl-*p*-phenylpiperidine derivative. Its chemical name is ethyl 1-methyl-4-phenylpiperidine-4-carboxylate. Phenobarbital is a barbiturate sedative. Chlorpromazine is a phenothiazine antipsychotic. Diazepam is a benzodiazepine anxiolytic. Imipramine is a tricyclic dibenzazepine antidepressant.

13. The answer is C *[XV C]*.
Unlike the salicylates, opioids do not possess anti-inflammatory activity. Opioids do suppress the cough reflex and are preeminent analgesics. Opioids cause constipation and are, thus, effective antidiarrheal agents. When used as preanesthetic medication, opioids permit a reduction in the amount of general anesthetic required for surgical anesthesia.

14. The answer is A *[XIII A 1, C 2]*.
Whereas many analeptics are useful in controlling more than one seizure type, trimethadione is effective primarily against absence (petit mal) seizures. Additionally, its side-effect profile is more extensive than the newer agents (e.g., lamotrigine, gabapentin, felbamate) that are effective in treating partial seizures.

15. The answer is C (I, II) *[V C 2]*.
Cholinesterase inhibitors are indirect-acting cholinergic agonists useful in treating myasthenia gravis and glaucoma. Their effects on gastrointestinal (GI) and urinary bladder smooth muscle would be to increase smooth-muscle tone, not decrease it.

16. The answer is D (II, III) *[VI C 1 g, h]*.
All three compounds listed in the question are antimuscarinic agents; however, only benztropine and trihexyphenidyl are used to control Parkinsonism and some neuroleptic-induced extrapyramidal disorders. Ipratropium is a newly approved agent for the treatment of bronchospasm.

17. The answer is D (II, III) *[III B 1 b, C 1, 2]*.
Dobutamine is a β_1-selective adrenergic agonist. It would be inappropriate to use dobutamine to decrease blood flow at the site of local anesthetic administration. Epinephrine is a nonselective α- and β-agonist, and phenylephrine is an α_1-selective agonist; both of these drugs can be used to limit the systemic absorption of local anesthetics and prolong their activity.

18. The answer is E (all) *[IX D 2]*.
Careful administration of a local anesthetic by a knowledgeable practitioner is essential to prevent systemic absorption and consequent toxicity. This is especially important when the patient has cardiovascular disease, poorly controlled diabetes, thyrotoxicosis, or peripheral vascular disease.

19. The answer is E (all) *[XII C 1, 2, 3]*.
Benzodiazepines can serve as induction agents for general anesthesia; they also have anxiolytic properties. In addition, intravenous diazepam is used to treat status epilepticus, whereas clonazepam is used orally for myoclonic and absence (petit mal) seizures. Benzodiazepines also diminish alcohol withdrawal symptoms.

20. The answer is B *[VI D]*.
This anticholinergic, if absorbed systemically, could cause classic anticholinergic effects, which include urinary retention.

21. The answer is A *[IV C 4]*.
Because this is a nonselective β-blocker, there could be some inhibition of β_2-receptors in the bronchial tree, causing bronchoconstriction and possible complication of his asthma.

22. The answer is C *[III C 6]*.
Propranolol is a nonselective β-blocker, and prazosin is a selective α_1-blocker. Neither ipratropium nor Proscar works through the adrenergic system. Metaproterenol is a selective β_2-agonist.

23. The answer is D *[V A 2, C 2]*.
Pilocarpine acts directly at the muscarinic receptor, whereas epinephrine and timolol both act directly at β-receptors. Isoflurophate inhibits the metabolism of acetylcholine, indirectly increasing levels of the endogenous neurotransmitter.

24. The answers are A and E *[IV B 3, D 4]*.
Metoprolol, a β_1-selective agent, can cause bradycardia alone. The addition of topical timolol, while limiting systemic absorption, could have an additive β-blocking effect to decrease heart rate (negative chronotropy).

25. The answers are B and D *[V C 1, 2]*.
Pilocarpine and isoflurophate could limit the effects of each other, because ultimately both act via cholinergic receptors. Pilocarpine acts directly on the receptor, while isoflurophate indirectly increases acetylcholine levels. Pilocarpine and acetylcholine could compete for each other at the receptor site, effectively decreasing the effects of both. Epinephrine and timolol are β-agonists and β-antagonists, respectively. Although both agents are effective in treating glaucoma alone, the use of both concomitantly could result in a pharmacological antagonism, effectively decreasing the effects of both.

26–28. The answers are: 26-C *[XII B 2]*, **27-B** *[XI C 2]*, **28-D** *[XI B 3, D 3]*.
Buspirone's mechanism of anxiolytic action is unknown. Unlike the benzodiazepines, buspirone lacks hypnotic and anticonvulsant properties. The tricyclic antidepressant imipramine is useful in the treatment of enuresis, because the compound blocks muscarinic receptors mediating micturition. Trazodone is categorized as an atypical antidepressant that selectively blocks serotonin reuptake.

29–31. The answers are: 29-B *[IX A; Figure 13-15]*, **30-D** *[XII A; Table 13-7]*, **31-C** *[XI A 2; Figure 13-19]*.
The structure shown in question 29 is that of procaine, which is a diethylaminoethyl *p*-aminobenzoate ester. It contains a hydrophilic amino group in the alcohol portion of the molecule and a lipophilic aromatic acid connected by the ester linkage. The procaine molecule is typical of ester-type local anesthetics.

The structure in question 30 is that of diazepam, which has a benzo-1,4-diazepine as its base nucleus. The widely used benzo-1,4-diazepine derivatives have significant anxiolytic, hypnotic, and anticonvulsant activities.

The structure in question 31 is that of desipramine, which has a dibenzazepine as its base nucleus. Dibenzazepine derivatives that have a methyl- or dimethylaminopropyl group attached to the ring nitrogen have significant antidepressant activity. Similarly substituted dibenzocycloheptadienes also have antidepressant activity. Together, these two chemical classes make up the majority of the tricyclic antidepressants.

32. The answer is A *[X C]*.
Clozapine, while therapeutically defined as a general antipsychotic, is used almost exclusively in the treatment of schizophrenia.

33. The answer is B *[XI A 3, C 2]*.
Fluoxetine is most likely being used in this patient in an attempt to treat his depression and obsessive-compulsive disorder with the same drug. Clinical trials have shown fluoxetine to improve both conditions. The use of a single agent for both conditions will minimize the risk of drug–drug interactions, as well as reduce the chances of adverse effects.

14
Autacoids and Their Antagonists, Nonnarcotic Analgesic–Antipyretics, and Nonsteroidal Anti-inflammatory Drugs

Scott F. Long

I. INTRODUCTION

A. Autacoids, also called autopharmacological agents or local hormones, have widely differing structures and pharmacological actions. Although the term remains poorly defined, the currently accepted criteria that defines a substance as an autacoid is local release and action limited to a specific site. Two of most extensively investigated autacoids are **histamine** and the **prostaglandins.** However, **serotonin, bradykinin, and kallidin** also function in a similar manner. While some autacoids (histamine and serotonin) function as neurotransmitters, their autacoid function will be the focus of this chapter. Currently, there are no agents that specifically modulate the function of bradykinin or kallidin; however, drugs or analogues that mimic, block, or modulate other autacoid functions have important therapeutic roles.

B. Non–narcotic analgesic–antipyretics have dissimilar structures but share certain therapeutic actions, including relief of pain, fever, and sometimes inflammation. Mechanistically, these agents act by inhibiting synthesis of prostaglandins.

C. Nonsteroidal anti-inflammatory drugs (NSAIDs) differ in structure and activity from the non-narcotic analgesic–antipyretics, but possess anti-inflammatory properties. Additionally, many of these agents also exhibit antipyretic and analgesic activity. NSAIDs also act by inhibition of prostaglandin synthesis.

II. AUTACOIDS AND THEIR ANTAGONISTS

A. Histamine and antihistaminics

  1. Chemistry
    a. Histamine (Figure 14-1) is a bioamine derived principally from dietary histidine, which is decarboxylated by L-histidine decarboxylase.
    b. Antihistaminics (histamine antagonists) can be classified as **H_1 or H_2-receptor antagonists.**
      (1) H_1-receptor antagonists, the classic antihistaminic agents, are chemically classified as **ethylenediamines** (e.g., pyrilamine, tripelennamine), **alkylamines** (e.g., brompheniramine, chlorpheniramine, acrivastine), **ethanolamines** (e.g., diphenhydramine, dimenhydrinate, clemastine, doxylamine), **piperazines** (e.g., meclizine, cyclizine, hydroxyzine, cetirizine), **phenothiazines** (e.g., promethazine), **dibenzocycloheptenes** (cyproheptadine), **phthalazinone** (azelastine), and **piperidines** (e.g., terfenadine, astemizole, levocabastine, loratidine, fexofenadine). The piperidines noted above, acrivastine, and cetirizine comprise the second-generation antihistaminics, which are less sedating than the older, first-generation drugs, due to their limited ability to cross the blood–brain barrier (Figure 14-2).

(2) H$_2$-receptor antagonists are heterocyclic congeners of histamine. These include cimetidine, ranitidine, famotidine, and nizatidine (Figure 14-3).

(3) Alternatives to the H$_2$-receptor antagonists include omeprazole, lansoprazole, rabeprazole, pantoprazole, and esomeptazole; **specific inhibitors of H$^+$,K$^+$-ATPase (proton pump inhibitors, or PPIs),** the ultimate mediator of gastric acid secretion.

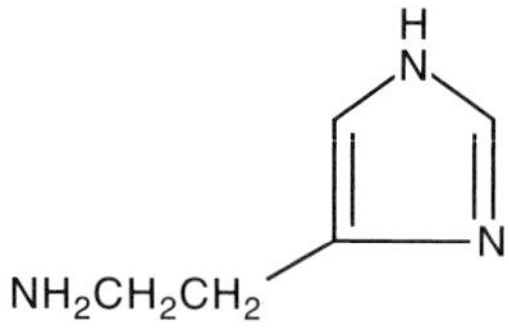

Figure 14-1. Structural formula of histamine, an autacoid.

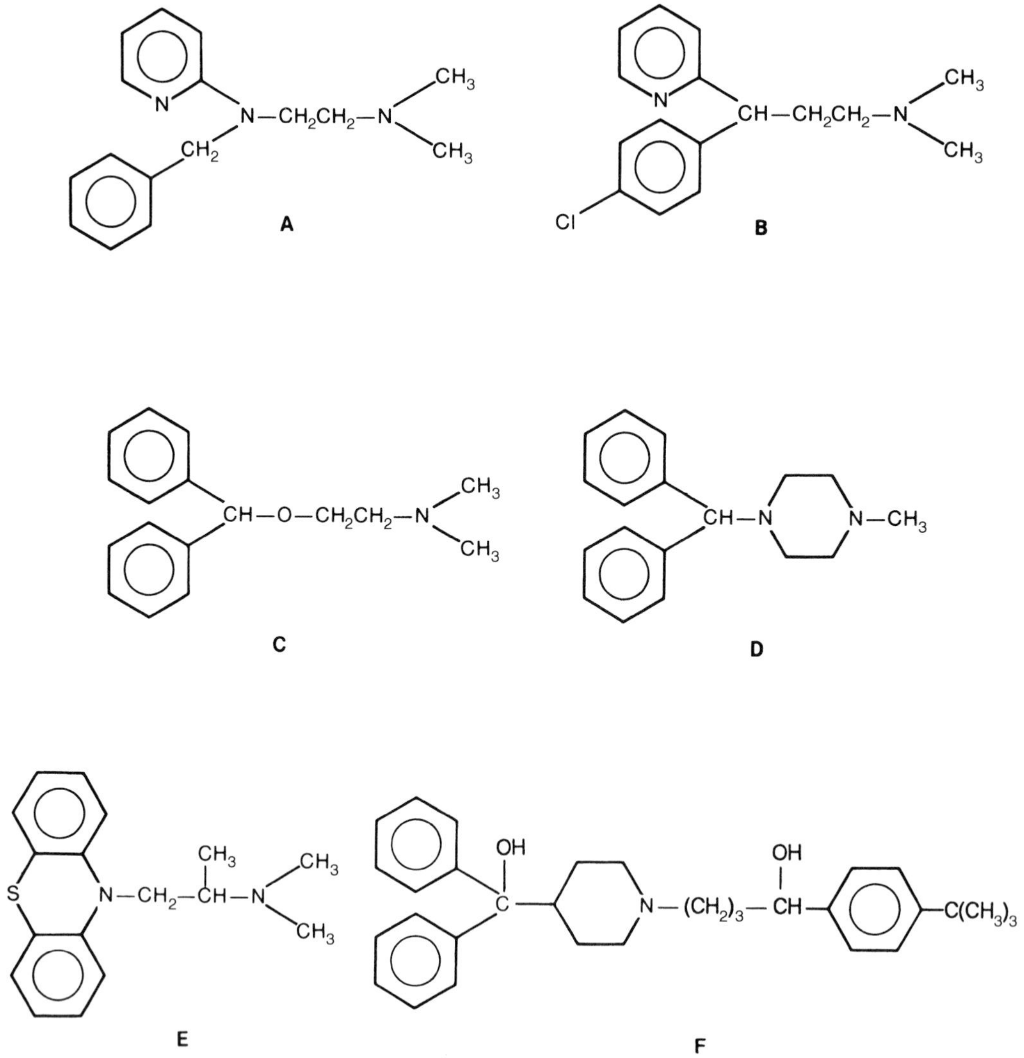

Figure 14-2. Structural formulas of (*A*) tripelennamine (Pyribenzamine), (*B*) chlorpheniramine (Chlor-Trimeton), (*C*) diphenhydramine (Benadryl), (*D*) cyclizine (Marezine), (*E*) promethazine (Phenergan), and (*F*) terfenadine (Seldane), representative H$_1$-receptor antagonists.

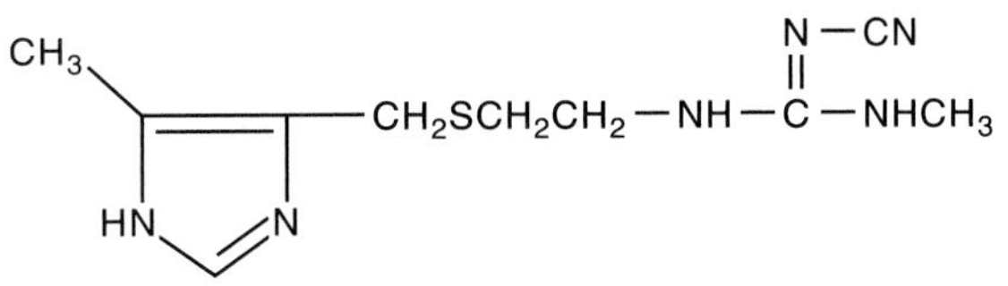

Figure 14-3. Structural formula of cimetidine, an H_2-receptor antagonist.

Table 14-1. Selected Actions of Endogenous Histamine

Site	Action	Receptor Type
Cardiovascular		
Vascular	Arterial contraction	H_1
	Arteriolar relaxation	H_1 and H_2
	Venule contraction	H_1
	Venule relaxation	H_2
	Endothelial cells, release of EDRF	H_1
	Endothelial cells, contraction	H_1
Heart	Increased heart rate	H_2
	Increased force of contraction	H_2
	Slowed atrioventricular conduction	H_1
Respiratory	Bronchiolar smooth-muscle contraction	H_1
Gastrointestinal		
Gastric mucosa	Increased secretion of acid and pepsin	H_2
GI smooth muscle	Contraction	H_1
Various		
Cutaneous nerves	Pain and itch	H_1

EDRF = Endothelium-derived relaxing factor.

Structurally, these agents are substituted **benzimidazoles** linked to a pyridine ring by a sulfinyl bridge that is required for H^+,K^+-ATPase inhibition.

2. Pharmacology

    a. Histamine has powerful pharmacological actions, mediated by two specific receptor types (Table 14-1). A third histamine receptor has been identified. Its function has yet to be elucidated, but it is believed to act, at least in part, as an autoreceptor.

        (1) H_1-**receptors mediate** typical allergic and anaphylactic responses to histamine, such as bronchoconstriction, vasodilation, increased capillary permeability, and spasmodic contractions of gastrointestinal (GI) smooth muscle.

        (2) H_2-**receptors mediate** other responses to histamine, such as increased secretion of gastric acid, pepsin, and Castle's factor (intrinsic factor).

    b. H_1-**receptor antagonists** competitively block H_1-receptors, thus limiting the histamine's effects on bronchial smooth muscle, capillaries, and GI smooth muscle. These antagonists also prevent histamine-induced pain and itching of the skin and mucous membranes.

    c. H_2-**receptor antagonists** competitively block H_2-receptors, thus limiting the effects of histamine on gastric secretions.

    d. The **PPIs** irreversibly inhibit the proton pump H^+,K^+-ATPase by covalently binding to the protein.

3. Therapeutic indications

    a. Exogenous histamine can be used as a **diagnostic agent** for testing gastric function. However, other stimulants of gastric secretion (pentagastrin) are more suitable and safer.

    b. H_1-**receptor antagonists** are used to provide symptomatic relief of **allergic symptoms,** such as seasonal rhinitis, conjunctivitis, and the symptoms of rhinoviral infections (common cold). Their antihistaminic effects also make them useful for symptomatic relief of urticaria. Agents with a high degree of anticholinergic activity (e.g., diphenhydramine, dimenhydrinate, meclizine, cyclizine) are sometimes used to treat nausea and vomiting associated with motion sickness and vertigo. Additionally, promethazine is sometimes used as an antiemetic, and hydroxyzine pamoate is occasionally employed as a mild anxiolytic. The second-generation drugs (i.e., terfenadine, astemizole, levocabastine, loratidine, fexofenadine, acrivastine, cetirizine, and azelastine) provide the added advantage of very little to negligible sedation, due to their relative inability to cross the blood–brain barrier. Note that the two older agents (terfenadine and astemizole) are no longer available due to a high incidence of life-threatening arrhythmias (torsades de pointes).

   c. **H₂-receptor antagonists** are used to treat **gastric hypersecretory** conditions, such as duodenal ulcer and Zollinger-Ellison syndrome. They are effective in reducing pain associated with gastroesophageal reflux disease, but note that they do not prevent actual reflux.

   d. The **proton pump inhibitors** are used to treat **duodenal ulcers** and are the drugs of choice for the treatment of **Zollinger-Ellison syndrome.**

4. **Adverse effects**
   a. **Histamine** may cause numerous adverse effects related to its basic pharmacology (see II A 2 a).
   b. **H₁-receptor antagonists** are associated with the following **adverse effects:**
      (1) Central nervous system (CNS) effects, such as CNS depression, sedation, fatigue, tinnitus, hallucinations, and ataxia
      (2) GI effects, such as nausea and vomiting
      (3) Antimuscarinic effects, such as dry mouth, urinary retention, and constipation
      (4) Teratogenic effects (possible with piperazine compounds)
   c. **Peripheral H₁-receptor antagonists,** terfenadine and astemizole, are devoid of significant sedative and antimuscarinic effects. However, elevated plasma levels of both astemizole and terfenadine have been associated with electrocardiographic QT prolongation, cardiac arrest, torsades de pointes, and other ventricular arrhythmias. It is thought that the QT lengthening effect is mediated through blockade of a delayed rectifying potassium channel by the parent compound that is independent of their histamine-blocking activity. Moreover, concomitant use of these agents with drugs or foods that inhibit their hepatic metabolism (including the antifungal ketoconazole, the macrolide antibiotics erythromycin and troleandomycin, and grapefruit juice) is contraindicated because such a combination results in significantly elevated antihistamine plasma levels. Note that the incidence of arrhythmias was great enough to warrant the removal of both drugs from the market. The newer agents lack the propensity to cause life-threatening arrhythmias.
   d. **H₂-receptor antagonists** are associated with these adverse effects:
      (1) CNS effects, such as confusion and dizziness
      (2) Hepatic and renal dysfunction
      (3) Inhibition of the hepatic microsomal drug-metabolizing enzyme system (with cimetidine)
      (4) Androgenic effects (with high doses of cimetidine), such as impotence and gynecomastia in men and galactorrhea in women
   e. The **H⁺,K⁺-ATPase inhibitors** have been reported to cause diarrhea, GI pain, and headache as their most frequent adverse effects. Additionally, they may interfere with the metabolism of diazepam, warfarin, phenytoin, and theophylline.

B. Serotonin

1. **Chemistry**
   a. **Serotonin** (5-hydroxytryptamine, Figure 14-4) is a bioamine that is synthesized from the amino acid tryptophan by a two-step enzymatic process catalyzed by tryptophan hydroxylase and L-amino acid decarboxylase.
   b. **Serotonin agonists**
      (1) **5-HT₁D–receptor agonists (i.e., sumatriptan, rizatriptan, naratriptan, zolmetriptan, almotriptan, and frovatriptan)** are indole derivatives structurally similar to serotonin (see Figure 14-4).
      (2) **Cisapride** (a **benzamide**) and **tegaserod** (an **indole** derivative) act as 5-HT₄–receptor agonists (see Figure 14-4).
      (3) **Ergot alkaloids (ergotamine)** have some activity as a serotonin agonist/partial agonist.

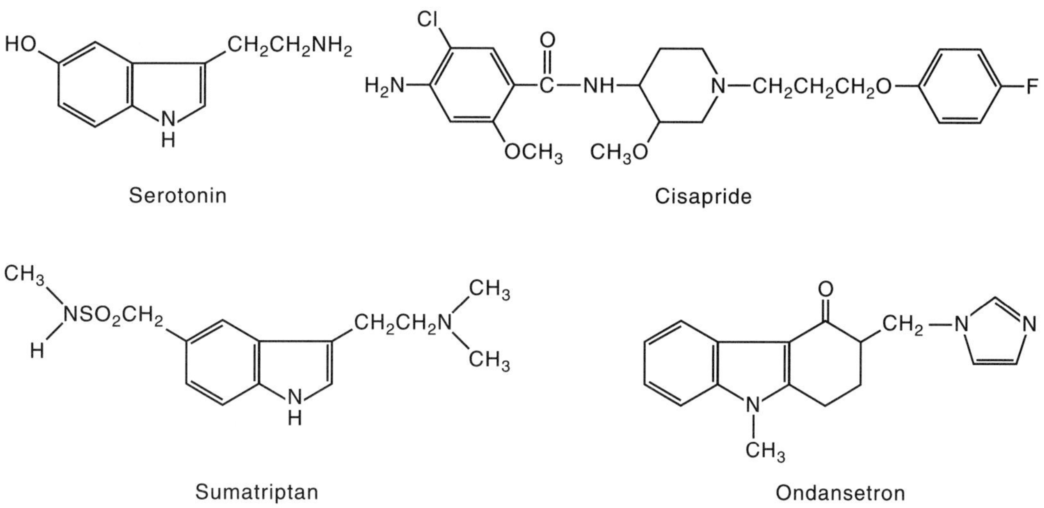

Figure 14-4. Structures of serotonin and representative serotonin agonists sumatriptan (Imitrex), cisapride (Propulsid), and the antagonist ondansetron (Zofran).

   c. Serotonin antagonists
   (1) Ergot alkaloids and derivatives with antagonist/partial agonist activity include **ergonovine, dihydroergotamine, methysergide, and bromocriptine.**
   (2) 5-HT$_3$–antagonists may be either **indole** derivatives **(ondansetron)** or **benzimidozoles (granisetron).** Other drugs of the class include **dolasetron** and **alosetron** (see Figure 14-4).

2. Pharmacology
   a. Serotonin exerts a wide range of effects via a family of receptors that includes at least seven types and several subtypes. Major physiological effects of serotonin include vasoconstriction (5-HT$_2$), platelet aggregation (5-HT$_2$), increased release of acetylcholine in the enteric region (5-HT$_4$), nausea/emesis (5-HT$_3$), and numerous behavioral actions that influence anxiety, depression, aggression, impulsivity, and appetite (5-HT$_1$, 5-HT$_2$, 5-HT$_3$). Additionally, the 5-HT$_{1D}$–receptor acts as an autoreceptor to inhibit presynaptic activity at both serotonergic and adrenergic neuron in the CNS. Serotonin may also produce numerous other effects, including the opposite of those stated above, depending on the specific receptor that mediates the event.
   b. Serotonin agonists
   (1) 5-HT$_{1D}$–agonists mimic the actions of serotonin at this autoreceptor to decrease presynaptic neurotransmitter release. This action results in decreased release of serotonin and/or noradrenaline. Consequently, serotonin/noradrenaline-induced vasoconstriction of cerebral vessels cannot occur.
   (2) Cisapride and **tegaserod (Zelnorm)** activate the serotonergic receptor (5-HT$_4$) to cause the release of acetylcholine, other neurotransmitters, and calcitonin gene-related peptide. These, in turn, increase gastric and intestinal motility and tone.
   (3) Ergot alkaloids produce a wide range of pharmacological effects, including both agonistic and antagonistic activity at adrenergic, dopaminergic, and serotonergic receptors. Specific actions are dependent upon drug and animal models.
   c. Serotonin antagonists such as **ondansetron** and related drugs block the ion-channel coupled 5-HT$_3$–receptor, thus inhibiting the ability of serotonin to cause nausea and/or emesis. This action appears to occur both locally at the GIT and centrally in the area postrema. Additionally, activation of peripheral 5-HT$_3$–receptors will increase pain, abdominal distention, and motor responses of the intestinal tract. Blockade of these actions by **alosetron** are responsible for its usefulness in certain cases of irritable bowel syndrome (IBS).

3. Therapeutic indications
   a. Serotonin agonists
   (1) Numerous CNS active drugs utilize the serotonergic system to modulate behavior, such as the anorexiants (dexfenfluramine), anxiolytics (buspirone), and selective

serotonin reuptake inhibitors for depression (fluoxetine). These drugs are acting more on the neurotransmitter function of serotonin and will not be discussed here.

(2) Some **ergot alkaloids, sumatriptan,** and similar drugs act to modulate the autacoid function of serotonin. They are used to prevent and treat pain associated with migraine headaches by altering serotonin's actions that result in changes in vascular tone.

(3) Additionally, some **ergot alkaloids** are used to prevent postpartum hemorrhaging (through both vasoconstrictive and uterine contractile actions) and to prevent postpartum breast engorgement (**bromocriptine,** through dopaminergic activity).

(4) Cisapride is used in the treatment of gastroesophageal reflux disease by increasing pyloric sphincter tone, which is mediated by acetylcholine release. The use of cisapride is extremely limited and is available only for investigational drug use, due to a high incidence of cardiac arrhythmias and death.

(5) Tegaserod is used in the treatment of women only with IBS whose primary symptom of the disease is constipation.

b. Serotonin antagonists. These agents **(e.g., ondasetron, granisetron, dolasetron)** are used to prevent and treat nausea and emesis secondary to antineoplastic therapy by blocking the actions of serotonin at the 5-HT$_3$–receptor. **Alosetron** is used for the treatment of women only with IBS whose primary symptom is diarrhea.

4. Adverse effects
a. Serotonin agonists

(1) 5-HT$_{1D}$–agonists may produce feelings of warmth, paresthesias, dizziness, and tightness or heaviness in the chest. Rarely, patients may experience chest pain. Since these agents may cause coronary vasoconstriction, they are contraindicated in angina patients and should be used cautiously in patients with hypertension or other risk factors for ischemic heart disease.

(2) Cisapride and **tegaserod** may produce diarrhea, abdominal cramping and pain, dizziness, and headache as side effects. Patients should be counseled to take cisapride with meals to increase its absorption. Additionally, cisapride may cause a lengthening of the QT interval and torsades de pointes by a mechanism similar to terfenadine.

(3) Ergot alkaloids may cause GI upset and cold extremities. As toxicity progresses, the patient may experience emesis, diarrhea, peripheral pain secondary to local ischemia, and hallucinations or delusions.

b. Serotonin antagonists. The 5-HT$_3$–antagonists will produce headache, constipation, and dizziness. Additionally, granisetron has been reported to produce somnolence and diarrhea. The use of **alosetron** in women with diarrhea-associated IBS has resulted in some cases of ischemic colitis and life-threatening complications from severe constipation.

C. Prostaglandins

1. Chemistry

a. Prostaglandins are **derivatives** of prostanoic acid, a 20-carbon fatty acid containing a 5-carbon ring (Figure 14-5). In the body, prostaglandins are principally synthesized from arachidonic acid, which has been formed from the membrane phospholipids by action of phospholipase A$_2$. Specifically, prostaglandins are synthesized from arachidonic acid by the enzyme cyclooxygenase, which exists as two isozymes, COX I and COX II. COX I appears to function constantly. Its role appears to be the daily synthesis of prostaglan-

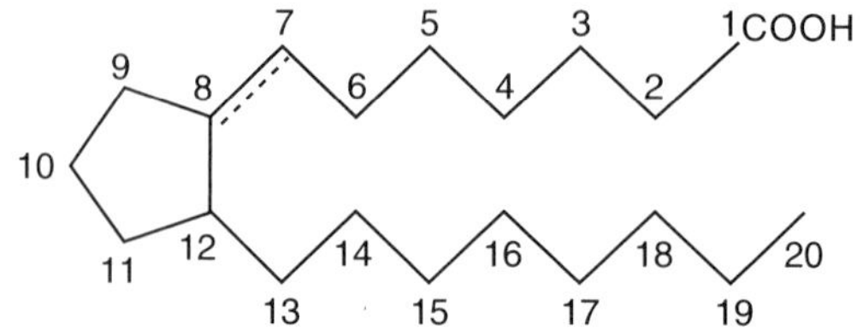

Figure 14-5. Structural formula of prostanoic acid, from which the prostaglandins are derived.

dins that contribute to normal homeostasis, includes protection of the gastric mucosa through prostaglandins and hemostasis through the synthesis of thromboxane. COX II is expressed only in response to inflammation or injury. Its role appears to be limited to the production of prostaglandins for their role in the inflammatory response. Note that the products of cyclooxygenase are then converted into either prostaglandins by prostaglandin synthase or thromboxanes by thromboxane synthase. The thromboxanes differ from the prostaglandins mainly by the substitution of a tetrahydropyran ring structure for the pentane ring found in prostaglandins. The only clinically relevant thromboxane currently identified is thromboxane A_2 (TXA$_2$), which causes platelet aggregation.

    b. Classification of prostaglandins as prostaglandin A (PGA), prostaglandin B (PGB), prostaglandin E (PGE), and so forth relates to the presence or absence of keto or hydroxyl groups at positions 9 and 11 (see Figure 14-5). Subscripts relate to the number and position of double bonds in the aliphatic chains (Figure 14-6).

2. Pharmacology
    a. Endogenous prostaglandins appear to affect numerous body functions. They are released in response to many chemical, bacterial, mechanical, and other insults, and they appear to contribute to the signs and symptoms of the inflammatory process, including pain and edema.
    b. Physiological responses to prostaglandins include vasodilation in most vascular beds, although vasoconstriction can occur in isolated areas. PGI inhibits platelet aggregation and stimulates gastric release of bicarbonate and mucus, both of which serve to protect the gastric epithelium. PGEs inhibit platelet aggregation, relax bronchial and GI smooth muscle, contract uterine smooth muscle, and inhibit gastric acid secretion. Alternatively, PGDs and PGFs contract bronchial and GI smooth muscle. Prostaglandins also increase renal blood flow, promote diuresis, natriuresis, and kaliuresis, but paradoxically increase renin secretion. They also possess diverse endocrine and metabolic effects.

3. Therapeutic indications
    a. PGE$_1$ analogues
       (1) Alprostadil (Prostin VR Pediatric) is used for temporary maintenance of a patent ductus arteriosus when awaiting corrective surgery for congenital heart defects.
       (2) Alprostadil (Caverject) is used in treating impotence due to erectile dysfunction.
       (3) Misoprostol (Cytotec) is used for the prevention of NSAID-induced GI ulcers (see Figure 14-6).
    b. PGE$_2$ analogues and derivative dinoprostone (Prostin E$_2$, Prepidil, Cervidil) are used for their abortifacient effects and to induce cervical-ripening in pregnancy.
    c. PGF$_{2\alpha}$ analogues
       (1) Carboprost (Hemabate), was used for its abortifacient effects. A high incidence of cardiovascular collapse caused its removal from the U.S. market.
       (2) Latanoprost (Xalatan), travoprost (Travatan), bimatoprost (Lumigan), and **unoprostone (Rescula)** are used topically to lower intraocular pressure in glaucoma.
    d. PGI analogue epoprostenol (prostacyclin, Flolan) is used primarily for the treatment of emergent pulmonary hypertension.

4. Adverse effects associated with PGE include:
    a. CNS effects, such as CNS irritability, fever, seizures, and headache
    b. Cardiovascular effects, such as hypotension, dysrhythmias, vasodilation, flushing, and cardiac arrest
    c. Respiratory effects, such as respiratory depression and distress

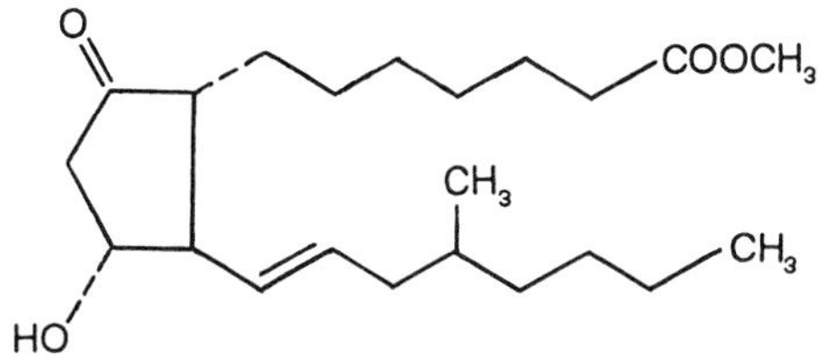

Figure 14-6. Structural formula of misoprostol (Cytotec), a derivative of prostaglandin E$_1$ (PGE$_1$).

 d. Hematological effects, such as anemia, thrombocytopenia, and disseminated intravascular coagulation (DIC)
 e. Diarrhea
 f. Decreased renal function
 g. Spotty bleeding and menstrual irregularities, abortion, and penile pain

D. Leukotrienes

 1. **Chemistry**
    a. **Leukotrienes:** The leukotrienes are 20-carbon derivatives of the fatty acids that are formed via the enzymatic pathway catalyzed by lipoxygenase. Unlike the prostaglandins, they contain no ring structure and are covalently linked to two or three amino acids. The two important leukotrienes identified to date (LTC_4 and LTD_4) differ only by the presence of glutamine. The nomenclature of the leukotrienes is similar to that used for the prostaglandins.
    b. **Leukotriene antagonists**
       (1) **Lipoxygenase inhibitors** such as **zilueton (Zyflo)** are benzothiophene derivatives.
       (2) **Leukotriene antagonists** such as **zafirlukast (Accolate)** and **montelukast (Singulair)** represent a diverse chemical group that is peptidomimetic-like in its structure.

 2. **Pharmacology**
    a. **Leukotrienes** play a role in numerous physiological functions. They have been identified as the slow-reacting substance of anaphylaxis. Specific actions of the leukotrienes include the following:
       (1) **Heart**
          (a) Negative inotropy
          (b) Smooth-muscle chemotaxis
       (2) **GI tract:** Neutrophil chemotaxis that has been correlated with inflammatory bowel disease
       (3) **Pulmonary:** The actions of the leukotrienes within the pulmonary system appear to be major. These actions are the most important pharmacologically.
          (a) Bronchoconstriction
          (b) Increased permeability
          (c) Increased mucus secretion
       (4) **Blood/lymph:** As noted previously, the leukotrienes act as chemotactic agents for neutrophils and eosinophils, and act to modify lymphocyte proliferation and differentiation.
    b. **Leukotriene antagonists**
       (1) **The lipoxygenase inhibitor zileuton** prevents the synthesis of leukotrienes by inhibiting the enzyme responsible for their formation, namely lipoxygenase. This action prevents the formation of all leukotrienes, thus preventing their contribution to various inflammatory processes.
       (2) The leukotriene antagonists **zafirlukast** and **montelukast** nonselectively and competitively inhibit the endogenous leukotrienes at their various receptor sites. This action blocks the effects of histamine, most notably the bronchoconstriction and pulmonary edema associated with asthma and allergic reactions.

 3. **Therapeutic indications for zileuton, zafirlukast, and montelukast** are limited to the treatment of asthma. These agents reduce bronchospasm and associated symptoms that are mediated through the leukotrienes.

 4. **Adverse Effects**
    a. **Zilueton** presents with relatively few side effects, predominantly gastrointestinal in nature (i.e., dyspepsia and nausea). However, it does cause transient increases in hepatic enzymes. This potential for hepatotoxicity has limited its use.
    b. **Zafirlukast** may produce GI upset and liver dysfunction (not as great as with zileuton), and may inhibit the metabolism of theophylline, warfarin, and potentially other drugs. Sudden withdrawal of corticosteroids in patients taking zafirlukast has precipitated a Churg-Strauss syndrome of eosinophilic vasculitis. Patients should be counseled to take zafirlukast with food to enhance its absorption.
    c. **Montelukast** presents with a side-effect profile similar to that for zafirlukast but typically with less incidence than with zafirlukast. Churg-Strauss syndrome has not been reported; however, this may simply reflect the relatively recent appearance of the drug on the market. Montelukast may be taken without regard to food.

III. NONNARCOTIC ANALGESIC–ANTIPYRETICS AND NSAIDS

A. Salicylates

1. **Chemistry**
   a. Salicylates are **derivatives of salicylic acid,** which is found as the glycoside salicin in willow bark. The prototypical drug is **aspirin,** the acetyl ester of salicylic acid (Figure 14-7). A simple ester, aspirin hydrolyzes easily, is unstable in aqueous media, and is affected by moisture.
   b. **More stable** salicylates include **diflunisal** and the topical agent **methyl salicylate** (wintergreen oil) [Figure 14-8]. Other salicylates include **salsalate, sodium thiosalicylate** (injectable), **choline salicylate** (oral liquid), and the salicylate **derivatives mesalamine, olsalazine,** and **sulphasalazine.**
   c. Most salicylates are **weak acids.** Their excretion is influenced by changes in urinary pH.

2. **Pharmacology**
   a. Salicylates **inhibit** the enzyme cyclooxygenase and, thus, inhibit local prostaglandin synthesis (see II C 1 a). As a result, they are analgesic for low-intensity integumental pain, antipyretic, and anti-inflammatory. Note that aspirin is the only salicylate that irreversibly inhibits cyclooxygenase by covalent acetylation of the enzyme.
   b. Salicylates also **block** platelet cyclooxygenase and subsequent formation of thromboxane A_2. As a result, they inhibit platelet aggregation and eventual thrombus formation.

3. **Therapeutic indications**
   a. Salicylates are indicated for use as:
      (1) **Analgesics,** for relief of musculoskeletal pain, headache, neuralgias, myalgias, and spasmodic dysmenorrhea
      (2) **Anti-inflammatory agents,** for relief of various arthritis symptoms and acute rheumatic fever
      (3) **Antipyretic agents,** for relief of fever. (Children with varicella or influenza-type viral infections should not be given salicylates because of the observed association between salicylate use in these situations and Reye's syndrome.)
   b. **Aspirin** is also indicated for **prophylaxis of myocardial infarction.**
   c. **Methyl salicylate** (wintergreen oil) is used topically as a **counterirritant.**
   d. **Sulphasalazine, olsalazine, and mesalamine** are used to reduce the inflammation associated with inflammatory bowel disease and Crohn's disease.

4. **Adverse effects**
   a. **Salicylates** are associated with the following effects:
      (1) GI effects, such as nausea, vomiting, and GI irritation, discomfort, ulceration, and hemorrhage

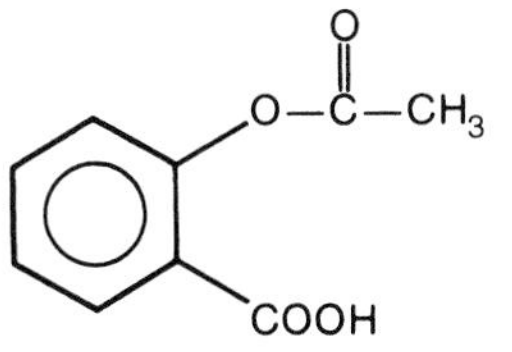

Figure 14-7. Structural formula of aspirin, the prototypical salicylate analgesic–antipyretic.

A   **B**

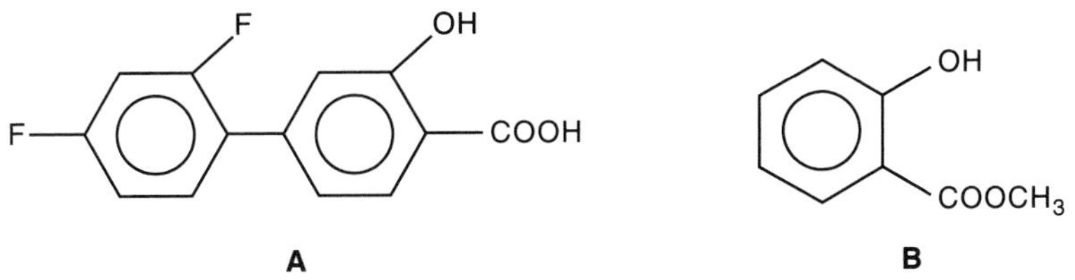

Figure 14-8. Structural formulas of (*A*) diflunisal (Dolobid) and (*B*) methyl salicylate (wintergreen oil), salicylate derivatives.

(2) Increased depth of respirations

(3) Excessive bleeding associated with inhibition of thromboxane synthesis

(4) Uncoupling of oxidative phosphorylation, hyperglycemia, glycosuria, and reduced lipogenesis

(5) Delayed onset of labor

(6) **Low daily doses** of salicylates (2 g) decrease renal urate excretion and increase serum uric acid levels. **High daily doses** (5 g) have the opposite effect.

b. Sulphasalazine has also been shown to have male reproductive effects, causing infertility.

c. Salicylism (salicylate toxicity, usually marked by tinnitus, nausea, and vomiting)

d. Ingestion of 1 tsp of the topical agent **methyl salicylate** (wintergreen oil) can cause **fatal intoxication.**

B. *p*-Aminophenol derivatives

1. **Chemistry.** The prototypical *p*-aminophenol derivative is **acetaminophen,** an active metabolite of phenacetin and acetanilid (Figure 14-9).

2. **Pharmacology**
   a. *p*-Aminophenol derivatives inhibit central prostaglandin synthesis (see II C I a). They are analgesic for low-intensity pain and are antipyretic.
   b. Because they are less effective than salicylates in blocking peripheral prostaglandin synthesis, they have no anti-inflammatory activity and do not affect platelet function.

3. **Therapeutic indications**
   a. Acetaminophen and **phenacetin** are indicated for use as **analgesics** and **antipyretics,** particularly in the patient unable to tolerate salicylates.
   b. Acetaminophen may be safely used as an **alternative antipyretic** in the child with varicella or an influenza-type viral infection [see III A 3 a (3)].

4. **Adverse effects**
   a. When given in therapeutic doses, adverse effects are limited to:
   (1) Skin rash
   (2) Hemolytic anemia (with long-term phenacetin use)
   (3) Methemoglobinemia
   (4) Renal dysfunction and tubular necrosis
   b. Acute acetaminophen overdose causes severe hepatotoxicity with necrosis and liver failure.

C. Pyrazolone derivatives

1. **Chemistry.** The most important pyrazolone derivatives are **phenylbutazone,** its metabolite **oxyphenbutazone,** and the uricosuric agent **sulfinpyrazone** (Anturane). Phenylbutazone is the prototypical agent (Figure 14-10).

2. **Pharmacology**
   a. Phenylbutazone, oxyphenbutazone, and **azapropazone** inhibit prostaglandin synthesis (see II C I a) and stabilize lysosomal membranes. As a result, they have analgesic, antipyretic, and anti-inflammatory effects. They also have good uricosuric activity.
   b. Sulfinpyrazone inhibits proximal tubular absorption of urate and has a uricosuric effect. However, it is devoid of analgesic, antipyretic, or anti-inflammatory effects.

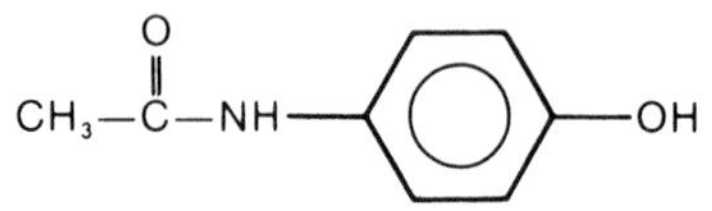

Figure 14-9. Structural formula of acetaminophen, the prototypical *p*-aminophenol derivative.

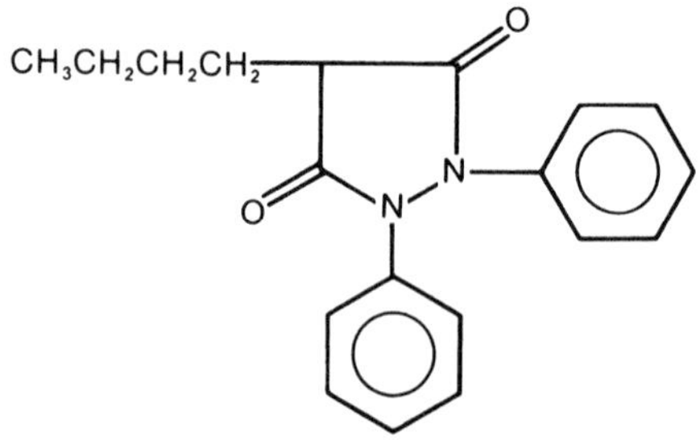

Figure 14-10. Structural formula of phenylbutazone (Butazolidin), a pyrazolone derivative.

3. Therapeutic indications

a. Phenylbutazone and **oxyphenbutazone** are used for short-term treatment of acute rheumatoid arthritic conditions and acute gout. However, they should be given only after other therapeutic measures have failed.

b. Sulfinpyrazone is used to control hyperuricemia in the treatment of intermittent and chronic gout.

4. Adverse effects

a. The adverse effects of **phenylbutazone, oxyphenbutazone,** and **azapropazone** (to a much less extent) often limit their use and include:

(1) GI effects, such as discomfort, nausea, vomiting, dyspepsia, and peptic ulceration
(2) Blood dyscrasias, such as agranulocytosis, aplastic anemia, hemolytic anemia, thrombocytopenia, and petechiae
(3) Cardiovascular effects, such as congestive heart failure with edema and dyspnea
(4) Renal effects, such as nephrotic lithiasis, renal necrosis, impaired renal function, and renal failure
(5) CNS effects, such as drowsiness, agitation, confusion, headache, lethargy, numbness, weakness, tinnitus, and hearing loss
(6) Hyperglycemia
(7) Skin rash

b. Sulfinpyrazone is associated with these adverse effects:

(1) GI effects, such as discomfort and upset
(2) Blood dyscrasias, as with phenylbutazone and oxyphenbutazone
(3) Renal failure

D. Agents used for the treatment of gout

1. Chemistry

a. Acute attacks of gout result from an inflammatory response to joint depositions of sodium urate crystals. Therapeutic agents counter this response by reducing plasma uric acid concentrations or inhibiting the inflammatory response.

b. Agents used for the treatment of gout have widely varying structures and include the pyrazolone derivative sulfinpyrazone (see III C 2 b, 3 b, 4 b); the alkaloid colchicine; isopurines, such as allopurinol; and benzoic acid derivatives, such as probenecid (Figure 14-11).

2. Pharmacology

a. Colchicine's mechanism of action is presumed to be related to its antimitotic activity. It inhibits tubulin synthesis, which is required for the movement of inflammatory cells. There, colchicine appears to inhibit chemotaxis of leukocytes and other inflammatory cells in the affected joint, thus reducing the inflammatory response to deposited urate crystals by inhibiting leukocyte migration and phagocytosis. It also interferes with kinin formation and reduces leukocyte lactic acid production.

b. Allopurinol reduces serum urate levels by blocking uric acid production. It competitively inhibits the enzyme xanthine oxidase, which converts xanthine and hypoxanthine to uric acid.

c. Probenecid, a uricosuric agent, inhibits the proximal tubular reabsorption of uric acid, increasing uric acid excretion, thus reducing plasma uric acid concentrations.

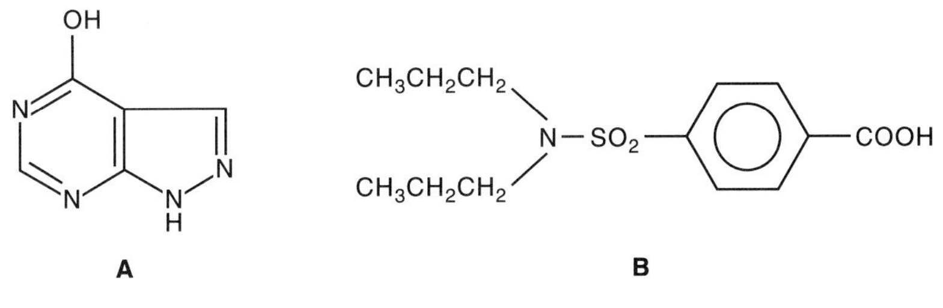

Figure 14-11. Structural formulas of (*A*) allopurinol (Zyloprim) and (*B*) probenecid (Benemid), agents used in the treatment of gout.

3. **Therapeutic indications**
   a. **Colchicine** is used principally for the treatment of acute gout attacks.
   b. **Allopurinol,** which reduces uric acid synthesis and facilitates the dissolution of tophi (chalky urate deposits), is used to prevent the development or progression of chronic tophaceous gout.
   c. **Probenecid** is used to treat chronic tophaceous gout. It is also used in smaller doses to prolong the effectiveness of penicillin-type antibiotics by inhibiting their tubular secretion.

4. **Adverse effects**
   a. Chronic use of **colchicine** is associated with these adverse effects:
      (1) Agranulocytosis, aplastic anemia, myopathy, hair loss, and peripheral neuritis
      (2) Nausea, vomiting, abdominal pain, and diarrhea (indications of impending toxicity)
   b. **Allopurinol** is associated with these adverse effects:
      (1) GI effects, such as GI distress, nausea, vomiting, and diarrhea
      (2) Skin rash, Stevens-Johnson syndrome, and hepatotoxicity
      (3) Precipitation of an acute gout attack (with initial allopurinol therapy due to initial mobilization of stored urate)
   c. **Probenecid** is associated with these adverse effects:
      (1) Headaches, nausea, vomiting, urinary frequency, sore gums, and dermatitis
      (2) Dizziness, anemia, hemolytic anemia, and renal lithiasis

E. **NSAIDs**

1. **Chemistry**
   a. The classic **NSAIDs** consist of many structurally diverse acids. These include **propionic acid** derivatives (fenoprofen, flurbiprofen, ibuprofen, ketoprofen, carprofen, naproxen, and oxaprozin), **acetic acid** derivatives (diclofenac, etodolac, indomethacin, ketorolac, nabumetone, sulindac, and tolmetin), **fenamates** or **anthranilic** acid derivatives (meclofenamate and mefenamic acid), and the **oxicams** (piroxicam) [Figure 14-12].

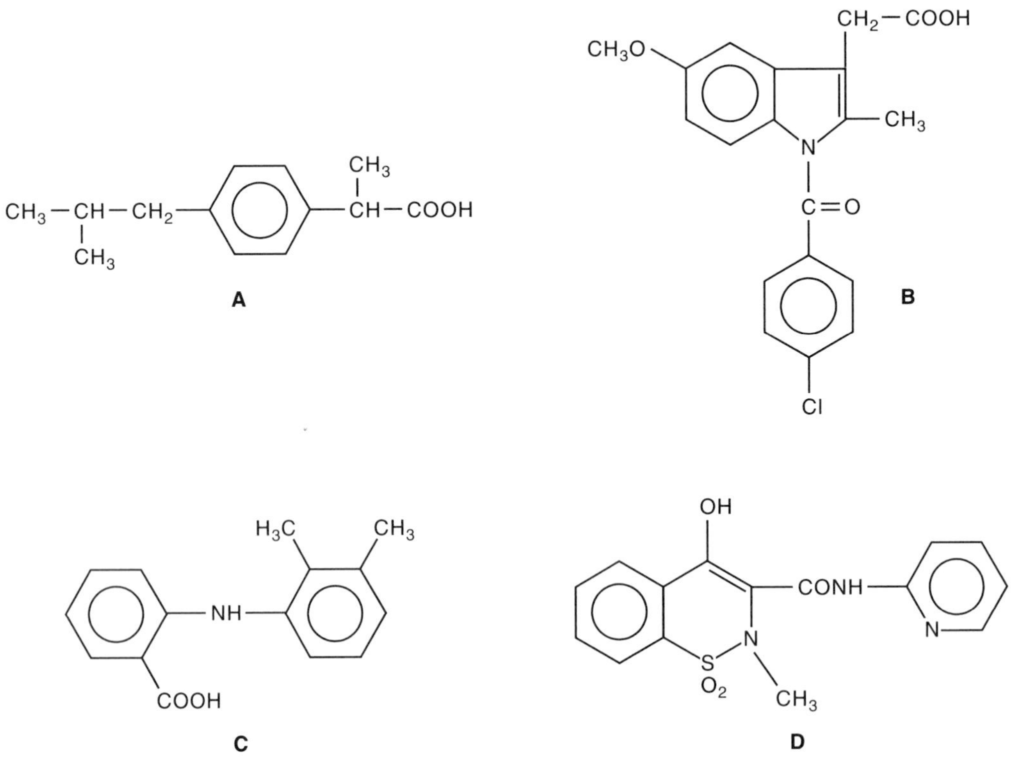

Figure 14-12. Structural formulas of (*A*) ibuprofen, (*B*) indomethacin, (*C*) mefenamic acid, and (*D*) piroxicam, representative nonsteroidal anti-inflammatory drugs (NSAIDs).

   b. Selective cyclooxygenase II inhibitors celecoxib (Celebrex) and rofecoxib (Vioxx), and valdecoxib (Bextra) are pyrazole derivatives (Figure 14-13).

2. Pharmacology

   a. Nonspecific NSAIDs have anti-inflammatory effects, resulting from their ability to inhibit the cyclooxygenase enzyme system and, thus, reduce local prostaglandin synthesis (see II C 1 a).

   b. NSAIDs also have analgesic and antipyretic effects. Additionally, some NSAIDs have mild uricosuric activity. Some agents also have weak inhibitory activity for lipoxygenase, mild selectivity for COX II, and weak to moderate ability to inhibit leukocyte proliferation and migration and to stabilize lysosomal membranes. The clinical relevance of these secondary actions has not been elucidated.

   c. COX II inhibitors exert anti-inflammatory effects by specifically inhibiting prostaglandin synthesis associated with the inflammatory response. Their ability to decrease pain and inflammation associated with arthritic diseases is approximately equal to that produced by the nonselective NSAIDs. Moreover, by virtue of their selectivity, their actions on gastric mucosa and platelet aggregation are theorized to be less than the nonselective NSAIDs.

3. Therapeutic indications

   a. NSAIDs, like aspirin, are agents of choice for the treatment of rheumatoid arthritis, osteoarthritis, and ankylosing spondylitis. They may also be used as secondary treatments in gouty arthritis.

   b. COX II inhibitors are approved for use in both rheumatoid arthritis and osteoarthritis.

4. Adverse effects

   a. NSAIDs are associated with these adverse effects:

      (1) GI effects, such as GI distress and irritation, erosion of gastric mucosa, nausea, vomiting, and dyspepsia

      (2) CNS effects, such as CNS depression, drowsiness, headache, dizziness, visual disturbances, ototoxicity, and confusion

      (3) Hematologic effects, such as thrombocytopenia, altered platelet function, and prolonged bleeding time

      (4) Skin rash

      (5) Nephrotoxicity

   b. COX II inhibitors do not appear to cause as great an incidence of adverse drug reactions as the nonselective NSAIDs. The most commonly reported side effects include GI upset at a lower incidence level. Despite the promise of minimal GI ulceration, some patients have experienced gastrointestinal bleeding with these drugs. This risk of gastric damage and potential ulceration appears to increase with chronic use of these drugs. The potential for nephrotoxicity does exist for these drugs, and patients should be monitored for changes in renal function.

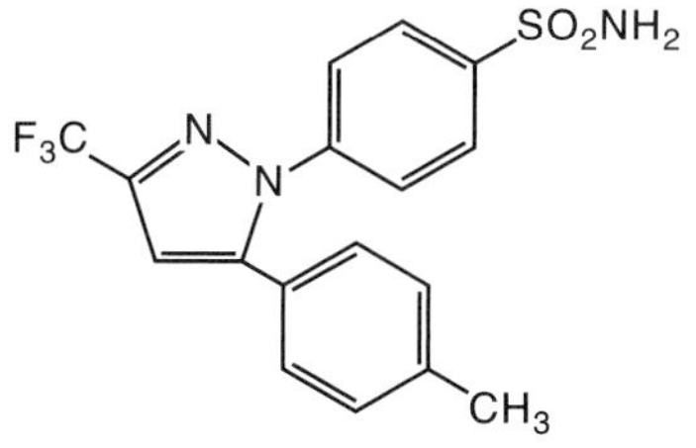

Celecoxib (Celebrex)

Figure 14-13. Structural formula of celecoxib (Celebrex), a COX II specific inhibitor.

STUDY QUESTIONS

Directions: Each of the numbered items or incomplete statements in this section is followed by answers or by completions of the statement. Select the **one** lettered answer or completion that is **best** in each case.

1. A 32-year-old forklift operator with a past history of cardiac arrhythmias is suffering from seasonal rhinitis. Which of the following choices is the best recommendation for this patient?

(A) Diphenhydramine
(B) Meclizine
(C) Astemizole
(D) Fexofenadine
(E) Famotidine

2. Mechanistically, which of the following drugs will decrease stomach acid secretion by blockade of H_2-histaminic receptors?

(A) Pyrilamine
(B) Hydroxyzine
(C) Cisapride
(D) Omeprazole
(E) Ranitidine

3. Lansoprazole would be effective in the treatment of

(A) gastroesophageal reflux disease
(B) peptic ulcer disease
(C) Zollinger-Ellison syndrome
(D) all of the above
(E) none of the above

4. Rizatriptan is contraindicated in which of the following migraine patients?

(A) A 28-year-old female 8 months pregnant
(B) A 48-year-old patient with a history of angina pectoris
(C) A 34-year-old patient with gastroesophageal reflux disease
(D) A 62-year-old patient with gouty arthritis
(E) A 55-year-old patient with a history of rheumatoid arthritis

5. Which of the following agents would decrease the pain associated with gastroesophageal reflux disease without appreciably altering gastric pH?

(A) Cimetidine
(B) Omeprazole
(C) Cisapride
(D) Ondansetron
(E) Sumatriptan

6. Which of the following is an appropriate indication for the drug tegaserod?

(A) A female patient with constipation-related IBS
(B) A female patient with diarrhea-related IBS
(C) A male patient with Crohn's disese
(D) A male patient with constipation-related IBS
(E) A patient with Zollinger-Ellison syndrome

7. Which of the following prostaglandin analogues is used specifically for the treatment of NSAID-induced gastrointestinal (GI) ulceration?

(A) Alprostadil
(B) Misoprostol
(C) Carboprost
(D) Dinoprostone
(E) Epoprostenol

8. Which of the following compounds is most likely to lower circulating levels of leukotrienes?

(A) Zileuton
(B) Montelukast
(C) Carprofen
(D) Aspirin
(E) Allopurinol

9. The action of aspirin that results in its greater efficacy as an antithrombotic (antiplatelet) drug is its ability to

(A) inhibit lipoxygenase as well as cyclooxygenase
(B) selectively inhibit cyclooxygenase I
(C) inhibit leukocyte migration
(D) promote uric acid excretion
(E) acetylate cyclooxygenase

10. A 6-year-old patient presents with the following symptoms. She is experiencing fever of 102°F, chills, sore throat, and rash. The best recommendation for treating the child's fever is

(A) pediatric aspirin, because it is flavored and will ensure patient compliance.
(B) choline salicylate, because it is in the liquid form and hence more easily swallowed.
(C) acetaminophen, since the specific disease state is not known.
(D) Any of the above recommendations are acceptable.
(E) None of the above recommendations is acceptable.

11. Which of the following drugs may be effective in the treatment of gouty arthritis by acting by two separate and distinct mechanisms?

(A) Allopurinol
(B) Probenecid
(C) Colchicine
(D) Indomethacin
(E) Sulfinpyrazone

12. Acute or chronic colchicine toxicity may be identified by which of the following signs/symptoms?

(A) Alopecia
(B) Blood dyscrasias
(C) Severe gastrointestinal (GI) upset
(D) All of the above
(E) None of the above

13. Patients taking chronic doses of nonselective NSAIDs should periodically be screened for which of the following toxicity(ies)?

(A) Nephrotoxicity
(B) Peripheral neuropathy
(C) Cardiotoxicity
(D) All of the above
(E) None of the above

14. Which of the following medications would represent arthritis therapy that is least likely to cause gastric ulceration?

(A) Aspirin
(B) Acetaminophen
(C) Piroxicam
(D) Meclofenamate
(E) Rofecoxib

15. In addition to their ability to decrease inflammatory prostaglandin synthesis, some NSAIDs may owe part of their effects to their ability to

(A) inhibit leukocyte migration
(B) inhibit leukotriene synthesis
(C) stabilize lysosomal membranes
(D) All of the above
(E) None of the above

Questions 16–20
J.D. is a 32-year-old female. Her medical history includes ongoing asthma, allergic rhinitis, gastroesophageal reflux disease, and juvenile arthritis. Her medication history indicates that she is currently taking the following medications:

1. Celecoxib
2. Cisapride
3. Zafirlukast
4. Ranitidine
5. Cetirizine

16. Which of the medications should be taken with food, to enhance their absorption?

(A) 2 and 3
(B) 1 and 4
(C) 2 and 4
(D) 3 and 5
(E) None of the above

17. Which medications are being taken for asthma and allergic reactions?

(A) 2 and 3
(B) 1 and 4
(C) 2 and 4
(D) 3 and 5
(E) None of the above

18. Which drugs are being used to treat her arthritis?

(A) 2 only
(B) 1 only
(C) 1 and 4
(D) 3 and 5
(E) None of the above

19. Which drugs are being used to treat her GERD?

(A) 2 and 3
(B) 1 and 4
(C) 2 and 4
(D) 3 and 5
(E) None of the above

20. Which drugs are acting by modulating the serotonergic autacoid system?

(A) 2 only
(B) 1 only
(C) 1 and 4
(D) 3 and 5
(E) None of the above

ANSWERS AND EXPLANATIONS

1. The answer is D *[I A 2 b, 4 b, c].*
Diphenhydramine and meclizine both possess strong anticholinergic activity. This will increase the risk of sedation, which could prove dangerous in a person who operates heavy machinery. Famotidine inhibits H_2, rather than H_1-receptors; hence, it would not be appropriate in this patient. Astemizole and fexofenadine both provide relief of allergic symptoms; however, astemizole may cause the prolonged QT interval associated with torsades de pointes arrhythmias. Fexofenadine lacks this effect, making it the best choice for this patient, who has a history of arrhythmias.

2. The answer is E *[I A 2 c].*
Pyrilamine and hydroxyzine are both inhibitors of the H_1-receptor, thus having no effect on gastric acid secretion (note that their anticholinergic effects could slightly decrease acid release, but this action is usually mild and a sufficient dose to provide the effect would also produce profound anticholinergic side effects). Cisapride is a serotonergic agonist and does not contribute to acid control. Omeprazole will reduce acid secretion to a greater extent than ranitidine. However, omeprazole does not act through the histaminergic receptor; rather, it directly inhibits the acid pump. Therefore, ranitidine, which competitively blocks histamine at the H_2-receptor, is the correct answer.

3. The answer is D *[II A 3].*
Since all three of these disease states represent some action of excessive acid secretion, lansoprazole, which also blocks the proton or acid pump, would be effective in reducing the acid-induced pain and damage associated with GERD, PUD, and Zollinger-Ellison syndrome.

4. The answer is B *[II B 4 a (1)].*
Rizatriptan and similar drugs act by blocking the effects of serotonin at its autoreceptor, thus reducing the actions of postsynaptic serotonin and possibly noradrenaline. In most areas, these neurotransmitters cause vasoconstriction. However, in the coronary vessels, serotonin normally causes vasodilation. Since this action is blocked by rizatriptan, vasoconstriction results, thus increasing the risk of an anginal attack, especially in patients with Prinzmetal's angina.

5. The answer is C *[II A 2 a, d, B 3 a, 4].*
Sumatriptan and ondansetron have no actions on gastric release of acid or on gastric tone. Cimetidine and omeprazole would both be effective in GERD by decreasing acid release, thus increasing gastric pH. Cisapride does not alter pH through changes in acid secretion or through neutralization of gastric acids. It exerts its action by serotonergically mediating acetylcholine release, which increases gastroesophageal sphincter tone, and by shortening gastric transit time, thus reducing sphincter pressure.

6. The answer is A *[II B 2, 3].*
Currently, drugs are available specifically for women with IBS characterized by either constipation or diarrhea. The intestinal inhibitory action of alosetron makes it useful for those patients with diarrhea-associated IBS, while the prokinetic actions of tegaserod support its use in those patients with constipation-associated IBS. There are currently no drugs available specifically for males with IBS. Tegaserod has no effect on gastric acid secretion and would, therefore, not be useful in Zollinger-Ellison syndrome.

7. The answer is B *[II C 3 a (3)].*
While most prostaglandin analogues are nonspecific in their sites of action and may produce similar physiological effects, misoprostol is specifically formulated and marketed for use in NSAID-induced PUD. This nonspecificity of effect is evident if one remembers that misoprostol may precipitate abortion or birth defects if sufficient exposure occurs during pregnancy.

8. The answer is A *[II D 1 a, b (1), (2)].*
Allopurinol will lower circulating levels of uric acid by preventing its formation from hypoxanthine, but it has no effect on leukotriene formation. Carprofen and aspirin both decrease prostaglandin formation. This action can cause a shift in the arachidonic pathway, actually increasing leukotriene formation.

Montelukast, while inhibiting the actions of leukotrienes at their receptors, does not alter the synthesis of the eicosanoid. Zileuton inhibits the enzyme lipoxygenase, thus reducing the synthesis of leukotrienes and decreasing their availability for circulation.

9. The answer is E *[III A 2 a].*
Although aspirin, like many other NSAIDs, inhibits cyclooxygenase, it is the only drug that irreversibly inhibits the enzyme. This action permits a longer duration of action, especially with the actions on thromboxane, which is the eicosanoid that is responsible for causing platelet aggregation. The ability of aspirin to inhibit lipoxygenase, selectively inhibit cyclooxygenase I, or inhibit leukocyte migration has never been demonstrated as clinically significant. It does act as a uricosuric at higher doses, but this action has no effect on platelet function.

10. The correct answer is C *[III A 3 a (3), B 3 b].*
The use of aspirin and presumably other salicylates has been correlated with a greater incidence of Reye's syndrome in children who suffer from certain viral infections. The potential risk outweighs the benefit of using aspirin as an antipyretic in these patients. Since acetaminophen is equally effective in the treatment of fever and has not been correlated with Reye's syndrome, most clinicians prefer it for fever of undiagnosed origin.

11. The answer is D *[III E 2 b].*
All of the agents listed are effective in the treatment of gout. Allopurinol inhibits xanthine oxidase, thus preventing uric acid formation. Probenecid is a uricosuric agent that promotes the excretion of uric acid. Colchicine inhibits the migration of inflammatory cells into the synovial spaces, thus preventing acute inflammation. While sulfinpyrazone is an NSAID-derivative, it has no anti-inflammatory activity. Its efficacy is due to its uricosuric actions. Indomethacin, like many other NSAIDs, will reduce prostaglandin formation, easing the pain associated with inflammation. Additionally, it inhibits leukocyte migration and stabilizes lysosomal membranes, thus inhibiting the inflammatory response, and possesses mild uricosuric activity, thus hastening the excretion of uric acid.

12. The correct answer is D *[III D 4 a].*
Alopecia and blood dyscrasias such as agranulocytosis and aplastic anemia are common with chronic administration of colchicine. Signs of acute intoxication include severe gastrointestinal upset, including nausea, emesis, and diarrhea. In acute attacks of gouty arthritis, the usual dose of colchicine is 0.5 mg every 2 hours for 4 doses or until GI upset begins. Therefore, mild forms of these symptoms are often used to signal the patient that therapy should be withdrawn.

13. The correct answer is A *[III E 4 a].*
As a class, the incidence of peripheral nerve damage or cardiac toxicity with NSAIDs is rare. However, NSAIDs produce a number of adverse reactions that affect the liver, GI tract, central nervous system, bone marrow, skin, and kidneys. As a class, almost all of these agents have the potential to produce nephrotoxicity.

14. The correct answer is E *[III 2 c].*
Acetaminophen is incorrect since it has relatively little peripheral anti-inflammatory activity. Aspirin, piroxicam, and meclofenamate are all effective in treating arthritis. However, the incidence of gastric damage is well documented for all three drugs. Rofecoxib, by virtue of its relative selectivity for the COX II enzyme, does not damage the gastric mucosa to the extent of nonselective NSAIDs. Although five patients to date have died from gastric bleeding after taking a selective COX II inhibitor, these reactions are rare, and most patients have little GI toxicity with these agents.

15. The correct answer is D *[III E 2 b].*
Many, but not all, NSAIDs have mechanisms that contribute to their ability to reduce inflammation, including inhibition of leukocyte and lymphocyte migration, inhibition of lipoxygenase, and stabilization of lysosomal membranes, thus preventing the release of inflammatory mediators such as the cytokines and eicosanoids.

16–20. The correct answers are: 16-A *[II A 4 a (2), D 4 b]*, **17-D** *[II A 3 b, D 4 b 2]*, **18-B** *[III E 3 b]*, **19-C** *[II A 3 c, B 3 a (4)]*, **20-A** *[II B 2 b (2)].*
The absorption of both zafirlukast and cisapride is limited if taken on an empty stomach. They should, therefore, be taken with food to enhance bioavailability. This patient is taking zafirlukast to reduce asthma-induced bronchoconstriction and cetirizine for her allergic rhinitis. While both of the agents in-

terfere with the inflammatory response, the zafirlukast is specific for bradykinin-induced bronchoconstriction, while the cetirizine provides nonsedating relief from the inflammatory response resulting from exposure to dusts and pollens. Celecoxib is the only medication in her profile that is approved for use in arthritis. It reduces pain and inflammation associated with the inflammatory prostaglandins by selectively inhibiting COX II. The patient is taking two medications for GERD. The ranitidine will reduce acid secretions, so that if reflux occurs, it will not be as painful or damaging to the esophageal mucosa. The cisapride, by acting at serotonergic receptors causing the release of acetylcholine, will increase esophageal sphincter tone and reduce sphincter pressure by hastening gastric transit time. This will reduce the likelihood of reflux.

15
Medicinal Chemistry and Pharmacology: Cardiovascular and Diuretic Drugs
J. Edward Moreton

I. INTRODUCTION. Many categories of drugs affect the cardiovascular (CV) and renal systems. Certain drugs can be used to treat heart failure (e.g., cardiac glycosides and diuretics), relieve angina pectoris (e.g., antianginal agents), and control dysrhythmias (e.g., antiarrhythmic agents). Others can reduce hypertension (e.g., antihypertensives, including a variety of diuretics, β-blocking agents, and arteriolar smooth-muscle dilators), treat the hyperlipidemias (e.g., antihyperlipidemic agents), reduce clotting and treat such conditions as venous thrombosis and pulmonary embolism (e.g., anticoagulants, thrombolytics), and treat anemias (e.g., antianemic agents).

II. CARDIAC GLYCOSIDES AND POSITIVE INOTROPES

A. Chemistry

1. Almost all of the cardiac glycosides (also called **cardiotonics**) are naturally occurring steroidal glycosides obtained from plant sources. **Digitoxin** is obtained from *Digitalis purpurea,* **digoxin** from *Digitalis lanata,* and **ouabain** from *Strophanthus gratus.*

2. The cardiac glycosides are closely related structurally, consisting of one or more sugars (i.e., **glycone portion**) and a steroidal nucleus (i.e., **aglycone or genin portion**) bonded through an **ether (glycosidic) linkage.** These agents also have an **unsaturated lactone substituent (cyclic ester)** on the genin portion. The prototypical agent is **digitoxin** (Figure 15-1).
   a. Digoxin (Lanoxin) has an additional hydroxyl group at position 12 (see Figure 15-1).
   b. Ouabain has a rhamnose glycone portion and additional hydroxyl groups at positions 1, 5, 11, and 19 (see Figure 15-1).

3. Removing the glycone portion causes decreased activity and increased toxicity from changes in polarity that cause erratic absorption from the gastrointestinal (GI) tract.

4. The **duration of action** of a cardiac glycoside is **inversely proportional to the number of hydroxyl groups,** which increase polarity. Increased polarity results in decreased protein binding, decreased liver biotransformation, and decreased renal tubular reabsorption.
   a. Digitoxin has a long duration of action and may accumulate.
   b. Ouabain, in contrast, has an extremely short duration of action and is effective only when given intravenously.

5. **Amrinone, inamrinone, and milrinone** are bipyridine derivatives with positive inotropic action (Figure 15-2).

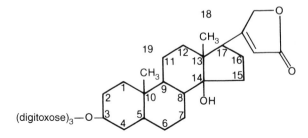

Figure 15-1. Structural formula of digitoxin (Crystodigin), the prototypical cardiac glycoside.

B. Pharmacology. Cardiac glycosides increase myocardial contractility and efficiency, improve systemic circulation, improve renal perfusion, and reduce edema. The electrophysiological effects of cardiac glycosides are summarized in Table 15-1. Angiotensin-converting enzyme (ACE) inhibitors and perhaps angiotensin AT_1-receptor antagonists, vasodilators such as nitroprusside, nitroglycerin, hydralazine, and diuretics may be important adjuncts to cardiac glycosides. ACE inhibitors may be considered as first-line treatment.

1. When given in therapeutic doses, cardiac glycosides produce positive inotropic effects by inhibiting membrane-bound Na^+/K^+-activated ATPase. These effects of cardiac glycosides increase the rate of tension development, the contractility, and the rate of relaxation of cardiac muscle. The effects include:
   a. Increase in intracellular sodium concentration
   b. Reduction in calcium transport from the cell by the sodium-calcium exchanger
   c. Facilitation of calcium entry via voltage-gated membrane channels
   d. Increased release of calcium from sarcoplasmic reticulum

2. Therapeutic doses of cardiac glycosides also cause:
   a. A negative chronotropic effect from increased vagal tone of the sinoatrial (SA) node
   b. Diminished central nervous system (CNS) sympathetic outflow from increased carotid sinus baroreceptor sensitivity
   c. Systemic arteriolar and venous constriction, which increases venous return and, thus, increases cardiac output

3. Amrinone and milrinone produce positive inotropic effects and vasodilation via selective inhibition of type III phosphodiesterase (PDE) isozyme, leading to an increase in cyclic adenosine monophosphate (cAMP) in cardiac and smooth muscle. Inhibition of type III PDE produces:
   a. Vasodilation and fall in vascular resistance
   b. Increased force of cardiac contraction
   c. Increased velocity of cardiac relaxation

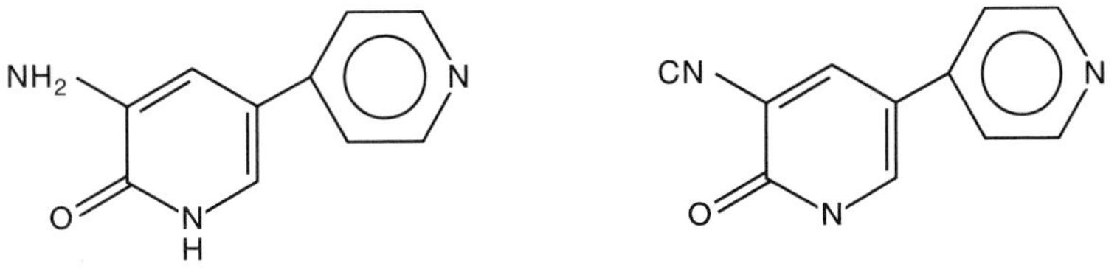

Figure 15-2. Structural formulas of bipyridine derivatives (*A*) amrinone (Inocor) and (*B*) milrinone (Primacor).

Table 15-1. Effects of Cardiac Glycosides on the Heart

	Atria	**AV Node**	**Ventricles**
Direct effects	Contractility ↑ ERP ↑ Conduction velocity ↓	ERP ↑ Conduction velocity ↓	Contractility ↑ ERP ↓ Automaticity ↑
Indirect effects	ERP ↓ Conduction velocity ↑	ERP ↑ Conduction velocity ↓	No effect
Effects on electrocardiogram	P changes	P-R interval ↑	Q-T ↓; T and ST depressed
Adverse effects	Extrasystole Tachycardia	AV depression or block	Fibrillation Extrasystole Tachycardia

AV = atrioventricular; ERP = effective refractory period. Arrows indicate changes: ↑ = increased; ↓ = decreased.
Reprinted with permission from Jacob LS: *Pharmacology*, 3rd ed. Malvern, PA, Harwal, 1992, p 96.

C. **Therapeutic indications**

   1. Congestive heart failure

   2. Atrial fibrillation

   3. Atrial flutter

   4. Paroxysmal atrial tachycardia

   5. Amrinone and milrinone are indicated for short-term treatment of congestive heart failure only.

D. **Adverse effects**

   1. **Early adverse effects** of cardiac glycosides represent the early stages of toxicity, including:
      a. GI effects such as anorexia, nausea, vomiting, and diarrhea
      b. CNS effects such as headache, visual disturbances (green or yellow vision), confusion, delirium, neuralgias, and muscle weakness

   2. **Later adverse effects** represent intoxication and include such serious cardiac disturbances as premature ventricular contractions, paroxysmal and nonparoxysmal atrial tachycardia, atrioventricular (AV) dissociation or block, ventricular tachycardia, and ventricular fibrillation.

III. DRUGS FOR TREATMENT OF MYOCARDIAL ISCHEMIA

A. **Chemistry**

   1. **Antianginal agents** include **nitrites** (i.e., organic esters of nitrous acid) such as amyl nitrite; **nitrates** (i.e., organic esters of nitric acid) such as nitroglycerin and isosorbide; **β-blockers** such as propranolol; and **calcium antagonists** such as verapamil and nifedipine (Figure 15-3).
      a. **Amyl nitrite** is a very volatile and flammable liquid administered by inhalation. It requires special precautions (especially restriction of smoking) during administration.

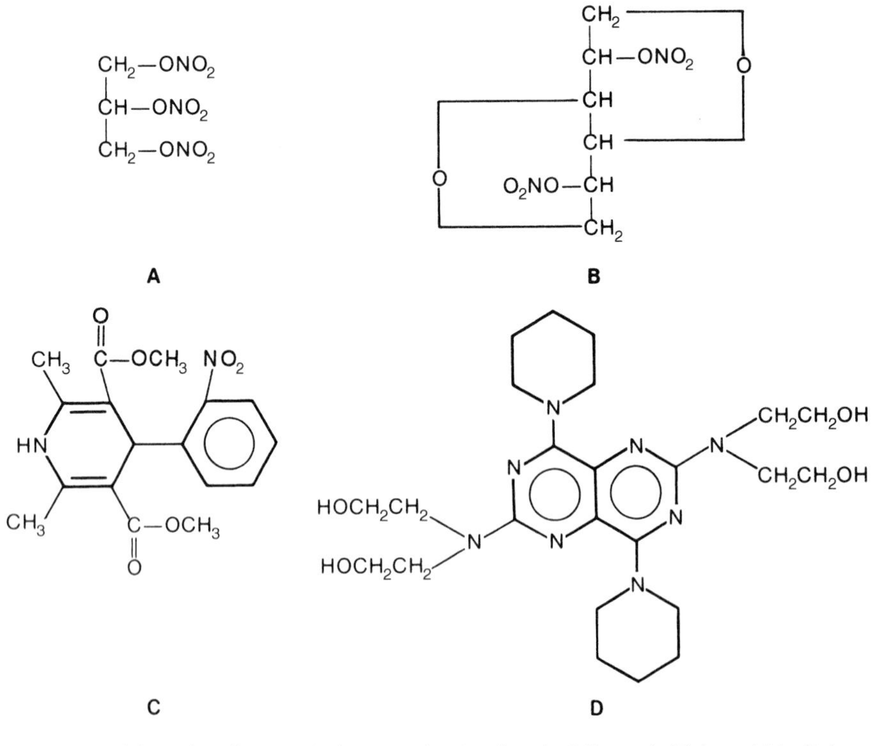

Figure 15-3. Structural formulas of antianginal agents (*A*) nitroglycerin (Nitrostat), (*B*) isosorbide dinitrate (Isordil), (*C*) nifedipine (Procardia), and (*D*) dipyridamole (Persantine).

    b. Nitroglycerin is also a very volatile and flammable liquid and requires great care during storage. It must be dispensed from its original glass containers and protected from body heat.

      (1) When given intravenously, nitroglycerin requires the use of special plastic administration sets to avoid absorption and loss of potency.

      (2) Nitroglycerin is metabolically unstable and undergoes extensive first-pass metabolism.

  2. Peripheral vasodilators include the dipiperidino-dipyrimidine dipyridamole (see Figure 15-3).

B. Pharmacology

  1. Nitrites and nitrates are fast-acting antianginal agents that directly relax vascular smooth muscle by formation of the free radical nitric oxide (NO), which is identical to endothelium-derived relaxing factor (EDRF). NO activates guanylyl cyclase to increase synthesis of cGMP within smooth muscle, resulting in dephosphorylation of light chain myosin and muscle relaxation. This causes peripheral pooling of the blood, diminished venous return (reduced preload), decreased systemic vascular resistance, and decreased arterial pressure (reduced afterload). These vascular effects:

    a. Reduce myocardial oxygen demand

    b. Cause redistribution of coronary blood flow along the collateral coronary arteries, improving perfusion of the ischemic myocardium

  2. β-Adrenergic blockers decrease sympathetic-mediated myocardial stimulation (see Chapter 13 V A 2, C 3). The resulting negative inotropic and negative chronotropic effects reduce myocardial oxygen requirements.

  3. Calcium antagonists (also known as **calcium channel blockers**) block calcium entry through the membranous calcium ion (Ca^{2+}) channels of coronary and peripheral vascular smooth muscle.

    a. Peripheral arterioles dilate and total peripheral resistance decreases, reducing afterload and reducing myocardial oxygen requirements.

    b. Calcium antagonists also increase oxygen delivery to the myocardium by dilating coronary arteries and arterioles.

  4. Dipyridamole relaxes smooth muscles, decreasing coronary vascular resistance and increasing coronary blood flow.

C. Therapeutic indications

  1. Nitrites and nitrates are used to relieve acute anginal attacks, as prophylaxis during anticipation of an acute anginal attack, and for long-term management of recurrent angina pectoris.

  2. β-Adrenergic blockers are used for adjunctive prophylaxis of chronic stable angina pectoris in combination with nitrites or nitrates.

  3. Calcium antagonists are used to treat chronic stable angina pectoris and variant (Prinzmetal's) angina.

  4. Dipyridamole is used primarily for prophylaxis of angina pectoris, although its beneficial effects are not well understood.

D. Adverse effects

  1. Nitrites and nitrates are associated with:

    a. CNS effects such as headache, apprehension, dizziness, and weakness

    b. CV effects such as hypotension, tachycardia, palpitations, and syncope

    c. Skin effects such as rash and dermatitis

    d. Methemoglobinemia

  2. β-Adrenergic blockers are associated with:

    a. Worsening of congestive heart failure

    b. Bradycardia and hypotension

    c. Reduced kidney blood flow and decreased glomerular filtration

  3. Calcium antagonists generally produce only mild adverse effects.

    a. When given in conjunction with β-adrenergic blockers, the CV effects of calcium antagonists may be enhanced, resulting in bradycardia, hypotension, peripheral edema, congestive heart failure, AV block, and asystole.

    b. Verapamil may also cause sleeplessness, muscle fatigue, nystagmus, and emotional depression. During the first week of therapy, verapamil increases serum digitalis concentrations and may cause digitalis toxicity.

  4. Dipyridamole is associated with:
    a. GI effects such as nausea, vomiting, and diarrhea
    b. CNS effects such as headache and dizziness
    c. CV effects such as hypotension (with excessive doses)

IV. ANTIARRHYTHMIC AGENTS

A. Chemistry. Antiarrhythmic agents have widely diverse chemical structures. They include representatives of these groups:

  1. Cinchona alkaloids (e.g., quinidine, an optical isomer of quinine)

  2. Amides [e.g., procainamide (Pronestyl), flecainide (Tambocor); disopyramide (Norpace)]

  3. Xylyl derivatives [e.g., lidocaine (Xylocaine), mexiletine (Mexitil)]

  4. Quaternary ammonium salts [e.g., bretylium (Bretylol)]

  5. Diiodobenzyloxyethylamines [e.g., amiodarone (Cordarone)]

  6. β-Blockers [e.g., nadolol (Corgard), propranolol (Inderal), esmolol (Brevibloc), acebutolol (Sectral)]

  7. Calcium antagonists [e.g., diltiazem (Cardizem), verapamil (Calan)]

  8. Hydantoins [e.g., phenytoin (Dilantin)]

B. Pharmacology. Antiarrhythmic agents are classified according to their ability to alter the action potential of cardiac cells (Tables 15-2 and 15-3).

  1. Class IA drugs (e.g., quinidine, procainamide, disopyramide) produce state-dependent sodium channel blockade to slow the rate of rise of phase 0 (the phase of rapid depolarization and reversal of transmembrane voltage) and prolong repolarization and effective refractory period.

  2. Class IB drugs (e.g., lidocaine, tocainide, mexiletine, phenytoin) have a minimal effect on the rate of rise of phase 0 and shorten repolarization.

  3. Class IC drugs (e.g., flecainide, propafenone) have a marked effect in slowing the rate of rise of phase 0 and in slowing conduction. They have little effect on repolarization. Encainide was withdrawn from the market but is available on a limited basis.

Table 15-2. Major Effects of Antiarrhythmic Drugs on Electrocardiogram

Drug	QRS	Q-T	P-R*
Quinidine Procainamide Amiodarone	↑	↑	→↑
Disopyramide	↑	↑	→
Lidocaine Phenytoin Tocainide Mexiletine	→	↓	→↑↓
Propranolol	→	↓	→↑

Arrows indicate changes: ↑ = increased; ↓ = decreased; → = no change.
*P-R intervals: All antiarrhythmic drugs have a variable response, usually with little observable effect. However, lidocaine hardly ever affects the P-R interval, whereas phenytoin and propranolol usually increase the P-R interval.
Reprinted with permission from Jacob LS: *Pharmacology,* 3rd ed. Malvern, PA, Harwal, 1992, p 102.

4. **Class II drugs** (e.g., propranolol, nadolol, esmolol, acebutolol) are β-adrenergic antagonists that competitively block catecholamine-induced stimulation of cardiac β-receptors and depress depolarization of phase 4.

5. **Class III drugs** (e.g., bretylium, amiodarone, sotalol, ibutilide, dofetilide) increase action potential duration by prolonging repolarization via blockade of the delayed rectifier potassium current I_{Kr}.

6. **Class IV drugs** (e.g., verapamil, diltiazem, bepridil) are calcium antagonists that block the slow inward current carried by calcium during phase 2 (i.e., long-sustained depolarization or the plateau of the action potential), increase the effective refractory period, and depress phase 4 depolarization.

7. **Digoxin and adenosine.** Digitalis glycosides (digoxin) elicit a vagotonic response that increases AV nodal refractoriness. Adenosine acts at G-protein–coupled adenosine receptors to increase AV nodal refractoriness.

8. **Moricizine** is a type I antiarrhythmic but not A, B, or C. It exhibits potent local anesthetic activity and myocardial membrane stabilizing activity. Moricizine reduces fast inward sodium current, decreasing the action potential duration and effective refractory period, and increases the PR, QRS, and QT_e interval.

C. **Therapeutic indications.** Antiarrhythmic agents are used to reduce abnormalities of impulse generation (ectopic pacemaker automaticity) and to modify the disturbances of impulse conduction within cardiac tissue. (For indications for specific agents, see Table 15-4.)

Table 15-3. Effects of Antiarrhythmic Drugs on Electrophysiologic Properties of the Heart

Drug Class	Automaticity		Effective Refractory Period		Membrane Responsiveness
	SA Node	**Purkinje Fibers**	**AV Node**	**Purkinje Fibers**	**Purkinje Fibers**
IA	→↑	↓→	↑→↓	↑↓	↓
IB	→	↓	→↓	↓	→↓
IC	→	↓	↑	↓	↓
II	↓	↓	↑	↓→↑	↓
III	↑↓	↑↓	↓→↑	↑	→
IV	↓	→↓	↑	→	→

Arrows indicate changes: ↑ = increased; ↓ = decreased; → = no change.

Table 15-4. Use of Antiarrhythmic Drugs in Common Cardiac Arrhythmias

Arrhythmia	Treatment of Choice	Alternatives
I. Supraventricular Atrial fibrillation or flutter	Digitalis to control ventricular rate, direct current (DC) shock for conversion	Quinidine to suppress recurrences after DC shock
Paroxysmal atrial or nodal tachycardia	Vagotonic maneuver; digitalis	Verapamil (quinidine, procainamide, disopyramide, and β-adrenergic antagonists may all be useful, especially prophylactically)
II. Ventricular Ventricular premature depolarization	Lidocaine	Procainamide, quinidine, or disopyramide for prolonged suppression
Ventricular tachycardia	DC shock	Lidocaine, procainamide, or mexiletine
III. Digitalis-induced	Lidocaine or phenytoin	Procainamide is somewhat useful; β-adrenergic antagonists are useful but have a high incidence of adverse effects

Reprinted with permission from Jacob LS: *Pharmacology*, 3rd ed. Malvern, PA, Harwal, 1992, p 102.

D. Adverse effects

1. **Class IA drugs** are associated with CV effects such as myocardial depression, AV block, ventricular dysrhythmias, asystole, and hypotension, and with GI effects such as GI upset, nausea, vomiting, and diarrhea. In addition:
   a. **Quinidine** can cause cinchonism, with tinnitus, confusion, photophobia, headache, and psychosis.
   b. **Procainamide** can cause systemic lupus erythematosus–like syndrome.
   c. **Disopyramide** can cause congestive heart failure and antimuscarinic effects.

2. **Class IB drugs** are associated with CNS effects, including CNS depression, drowsiness, disorientation, and paresthesias; CV effects, including hypotension and circulatory collapse; and hepatitis. In addition:
   a. **Lidocaine** can cause seizures and respiratory arrest.
   b. **Tocainide** can cause pneumonitis and blood dyscrasias.
   c. **Mexiletine** can cause hepatic injury and blood dyscrasias.
   d. **Phenytoin** can cause nystagmus, decreased mental function, and blood dyscrasias.

3. **Class IC drugs** are associated with:
   a. CV effects, including worsening of arrhythmias in patients with ventricular arrhythmias, particularly patients with a history of myocardial infarction (MI). They can worsen sinus node dysfunction and heart failure.
   b. Visual disturbances such as blurred or double vision

4. **Class II drugs** are associated with:
   a. CV effects such as hypotension, AV block, and asystole
   b. Respiratory effects such as bronchospasm

5. **Class III drugs** are associated with:
   a. CV effects such as hypotension and initially increased dysrhythmias
   b. GI effects such as nausea and vomiting

6. **Class IV drugs** are associated with CV adverse effects such as hypotension, bradycardia, AV block, congestive heart failure, and asystole.

7. **Cardiac glycosides** (see II D). **Adenosine** causes asystole lasting less than 5 seconds and is the therapeutic objective.

8. Because of its proarrhythmic activity, **moricizine** is reserved for patients with life-threatening ventricular arrhythmias.

V. ANTIHYPERTENSIVE AGENTS

A. **Chemistry.** Antihypertensive agents vary so widely in chemical structure that they are usually classified by mechanism of action rather than chemical class (Table 15-5).

B. **Pharmacology.** Antihypertensive agents lower blood pressure by reducing total peripheral resistance or cardiac output through a variety of mechanisms (see Table 15-5).

1. **Diuretics** such as thiazides create a negative sodium balance, reduce blood volume, and decrease vascular smooth-muscle responsiveness to vasoconstrictors (see VI C).

2. **Vasodilators** such as diazoxide and minoxidil are potassium channel activators that produce membrane hyperpolarization, while hydralazine may stimulate formation of EDRF (NO) to decrease arterial resistance. Sodium nitroprusside releases NO to relax both arterioles and veins.

3. **Peripheral sympatholytics** interfere with adrenergic function by blocking postganglionic adrenergic receptors (e.g., propranolol, prazosin), limiting the release of neurotransmitters from adrenergic neurons (e.g., guanethidine), or depleting intraneuronal catecholamine storage sites (e.g., reserpine).

4. **Central α_2-sympathomimetics** (e.g., clonidine, methyldopa) appear to mediate their effects by stimulating presynaptic α_2-inhibitory receptors, resulting in a negative sympathetic outflow and lowered peripheral resistance.

Table 15-5. Classification of Antihypertensive Agents by Their Mechanism of Action

Mechanism of Action	Drug
Vasodilators	
Arteriolar	Diazoxide (Hyperstat IV)
	Hydralazine (Apresoline)
	Minoxidil (Loniten)
Arteriolar and venous	Nitroprusside (Nipride)
Peripheral sympatholytics	Acebutolol (Sectral)
	Atenolol (Tenormin)
	Betaxolol (Kerlone)
	Bisoprolol (Zebeta)
	Carteolol (Cartrol)
	Carvediolol (Coreg)
	Doxazosin (Cardura)
	Guanadrel (Hylorel)
	Guanethidine (Ismelin)
	Labetalol (Trandate)
	Metoprolol (Lopressor)
	Nadolol (Corgard)
	Penbutolol (Levatol)
	Pindolol (Visken)
	Prazosin (Minipress)
	Propranolol (Inderal)
	Reserpine (Serpasil)
	Terazosin (Hytrin)
	Timolol (Blocardren)
Central α_2-sympathomimetics	Clonidine (Catapres)
	Guanabenz (Wytensin)
	Guanfacine (Tenex)
	Methyldopa (Aldomet)
Calcium channel blockers	Amlodipine (Norvasc)
	Diltiazem (Cardizem) SR
	Felodipine (Plendil)
	Isradipine (DynaCirc)
	Nicardipine (Cardene)
	Nifedipine (Procardia) SR
	Verapamil (Calan)
Angiotensin II–receptor antagonists	Candesartan (Atacand)
	Ibersartan (Avopro)
	Losartan (Cozarr)
	Telmisartan (Micardis)
	Valsartan (Diovan)
Angiotensin-converting enzyme inhibitors	Benazepril (Lotensin)
	Captopril (Capoten)
	Enalapril (Vasotec)
	Fosinopril (Monopril)
	Lisinopril (Prinivil)
	Moexipril (Univasc)
	Perindopril (Aceon)
	Quinapril (Accupril)
	Ramipril (Altace)
	Trandolapril (Mavik)

5. **Calcium channel blockers** (e.g., amlodipine, diltiazem, felodipine, isradipine, nicardipine, nifedipine, verapamil) lower vascular resistance and blood pressure via blockade of voltage-gated calcium channels. Arterioles are more sensitive than veins.

6. **ACE inhibitors** (e.g., captopril) block the conversion of inactive angiotensin I to the potent vasoconstrictor angiotensin II. The reduced angiotensin II concentration also lowers aldosterone concentration, which limits sodium retention.

7. **Angiotensin II–receptor antagonists** (e.g., losartan) are nonpeptide antagonists of the AT_1 angiotensin II–receptor subtype located in vasculature, myocardium, brain, kidney, and adrenal glomerulosa. They produce vasodilation, cause loss of salt and water to decrease plasma volume, and decrease myogenic activity.

C. **Therapeutic indications**

1. Antihypertensive agents are used separately or in combination to **treat high blood pressure.**

2. These agents may also be administered parenterally to **treat hypertensive emergencies** such as malignant hypertension, eclampsia, or the severe hypertension associated with excess catecholamines. Parenteral therapy may include some combination of these agents:
   a. **Arteriolar and venous vasodilator** such as nitroprusside
   b. **Arteriolar vasodilator** such as diazoxide or hydralazine
   c. **Dual α-adrenergic– and β-adrenergic–receptor blockers** such as labetalol
   d. **β-Blocking agent** such as propranolol
   e. **Ganglionic blocking agent** such as trimethaphan

D. **Adverse effects**

1. **Diuretics (thiazides)** can cause:
   a. Fluid and solute imbalances such as hypokalemia, hypercalcemia, hyperuricemia, hypomagnesemia, hyponatremia, and hyperglycemia
   b. Increased serum low-density lipoprotein cholesterol and triglyceride concentrations
   c. Other effects (see VI C 4)

2. **Vasodilators** are associated with:
   a. GI upset
   b. CNS effects such as headache and dizziness
   c. CV effects such as tachycardia, fluid retention, and worsening of angina
   d. Other effects such as nasal congestion, hepatitis, glomerulonephritis, and systemic lupus erythematosus–like syndrome

3. **Peripheral sympatholytics** are associated with a variety of adverse effects, depending on the specific agent.
   a. **β-Blockers** (e.g., propranolol) are associated with:
      (1) CV effects such as bradycardia, congestive heart failure, and Raynaud's phenomenon
      (2) GI upset
      (3) Blood dyscrasias
      (4) CNS effects such as depression, hallucinations, organic brain syndrome, and transient hearing loss
      (5) Other effects such as increased airway resistance, increased serum triglyceride concentrations, decreased high-density lipoprotein cholesterol concentrations, and psoriasis
      (6) Cardiac arrhythmias if withdrawal is abrupt
   b. **Prazosin** is associated with:
      (1) CV effects such as sudden syncope with the first dose, palpitations, and fluid retention
      (2) CNS effects such as headache, drowsiness, weakness, dizziness, and vertigo
      (3) Antimuscarinic effects and priapism
   c. **Guanethidine** is associated with:
      (1) CV effects such as bradycardia, orthostatic hypotension, and sodium and water retention
      (2) Diarrhea
      (3) Aggravation of bronchial asthma

    d. Reserpine is associated with:
- **(1)** CNS effects such as nightmares, depression, and drowsiness
- **(2)** CV effects such as bradycardia
- **(3)** GI effects such as GI upset and activation of peptic ulcer
- **(4)** Nasal stuffiness

4. Central α_2-sympathomimetics also have adverse effects that vary with the specific agent.
    a. Clonidine is associated with:
- **(1)** CNS effects such as sedation and drowsiness
- **(2)** Dry mouth and severe rebound hypertension
- **(3)** Insomnia, headache, and cardiac dysrhythmias (with sudden withdrawal)

    b. Methyldopa is associated with:
- **(1)** CV effects such as orthostatic hypotension and bradycardia
- **(2)** CNS effects such as sedation and fever
- **(3)** GI effects such as colitis
- **(4)** Other effects such as hepatitis, cirrhosis, Coombs'-positive hemolytic anemia, and systemic lupus erythematosus–like syndrome

5. Calcium channel blockers are associated with CV effects resulting in hypotension, dizziness, headache, and flushing. When given with β-adrenergic blockers, their effects may be enhanced, resulting in bradycardia, hypotension, peripheral edema, congestive heart failure, AV block, and asystole.

6. ACE inhibitors are associated with:
- **a.** CV effects such as hypotension and syncope
- **b.** Hematologic effects such as neutropenia and agranulocytosis
- **c.** Other effects such as chronic cough, anorexia, polyuria, oliguria, acute renal failure, cholestatic jaundice, and (rarely) angioedema

7. Angiotensin II–receptor antagonists are associated with adverse effects similar to ACE inhibitors, except that cough and angioedema, which are independent of angiotensin antagonism, occur less frequently.

VI. DIURETICS

A. Osmotic diuretics

1. Chemistry. Osmotic diuretics (e.g., mannitol, urea, glycerin, isosorbide) are highly polar, water-soluble agents with a low renal threshold (Figure 15-4).

2. Pharmacology
- **a.** Osmotic diuretics are relatively inert chemicals that are freely filtered at the glomerulus and poorly reabsorbed from the renal tubule. By increasing the osmolarity of the glomerular filtrate, they **limit tubular reabsorption of water** and, thus, **promote diuresis.**
- **b.** Because these agents increase water, sodium, chloride, and bicarbonate excretion, they cause an **increase in urinary pH.**

3. Therapeutic indications. Osmotic diuretics are used to:
- **a.** Help prevent and treat oliguria and anuria
- **b.** Reduce cerebral edema and decrease intracranial pressure
- **c.** Reduce intraocular pressure

4. Adverse effects. Osmotic diuretics are associated with:
- **a.** Headache and blurred vision
- **b.** Increased blood volume that worsens congestive heart failure

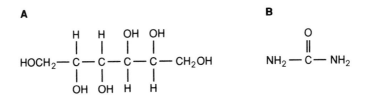

Figure 15-4. Structural formulas of osmotic diuretics (*A*) mannitol (Osmitrol) and (*B*) urea (Ureaphil).

B. Carbonic anhydrase inhibitors

1. **Chemistry.** Carbonic anhydrase inhibitors are aromatic or heterocyclic sulfonamides with a prominent thiadiazole nucleus. **Acetazolamide** is the prototypical agent (Figure 15-5).

2. **Pharmacology**
   a. Carbonic anhydrase inhibitors **noncompetitively inhibit the enzyme carbonic anhydrase.** This prevents the enzyme from providing the tubular hydrogen ions needed for exchange with sodium in the proximal tubule, resulting in sodium bicarbonate diuresis.
   b. Because these agents increase water, sodium, potassium, and bicarbonate excretion, they cause an **alkaline urinary pH.**

3. **Therapeutic indications.** Carbonic anhydrase inhibitors are used to:
   a. Reduce edema (as adjunct diuretic therapy)
   b. Reduce intraocular pressure (retard aqueous humor formation)
   c. Alkalinize the urine, enhancing excretion of acidic drugs and their metabolites
   d. Treat motor disorders such as petit mal epilepsy, paroxysmal chorea and dystonia, periodic ataxia, and some cases of essential tremor

4. **Adverse effects.** Carbonic anhydrase inhibitors are associated with:
   a. CNS effects such as CNS depression, drowsiness, sedation, fatigue, disorientation, and paresthesia
   b. GI effects such as GI upset, nausea, vomiting, and constipation
   c. Hematologic effects such as bone marrow depression, thrombocytopenia, hemolytic anemia, leukopenia, and agranulocytosis
   d. Hyperchloremic metabolic acidosis
   e. Sulfonamide-type hypersensitivity reactions

C. Benzothiadiazide diuretics

1. **Chemistry**
   a. The commonly used thiazide diuretics are primarily closely related **benzothiadiazides with variable substituents.** The prototypical agent is chlorothiazide (Figure 15-6*A*).
   b. Optimal diuretic activity depends on certain **structural features.**
      (1) The benzene ring must have a **sulfonamide** group (preferably unsubstituted) in position 7 and a **halogen** (usually a chloro group) or a **trifluoromethyl group** in position 6 (see Figure 15-6).
      (2) **Saturation of the 3,4-double bond** increases potency as with hydrochlorothiazide (see Figure 15-6*B*).
      (3) **Lipophilic substituents** at position 3 or **methyl groups** at position 2 enhance potency and prolong activity as with cyclothiazide (see Figure 15-6*C*) and bendroflumethiazide.
      (4) **Replacement of the sulfonyl group** in position 1 by a **carbonyl group** prolongs activity as with quinethazone (see Figure 15-6*D*).
   c. A few **sulfamoylbenzamides** (e.g., indapamide, chlorthalidone) have activity similar to that of the benzothiadiazides (Figure 15-7).
   d. **Benzothiadiazines without the sulfonamide group** (e.g., diazoxide) exhibit antihypertensive activity but lack diuretic activity (Figure 15-8).

2. **Pharmacology**
   a. Benzothiadiazides **directly inhibit sodium and chloride reabsorption** on the luminal membrane of the early segment of the distal convoluted tubule.
   b. These agents increase water, sodium, chloride, potassium, and bicarbonate excretion and decrease calcium excretion and uric acid secretion. They may cause an **alkaline urinary pH** by inhibiting carbonic anhydrase.

3. **Therapeutic indications.** Benzothiadiazides are used to treat:
   a. Chronic edema
   b. Hypertension
   c. Congestive heart failure (as adjunctive edema therapy)

4. **Adverse effects.** Benzothiadiazides are associated with:
   a. CNS effects such as headache, dizziness, paresthesias, drowsiness, and restlessness
   b. GI effects such as GI irritation, nausea, vomiting, abdominal bloating, and constipation
   c. Cardiovascular effects such as orthostatic hypotension, palpitations, hemoconcentration, and venous thrombosis

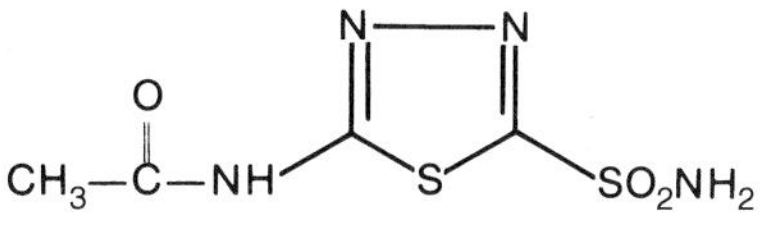

Figure 15-5. Structural formula of acetazolamide (Diamox), the prototypical carbonic anhydrase inhibitor.

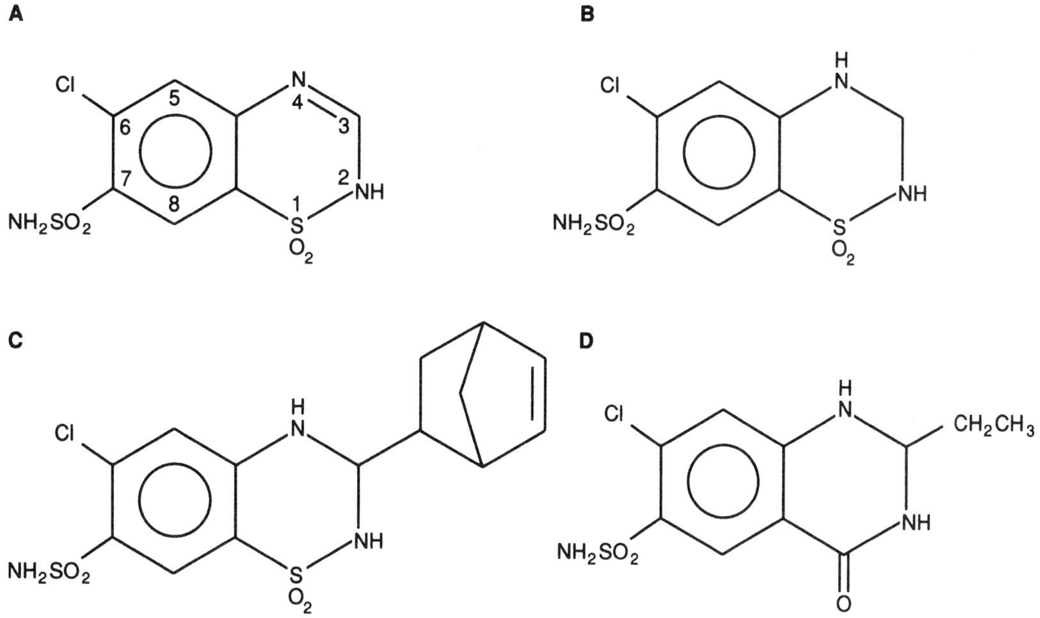

Figure 15-6. Structural formulas of (*A*) chlorothiazide (Diuril), the prototypical benzothiadiazide diuretic, and (*B*) hydrochlorothiazide (Hydrodiuril), as well as (*C*) cyclothiazide (Anhydron) and (*D*) quinethazone (Hydromox), related compounds with substituents that prolong activity and enhance potency.

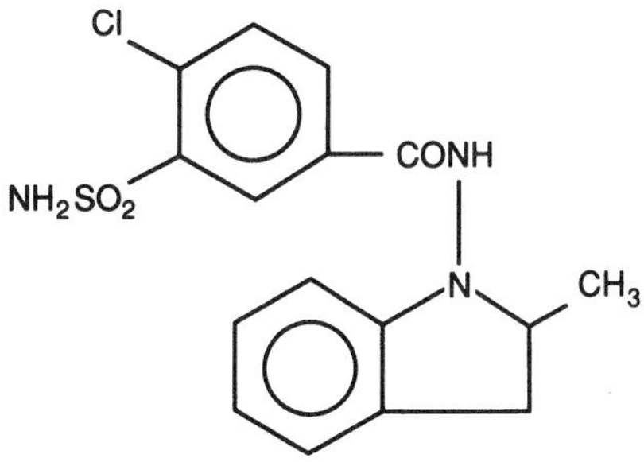

Figure 15-7. Structural formula of indapamide (Lozol), a sulfamoylbenzamide with pharmacological activity similar to that of the benzothiadiazide diuretics.

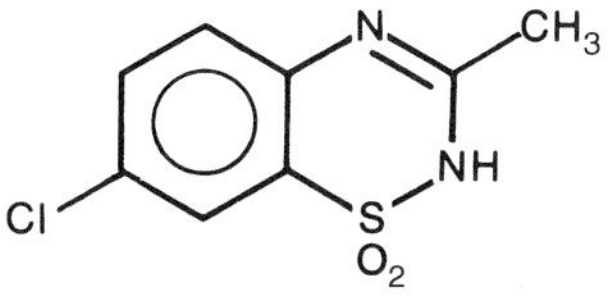

Figure 15-8. Structural formula of diazoxide (Hyperstat), a benzothiadiazine lacking a sulfonamide group and diuretic action.

   d. Hematologic effects such as blood dyscrasias, leukopenia, thrombocytopenia, agranu-
      locytosis, aplastic anemia, hemolytic anemia, and rash
   e. Fluid and electrolyte imbalances such as hypokalemia, hyponatremia, and hypercalcemia
   f. Muscular cramps
   g. Hyperuricemia and acute gout attacks
   h. Hypercholesterolemia and hypertriglyceridemia
   i. Sulfonamide-type hypersensitivity reaction

D. Loop diuretics

1. **Chemistry.** Loop diuretics are anthranilic acid derivatives with a sulfonamide substituent
   (e.g., furosemide, bumetanide) or aryloxyacetic acids without a sulfonamide substituent (e.g.,
   ethacrynic acid) [Figure 15-9].

2. **Pharmacology**
   a. These agents act principally at the thick ascending limb of the loop of Henle, where
      they **inhibit the cotransport of sodium, potassium, and chloride from the luminal fil-
      trate.**
   b. Loop diuretics increase excretion of water, sodium, potassium, calcium, and chloride;
      decrease uric acid secretion; and cause **no change in urinary pH.**

3. **Therapeutic indications.** Loop diuretics are used to treat:
   a. Edema from congestive heart failure, hepatic cirrhosis, and renal disease
   b. Pulmonary edema and ascites

4. **Adverse effects.** Loop diuretics are associated with:
   a. Fluid and solute imbalances such as dehydration, hypokalemia, hyperuricemia, hyper-
      calciuria, and azotemia
   b. CNS effects such as headache, vertigo, blurred vision, tinnitus, and (rarely) irreversible
      hearing loss
   c. Hematologic effects such as thrombocytopenia and agranulocytosis
   d. Cardiovascular effects such as orthostatic hypotension
   e. GI effects such as nausea, vomiting, and diarrhea
   f. Leg cramps
   g. Hypercholesterolemia and hypertriglyceridemia
   h. Sulfonamide-type hypersensitivity reaction

E. Potassium-sparing diuretics

1. **Chemistry.** The potassium-sparing diuretics are pteridine or pyrazine derivatives (e.g.,
   triamterene, amiloride) or steroid analogue antagonists of aldosterone (e.g., spironolactone) [Figure 15-10].

2. **Pharmacology**
   a. Spironolactone and **eplerenone** act as **competitive inhibitors of aldosterone** at miner-
      alocorticoid receptors in the late distal tubule and collecting duct. They interfere with al-
      dosterone-mediated sodium–potassium exchange, decreasing potassium secretion.
   b. Triamterene and amiloride, which are not aldosterone antagonists, act directly on the
      late distal tubule and collecting duct. They disrupt sodium exchange with potassium
      and hydrogen by blocking sodium channels and decreasing the driving force for secre-
      tion of potassium and hydrogen.
   c. The potassium-sparing diuretics increase bicarbonate excretion and cause an **alkaline
      urinary pH.**

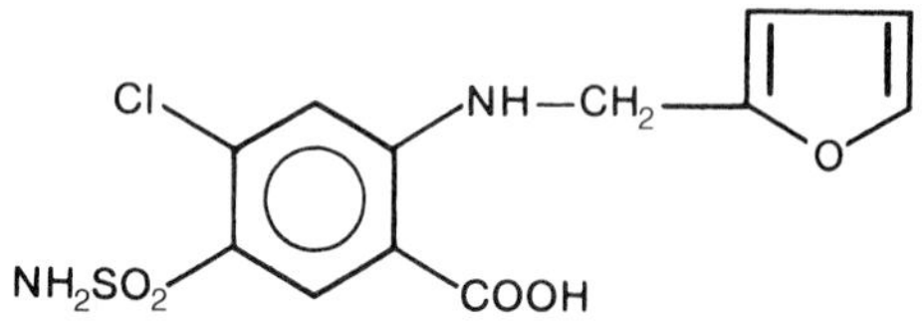

A 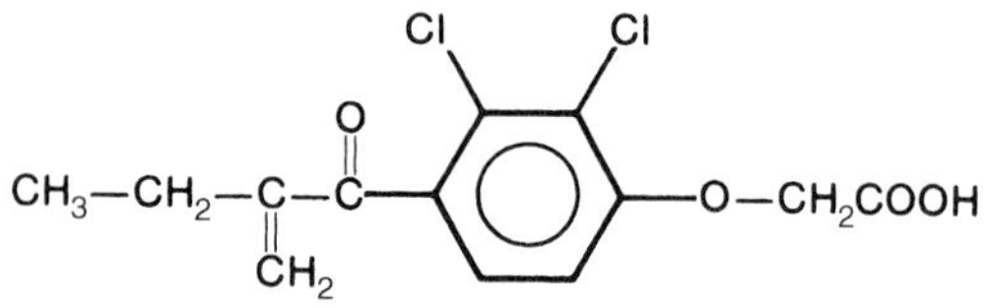   **B**

Figure 15-9. Structural formulas of loop diuretics (*A*) furosemide (Lasix) and (*B*) ethacrynic acid (Edecrin).

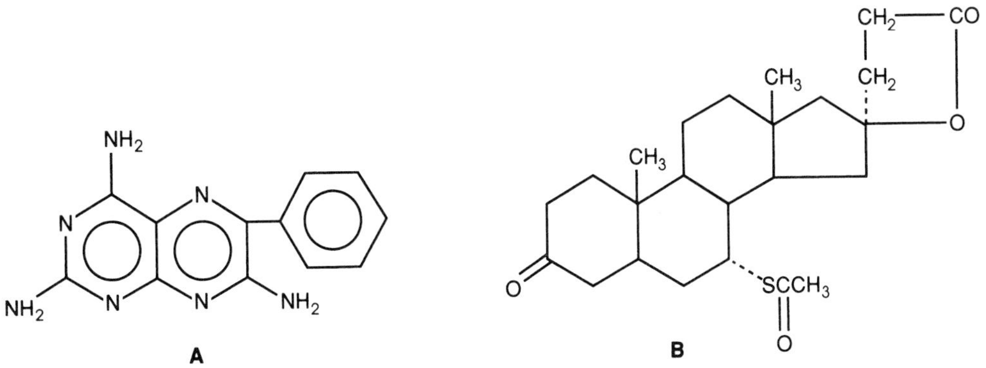

Figure 15-10. Structural formulas of potassium-sparing diuretics (*A*) triamterene (Dyrenium) and (*B*) spironolactone (Aldactone).

   3. Therapeutic indications. Potassium-sparing diuretics are used:
   a. As adjunctive therapy to treat edema from congestive heart failure, hepatic cirrhosis, nephrotic syndrome, and hyperaldosteronism (primary and secondary)
   b. As adjunctive therapy (with thiazides and loop diuretics) to treat hypertension
   c. To treat or prevent hypokalemia

   4. Adverse effects
   a. Spironolactone is associated with:
      (1) Hyperkalemia
      (2) GI effects such as GI upset, GI bleeding, gastritis, nausea, abdominal cramps, and diarrhea
      (3) Endocrine effects such as gynecomastia, menstrual irregularities, and hirsutism
      (4) CNS effects such as mental confusion and lethargy
   b. Triamterene and **amiloride** are associated with:
      (1) Hyperkalemia
      (2) GI effects such as GI upset, GI bleeding, nausea, and vomiting
      (3) CNS effects such as headache and dizziness
      (4) Increased uric acid levels in patients with gouty arthritis (with triamterene)
      (5) Methemoglobinemia in patients with alcoholic cirrhosis (with triamterene, which inhibits dihydrofolate reductase)

VII. ANTIHYPERLIPIDEMIC AGENTS

   A. Chemistry. Antihyperlipidemic agents vary in chemical structure and are usually classified by their site of action—locally in the intestine (nonabsorbable agents) or systemically (absorbable agents).

   1. Nonabsorbable agents are **bile acid sequestrants.** These agents are hydrophilic, water-insoluble resins that bind to bile acids in the intestine. Examples include **cholestyramine chloride,** a basic anion-exchange resin consisting of trimethylbenzylammonium groups in a large copolymer of styrene and divinylbenzene, and **colestipol hydrochloride,** a copolymer of diethylpentamine and epichlorohydrin (Figure 15-11).

   2. Absorbable agents include **nicotinic acid** (but not the structurally similar nicotinamide), the aryloxyisobutyric acid derivatives **clofibrate** and **fenofibrate** (prodrugs) and **gemfibrozil,** the sulfur-containing bis-phenol **probucol,** the 3-hydroxy-3-methylglutaryl-coenzyme A (HMG-CoA) reductase inhibitor **lovastatin,** and the fatty fish oils containing large amounts of **eicosapentaenoic acid (EPA)** and **docosahexaenoic acid (DHA)** [Figure 15-12].

   B. Pharmacology. Antihyperlipidemic agents **increase catabolism** or **reduce lipoprotein production** (e.g., lovastatin, clofibrate, gemfibrozil) or **increase the efficiency of lipoprotein removal** (e.g., cholestyramine, colestipol).

   C. Therapeutic indications. These agents are used (in conjunction with appropriate diet and exercise) to reduce plasma lipoprotein concentrations.

D. Adverse effects

1. **Nonabsorbable agents** (e.g., cholestyramine, colestipol) are associated with GI distress, including abdominal bloating, nausea, dyspepsia, steatorrhea, and constipation or diarrhea.

2. **Absorbable agents** (e.g., statins, fibrates) are associated with GI distress, skin rash, and leukopenia.
   a. **Lovastatin** and other statins (e.g., simvastatin, pravastatin, fluvastatin, atorvastatin, cerivastatin) may increase blood transaminase and creatinine phosphokinase activity associated with myopathy, especially when combined with fibrates or cyclosporins.
   b. **Clofibrate** may cause nausea, vomiting, dysphagia, weight gain, alopecia, and breast tenderness. Clofibrate carries a warning of hepatic **tumorigenesis** and cholelithiasis.
   c. **Gemfibrozil** may also cause skeletal muscle pain, blurred vision, and anemia.
   d. **Nicotinic acid** produces flushing associated with pruritus, which may be alleviated by one aspirin per day. Tolerance to nicotinic acid develops in 1–2 weeks. High doses of nicotinic acid (2 g/day) may produce hepatic damage.
   e. **Probucol** may be associated with prolonged QT interval, syncope, ventricular arrhythmia, and sudden death and should not be given to patients with a history of myocardial infarction or to patients taking Class I or Class II antiarrhythmic drugs, tricyclic antidepressants, or phenothiazines.

VIII. ANTICOAGULANT, ANTIPLATELET, AND THROMBOLYTIC AGENTS

A. **Anticoagulants.** The major anticoagulant agents are **heparin** and the **oral anticoagulants.**

1. **Chemistry**
   a. **Heparin** is a large, highly acidic mucopolysaccharide composed of sulfated D-glucosamine and D-glucuronic acid molecules (Figure 15-13).
   b. **Low–molecular-weight heparin (LMWH) fragments** (1–10 kDa) **enoxaparin, dalteparin, tinzaparin, and ardeparin** are produced through controlled depolymerization of heparin, but they are not interchangeable with heparin in their actions and use.
   (1) Because they are highly acidic, heparin and LMWH fragments exist as anions at physiologic pH and are very poorly absorbed from the GI tract. Thus, they are usually administered parenterally as the sodium salt.

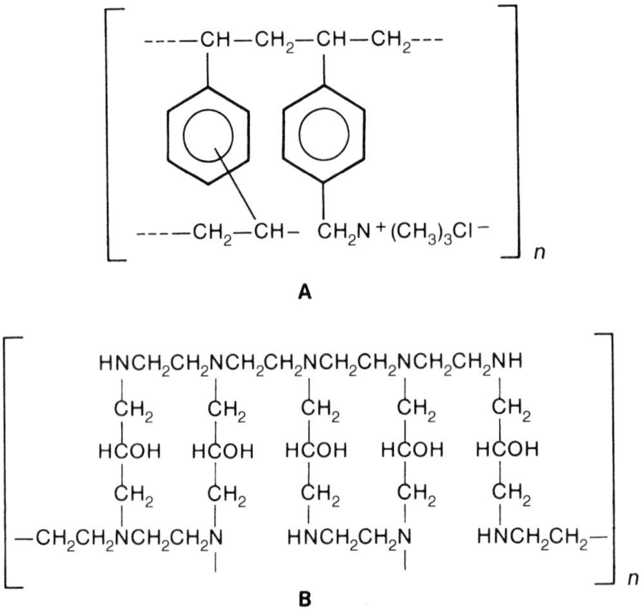

Figure 15-11. Structural formulas of nonabsorbable antihyperlipidemic agents (*A*) cholestyramine chloride (Questran) and (*B*) colestipol hydrochloride (Colestid).

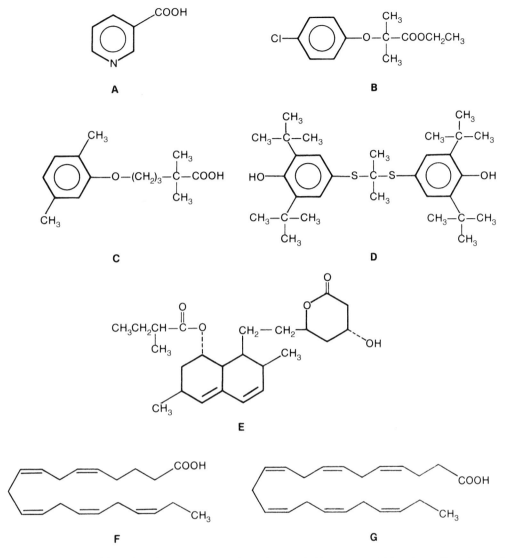

Figure 15-12. Structural formulas of (*A*) nicotinic acid (niacin), (*B*) clofibrate (Atromid-S), (*C*) gemfibrozil (Lopid), (*D*) probucol (Lorelco), (*E*) lovastatin (Mevacor), (*F*) eicosapentaenoic acid (found in Promega, Proto-Chol, and others), and (*G*) docosahexaenoic acid (found in Promega, Proto-Chol, and others). These agents are absorbable anti-hyperlipidemics.

(**2**) The action of heparin and LMWH fragments is quickly terminated by **protamine sulfate,** a highly basic protein that combines chemically with them in approximately equal amounts (mg:mg).

c. Low–molecular-weight heparinoids (danaparoid) are **glycosaminoglycans** extracted from porcine mucosa.

d. Lepirudin is a recombinant deoxyribonucleic acid (DNA)-derived 65 amino acid polypeptide nearly identical to hirudin, which belongs to the group of isopolypeptides of the leech *Hirudo medicinalis.* **Argatroban** and **bivalirudin** are synthetic thrombin inhibitors.

e. Oral anticoagulants consist of the highly effective **coumarin derivatives** and the relatively unimportant **indanedione derivatives.**

(**1**) The **coumarin derivatives** (e.g., **warfarin, dicumarol**) are water-insoluble, weakly acidic 4-hydroxycoumarin lactones (Figure 15-14).

(**a**) These agents are **chemically related to vitamin K,** and their mechanism of action is directly related to their antagonism of the reductase responsible for reducing vitamin K epoxide to the reduced hydroquinone.

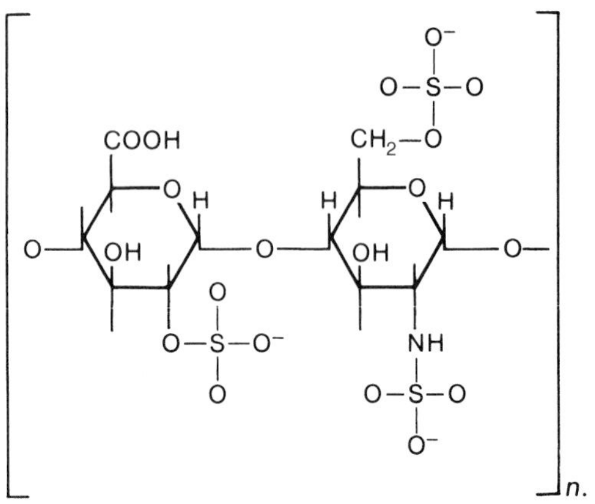

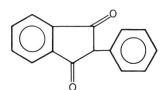

Figure 15-13. Structural formula of heparin, a muco-polysaccharide anticoagulant agent.

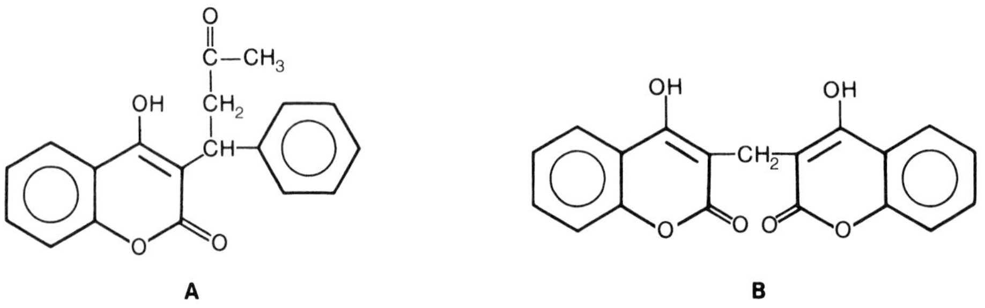

A

B

Figure 15-14. Structural formulas of coumarin-derivative oral anticoagulants (*A*) warfarin (Coumadin) and (*B*) dicumarol.

Figure 15-15. Structural formula of the indanedione-derivative oral anticoagulant phenindione (Hedulin).

   (b) These agents are also highly protein bound and extensively metabolized in the liver. These characteristics, in addition to their relatively narrow therapeutic index, make them very susceptible to significant drug interactions.
   (2) Phenindione represents a typical **indanedione derivative** (Figure 15-15).

2. Pharmacology
   a. Heparin catalyzes the inhibition of thrombin by antithrombin III (heparin cofactor), preventing the conversion of fibrinogen to fibrin.
   b. LMWH fragments are unable to catalyze inhibition of thrombin, but they catalyze inhibition by antithrombin III of factor Xa, which is responsible for conversion of prothrombin to thrombin. Heparin prolongs blood-clotting time both *in vivo* and *in vitro*, while LMWH fragments have minimal *in vitro* effect.
   c. Glycosaminoglycans (Danaparoid) inhibit fibrin formation by inhibition of clotting factors Xa and IIa (lesser effect).
   d. Lepirudin, argatroban, and **bivalirudin** bind to and block the thrombogenic activity of thrombin.
   e. Oral anticoagulants interfere with the vitamin K–dependent hepatic synthesis of the active clotting factors II (prothrombin), VII, IX, and X and the anticoagulant proteins C and S. These agents prolong blood-clotting time *in vivo* only.

3. **Therapeutic indications**
   a. **Heparin** is indicated:
      (1) For the prophylaxis and treatment of venous thrombosis, pulmonary embolism, peripheral arterial embolism, and atrial fibrillation with embolization
      (2) To prevent clotting during arterial surgery and cardiac surgery
      (3) To diagnose and treat disseminated intravascular coagulation (DIC)
      (4) To prevent postoperative venous thrombosis and pulmonary embolism (in low-dose form)
      (5) To prevent cerebral thrombosis during an evolving stroke
      (6) As adjunct therapy to prevent coronary occlusion with acute MI
   b. **LMWH** fragments are approved for treatment of thromboembolic complications associated with surgery, unstable angina, and MI.
   c. **Danaparoid** is approved for prevention of deep vein thrombosis.
   d. **Lepirudin** and **argatroban** are indicated for treatment of heparin-induced thrombocytopenia.
   e. **Warfarin sodium,** an oral anticoagulant, is indicated:
      (1) For the prophylaxis and treatment of venous thrombosis, pulmonary embolism, and atrial fibrillation with embolization
      (2) As adjunct therapy to prevent coronary occlusion with acute MI

4. **Adverse effects**
   a. **Heparin**
      (1) Heparin is associated with:
         (a) Hematologic effects such as hemorrhage, local irritation, thrombocytopenia, hematoma, ulceration, erythema, and pain
         (b) Other effects such as hypersensitivity reactions, fever, chills, and urticaria
      (2) Severe adverse effects may be treated by administering protamine sulfate, the specific antidote for heparin.
   b. **LMWH** fragments are absorbed more uniformly than heparin, have a longer biological half-life, and may be associated with a lower incidence of side effects than heparin.
   c. **Danaparoid** is contraindicated in various bleeding disorders and patients hypersensitive to pork products. Danaparoid contains sodium sulfite, which may cause life-threatening allergic reactions.
   d. **Lepirudin** may be associated with cerebral bleeding and allergic, skin, and anaphylactic reactions.
   e. **Warfarin**
      (1) The oral anticoagulant warfarin sodium is associated with these adverse effects:
         (a) Hemorrhage
         (b) Anorexia, urticaria, purpura, and alopecia
      (2) Bleeding may be treated by administering vitamin K (phytonadione), the specific antidote for warfarin sodium.

B. Antiplatelet agents

1. **Chemistry.** Antiplatelet drugs include aspirin, a salicylate; ticlopidine, a thienopyridine; dipyridamole, a dipiperidino-dinitro pyrimidine; and the Fab fragments of human monoclonal antibody to the GPIIb/IIIa receptor.

2. **Pharmacology**
   a. **Aspirin** in low doses inhibits platelet cyclooxygenase production of thromboxane A_2, preventing platelet aggregation. Cyclooxygenase is permanently inhibited for the life of the platelet (7–10 days).
   b. **Ticlopidine** and **clopidogrel** interfere with adenosine diphosphate (ADP)-induced membrane-mediated platelet–fibrinogen binding, leading to inhibition of platelet–platelet aggregation.
   c. **Fab fragments** (e.g., Abciximab) are monoclonal antibodies against the glycoprotein IIb/IIIa (GPIIb/IIIa)–receptor that permanently inhibit platelet–platelet interaction.
   d. **GPIIb/IIIa-receptor antagonists (e.g., tirofiban, eptifibatide)** are reversible antagonists of fibrinogen, von Willebrand's factor, and other adhesion ligands at the GPIIb/IIIa receptor, leading to inhibition of platelet aggregation.
   e. **Anagrelide** decreases platelet production.

    f. Cilostazol and its metabolites are PDE III inhibitors that increase cAMP, leading to vasodilation and decreased platelet aggregation.

    g. Dipyridamole may inhibit platelet aggregation via inhibition of:

        (1) Red blood cell adenosine, which acts on A_2 receptors of platelets

        (2) Phosphodiesterase to increase intracellular concentrations of cAMP

        (3) Thromboxane A_2 formation

  3. Therapeutic indications

    a. Aspirin is indicated for reduction of mortality in post-MI, prophylactic treatment of MI to prevent reinfarction, and prophylaxis following transient ischemic attacks and minor stroke.

    b. Ticlopidine is approved to reduce the risk of thrombotic stroke in patients with demonstrated risk but who cannot tolerate aspirin. **Clopidogrel** is approved to reduce MI, stroke, and vascular deaths.

    c. Abciximab is indicated for use with aspirin and heparin in patients undergoing percutaneous transluminal coronary angioplasty (PTCA) or atherectomy.

    d. Tirofiban and eptifibatide are approved for treatment of acute coronary syndrome and patients undergoing PTCA.

    e. Anagrelide is approved to reduce platelet count in patients with essential thrombocythemia.

    f. Cilostazol is approved for treatment of intermittent claudication.

    g. Dipyridamole is indicated for prophylaxis against thromboembolism after cardiac valve replacement.

  4. Adverse effects

    a. Aspirin in doses used for treatment of thrombotic disease is associated with epigastric pain, heartburn, nausea, rash, nasal polyps, gout, and anaphylactic reactions in sensitive individuals.

    b. Ticlopidine is associated with a high incidence of adverse reactions, including diarrhea, rash, nausea, vomiting, GI pain, and neutropenia.

    c. Abciximab is associated with major and minor bleeding events, thrombocytopenia, human antichimeric antibody formation, cardiac arrhythmias, AV block, bradycardia, diarrhea, abnormal thinking, and dizziness.

    d. Tirofiban and eptifibatide are associated with bleeding events and bleeding complications, nausea, fever, and headaches, and in the case of eptifibatide with hypotension.

    e. Anagrelide carries a warning for use in patients with heart disease and may lead to serious adverse effects, including congestive heart failure, myocardial infarction, heart block, fibrillation, and others.

    f. Cilostazol is contraindicated in patients with congestive heart failure. In dogs, cilostazol produced cardiovascular lesions, including endocardial hemorrhage and hemosiderin deposition, necrosis of smooth muscle, intimal thickening, and arteritis in the coronary artery.

    g. Dipyridamole is associated with nausea, epigastric pain, dizziness, headache, and rash.

C. Thrombolytic agents

  1. Chemistry

    a. Alteplase, reteplase, and tenecteplase are recombinant DNA-derived **tissue plasminogen activators (t-PA)** consisting of 527 and 355 amino acids, respectively, of the natural tissue plasminogen activator, which catalyzes conversion of plasminogen to plasmin.

    b. Streptokinase is a nonenzymatic 47-kDa protein derived from cultures of Group C β-hemolytic streptococci.

    c. Anistreplase (anisoylated plasminogen streptokinase activator complex, APSAC) is a complex of human lys-plasminogen and streptokinase with an anisoyl group blocking the catalytic site.

    d. Urokinase is a two-chain serine protease obtained from cultured human kidney cells.

  2. Pharmacology. Thrombolytic agents facilitate the conversion of plasminogen to plasmin that subsequently hydrolyzes fibrin to dissolve clots.

    a. Alteplase and **reteplase** are referred to as clot selective because conversion of plasminogen to plasmin by t-PA is enhanced several hundred-fold in the presence of fibrin.

   b. Streptokinase, which has no enzymatic activity, forms a 1 to 1 complex with plasminogen, resulting in a conformational change that exposes the catalytic site of plasminogen.
   The stable activated complex subsequently cleaves free plasminogen to form plasmin.
   c. Anistreplase is a prodrug activated *in vivo* by deacylation of the anisole moiety from the
   active site of the plasminogen-streptokinase complex. The activated complex converts
   plasminogen to plasmin in the bloodstream or thrombus.
   d. Urokinase, in contrast to streptokinase, is enzymatic and directly converts plasminogen
   to plasmin.

3. Therapeutic indications
   a. Alteplase and reteplase are indicated for treatment of acute MI and acute massive pulmonary embolism.
   b. Streptokinase is indicated for acute MI, deep vein thrombosis, arterial thrombosis, and
   arterial emboli, except those originating from the left side of the heart.
   c. Anistreplase is indicated for treatment of acute MI and lysis of coronary arterial thrombi.
   d. Urokinase is indicated for treatment of coronary artery thrombosis and pulmonary emboli.

4. Adverse effects
   a. t-PAs are associated with:
      (1) Internal bleeding of the GI and genitourinary tract, retroperitoneal bleeding, and
      intracranial bleeding
      (2) Superficial bleeding at catheter insertion sites, arterial punctures, and surgical sites
      (3) Other adverse effects, including hypersensitivity reactions, nausea, vomiting, hypo-
      tension, and fever
   b. Streptokinase may be associated with:
      (1) Internal and superficial bleeding as above
      (2) Allergic reactions, including bronchospasm, angioneurotic edema, urticaria, head-
      ache, and delayed hypersensitivity reactions
   c. Anistreplase may be associated with:
      (1) Internal and superficial bleeding as above
      (2) Cardiac arrhythmias and hypotension
      (3) Allergic type reactions such as bronchospasm, angioneurotic edema, urticaria, and
      delayed purpuric rash
   d. Urokinase may be associated with:
      (1) Internal and superficial bleeding as above
      (2) Allergic reactions leading to bronchospasm and skin rash

IX. ANTIANEMIC AGENTS

A. Chemistry. The major antianemic agents are iron preparations, cyanocobalamin (vitamin B_{12}),
folic acid, and hematopoietic growth factors **(erythropoietin, colony-stimulating factors, and
interleukins-11).**

   1. Most iron preparations consist of ferrous salts, which are better absorbed from the GI tract
   than ferric salts or elemental iron.
      a. Typical oral preparations include **ferrous sulfate** (e.g., Feosol), **ferrous gluconate** (e.g.,
      Fergon), and **ferrous fumarate** (e.g., Feostat).
      b. When parenteral administration is indicated, **iron dextran** (e.g., Imferon) may be used.
      This preparation consists of a complex of ferric hydroxide and low–molecular-weight
      dextrans, forming a colloidal solution.

   2. Cyanocobalamin (vitamin B_{12}) is a nucleotide-like macromolecule with a modified porphyrin unit (a corrin ring) containing a trivalent cobalt atom. A cyanide ion is also coordi-
   nated to the cobalt atom, as is a benzimidazole group. The benzimidazole group is bonded
   to an α-ribosyl phosphate.

   3. Folic acid consists of three major components: a pteridine nucleus bonded to the nitrogen
   of *p*-aminobenzoic acid, which is bonded through an amide linkage to glutamic acid
   (Figure 15-16).

   4. Epoetin alfa and **darbepoetin alfa** are glycoproteins produced via recombinant DNA technology. Epoetin alfa (165 amino acid, 30.4 kDa) is identical to natural erythropoietin.

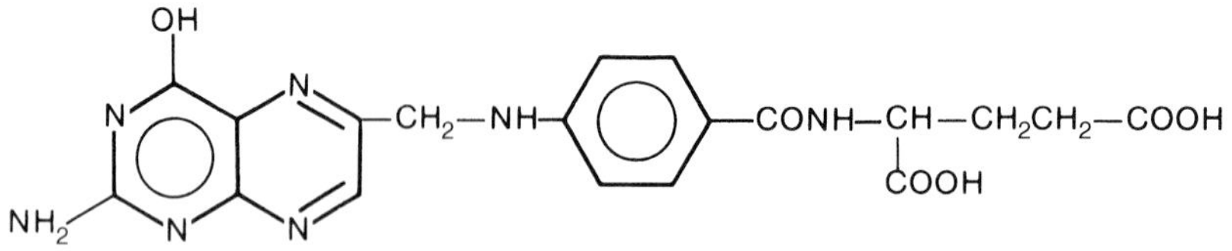

Figure 15-16. Structural formula of folic acid, an antianemic agent.

5. Colony-stimulating factors **filgrastim** and **pegfilgrastim** (granulocyte–colony-stimulating factor; G-CSF) and **sargramostim** (granulocyte macrophage–colony-stimulating factor; GM-CSF) are glycoproteins produced via recombinant DNA technology.

6. **Oprelvekin (interleukin-11)** is a recombinant DNA-produced nonglycosylated polypeptide growth factor differing from the natural cytokine by one amino acid.

B. **Pharmacology**

1. **Iron preparations** (ferrous salts) are readily absorbed from the GI tract and stored in the bone marrow, liver, and spleen as **ferritin** and **hemosiderin.** They are subsequently incorporated as needed into hemoglobin, where the iron reversibly binds molecular oxygen. A lack of body iron causes iron-deficiency anemia with hypochromic, microcytic red blood cells, which transport oxygen poorly.

2. **Cyanocobalamin** is readily absorbed from the GI tract in the presence of intrinsic factor (Castle's factor), a glycoprotein produced by gastric parietal cells, which is necessary for GI absorption of cyanocobalamin.
   a. Cyanocobalamin is transported to tissue by transcobalamin II. It is essential for cell growth, for maintaining normal nerve cell myelin, and for the metabolic functions of folate.
   b. Lack of dietary cyanocobalamin (or lack of intrinsic factor) causes a vitamin B_{12} deficiency and megaloblastic anemia with hyperchromic, macrocytic, immature red blood cells. Demyelination of nerve cells also occurs, causing irreversible CNS damage.

3. **Folic acid** is readily absorbed from the GI tract, transported to tissue, and stored intracellularly. It is a precursor of several coenzymes (derivatives of tetrahydrofolic acid) that are involved in single-carbon–atom transfers. A lack of dietary folic acid causes folic acid deficiency and megaloblastic anemia with hyperchromic, macrocytic, immature red blood cells. However, folic acid deficiency causes no neurologic impairment.

4. Endogenous erythropoietin, whose production in the kidneys is stimulated by blood loss, anemia, and hypoxia, is mimicked by **epoetin alfa** and **darbepoetin alfa** to increase proliferation and differentiation of erythroid progenitor cells.

5. **Filgrastim** and **pegfilgrastim** increase proliferation, differentiation, and activation of neutrophils in patients exhibiting neutropenia subsequent to myelosuppressive chemotherapy. **Sargramostim** stimulates maturation of granulocytes and macrophages and activation of mature cells via cell surface receptors.

6. **Oprelvekin** increases platelet production via stimulation of hematopoietic stem cells, megakaryocytes progenitor cells, and maturation of megakaryocytes.

C. **Therapeutic indications**

1. **Iron preparations** (ferrous salts) are used to treat iron-deficiency anemia.

2. **Cyanocobalamin** is used to treat megaloblastic anemia resulting from vitamin B_{12} deficiency.

3. **Folic acid** is used to treat megaloblastic anemia resulting from folic acid deficiency.

4. **Epoetin alfa** and **darbepoetin alfa** are approved for treatment of anemia resulting from chronic renal failure.

5. **Filgrastim** and **pegfilgrastim** are approved for treatment of chronic and chemotherapy-induced neutropenia. Sargramostim is approved for myeloid reconstitution in patients with

non-Hodgkin's or Hodgkin's disease or who have undergone bone marrow transplantations.

    6. Oprelvekin is approved for prevention of chemotherapy-related thrombocytopenia.

D. Adverse effects

    1. Iron preparations are associated with GI effects such as GI distress, nausea, heartburn, diarrhea, and constipation.

    2. Cyanocobalamin only rarely produces adverse effects.

    3. Folic acid is associated only with rare allergic reactions after parenteral administration.

    4. Epoetin alfa and **darbepoetin alfa** may increase blood pressure, which should be monitored and effectively managed.

    5. Filgrastim may produce allergic reactions involving skin, respiratory, or cardiovascular systems after initial or subsequent dosing. **Filgrastim** and **pegfilgrastim** are contraindicated in patients allergic to Escherichia coli–derived proteins.

    6. Oprelvekin produces fluid retention, which may lead to peripheral edema and dyspnea.

STUDY QUESTIONS

Directions: Each of the numbered items or incomplete statements in this section is followed by answers or by completions of the statement. Select the **one** lettered answer or completion that is **best** in each case.

1. Calcium channel blockers have all of the following characteristics EXCEPT

(A) they block the slow inward current carried by calcium during phase 2 of the cardiac action potential
(B) they dilate peripheral arterioles and reduce total peripheral resistance
(C) they constrict coronary arteries and arterioles and decrease oxygen delivery to the myocardium
(D) they are useful in treating stable angina pectoris and Prinzmetal's angina
(E) adverse effects include aggravation of congestive heart failure

2. The termination of heparin activity by protamine sulfate is due to

(A) a chelating action
(B) the inhibition of gastrointestinal absorption of heparin
(C) the displacement of heparin–plasma protein binding
(D) an acid–base interaction
(E) the prothrombin-like activity of protamine

3. Which of the following cardiovascular agents is classified chemically as a glycoside?

(A) Nifedipine
(B) Digoxin
(C) Flecainide
(D) Cholestyramine
(E) Warfarin

4. Cardiac glycosides may be useful in treating all of the following conditions EXCEPT

(A) atrial flutter
(B) paroxysmal atrial tachycardia
(C) congestive heart failure
(D) ventricular tachycardia
(E) atrial fibrillation

5. Ingestion of which of the following vitamins should be avoided by a patient taking an oral anticoagulant?

(A) Vitamin A
(B) Vitamin B
(C) Vitamin D
(D) Vitamin E
(E) Vitamin K

6. The structure shown below is characteristic of which of the following agents?

(A) Osmotic diuretics
(B) Carbonic anhydrase inhibitors
(C) Thiazides
(D) Loop diuretics
(E) Potassium-sparing diuretics

7. Which of the following diuretics is most similar in chemical structure to the antihypertensive agent diazoxide?

(A) Furosemide
(B) Spironolactone
(C) Mannitol
(D) Acetazolamide
(E) Chlorothiazide

Directions: Each item below contains three suggested answers, of which **one or more** is correct. Choose the answer:

A	if **I only** is correct
B	if **III only** is correct
C	if **I and II** are correct
D	if **II and III** are correct
E	if **I, II, and III** are correct

8. In the oral treatment of iron-deficiency anemias, iron is preferably administered as

  I. ferrous iron
  II. ferric salts
  III. elemental iron

9. Parenterally administered antihypertensive agents used in treating hypertensive emergencies include the

  I. centrally acting antiadrenergic clonidine
  II. arteriolar and venous vasodilator nitroprusside
  III. ganglionic-blocking agent trimethaphan

10. Certain factors contribute to the longer duration of action of digitoxin when compared with that of digoxin. These include

  I. greater protein binding
  II. reduced polarity
  III. greater tubular reabsorption

11. Oral anticoagulants have the following properties:

  I. They interfere with vitamin K–dependent synthesis of active clotting factors II, VII, IX, and X.
  II. They have adverse effects that include hemorrhage, urticaria, purpura, and alopecia.
  III. They prolong the clotting time of blood both in vivo and in vitro.

Directions: The group of items in this section consists of lettered options followed by a set of numbered items. For each item, select the **one** lettered option that is most closely associated with it. Each lettered option may be selected once, more than once, or not at all.

Questions 12–14

For each group of adverse effects, select the class of drug that most closely relates to it.

(A) Cardiac glycosides
(B) Calcium channel blockers
(C) Angiotensin-converting enzyme (ACE) inhibitors
(D) β-Adrenergic blockers
(E) Nitrites and nitrates

12. Bradycardia, hypotension, increased airway resistance, and congestive heart failure

13. Visual disturbances (yellow or green vision), confusion, anorexia, vomiting, atrioventricular (AV) block, and ventricular tachycardia

14. Hypotension, acute renal failure, cholestatic jaundice, and agranulocytosis

Questions 15–17

For each statement listed below, select the drug that it most closely characterizes.

(A) Furosemide
(B) Hydrochlorothiazide
(C) Spironolactone
(D) Mannitol
(E) Acetazolamide

15. It interferes with distal tubular aldosterone-mediated sodium–potassium exchange, renders the urine alkaline, and may cause hyperkalemia, gynecomastia, and menstrual irregularities.

16. Freely filtered, this drug limits tubular reabsorption of water and is useful in reducing cerebral edema and intracranial pressure.

17. The principal site of action of this drug is on the thick ascending limb of Henle's loop; it is useful in treating pulmonary edema and ascites.

ANSWERS AND EXPLANATIONS

1. The answer is C *[III B 3, C 3, D 3].*
Calcium channel blockers are used in the treatment of angina because they dilate coronary arteries and arterioles, thus decreasing coronary vascular resistance and increasing coronary blood flow.

2. The answer is D *[VIII A 1, 4; Figure 15-13].*
Heparin is a highly acidic mucopolysaccharide, whereas protamine is a highly basic protein. When administered subsequently to heparin, protamine chemically combines with it (presumably by an acid–base interaction) and inactivates its anticoagulant effect. Hence, it is an effective antidote for heparin. Caution must be employed when using protamine because an excess of protamine can cause an anticoagulant effect itself.

3. The answer is B *[II A 1].*
Most glycosides are natural products obtained from plant material. Although there are very few medicinal agents that are glycosides, the group known as the cardiac glycosides is extremely important and is widely used for treating congestive heart failure. Digoxin is a cardiac glycoside obtained from *Digitalis ianata.* Other cardiac glycosides include digitoxin, which is obtained from *Digitalis purpurea,* and ouabain, which is obtained from *Strophanthus gratus.*

4. The answer is D *[II C; Table 15-4].*
Ventricular tachycardia is produced by toxic cardiac glycoside dosage and would not be a therapeutic indication for the agents. Cardiac glycosides increase systolic contraction velocity and increase the refractory period of the atrioventricular (AV) node. They also have a positive inotropic effect.

5. The answer is E *[VIII A 2 e, 4 e].*
The oral anticoagulants, such as warfarin, act by inhibiting the liver biosynthesis of prothrombin, which is the precursor of the enzyme thrombin that catalyzes the conversion of soluble fibrinogen to the insoluble polymer fibrin, which results in clot formation. One of the principal factors in the biosynthesis of prothrombin is vitamin K, with which warfarin competes to inhibit this process. Since this is a reversible competition, vitamin K acts as an antagonist to the oral anticoagulants.

6. The answer is C *[VI A; Figure 15-6].*
The structure can be recognized as a benzothiadiazine, which is known also as a thiazide. It represents the structure of hydrochlorothiazide, a sulfonamide diuretic. Other sulfonamide diuretics include the carbonic anhydrase inhibitors, such as acetazolamide, and the loop diuretics, such as furosemide. Neither of these subclasses contains drugs with a benzothiadiazine nucleus.

7. The answer is E *[VI C; Figures 15-6, 15-8].*
Diazoxide is a benzothiadiazine derivative; therefore, it would be most similar to chlorothiazide, which is also a benzothiadiazine. While both the thiazides and the diazoxides have antihypertensive activity, only the thiazides have significant diuretic activity. One of the structural requirements of the thiazide diuretics is an electron-withdrawing group, such as a halogen, ortho to the sulfonamide group on the benzene nucleus. The diazoxide molecule lacks such a group.

8. The answer is A (I) *[IX A 1].*
Absorption of orally administered iron is significantly improved with ferrous iron than with either ferric salts or elemental iron, presumably because of its better solubility characteristics. Iron preparations (ferrous salts) are more readily absorbed from the gastrointestinal tract and are stored in the bone marrow, liver, and spleen as ferritin and hemosiderin.

9. The answer is D (II, III) *[V B 4, C 2 a, e].*
Clonidine is not recognized as a drug of choice for hypertensive emergencies, possibly because of its central mechanism of action and the latent period required for its effect, compared with other peripheral agents.

10. The answer is E (all) *[II A; Figure 15-1].*
Structurally, digitoxin has only one alcohol group on its steroidal nucleus, whereas digoxin has two. This slight difference in structure has a significant effect on the polarity of the molecule. Owing to its greater liposolubility, digitoxin is more likely to undergo tubular reabsorption, to undergo enterohepatic cycling,

to penetrate into the liver microsomes and undergo metabolism, and to be protein-bound, all of which contribute to its longer duration of action and potential cumulative effects.

11. The answer is C (I, II) *[VIII A 2 e, 4 e (1)]*.
Oral anticoagulants are only effective *in vivo* since they block hepatic synthesis of vitamin K–dependent coagulation factors (factors II, VII, IX, and X). This also explains the latency period associated with initiation of oral anticoagulant therapy.

12–14. The answers are: 12-D *[III D 2]*, **13-A** *[II D]*, **14-C** *[V D 6]*.
Nonselective β-adrenergic blockers (e.g., propranolol) produce adverse effects associated with their mechanism of action on the autonomic nervous system. Thus, bronchospasm, lowering of blood pressure, and reduced heart rate result from blockade of autonomic β-adrenergic receptors. Visual disturbances (yellow or green vision) are peculiar to cardiac glycoside overdose. AV dissociation and ventri-cular tachycardia are obviously more significant adverse effects. (ACE) inhibitors reportedly may cause blood dyscrasias in addition to cholestatic jaundice and acute renal failure.

15–17. The answers are: 15-C *[VI E 2 a, 4 a]*, **16-D** *[VI A 2 a, 3 b]*, **17-A** *[VI D 2 a, 3 a]*.
Spironolactone interferes with aldosterone-mediated sodium–potassium exchange, reducing the amount of potassium excreted, and is often used with other diuretics that promote the excretion of potassium, such as the benzothiadiazides. Mannitol increases the osmolarity of the glomerular filtrate since it is reabsorbed poorly. By increasing the osmolarity of the glomerular filtrate, mannitol limits tubular reabsorption of water, thus promoting diuresis. In this way, it reduces cerebral edema and decreases intracranial pressure. Furosemide is a diuretic of choice for treating acute congestive heart failure because it promotes a significant rapid excretion of water and sodium.

16
Medicinal Chemistry and Pharmacology: Endocrinology and Related Drugs

Marc W. Harrold
Pui-Kai Li

I. INTRODUCTION. Hormones are substances secreted by specific tissues and transported to other specific tissues, where they exert their effects. They can be classified pharmacologically as drugs. Hormones can be obtained from natural substances (animal preparations), or they may be synthetic or semisynthetic compounds resembling the natural products. They are often used for replacement therapy (e.g., exogenous insulin for treatment of diabetes mellitus). However, they can also be used for a variety of other therapeutic and diagnostic purposes. Certain drugs (e.g., thyroid hormone inhibitors, oral antidiabetic agents), while not hormones themselves, influence the synthesis or secretion of hormones. Therapeutically useful hormones and related drugs include the pituitary hormones, the gonadal hormones, the adrenocorticosteroids, the thyroid hormones and inhibitors, and the antidiabetic agents.

II. PITUITARY HORMONES

A. Chemistry. Pituitary hormones are divided into two groups by their site of secretion.

1. **Posterior pituitary hormones.** The two posterior pituitary hormones, **oxytocin** (Pitocin) and **vasopressin** (Pitressin), are closely related octapeptides. They differ from each other in only two of their eight amino acids but have different biological actions.

2. **Anterior pituitary hormones**
   a. **Protein molecules** are anterior pituitary hormones that are used therapeutically.
      (1) **Corticotropin** (Acthar), known as **adrenocorticotropic hormone (ACTH),** is a single-chain polypeptide containing 39 amino acids. It has a molecular weight (mol wt) of 4600.
      (2) **Thyrotropin** (Thytropar), known as **thyroid-stimulating hormone (TSH),** is a glycoprotein with a mol wt of 28,000.
      (3) **Thyrotropin-releasing hormone (TRH)** [Relefact], known as protirelin, is a tripeptide with a mol wt of 363.
      (4) **Growth hormone** (Asellacrin), known as somatotropin, consists of 191 amino acids and has a mol wt of 21,500.
   b. **Pituitary gonadotropins** are anterior pituitary hormones that are not available for therapeutic use. These include **follicle-stimulating hormone (FSH), luteinizing hormone (LH),** and **prolactin [luteotropic hormone (LTH)].** However, several related nonpituitary gonadotropins have FSH-like or LH-like actions and are used therapeutically. These include:
      (1) **Menotropins** (Pergonal), known as human menopausal gonadotropin (hMG), are high in FSH-like and LH-activity and are obtained from the urine of postmenopausal women.
      (2) **Urofollitropin** (Metrodin) is high in FSH-like activity and is obtained from the urine of postmenopausal women.
      (3) **Human chorionic gonadotropin (hCG)** [Follutein] has LH-like activity and is obtained from the urine of pregnant women.

B. Pharmacology. The therapeutically important pituitary hormones include the **anterior pituitary agents** (corticotropin), **growth hormone** (somatotropin), and **menotropins** (gonadotropin), and the **posterior pituitary agents** (vasopressin and oxytocin).

1. **Corticotropin** is secreted from the anterior pituitary, stimulating the adrenal cortex to produce and secrete adrenocorticosteroids (see IV).

2. **Growth hormone** stimulates protein, carbohydrate, and lipid metabolism to promote increased cell, organ, connective tissue, and skeletal growth, causing a rapid increase in the overall rate of linear growth.

3. **Menotropins** produce ovarian follicular growth and induce ovulation by means of FSH-like and LH-like actions.

4. **Vasopressin** has vasopressor and antidiuretic hormone (ADH) activity. It acts primarily on the distal renal tubular epithelium, where it promotes the reabsorption of water.

5. **Oxytocin** stimulates uterine contraction and plays an important role in the induction of labor.

C. **Therapeutic indications**

1. **Corticotropin** is used primarily for the diagnosis and differentiation of primary and secondary adrenal insufficiency.

2. **Growth hormone** is used for the long-term treatment of children whose growth failure is the result of lack of endogenous growth hormone secretion.

3. **Menotropins** are used to induce ovulation and pregnancy in anovulatory infertile women whose anovulation is not the result of primary ovarian failure. In men, menotropins are used to induce spermatogenesis.

4. **Vasopressin** is used to treat neurogenic diabetes insipidus and to treat postoperative abdominal distention.

5. **Oxytocin** is used to promote delivery by initiating and improving uterine contractions and to control postpartum bleeding or hemorrhage.

D. **Adverse effects**

1. **Corticotropin** is only rarely associated with adverse effects, which represent hypersensitivity reactions or corticosteroid excess.

2. **Growth hormone** is associated with adverse effects primarily related to the development of antibodies to growth hormone. The antibodies are nonbinding in most cases and do not interfere with continued growth hormone treatment.

3. **Menotropins** are associated with:
   a. **Hypersensitivity,** arterial thromboembolism, febrile reactions, ovarian enlargement hyperstimulation syndrome, hemoperitoneum, and (rarely) birth defects in women
   b. **Gynecomastia** in men

4. **Vasopressin** is associated with:
   a. Gastrointestinal (GI) effects, such as abdominal cramps, flatulence, nausea, and vomiting
   b. Central nervous system (CNS) effects, such as tremor, sweating, vertigo, and headache
   c. Other effects, such as urticaria, bronchoconstriction, and anaphylaxis

5. **Oxytocin** is associated with:
   a. Severe water intoxication with convulsions and coma after slow (24-hour) infusion
   b. Uterine hypertonicity, with spasm, tetanic contraction, or uterine rupture
   c. Postpartum hemorrhage
   d. Nausea, vomiting, and anaphylaxis
   e. Fetal effects, such as bradycardia, neonatal jaundice, cardiac dysrhythmias, and premature ventricular contractions

III. **GONADAL HORMONES.** Most natural and synthetic gonadal hormones are derivatives of cyclopentanoperhydrophenanthrene (Figure 16-1). All hormones having this fused reduced 17-carbon-atom ring system are classified as steroids.

A. **Estrogen**

1. **Natural and semisynthetic estrogens.** The basic nucleus of the natural estrogens has a methyl group designated as C-18 on position C-13 of cyclopentanoperhydrophenanthrene. This basic nucleus is known as **estrane.**
   a. Unlike other steroid hormones, all estrogens have an aromatic A ring (see Figure 16-2).

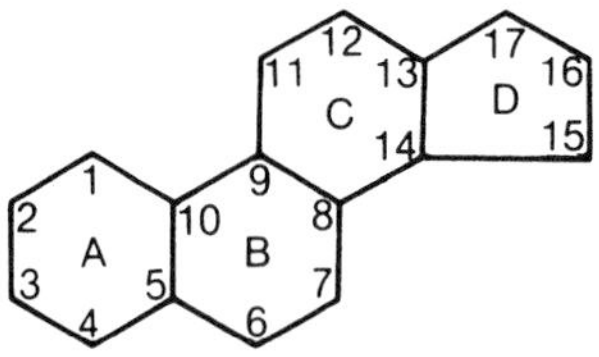

Figure 16-1. Structural formula of cyclopentanoperhydrophenanthrene, from which the gonadal hormones are derived. The letters *A* through *D* indicate the rings, which may be modified during subsequent conversions; the numbers 1 through 17 refer to carbon atom positions on the rings.

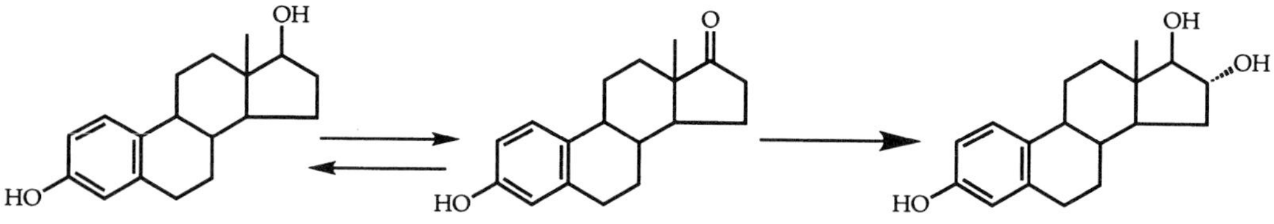

Figure 16-2. Structural formulas of (*A*) estradiol, which exists in the body in equilibrium with (*B*) estrone, which in turn is converted to (*C*) estriol before excretion.

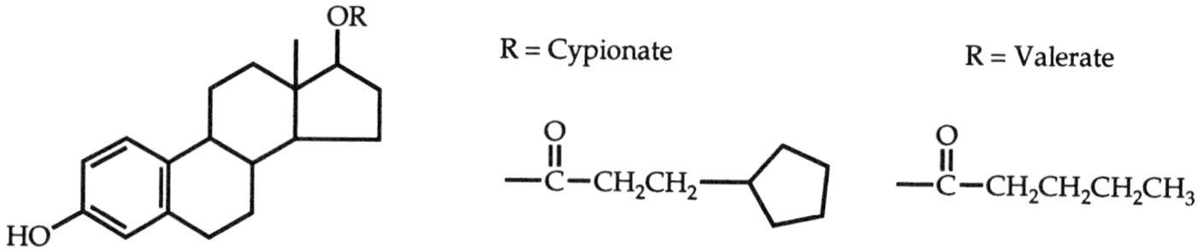

Figure 16-3. Structural formulas of estradiol cypionate and valerate.

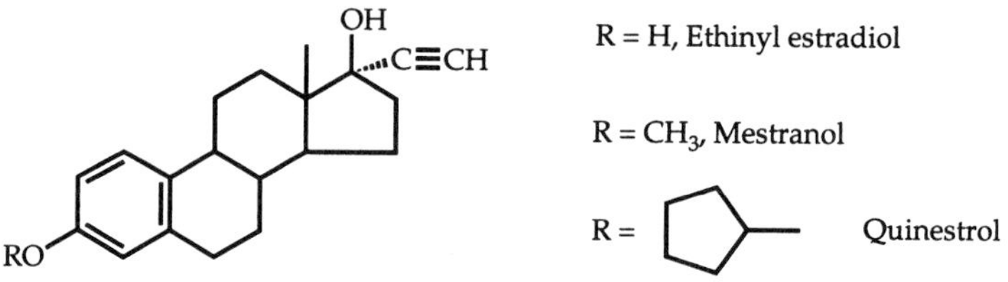

Figure 16-4. Structural formulas of ethinyl estradiol, mestranol, and quinestrol.

    b. Estradiol (Estrace), the principal estrogenic hormone, exists in the body in equilibrium with estrone, which is converted to estriol prior to excretion (Figure 16-2).
    c. Several estradiol esters, such as estradiol cypionate and estradiol valerate (Figure 16-3), are prepared as intramuscular injections in oil, to prolong their action. These estradiol esters are slowly hydrolyzed in muscle tissues to estradiol before absorption and, thus, are considered to be prodrugs.
    d. Several 17α-substituted estradiols increase resistance to first-pass metabolism and enhance oral effectiveness. Two of these estradiol derivatives, ethinyl estradiol and its 3-methyl ether mestranol, are used principally as the estrogenic components of serial-type oral contraceptives (Figure 16-4). Another, quinestrol (Estrovis), is used principally for estrogen-replacement therapy.

2. **Nonsteroidal synthetic estrogens** (e.g., diethylstilbestrol, dienestrol, chlorotrianisene) are nonsteroidal stilbene derivatives that appear to assume an estradiol-like conformation in vivo (Figure 16-5).

3. **Estrogen antagonists** (antiestrogens). The antiestrogens clomiphene, tamoxifen citrate, and toremifene citrate are stilbene derivatives that are structurally related to chlorotrianisene (Figure 16-6). Fulvestrant (Faslodex) is the newest potent steroidal anti-estrogen (Figure 16-6). However, these agents have different in vivo binding sites and activities.

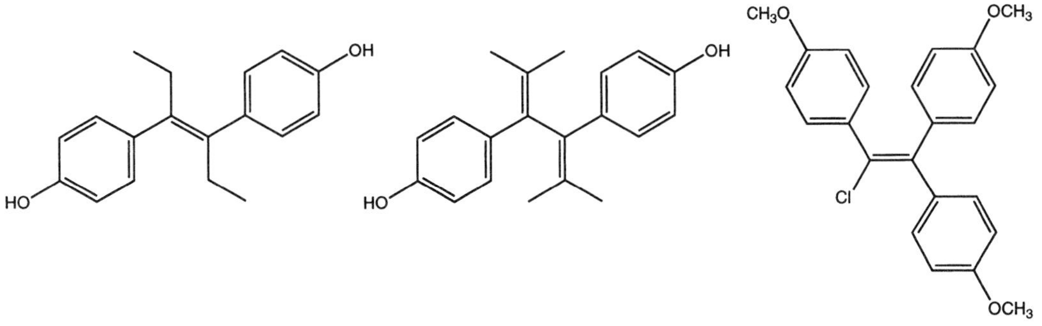

A   B   C

Figure 16-5. Structural formulas of (*A*) diethylstilbestrol (*DES*), (*B*) dienestrol, and (*C*) chlorotrianisene (Tace), synthetic estrogens derived from stilbene.

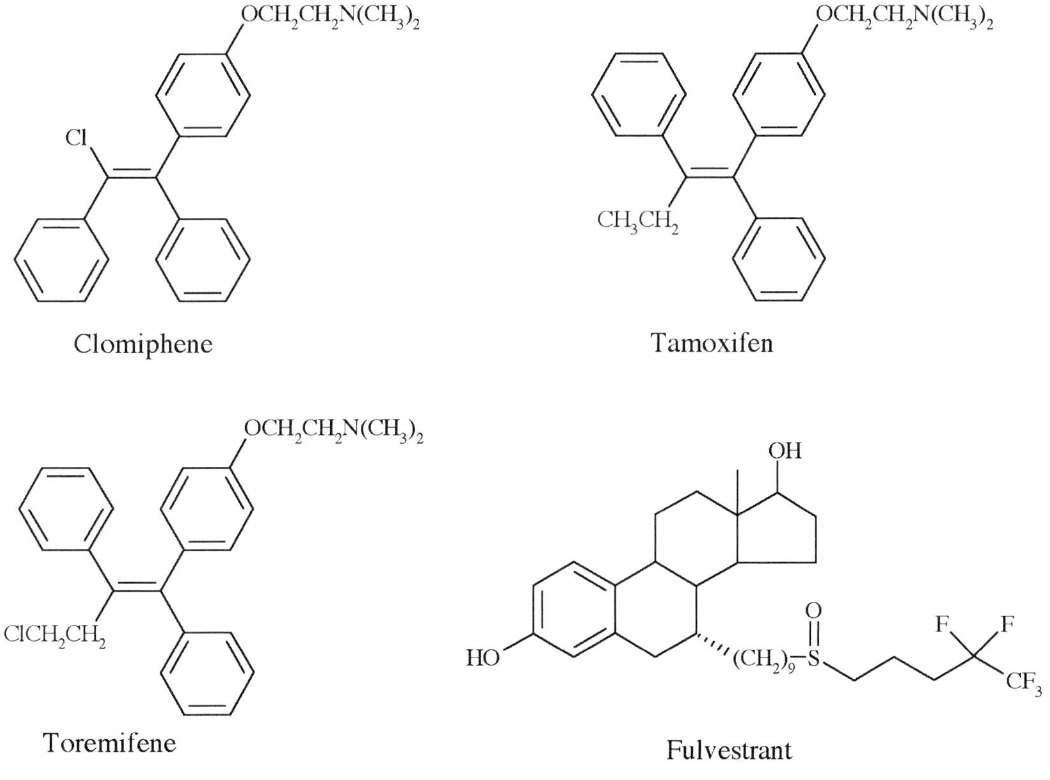

Clomiphene   Tamoxifen

Toremifene   Fulvestrant

Figure 16-6. Structural formulas of the antiestrogens clomiphene, tamoxifen, toremifene, and fulvestrant. Clomiphene, tamoxifen, and toremifene are structurally similar to chlorotrianisene, while fulvestrant is a larger and more lipid soluble analogue of estradiol.

4. Pharmacology (estrogen). The specificity of estrogen actions is due to the presence of estrogen receptors in estrogen-responsive tissues (e.g., vagina, uterus, mammary glands, anterior pituitary, hypothalamus). The receptors are located in the nucleus. When the estrogen has bound to the estrogen receptor, the receptor undergoes a conformational change that activates the estrogen-receptor complex, increases its affinity for DNA, and alters the production of messenger RNA (mRNA). This ultimately leads to either an increase or decrease in enzyme or protein synthesis.

5. Therapeutic uses
   a. Estrogens
      (1) Oral contraceptives (in combination with progestins)
      (2) Treatment of menopausal symptoms
         (a) Vasomotor disorder
         (b) Urogenital atrophy
         (c) Psychological disorder
      (3) Acne
      (4) Osteoporosis, both senile and postmenopausal osteoporosis
      (5) Prostate cancer
   b. Antiestrogens
      (1) Tamoxifen, toremifene, and fulvestrant are used to treat estrogen-dependent breast cancer.
      (2) Clomiphene is used to induce ovulation in women who have ovulation failure.

6. Adverse effects of estrogens
   a. GI effects, such as GI distress, nausea, vomiting, anorexia, and diarrhea
   b. Cardiovascular effects, such as hypertension and an increased incidence of thromboembolic diseases, stroke, and myocardial infarction
   c. Fluid and electrolyte disturbances, such as increased fluid retention and increased triglyceride level
   d. An increased incidence of endometrial cancer and hepatic adenomas (associated with long-term use)

7. Aromatase inhibitors and selective estrogen receptor modulators
   a. Pharmacology
      (1) Anastrozole and **letrozole** (Figure 16-7) are potent and selective nonsteroidal **inhibitors of aromatase.** Exemestane is the only steroidal irreversible inhibitor of aromatase (Figure 16-7), an enzyme responsible for the conversion of androgens (e.g., androstenedione and testosterone) to estrogens (e.g., estrone and estradiol).
      (2) Raloxifene (see Figure 16-7) is a **selective estrogen receptor modulator** (SERM). It reduces bone resorption and decreases bone turnover. Its biological actions, like those of estrogen, are mediated through binding to the estrogen receptor. Clinical data indicate that raloxifene has estrogen-like effects on bone and lipid metabolism, but exhibits estrogen antagonist effects on uterine and breast tissue.
   b. Therapeutic uses
      (1) Aromatase inhibitors are used to treat advanced breast cancer.
      (2) SERMs are used for the prevention of osteoporosis.

B. Progestins

1. The **naturally occurring** progestin progesterone is a C-21 steroid. Its basic nucleus is known as pregnane (Figure 16-8).

2. Synthetic progestins, which are also steroids, consist of two types.
   a. The 17α-hydroxyprogesterone derivatives (e.g., medroxyprogesterone acetate, megestrol acetate) typically introduce a methyl group at position C-6 of progesterone and an acetoxyl group at position C-17. These substitutions increase lipid solubility and decrease first-pass metabolism, enhancing oral activity and the progestin effect (Figure 16-9).
   b. The 17α-ethinylandrogens are structurally classified as androgens but contain progestational activities.
      (1) The 17α-ethinylandrogens are more liposoluble than progesterone and undergo less first-pass metabolism.
      (2) These agents have potent oral activity and are extensively used as oral contraceptives. Other 17α-ethinylandrogens include the positional isomer of norethindrone,

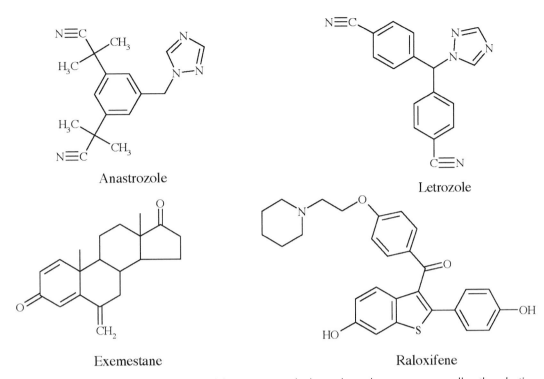

Anastrozole

Letrozole

Exemestane

Raloxifene

Figure 16-7. Structures of the aromatase inhibitors anastrozole, letrozole, and exemestane as well as the selective estrogen receptor modulator (SERM), raloxifene.

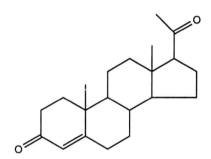

Figure 16-8. Structural formula of progesterone, which is a derivative of pregnane.

norethynodrel, its 18-methyl homologue norgestrel, and its 3,17-diacetate analogue ethynodiol diacetate (Figure 16-10).

3. **Pharmacology.** The mechanism of action of progestins is similar to estrogen. Progestins bind to progesterone receptor located in the nucleus of progestin-responsive tissues. The formation of progestin-receptor complex results in the increase in the synthesis of mRNA and specific enzyme or protein synthesis.

4. **Therapeutic uses**
   a. Oral contraceptives (alone or in combination with estrogens)
   b. Menstrual disorder (dysfunctional uterine bleeding, dysmenorrhea)
   c. Endometriosis

5. **Adverse effects**
   a. Gynecological effects, such as irregular menses, breakthrough bleeding, and amenorrhea
   b. Weight gain and edema
   c. Exacerbation of breast carcinoma

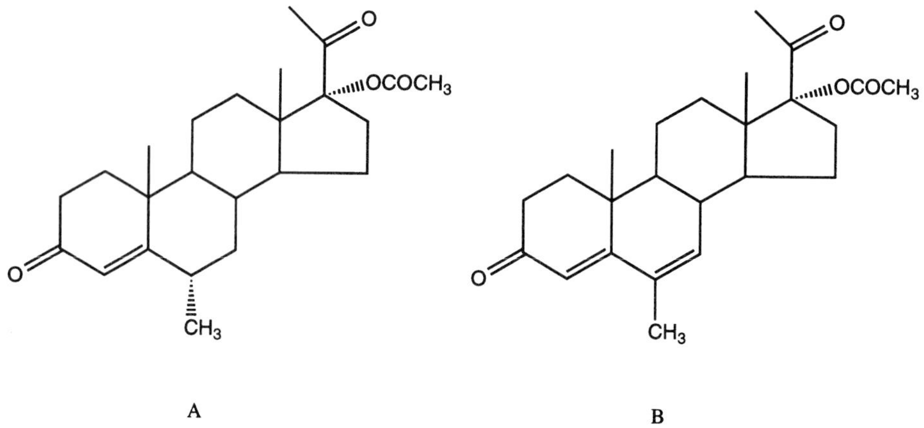

Figure 16-9. Structural formulas of (*A*) medroxyprogesterone acetate (Provera) and (*B*) megestrol acetate (Megace), synthetic progestins.

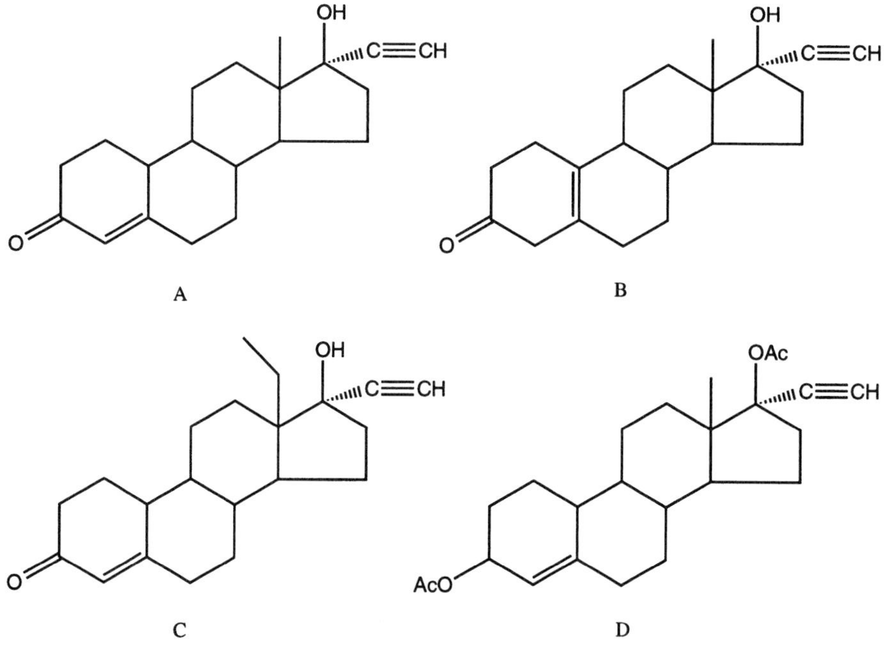

Figure 16-10. Structural formulas of (*A*) norethindrone, (*B*) norethynodrel, (*C*) norgestrel, and (*D*) ethynodiol diacetate.

C. Androgens and anabolic steroids

1. The primary natural androgen is **testosterone,** a C-19 steroid (Figure 16-11). Testosterone has two physiological effects, androgenic and anabolic effects.

   a. Compounds used for **androgenic effects**

   (1) Esters of testosterone, such as testosterone 17-enanthate (Delatestryl), resemble estradiol esters in that they provide increased duration of action when administered intramuscularly (Figure 16-12).

   (2) Introduction of a methyl group at position C-17 results in potent, orally active androgens, such as fluoxymesterone (see Figure 16-12).

   b. Compounds used for **anabolic effects** include drugs resulting from structural modifications of testosterone. These drugs have a much-enhanced anabolic–androgenic activity

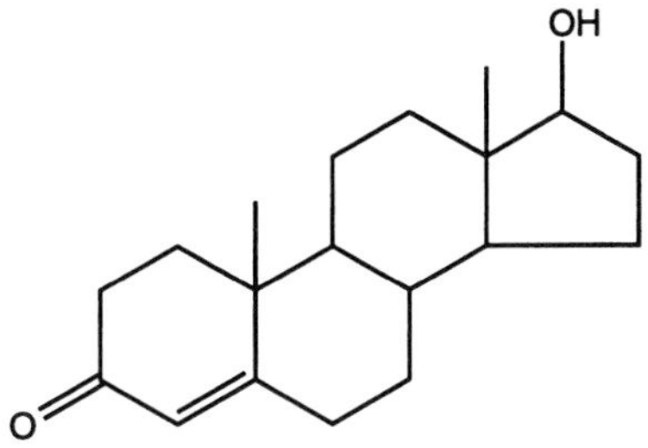

Figure 16-11. Structural formula of testosterone.

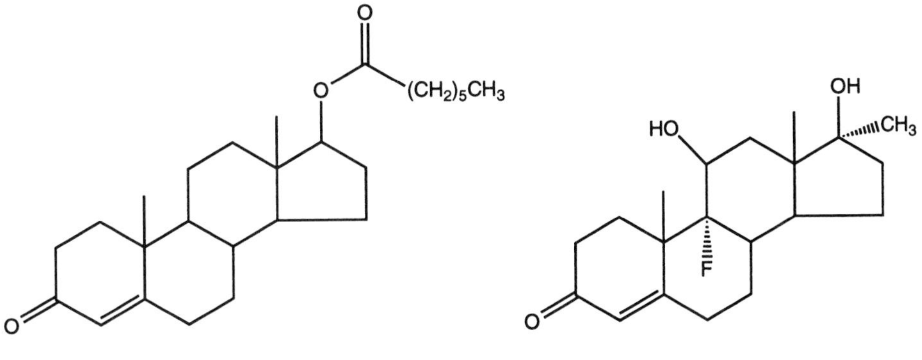

Figure 16-12. Structural formulas of (*A*) testosterone enanthate and (*B*) fluoxymesterone.

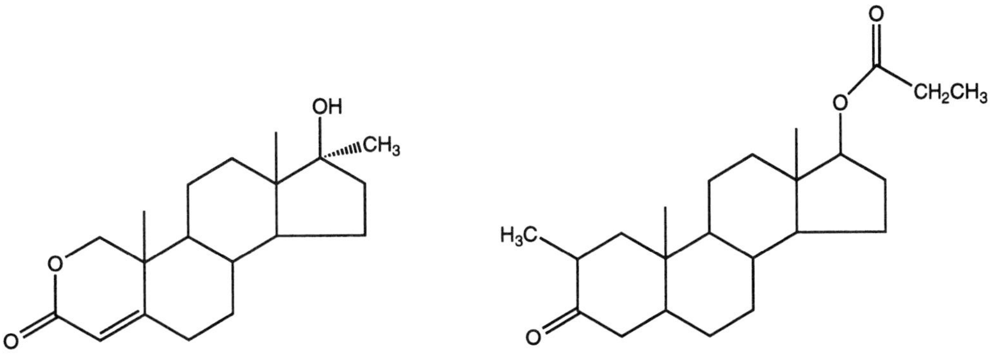

Figure 16-13. Structural formulas of (*A*) oxandrolone and (*B*) dromostanolone.

ratio (e.g., oxandrolone, dromostanolone) [Figure 16-13]. Agents with 17-methyl groups are orally active.

2. **Pharmacology** (androgen). Androgen's mechanism of action is similar to that of estrogen. However, the molecule that binds to an androgen receptor is not testosterone. Testosterone is converted to dihydrotestosterone in the cytoplasm of androgen-responsive tissue by the enzyme 5α-reductase. Dihydrotestosterone binds to an androgen receptor in the nucleus.

The formation of androgen-receptor complex results in the increase in the synthesis of mRNA and specific enzyme or protein synthesis.

3. **Therapeutic uses**
   a. Androgen-replacement therapy
   b. Breast cancer and endometriosis
   c. Female hypopituitarism, in combination with estrogen therapy
   d. Anabolic therapy, use in patients with negative nitrogen balance
   e. Anemia

4. **Adverse effects**
   a. Fluid retention
   b. Increased low-density lipoprotein (LDL) and decreased high-density lipoprotein (HDL) cholesterol levels
   c. Psychological changes
   d. Liver disorders
   e. Development of masculine features in female
   f. Decreased fertility in male

D. **Antiandrogens**

   1. Most of the antiandrogens are **nonsteroidal** in nature. They include **flutamide, bicalutamide,** and **nilutamide** (Figure 16-14).

   2. **Pharmacology.** Flutamide, bicalutamide, and nilutamide inhibit the action of androgens by competitively binding to androgen receptors in the target tissue.

   3. **Therapeutic use.** They are used in the treatment of prostate cancer, in combination with luteinizing hormone–releasing hormone (LH-RH) agonists.

E. **5α-Reductase inhibitors**

   1. Currently available agents include finasteride and dutasteride.

   2. **Pharmacology.** Finasteride is a competitive inhibitor of 5α-reductase, an enzyme that converts testosterone to the potent androgen, **5α-dihydrotestosterone (DHT).**

   3. **Therapeutic uses**
      a. Benign prostatic hyperplasia (BPH)
      b. Androgenic alopecia (1/5 the dose used in BPH)

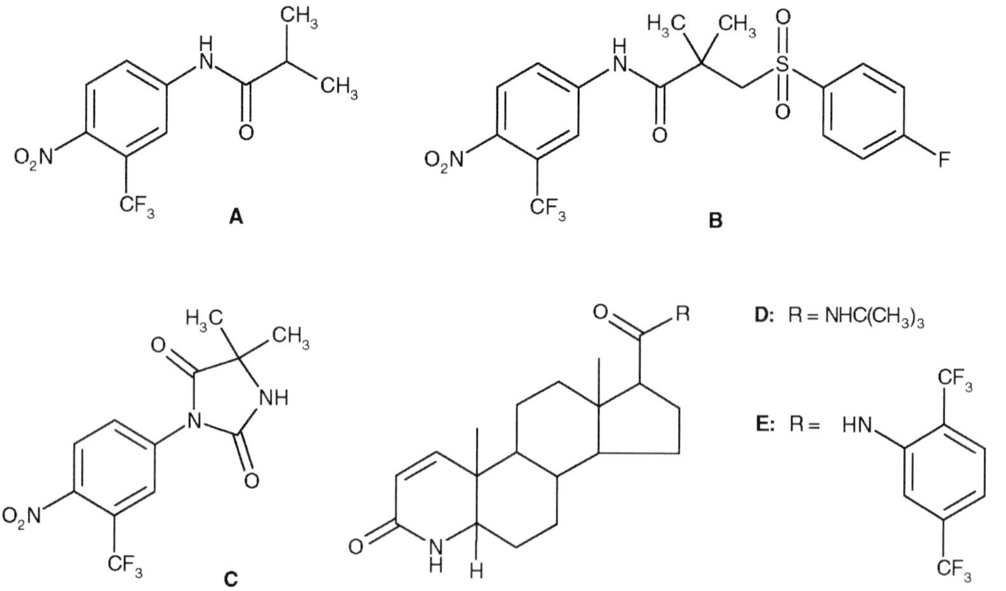

Figure 16-14. Structures of antiandrogens (*A*) flutamide, (*B*) bicalutamide, and (*C*) nilutamide, and the 5α-reductase inhibitors (*D*) finasteride, and (*E*) dutasteride.

IV. ADRENOCORTICOSTEROIDS

A. Chemistry. The adrenal cortex synthesizes adrenocorticosteroids. Adrenocorticoids are divided into two classes. The first class is **mineralocorticoids,** possessing sodium-retaining and potassium-excreting effects, and the second class is **glucocorticoids,** possessing anti-inflammatory, protein-catabolic, and immunosuppressant effects. However, most naturally occurring adrenocorticosteroids have some degree of both mineralocorticoid and glucocorticoid activity. All adrenocorticosteroids are derived from the C-21 pregnane steroidal nucleus.

1. **Cortisone** and **hydrocortisone,** which are formed in the middle (fascicular) layer of the adrenal cortex (Figure 16-15), are the prototypical glucocorticoids.
    a. The 17 β-ketol side chain (—COCH₂OH), the 4-ene, and the 3-ketone structures are found in all clinically useful adrenocorticosteroids (see Figure 16-15).
    b. Many natural, semisynthetic, and synthetic glucocorticoids are available. **Modifications** of the prototypes cortisone and hydrocortisone represent attempts to increase glucocorticoid activity while decreasing mineralocorticoid activity.
       (1) The oxygen atom at position C-11 is essential for glucocorticoid activity.
       (2) A double bond between positions C-1 and C-2 increases glucocorticoid activity without increasing mineralocorticoid activity as with prednisolone (Figure 16-16).
       (3) Fluorination at position C-9 greatly increases both mineralocorticoid and glucocorticoid activity, as with fludrocortisone; whereas fluorination at position C-6

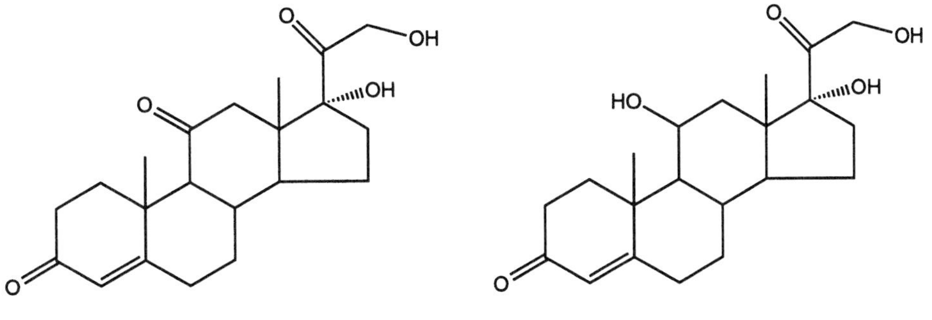

Figure 16-15. Structural formulas of (A) cortisone and (B) hydrocortisone.

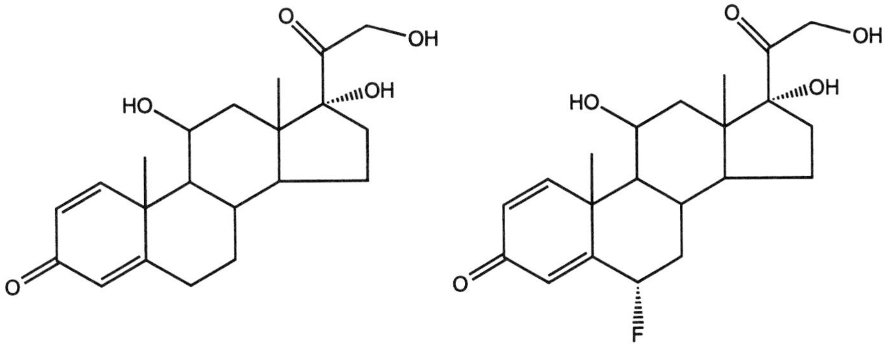

Figure 16-16. Structural formulas of (A) prednisolone, and (B) fluprednisolone.

increases glucocorticoid activity with less effect on mineralocorticoid activity, as with fluprednisolone (see Figure 16-16).

(4) A hydroxyl group at position C-17 and a hydroxyl group (as with triamcinolone) or a methyl group (as with dexamethasone) at position C-16 enhance glucocorticoid activity and abolish mineralocorticoid activity (Figure 16-17).

(5) An acetate ester at position C-21 or a 16α-, 17α-isopropylidenedioxy group (also known as an acetonide group) enhances topical absorption, as with fluocinonide (see Figure 16-17).

2. Aldosterone, which is formed in the outer (glomerular) layer of the adrenal cortex, is the prototypical mineralocorticoid. The two clinically useful mineralocorticoids are **desoxycorticosterone acetate** and **fludrocortisone acetate** (Figure 16-18).

B. Pharmacology

1. Therapeutically useful adrenocorticosteroids mimic the activity of the natural glucocorticoids and have metabolic, anti-inflammatory, and immunosuppressive activity.

2. Adrenocorticosteroids require cytoplasmic receptors for transportation to the nuclei of target tissue cells, where they stimulate production of messenger and ribosomal RNA. Adrenocorticosteroids also act in the feedback regulation of pituitary corticotropin.

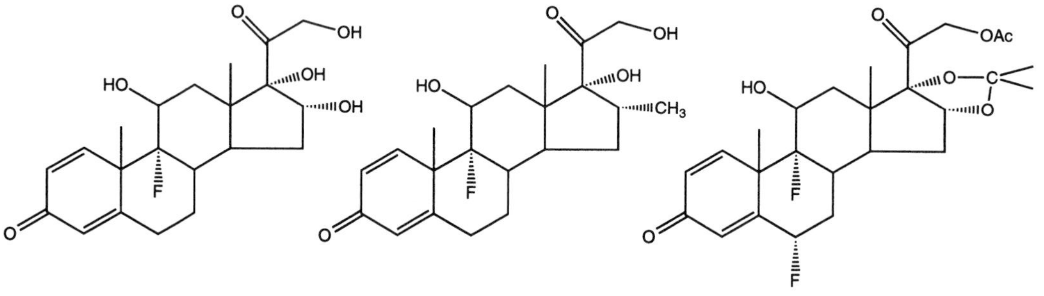

Figure 16-17. Structural formulas of (*A*) triamcinolone, (*B*) dexamethasone, and (*C*) fluocinonide.

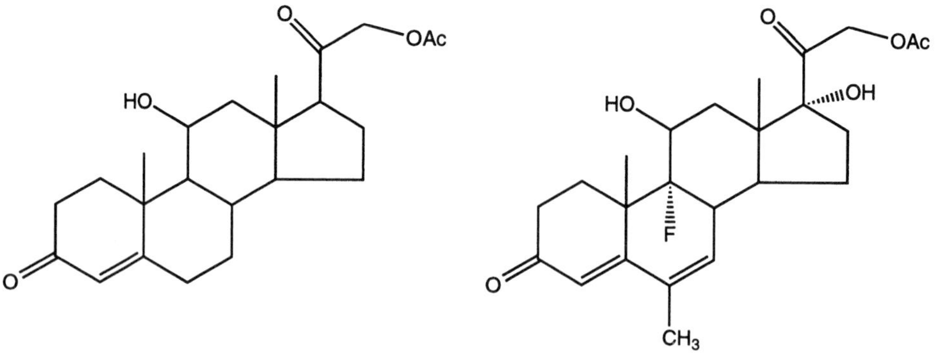

Figure 16-18. Structural formulas of (*A*) desoxycorticosterone acetate and (*B*) fludrocortisone acetate, the clinically useful mineralocorticoids.

C. Therapeutic indications. Adrenocorticosteroids are used:

1. As replacement therapy, to treat acute and chronic adrenal insufficiency

2. As the therapy of last resort, to treat severe, disabling arthritis

3. To treat severe allergic reactions

4. To treat chronic ulcerative colitis

5. To treat rheumatic carditis

6. To treat renal diseases, including nephrotic syndrome

7. To treat collagen vascular diseases

8. To treat cerebral edema

9. As topical agents, to treat skin disorders and inflammatory ocular disorders

D. Adverse effects. Adrenocorticosteroids are associated with:

1. Suppression of pituitary-adrenal integrity

2. GI effects, such as peptic ulcer, GI hemorrhage, ulcerative esophagitis, and acute pancreatitis

3. CNS effects, such as headache, vertigo, increased intraocular and intracranial pressures, muscle weakness, and psychological disturbances (euphoria or dysphoria, depression, suicidal tendencies)

4. Cardiovascular effects, such as edema and hypertension

5. Other effects, including weight gain, osteoporosis, hyperglycemia, flushed face and neck, acne, hirsutism, cushingoid "moon face" and "buffalo hump," and increased susceptibility to infection

V. THYROID HORMONES AND INHIBITORS

A. Chemistry

1. **Synthesis of thyroid hormones** is a four-step process beginning with the concentration of iodide in the thyroid gland. The enzyme iodoperoxidase then catalyzes steps two and three: iodination of tyrosine residues located on thyroglobulin, a 650,000 mol wt glycoprotein located within the thyroid gland; and coupling of the iodinated tyrosine precursors. Finally, proteolysis of thyroglobulin produces the two naturally occurring thyroid hormones, **thyroxine (levothyroxine, T_4)** and **triiodothyronine (liothyronine, T_3)** in a ratio of 4 to 1.
   a. Levothyroxine is less potent than liothyronine but possesses a longer duration of action (6–7 days versus 1–2 days).
   b. Peripheral deiodination by **5'-deiodinase** converts T_4 to T_3.
   c. **Regulation** of thyroid hormone production involves a hypothalamic-pituitary-thyroid feedback system. **Thyrotropin-releasing hormone (TRH)** is secreted by the hypothalamus and stimulates the release of **thyroid-stimulating hormone (TSH, thyrotropin)** from the anterior pituitary. Thyrotropin stimulates the thyroid gland to produce T_4 and T_3. These hormones then regulate their own synthesis by binding to specific sites in the anterior pituitary and inhibiting the release of TSH.

2. **Available thyroid preparations**
   a. The **sodium salts** of T_3 and T_4 are used therapeutically (Figure 16-19). Due to peripheral conversion, the administration of levothyroxine sodium alone will produce the natural 4 to 1 ratio of T_4 to T_3.
   b. **Liotrix** (Thyrolar) is a 4 to 1 mixture of levothyroxine sodium to liothyronine sodium, which is equivalent to, but offers no advantages over, levothyroxine only.
   c. **Thyroid USP** is made from dried, defatted thyroid glands of domestic animals and is standardized based on iodine content.
   d. **Thyroglobulin** (Proloid) is a partially purified extract of frozen porcine or bovine thyroid gland. It contains both T_3 and T_4 and conforms to USP iodine content requirements.
   e. **Thyrotropin** (TSH) is a highly purified and lyophilized thyrotropic hormone isolated from bovine anterior pituitary glands.

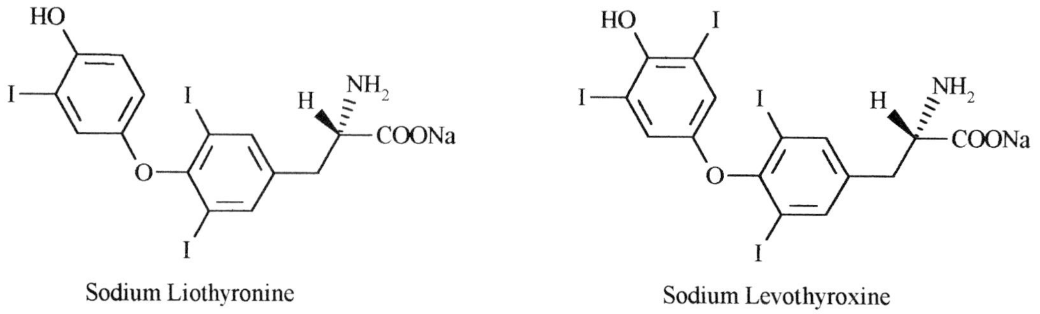

Sodium Liothyronine   Sodium Levothyroxine

Figure 16-19. Sodium salt forms of the naturally occurring thyroid hormones, liothyronine (T$_3$) and levothyroxine (T$_4$).

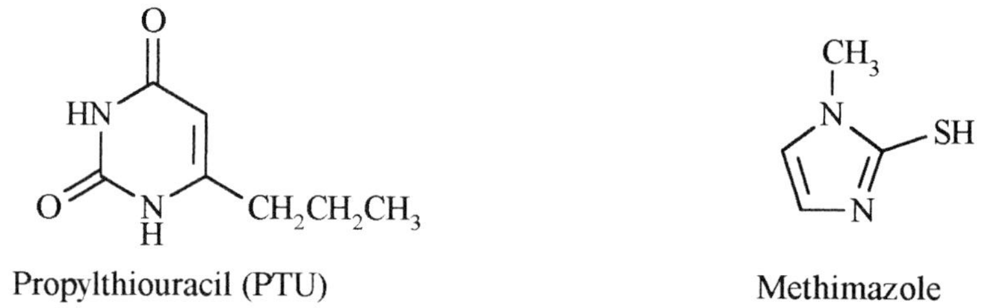

Propylthiouracil (PTU)   Methimazole

Figure 16-20. Structures of the thiourylene class of antithyroid hormones.

3. **Inhibitors** of thyroid function directly or indirectly interfere with the synthesis of thyroid hormones. These agents include ionic inhibitors, potassium or sodium iodide, radioactive iodine (e.g., Na^{131}I), and the thiourylenes (e.g., propylthiouracil, methimazole) [Figure 16-20].

B. **Pharmacology**

1. **Thyroid hormone preparations** mimic the activity of endogenous and thyroid hormones. These hormones regulate growth and development, have calorigenic and metabolic activity, and (through sensitization of β-adrenergic receptors) have positive inotropic and chronotropic effects on the myocardium.

2. **Thyroid inhibitors** act via several different mechanisms.
   a. **Ionic inhibitors,** such as thiocyanate (SCN$^-$) and perchlorate (ClO$_4^-$), are inorganic, monovalent anions that interfere with the concentration of iodide ion by the thyroid gland.
   b. **Iodides in high concentrations** (e.g., Lugol's solution) have profound effects in all aspects of thyroid synthesis, release, and metabolism. Iodides limit their own transport, inhibit the synthesis of both iodotyrosine and iodothyronine, and most importantly, inhibit the release of thyroid hormones.
   c. **Radioactive iodine (**^{131}**I)** is administered as a sodium salt, is rapidly trapped by the thyroid gland, and is incorporated into both tyrosine precursors and mature thyroid hormones. Radioactive β-particle decay produces localized destruction of thyroid cells and the desired therapeutic effect.
   d. **Thiourylenes** inhibit the enzyme iodoperoxidase, thereby inhibiting two crucial steps in thyroid synthesis: the incorporation of iodine into tyrosine precursor molecules and the coupling of iodinated tyrosines to form T$_4$ and T$_3$. Additionally, propylthiouracil inhibits the conversion of T$_4$ to T$_3$.

C. **Therapeutic indications**

1. The major indications for **thyroid hormone preparations** are hypothyroidism (i.e., myxedema), myxedema coma, cretinism, and simple goiter. Other indications include endemic goiter and thyrotropin-dependent carcinoma.

2. **Thyrotropin** is used as an adjunct in the detection and treatment of thyroid cancer.

3. **Thyroid inhibitors** are used to treat hyperthyroidism. The two most common types of hyperthyroidism are **Graves' disease** and **toxic adenoma.** Less common causes are toxic multinodular goiter, thyroiditis, and single hyperfunctioning thyroid nodules.

   a. **Ionic inhibitors** are rarely used therapeutically; however, the metabolism of some foods (e.g., cabbage) and drugs (e.g., sodium nitroprusside) can produce significant amounts of thiocyanate.

   b. **High concentrations of iodide** (Lugol's solution) are used before thyroid surgery to make the thyroid gland firmer and reduce its size.

   c. ^{131}I is useful particularly in treating hyperthyroidism in older patients and in patients with heart disease.

   d. **Thiourylenes** (e.g., propylthiouracil, methimazole) are used to control mild cases of hyperthyroidism, in conjunction with ^{131}I, and to prepare patients before thyroid surgery. They are less effective in producing permanent remission of Graves' disease.

D. Adverse effects

1. **Thyroid hormone preparations** are only **rarely associated** with adverse effects. Overdosage can cause palpitations, nervousness, insomnia, and weight loss.

2. **Thyrotropin** is associated with nausea, vomiting, headache, urticaria, anaphylaxis, thyroid gland swelling, transient hypotension, tachycardia, and arrhythmias.

3. **Thyroid inhibitors** are associated with adverse effects that depend on the agent used.

   a. **Ionic inhibitors,** specifically perchlorate, can cause fatal aplastic anemia when used in excessive amounts (i.e., 2–3 g/day).

   b. **Iodides** are associated with these adverse effects.

      (1) Iodism, including increased salivation, brassy taste, sore teeth and gums, swollen eyelids, inflamed larynx and pharynx, frontal headache, skin lesions, and skin eruptions

      (2) Hypersensitivity reactions with fever, arthralgia, eosinophilia, and angioedema

      (3) Large doses of iodides given over long periods can cause goiter and hypothyroidism, which can be corrected by the administration of thyroid hormone.

   c. ^{131}I is associated with:

      (1) Delayed hypothyroidism (relatively high incidence)

      (2) Possible effects on the future offspring of young adults

   d. **Thiourylenes** are associated with:

      (1) Dermatological effects such as urticarial papular rash and dermatitis

      (2) Hematological effects such as agranulocytosis, thrombocytopenia, and granulocytopenia

      (3) GI effects such as nausea, vomiting, and GI distress

      (4) Pain, stiffness in the joints, headache, and paresthesias

      (5) Other effects such as drug fever, hepatitis, nephritis, and systemic lupus erythematosus–like syndrome are rare.

E. Drug interactions with thyroid hormones

1. Bile acid sequestrants (BAS), calcium, ferrous sulfate, sucralfate, iron, and aluminum hydroxide antacids can **decrease the absorption** of thyroid hormones. An appropriate solution to this problem is to adequately space the administration of these agents (e.g., take the thyroid hormone 1 hour before or 4 hours after taking the BAS).

2. A number of drugs, including phenytoin, carbamazepine, and rifampin, **accelerate thyroid metabolism.** An appropriate solution to this problem is to increase the dose of the thyroid hormone.

VI. ANTIDIABETIC AGENTS

A. Chemistry. Antidiabetic agents include insulin preparations and oral hypoglycemic agents.

1. **Insulin** is an endocrine hormone secreted by the β cells of the pancreas. It is a 51–amino acid protein composed of **two polypeptide chains:** an A chain of 21 amino acids and a B chain of 30 amino acids. Two interchain disulfide bonds connect the A and B chains, and

a third intrachain disulfide bond is found between Cys_6 and Cys_{11} of the A chain. Insulin is derived from an 86–amino acid precursor known as proinsulin.

a. **Source.** Insulin is available as bovine insulin (which differs from human insulin by three amino acids), porcine insulin (which differs from human insulin only in the terminal amino acid), and human insulin. Additionally, several synthetic insulin analogues—**lispro insulin** (Humalog), **insulin aspart** (NovoLog), and **insulin glargine** (Lantus)—are available.

   (1) **Single-species** insulins contain only bovine or only porcine insulin.

   (2) **Mixed** insulins contain both bovine and porcine insulin.

   (3) **Human** insulins are prepared either by enzymatic conversion of the terminal amino acid of porcine insulin (Novolin) or by means of recombinant DNA technology (Humulin).

b. **Categories.** Preparations of insulin are divided into three categories according to their on-set, duration, and intensity of action following subcutaneous (SQ) administration: fast-acting, intermediate-acting, and long-acting. Insulin solubility at the injection site depends on the physical state, the zinc content, the nature of the buffer, and the protein content.

   (1) **Short-acting** insulins include lispro insulin, insulin aspart, regular insulin, and semi-lente insulin.

   (a) **Lispro insulin** differs from normal insulin in that the Lys_{29} and Pro_{28} residues of the β-chain are reversed. This structural alteration provides for a shorter onset (30–60 minutes) and duration (3–4 hours) than that of regular insulin.

   (b) **Insulin aspart** differs from normal insulin in that the Pro_{28} residue of the β-chain is replaced with an aspartic acid (Asp). This structural change reduces the ten-dency of insulin to self-associate as hexamers and thus provides for a rapid on-set and short duration, similar to that described for lispro insulin. Both lispro in-sulin and insulin aspart should be administered immediately (5–10 minutes) before a meal.

   (c) **Regular insulin** (also called insulin injection or crystalline zinc insulin) is a sol-uble insulin prepared at neutral pH. It is the only type of insulin that can be mixed with all other insulins (except glargine) and also the only type forming a clear solution, which can be given intravenously.

   (d) **Semilente insulin** is a finely divided, amorphous preparation also called prompt insulin zinc suspension. The lente insulins [see VI A 1 b (2) (b), (3) (b)] contain no modifying protein and are prepared with an acetate buffer. Lente insulins can be mixed with each other but cannot be mixed with either NPH insulin (iso-phane insulin) or protamine zinc insulin (PZI). These latter insulins are prepared with a phosphate buffer, which is incompatible with the acetate buffer of the lente insulins. Semilente insulin has a duration of action comparable to that of regular insulin.

   (2) **Long-acting** insulins include PZI, ultralente insulin, and insulin glargine.

   (a) PZI consists of insulin complexed with zinc and an excess of protamine in a phosphate buffer.

   (b) Ultralente insulin is a large, crystalline form, also known as extended insulin zinc suspension. Its duration of action is comparable to that of PZI.

   (c) **Insulin glargine** differs from normal insulin in that Gly replaces the Asn_{21} residue of the α-chain and a basic Arg-Arg dipeptide replaces the Thr_{30} of the β-chain. These structural alterations cause a decreased solubility at physiological pH, precipitation and delayed absorption following subcutaneous injection, and an increased duration of action.

   (3) **Intermediate-acting** insulins include NPH and lente insulin.

   (a) NPH is similar to PZI but contains stoichiometric amounts of protamine and in-sulin (no excess).

   (b) Lente insulin, also known as insulin zinc suspension, is a mixture of 70% ultra-lente crystals and 30% semilente powder. Its duration of action is comparable to that of NPH.

2. **Oral antidiabetic agents** can be classified as either sulfonylureas, biguanides, meglitinides, thiazolidinediones, or β-glucosidase inhibitors.

   a. **Sulfonylureas,** shown in Table 16-1, are acidic compounds and include both first- and second-generation agents. Second-generation agents (**glyburide, glipizide,** and **glime-pride**) have larger groups attached to the aromatic ring (i.e., larger R_1 substituents), are more lipid soluble, and are more potent as compared to first-generation agents (**tolbu-tamide, chlorpropamide, tolazamide,** and **acetohexamide**).

Table 16-1. Oral Hypoglycemic Agents: The Sulfonylureas

General Sulfonylurea Structure

$$R_1 \!-\! \langle\text{phenyl}\rangle \!-\! \overset{\overset{O}{\|}}{\underset{\underset{O}{\|}}{S}} \!-\! \overset{H}{N} \!-\! \overset{\overset{O}{\|}}{C} \!-\! \overset{H}{N} \!-\! R_2$$

Drug	R_1 Substituent	R_2 Substituent
First-generation agents		
Tolbutamide (Orinase)	CH_3	$CH_2CH_2CH_2CH_3$
Chlorpropamide (Diabinese)	Cl	$CH_2CH_2CH_3$
Tolazamide (Tolinase)	CH_3	$-N\langle\text{azepane ring}\rangle$
Acetohexamide (Dymelor)	$H_3C-\overset{\overset{O}{\|}}{C}$	$\langle\text{cyclohexyl}\rangle$
Second-generation agents Glyburide (DiaBeta, Micronase)	$Cl\langle\text{benzene, }OCH_3\rangle\text{C}(=O)NHCH_2CH_2$	$\langle\text{cyclohexyl}\rangle$
Glipizide (Glucotrol)	$H_3C\langle\text{pyrazine}\rangle\text{C}(=O)NHCH_2CH_2$	$\langle\text{cyclohexyl}\rangle$
Glimepride (Amaryl)	$H_3C,\ H_3C\langle\text{cyclopentenone}\rangle\text{C}(=O)NHCH_2CH_2$	$\langle\text{methyl-cyclohexyl}\rangle-CH_3$

  b. **Metformin,** a **biguanide,** is a basic compound and is currently the only available agent in its chemical class (Figure 16-21). An additional agent, **phenformin,** was withdrawn from the market in 1977 because of a high incidence of fatal lactic acidosis.
  c. **Meglitinides** are acidic compounds. Currently available compounds in this chemical class include **repaglinide** and **nateglinide** (see Figure 16-21).
  d. **Rosiglitazone** and **pioglitazone** are acidic compounds and can be chemically classified as **thiazolidinediones.** A third agent, **troglitizone,** was withdrawn from the market because of rare but severe hepatic toxicity (see Figure 16-21).

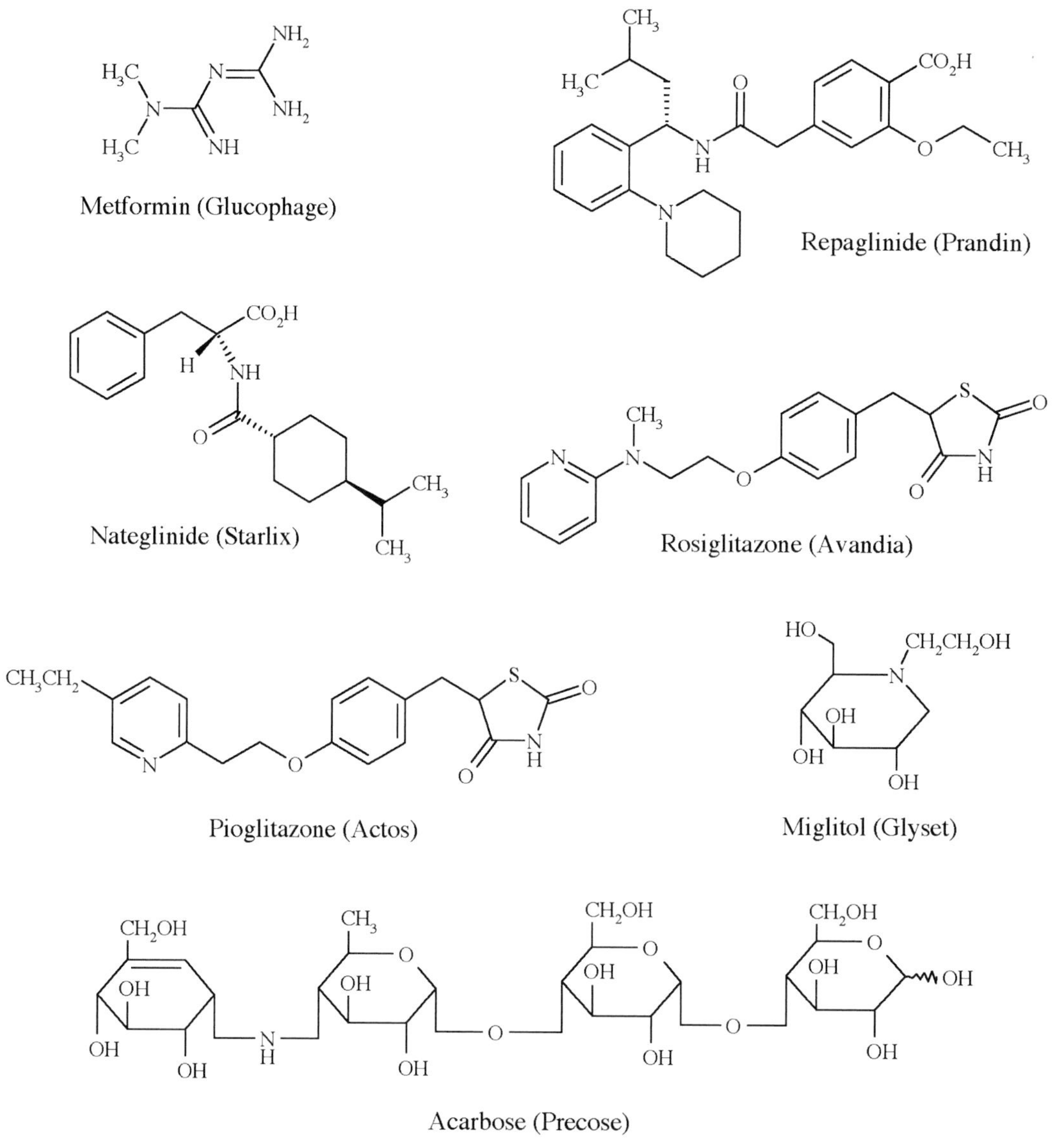

Figure 16-21. Structures of oral hypoglycemic agents: biguanides (metformin), meglitinides (repaglinide and nateglinide), thiazolidinediones (pioglitazone and rosiglitazone) and α-glucosidase inhibitors (miglitol and acarbose).

   e. Inhibitors of α-glucosidase are basic analogues of either monosaccharides or polysaccharides. The monosaccharide **miglitol** has better oral absorption than the α-1-4 linked tetrasaccharide **acarbose** (see Figure 16-21).

B. Pharmacology

1. **Insulin preparations** mimic the activity of endogenous insulin, which is required for the proper utilization of glucose in normal metabolism. Insulin interacts with a specific cell-surface receptor to facilitate the transport of glucose and amino acids.

2. **Oral antidiabetic agents** act through a variety of mechanisms.
   a. **Sulfonylureas** block adenosine triphosphate (ATP)-sensitive potassium channels, which stimulates the release of insulin from pancreatic β cells. Thus, sulfonylureas can also be

classified as potassium channel blockers (or closers). Additionally, sulfonylureas can enhance the peripheral response to a given amount of insulin by increasing the number or affinity of cell-surface insulin receptors. The clinical significance of this extrahepatic effect has been questioned.

b. Biguanides do not stimulate the release of insulin, do not cause hypoglycemia, and thus are best described as antihyperglycemic agents. The reduction in glucose levels seen with these agents is thought to be caused by an increase in insulin action in peripheral tissues as well as an inhibition of gluconeogenesis. It has been proposed that these compounds increase glucose transport across skeletal muscle cell membranes.

c. Meglitinides are similar to the sulfonylureas in that they lower glucose levels by stimulating the release of insulin. They differ from the sulfonylureas in that they have a more rapid onset of action and a shorter duration of action.

d. Thiazolidinediones do not stimulate insulin secretion, but instead bind to nuclear peroxisome proliferator-activated receptors (PPARs) involved in transcription of insulin-responsive genes and in regulation of adipocyte differentiation and lipid metabolism. This decreases insulin resistance and improves target cell response to insulin. These compounds are active only when insulin is present.

e. α-Glucosidase inhibitors inhibit the digestion of carbohydrates in the small intestine and therefore decrease the postprandial rise in glucose levels.

C. Therapeutic indication

1. Insulin preparations are used to treat insulin-dependent diabetes mellitus (IDDM) that cannot be controlled by diet alone. They can also be used in patients with non–insulin-dependent diabetes mellitus (NIDDM) in patients who are not adequately controlled by either diet or oral antidiabetic agents.

2. Oral antidiabetic agents are used as an adjunct to diet in treating NIDDM that cannot be controlled by diet alone. Each class of compounds can be used either as monotherapy or in combination with one another.

D. Adverse effects

1. Insulin preparations are associated with these adverse effects.
   a. Hypoglycemia, with sweating, tachycardia, and hunger; possibly progressing to insulin shock with hypoglycemic convulsions
   b. Hypersensitivity reactions
   c. Local irritation at the injection site

2. **Oral antidiabetic agents** produce a variety of adverse effects, which depend on both the class and mechanism of the compounds.
   a. Sulfonylureas are associated with the following adverse effects.
   (1) Hypoglycemia, particularly in patients with renal or hepatic insufficiency who are taking longer-acting agents (e.g., chlorpropamide)
   (2) GI effects, such as nausea, vomiting, diarrhea, and constipation
   (3) Hypersensitivity reactions, such as skin rash and photosensitivity. Cross-sensitivity may occur among classes of compounds that also contain the benzene sulfonamide functional group (e.g., **sulfanilamide antibacterials, thiazides, loop diuretics,** and **carbonic anhydrase inhibitors**).
   (4) Blood dyscrasias, such as leukopenia, thrombocytopenia, agranulocytosis, and hemolytic anemia
   (5) Cholestatic jaundice
   (6) Hyponatremia due to a potentiation of the effects of antidiuretic hormone (seen primarily with chlorpropamide)
   b. Biguanides do not cause hypoglycemia but have been associated with the following adverse effects.
   (1) Fatal lactic acidosis. Phenformin was withdrawn from the United States market in 1977 because of a high incidence of this serious adverse effect. The frequency of this effect in metformin is considerably less than that seen with phenformin, and in most if not all reported cases, the lactic acidosis occurred in patients in whom metformin was contraindicated.
   (2) Metallic taste
   (3) GI effects, such as epigastric distress, nausea, vomiting, diarrhea, and anorexia

    c. **Repaglinide** is associated with the following adverse effects. **Nateglinide,** the other commercially available **meglitinide,** is only associated with hypoglycemia.

        (1) **Hypoglycemia.** Due to its shorter duration of action, it is not as likely as the sulfonylureas to cause severe hypoglycemia.

        (2) **Upper respiratory infection, rhinitis,** and **bronchitis**

        (3) **Headache** and **back pain**

    d. **Thizaolidinediones** used alone, have a low probability of producing hypoglycemia. This probability increases when they are used in combination with either insulin or sulfonylureas. Other adverse effects associated with this class of agents include:

        (1) **Hepatotoxicity,** although rare, can be severe and fatal. To date, this has only occurred with troglitazone, resulting in its removal from the market. As a result, strict monitoring is used during the first year of therapy and then periodically afterwards.

        (2) **GI effects,** such as nausea and vomiting, abdominal fullness, epigastric discomfort, and diarrhea

        (3) An initial and reversible decrease in hemoglobin and white blood count during the first 4–8 weeks of therapy

        (4) **Weight gain** and **edema**

        (5) **Headache**

        (6) **Upper respiratory infection**

    e. **α-Glucosidase inhibitors** do not cause hypoglycemia but have been associated with **GI distress** due to the presence of undigested carbohydrates in the lower GI tract. Smaller compounds such as the monosaccharide **miglitol** are better absorbed and produce fewer GI effects than larger compounds such as **acarbose.**

E. Drug interactions for oral antidiabetic agents can be separated into two major groups: those that alter glucose levels and those that are agent or class specific.

    1. There are a number of compounds that alter glucose levels and thus require changes in drug therapy. These interactions do not specifically interfere with the absorption, distribution, mechanism, or elimination of any specific oral antidiabetic drug and have been referred to as pharmacodynamic drug interactions.

        a. **Thiazide diuretics** can cause an increase in blood glucose levels by altering carbohydrate metabolism.

        b. **β-Blockers** can have varying effects on glucose levels. They can potentiate hypoglycemia by inhibiting glycogenolysis and glucagon release; however, they can also promote hyperglycemia by inhibiting insulin secretion and decreasing tissue sensitivity to insulin. Additionally, these compounds can mask the signs of hypoglycemia by blunting the reflex tachycardia.

        c. **Oral contraceptives and glucocorticoids** can decrease the efficacy of antidiabetic agents by promoting insulin resistance. Additionally, glucocorticoids produce metabolic effects that are opposite those of insulin.

        d. A number of other drugs can also decrease the glucose-lowering effects of antidiabetic agents. These include **phenytoin, sympathomimetics, corticotropoin, ACTH, salicylates, and isoniazid.**

        e. Some **androgens and anabolic steroids** can cause hypoglycemia in diabetic patients, but not in nondiabetic individuals.

        f. **Monoamine oxidase inhibitors** (MAOIs) can stimulate insulin secretion and can contribute to hypoglycemic.

        g. **4-Fluoroquinolones** (e.g., ciprofloxacin, ofloxacin) have been reported to cause alterations in blood glucose levels—hypoglycemia in some individuals and hyperglycemia in others.

    2. **Drug or drug class specific interactions**

        a. **Sulfonylureas** are highly plasma protein bound, cause the release of insulin by blocking potassium channels in pancreatic cells, and with the exception of acetohexamide, are oxidatively metabolized by CYP450 enzymes. As a result, drug interactions will occur with:

            (1) Drugs capable of causing **plasma protein displacement** (e.g., fibrates, sulfonamides, phenylbutazone).

            (2) The **potassium channel openers** minoxidil and diazoxide.

            (3) Drugs capable of **inducing or inhibiting** CYP450 enzymes. Glimepride is metabolized by the CYP2C9 isoform; however, literature references do not provide specific isoform designations for other sulfonylureas.

b. Biguanides. An increased risk of lactic acidosis and acute renal failure can occur if metformin is coadministered with any of the following agents.

    (1) Cationic drugs eliminated by renal tubular secretion (e.g., amiloride, cimetidine, dofetilide, midodrine, morphine, procainamide, quinidine, quinine, ranitidine, triamterene, trimethoprim, or vancomycin). These compounds may interfere with the renal tubular secretion of metformin.

    (2) Iodinated contrast materials

    (3) Corticosteroids

c. Meglitinides have the same drug interaction profile as the sulfonylureas. Nateglinide is oxidatively metabolized by the CYP2C9 and CYP3A4 isozymes, while repaglinide is metabolized solely by CYP3A4. Drug interactions involving metabolism would therefore be limited to those capable of inducing or inhibiting these two isozymes.

d. Thiazolidinediones. Pioglitazone requires CYP3A4 for oxidative metabolism and therefore has possible drug interactions with other compounds that inhibit or induce this isozyme. Additionally, pioglitazone can induce CYP3A4 and may decrease the bioavailability of oral contraceptives and other compounds requiring its activity. In contrast, rosiglitazone is metabolized by CYP2C8 and has no clinically significant drug interactions involving CYP450 enzymes.

e. α-Glucosidase inhibitors may impair the oral absorption of digoxin.

STUDY QUESTIONS

Directions: Each of the numbered items or incomplete statements in this section is followed by answers or by completions of the statement. Select the **one** lettered answer or completion that is **best** in each case.

1. The following structure is a hormone. It would be classified best as

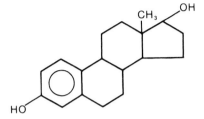

(A) an estrogen
(B) a progestin
(C) an androgen
(D) a gonadotropin
(E) an adrenocorticosteroid

2. All of the following substances are endogenous tropic hormones secreted by the pituitary gland EXCEPT

(A) somatotropin
(B) human chorionic gonadotropin (hCG)
(C) follicle-stimulating hormone (FSH)
(D) thyroid-stimulating hormone (TSH)
(E) adrenocorticotropic hormone (ACTH)

3. Which of the following substances when present in urine is the most likely positive sign of pregnancy?

(A) Thyroid-stimulating hormone (TSH)
(B) Corticotropin (ACTH)
(C) Human chorionic gonadotropin (hCG)
(D) Interstitial cell-stimulating hormone (ICSH)
(E) Protamine zinc insulin (PZI)

4. All of the following hormonal drugs possess a steroidal nucleus EXCEPT

(A) ethinyl estradiol
(B) norethindrone
(C) liothyronine
(D) prednisolone
(E) fluoxymesterone

5. Which of the following glucocorticoids produces the least sodium retention?

(A) Cortisone
(B) Hydrocortisone
(C) Prednisolone
(D) Dexamethasone
(E) Fludrocortisone

6. Which of the following insulins can be administered intravenously?

(A) Regular insulin
(B) Isophane insulin (NPH)
(C) Protamine zinc insulin (PZI)
(D) Semilente insulin
(E) Ultralente insulin

7. In comparing levothyroxine to liothyronine, which of the following statements is NOT correct?

(A) Both levothyroxine and liothyronine are naturally occurring thyroid hormones.
(B) Liothyronine can be converted in the peripheral circulation to levothyroxine.
(C) Liothyronine is more potent than levothyroxine.
(D) The plasma concentration of liothyronine is less than that of levothyroxine.
(E) Liothyronine has a shorter duration of action than levothyroxine.

8. Which of the following classes of compounds stimulates the release of insulin from pancreatic β-cells?

(A) Progestins
(B) Biguanides
(C) α-Glucosidase inhibitors
(D) Thiourylenes
(E) Sulfonylureas

9. Which of the following compounds is incorrectly matched with its mechanism of action?

(A) Flutamide: competitively blocks the binding of androgens to their receptor
(B) Finasteride: inhibits 5α-reductase
(C) Miglitol: inhibits α-glucosidase
(D) Pioglitazone: competitively blocks the binding of estrogens to their receptor
(E) Anastrazole: inhibits aromatase

10. Which of the following compounds is incorrectly matched with one of its therapeutic uses?

(A) Raloxifene: advanced breast cancer
(B) Metformin: non–insulin-dependent diabetes mellitus (NIDDM)
(C) Finasteride: benign prostatic hyperplasia
(D) Propylthiouracil: hyperthyroidism
(E) Tamoxifen: estrogen-dependent breast cancer

Directions: Each question below contains three suggested answers, of which **one or more** is correct. Choose the answer

A	if **I only** is correct
B	if **III only** is correct
C	if **I and II** are correct
D	if **II and III** are correct
E	if **I, II, and III** are correct

11. Hormones that form lipophilic esters without prior structural modifications include

I. hydrocortisone
II. testosterone
III. progesterone

12. Insulin preparations that contain a modifying protein include

I. lente insulin
II. regular insulin
III. isophane insulin (NPH)

Directions: Each group of items in this section consists of lettered options followed by a set of numbered items. For each item, select the **one** lettered option that is most closely associated with it. Each lettered option may be selected once, more than once, or not at all.

Questions 13–15
For each pharmacological property, select the hormone that most closely relates to it.

(A) Testosterone
(B) Insulin
(C) Corticotropin
(D) Estradiol
(E) Vasopressin

13. Secreted by pancreatic β cells to facilitate glucose and amino acid transport for normal cellular metabolic processes

14. Initiates and controls male sexual development and maintains the integrity of the male reproductive system

15. Promotes the resorption of water at the renal distal convoluted tubule

Questions 16–18
For each adverse effect, select the class of drug that most closely relates to it.

(A) Antithyroid agents
(B) Sulfonylurea oral hypoglycemics
(C) Adrenocorticosteroids
(D) Progestins
(E) Androgens

16. Peptic ulceration and gastrointestinal hemorrhage; hyperglycemia, hypertension, and edema; "buffalo hump" and "moon face"; psychological disturbances; and increased susceptibility to infection

17. Agranulocytosis and other blood dyscrasias, cholestatic jaundice, nausea and vomiting, hypoglycemia, and photosensitivity

18. Hepatotoxicity and jaundice, urinary retention and azoospermia, prostatic hypertrophy and priapism, and paradoxical gynecomastia

ANSWERS AND EXPLANATIONS

1. The answer is A *[III A 1 a; Figure 16-1].*
Ring A is aromatic. Because the only type of steroidal hormone that has an aromatic A ring is an estrogen, this structure represents an estrogen. Other structural characteristics of estrogens include the fact that the structure contains 18 carbon atoms; thus, it is an estrane and contains a β-alcohol group in position 17.

2. The answer is B *[II A 2 a, b].*
Human chorionic gonadotropin (hCG) is produced by placental tissue and serves to stimulate the secretion of progesterone during pregnancy. Growth hormone (somatotropin), follicle-stimulating hormone (FSH), thyroid-stimulating hormone (TSH), and corticotropin (ACTH) are all secreted by the anterior pituitary gland.

3. The answer is C *[II A 2 b (3)].*
Human chorionic gonadotropin (hCG) is a proteinaceous tropic hormone that is secreted by chorionic (e.g., placental) tissue. Thus, hCG is present in the urine only after conception has occurred.

4. The answer is C *[V A 1; Figures 16-4, 16-10, 16-12, 16-16, 16-19].*
Liothyronine is a thyroid hormone. Thyroid hormones consist of iodinated aromatic amino acids and are not steroidal in nature. Ethinyl estradiol is a steroidal estrogen, norethindrone is a steroidal 19-norprogestin, prednisolone is an adrenocorticosteroid, and fluoxymesterone is a steroidal androgen.

5. The answer is D *[IV A 1 b (4); Figure 16-17].*
Glucocorticoids have varying degrees of mineralocorticoid activity. This mineralocorticoid activity, which can result in sodium and fluid retention, can be blocked by the introduction of a methyl or hydroxyl group in position 16 of the steroidal nucleus. Dexamethasone has a 16 α-methyl substituent.

6. The answer is A *[VI A 1 b].*
Most insulin preparations are suspensions; thus, they contain particulate matter. Only clear solutions may be administered intravenously. Regular insulin, which consists of water-soluble crystalline zinc insulin is therefore suitable for intravenous administration. Insulin preparations normally are injected subcutaneously.

7. The answer is B *[V A 1 a, b].*
The thyroid gland produces both levothyroxine (T_4) and liothyronine (T_3). The natural ratio of these compounds is 4 to 1 in favor of levothyroxine; therefore, liothyronine is normally present at a lower concentration than levothyroxine. Liothyronine is more potent than levothyroxine, but has a shorter duration of action. Peripheral conversion involves deiodination, thus levothyroxine is converted to liothyronine. The reverse process is not possible.

8. The answer is E *[VI B 2 a, b, e].*
Of the five classes of compounds listed, only biguanides, α-glucosidase inhibitors, and sulfonylureas are used in the treatment of non–insulin-dependent diabetes mellitus (NIDDM). These classes provide their beneficial effects through different mechanisms of action. Biguanides enhance the peripheral use of insulin, suppress gluconeogenesis, and are often referred to as antihyperglycemic agents. α-Glucosidase inhibitors decrease the absorption of glucose. Sulfonylureas and the structurally unrelated compounds, repaglinide and nateglinide, stimulate the secretion of insulin from pancreatic β cells.

9. The answer is D *[III A 7, D 2, E 2; VI A 2 d, B 2 d].*
Pioglitazone does not interact with estrogen receptors. It is an oral hypoglycemic agent that produces its effects by binding to nuclear peroxisome proliferator-activated receptors (PPARs) involved in transcription of insulin-responsive genes and in regulation of adipocyte differentiation and lipid metabolism. The other four agents are correctly matched to their mechanisms.

10. The answer is A *[III A 5 b, 7, E 3; V C 3 d; VI A 2, C 2].*
Raloxifene is a selective estrogen receptor modulator (SERM) and is not used to treat breast cancer. Instead, because of its ability to reduce bone resorption and decrease bone turnover, it is used for the prevention of osteoporosis. All of the other four compounds are correctly matched to their therapeutic use. Finasteride is also used to treat androgenic alopecia.

11. The answer is C (I, II) *[III C 1; Figures 16-8, 16-11, 16-15].*
Hydrocortisone has a 21-hydroxyl group, and testosterone has a 17-hydroxyl group; therefore, both of these agents can form esters (e.g., hydrocortisone acetate, testosterone propionate). Progesterone does not have any alcohol groups in its molecule; therefore, it cannot directly form any esters.

12. The answer is B (III) *[VI A 1 b].*
Regular insulin, which is a rapid-acting insulin preparation, contains only zinc insulin crystals. All lente insulins are free of modifying proteins, which contributes to their hypoallergenic properties. Isophane insulin is NPH insulin, which contains protamine, a strongly basic protein. The protamine reduces the water solubility of zinc insulin and lengthens its duration of action. Isophane insulin is classified as an intermediate-acting insulin preparation, having a duration of action of about 24 hours.

13-15. The answers are: 13-B *[VI A 1, B 1],* **14-A** *[III C 2],* **15-E** *[II B 4].*
Insulin is required for the proper utilization of glucose and the transport of glucose and amino acids across cell membranes. Testosterone, which is produced principally from the Leydig cells of the testes, is responsible for male sexual characteristics. Vasopressin is secreted from the posterior pituitary and is sometimes referred to as an antidiuretic hormone.

16-18. The answers are: 16-C *[IV D],* **17-B** *[VI D 2 a],* **18-E** *[III C 4].*
Exogenously administered adrenocorticosteroids are effective anti-inflammatory agents but give rise to a wide range of metabolic and immunosuppressive effects that result in severe adverse effects. Oral antidiabetic agents of the sulfonylurea type can cause blood dyscrasias, impaired liver function, and photosensitivity. Exogenously administered androgens suppress sperm formation and cause paradoxical gynecomastia. Most significant is the hepatotoxicity produced by alkyl-substituted androgen compounds.

17

Drug Metabolism, Prodrugs, and Pharmacogenetics

Marc W. Harrold

I. INTRODUCTION TO DRUG METABOLISM. Drug metabolism (also called **biotransformation**) refers to the biochemical changes that drugs and other foreign chemicals **(xenobiotics)** undergo in the body, leading to the formation of different metabolites with different effects. Xenobiotics can undergo a variety of biotransformation pathways, resulting in the production of a mixture of intermediate metabolites and excreted products, including unchanged parent drug. Rarely is only one metabolite produced from a single drug.

    A. Inactive metabolites. Some metabolites are inactive (i.e., their pharmacologically active parent compounds become inactivated or detoxified).

        1. The hydrolysis of **procaine** to *p*-aminobenzoic acid and diethylethanolamine results in a loss of anesthetic activity.

        2. The oxidation of **6-mercaptopurine** to 6-mercapturic acid results in a loss of anticancer activity.

    B. Metabolites that retain similar activity. Certain metabolites retain the pharmacological activity of their parent compounds to a greater or lesser degree.

        1. Imipramine is demethylated to the essentially equiactive antidepressant, **desipramine.**

        2. Acetohexamide is reduced to the more active hypoglycemic, **l-hydroxyhexamide.**

        3. Codeine is demethylated to the more active analgesic, **morphine.**

    C. Metabolites with altered activity. Some metabolites develop activity different from that of their parent drugs.

        1. The antidepressant **iproniazid** is dealkylated to the antitubercular, **isoniazid.**

        2. The vitamin **retinoic acid** (vitamin A) is isomerized to the anti-acne agent, **isoretinoic acid.**

    D. Bioactivated metabolites. Some pharmacologically inactive parent compounds are converted to active species within the body. These parent compounds are known as **prodrugs.**

        1. The prodrug **enalapril** is hydrolyzed to **enalaprilat,** a potent antihypertensive.

        2. The prodrug **sulindac,** a sulfoxide, is reduced to the active sulfide.

        3. The antiparkinsonian **levodopa (L-dopa)** is decarboxylated in the neuron to active **dopamine.**

II. BIOTRANSFORMATION PATHWAYS

    A. Phase I reactions are those in which polar functional groups are introduced into the molecule or unmasked by oxidation, reduction, or hydrolysis.

        1. Oxidation is the most common phase I biotransformation.
            a. The majority of oxidations occur in the **liver;** however, extrahepatic tissues, such as the **intestinal mucosa, lungs,** and **kidney,** can also serve as metabolic sites.
            b. The vast majority of oxidations are catalyzed by a group of mixed-function oxidases known as **cytochrome P$_{450}$ (CYP450).** These oxidases are bound to the smooth endoplastic reticulum of the liver and require both NADPH and a porphyrin prosthetic group. Unlike most enzymes, CYP450 uses a variety of oxidative biotransformations to metabolize a diverse group of substrates.

c. CYP450 exists in **multiple isoforms** or families. The presence of these different isoforms is responsible for the large substrate variation seen with CYP450.
   (1) CYP450 isoforms are named using the root "CYP" followed by an arabic number designating the family, a letter designating the subfamily, and a second arabic number indicating the individual gene (e.g., CYP3A4).
   (2) Six mammalian families are involved in steroid and bile acid metabolism: CYP7, CYP11, CYP17, CYP19, CYP21, and CYP27.
   (3) Four mammalian families are involved in xenobiotic, or drug, metabolism: CYP1, CYP2, CYP3, and CYP4. Examples of drugs metabolized by these families and subfamilies are shown in Table 17-1. Note that some drugs (e.g., theophylline, dextromethorphan) are metabolized by multiple isoforms.

Table 17-1. Examples of Drugs Metabolized by Specific CYP450 Isoforms

CYP1A
Acetaminophen
Estradiol
Fluoroquinolones
Imipramine
Theophylline

CYP2C
Chloramphenicol
Chlorpheniramine
Diazepam
Diclofenac
Ibuprofen
Imipramine
Loratadine
Methobarbital
Naproxen
Omeprazole
Phenylbutazone
Phenytoin
Propranolol
Retinoic Acid and Retinol
Testosterone
Tolbutamide
Warfarin

CYP2D
Amitriptyline and Other TCAs
β-Blockers
Captopril
Chlorpheniramine
Clemastine
Clozapine
Codeine
Dextromethorphan
Diphenhydramine
Dolasetron and Ondansetron
Fluoxetine and Other SSRIs
Haloperidol
Hydroxyzine
Imipramine
Lidocaine
Mexilitene
Quinidine
Thioridazine

CYP2E
Acetaminophen
General Anesthetics
   (Fluorinated Hydrocarbons)
Theophylline

CYP3A
Amiodarone
Carbamazepine
Clotrimazole
Codeine
Cyclosporin
Dapsone
Dexamethasone
Dextromethorphan
Diazepam
Dihydroergotamine
1,4-Dihydropyridines (e.g., Nifedipine)
Diltiazem
Dolasetron
Estradiol
Erythromycins and Clarithromycin
Hydrocortisone
Itraconazole
Ketoconazole
Lidocaine
Lovastatin
Norethisterone
Prednisone and Prednisolone
Quinidine
Rifampin and Analogues
Tamoxifen
Testosterone
Theophylline
Trazolam
Valproic Acid
Verapamil

CYP4B
Prostaglandins

d. Additional oxidations (e.g., ethanol to acetaldehyde) are catalyzed by nonmicrosomal oxidases located in cytosol and mitochondria of extrahepatic tissues.

e. CYP450 and nonmicrosomal oxidases catalyze aromatic, aliphatic, olefinic, benzylic, allylic, and α-hydroxylations; *N*-, *O*-, and *S*-dealkylations; oxidative deamination; *N*- and *S*-oxidations; desulfuration; dehalogenation; and oxidations of alcohols and aldehydes (Table 17-2).

f. The **increased polarity** of the oxidized products (metabolites) enhances their water solubility and reduces their tubular reabsorption to some extent, thus favoring their excretion in the urine. These metabolites are somewhat **more polar** than their parent compounds and very commonly undergo further biotransformation by phase II pathways (see II B).

2. Reduction is less commonly encountered than oxidation; however, the overall goal is the same: to create polar functional groups that can be eliminated in the urine. There is evidence suggesting that the CYP450 system might be involved in some reductions. Additionally, bacteria resident in the GI tract are known to be involved in azo and nitro reductions. Reactions catalyzed by reductases are shown in Table 17-3.

3. Enzymatic hydrolysis, the addition of water across a bond, also results in more polar metabolites (see Table 17-3).

a. Esterase enzymes, usually present in plasma and various tissues, are nonspecific and catalyze de-esterification, hydrolyzing relatively nonpolar esters into two polar, more water-soluble compounds: an alcohol and an acid. Esterases are responsible for converting many prodrugs into their active forms.

b. Amidase enzymes hydrolyze amides into amines and acids (deamidation). Deamidation occurs primarily in the liver.

c. Ester drugs susceptible to plasma esterases (e.g., procaine) are usually shorter acting than structurally similar **amide drugs** (e.g., procainamide), which are not significantly hydrolyzed until they reach the liver.

d. Lactones and **lactams** are cyclic esters and amides, respectively, and are thus also susceptible to hydrolytic metabolism.

B. Phase II reactions are those in which the functional groups of the original drug (or metabolite formed in a phase I reaction) are masked by a **conjugation reaction.** Most phase II conjugates are very polar, resulting in rapid drug elimination from the body.

1. Conjugation reactions combine the **parent drug** (or its metabolites) with certain **natural endogenous constituents,** such as glucuronic acid, glycine, glutamine, sulfate, glutathione, the two-carbon acetyl fragment, or the one-carbon methyl fragment. These reactions generally require both a **high-energy molecule** and an **enzyme.**

a. The **high-energy molecule** consists of a **coenzyme** bound to the endogenous substrate, the parent drug, or the drug's phase I metabolite.

b. The **enzymes** (called **transferases**) that catalyze conjugation reactions are found mainly in the liver and, to a lesser extent, in the intestines and other tissues.

c. Most conjugates are **highly polar** and **unable to cross cell membranes,** making them almost always **pharmacologically inactive** and of little or no toxicity. Exceptions to this are acetylated and methylated conjugates. These conjugates do not possess increased polarity; however, they are usually pharmacologically inactive.

2. There are **six conjugation pathways** (Table 17-4).

a. Glucuronidation is the **most common** conjugation pathway because of a readily available supply of glucuronic acid as well as a large variety of functional groups, which can enzymatically react with this sugar derivative.

(1) The high-energy form of glucuronic acid, **uridine diphosphate glucuronic acid,** reacts with a variety of functional groups under the influence of glucuronyl transferase.

(2) Drugs that possess **hydroxyl** or **carboxyl** functional groups readily undergo glucuronidation to form ethers and esters, respectively. In addition, *N*-, *S*-, and *C*-glucuronides are also possible.

(3) As shown in Table 17-4, the addition of glucuronic acid to a drug molecule adds three hydroxyl groups and one carboxyl group. This addition greatly increases the **hydrophilicity** of the drug molecule. As a result, it is unlikely to penetrate cell membranes and elicit pharmacological activity. It is also poorly reabsorbed by the renal tubules and, thus, is readily excreted.

Table 17-2. Phase I Metabolism: Oxidative Pathways

Type of Reaction (Examples)	Reaction Pathway
1. Aromatic Hydroxylation (phenytoin, phenylbutazone)	1. R–(benzene) $\longrightarrow$ R–(benzene)–OH
2. Aliphatic Hydroxylation (pentobarbital, meprobamate)	2. R–CH$_2$–CH$_3$ $\longrightarrow$ R–CH(OH)–CH$_3$
3. Olefinic Hydroxylation (carbamazepine, cyproheptadine)	3. R–CH=CH–R $\longrightarrow$ R–CH(OH)–CH(OH)–R
4. Benzylic Hydroxylation (tolbutamide, imipramine)	4. R–(benzene)–CH$_3$ $\longrightarrow$ R–(benzene)–CH$_2$OH
5. Allylic Hydroxylation (pentazocine, hexobarbital)	5. R–CH$_2$–CH=CH–CH$_3$ $\longrightarrow$ R–CH=CH–CH$_2$OH
6. Hydroxylation-α to a Carbonyl (diazepam, ketamine)	6. R_1–NH–C(=O)–CH$_2$–R_2 $\longrightarrow$ R_1–NH–C(=O)–CH(OH)–R_2
7. Oxidative Deamination (amphetamine, dopamine)	7. R–CH$_2$–CH(NH$_2$)–CH$_3$ $\longrightarrow$ R–CH$_2$–C(=O)–CH$_3$
8. N-Dealkylation (morphine, ephedrine)	8. R–NH–CH$_3$ $\longrightarrow$ R–NH$_2$
9. N-Oxidation (acetaminophen, guanethidine)	9. Ar–NH–CH$_3$ $\longrightarrow$ Ar–N(OH)–CH$_3$
10. O-Dealkylation (codeine, papaverine)	10. R–O–CH$_3$ $\longrightarrow$ R–OH
11. S-Dealkylation (6-methylmercaptopurine)	11. R–S–CH$_3$ $\longrightarrow$ R–SH
12. S-Oxidation (chlorpromazine, mesoridazine)	12. Ar–S–R $\longrightarrow$ Ar–S(=O)–R
13. Desulfuration (thiopental)	13. R_1–C(=S)–R_2 $\longrightarrow$ R_1–C(=O)–R_2
14. Dehalogenation (halothane, chloramphenicol)	14. CF$_3$–CHClBr $\longrightarrow$ CF$_3$–CHO
15. Oxidation of Alcohols (ethanol, estradiol)	15. R–CH$_2$OH $\longrightarrow$ R–CHO
16. Oxidation of Aldehydes (acetaldehyde, PGE$_2$)	16. R–CHO $\longrightarrow$ R–CO$_2$H

Table 17-3. Phase I Metabolism: Reductive and Hydrolytic Pathways

Type of Reaction (Examples)	Reaction Pathway
Reduction	
1. Carbonyl Reduction (acetohexamide)	1. $R_1-\overset{O}{\overset{\|}{C}}-R_2 \longrightarrow R_1-\overset{OH}{\underset{\|}{C}}-R_2$
2. Azoreduction (sulfasalazine, olsalazine)	2. $R_1-C_6H_4-N=N-C_6H_4-R_2 \longrightarrow R_1-C_6H_4-NH_2 + HN_2-C_6H_4-R_2$
3. Nitroreduction (chloramphenicol, clonazepam)	3. $O_2N-C_6H_4-R \longrightarrow H_2N-C_6H_4-R$
Hydrolysis	
4. Ester Hydrolysis (procaine, meperidine)	4. $R_1-\overset{O}{\overset{\|}{C}}-O-R_2 \longrightarrow R_1-\overset{O}{\overset{\|}{C}}-OH + HO-R_2$
5. Amide Hydrolysis (lidocaine, indomethacin)	5. $R_1-\overset{O}{\overset{\|}{C}}-\overset{}{\underset{H}{N}}-R_2 \longrightarrow R_1-\overset{O}{\overset{\|}{C}}-OH + H_2N-R_2$

(4) Glucuronides with **high molecular weight** (more than 500) are often excreted into the bile and, eventually, into the intestines. The intestinal enzyme β-glucuronidase can then hydrolyze the conjugate, releasing the unaltered drug (or its primary metabolite) for reabsorption by the intestine.

b. **Sulfate conjugation** is much less common than glucuronide conjugation because there is no available pool of endogenous sulfate. Additionally, there are fewer functional groups capable of forming sulfate conjugates. The high-energy form of sulfate, **3′-phosphoadenosine-5′-phosphosulfate (PAPS),** reacts with phenols, alcohols, arylamines, and N-hydroxyl compounds under the influence of **sulfotransferase** to form highly polar metabolites.

c. **Amino acid conjugation** involves the reaction of either glycine or glutamine with aliphatic or aromatic acids to form amides. A drug molecule is first converted to an acyl coenzyme A intermediate. An N-acyltransferase enzyme then catalyzes the conjugation of the activated drug molecule with the amino acid.

d. **Glutathione conjugation** is extremely important in preventing toxicity from a variety of harmful electrophilic agents. Glutathione, a tripeptide containing a nucleophilic sulfhydryl group, is present in almost all mammalian tissues. Under the influence of **glutathione S-transferase,** glutathione can react with halides, epoxides, and other electrophilic compounds to form harmless inactive products. When glutathione has reacted with an electrophile, it undergoes a series of reactions to produce a mercapturic acid derivative, which is eliminated.

e. **Methylation** of oxygen-, nitrogen-, and sulfur-containing functional groups results in metabolites that are usually less polar than the unaltered drugs. Methylation can inactivate certain compounds [e.g., catechol O-methyl transferase (COMT) methylates a number of catecholamine neurotransmitters], but overall it plays a minor role in the elimination of drugs. Its major role is in the biosynthesis of endogenous compounds (e.g., epinephrine). The high-energy form required for methyltransferase enzymes is S-adenosylmethionine (SAM).

f. **Acetylation** can occur with primary amines, hydrazides, sulfonamides, and, occasionally, amides. It leads to the formation of N-acetylated products. These products are usually less polar than the unaltered drug and can retain pharmacological activity.

Table 17-4. Phase II Metabolism: Conjugation Pathways

Type of Conjugate	Reaction Pathway R = Drug Molecule; X = Functional Group
1. Glucuronide (X = OH, NR_2, CO_2H, SH, acidic carbon atoms)	1. HO_2C ... HO, HO, HO, O, H + R–X ⟶ HO_2C ... HO, HO, HO, O, X–R, H (UDP)
2. Sulfate (X = OH, arylamines, NH-OH)	2. $HO{-}S{-}O{-}P{-}O$ — Adenine — H_2O_3PO OH + R–X ⟶ $HO{-}S{-}X{\diagdown}R$
3. Amino Acid (Occurs only with acid functional groups)	3. $R{-}C({=}O){-}S{-}CoA$ + $H_2N{-}C(H)(Y){-}CO_2H$ ⟶ $R{-}C({=}O){-}N(H){-}C(H)(Y){-}CO_2H$ Y = H or $CH_2CH_2CO_2H$
4. Glutathione (X = electrophilic center such as halide, epoxide, or Michael acceptor)	4. γ-Glu–N(H)–...–SH ...–Gly + R–X ⟶ γ-Glu–N(H)–...–S–R ...–Gly
5. Methyl (X = OH, NH_2, SH)	5. HO_2C–...–NH_2–...–S^+(CH_3)– Adenine — H_2O_3PO OH + R–X ⟶ $R{-}X{-}CH_3$
6. Acetylation (X = NH_2, $NHNH_2$, SO_2NH_2, CO-NH_2)	6. $H_3C{-}C({=}O){-}S{-}CoA$ + R–X ⟶ $H_3C{-}C({=}O){-}X{\diagdown}R$

(1) *N*-acetylated metabolites can accumulate in tissue or in the kidneys, as in the case of certain antibacterial sulfonamides. Crystalluria and subsequent tissue damage may result.

(2) The high-energy molecule for acetylation is acetyl-CoA. The reaction is catalyzed by *N*-acetyltransferase.

III. FACTORS INFLUENCING DRUG METABOLISM

A. **Chemical structure** specifically influences a drug's metabolic pathway. The presence or absence of certain functional groups will determine the necessity, route, and extent of metabolism.

B. **Species differences**

1. **Qualitative differences** in the actual metabolic pathway. Such a variation can result from a genetic deficiency of a particular enzyme or a difference in a particular endogenous substrate. In general, qualitative differences occur primarily with **phase II reactions.**

2. **Quantitative differences** are differences in the extent to which the same type of metabolic reaction occurs. Such a variation can result from a difference in the enzyme level, the presence of species specific isozymes, a difference in the amount of endogenous inhibitor or inducer, or a difference in the extent of competing reactions. In general, quantitative differences occur primarily with **phase I reactions.**

C. **Physiological or disease state**

1. Because the liver is the major organ involved in biotransformation, **pathological factors** that **alter liver function** can affect a drug's hepatic clearance.

2. **Congestive heart failure** decreases hepatic blood flow by reducing cardiac output, which alters the extent of drug metabolism.

3. An **alteration in albumin production** (the plasma's major drug-binding protein) can alter the fraction of bound to unbound drug. Thus, a decrease in plasma albumin can increase the fraction of unbound (free) drug, which then becomes available to exert a more intense pharmacological effect. The reverse is true when plasma albumin increases.

D. **Genetic variations**

1. The **acetylation rate** depends on the amount of N-acetyltransferase present, which is determined by genetic factors. The general population can be divided into **fast acetylators** and **slow acetylators.** For example, fast acetylators are more prone to **hepatotoxicity** from the antitubercular agent isoniazid than slow acetylators, whereas slow acetylators are more prone to isoniazid's other toxic effects (see VII B 4d).

2. The discovery of isoforms and families of CYP450 enzymes has shown that genetic variations exist in isoforms that oxidize **debrisoquine.** Individuals who are poor metabolizers of this compound **(PM phenotype)** also exhibit impaired metabolism of more than 20 other therapeutic agents, including β-blockers, antiarrhythmics, opioids, and antidepressants. Approximately 5%–10% of whites, 2% of Asians, and 1% of Arabs express the PM phenotype and are at risk for adverse drug reactions.

E. **Drug dosage**

1. An **increase** in drug dosage results in increased drug concentrations and can saturate certain metabolic enzymes. As drug concentration exceeds 50% saturation for a particular enzyme, drug elimination via this path no longer follows solely first-order kinetics, but rather is a mix of zero- and first-order kinetics. At 100% saturation, metabolism via this enzyme follows zero-order kinetics.

2. **When the metabolic pathway is saturated** (either because of an exceedingly high drug level or because the supply of an endogenous conjugated agent is exhausted), an alternative pathway may be pursued. For example, at normal doses, 98% of a dose of acetaminophen undergoes conjugation with either glucuronic acid or sulfate; however, at toxic doses, conjugation pathways become saturated and acetaminophen undergoes extensive N-hydroxylation, which can lead to hepatotoxicity.

F. **Nutritional status**

1. The levels of some **conjugating agents** (or endogenous substrates), such as sulfate, glutathione, and (rarely) glucuronic acid, are sensitive to body nutrient levels. For example, a **low-protein diet** can lead to a deficiency of certain amino acids, such as glycine. Low-protein diets also decrease oxidative drug metabolism capacity.

2. Diets **deficient in essential fatty** acids (particularly linoleic acid) reduce the metabolism of ethyl-morphine and hexobarbital by decreasing synthesis of certain drug-metabolizing enzymes.

3. A **deficiency of certain dietary minerals** also affects drug metabolism. Calcium, magnesium, and zinc deficiencies decrease drug-metabolizing capacity, whereas iron deficiency appears to increase it. A copper deficiency leads to variable effects.

4. **Deficiencies of vitamins** (particularly vitamins A, C, E, and the B group) affect drug-metabolizing capacity. For example, a vitamin C deficiency can result in a decrease in oxidative pathways, whereas a vitamin E deficiency can retard dealkylation and hydroxylation.

G. Age

1. Metabolizing enzyme systems are not fully developed at birth; thus, **infants** and **young children** need to receive smaller doses of drugs than adults to avoid toxic side effects. This is particularly true of drugs that require glucuronide conjugation.

2. In **older children,** some drugs may be less active than in adults, particularly if the dosage is based on weight. The liver develops faster than the increase in general body weight and, thus, represents a greater fraction of total body weight.

3. In the **elderly,** metabolizing enzyme systems decline. The lowered level of enzyme activity slows the rate of drug elimination, causing higher plasma drug levels per dose than in young adults.

H. Gender.
Metabolic differences between the sexes have been observed for a number of compounds, suggesting that androgen, estrogen, and/or adrenocorticoid activity might affect the activity of certain CYP450 enzyme isozymes.

1. Metabolism of diazepam, prednisolone, caffeine, and acetaminophen is **slightly faster in women.**

2. Oxidative metabolism of propranolol, chlordiazepoxide, lidocaine, and some steroids occurs **faster in men** than in women.

I. Circadian rhythms.
The **nocturnal plasma levels** of drugs, such as theophylline and diazepam, are lower than the **diurnal plasma levels.**

J. Drug administration route

1. **Oral administration.** The drug is absorbed from the GI tract and transported to the liver through the hepatic portal vein before entering the systemic circulation. Thus, the drug is subject to hepatic metabolism before it reaches its site of action. This is an effect known as the **first-pass effect, or presystemic elimination** (Table 17-5).
   a. The first-pass effect can cause **significant clinical problems.** Because drugs are metabolized in the liver from their active forms to inactive forms, this effect must be counteracted to achieve the desired plasma or tissue drug level.
   b. A common approach is to **increase the oral dose,** offsetting the loss of drug activity from the first-pass effect.

Table 17-5. Examples of Drugs That Undergo First-Pass Metabolism

Acetaminophen	Fluorouracil	Oxprenolol
Albuterol	Imipramine	Pentazocine
Alprenolol	Isoproterenol	Progesterone
Aspirin	Lidocaine	Propoxyphene
Cortisone	Meperidine	Propranolol
Cyclosporin	Methyltestosterone	Salbutamol
Desipramine	Metoprolol	Terbutaline
Dihydropyridines	Nortriptyline	Testosterone
Estradiol	Organic Nitrates	Verapamil

2. **Intravenous administration** bypasses the first-pass effect because the drug is delivered directly to the bloodstream without being metabolized in the liver. Thus, intravenous doses of drugs undergoing considerable first-pass effects are much smaller than oral doses.

3. **Sublingual administration** and **rectal administration** also bypass first-pass effects, although rectal administration can produce variable effects.

IV. EXTRAHEPATIC METABOLISM

A. Definition. Extrahepatic metabolism refers to drug biotransformation that takes place in **tissues other than the liver.** The most common sites include the **portals of entry** (e.g., GI mucosa, nasal passages, lungs) and the **portals of excretion** (e.g., kidneys). However, metabolism can occur throughout the body.

B. Metabolism sites

1. **Plasma** contains **esterases,** which are responsible primarily for hydrolysis of esters. **Simple esters** (e.g., procaine, succinylcholine) are rapidly hydrolyzed in the blood. Additionally, plasma esterases can activate a variety of ester prodrugs.

2. Metabolizing enzymes in the **intestinal mucosa** are especially important for drugs undergoing microsomal oxidation, glucuronide conjugation, and sulfate conjugation.
   a. As a lipid-soluble drug passes through the intestinal mucosa during drug absorption, it can be metabolized into polar or inactive metabolites before entering the blood. The result is **comparable to a first-pass effect.**
   b. The intestinal mucosa's drug-metabolizing capacity compares to that of the liver. However, it shows much greater individual variation because of its greater exposure to the environment.

3. **Intestinal bacterial flora** secrete a number of enzymes capable of metabolizing drugs and other xenobiotics.
   a. Any factor that **modifies the intestinal flora** may also **modify drug activity.** Age, diet, disease state, and exposure to environmental chemicals or drugs may all be important.
      (1) Certain **diseases,** particularly **intestinal disease,** affect intestinal flora. Ulcerative colitis, for example, promotes bacterial growth. Diarrhea reduces the number of bacteria.
      (2) Certain **environmental chemicals** and **drugs** also act on intestinal flora. Antibiotics, for example, decrease the number of bacteria.
   b. Bacterial flora **secrete** β-glucuronidase, which hydrolyzes the polar glucuronide conjugates of bile and allows the free, nonpolar bile acids to be reabsorbed. This **enterohepatic circulation** partially maintains the pool of bile acids. This same principle applies to certain glucuronide conjugates of drugs.
   c. Certain bacterial flora **convert** vitamin precursors to their **active forms,** as with vitamin K.
   d. Bacterial flora can also **convert** certain substances to their **toxic forms,** as with the conversion of the artificial sweetener cyclamate to cyclohexylamine, a suspected carcinogen.
   e. Intestinal bacteria produce **azoreductase,** which reduces the prodrug sulfasalazine to the active anti-inflammatory aminosalicylic acid and the active antibacterial sulfapyridine. Sulfasalazine is one of the few agents effective in the treatment of ulcerative colitis.

4. The **acidic environment** of the **stomach** produces nonenzymatic degradation of a number of drug molecules, including penicillin G, carbenicillin, erythromycin, and tetracycline. Additionally, gastric acid assists in the degradation of proteins and peptides (e.g., insulin).

5. The **nasal mucosa** provides a high level of CYP450 activity, which can significantly alter the amount of drug that reaches the systemic circulation. Nasal decongestants, anesthetics, nicotine, cocaine, and other compounds have been shown to undergo nasal metabolism.

6. The **lung** is responsible for first-pass metabolism of drugs administered intravenously, intramuscularly, transdermally, or subcutaneously.
   a. The **total amount** of **metabolizing enzymes** present in the lungs is less than that in the liver; however, the specific activities of the enzymes are comparable to those in the liver.
   b. The lungs provide **second-pass metabolism** for drugs leaving the liver.

C. Placental and fetal metabolism

1. **Placenta.** In general, if a drug or other xenobiotic is lipid soluble enough to be absorbed into the circulation when administered to a pregnant woman, it will likely also pass through the placenta.

   a. The placenta is not a physical or metabolic barrier to xenobiotics. Very little xenobiotic-metabolizing enzyme activity has been demonstrated in the placenta.

   b. Drugs present in their **active form** in the maternal circulation likely pass **unchanged** into the fetal circulation.

   c. An exception to this lack of enzyme activity in the placenta is the presence of a small amount of **aryl aromatic hydroxylase,** which is **inducible in pregnant women who smoke cigarettes.** A potential consequence is an increase in the production of penultimate carcinogens from the action of this enzyme on the polycyclic aromatic hydrocarbons present in cigarette smoke and other environmental sources.

2. **Fetus.** In terms of fetal metabolism, there are varying degrees of drug-metabolizing activity dependent upon a number of factors including fetal age.

   a. A **major deficiency** is that of **glucuronic acid conjugating activity** both in the **fetus and the neonate.**

   b. Two consequences of this are the **gray baby syndrome,** resulting from decreased chloramphenicol glucuronidation, and **neonatal hyperbilirubinemia,** resulting from a decrease in bilirubin glucuronide formation.

V. STRATEGIES TO MANAGE DRUG METABOLISM.

A variety of methods have been used to circumvent the rapid metabolism of certain drugs. These methods seek to improve drug therapy by decreasing the overall extent of metabolism and increasing the duration of action. In some instances, these methods have provided increased site specificity.

A. Pharmaceutical strategies involve the use of different **dosage forms** to either avoid or compensate for rapid metabolism.

1. **Sublingual tablets** are useful for delivering drugs directly into the systemic circulation and bypassing hepatic first-pass metabolism. **Nitroglycerin,** a rapidly acting antianginal agent, is essentially ineffective when administered orally due to an extremely high first-pass effect but is very effective in treating acute attacks of angina if given sublingually.

2. **Transdermal patches** and **ointment formulations** provide a continuous supply of drug over an extended period of time and are useful for rapidly metabolized compounds such as nitroglycerin. These delivery systems, while not suited to treat acute anginal symptoms, are effective in providing prophylactic concentrations of nitroglycerin.

3. **Intramuscular depot injections** also provide a continuous supply of drug over an extended period of time. Highly lipid soluble esters of **estradiol** and **testosterone** (e.g., estradiol benzoate, testosterone enanthate) are slowly absorbed from their administration site. Hydrolysis of these prodrugs (see VI) produces a steady supply of these rapidly metabolized hormones.

4. **Enteric-coated formulations** can protect acid-sensitive drugs as they pass through the acidic environment of the stomach. **Methenamine, erythromycin,** and **omeprazole** are examples of acid-sensitive agents that are available as enteric-coated preparations.

5. **Nasal administration** allows for the delivery of peptides, such as **calcitonin salmon,** which have very low (if any) oral bioavailability. Characteristics of the lung make it ideal for the administration of peptides. Aerosolized drugs only need to penetrate a thin epithelial layer to reach abundant capillary beds. Additionally, the lungs contain protease inhibitors, which allow for greater stability of the peptides.

B. Pharmacological strategies involve the concurrent use of enzyme inhibitors to decrease drug metabolism. In some instances, the concurrent use of an additional agent does not prevent metabolism but rather prevents the toxicity caused by metabolites of the therapeutic agent.

1. **Levodopa (L-dopa),** the amino acid precursor of dopamine, is used in the treatment of parkinsonism. Unlike dopamine, L-dopa can penetrate the blood–brain barrier and reach

the central nervous system (CNS). When in the brain, it is decarboxylated to dopamine. To ensure that adequate concentrations of L-dopa reach the CNS, peripheral metabolism of the drug must be blocked. The concurrent administration of **carbidopa,** a dopa decarboxylase inhibitor that cannot penetrate the blood–brain barrier, prevents peripheral formation of dopamine and allows site-specific delivery of dopamine to the CNS.

2. **β-Lactam antibiotics.** The antibacterial activity of a number of β-lactam antibiotics is reduced by microorganisms capable of secreting the enzyme β-lactamase. This enzyme hydrolyzes the β-lactam ring and inactivates the antibiotic. To counter this resistance mechanism, a β-lactamase inhibitor, such as **clavulanic acid,** is used in conjunction with a penicillin, such as **amoxicillin,** to successfully treat infections caused by β-lactamase–producing bacteria.

3. **Ifosfamide** is an alkylating agent that must undergo in vivo metabolism to produce an active nitrogen mustard. In the process of this metabolic activation, significant concentrations of **acrolein** are produced. These acrolein molecules react with nucleophiles on renal proteins and produce hemorrhagic cystitis. To prevent this toxicity, ifosfamide is always coadministered with **mesna,** a sulfhydryl-containing compound that reacts with and neutralizes any acrolein that is present in the kidney.

4. **HIV protease inhibitors** are extensively metabolized by CYP3A isozymes. In addition, compounds within this class can inhibit these same isozymes. This latter action has been used to optimize therapy. **Ritonavir** is an HIV protease inhibitor that is known to cause hepatotoxicity at therapeutic doses. **Lopinavir** is an HIV protease inhibitor that is ineffective if used alone due to rapid CYP3A oxidation. A new strategy combines a low dose of ritonavir with a therapeutic dose of lopinavir. This results in an inhibition of CYP3A, the establishment of adequate plasma levels of lopinavir, and therapeutic efficacy without hepatotoxicity.

C. **Chemical strategies** involve the addition, deletion, or isosteric modification of key functional groups. These molecular modifications hinder or completely eliminate metabolic transformations (Figure 17-1).

1. **Testosterone** is not orally active due to rapid oxidation of its 17-hydroxyl group to a ketone. Addition of a 17α-methyl group converts the labile secondary alcohol to a stable tertiary alcohol. The resulting compound, **methyltestosterone,** is only half as potent as testosterone; however, it is not subject to rapid first-pass metabolism and can be used orally. A similar strategy has been used to make orally active estradiol analogues.

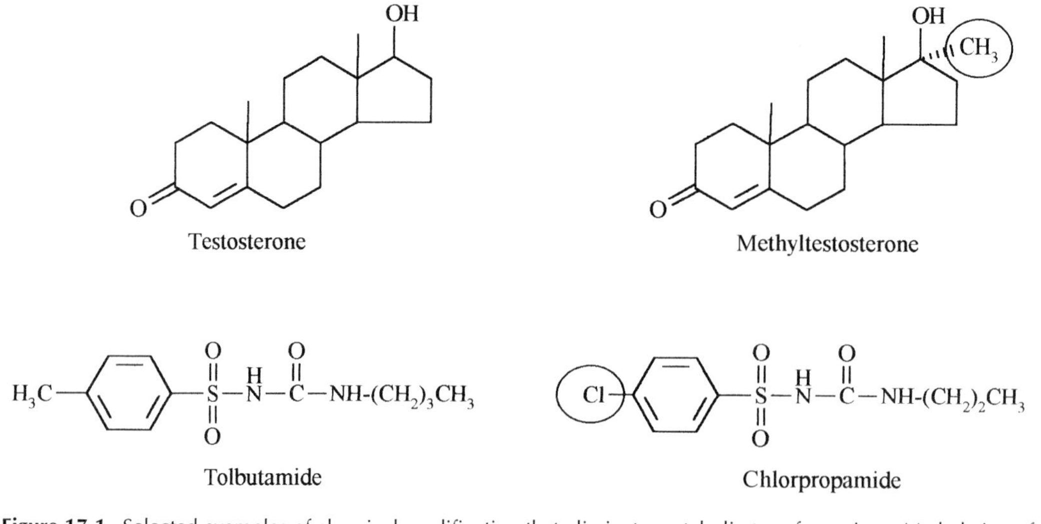

Testosterone

Methyltestosterone

Tolbutamide

Chlorpropamide

Figure 17-1. Selected examples of chemical modification that eliminate metabolic transformations. Methylation of testosterone blocks the rapid oxidation of the 17-hydroxyl group and allows oral activity, whereas replacement of the metabolically labile *para*-methyl group on tolbutamide with a chloro group allows for a much longer duration of action.

2. **Tolbutamide** is an oral hypoglycemic with a short duration of action. This sulfonylurea rapidly undergoes oxidation of its para-methyl group. A structurally similar compound, **chlorpropamide,** has a nonmetabolizable para-chloro group and, as a result, has a much longer duration of action.

3. **Isoproterenol** is a potent β-adrenergic agonist used for the relief of bronchospasm associated with bronchial asthma. Because it is a catechol (i.e., 3,4-dihydroxy–substituted benzene ring), isoproterenol is subject to rapid metabolism by catechol O-methyl transferase (COMT) and, thus, has poor oral activity. Alteration of the 3,4-dihydroxy substitution to a 3,5-dihydroxy substitution produces **metaproterenol,** a bronchodilator that is not susceptible to COMT, is orally active, and has a longer duration of action than isoproterenol.

4. **Octreotide** is a synthetic octapeptide used to suppress or inhibit severe diarrhea associated with certain tumors. Octreotide mimics the actions of **somatostatin,** a naturally occurring, 14–amino acid peptide. Somatostatin undergoes rapid proteolysis, has a half-life of 1–3 minutes, and must be administered as a continuous intravenous infusion. Octreotide contains the amino acids essential for clinical efficacy but replaces two of the amino acids with their D-enantiomers. These unnatural D–amino acids are more resistant to hydrolysis. As a result, octreotide has an increased half-life and can be administered as a subcutaneous injection.

VI. PRODRUGS.
These drugs are molecules that are either inactive or very weakly active and require in vivo biotransformation to produce the physiologically active drug. The phase I metabolic processes discussed previously are used to activate prodrugs. A variety of **advantages** can be gained by using a prodrug instead of the active form of the drug.

A. An **increase in water solubility** is useful for the preparation of ophthalmic and parenteral formulations. **Sodium succinate esters** and **sodium phosphate esters** have been used to make a number of water-soluble steroid prodrugs.

B. An **increase in lipid solubility** is useful for a variety of reasons.

1. **Increased duration of action.** Lipid-soluble esters of estradiol, such as benzoate, valerate, and cypionate, are used to prolong estrogenic activity. IM injections of these esters in oil result in a deposit of drug that is slowly hydrolyzed, thereby releasing free estradiol over a prolonged period of time (see V A 3).

2. **Increased oral absorption** is obtained by converting carboxylic acid groups to esters. These esters can then be rapidly converted to the active acids by plasma esterases. **Enalaprilat** is a potent angiotensin-converting enzyme (ACE) inhibitor that is used for parenteral administration, but, due to its high polarity, it is orally inactive. Its monomethyl ester, **enalapril,** is considerably more lipophilic and, thus, provides good oral absorption. This strategy has been successfully used for a variety of other compounds, including additional ACE inhibitors, fibric acid derivatives, ampicillin, and several cephalosporins.

3. **Increased topical absorption** of steroids is obtained by masking hydroxyl groups as esters or acetonides. These prodrugs are much less polar than the parent compounds and allow increased dermal permeability for the treatment of inflammatory, allergic, and pruritic skin conditions. Examples include **triamcinolone acetonide, diflorasone diacetate,** and **betamethasone valerate.**

4. **Increased palatability.** Antibiotics such as **sulfisoxazole** have a bitter taste and are not suitable for administration to young children who cannot yet swallow tablets or capsules. Esterification to produce **sulfisoxazole acetyl** decreases the water solubility of the antibiotic and, thus, decreases its interaction with bitter taste receptors on the tongue. This compound is marketed as a flavored suspension. Similar strategies have been used to mask the bitter taste of **chloramphenicol** and other antibiotics.

C. **A decrease in GI irritation.** Nonsteroidal anti-inflammatory agents (NSAIDs) produce gastric irritation and ulceration via two mechanisms: a direct irritant effect of the acidic molecule and inhibition of gastroprotective prostaglandin production. The prodrugs **sulindac** and **nabumetone** produce less GI irritation because the gastric and intestinal mucosa are not exposed to high concentrations of active drug during oral administration. Additionally, nabumetone is a ketone, not an acid, and lacks any direct irritant effects.

D. Site specificity is useful for increasing the concentration of drug at the active site and for decreasing side effects.

1. **Methyldopa** is a prodrug that is structurally similar to L-dopa. As a result, methyldopa is transported into the CNS and metabolized to the active compound, **α-methyldopamine,** via the same path used for the synthesis of dopamine. This allows a significant amount of α-methyldopamine to reach the CNS and bind to central α_2-adrenergic receptors.

2. **Omeprazole** is used to treat gastric ulcers and other hypersecretory disorders. After oral absorption, it is selectively activated at the acidic pH levels (pH less than 1) seen in gastric parietal cells. This allows the active form of the drug to be produced in close proximity to the enzyme H^+/K^+-ATPase (proton pump), resulting in irreversible inhibition of the enzyme and a decrease in gastric acid secretion. Activation in the stomach prior to absorption can be prevented by the use of enteric-coated formulations (see V A 4).

3. **Formaldehyde** is an effective urinary tract antiseptic; however, oral administration results in significant toxicity. To avoid this problem, the prodrug **methenamine** is administered instead. Methenamine is stable and nontoxic at normal physiological pH, but is selectively hydrolyzed to formaldehyde and ammonium ions in the acidic urine (pH less than 5.5). As with omeprazole, activation before absorption can be prevented by the use of enteric-coated formulations (see V A 4).

4. **Olsalazine** is a highly polar dimer of 5-aminosalicylic acid that is poorly absorbed after oral administration. On reaching the large intestine, colonic bacteria cleave the azo bond and liberate the active anti-inflammatory agent. Olsalazine and a related compound, **sulfasalazine,** are useful in treating inflammatory bowel disease.

5. **Diethylstilbestrol** is a synthetic estrogen that can produce undesirable, feminizing side effects when used in the treatment of prostate cancer. These side effects can be avoided by the use of the ester prodrug, **diethylstilbestrol diphosphate.** This prodrug is inactive until dephosphorylated by acid phosphatase, an enzyme that is highly active in prostate tumor cells. This allows for a localized release of active compound and a decrease in systemic side effects.

E. Increased shelf life of both solids and parenteral admixtures can be obtained by the use of prodrugs.

1. **Cefamandole** is a second-generation cephalosporin that is unstable in solid dosage forms. Esterification of the α-hydroxyl group with formic acid produces **cefamandole nafate,** a stable prodrug that is hydrolyzed by plasma esterases to produce the parent antibiotic.

2. **Cyclophosphamide** is a prodrug that requires in vivo oxidation, followed by nonenzymatic decomposition, to produce the active phosphoramide mustard. As a result, aqueous solutions of cyclophosphamide are much more stable than those of other nitrogen mustards (i.e., mechlorethamine). **Mechlorethamine** is highly reactive, does not require in vivo activation, and can rapidly decompose in aqueous environments before administration.

VII. PHARMACOGENETICS

A. Genes and their involvement in drug response and toxicity

1. **Genes** can be defined as discrete segments of DNA that are capable of reproduction during cell replication and that are responsible for guiding the biosynthesis of specific proteins and enzymes.

2. Genes encode proteins involved in the **absorption, transport, metabolism, and elimination** of drug molecules. Additionally, they encode proteins that serve as **drug receptors.** It is obvious then that a genetic disposition that would result in either an **over- or an underexpression of these genes** could significantly alter drug response and toxicity.

3. Assuming that a patient has been prescribed a medication that is indicated for his or her condition or disease state, there are several reasons why a patient may not respond or may suffer severe adverse effects:
   a. **Inappropriate dosing**
   b. **Drug–drug interactions**
   c. **Drug allergies**

d. Medication errors
e. Genetic predisposition

4. In its most simplistic form, **pharmacogenetics** can be defined as the use of genetic information to select the "right drug for the right patient." This area of study primarily seeks to identify the individual genetic differences and predispositions that influence drug response and safety.

B. **Genetic variation** in the DNA sequence can cause certain populations of individuals to be **more likely to develop specific disease states,** to be **more likely to follow a specific path of disease progression,** to be **more likely to respond to specific drug therapy,** and/or to be **more likely to develop certain adverse drug effects.**

1. The genetic variation between any two unrelated individuals is approximately one base pair change in every 1000 base pairs.

2. These changes are referred to as **single nucleotide polymorphisms (SNPs)** and are the most common form of genetic variation.

3. **The effects of SNPs vary** based upon the **type and location** of the variation.
   a. **An SNP located within the coding region** of a gene could produce no discernable effects, negligible effects, or a significant alteration in effects depending upon how the SNP affected the amino acid coding.
      (1) An SNP that **did not alter** the amino acid sequence in a protein would produce **no discernable effects.**
      (2) An SNP that resulted in one amino acid being replaced by a **similar amino acid** would have a **negligible effect** (e.g., changing a portion of the genetic code from AUU to GUU would result in isoleucine being replaced by valine, a similar hydrophobic amino acid).
      (3) An SNP that resulted in one amino acid being replaced by one with **significantly different chemical properties** would cause **a significant alteration of effects** (e.g., changing a portion of the genetic code from GUU to GAU would result in valine being replaced with the acidic, and more hydrophilic, aspartic acid).
   b. **An SNP in a splicing control region** could result in the formation of a novel protein that is either larger or smaller in size than that which is naturally occurring.
   c. **An SNP in a promoter region** could alter the transcription rate, resulting in either an increase or a decrease in the production of the target protein.
   d. An SNP residing outside of any of the above locations is **genetically silent** and does not produce any observable effects.

4. **Examples of known genetic variations and their effects on drug efficacy and safety**
   a. **Warfarin.** Patients with specific variations in the gene for the metabolizing enzyme CYP2C9 require lower doses and are at an increased risk of bleeding.
   b. **Salmeterol and albuterol.** Genetic variations in the gene coding for the β_2-adrenergic receptor (ADBR2) can result in a decreased efficacy.
   c. **6-Mercaptopurine.** Genetic variations affecting the enzyme thiopurine methyltransferase are known to produce increased toxicity.
   d. **Procainamide, hydralazine, and isoniazid.** Genetic variations affecting the rate of N-acetylation affect both the efficacy and adverse effect profiles of these agents. The identification of fast and slow acetylators is one of the best known examples of how genetic variation can affect therapeutic safety and efficacy.
   e. **Quinidine, cisapride, and clarithromycin.** Genetic variations in the gene coding for potassium channels can result in increased risk and prevalence of QT-syndrome and arrhythmias.
   f. **Zileuton.** Patients with genetic variations in the gene coding for the enzyme 5-lipoxygenase do not respond to this drug.

C. **Clinical pharmacogenetic assays**

1. The **goal** of a clinical pharmacogenetic assay is to place patients into one of four categories.
   a. Individuals who are most likely to respond and are at a low risk for adverse effects
   b. Individuals who are most likely to respond and are at a high risk for adverse effects
   c. Individuals who are less likely to respond and are at a low risk for adverse effects
   d. Individuals who are less likely to respond and are at a high risk for adverse effects

2. Issues in the development of pharmacogenetic assays include:
   a. Improvement in a medically important response (i.e., the assay should allow health-care providers to make a better decision than would otherwise be possible).
   b. **False positives for efficacy-based assays should be kept at a minimum** in order to prevent nonresponders from being prescribed drugs that will not provide the desired therapeutic outcomes. False negatives (i.e., responders identified as nonresponders) are not as crucial since they would be prescribed appropriate alternative therapy.
   c. **False negatives for safety-based assays should be kept at a minimum** in order to prevent at-risk patients from being exposed to potential serious adverse effects. A higher rate of false positives (i.e., patients identified as "at risk") is acceptable. Excluding a certain percentage of patients in order to avoid serious adverse effects has been proposed to be a reasonable trade-off.
   d. The results for the assays must be both interpretable and provide clinically useful results. The assays should be simple to use in a clinical setting and should provide results that are easily understood by the patient, physician, pharmacist, and other health-care providers.
   e. Analytical and clinical validation of the assay must meet FDA approval standards.

3. As defined here, pharmacogenetic assays do not test for the presence or absence of a disease-specific mutation, nor do they provide any information that could be used to predict disease states in an individual or his or her family. As such, it has been suggested that legal and ethical issues surrounding disease-specific gene tests should not apply to predictions of safety and efficacy of drugs (i.e., the primary focus of pharmacogenetics).

D. SNP maps and their potential use

1. An SNP map for an individual contains the specific number and locations of base pair variations. Such a map could be used to predict patient response and susceptibility to serious adverse reactions.

2. **A simplified example of this is shown in Figure 17-2.** A large database would initially be used to identify SNPs that could be used as predictors of efficacy and safety. At the top of Figure 17-2, the two outside, shaded regions in this **hypothetical model** should be regarded as SNPs that would predict that a patient would favorably respond to the drug. Sim-

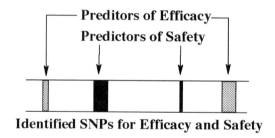

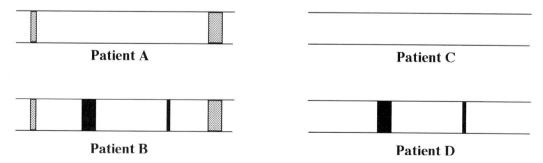

Figure 17-2. Hypothetical single nucleotide polymorphism (SNP) maps. At the top is a composite SNP profile developed by using genetic information from a large database of patients/volunteers. This overall SNP can then be compared to individual SNP maps (i.e., **Patients A–D**) to help determine the overall benefit/risk for the given drug in each of these four patients.

ilarly, the two inner, black regions should be regarded as SNPs that would indicate that a patient was more prone to the development of serious adverse effects. Other SNPs (i.e., the nonhighlighted rectangles shown for the four patients) should be regarded as irrelevant here (i.e., they do not predict either efficacy or safety for the drug in question).

a. Patient A would be predicted to respond to treatment without the development of any serious adverse effects.

b. Patient B would be predicted to respond to treatment but would also be expected to develop serious adverse effects.

c. Patient C would be predicted to be a nonresponder to treatment but would be unlikely to experience any serious adverse effects.

d. Patient D would be predicted to be a nonresponder to treatment but would be expected to develop serious adverse effects.

STUDY QUESTIONS

Directions: Each of the numbered items or incomplete statements in this section is followed by answers or by completions of the statement. Select the one lettered answer or completion that is **best** in each case.

1. Which of the following statements concerning drug metabolism is true?

(A) Generally, a single metabolite is excreted for each drug administered.
(B) Often, a drug may undergo a phase II reaction followed by a phase I reaction.
(C) Drug-metabolizing enzymes are found only in the liver.
(D) All metabolites are less active pharmacologically than their parent drugs.
(E) Phase I metabolites more likely are able to cross cellular membranes than phase II metabolites.

2. Which of the following metabolites would be the least likely excretion product of orally administered aspirin (see structure below)?

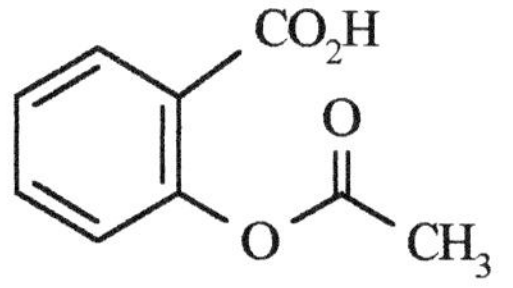

(A) Glycine conjugate
(B) Ester glucuronide
(C) Unchanged drug
(D) Ether glucuronide
(E) Hydroxylated metabolite

3. Sulfasalazine (see structure below) is a prodrug that is activated in the intestine by bacterial enzymes. The enzyme most likely responsible is

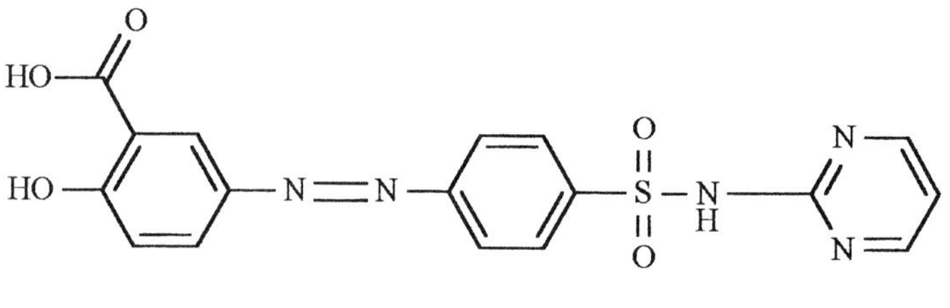

(A) azoreductase
(B) pseudocholinesterase
(C) N-acetyltransferase
(D) β-glucuronidase
(E) methyltransferase

4. Chloramphenicol (see structure below) is considered to be toxic in infants (gray baby syndrome). This is due to tissue accumulation of unchanged chloramphenicol, resulting from an immature metabolic pathway. Which of the following enzymes would most likely be deficient?

(A) Pseudocholinesterase
(B) Glucuronyl transferase
(C) N-Acetyltransferase
(D) Azoreductase
(E) Methyltransferase

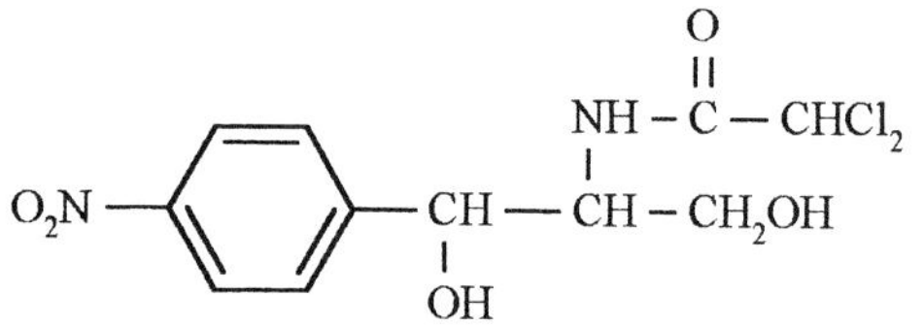

5. Which of the following therapeutic advantages cannot be obtained by the use of prodrugs? Increased

(A) oral absorption
(B) water solubility
(C) duration of action
(D) potency
(E) palatability

6. Which of the following statements regarding pharmacogenetics is INCORRECT?

(A) Single nucleotide polymorphisms (SNPs) in a promoter region can result in a decreased production of a target protein.

(B) It is crucial that false positives for safety-based assays be kept at a minimum.

(C) The area of pharmacogenetics focuses primarily on the genetic variations that affect drug efficacy and safety.

(D) The effects of SNPs vary based upon the type and location of the variation.

(E) Genetic variation occurs whenever there is a change in the DNA nucleotide base pair sequence.

Directions: Each question below contains three suggested answers, of which **one or more** is correct. Choose the answer

A	if **I only** is correct
B	if **III only** is correct
C	if **I and II** are correct
D	if **II and III** are correct
E	if **I, II, and III** are correct

7. Terms that may be used to describe the following metabolic reaction include

I. *N*-dealkylation
II. oxidative deamination
III. phase I metabolism

8. Which of the following reactions can be classified as phase II metabolism?

I.

II.

III.

9. Conditions that tend to increase the action of an orally administered drug that undergoes phase II metabolism include

I. enterohepatic circulation
II. enzyme saturation
III. first-pass effect

10. Which of the following statements concerning CYP450 are correct?

I. The CYP7, CYP11, and CYP27 subfamilies are involved in cholesterol metabolism.
II. A single drug may be metabolized by multiple isoforms of CYP450.
III. The majority of xenobiotics, or drugs, are metabolized by the CYP4B and CYP1A subfamilies.

11. Metabolic reactions likely to be affected by a protein-deficient diet include

I. glycine conjugation
II. hydrolysis
III. glucuronidation

Directions: The group of items in this section consists of lettered options followed by a set of numbered items. For each item, select the **one** lettered option that is most closely associated with it. Each lettered option may be selected once, more than once, or not at all.

Questions 12–15

For each drug, select its most likely metabolic pathway.

(A) Ether glucuronidation
(B) Ester glucuronidation
(C) Nitroreduction
(D) Oxidative deamination
(E) Ester hydrolysis

12. Benzoic acid

13. Procaine

14. Acetaminophen

15. Amphetamine

ANSWERS AND EXPLANATIONS

1. The answer is E *[I; II A 1, B].*
Phase I metabolites are often somewhat more polar than their parents. With the exception of acetylated and methylated metabolites, phase II metabolites are always much more polar than their parents. Thus, phase I metabolites are more likely to retain some liposolubility and are more likely to cross cellular membranes.

It is unusual for a single metabolite to be excreted for a given drug. Most drugs yield a mixture of metabolites. Because of the high polarity and subsequent high excretion of phase II metabolites, they are not likely to undergo further metabolism. Phase I metabolites, on the other hand, are less polar and are very likely to undergo further phase II metabolic reactions.

Whereas the major site of metabolism is the liver, there are many extrahepatic sites that secrete drug-metabolizing enzymes. Although many metabolites are less pharmacologically active than their parents, there are many drugs whose metabolites have equal or greater pharmacological activity and sometimes greater toxicity as well. Prodrugs (i.e., drugs inactive in the form administered) always form at least one active metabolite.

2. The answer is C *[II A 1 e, 3 a, B 2 a (2), c; Tables 17-2, 17-3, and 17-4].*
Because of the types of functional groups present, aspirin may undergo a number of different metabolic reactions. These include hydroxylation of the aromatic nucleus, conjugation of the carboxyl group with glycine, conjugation of the carboxyl group with glucuronic acid with the formation of an ester glucuronide, hydrolysis of the acetate ester, and conjugation of the phenol group (resulting from hydrolysis of the acetate ester) with glucuronic acid to form an ether glucuronide.

Because the acetate ester is a simple ester, aspirin is susceptible to hydrolysis in the acid media of the stomach before absorption takes place. In addition, any acetylated molecules that are absorbed are subjected to hydrolysis and are catalyzed by the many esterases present in the circulation. Any acetylated molecules not hydrolyzed in the circulation are subject to hydrolysis in the liver. All of these processes occur before the drug reaches the glomerular filtrate; therefore, excretion of the unchanged acetylated drug is highly unlikely.

3. The answer is A *[II A 2; Table 17-3].*
Sulfasalazine has both anti-inflammatory and antibacterial activity when converted to aminosalicylic acid and sulfapyridine in the body. This reaction occurs by reductive cleavage of the "azo" linkage contained in the sulfasalazine molecule and is catalyzed in the intestine by bacterial azoreductase. This is a form of site-specific delivery because the intact drug is not absorbed from the stomach or upper intestine and reaches the colon, where it is metabolized. Sulfasalazine is one of a few drugs that is effective for the treatment of ulcerative colitis.

4. The answer is B *[II B 2 a (2); III G 1; Tables 17-2, 17-3, and 17-4].*
The chloramphenicol molecule contains an aromatic nucleus, which would be subject to hydroxylation, a nitro group that is subject to reduction, an amide group that is subject to liver hydrolysis, and alcohol groups that are subject to glucuronidation. Of all the enzyme systems responsible for these reactions, the system responsible for glucuronidation is developed poorly in premature infants and infants up to approximately 6–8 weeks of age.

5. The answer is D *[VI A, B 1–4].*
By definition, prodrugs are inactive or very weakly active molecules that require in vivo activation to the parent molecule. Thus, conversion of a drug molecule to a prodrug does not increase potency because the original molecule, with whatever potency it contains, is produced after administration. A variety of advantages, including increased water solubility, duration of action, oral absorption, and palatability, can be obtained through the use of prodrugs, but none of these advantages results in an increase in potency of the parent molecule.

6. The answer is B *[VII A 4, B 1–3, C 2 c].*
While keeping false positives and false negatives at a minimum is always desirable, it is most crucial that false negatives be kept at a minimum for safety-based assays in order to prevent at-risk patients from being exposed to potential serious side effects. A higher rate of false positives is acceptable since preventing serious adverse effects is perceived to be more important than excluding some patients from therapy.

Genetic variation occurs whenever there are base pair changes in the DNA nucleotide sequence. The most common form of genetic variation is a single nucleotide polymorphism (SNP). The cumulative effects of these variations vary based on the types and locations of the SNPs. Variations in coding regions can alter protein function, while those in splicing and promoter regions can alter protein size and protein production, respectively. Some SNPs produce no discernable changes and are therefore genetically silent. Pharmacogenetics primarily seeks to use SNPs and other genetic information to predict predispositions that influence drug response and safety in individual patients.

7. The answer is D (II, III) *[II A; Table 17-2].*
The reaction shown in the question involves the conversion of one functional group to another (amine to carbonyl); thus, it is classified as a phase I reaction. The introduction of oxygen into the molecule indicates oxidation, and the loss of the amino group signifies deamination; thus, the reaction also can be classified as oxidative deamination. *N*-Dealkylation implies the removal of an alkyl group from a nitrogen. The nitrogen in the parent molecule does not have an alkyl group attached to it.

8. The answer is C (I, II) *[II A, B; Table 17-4].*
Phase II metabolic reactions involve masking an existing functional group with a natural endogenous constituent. The formulas shown in choices I and II represent this type of reaction, with choice I being an acetylation reaction and choice II, a glycine conjugation reaction. Choice III represents a change in an existing functional group and, thus, represents a phase I reaction. It is an oxidative deamination reaction.

9. The answer is C (I, II) *[II B 2 a (4), III E 1, 2; IV B 3 b].*
Enterohepatic circulation refers to the process by which glucuronides, which are secreted into the intestine with the bile, are hydrolyzed by intestinal bacterial β-glucuronidase. The hydrolyzed free drug, which is no longer polar, becomes available for intestinal reabsorption into the system and subsequent penetration to its active site.
    If an enzyme system becomes saturated, then the active drug cannot be inactivated by that pathway. If the drug cannot undergo an alternative pathway, the increased plasma levels of an unchanged active drug can result in increased activity or toxicity.
    The first-pass effect results in metabolism of a drug by the liver before the drug reaches its site of action, resulting in an overall decrease in its activity. Drugs that undergo first-pass metabolism generally are effective in much smaller intravenous doses as compared to oral doses.

10. The answer is C (I, II) *[II A 1 c; Table 17-1]*
There are six mammalian families involved in steroid and bile acid metabolism. These are CYP7, CYP11, CYP17, CYP19, CYP21, and CYP27. Since cholesterol is the common intermediate for the biosynthesis of all endogenous steroids, some of these enzymes are directly involved in cholesterol metabolism. The families listed, CYP7, CYP11, and CYP27, all metabolize cholesterol, while the other three families catalyze additional oxidations of the initial metabolites.
    As is evident from Table 17-1, multiple isoforms of CYP450 can metabolize a single drug. An example of this is seen with imipramine, an antidepressant that is metabolized by CYP1A, CYP2C, and CYP2D isoforms. Additionally, Table 17-1 indicates that the subfamilies CYP2C, CYP2D, and CYP3A metabolize the majority of drugs, or xenobiotics.

11. The answer is A (I) *[III F 1].*
Phase II metabolic reactions require natural endogenous substrates, which normally are supplied in the diet. A deficiency of these substances results in a decrease in the biotransformation of drugs that use these pathways. Glycine conjugation is a phase II reaction. Glycine is an amino acid that requires dietary protein. A diet deficient in protein, therefore, could lead to a deficiency of glycine and, thus, a decrease in glycine conjugation. Glucuronidation is also a phase II reaction that requires endogenous glucuronic acid, but this substance is supplied by dietary carbohydrates. Hydroxylation is a phase I metabolic reaction and does not require dietary protein.

12–15. The answers are: 12-B *[II B 2 a (2)],* **13-E** *[II A 3 a],* **14-A** *[II B 2 a (2)],* **15-D** *[II A 1 e].*
Benzoic acid contains a carboxylic acid, a functional group that commonly undergoes conjugation with glucuronic acid. The resulting conjugation produces an ester. Carboxylic acids can also undergo conjugation with the amino acids glycine and glutamine. Additionally, benzoic acid can undergo aromatic hydroxylation, a common phase I pathway for drugs containing unsubstituted aromatic rings. Of these options, ester glucuronidation is the only answer available here.
    Procaine is an ester-containing local anesthetic. Due to the wide physiological distribution of esterase enzymes, it is extremely susceptible to in vivo hydrolysis. This susceptibility to hydrolysis is the major reason why ester-containing local anesthetics have shorter durations of action as compared to those in other chemical classes.

One of the principal functional groups in acetaminophen is the phenol group. Similar to the carboxylic acid in benzoic acid, the phenol commonly undergoes glucuronide conjugation. The one difference is that a phenol (or an alcohol) produces an **ether** glucuronide, while a carboxylic acid produces an **ester** glucuronide. Phenols also commonly undergo sulfate conjugation reactions and occasionally undergo O-methylation reactions.

The principal functional group in amphetamine is its primary amine. Oxidative deamination is a very common metabolic path for primary amines. Occasionally, primary amines undergo phase II acetylation; however, this is a less common pathway. Aromatic hydroxylation, similar to that discussed above for benzoic acid, is also possible for amphetamine.

18
Drug–Drug and Drug–Nutrient Interactions

Alice C. Engelbrecht
Leon Shargel

I. INTRODUCTION

A. Types of drug interaction

1. **Drug interaction** refers to an **adverse** drug response produced by the administration of a drug or coexposure of the drug with another substance, which modifies the patient's response to the drug. Some drug interactions are intentional in order to provide improved therapeutic response or to decrease adverse drug effects. A **precipitant** drug is the drug, chemical, or food element causing the interaction. An **object** drug is the drug affected by the interaction.

2. Drug interactions include:
   a. **Drug–drug** interactions
   b. **Drug–herbal** interactions
   c. **Food–drug** interactions
   d. **Chemical–drug** interactions, such as the interaction of a drug with alcohol or tobacco
   e. **Drug–laboratory** test interactions (alterations in diagnostic laboratory test results caused by the drug) [see Chapter 37]

B. Classification of drug interactions. Drug interactions that occur *in vivo* are generally classified as **pharmacokinetic** or **pharmacodynamic** interactions.

1. **Pharmacokinetic** or **biopharmaceutical** interactions occur when the absorption, distribution (protein and tissue binding), or elimination (excretion and/or metabolism) of the drug is affected by another drug, chemical, or food element.

2. **Pharmacodynamic** interactions occur when the pharmacodynamic effect of the drug is altered by another drug, chemical, or food element, producing an antagonistic, synergistic, or additive effect.

3. **Pharmaceutical** interactions are caused by a chemical or physical incompatibility when two or more drugs are mixed together. Pharmaceutical interactions can occur during the extemporaneous compounding of drugs, including the preparation of intravenous (IV) solutions. For example, an IV solution of aminophylline has an alkaline pH and should not be mixed with such drugs as epinephrine, erythromycin gluceptate, or cephalothin sodium, which decompose in alkaline pH. Phenytoin sodium will precipitate from a solution that has an acid pH, such as dextrose 5%. Pharmaceutical interactions are usually considered during the development, manufacturing, and marketing of the drug product. Only drug interactions causing pharmacokinetic or pharmacodynamic changes of the object drug will be considered in this chapter.

II. PHARMACOKINETIC INTERACTIONS

A. Absorption

1. Drug interactions can affect the **rate** and the **extent** of systemic drug absorption (bioavailability) from the absorption site, resulting in increased or decreased drug bioavailability (Table 18-1).

Table 18-1. Drug Interactions That Affect the Bioavailability of the Drug from the Gastrointestinal (GI) Tract

Drug Interaction	Examples (Precipitant drugs)	Effect (Object drugs)
Complexation/chelation	Calcium, magnesium, or aluminum and iron salts	Levofloxacin complexes with divalent cations, causing a decreased bioavailability
	Sodium polystyrene sulfonate	Cations in antacids bind to sodium polystyrene sulfonate, causing reduced renal clearance of bicarbonate, resulting in systemic acidosis
Adsorption	Cholestyramine	Decreased bioavailability of digoxin, thyroxine
	Kaolin	Decreased bioavailability of digoxin
	Activated charcoal	Decreased bioavailability of many drugs
Increased GI motility	Laxatives, cathartics	Increases GI motility, decreases bioavailability for drugs that are absorbed slowly. May also affect the bioavailability of drugs from controlled-release products
Decreased GI motility	Anticholinergic agents	Propantheline decreases the gastric emptying of acetaminophen (APAP), delaying APAP absorption from the small intestine.
Alteration of gastric pH	H-2 blockers and antacids	Both H-2 blockers and antacids increase gastric pH. The dissolution of drugs like ketoconazole and omeprazole are reduced, causing decreased drug absorption.
Alteration of intestinal flora	Antibiotics (e.g., tetracyclines, penicillin)	Digoxin has better bioavailability after erythromycin. Erythromycin administration reduces bacterial inactivation of digoxin.
Inhibition of drug metabolism in intestinal cells	Monoamine oxidase inhibitors (MAO-Is) (e.g., tranylcypromine, phenelzine)	MAO-Is inhibit metabolism of tyromine-containing foods in the intestine, leading to hypertension caused by high tyromine levels.

2. The most common drug absorption **site** is in the **gastrointestinal (GI) tract.** However, drug bioavailability from other absorption sites, such as the skin, can be affected by drug interactions. For example, epinephrine, a vasoconstrictor, will decrease the percutaneous absorption of lidocaine, a local anesthetic agent.

3. Other **potential** drug interactions that affect bioavailability in the GI tract could be due to:
   a. **Competition** for carrier-mediated drug absorption in which the participant drug (e.g., purine, pyrimidine) competes for the same carrier as the object drug (e.g., purine or pyrimidine antimetabolite).
   b. **Alteration** of intestinal blood flow caused by the precipitant drug. In congestive heart disease, the blood flow to the GI tract is poor and an orally administered drug can have a slower rate of bioavailability. After digoxin therapy, the perfusion of the GI tract is improved along with bioavailability of the object drug.

B. **Distribution.** The distribution of the drug may be affected by plasma protein binding and displacement interactions or tissue and cellular interactions.

   1. **Plasma protein binding and displacement**
      a. **Valproic acid** displaces phenytoin from plasma protein–binding sites and reduces hepatic phenytoin clearance by inhibiting the liver's metabolism of phenytoin.
      b. **Aspirin** decreases protein binding and inhibits the metabolism of valproate.

   2. **Tissue and cellular interactions.** Digoxin toxicity can be enhanced by concurrent administration of quinidine. Quinidine reduces digoxin clearance and displaces digoxin from tissue-binding sites, leading to a higher plasma digoxin concentration and a reduced distribution volume.

C. Drug elimination and clearance

1. Drug metabolism and hepatic clearance

a. Drug metabolism (hepatic clearance) can be affected by enzyme induction, enzyme inhibition, substrate competition for the same enzyme, and changes in hepatic blood flow (Table 18-2).

b. Many drugs that share the same drug-metabolizing enzymes have a potential for a drug interaction. For example, erythromycin inhibits the hepatic metabolism of cisapride, causing clinically significant cardiac arrhythmias. Fluconazole inhibits the metabolism of phenytoin, saquinavir, and cisapride. Phenytoin, carbamazepine, and phenobarbital elevate levels of glucuronyl transferase, increasing the clearance of valproate (Table 18-3).

c. Over-the-counter (OTC) drugs and herbal preparations can also be involved in CYP450 isoenzyme metabolism and can cause serious drug–herbal interactions. For example, St. John's wort may induce CYP3A4 isoenzymes and decrease cyclosporin to subtherapeutic levels.

d. Foods may also interfere with hepatic drug metabolism. For example, grapefruit juice is a powerful inhibitor of the CYP3A4 isoenzyme, and will increase blood levels of saquinavir if taken together.

e. Nonhepatic enzymes can be involved in drug interactions. For example, serious drug interactions have been reported in patients receiving antidepressants similar to nefazodone hydrochloric acid (HCl) in combination with a monamine oxidase inhibitor. A considerable portion of the CYP3A4 enzymes are found in the GI tract, where some of these substrates are metabolized.

f. A decrease in the hepatic blood flow can decrease the hepatic clearance for high extraction drugs, such as propranolol and morphine.

2. Renal drug clearance can be affected by changes in glomerular filtration, tubular reabsorption, active drug secretion, and renal blood flow and nephrotoxicity (Table 18-4).

Table 18-2. Drug Interactions That Affect the Drug Metabolism

Drug Interaction	Examples (Precipitant drugs)	Effect (Objective drugs)
Enzyme induction		
	Smoking (polycyclic aromatic hydrocarbons)	Smoking increases theophylline clearance
	Barbiturates	Phenobarbital increases the metabolism of warfarin
Enzyme inhibition		
Mixed function oxidase	Cimetidine	Decreased theophylline clearance
Other enzymes	Monoamine oxidase inhibitors, MAO-Is (e.g., pargyline, tranylcypromine)	Serious hypertensive crisis can occur following ingestion of foods with a high content of tyramine or other pressor substances (e.g., cheddar cheese, red wines).

D. Herbal–drug interactions

1. Herbal preparations are various combinations of herbs, sometimes being one herb, or a combination of herbs. Some herbal preparations represent a single herb containing a variety of alkaloids or constituents that may exhibit a variety of pharmacological activities.

a. Some herbs contain a number of different pharmacologically active constituents. St. John's wort has at least six different constituents: hyperforin, biapigenin, hypericin, quercitin, chlorogenic acid, and pseudohypericin. St. John's wort appears to be an inducer of an important metabolic pathway, CYP450.

b. Traditional Chinese medicine (TCM) may contain a combination of herbs. Some imported TCM products have been found to contain unlisted legend drugs.

Table 18-3. Drug Actions with Cytochrome P450 Enzymes

Enzyme	Inhibitor	Inducer	Substrate
CYP1A2	Ciprofloxacin Fluoxetine Nefazodone Fluvoxamine	Phenobarbital Carbamazepine Phenytoin	Theophylline Amitriptyline Verapamil Propranolol Clozaril
CYP2C9	Miconazole Clopidogrel Fluvastatin Fluconazole	Rifampin Carbamazepine Phenytoin	Amitriptyline Losartan Warfarin Celecoxib Phenytoin
CYP2C19	Ketoconazole Omeprazole Isoniazid	Rifampin	Diazepam Phenytoin Lansoprazole
CYP2D6	Quinidine Cimetidine Fluoxetine Ritonavir Haloperidol	None known	Amitriptyline Metoprolol Propafenone Codeine
CYP2E1	Cimetidine	Ritonavir Isoniazid Alcohol	Acetaminophen Caffeine Venlafaxine
CYP3A family	Erythromycin Ketoconazole Saquinavir Verapamil Omeprazole	Carbamazepine Phenobarbital Prednisone Troglitazone	Cisapride Caffeine Lidocaine Ethylestradiol Terfenadine Triazolam Amitriptyline Theophylline Cyclosporin Amlopdipine Indinavir Saquinavir

Table 18-4. Drug Interactions That Affect the Renal Clearance

Drug Interaction	Examples	Effect
Glomerular filtration rate (GFR) and renal blood flow	Methylxanthines (e.g., caffeine, theobromine)	Increased renal blood flow and GFR will decrease time for reabsorption of various drugs, leading to more rapid urinary drug excretion.
Active tubular secretion	Probenecid	Probenecid blocks the active tubular secretion of penicillin and some cephalosporin antibiotics.
Tubular reabsorption and urine pH	Antacids, sodium bicarbonate	Alkalinization of the urine increases the reabsorption of amphetamine and decreases its clearance. Alkalinization of urine pH increases the ionization of salicylates, decreases reabsorption, and increases its clearance.

   c. Some herbal preparations may contain unrecognized contaminants such as heavy metals, or a similar-appearing herb mistakenly harvested. These are quality control issues that are to a large extent unregulated by government agencies.

   d. Drug–herbal interactions are of greatest concern when patients are taking drugs with a narrow therapeutic window. For example, coenzyme Q10 has a chemical structure related to vitamin K. Patients on warfarin therapy will have increased bleeding due to coenzyme Q10. Wheat grass is high in vitamin K and should also be avoided by patients taking warfarin. Ginger, garlic, and feverfew also increase bleeding in patients taking warfarin.

  2. The predominant effect or interaction depends upon the relative potency of each constituent in the herb. Potency is influenced by a variety of factors:
   a. The stage of growth during which the herb was harvested
   b. The drying time
   c. The solvents used in extraction of the herb
   d. The shelf life and storage conditions of the herbal extract

E. Food–drug interactions

  1. Food can increase, decrease, or not effect the absorption of drugs (Table 18-5).

  2. Food can influence the bioavailability of a drug from a modified-release dosage form [e.g., controlled release, delayed release (enteric coated)] rather than from an immediate-release dosage form.

  3. Complexation and adsorption of the drug in the GI tract with another food element is a common drug interaction that reduces the extent of drug absorption. For example, quinolone antibiotics and tetracycline complex with calcium (found in milk products).

  4. Food can be metabolized by the same liver enzymes that metabolize drugs, causing enzyme inhibition or induction, and resulting in toxic or subtherapeutic drug levels. For example, grapefruit and valencia oranges inhibit the CYP3A4 isoenzyme system, causing increased levels of substrate drugs such as saquinavir, indinavir, midazolam, nimodipine, nifedipine, lovastatin, cyclosporin, carbamazepine, and verapamil.

  5. Food can pharmacodynamically antagonize the effect of some drugs. For example, spinach and broccoli provide dietary sources of vitamin K, which antagonizes the effect of warfarin.

F. Chemical–drug interactions

  1. Smoking by inhaling aromatic polycyclic hydrocarbons can increase the intrinsic clearance (enzyme induction) of drugs such as theophylline, diazepam, and tricyclic antidepressants.

  2. Alcohol can increase or decrease the activity of hepatic drug metabolizing enzymes.
   a. Chronic alcoholism can increase the rate of metabolism of tolbutamide, warfarin, and phenytoin.
   b. Acute alcohol intoxication can inhibit hepatic enzymes in nonalcoholic individuals.

Table 18-5. Affect of Food on Drug Bioavailability

Reduced or delayed	Increased	Not affected by food
NSAIDs (nonsteroidal anti-inflammatory drugs) naproxen, naproxen sodium Aspirin Acetaminophen Antibiotics (tetracycline and penicillin) Ethanol	Griseofulvin Metoprolol Phenytoin Propoxyphene Dicumarol Morphine	Theophylline[1] Metronidazole

[1]Food does not significantly affect drug absorption of theophylline in an immediate-release dosage form. However, food may affect theophylline absorption from a controlled-release formulation.

III. PHARMACODYNAMIC INTERACTIONS

A. Drugs that have similar pharmacodynamic actions may produce an excessive pharmacological or **toxic response.** For example, central nervous system depressants, such as the combination of alcohol and antihistamines (e.g., diphenhydramine, chlorpheniramine) can produce increased drowsiness in the patient. Drugs having anticholinergic effects, such as promethazine and OTC antihistamines, can cause dryness of the mouth, blurred vision, and urinary retention.

B. The alteration of **electrolyte concentrations** produced by a diuretic, such as a thiazide derivative, will deplete potassium, resulting in sensitization of the heart to digoxin therapy. Depletion of sodium can also result in lithium toxicity.

C. By inhibiting platelet aggregation, aspirin increases the risk of bleeding in patients on anticoagulant (e.g., warfarin, dicumarol, clopidogrel) therapy.

IV. CLINICAL SIGNIFICANCE AND MANAGEMENT OF DRUG INTERACTIONS

A. Potential drug interactions

1. **Multiple-drug therapy,** including both **prescription** and **nonprescription** (OTC) medication, can potentially lead to drug interactions. The more drugs used by a patient, the greater the potential for a drug interaction in the patient.

2. **Multiple prescribers.** Patients can be seen by different prescribers who prescribe interacting medication.

3. **Patient compliance.** Patients need to follow proper instructions for taking medications. For example, a patient might take tetracycline with food rather than before meals.

4. **Patient risk factors**
   a. Older patients are at more risk for drug interactions than younger patients. Older patients might have changes in their physiological and pathophysiological condition that lead to altered body composition, altered GI transit time and drug absorption, decreased protein binding, altered distribution, and decreased drug clearance.
   b. Patients with predisposing illness (diabetes, asthma, AIDS, and alcoholism) and patients who are clinically hypersensitive (atopic) are more at risk for drug interactions than nonatopic patients.

B. Clinical significance

1. Not all drug interactions are clinically significant or cause an adverse effect. In some cases, interacting drugs can be prescribed for patients as long as the patient is given proper instructions and is compliant. For example, cimetidine and an antacid might be prescribed to the patient, but the patient should be instructed to not take both medications at the same time.

2. Combination drug therapy can have beneficial effects. Drug combinations are used to improve the therapeutic objective or to decrease adverse events. Some examples include:
   a. Trimethoprim and sulfamethoxazole—combination antibiotic for increased efficacy in urinary tract infections
   b. Amoxicillin and clavulanate potassium—combination containing a β-lactamase inhibitor (clavulanate) to inhibit the breakdown of amoxicillin
   c. Hydrochlorothiazide and triamterene—combination diuretic and antihypertensive to minimize potassium excretion

3. Some drug–food and drug–drug interactions are utilized for their beneficial effects.
   a. Saquinavir is given with food to increase its bioavailability through enhanced absorption.
   b. Probenecid inhibits renal tubular secretion of penicillin, thereby prolonging the plasma half-life of the antibiotic.

4. The determination of the clinical significance of a potential drug interaction should be documented in the literature. The likelihood of a drug interaction can be classified as follows:
   a. **Established**—a drug interaction supported by well-proven clinical studies
   b. **Probable**—a drug interaction that is very likely but might not be proven clinically

      c. Suspected—a drug interaction that might occur; some data might be available

      d. Possible—a drug interaction that could occur; limited data are available

      e. Unlikely—a drug interaction that is doubtful; no good evidence of an altered clinical effect is available

   5. The clinical relevance of a potential drug interaction should also consider the:

      a. Size of the dose and the duration of therapy

      b. Onset (rapid, delayed) and **severity** (major, moderate, minor) of the potential interaction

      c. Extrapolation to related drugs

C. Management of drug interactions

   1. Review the patient profile, including drug history and patient risk factors.

   2. Avoid complex therapeutic drug regimens.

   3. Determine the probability of a clinically significant drug interaction.

   4. Suggest a different drug if there is a high probability for a clinically significant drug interaction. For example, acetaminophen can be used for headache instead of aspirin for a patient on anticoagulant therapy.

   5. Carefully instruct the patient as to the timing of the medication. For example, the antacid and H-2 blocker should not be taken at the same time. The patient should use maximum spacing between drugs.

   6. Monitor the patient for adverse events. Sulfonamides, such as sulfisoxazole and sulfamethoxazole, can prolong prothrombin time in patients given warfarin therapy. The prothrombin times should be monitored in these patients.

   7. Reevaluate the patient profile and drug history when changing drug therapy. For example, when discontinuing the diuretic of a congestive heart failure patient on digoxin, a review of the profile may reveal a potassium supplement that should be discontinued as well.

V. REFERENCES. A vast number of drug interactions are reported in the literature. Some general references that are updated periodically include:

A. *Drug Interaction Facts,* Facts and Comparisons, St. Louis, MO.

B. Hansten PD, Horn JR (eds). *Drug Interactions & Updates.* Applied Therapeutics, Inc., Vancouver, WA.

C. Zucchero FJ, Hogan MJ, Schultz CD (eds). *Evaluations of Drug Interactions.* Professional Drug Systems, St. Louis, MO.

D. *PDR Guide to Drug Interactions, Side Effects, and Indications.* Medical Economics Data, Montvale, NJ.

E. *MICROMEDEX® Systems, DRUGDEX® System, Drug Evaluations,* Englewood, CO.

STUDY QUESTIONS

Directions: Each question below contains three suggested answers, of which **one** or more is correct. Choose the answer

A	if **I only** is correct
B	if **III only** is correct
C	if **I and II** are correct
D	if **II and III** are correct
E	if **I, II, and III** are correct

1. Drug interactions may be classed as

 I. pharmacokinetic interactions
 II. pharmacodynamic interactions
 III. pharmaceutical interactions

2. Situations that can potentially lead to drug interactions include

 I. multiple-drug therapy
 II. multiple prescribers
 III. patient compliance

Directions: The question below is followed by five suggested answers. Select the **one** lettered answer that is the **best** response to the question.

3. Which of the following statements regarding drug interactions is true?

(A) All drug interactions can potentially cause an adverse response in the patient.

(B) The clinical significance for each potential drug interaction must be considered individually.

(C) A precipitant drug that inhibits the metabolism of the object drug causes a more serious drug interaction compared to a precipitant drug causing an increase in the bioavailability of the object drug.

(D) If the patient is prescribed drugs that can potentially interact, the prescriber should be called, and a different precipitant drug should be suggested.

(E) Food–drug interactions are unlikely to have clinical significance.

ANSWERS AND EXPLANATIONS

1. The answer is E *[I B]*.
Most drug interactions in vivo are caused by pharmacokinetic and pharmacodynamic interactions. Pharmaceutical interactions can occur during extemporaneous compounding, preparation of intravenous (IV) admixtures, and improper dosing, as in the case of giving aspirin with acidic juices (e.g., orange, cranberry).

2. The answer is E *[IV A 1–3]*.
Patient profiles might not contain all the drug history information of the patient. Patients who take non-prescription (OTC) medications, go to several different physicians, or purchase drugs at various pharmacies may neglect to inform the pharmacist of all the medications being taken.

3. The answer is B *[IV B]*.
Not all drug interactions are clinically significant. Some potential clinically significant drug interactions can be prevented by proper patient instruction and compliance. The potential for a clinically significant drug interaction should be documented before calling a physician concerning the prescribed medication.

19
Nuclear Pharmacy

Stephen C. Dragotakes
Jeffrey P. Norenberg

I. INTRODUCTION

A. Overview

1. **Nuclear pharmacy** is defined as a "patient-oriented service that embodies the scientific knowledge and professional judgment required to improve and promote health through the safe and efficacious use of radioactive drugs for diagnosis and therapy."*

2. **Radiopharmaceuticals** are drug products that contain a biological moiety and a radioactive element. The biological construct targets a physiological or pathophysiological process of interest, allowing the localization of radiation that in turn may be imaged or used to effect therapy. Most radiopharmaceuticals are used in diagnostic medical imaging; however, they are also used in therapeutic applications, such as in the treatment of hyperthyroidism, thyroid cancer, polycythemia vera, and in the alleviation of bone pain.

3. **Nuclear pharmacy practice** entails the:
   a. Procurement of radiopharmaceuticals
   b. Compounding of radiopharmaceuticals
   c. Performance of routine quality control procedures
   d. Dispensing of radiopharmaceuticals
   e. Distribution of radiopharmaceuticals
   f. Implementation of basic radiation protection procedures and practices
   g. Consultation and education of the nuclear medicine community, patients, pharmacists, other health professionals, and the general public regarding:
      (1) Physical and chemical properties of radiopharmaceuticals
      (2) Pharmacokinetics and biodistribution of radiopharmaceuticals
      (3) Drug interactions and other factors that alter patterns of distribution
   h. Monitoring of patient outcomes
   i. Research and development of radiopharmaceuticals

B. Properties of radiopharmaceuticals

1. **Pharmacological effects.** Typically, radiopharmaceuticals lack pharmacological effects because the mass quantities range from picogram (pg) to nanogram (ng) per kilogram (kg) of administered dose.

2. **Route of administration.** Most radiopharmaceuticals are prepared as sterile, pyrogen-free intravenous (IV) solutions or suspensions to be administered directly to the patient. Other routes of administration include intradermal, oral, interstitial, and inhalation (e.g., radioactive gases, aerosols).

3. **Radionuclides**
   a. The radioactive component of a radiopharmaceutical is referred to as a radionuclide. Nuclides are identified as atoms having a specific number of protons and neutrons in the nucleus. A nuclide is typically identified by the chemical symbol of the element with a mass number to the upper left superscript, indicating the sum of protons and neutrons (e.g., iodide-131 is indicated ^{131}I). When the atom is radioactive, it is called a radionuclide.
   b. Radionuclides undergo spontaneous radioactive decay accompanied by the release of energy. The distribution, metabolism, and elimination of the radiopharmaceutical

---

*American Pharmaceutical Association. Nuclear Pharmacy Practice Guidelines. Academy of Pharmacy Practice, 1995.

can be determined by measuring this energy with imaging equipment. There are four major types of radiation emitted through this process: alpha, beta, gamma, and x-rays. Alpha and beta radiations are not useful in medical imaging and are therefore undesirable in diagnostic applications. Most diagnostic radiopharmaceuticals use penetrating gamma radiation, which can be easily detected and converted into imaging data.

4. Half-lives of radiopharmaceuticals

a. Physical half-life of a radiopharmaceutical is the amount of time necessary for the radioactive atoms to decay to one-half their original number. Each radionuclide is characterized by a specific half-life that is a physical constant.

b. Biological half-life of a radiopharmaceutical is the amount of time required for the body to metabolize or eliminate one-half of the administered dose of any substance through biological processes.

c. Effective half-life of a radiopharmaceutical is the time required for an administered radiopharmaceutical dose to be reduced by one-half due to both physical decay and biological mechanisms. It is defined as:

$$T_e = (T_p) + (T_b)/(T_p) \times (T_b)$$

where T_e = effective half-life, T_p = physical half-life, and T_b = biological half-life.

C. Optimal radiopharmaceuticals

1. Optimal diagnostic radiopharmaceuticals

a. They should contain a radionuclide with a half-life short enough to minimize radiation exposure to the patient, yet long enough to allow for collection of imaging information. The optimal relationship is a physical half-life equal to approximately 67% of the biological process of interest.

b. They should incorporate a gamma-emitting radionuclide, which decays with the emission of a photon energy between 100–300 kiloelectron volts (keV), which is efficiently detected with current instrumentation.

c. Radiopharmaceuticals should contain a biological component that allows rapid localization in the organ system of interest and be metabolized or excreted from the non-target tissues to maximize contrast and minimize the radiation absorbed dose to non-target organs.

d. They should be readily available and cost-effective.

2. Optimal therapeutic radiopharmaceuticals

In addition to c. and d. above, they should contain alpha- or beta-emitting radionuclides that can effectively deliver radiation in quantities sufficient to cause the desired therapeutic effect. These effects include apoptosis, DNA damage, or irreparable cell damage leading to tissue effects.

II. SODIUM PERTECHNETATE TECHNETIUM-99m (^{99m}Tc) GENERATOR

A. Overview

1. ^{99m}Tc is the most commonly used radionuclide in diagnostic imaging today. This radionuclide is produced by the radioactive decay of molybdenum-99 (^{99}Mo).

a. ^{99m}Tc is obtained via commercially supplied, sterile, pyrogen-free generator systems. A generator is a device used to separate a short half-life radionuclide from the longer-lived parent nuclide, while retaining the parent to produce more of the daughter nuclide. In this way, short half-life nuclides can be made available continuously at great distances from the sites of generator production.

b. All of the commercially supplied generators currently use ^{99}Mo obtained from the fission of uranium-235 (^{235}U). This ^{99}Mo parent is absorbed on an alumina ion (Al_2O_3) exchange column, and the ^{99m}Tc formed from its decay is exchanged for the chloride ion (Cl^-) available in the 0.9% saline eluate solution washed through the column, as the sodium pertechnetate $Na^+(^{99m}TcO_4)^-$ form.

2. The chemical valence state of $Na^{+99m}TcO_4^-$ as it is eluted from the column is $^{+7}$. Typically, it must be reduced to a lower valence state before it is able to react with other compounds.

Although many processes can reduce ^{99m}Tc, the stannous ion (Sn^{2+}) reduction method is most commonly used in ^{99m}Tc radiopharmaceutical kits.

    a. A radiopharmaceutical kit consists of sterile, pyrogen-free vials containing a reducing agent, the biological compound to be labeled, and any additional adjutants necessary to effect the reaction or to stabilize the labeled product.

    b. In most cases, they are lyophilized under inert atmospheres, so as to minimize oxidation of the reducing agent (e.g., Sn^{2+}).

B. Sodium pertechnetate Tc-99m USP [United States Pharmacopeia] ($Na^{+99m}TcO_4^-$) as eluted from a generator in 0.9% sodium chloride (NaCl) solution is an isotonic, sterile, nonpyrogenic, diagnostic radiopharmaceutical suitable for IV injection, oral administration, and direct instillation.

    1. Physical properties

        a. The solution should be clear, colorless, and free of visible foreign material. The pH is 4.5–7.0.

        b. $Na^{+99m}TcO_4^-$ is itself a radiopharmaceutical, or it may be used to radiolabel all other ^{99m}Tc radiopharmaceuticals.

    2. Biodistribution

        a. $^{99m}TcO_4^-$ is handled by the body in a fashion similar to ^{131}I; that is, it is taken up and released but not organified by the thyroid.

        b. After IV administration, $^{99m}TcO_4^-$ concentrates in the choroid plexus, thyroid gland, salivary gland, and stomach, but remains in the circulation long enough for first-pass blood-pool studies, organ perfusion, and major vessel studies.

        c. It is primarily excreted by the kidneys unchanged and is expressed in the urine 15–50% by 24 hours.

        d. Approximately 10–55% of the administered dose is eliminated via feces within 3 days.

    3. Decay data

        a. ^{99m}Tc decays by isomeric transition with a physical half-life of 6 hours.

        b. The primary radiation emissions are 140 keV gamma energy photons.

    4. Purity

        a. USP radionuclidic purity requires a ^{99}Mo breakthrough limit of less than 0.15 μCi/mCi of ^{99m}Tc at the time of patient administration.

        b. USP chemical purity requires an aluminum ion (Al^{+3}) test result of less than 10 μg/mL.

    5. Administration and dosage. All of the following imaging studies are administered via IV except nasolacrimal imaging, which is instilled into the lacrimal canal.

        a. Brain imaging: 10–20 mCi [370–740 megabecquerels (MBq)]

        b. Thyroid imaging: 1–10 mCi (37–370 MBq)

        c. Salivary gland imaging: 1–5 mCi (37–185 MBq)

        d. Placenta localization: 1–3 mCi (37–111 MBq)

        e. Blood-pool imaging: 10–30 mCi (370–740 MBq)

        f. Urinary bladder imaging: 0.5–1 mCi (18–37 MBq)

        g. Nasolacrimal imaging: less than 100 μCi (less than 3.7 MBq)

III. RADIOPHARMACEUTICALS FOR CARDIOVASCULAR IMAGING

    A. Perfusion agents for cardiac imaging. Radiopharmaceuticals are useful in cardiac imaging as agents that provide information on the regional myocardial blood perfusion. They typically are administered as part of a cardiac stress test so as to provide information at peak cardiac output. The patient will run on a treadmill to "stress" the heart. IV coronary vessel dilating agents are used in place of the treadmill when the patient is not physically able to exercise. Examples of these pharmacological agents are dipyridamole, adenosine, and dobutamine. The patient will also be imaged when the heart is at "rest."

        1. Thallous chloride Tl-201 (^{201}Tl) is a radionuclide that is produced by a cyclotron. It is used for myocardial perfusion imaging in the diagnosis of coronary artery disease and localization of myocardial infarction.

a. Biodistribution

(1) ^{201}Tl is a monovalent cation with distribution analogous to a potassium ion (K^+); myocardial uptake is by active transport via the Na^+/K^+-adenosine triphosphatase (ATPase) pump.

(2) Biodistribution is generally proportional to organ blood flow at the time of injection with blood clearance by myocardium, kidneys, thyroid, liver, and stomach. The remainder is distributed uniformly throughout the rest of the body.

(3) ^{201}Tl is excreted slowly and equally in both urine and feces.

b. Decay data

(1) The **physical half-life** is 73 hours.

(2) The **effective half-life** is 2.4 days.

(3) The **biological half-life** is 11 days.

(4) The **primary radiation emissions** are 68–80 keV x-rays and 167 and 135 keV gamma energy photons.

c. Administration and dosage. IV, 2–4 mCi (74–148 MBq)

2. Technetium Tc-99m sestamibi (Tc-MIBI) exists as a sterile, pyrogen-free IV injection after kit reconstitution with $Na^{+99m}TcO_4^-$ and heating at 100°C for 10 minutes.

a. Biodistribution

(1) ^{99m}Tc sestamibi is a cation complex that has been found to accumulate in viable myocardium by passive diffusion into the myocyte with subsequent binding to the mitochondria within the cell.

(2) The major pathway for clearance of ^{99m}Tc sestamibi is the hepatobiliary system. This agent is excreted without any evidence of metabolism via urine and feces.

b. Decay data

(1) The **effective half-life** is 3 hours.   (Myocardium)

(2) The **biological half-life** is 6 hours.   (Myocardium)

c. Administration and dosage. IV, 10–30 mCi (370–1110 MBq)

3. Technetium Tc-99m tetrofosmin exists as a sterile and pyrogen-free IV injection after kit reconstitution with sodium pertechnetate ^{99m}Tc injection USP.

a. Description. ^{99m}Tc tetrofosmin is a lipophilic, cationic ^{99m}Tc complex that has been found to accumulate in viable myocardium.

b. Biodistribution. The major pathways for clearance of ^{99m}Tc tetrofosmin are the renal system and the hepatobiliary system with 26% of the administered dose excreted in the feces and 40% excreted in the urine within 48 hours.

c. Physical properties (see II A, II B 3)

d. Administration and dosage. IV during exercise, 5–8 mCi (185–296 MBq); during rest, 15–24 mCi (555–1443 MBq)

4. Technetium Tc-99m teboroxime (no longer available)

5. Rubidium chloride Rb-82 (^{82}Rb) is a generator-produced radiopharmaceutical obtained by the decay of its accelerator-produced parent strontium (^{82}Sr; half-life is 25 days) adsorbed on a stannous oxide column.

a. Biodistribution

(1) When eluted with 0.9% NaCl at a rate of 50 mL/min, a solution of the short-lived daughter ^{82}Rb is eluted from the generator for direct IV administration.

(2) After IV administration, ^{82}Rb rapidly clears from the blood and is extracted by the myocardial tissue in a manner analogous to K^+.

(3) Myocardial activity is visualized within 1 minute after administration.

b. Decay data

(1) The **physical half-life** is 75 seconds.

(2) The **decay mode** is by positron emission.

(3) The **primary radiation emissions** are annihilation 511 keV gamma energy photons.

(4) Parent ^{82}Sr and contaminant ^{85}Sr breakthrough must be closely monitored. Acceptable levels of strontium breakthrough are less than 0.02 μCi ^{82}Sr/mCi ^{82}Rb, and less than 0.2 μCi ^{85}Sr/mCi ^{82}Rb.

c. Administration and dosage. IV, 30–60 mCi (1110–2220 MBq)

6. Ammonia N-13 exists under a USP monograph as an on site cyclotron produced, sterile IV solution of $^{13}NH_3$, useful as a myocardial perfusion agent.

a. Decay data

(1) Physical half-life is 10 minutes.

(2) Decay mode is positron emission resulting in the production of two 511 keV annihilation gamma photons.

  b. Biodistribution

    (1) After IV injection, it circulates as $^{13}NH_3$ but localizes into the myocytes via diffusion as $^{13}NH_3$. It is then metabolized to glutamine and retained by the myocytes.

    (2) After IV injection, it is cleared rapidly from the blood, with less than 2% of the administered dose remaining after 5 minutes postinjection.

    (3) It is predominantly metabolized to ^{13}N-glutamine by different organs of the body.

    (4) Ten percent to twenty percent is excreted via the renal system.

  c. Administration and dosage. IV, 15–20 mCi (555–740 MBq)

B. Agents used to measure cardiac function (regional myocardial wall motion)

  1. Technetium-Tc-99m-labeled red blood cells (Tc-RBCs) are used for blood-pool imaging, including cardiac first-pass and gated equilibrium imaging (regional cardiac wall motion).

    a. Physical properties. Autologous RBCs can be labeled by a number of techniques that use the Sn^{2+} radiolabeling method with three general steps.

      (1) The cells are treated with Sn^{2+} to provide an intracellular source of the reducing agent. This step can be carried out with either in vivo or in vitro labeling procedures.

      (2) The next step is the removal of excess Sn^{2+} either by chemical oxidation (in vitro method) or by biological clearance (in vivo method).

      (3) All of the methods include the addition of sodium pertechnetate ($^{99m}TcO_4^-$). This ^{99m}Tc, while in the $^{+7}$ valence state, crosses the intact erythrocyte membrane and binds to intracellular hemoglobin (Hb) after being reduced by the available intracellular Sn^{2+}.

    b. Biodistribution. After IV injection, the labeling RBCs distribute within the blood pool and are well maintained in the blood pool with a bi-exponential whole body clearance of 2.5–2.7 hours and 75–176 hours (e.g., major route of excretion is via the urine).

    c. Administration and dosage. IV, 10–20 mCi (370–740 MBq)

  2. Pyrophosphate injection USP and phosphates USP. The major use for these agents in nuclear medicine is as convenient and stable sources of Sn^{2+} for the labeling of autologous RBCs. In this application, the kits are reconstituted with normal saline and injected via IV.

  3. Technetium Tc-99m albumin (99mTc-HSA) injection

    a. Biodistribution

      (1) ^{99m}Tc albumin distributes initially within the intravascular space and leaves this space at a rate slow enough to permit imaging of the blood pool.

      (2) Plasma clearance is bi-exponential: a fast component clearing with a half-life of 2 hours and a slow component clearing with a half-life of 10–16 hours.

      (3) The major route of elimination is via the urine.

    b. Administration and dosage. IV, 20 mCi (740 MBq)

C. Agents for imaging myocardial infarction include **pyrophosphate injection USP and phosphates USP.**

  1. Mechanism of localization. The skeletal localizing radiopharmaceutical pyrophosphate has been shown to accumulate also in zones of myocardial infarction. This localization is thought to be due to binding of the pyrophosphate to microcalcification with hydroxyapatite crystals found in infarcted tissue.

  2. Biodistribution of labeled pyrophosphate depends on the ability of phosphates to become involved with calcium ion (Ca^{2+}) deposition in necrotic cardiac tissue.

IV. SKELETAL IMAGING

A. Skeletal imaging agents

  1. Overview. ^{99m}Tc-labeled bone agents are useful in the detection of bone lesions that are associated with metastatic neoplasms, metabolic disorders, and infections of the bone. The imaging advantages of ^{99m}Tc, coupled with the sensitivity of bone agent localization in skeletal bone hydroxyapatite, allows for detection of bone pathology before evidence is shown by conventional x-rays.

2. ^{99m}Tc bone agents. There are many different forms of ^{99m}Tc bone agents with minor differences in their individual chemical structure. Currently used bone-imaging agents are based on either the P—C—P diphosphonate structure, including ^{99m}medronate disodium, and ^{99m}Tc oxidronate, or the inorganic P—O—P phosphate structure such as ^{99m}Tc pyrophosphate. These bone agents are Sn^{2+} reduction method kits, which exist as sterile, pyrogen-free IV radiopharmaceuticals after reconstitution with $Na^{+99m}TcO_4^-$.

a. Physical properties

(1) All of the ^{99m}Tc bone-imaging agents are susceptible to radiological decomposition with reoxidation of the ^{99m}Tc tto a higher valence state. These agents sometimes include antioxidants (e.g., ascorbic or gentisic acid) in their formulation to improve the in vitro stability of these products.

(2) They should be stored at room temperature before and after reconstitution.

b. Biodistribution

(1) It is believed that the localization of the diphosphonates occurs by chemisorption onto the hydroxyapatite mineral matrix of skeletal bone with uptake related to bone metabolic activity and bone blood flow.

(2) For ^{99m}Tc medronate disodium and ^{99m}Tc oxidronate, approximately 50% of the administered dose localizes in the skeleton, and 50% is excreted by the kidneys within the first 4–6 hours after IV injection.

c. Administration and dosage. IV, 10–20 mCi (370–740 MBq)

B. Bone marrow imaging (see VI A 1, VI A 3, VI B)

V. LUNG IMAGING.
Radiopharmaceuticals are used to evaluate both pulmonary perfusion and pulmonary ventilation, to detect pulmonary embolism, and to assess pulmonary function before pneumonectomy.

A. Pulmonary perfusion imaging

1. Technetium Tc-99m albumin aggregated (^{99m}Tc-MAA)

a. Physical properties

(1) The ^{99m}Tc albumin aggregated kit contains human serum albumin that has been aggregated by heat denaturation.

(2) This Sn^{2+} reduction method kit exists as a sterile, pyrogen-free suspension of radiolabeled aggregated particles after reconstitution with $Na^{+99m}TcO_4^-$.

(3) It should be stored at 2°C–8°C after reconstitution.

b. Biodistribution

(1) After IV administration of ^{99m}Tc albumin aggregated, 80% of the radiolabeled albumin particles become trapped by capillary blockade in the pulmonary circulation.

(2) After trapping, the particles are cleared from the lungs mainly by mechanical breakup. These smaller particles are ultimately cleared from the circulation by the reticuloendothelial system.

(3) Particle size should be controlled; that is, 90% of the particles should be between 10 and 90 μm, and none should be greater than 150 μm to ensure adequate trapping by the lung capillary bed but no occlusion of the large-bore vessels.

(4) Particle number should be between 200,000 and 700,000 particles per adult dose to obtain uniform imaging data without compromising capillary blood flow. Neonates should receive <125,000 particles.

c. Decay data. Biological half-life in the lung is 2–3 hours.

d. Administration and dosage. IV, 1–4 mCi (37–148 MBq)

B. Pulmonary ventilation imaging with radioactive gases is a routine nuclear medicine procedure that can provide valuable information about regional lung ventilation. Radiopharmaceuticals that are used are either radioactive gases or radioaerosols.

1. Xenon Xe-133 (^{133}Xe) is supplied as a radioactive gas contained in glass septum vials to be administered by inhalation through a closed respiratory system or a spirometer. It is a byproduct of ^{235}U fission.

a. Biodistribution

(1) ^{133}Xe is a readily diffusible gas, which is neither used nor produced by the body. It passes through membranes and freely exchanges between blood and tissue, tending to concentrate more in body fat.

(2) Inhaled ^{133}Xe distributes within the alveoli and enters the pulmonary venous circulation via the capillaries with most of the absorbed ^{133}Xe returned and exhaled from the lungs after a single pass through the peripheral circulation.

(3) In concentrations used for diagnosis, the gas is physiologically inactive.

b. Decay data
(1) The **effective half-life** in the lung is 2 minutes.
(2) The **physical half-life** is 5.2 days.
(3) The **decay mode** is by beta minus and gamma decay.
(4) The **primary radiation emissions** are 100 keV beta energy and 81 keV gamma energy photons.

c. Administration and dosage. Inhalation, 2–30 mCi (74–1110 MBq)

2. Xenon Xe-127 (^{127}Xe) is supplied as a radioactive gas contained in glass septum vials to be administered by inhalation through a closed respiratory system or a spirometer. It is produced by a cyclotron.

a. Biodistribution. Localization is the same as ^{133}Xe.

b. Decay data
(1) The **physical half-life** is 36.4 days.
(2) The **decay mode** is by electron capture.
(3) The **primary radiation emissions** are 203 keV, 190 keV, 172 keV, and 375 keV gamma energy photons.

c. Administration and dosage. Inhalation, 5–10 mCi (185–370 MBq)

3. Krypton Kr-81m (^{81m}Kr) is generator produced by the decay of its parent radionuclide ^{81}Rb. It is supplied as a radioactive gas in the form of humidified oxygen eluted continuously through the generator and inhaled by the patient.

a. Decay data
(1) The **physical half-life** of ^{81m}Kr is 13 seconds.
(2) The **parent** ^{81}Rb half-life is 4.6 hours.
(3) The **primary radiation emissions** are 190 keV gamma energy photons.

b. Administration and dosage. Inhalation, 1–10 mCi (37–370 MBq)

4. Radioaerosols have become increasingly used with the advent of nebulizers that produce particles of a consistent size necessary for uniform lung distribution.

a. Biodistribution
(1) ^{99m}Tc pentetate (DTPA) radioaerosols of approximately 0.25 μm mass median aerodynamic diameter are useful in determining lung ventilation.
(2) After deposition of the nebulized droplets within the airways, the ^{99m}Tc pentetate is absorbed into the pulmonary circulation.
(3) The material is subsequently excreted by the kidneys. Clearance from the lungs is sufficiently slow to allow for imaging of the lungs in multiple projections from a single administration.

b. Physical properties (see II B 3)

c. Administration and dosage. Inhalation, 30 μCi (1110 MBq)

VI. HEPATIC IMAGING

A. Overview. Hepatic imaging requires the use of two different classes of radiopharmaceuticals to evaluate the two cell types responsible for hepatic function.

1. Reticuloendothelial system imaging. The liver, spleen, and bone marrow are evaluated with radiolabeled colloidal material, ranging in size from 0.1–3.0 μm. These particles are rapidly cleared from the blood by phagocytosis by the Kupffer cells or trapped in the space of Disse that is found between the polygonal hepatocytes and the Kupffer cells.

2. Liver spleen imaging. Radiopharmaceuticals are useful in imaging space occupying primary tumors and metastatic neoplasms, as well as hepatic defects caused by abscesses, cysts, and trauma.

3. Bone marrow imaging. Images that localize in the bone marrow are useful in the evaluation of pathologies that affect bone marrow.

4. Hepatobiliary imaging. Hepatocyte function can be evaluated by substances meeting requirements of molecular weight, lipophilicity, and chemical structure, to be excreted by the polygonal cells into the hepatobiliary system. Hepatobiliary imaging radiopharmaceuticals are useful in the diagnosis of cystic duct obstruction in acute cholecystitis as well as defining postcholecystectomy anatomy and physiology.

B. Reticuloendothelial imaging agents

1. **Technetium Tc-99m sulfur colloid (Tc_2S_7)** is a sterile, pyrogen-free IV radiopharmaceutical formed via a chemical reaction between $^{99m}TcO_4^-$ and an acidified solution of sodium thiosulfate at 100°C.

   a. **Physical properties**

      (1) Tc_2S_7 is thought to remain in the $^{+7}$ valence state as the heptasulfide coprecipitate of elemental sulfur that occurs during the reaction.

      (2) The use of $Na^{+99m}TcO_4^-$ with Al^{3+} levels over 10 µg/mL can lead to the formation of particles greater than 5 µm, which can result in lung uptake.

      (3) Heating times should be controlled to preclude large particle formation.

   b. **Biodistribution.** After administration, approximately 80%–90% of the dose is phagocytized by the Kupffer cells of the liver or trapped in the space of Disse that is found between the polygonal hepatocytes and the Kupffer cells, 5%–10% by the spleen, and the balance by the bone marrow. The blood clearance half-life is approximately 2.5 minutes. Particles are not metabolized and reside in the reticuloendothelial system for a prolonged period.

   c. **Administration and dosage.** IV, liver/spleen: 1–8 mCi (37–296 MBq); bone marrow: 3–12 mCi (111–444 MBq)

C. Hepatobiliary imaging agents

1. **Overview**

   a. **Iminodiacetic acid (IDA) derivatives,** which are lidocaine analogues, are useful as hepatobiliary imaging agents because of their lypophyllicity that allows them to be selectively cleared by carrier-mediated hepatocyte metabolic pathways. Because these agents share the same excretion pathway as bilirubin, patients who have increased bilirubin levels exhibit decreased hepatic clearance and an increased renal clearance. Lack of gallbladder visualization is an abnormal finding suggestive of acute cholecystitis.

   b. **Cholecystokinetic agents,** such as sincalide and cholecystokinin, may be used to empty the contents of the gallbladder in fasting patients prior to injection of IDA compounds in an attempt to promote gallbladder filling and visualization. These agents can also be injected after the injection of the IDA compound to cause a visualized gallbladder to empty. Cholecystokinetic agents are used to increase the specificity and sensitivity of the imaging procedure.

   c. **Narcotic analgesics,** such as morphine, have been used to constrict the sphincter of Oddi to produce increased intraductal pressures to promote retrograde gallbladder filling.

2. **Technetium Tc-99m disofenin (^{99m}Tc-DISIDA)**

   a. **Physical properties** (see II B 3)

   b. **Biodistribution**

      (1) ^{99m}Tc-DISIDA is rapidly cleared from the blood, with 8% remaining in the blood after 30 minutes.

      (2) Approximately 9% of the administered activity is excreted in the urine during the first 2 hours. The remainder of the activity is cleared through the hepatobiliary system.

      (3) Peak liver uptake is within 10 minutes, with peak gallbladder uptake by 30–40 minutes.

      (4) Gallbladder and intestinal visualization occurs within 60 minutes postadministration.

   c. **Administration and dosage.** IV, nonjaundiced patient: 1–5 mCi (37–185 MBq); jaundiced patient: 3–8 mCi (111–296 MBq)

3. **Technetium Tc-99m lidofenin (^{99m}Tc-HIDA)**

   a. **Physical properties** (see II B 3)

   b. **Biodistribution**

      (1) After administration, ^{99m}Tc-HIDA is rapidly cleared from the blood circulation, with 7% remaining after 26 minutes.

(2) Approximately 14%–22% of the administered activity can be excreted in the urine within the first 90 minutes, with the remainder of the activity clearing through the hepatobiliary system.
(3) Peak liver uptake occurs within 10–15 minutes, with visualization of the hepatic duct and gallbladder within 20–30 minutes.
(4) Intestinal activity can be visualized within 30 minutes.
c. Administration and dosage. IV, nonjaundiced patient: 2–5 mCi (74–185 MBq); jaundiced patient: 3–10 mCi (111–370 MBq)

4. Technetium Tc-99m mebrofenin
   a. Physical properties (see II B 3)
   b. Biodistribution
      (1) ^{99m}Tc mebrofenin is rapidly cleared from the blood, with 17% remaining after 10 minutes. Only 1% of the administered activity is excreted in the urine within the first hours, with the remainder of the activity clearing through the hepatobiliary system.
      (2) Peak liver uptake occurs within 10 minutes, with visualization of the hepatic duct and gallbladder within 10–15 minutes, then intestinal activity within 30–60 minutes.
   c. Administration and dosage. IV, nonjaundiced patient: 2–5 mCi (74–185 MBq); jaundiced patient: 3–10 mCi (111–370 MBq)

VII. RENAL IMAGING

A. Overview

1. Radiopharmaceuticals are used in renal imaging to determine renal function, renal vascular flow, and renal morphology. They are also useful for the evaluation of renal function in posttransplant patients for complications such as obstruction, infarction, leakage, tubular necrosis, and rejection.

2. The use of radiopharmaceuticals to determine renal function or renal morphology is based on the two physiological mechanisms responsible for excretion: glomerular filtration and tubular secretion.

B. Agents cleared by glomerular filtration are useful in determining the glomerular filtration rate (GFR), renal artery perfusion, and the visualization of the collecting system.

1. **Technetium Tc-99m pentetate (^{99m}Tc-DTPA)**
   a. Physical properties (see II B 3)
   b. Biodistribution
      (1) After administration, ^{99m}Tc pentetate rapidly distributes throughout extracellular fluid space from which it is rapidly cleared by glomerular filtration only.
      (2) Up to 10% may be protein bound, leading to a decrease in measured GFR.
      (3) After administration, 50% of the dose is cleared by the kidneys within 2 hours, and up to 95% is cleared by 24 hours.
   c. Administration and dosage. IV, 10–20 mCi (370–740 MBq)

2. **Sodium iothalamate I-125 injection** is a commercially supplied, sterile, pyrogen-free injection containing 1 mg sodium iothalamate per milliliter.
   a. Biodistribution
      (1) Sodium iothalamate ^{125}I is used for determination of the GFR but not for imaging due to poor imaging emissions of ^{125}I.
      (2) Thyroid blockade with oral potassium iodide (KI) is suggested.
   b. Decay data
      (1) The **physical half-life** is 59 days.
      (2) The **decay mode** is by electron capture.
      (3) The **primary radiation emissions** are 35 keV gamma energy photons and x-rays.
   c. Administration and dosage. IV, 10–50 μCi (3.7–18.5 MBq)

C. Tubular secretion agents are used to evaluate renal tubular function and measure effective renal plasma flow.

1. **Iodohippurate I-131 hippuran** is a commercially supplied, sterile, pyrogen-free, IV solution, produced by a reactor.

 a. Biodistribution
  (1) Iodohippurate ^{131}I hippuran is excreted 80% by tubular secretion and 20% by glomerular filtration.
  (2) Whole body biological half-life, excluding the bladder, is less than 1 hour.
  (3) Approximately 50% of an administered dose is excreted within 30 minutes, with 90% excreted within 8 hours.
  (4) Thyroid blockade with KI is suggested to reduce the radiation exposure to the thyroid.
 b. Decay data and dosage
  (1) The **physical half-life** is 8 days.
  (2) The **decay mode** is by beta minus decay.
  (3) The **primary radiation emissions** are 197 keV beta energy and 364 keV gamma energy photons.
  (4) **Administration and dosage.** IV, 10–100 μCi (0.4–3.7 MBq)

 2. Technetium Tc-99m mertiatide (^{99m}Tc-MAG3)
  a. Description
   (1) Supplied as a sterile, pyrogen-free, lyophilized kit containing betiatide, precursor of mertiatide, and chelation adjutants.
   (2) After the sodium pertechnetate is added to the kit, it must be heated in a hot water bath or heating block at 100°C for 10 minutes to form ^{99m}Tc mertiatide from the betiatide precursor.
  b. Biodistribution
   (1) Mertiatide is renally excreted, with 90% of administered dose excreted within 3 hours postinjection.
   (2) It is primarily cleared via active tubular secretion and to a small extent via glomerular filtration.
  c. Physical properties (see II B 3)
  d. Administration and dosage. IV, 5–10 mCi (185–370 MBq)

D. Renal cortical imaging agents are used to evaluate renal anatomy because of their ability to accumulate in the kidney and provide anatomical imaging data.

 1. Technetium Tc-99m gluceptate (^{99m}Tc-GLH)
  a. Physical properties (see II B 3)
  b. Biodistribution
   (1) ^{99m}Tc-GLH rapidly distributes throughout the body, with rapid blood clearance via glomerular filtration and tubular secretion and reabsorption.
   (2) Approximately 25% of the administered dose is excreted within the first hour, 65% within 6 hours, and 70% within 24 hours.
   (3) After 3–6 hours, a maximum of 5%–15% of the dose administered is concentrated in the proximal renal tubular cells of the renal cortex.
  c. Administration and dosage. IV, 10–20 mCi (370–740 MBq)

 2. Technetium Tc-99m succimer (^{99m}Tc-DMSA)
  a. Physical properties (see II B 3). ^{99m}Tc succimer complex must be allowed to incubate for 10 minutes postreconstitution and must be used within 4 hours postincubation.
  b. Biodistribution
   (1) Within 3–6 hours postadministration, 40%–50% of the dose localizes in the renal cortex, where it is taken up by the tubular cells.
   (2) Excretion into the urine is slow, with 5%–20% being excreted within the first 2 hours, 10%–30% by 6 hours, and less than 40% by 24 hours.
  c. Administration and dosage. IV, 2–6 mCi (74–222 MBq)

VIII. THYROID IMAGING

A. Overview

 1. The basic function of the thyroid gland is the production of thyroid hormone for the regulation of metabolism. The thyroid hormones are produced within the gland through the organification of iodine obtained from the oxidation of available iodide circulating in the blood. The inability of the body to distinguish between the isotopes of iodine provides a perfect metabolic tracer for the thyroid biochemical system.

2. The function of the thyroid gland can be evaluated by the uptake of ^{131}I or ^{123}I, allowing the detection of hypothyroidism with decreased uptake and hyperthyroidism with increased uptake.

3. $^{99m}TcO_4^-$ is a monovalent anion with an ionic radius similar to iodide. As a result, the pertechnetate ion is trapped by the thyroid gland in a fashion similar to iodide. The two species are sufficiently different in that $^{99m}TcO_4^-$ is not organified nor incorporated into thyroid hormone, and it is subsequently released unchanged.

B. Thyroid imaging agents

1. **Sodium iodide I-123 (^{123}I)** is a radiopharmaceutical available in either solution or capsule form for oral administration. It is produced by a cyclotron.
   a. Biodistribution
      (1) Orally administered iodine is rapidly absorbed from the gastrointestinal (GI) tract with thyroid gland uptake evident within minutes.
      (2) Sodium iodide ^{123}I is considered an ideal radiopharmaceutical for iodine uptake and imaging studies because of its short half-life and useful 159 keV primary gamma emissions.
   b. Decay data
      (1) The **physical half-life** is 13 hours.
      (2) The **biological half-life** is 3.5 days.
      (3) The **decay mode** is by electron capture.
      (4) The **primary radiation emissions** are 159 keV, 27 keV, and 529 keV gamma energy photons.
   c. Administration and dosage. Oral thyroid uptake: 100–200 μCi (3.7–7.4 MBq); thyroid image: 100–500 μCi (3.7–18.5 MBq)

2. **Sodium iodide I-131 (^{131}I)** is used for thyroid uptake and imaging studies; however, it is now used less often because of the high radiation dose absorbed.
   a. Biodistribution
      (1) Orally administered iodine is rapidly absorbed from the GI tract, with thyroid gland uptake within minutes.
      (2) Sodium iodide ^{131}I is not considered an ideal radioiodine radiopharmaceutical for iodine uptake and imaging studies because of its long half-life, poor imaging properties, and the high radiation dose to the thyroid from its beta decay component.
      (3) The radiation dose from the high energy beta particle with the imaging potential of its gamma emissions make this radionuclide the agent of choice for therapeutic treatment of hyperthyroidism and thyroid cancer.
   b. Decay data
      (1) The **physical half-life** is 8.08 days.
      (2) The **decay mode** is by beta decay.
      (3) The **primary radiation emissions** are 606 keV and 333 keV beta energy and 364 keV, 637 keV, and 284 keV gamma energy photons.
   c. Administration and dosage. Sodium iodide ^{131}I is available as either a capsule or in solution for oral administration.
      (1) **Diagnostics**
         (a) Thyroid uptake: 2–15 μCi (0.074–0.555 MBq)
         (b) Thyroid image: 30–50 μCi (1.11–1.85 MBq)
         (c) Whole body image: 1–5 mCi (37–185 MBq)
      (2) **Therapeutics**
         (a) Hyperthyroidism: 10–30 mCi (370–1110 MBq)
         (b) Thyroid carcinoma: 50–200 mCi (1850–7400 MBq)

3. **Na^{+99m}TcO$_4^-$** (see II B)

4. **^{201}Tl** (parathyroid imaging)
   a. Biodistribution. ^{201}Tl concentrates in the thyroid and also in parathyroid adenomas, which can be detected by a dual isotope subtraction technique of subtracting thyroid uptake counts from Na^{+99m}TcO$_4^-$ to unmask nonthyroid thallium uptake counts (see III A 1).
   b. Administration and dosage. IV, 2 mCi (74 MBq)

IX. BRAIN IMAGING

A. **Cerebral perfusion brain-imaging agents.** Radiopharmaceuticals for evaluating brain perfusion must possess a lipophilic partition coefficient sufficient to diffuse passively across the blood–brain barrier (BBB) almost completely within one pass of the cerebral circulation, as well as being sufficiently retained to permit data collection. The regional uptake of these agents is proportional to cerebral blood flow. This class of radiopharmaceuticals is useful in the diagnosis of altered regional blood perfusion in stroke.

1. **Technetium Tc-99m exametazime (^{99m}Tc-HMPAO)** exists as a sterile, pyrogen-free IV injection after reconstitution with sodium pertechnetate USP, which may be stabilized with the addition of a methylene blue/phosphate buffer stabilizing solution.
   a. **Description**
      (1) ^{99m}Tc exametazime is a neutral, lipid-soluble complex that freely crosses the BBB. This is a relatively unstable complex, which rapidly converts to a secondary, less lipophilic complex incapable of penetrating into the brain. The in vitro addition of a methylene blue/phosphate buffer stabilizing solution after preparing the ^{99m}Tc exametazime will stabilize the lipid-soluble complex for 4 hours.
      (2) Additional limitations on kit preparation parameters require the use of high mole fraction technetium generator eluates of less than 2 hours postelution from a generator previously eluted within 24 hours.
   b. **Biodistribution**
      (1) ^{99m}Tc exametazime rapidly clears from the blood, with a maximum brain uptake of 3.5%–7%, and up to 2.5% remaining after 24 hours.
      (2) The activity is widely distributed throughout the body, with 30% distributing to the GI tract.
      (3) Within 48 hours, 40% of the dose is excreted through the urine and 15% eliminated via the feces.
   c. **Physical properties** (see II B 3)
   d. **Administration and dosage.** IV, 10–20 mCi (370–740 MBq)

2. **Technetium Tc-99m bicisate (^{99m}Tc-ECD)**
   a. **Description**
      (1) ^{99m}Tc bicisate exists as a sterile, pyrogen-free IV injection after reconstitution with sodium pertechnetate ^{99m}Tc USP and the addition of a phosphate buffer.
      (2) After reconstitution, a stable lipophilic ^{99m}Tc bicisate complex is formed, which is able to cross the BBB by passive diffusion.
   b. **Biodistribution**
      (1) ^{99m}Tc bicisate is rapidly cleared from blood, with a maximum of 6.5% of administered dose localized in the brain, and 5% left in the blood after 1 hour.
      (2) Once located in the brain cells, ^{99m}Tc bicisate is metabolized by endogenous enzymes to a polar compound that is unable to diffuse out of the brain cells.
      (3) ^{99m}Tc bicisate is primarily eliminated via the kidneys, with 50% excreted within 2 hours, and 74% in 24 hours. Hepatobiliary excretion accounts for approximately 12.5% of the administered dose after 48 hours.
   c. **Radionuclide properties** (see II B 3)
   d. **Administration and dosage.** IV, 10–30 mCi (370–1110 MBq)

3. **Iofetamine hydrochloride I-123** is not commercially available.

B. **Carrier-mediated transport (cerebral metabolism) mechanisms.** These are responsible for transporting glucose across the BBB. Agents such as ^{18}F **fludeoxyglucose** aid in the evaluation of cerebral function by mapping the distribution of glucose metabolism. ^{18}F fludeoxyglucose is produced by a cyclotron.

1. **Biodistribution.** Currently, there is a USP monograph for on-site cyclotron produced ^{18}F fludeoxyglucose, which is a glucose analogue. ^{18}F fludeoxyglucose concentrates in the brain, where it is phosphorylated but does not undergo subsequent metabolism because of the replacement of the hydroxyl group in the 2 position with a fluorine atom. It is then metabolically trapped for a sufficient time to allow imaging.

2. **Decay data**
   a. The **physical half-life** is 109 minutes.
   b. The **decay mode** is by positron emission.

c. The **primary radiation emissions** are 633 keV energy positrons and 511 keV gamma energy photons.

3. **Administration and dosage.** IV, 5–10 mCi (185–370 MBq)

C. **Cerebral neurotransmitter imaging: Fluorodopa F-18 injection**
1. **Description**
a. Cerebral neurotransmitter synthesis can be studied with fluorodopa F-18 injection. The intracerebral distribution of this neurotransmitter tracer can be used in the assessment of neurodegenerative diseases such as parkinsonism.
b. Fluorodopa F-18 injection exists under a USP monograph as an on-site–produced sterile IV solution of a levodopa analogue in which a portion of the molecule has been replaced with ^{18}F, a positron-emitting radionuclide.

2. **Biodistribution**
a. After IV injection, plasma activity decreases to 10% of the administered dose within 5 minutes after injection.
b. Fluorodopa F-18 injection is predominantly metabolized in periphery via dopa decarboxylase, and catechol-O-methyl transferase. To maximize brain uptake, carbidopa may be used to decrease peripheral metabolism.
c. Rapid excretion via renal system as dopamine metabolites

3. **Radionuclide data** (see IX B 2)

4. **Administration and dosage.** IV, 10–20 mCi (370–740 MBq)

D. **Cerebrospinal fluid (CSF) dynamics.** Radionuclide cisternography is useful in the evaluation of hydrocephalus and in detecting CSF leaks. In CSF imaging, the radiopharmaceutical **indium In-111 pentetate (^{111}In-DTPA)** is introduced intrathecally into the spinal subarachnoid space, ascends through the basal cisterns, proceeds over the cerebral hemispheres, and drains eventually into the superior sagittal sinus. ^{111}In pentetate is commercially supplied as a sterile, pyrogen-free unit dose injection. It is produced by a cyclotron.

1. **Biodistribution**
a. After intrathecal injection, this radiopharmaceutical normally ascends to the parasagittal region within 24 hours.
b. After absorption into the bloodstream via the arachnoid villi, the major route of elimination is by kidney, with 65% of the dose excreted within 48 hours, and 85% within 72 hours.

2. **Decay data**
a. The **physical half-life** is 67 hours.
b. The **CSF biological half-life** is 12 hours.
c. The **effective half-life** is 10 hours.
d. The **decay mode** is by electron capture.
e. The **primary radiation emissions** are 245 keV and 171 keV gamma energy photons.

3. **Administration and dosage.** Intrathecal, 500 µCi (18.5 MBq)

X. **INFECTION AND INFLAMMATION.** Evaluation of sites of infection include the use of agents that can associate with components of the natural defense mechanisms and can accumulate where they localize.

A. **Gallium citrate Ga-67 (^{67}Ga)**
1. **Description**
a. It is supplied as a sterile, pyrogen-free radiopharmaceutical with preservatives.
b. The mechanism of localization is thought to be dependent on the formation of a gallium transferrin complex in the blood and on binding to transferrin receptors associated with infection and inflammation.
c. It accumulates in areas of white blood cell (WBC) localization.

2. **Biodistribution**
a. After administration, the highest concentration of ^{67}Ga citrate other than at the site of infection is in the renal cortex. After 24 hours, the maximum concentration shifts to bone and lymph nodes, but after 1 week, it is mainly concentrated in the liver and spleen.

b. ^{67}Ga citrate is excreted slowly from the body, with 26% via urine, and 9% via feces, and a whole body retention of 65% after 7 days.

3. Radionuclide data
   a. The **mode of production** is by cyclotron.
   b. The **decay mode** is by electron capture.
   c. The **physical half-life** is 78 hours.
   d. The **decay emissions** are 93 keV, 185 keV, 300 keV, and 393 keV gamma photons.

4. Administration and dosage. IV, for infection, 3–8 mCi (111–300 MBq). A daily laxative or an enema should be used by the patient after the injection and before the images to cleanse the bowel of radioactivity that may interfere with the images and possibly lead to a false positive.

B. WBC labeling agents. Radiolabeled WBCs are used in the detection of a wide variety of infectious and inflammatory processes. Current use includes the diagnosis of intra-abdominal abscesses, inflammatory bowel disease, appendicitis, fever of unknown origin, and osteomyelitis. WBCs can be radiolabeled with In-111 oxine or Tc-99m exametazime.

1. In-111 oxyquinolone solution (^{111}In oxine)
   a. Description
      (1) ^{111}In oxyquinolone is supplied as a sterile preservative-free, pyrogen-free, radiopharmaceutical solution for use in the radiolabeling of autologous leukocytes.
      (2) ^{111}In forms a saturated (a ratio of 1 to 3) neutral lipophilic complex with oxyquinoline, which enables it to penetrate a cell membrane.
      (3) After incubation of ^{111}In oxyquinoline with a population of autologous leukocytes, the ^{111}In is thought to become firmly bound to cytoplasmic components, thereby allowing the free oxine to be released by the cell.
   b. Biodistribution
      (1) After radiolabeling, the autologous leukocytes are reinjected, with 30% taken up by the spleen, and 30% taken up by the liver, reaching peak at 2–4 hours postinjection.
      (2) Pulmonary uptake is immediately evident postinjection, but it clears with minimal activity visible after 4 hours.
      (3) There is a biexponential blood clearance, with 9%–24% clearing with a biological half-life of 2–5 hours, and the remainder of 13%–18% clearing with a biological half-life of 64–116 hours.
      (4) Elimination is mainly through radioactive decay, with less than 1% excreted in feces and urine during the first 24 hours.
   c. Radionuclide data
      (1) The **mode of production** is by cyclotron.
      (2) The **decay mode** is by electron capture.
      (3) The **physical half-life** is 67 hours.
      (4) The **decay emissions** are 245 keV and 171 keV.
   d. Administration and dosage. IV, 200–500 μCi (7.4–8.5 MBq)

2. Technetium Tc-99m exametazime. As a sterile and pyrogen-free IV injection after reconstitution with sodium pertechnetate, ^{99m}Tc exametazime may be used to radiolabel leukocytes.
   a. Description
      (1) ^{99m}Tc exametazime is a neutral, lipid-soluble complex that is able to penetrate the WBC membrane. This lipophilic complex is relatively unstable and rapidly converts to a secondary complex incapable of penetrating the WBCs.
      (2) The methylene blue/phosphate buffer stabilized solution is not able to radiolabel cells and should not be used.
      (3) Additional limitations on kit preparation parameters require the use of high mole fraction technetium generator elutes of less than 2 hours postelution from a generator previously eluted within 24 hours.
   b. Biodistribution
      (1) After IV injection, the radiolabeled cells localize in the lungs, liver, spleen, blood pool, bone marrow, and bladder.
      (2) Elimination is primarily via the liver.
   c. Radionuclide data (see II B 1 b, 3 a, b)
   d. Administration and dosage. IV, for infection, 7–25 mCi (260–925 MBq)

XI. BREAST IMAGING

A. Technetium Tc-99m sestamibi (^{99m}Tc-MIBI)

1. **Description**
   a. ^{99m}Tc sestamibi is used for both breast and cardiac imaging.
   b. ^{99m}Tc sestamibi is indicated for planar imaging as a second line of evaluating breast lesions in patients with an abnormal mammogram or a palpable breast mass.
   c. ^{99m}Tc sestamibi may not be used to screen for breast cancer, to confirm the presence or absence of malignancy, or to replace a biopsy.

2. **Biodistribution.** ^{99m}Tc sestamibi is primarily excreted by the hepatobiliary system.

3. **Physical properties** (see II B 3)

4. **Administration and dosage.** IV, 20–30 mCi (740–1110 MBq)

XII. DEEP VEIN THROMBOSIS (DVT) IMAGING

A. Technetium Tc-99m apcitide injection

1. **Overview**
   a. ^{99m}Tc apcitide can be used to image acute venous thrombosis in the lower extremities of patients who have the signs and symptoms of acute venous thrombosis.
   b. ^{99m}Tc apcitide acts by detecting the thrombolytic process of DVT in contrast with ultrasound, which detects the effects of a DVT.
   c. Mechanism of action of ^{99m}Tc apcitide is based on the binding of the peptide apcitide to the GPIIb/IIa receptors found on the surface of activated platelets involved in active thrombus formation.

2. **Description**
   a. ^{99m}Tc apcitide is supplied as a vial containing a sterile, nonpyrogenic, freeze-dried mixture of bibapcitide, stannous chloride dihydrate and sodium glucoheptonate dihydrate.
   b. Bibapcitide is composed of two apcitide monomers; after sodium pertechnetate Tc-99m is added and the vial is heated, the bibapcitide is split and forms a Tc-99m complex of apcitide.
   c. ^{99m}apcitide exists as a sterile, pyrogen-free IV injection after kit reconstitution with Na^{+99m}TcO$_4^-$ and heating at 100°C for 15 minutes.

3. **Biodistribution**
   a. Fifty percent of the dose is excreted in the urine in the first 2 hours. Seventy-five percent is excreted through the urine after 8 hours.
   b. Ten percent of the dose is excreted via hepatobiliary clearance within 22–24 hours post-administration.
   c. Apcitide has two metabolites; both are more polar than the parent drug.
      (1) Metabolite A is present in the blood and urine, and metabolite B is only present in the urine.
      (2) Metabolite A represents approximately 10% of the total radioactivity administered, and metabolite B represents 30% of the total radioactivity administered.
   d. Highest localization of radioactivity is in the liver and kidneys.

4. **Radionuclide data** (see II B 3)

5. **Administration and dosage.** IV, 20 mCi (740 MBq)

XIII. TUMORS

A. The usefulness of radiopharmaceuticals in the detection of tumors varies in sensitivity and specificity, with differences in tumor location and type.

1. **Gallium citrate Ga-67 (^{67}Ga)**
   a. **Description**
      (1) Gallium citrate ^{67}Ga is supplied as a sterile, pyrogen-free radiopharmaceutical with preservatives.

(2) The mechanism of localization is thought to be dependent on the formation of a gallium transferrin complex, or binding to transferrin receptors on tumor cells.

(3) It accumulates in primary metastatic tumor sites and may detect the presence of Hodgkin's disease, lymphoma, and bronchogenic carcinoma.

b. Biodistribution (see X A 2)

c. Radionuclide data (see X A 3)

d. Administration and dosage. IV, for tumor, 10 mCi (370 MBq)

2. Indium In-111 pentetreotide

a. Description

(1) It is supplied as a sterile, pyrogen-free kit for the preparation of ^{111}In pentetreotide. The two-component kit consists of a reaction vial containing a lyophilized mixture of pentetreotide with stabilizer adjutants, and a second vial containing an indium ^{111}In chloride/ferric chloride solution.

(a) The pentetreotide molecule is a conjugate of pentetate [diethylenetriamine penta-acetic acid (per Dorland's) (DTPA)] and octreotide, which is a somatostatin analogue.

(b) ^{111}In pentetreotide is prepared by adding the ^{111}In/Fe chloride solution to the vial containing the pentetreotide. The pentetate portion of the molecule acts as a bifunctional chelate linking the ^{111}In radionuclide to the biological active octreotide portion of the agent.

(2) ^{111}In pentetreotide is indicated for localization of primary and metastatic neuroendocrine tumors expressing somatostatin receptors.

b. Biodistribution

(1) Within 1 hour after IV injection, ^{111}In pentetreotide distributes from the plasma to extravascular space, with less than one-third of the administered dose remaining in the plasma 10 minutes postinjection.

(2) ^{111}In pentetreotide localizes as a function of somatostatin receptor density, with accumulation in normal pituitary, thyroid, liver, spleen, and the urinary bladder.

(3) Elimination is primarily renal, with 50% of the administered dose excreted within 6 hours postinjection, 85% after 24 hours, and less than 90% after 48 hours. Less than 2% of the administered dose is cleared via the feces within 72 hours postinjection.

c. Radionuclide data

(1) The **mode of production** is by cyclotron.

(2) The **decay mode** is by electron capture.

(3) The **physical half-life** is 67 hours.

(4) The **decay emissions** are 245 keV and 171 keV.

d. Administration and dosage. IV, 3–6 mCi (111–222 MBq)

3. Iobenguane I-131 injection (^{131}I-MIBG)

a. Description

(1) It is supplied as a sterile, pyrogen-free radiopharmaceutical for use as an adjunctive diagnostic agent for the localization of primary and metastatic pheochromocytomas and neuroblastomas.

(2) Iobenguane (meta-iodobenzylguanidine) labeled with ^{131}I acts as a physiological analogue of norepinephrine and is transported and accumulated in the adrenal medulla. This allows for the detection of neuroendocrine tumors via the specific uptake of labeled iobenguane.

(3) Because of its physiological similarities to norepinephrine, many classes of drugs that interfere with catecholamine transport and function may affect the uptake and localization of labeled iobenguane.

b. Biodistribution

(1) After IV injection, there is rapid uptake in the liver, with lesser amounts accumulating in the lungs, heart, and spleen.

(2) Normal adrenal gland uptake is low, but for tumors such as pheochromocytomas and neuroblastomas, the uptake is relatively higher.

(3) Elimination is renal, with most of the drug excreted mainly unchanged. Forty percent to fifty percent of the administered dose is excreted within 24 hours, and 70%–90% is excreted within 4 days postinjection.

(4) Administration of potassium iodide 1 day before and for 10 days after administration is suggested to reduce thyroid uptake of potential radioiodide contaminants.

c. Physical data (see VIII B 2 b)
d. Administration and dosage. IV, 0.5–1 mCi (18.5–37 MBq)

4. Thallous chloride T1-201. This agent has utility as a tumor-imaging agent because of its accumulation in the rapidly metabolizing cells of certain tumors in accordance with its mechanism of localization (see III A 1).
  a. Administration and dosage. IV, 1.5–3 mCi (55–111 MBq)

5. Fludeoxyglucose F-18 USP. This agent has utility as a tumor-imaging agent because of an increased demand for glucose by tumors with an advanced state of malignancy. Not only can fludeoxyglucose F-18 locate and differentiate tumors, but it can also help to distinguish between recurrent brain tumor and radiation necrosis in patients receiving radiation therapy (see IX B).
  a. Administration and dosage. IV, 5–10 mCi (185–370 MBq)

6. Technetium Tc-99m depreotide
  a. Description
    (1) ^{99m}Tc depreotide is based on a synthetic peptide with a high binding affinity for somatostatin receptors in normal and abnormal tissues. ^{99m}Tc depreotide is used to identify somatostatin-receptor–bearing pulmonary masses in patients presenting with pulmonary lesions and who are known to have had a malignancy or have a history highly suspect for malignancy.
    (2) ^{99m}Tc depreotide is supplied as a vial containing a sterile, nonpyrogenic, freeze-dried mixture of depreotide, stannous chloride dihydrate, sodium glucoheptonate dihydrate, and edetate disodium dihydrate.
    (3) ^{99m}Tc depreotide exists as a sterile, pyrogen-free IV injection after kit reconstitution with $Na^{+99m}TcO_4{}^-$ and heating at 100°C for 10 minutes.
    (4) Caution should be exercised when giving this drug to patients with insulinomas, as depreotide exists as a somatostatin analogue that can produce severe hypoglycemia in patients with insulinomas.
  b. Biodistribution. Twelve percent of the administered dose is excreted through the urine within 4 hours.
  c. Radionuclide data. (see II B 3)
  d. Administration and Dosage. Peripheral IV injection, 15–20 mCi (555–740 MBq)

B. Antibodies

1. Indium In-111 satumomab pendetide
  a. Description
    (1) It is supplied as a sterile, pyrogen-free kit for the preparation of In-111 satumomab pendetide. The kit consists of a single-dose reaction vial containing 1 mg of satumomab pendetide, a monoclonal antibody (MoAb) conjugate, in a sodium phosphate–buffered saline solution. A second vial containing a sodium acetate solution is to be used for buffering an indium ^{111}In chloride solution used to label the satumomab pendetide.
      (a) The satumomab portion of the conjugate is a murine MoAb that binds specifically to the TAG-72 glycoprotein, which is expressed at high levels on colorectal and ovarian adenocarcinomas. The pendetide portion of the conjugate is a linker chelator, which is attached to the F_c carbohydrate portion of the satumomab antibody.
      (b) The agent is prepared by adding a buffered solution of ^{111}In chloride solution to the single-dose vial and allowing the mixture to sit for 30 minutes to allow the labeling reaction to occur.
    (2) Indium In-111 satumomab is indicated for determining the extent and location of extrahepatic malignant disease in patients who have known colorectal or ovarian cancer.
    (3) As a foreign protein, this product may produce human antimurine antibodies (HAMA) with accompanying potentially serious allergic reactions.
  b. Biodistribution
    (1) After IV injection, ^{111}In satumomab pendetide localizes in colorectal adenocarcinomas and ovarian epithelial carcinomas. It exhibits a slow plasma clearance and a mono-exponential or bi-exponential clearance, with a terminal phase half-life of 56 hours.

(2) Elimination is renal, with 10% of the administered dose excreted within the first 72 hours postinjection as a small–molecular-weight product of the catabolized In-111 satumomab pendetide.

c. Radionuclide data

  (1) The **mode of production** is by cyclotron.

  (2) The **decay mode** is by electron capture.

  (3) The **physical half-life** is 67 hours.

  (4) The **decay emissions** are 245 keV and 171 keV.

d. Administration and dosage. IV (slow), 5 mCi (185 MBq)

2. Indium In-111 capromab pendetide

  a. Description

  (1) ^{111}In capromab pendetide is an immunoglobulin G1 (IgG1) murine monoclonal antibody conjugated to the ^{111}In chelator GYK DTPA.

  (2) A ^{111}In capromab pendetide scan is indicated for use in preoperative staging in patients with moderate to high probability of extraprostatic metastasis.

  (3) Caution should be used in a patient who has received a murine-based antibody previously because there is a possibility for a HAMA (human anti-murine antibody) reaction.

  b. Radionuclide data (see XIII B 1 c)

  c. Administration and dosage

  (1) IV, 0.5 mg of capromab pendetide with 5 mCi ^{111}In chloride.

  (2) Note: The final dose must be filtered using a 0.22 μm GV filter.

3. Technetium Tc-99m arcitumomab

  a. Description

  (1) ^{99m}Tc arcitumomab is a murine monoclonal antibody Fab fragment.

  (2) It is indicated in conjunction with standard diagnostic evaluations for the detection of recurrent and/or metastatic colorectal cancer involving the liver, extrahepatic abdomen, and pelvis in patients with confirmed colorectal cancer.

  (3) The use of a Fab fragment helps to reduce the HAMA reaction.

  b. Biodistribution

  (1) Twenty-eight percent of the dose is excreted in the urine over the first 24 hours.

  (2) Ninety-three percent of the dose has been eliminated from the blood after 24 hours.

  (3) The Fab fragment minimizes liver metabolism and facilitates rapid blood clearance.

  c. Radionuclide data (see II B 3)

  d. Administration and dosage. IV, 1 mg arcitumomab with 20–30 mCi of ^{99m}Tc (740–1110 MBq)

XIV. THERAPEUTIC AGENTS.
The therapeutic use of radiopharmaceuticals is based on the concept of selective localization of radiopharmaceuticals coupled with the lethality of the same because of the tissue damage resulting from highly ionizing particulate emissions such as beta particles.

A. Chromic phosphate P-32 suspension (^{32}P)

  1. Description. Available as a sterile, pyrogen-free aqueous suspension used in the treatment of peritoneal or pleural effusions caused by metastatic disease. Also used in the treatment of ovarian and prostate cancer.

  2. Biodistribution

  a. Colloidal suspension of ^{32}P is rapidly taken up by macrophages adhering to the cavity wall, thereby concentrating and localizing the irradiation effect of the ^{32}P radionuclide beta particulate emission.

  b. After infusion, the suspension rapidly distributes from within the cavity and may localize in the lungs, adrenal glands, kidneys, lymph nodes, liver, spleen, bone marrow, plasma, erythrocytes, and leukocytes, depending on colloidal particle size.

  c. Elimination is primarily renal.

  3. Radionuclide data

  a. The **mode of production** is by reactor.

  b. The **decay mode** is beta.

  c. The **physical half-life** is 14.3 days.

  d. The **decay emissions** are 695 keV mean energy beta, 100% abundance.

4. Administration and dosage
   a. Intraperitoneal instillation: 10–20 mCi (370–740 MBq)
   b. Intrapleural instillation: 6–12 mCi (222–444 MBq)
   c. Carcinoma interstitial: 0.1–0.5 mCi (3.7–18.5 MBq)
   d. Caution is advised for visual inspection to prevent misadministration of the sodium phosphate form (clear, colorless), which is designated for intravascular use only.

B. Sodium phosphate P-32 solution (^{32}P)

1. Description
   a. It is available as a commercially supplied, sterile, pyrogen-free radiopharmaceutical.
   b. It is primarily used as an antineoplastic for the treatment of polycythemia rubra vera and is selectively used for the palliative treatment of metastatic bone pain.
   c. Its therapeutic effect is due to cell damage resulting from irradiation produced by beta particulate emission.

2. Biodistribution
   a. It concentrates as phosphate within the DNA of rapidly dividing hematopoietic cells in the treatment of polycythemia rubra vera and as phosphate in areas of increased bone formation.
   b. After IV administration, it diffuses rapidly into extracellular and intracellular space, concentrating in the bone marrow, spleen, and liver.
   c. Elimination is primarily renal, with 5%–10% excreted within 24 hours, and 20% within 1 week.
   d. Whole body biological half-life is approximately 39 days.

3. Radionuclide data
   a. The **mode of production** is by reactor.
   b. The **decay mode** is by beta.
   c. The **physical half-life** is 14.3 days.
   d. The **decay emissions** are 695 keV mean energy beta, 100% abundance.

4. Administration and dosage
   a. Polycythemia rubra vera: IV, 3–5 mCi (111–185 MBq)
   b. Metastatic bone lesions: IV, 10–21 mCi (370–777 MBq)
   c. Caution is advised for visual inspection to prevent misadministration of the chromic phosphate form (green, cloudy), which is designated for interstitial use only.

C. Sodium iodide I-131 (therapeutic)

1. Description
   a. It is indicated for treatment of hyperthyroidism and thyroid carcinoma.
   b. Its therapeutic action is due to the accumulation and retention of iodine and its isotope ^{131}I.

2. Biodistribution (see VIII A, B 2). Biological half-life in the thyroid: euthyroid patient, 80 days; hyperthyroid patient, 5–40 days

3. Radionuclide data (see VIII B 2 b)

4. Administration and dosage. Oral capsule or oral solution
   a. Hyperthyroidism, 10–30 mCi (370–1110 MBq)
   b. Thyroid carcinoma, 30–200 mCi (1110–7400 MBq)

D. Strontium Sr-89 chloride (^{89}Sr)

1. Description
   a. It is indicated for the alleviation of bone pain arising from metastatic bone disease.
   b. As a metabolic analogue of calcium, ^{89}Sr concentrates selectively in areas of increased osteogenesis, thus delivering a radiation dose sufficient to provide a palliative effect.
   c. Pain relief begins 7 to 21 days after administration, with maximum relief by 6 weeks and an average duration of 6 months.
   d. Reduction in patient analgesic usage occurs in up to 75% of patients treated, with complete pain relief in 20% of treated patients, and no pain relief in 20%–25% of treated patients.
   e. Bone marrow suppression effects limit ^{89}Sr use to patients with initial WBC counts >2,400 and platelet counts >60,000.

2. **Biodistribution**
   a. After administration, ^{89}Sr clears rapidly from blood and localizes in the bone hydroxy-apatite.
   b. Initial biological half-life in normal bone is 14 days, with longer retention in metastatic bone lesions. Between 12%–90% of the administered dose is retained for up to 3 months after administration.
   c. Elimination is primarily renal, with 66% of administered dose cleared via GFR within the first 2 days, and 33% is excreted via feces.

3. **Radionuclide data**
   a. The **mode of production** is by accelerator.
   b. The **decay mode** is by beta.
   c. The **emission data** are 1.46 MeV maximum beta energy, 100% abundance.
   d. The **physical half-life** is 50.5 days.

4. **Administration and dosage.** IV, 4 mCi (148 MBq), 40–60 μCi/kg (1.5–2.2 MBq/kg)

E. **Samarium Sm-153 lexidronam**

1. **Description**
   a. [153]Sm is indicated for the relief of pain in patients who have confirmed metastatic cancer of the bone.
   b. [153]Sm concentrates in areas of high bone turnover, and it accumulates more in osteoblastic lesions than in the normal bone.
   c. The goal of [153]Sm therapy is for patients to be able to reduce the amount of narcotic analgesics that they need to control their pain.

2. **Biodistribution**
   a. The lesion to normal bone ratio is 5:1.
   b. The percentage of uptake of [153]Sm is directly proportional to the number of lesions the patient has.
   c. Less than 1% of the dose remains in the blood 5 hours postinjection.
   d. [153]Sm is 100% renally excreted over 12 hours.
   e. The onset is approximately 1 week.

3. **Radionuclide data**
   a. The **mode of production** is by cyclotron.
   b. The **decay mode** is by beta and gamma decay.
   c. The **physical half-life** is 46.3 hours.
   d. The **decay emissions** are 640 keV, 710 keV, and 840 keV beta energy and 103 keV gamma energy photons.

4. **Precautions.** [153]Sm may cause bone marrow suppression, which should return to baseline within 8 weeks postinjection.

5. **Administration and dosage.** IV, 1 mCi/kg (37 MBq/kg)

F. **Yttrium Y-90 ibritumomab tiuxetan and indium in-111 ibritumomab tiuxetan**

1. **Overview**
   a. Indium In-111 ibritumomab tiuxetan and yttrium Y-90 ibritumomab tiuxetan are part of a therapeutic regimen used in the treatment of non–Hodgkin's lymphoma (NHL) patients with relapsed refractory low-grade, follicular, or transformed B-cell NHL and patients with rituximab refractory NHL.
   b. Ibritumomab tiuxetan is an immunoconjugate consisting of a monoclonal antibody ibritumomab, which is linked to the chelator tiuxetan.
   c. The ibritumomab antibody is a murine IgG1 kappa monoclonal antibody produced in Chinese hamster ovary (CHO) cells. The ibritumomab antibody is directed against the CD20 antigen, which is expressed on the surface of normal and malignant B lymphocytes.
   d. The linker chelator tiuxetan provides a high-affinity chelation site for ^{111}In, in the case of the imaging dose, and for ^{90}Y, in the case of the therapeutic dose.
   e. The therapeutic regimen is administered in two separate doses. This allows for the qualitative evaluation of the biodistribution in order to avoid potential toxicities such as abnormally high bone marrow localization or prolonged renal excretion. In each administration, patients must be premedicated with diphenhydramine 50 mg and acetaminophen

650 mg one half hour before receiving the rituximab infusion required prior to administering the radiolabeled antibody.

  (1) Step 1 is the administration of rituximab followed by the ^{111}In ibritumomab tiuxetan diagnostic imaging dose.

  (2) Step 2 follows Step 1 by 7–9 days and consists of a second rituximab infusion followed by the ^{90}Y ibritumomab therapy dose.

2. Description

  a. Supplied as two separate kits to produce a single dose of ^{111}In ibritumomab tiuxetan and a single dose of ^{90}Y ibritumomab tiuxetan

  b. Each kit consists of four vials containing:

   (1) 3.2 mg of ibritumomab tiuxetan in saline

   (2) 50 mM of sodium acetate

   (3) Formulation buffer (contains human serum albumin)

   (4) One empty reaction vial

  c. Exists as a sterile, nonpyrogenic IV solution after formulation with either ^{111}In or ^{90}Y

3. Biodistribution

  a. The mean half-life for ^{90}Y ibritumomab tiuxetan in the blood is 30 hours.

  b. 7.8% of the administered dose is excreted in the urine over 7 days.

  c. The estimated biological half-life is 48 hours.

4. Radionuclide data

  a. Indium In-111 (see XIII B 1 c)

  b. Yttrium Y-90

   (1) The mode of **production** is by reactor.

   (2) The **decay mode** is by beta.

   (3) The **physical half-life** is 64.1 hours.

   (4) The **decay emission** is 935 mean keV, 100% emission.

5. Precautions

  a. ^{90}Y ibritumomab tiuxetan should not be administered to patients with altered biodistributions of the ^{111}In ibritumomab tiuxetan imaging and dosimetry dose.

  b. ^{90}Y ibritumomab tiuxetan should not be administered to patients with:

   (1) ≤25% lymphoma marrow involvement

   (2) Platelet counts <100,000 cell/mm^3

   (3) Neutrophil count <1,500 cells/mm^3

   (4) Hypocellular bone marrow

   (5) History of failed stem cell collection

  c. Ibritumomab tiuxetan is contraindicated in patients with known hypersensitivity or anaphylactic reactions to murine proteins.

  d. Patients who have previously received murine-based protein therapy should be screened for human antimouse antibodies.

  e. Infusion-related adverse events, including asthenia, chills, and nausea, are common and are usually self-limited. Tumor lysis syndrome has been reported following rituximab infusions, which are part of ^{90}Y ibritumomab tiuxetan therapy. Patients should be monitored closely for this potentially fatal adverse event.

XV. REFERENCES

  A. American Pharmaceutical Association Nuclear Pharmacy Practice Guidelines. Academy of Pharmacy Practice, 1995.

  B. Bernier DR, Christian PE, Langan JK: *Nuclear Medicine Technology and Techniques.* St. Louis, Mosby 1994.

  C. Chilton HM, Witcofski R: *Nuclear Pharmacy: An Introduction to the Clinical Applications of Radiopharmaceuticals.* Philadelphia, Lea and Febiger 1986.

  D. Swanson DP, Chilton HM, Thrall JH: *Pharmaceuticals in Medical Imaging.* New York, Macmillan 1990.

  E. United States Pharmacopeia Drug Information (USPDI) 2002.

STUDY QUESTIONS

Directions: Each of the numbered items or incomplete statements in this section is followed by answers or by completions of the statement. Select the **one** lettered answer or completion that is **best** in each case.

1. Which of the following emissions from the decay of radionuclides is most commonly used in nuclear medicine diagnostic imaging?

(A) X-ray
(B) Beta
(C) Alpha
(D) Gamma
(E) Positron

2. Which of the following radionuclides is most commonly used in nuclear pharmacy practice?

(A) ^{67}Ga
(B) ^{201}Tl
(C) ^{99m}Tc
(D) ^{123}I
(E) ^{133}Xe

3. Which of the following radionuclides is produced using a generator?

(A) ^{99m}Tc
(B) ^{201}Tl
(C) ^{67}Ga
(D) ^{133}Xe
(E) ^{123}I

4. Which of the following radiopharmaceuticals can be used in skeletal imaging?

(A) ^{99m}Tc albumin aggregated
(B) ^{99m}Tc medronate disodium
(C) Xenon gas ^{133}Xe USP
(D) Thallous chloride ^{201}Tl USP
(E) ^{99m}Tc disofenin

5. Which of the following radiopharmaceuticals is used in the diagnosis of acute cholecystitis?

(A) ^{99m}Tc sulfur colloid
(B) ^{99m}Tc medronate disodium
(C) ^{99m}Tc albumin
(D) ^{99m}Tc exametazime
(E) ^{99m}Tc disofenin

6. Which of the following cyclotron-produced radiopharmaceuticals is used for assessing regional myocardial perfusion as part of an exercise stress test?

(A) Thallous chloride ^{201}Tl USP
(B) Sodium iodide ^{123}I
(C) Gallium citrate ^{67}Ga USP
(D) Indium ^{111}In pentetate
(E) Cobalt ^{57}Co cyanocobalamin

7. Glomerular filtration and the urinary collection system can best be evaluated using which of the following agents?

(A) ^{99m}Tc sulfur colloid
(B) ^{99m}Tc albumin
(C) ^{99m}Tc sestamibi
(D) ^{99m}Tc disofenin
(E) ^{99m}Tc pentetate

Directions: Each item below contains three suggested answers, of which **one or more** is correct. Choose the answer

> **A**   if **I only** is correct
> **B**   if **III only** is correct
> **C**   if **I and II** are correct
> **D**   if **II and III** are correct
> **E**   if **I, II, and III** are correct

8. The definition of the optimal radiopharmaceutical includes which of the following attributes?

  I. Short half-life
  II. Gamma photon with a 100–300 keV energy
  III. Rapid localization in target tissue and quick clearance from nontarget tissue

9. Which of the following statements are true for sodium pertechnetate ^{99m}Tc USP?

  I. It is used to radiolabel all other ^{99m}Tc radiopharmaceuticals.
  II. The molybdenum-99 (^{99}Mo) breakthrough limit is less than 0.15 μCi ^{99}Mo/mCi ^{99m}Tc (less than 0.15 kBq/MBq).
  III. It has a physical half-life of 16 hours.

10. Which of the following organs can be imaged with ^{99m}Tc sulfur colloid?

  I. Liver
  II. Spleen
  III. Bone marrow

11. Which of the following radiopharmaceuticals may be used to image the thyroid gland?

  I. Sodium iodide ^{131}I
  II. Sodium pertechnetate ^{99m}Tc USP
  III. Sodium iodide ^{123}I

Directions: The group of items in this section consists of lettered options followed by a set of numbered items. For each item, select the **one** lettered option that is most closely associated with it. Each lettered option may be selected once, more than once, or not at all.

Questions 12–16

Match each radiopharmaceutical with its mechanism of localization.

(A) Metabolic trapping
(B) Phagocytosis
(C) Capillary blockade
(D) Active transport
(E) Passive diffusion

12. Thallous chloride ^{201}Tl USP

13. ^{99m}Tc albumin aggregated USP

14. ^{99m}Tc sulfur colloid

15. ^{99m}Tc exametazime

16. ^{18}F fludeoxyglucose

ANSWERS AND EXPLANATIONS

1. The answer is D *[I B 3 b]*.
Current camera technology most efficiently detects gamma radiation. Alpha and beta emissions are not useful in nuclear medicine imaging because of their harmful particulate emissions and low tissue penetration. Although x-ray emissions can be used as in the case of the mercury daughter of the thallous chloride ^{201}Tl parent, they are not efficiently detected. Annihilation radiation associated with positron decay can be imaged, but this technology is currently limited to a few specialized centers.

2. The answer is C *[II A 1]*.
Technetium Tc-99m has become the radionuclide of choice in current nuclear pharmacy practice since its introduction in the mid-1960s. ^{99m}Tc fulfills all of the requirements of the optimal radiopharmaceutical with its physical half-life of 6 hours, 140 keV gamma energy emission, ready availability, cost, and ability to be radiolabeled to a wide variety of biologically active compounds.

3. The answer is A *[II A 1 a]*.
Technetium Tc-99m is obtained via commercially supplied, sterile, pyrogen-free generator systems. A generator is a device used to separate a short half-life radionuclide from the longer-lived parent nuclide, while retaining the parent to produce more of the daughter nuclide. In this way, short–half-life nuclides can be made available on a continuous basis at great distances from the sites of generator production.

4. The answer is B *[IV A 2]*.
The technetium Tc-99m diphosphonate compounds are the most popular bone imaging agents currently used in nuclear medicine imaging. They are rapidly taken up by skeletal bone, with 50% of the administered dose adsorbed onto bone hydroxyapatite and with the remainder excreted by the kidneys. The imaging advantages of the ^{99m}Tc, coupled with the sensitivity of bone agent localization in skeletal bone hydroxyapatite, allows for detection of bone pathology before evidence of pathology can be shown by conventional x-ray.

5. The answer is E *[VI C 1, 2]*.
^{99m}Tc disofenin is an iminodiacetic acid derivative, which is useful for hepatobiliary imaging due to its ability to be selectively cleared by a carrier-mediated hepatocyte pathway. Lack of gallbladder visualization is an abnormal finding suggestive of acute cholecystitis.

6. The answer is A *[III A 1]*.
Regional uptake of thallous chloride ^{201}Tl USP is proportional to myocardial blood supply. The injection of ^{201}Tl in concert with a treadmill exercise stress test determines myocardial perfusion at maximum cardiac output when cardiac demand outstrips supply and the distribution of ^{201}Tl is less after affected by collateral blood supply within the myocardium. Regions that do not take up ^{201}Tl are interpreted as areas of infarct or ischemia. If these focal areas of decreased uptake subsequently fill in with redistributed ^{201}Tl, they are interpreted to be areas of ischemia, in contrast with areas of infarct, which remain as diminished areas of activity.

7. The answer is E *[VII B 1]*.
^{99m}Tc pentetate is cleared through glomerular filtration in the same manner as inulin and can be used to determine the glomerular filtration rate (GFR) as well as in the evaluation of obstruction of vascular supply and renal morphology.

8. The answer is E (all) *[I C]*.
The optimal radiopharmaceutical has a half-life short enough to minimize radiation exposure to the patient yet long enough to allow for collection of imaging information. It should incorporate a gamma-emitting radionuclide, which decays with the emission of a photon energy between 100–300 keV, which is efficiently detected with current instrumentation. The radiopharmaceutical should localize rapidly in the organ system of interest and be metabolized, excreted, or both from the nontarget tissues to maximize contrast and minimize radiation-absorbed dose.

9. The answer is C (I, II) *[II A, B]*.
Sodium pertechnetate ^{99m}Tc USP decays by isomeric transition and has a physical half-life of 6 hours. The emission of a gamma photon has the energy of 140 keV.

10. The answer is E (all) *[VI B 1]*.
Technetium ^{99m}Tc sulfur colloid localizes within the reticuloendothelial system, with approximately 80%–90% of the dose phagocytized by the Kupffer cells of the liver, 5%–10% by the spleen and the balance by the bone marrow.

11. The answer is E (all) *[VIII B]*.
Although all of the listed agents accumulate in the thyroid gland, only sodium iodide ^{123}I possesses ideal imaging characteristics and organification into thyroid hormone. While the imaging properties of sodium pertechnetate ^{99m}Tc USP are good, the pertechnetate ion is only trapped by the thyroid and not organified, thus limiting the information provided by the image.

12–16. The answers are: 12-D *[III A 1]*, **13-C** *[V A 1]*, **14-B** *[VI B 1]*, **15-E** *[IX A 1]*, **16-A** *[IX B 1]*.
Thallous chloride ^{201}Tl USP is a monovalent cation with distribution analogous to potassium ion (K$^+$). Myocardial uptake is by active transport via the Na$^+$-K$^+$/ATPase pump.

After intravenous (IV) administration of ^{99m}Tc albumin aggregated USP, 80% of the radiolabeled albumin particles become trapped by capillary blockade in the pulmonary circulation.

After the administration of ^{99m}Tc sulfur colloid, approximately 80%–90% of the dose is phagocytized by the Kupffer cells of the liver, 5%–10% by the spleen, and the balance by the bone marrow.

^{99m}Tc exametazime is used for evaluating brain perfusion. It possesses a lipophilic partition coefficient that is sufficient to diffuse passively across the blood–brain barrier (BBB) almost completely within one pass of the cerebral circulation and that is sufficiently retained to permit data collection.

^{18}F fludeoxyglucose is used in evaluating cerebral function by mapping the distribution of cerebral glucose metabolism. As an analogue of glucose, ^{18}F fludeoxyglucose is transported into the brain by carrier-mediated transport mechanisms responsible for transporting glucose across the BBB. Because the presence of the F atom in the 2 position prevents metabolism beyond the phosphorylation step, ^{18}F fludeoxyglucose becomes metabolically trapped within the brain.

20
Pharmaceutical Care and Disease State Management

Peggy C. Yarborough

I. INTRODUCTION

A. The **practice of pharmacy** embraces a variety of settings, patient populations, and specialist as well as generalist pharmacists. Central to the practice of pharmacy, however, is the provision of clinical services directly to, and for the benefit of, **patients.**

B. Definition. The term **pharmaceutical care** (sometimes called **pharmacist care**) describes specific activities and services through which an individual pharmacist "cooperates with a patient and other professionals in designing, implementing and monitoring a therapeutic plan that will produce specific therapeutic outcomes for the patient."[1]

C. Pharmaceutical care is increasingly being augmented by activities that may be described as **focused areas of practice**—wherein the pharmacist is engaged in:

1. **Drug monitoring,** for a specific drug or for therapy for a specific disease state

2. **Disease monitoring,** for a specific disease state

3. **Drug/disease management,** by protocol

A pharmacist may incorporate one or more areas of focused practice into a general practice of pharmacy, or may specialize within a narrow field of practice. Examples of highly specialized practice include pharmacist-directed diabetes management clinics, hypertension clinics, anticoagulation clinics, and hospital-based infectious disease services.

II. SCOPE OF PRACTICE WITHIN PHARMACEUTICAL CARE

A. Role. Pharmaceutical care has evolved from an emphasis on prevention of drug-related problems (basically **drug management**) to the expanded roles of pharmacists in the **triage of patients, treatment of routine acute illnesses, management of chronic diseases,** and **primary disease prevention.**

B. Function. The provision of pharmaceutical care does not imply that the pharmacist is no longer responsible for dispensing functions. In many instances, however, implementation of pharmaceutical care services necessitates a redesign of the professional work flow (see VII), with assignment of technical functions to technical personnel under the direct supervision and responsibility of the pharmacist.

---

[1]Hepler CD, Strand LM. Opportunities and responsibilities in pharmaceutical care. *Am J Hosp Pharm* 1990; 47:533–543.

Table 20-1. Uniqueness of Pharmaceutical Care

	Traditional Pharmacy	**Clinical Pharmacy**	**Pharmaceutical Care**
Primary focus	Prescription order or OTC request	Physicians or other health professionals	Patient
Continuity	Upon demand	Discontinuous	Continuous
Strategy	Obey	Find fault or prevention	Anticipate or improve
Orientation	Drug product	Process	Outcomes

III. UNIQUENESS OF PHARMACEUTICAL CARE. Provision of pharmaceutical care overlaps somewhat with other aspects of pharmacy practice (Table 20-1). However, pharmaceutical care is not the same as these other areas, which include:

A. Clinical pharmacy

B. Patient counseling

C. Pharmaceutical services; when the activities of a pharmacy or pharmacy department are performed for "faceless" patients or charts, the activity is one of pharmacy service, not pharmaceutical care (e.g., chart or drug profile reviews without input from the patient or caregiver is not pharmaceutical care).

IV. ESSENTIAL COMPONENTS OF PHARMACEUTICAL CARE

A. Pharmacist–patient relationship. The importance of putting a face and personality with the clinical picture is a key component of pharmaceutical care. A pharmacist can have a caring relationship with a patient but not with a chart or drug profile. A pharmacist cannot have empathy for words on a page or on a computer screen. Pharmaceutical care is based upon a collaborative effort between pharmacist and patient.

B. Pharmacist's workup of drug therapy (PWDT). The provision of pharmaceutical care is often centered around a process described as the PWDT.[2] The PWDT contains the *thought processes* necessary for pharmaceutical care. The PWDT is too lengthy to be used as the chart note for pharmacist interventions; an abbreviated format known as a FARM (Table 20-2) note or a SOAP note is more appropriate for a chart notation (see Table 20-2). Nonetheless, it is helpful to the pharmacy student, or to a pharmacist entering a new field of pharmacy practice, to write out complete PWDTs for a variety of patients as a training or orientation exercise. Although the forms or methods used for the PWDT may vary, the components are essentially the same.

    1. Data collection. Collect, synthesize, and interpret relevant information, such as:
        a. Patient demographic data: age, race, sex
        b. Pertinent medical information
            (1) Current and past medical history
            (2) Family history
            (3) Social history
            (4) Dietary history
            (5) Medication history (prescription, OTC, social drugs; allergies)
            (6) Physical findings (e.g., weight, height, blood pressure, edema)
            (7) Laboratory or other test results (e.g., serum drug levels, potassium level, serum creatinine as relevant to drug therapy)
        c. Patient complaints, symptoms, signs

---

[2]Strand LM, Morley PC, Cipolle RJ, et al. Drug-related problems: their structure and function. *Ann Pharmacother* 1990;24:1093–1097.

Table 20-2. Components of a FARM Note and a SOAP Note

PWDT Component	FARM NOTE	SOAP NOTE
I. FINDINGS	The identified or suggestive patient-specific information that gives a basis for, or leads to, the recognition of a pharmacotherapy problem or indication for pharmacist intervention.	
	Findings **(F)** Subjective and objective data incorporated into same section	Subjective data **(S)** separated from objective data **(O)**
II. DESIRED OUTCOMES	Assessment **(A)** *An assessment is your clinical judgment based upon your findings.* As such, it is no better than your database (the findings)! The assessment forms the basis for your intervention plan.	
III. DESIRED END POINTS		
IV. DRUG-RELATED PROBLEMS		
V. THERAPEUTIC SELECTION	Resolutions/Recommendation **(R)**	Plan **(P)**
VI. MONITORING PARAMETERS	Monitoring **(M)**	
VII. FOLLOW-UP		

2. Develop or identify the **CORE pharmacotherapy plan**[3]
   a. **C = Condition** or patient need
   b. **O = Outcome(s)** desired for that condition
      (1) *Patient outcomes* (POEMS: Patient-Oriented Evidence that Matters). There are generally five categories of patient outcomes.
         • Mortality
         • Morbidity
            (i) Related to disease process
            (ii) Related to medication/treatment plan
         • Behavior
         • Economic
         • Quality of life
      (2) *Therapeutic end points* (surrogate markers; DOES: Disease-Oriented Evidence)
         • A therapeutic end point represents the pharmacological/therapeutic effect that is expected, ultimately, to achieve the desired outcome(s).
         • Most commonly, more than one end point will be needed to achieve an outcome. For example, near-normal glycemic control *and* normalization of blood pressure would be necessary to significantly reduce the risk of end-stage renal disease.
   c. **R = Regimen** to achieve the desired outcome(s)
      (1) *Existing therapy*—for example, a pharmacist is asked to work with a patient with one or more agents already prescribed for the disease process or problem.
         • Evaluate the current drug regimen for its potential to achieve desired end points and to meet the patient's individual needs.
         • Revise regimen as appropriate.
      (2) *Initial therapy*—a pharmacist is asked to work with a patient with a new diagnosis or is asked to develop an initial treatment plan.
         • List therapeutic options (drug and regimen) most likely to achieve the desired end points
         • Select the option best suited for the patient's medical, physical (e.g., handicap), psychosocial (e.g., support system), mental (motivation, denial, fear), and financial well-being.
   d. **E = Evaluation** parameters to assess outcome achievement
      (1) *Efficacy parameters.* What should be monitored, how often, and by whom—to ensure that therapeutic end points or patient outcomes are being achieved

[3]Canaday BR, Yarborough PC. Documenting pharmaceutical care: creating a standard. *Ann Pharmacother* 1994; 28:1292–1296.

Table 20-3. PRIME Pharmacotherapy Problem Types[3]

P = Pharmaceutical-based problems
  - Patient not receiving a prescribed drug, device, or intervention
  - Routine monitoring (labs, screenings, exams) missing

R = Risks to patient
  - Adverse drug reaction/drug allergy
  - Potential for overlap of adverse effects. These must be kept in mind as part of the workup or evaluation of any new complaint or problem reported by patient

I = Interactions
  - Drug–drug, drug–disease, drug–food interactions

M = Mismatch between medications and condition or patient needs
  - No indication for a current drug, device, or intervention
  - Indication for a drug, device, or intervention but none prescribed

E = Efficacy issues
  - Too much of the correct drug
  - Too little of the correct drug
  - Wrong drug, device, intervention, or regimen prescribed/More efficacious choice possible

---

(2) *Toxicity parameters.* What should be monitored, how often, and by whom—to ensure that adverse effects, allergic reactions, or toxicity is not occurring.

3. Identify the **PRIME pharmacotherapy problems** or indications for pharmacist interventions.[3] The goal is to identify actual or potential problems that could compromise the desired patient outcomes (Table 20-3).
   a. **P = Pharmaceutical**-based problems
      - Patient not receiving a prescribed drug, device, or intervention
      - Routine monitoring (labs, screenings, exams) missing
   b. **R = Risks** to patient
      - Adverse drug reaction/drug allergy
      - Potential for overlap of adverse effects. These must be kept in mind as part of the workup or evaluation of any new complaint or problem reported by patient
   c. **I = Interactions**
      - Drug–drug, drug–disease, drug–food interactions
   d. **M = Mismatch** between medications and condition or patient needs
      - No indication for a current drug, device, or intervention
      - Indication for a drug, device, or intervention but none prescribed
   e. **E = Efficacy** issues
      - Too much of the correct drug
      - Too little of the correct drug
      - Wrong drug, device, intervention, or regimen prescribed/More efficacious choice possible

C. **Documentation of pharmaceutical care.** Formulate a **FARM** or **SOAP progress note** to describe and document the interventions intended or provided by the pharmacist.[3] Some healthcare facilities may specify one format over the other; pharmacists need to become proficient in each.

   Format of a FARM note
   a. **F = Findings:** the patient-specific information that gives a basis for, or leads to, the recognition of a pharmacotherapy problem or indication for pharmacist intervention. Within the FARM format, "findings" include subjective as well as objective information about the patient.
   b. **A = Assessment:** the pharmacist's evaluation of the findings, including a statement of:
      (1) Any additional information that is needed to best assess the problem in order to make recommendations
      (2) The severity, priority, or urgency of the problem
      (3) The short-term and long-term goals of the intervention proposed or provided

422 Chapter 20 IV C

    (4) Examples of **short-term goals** include: eliminate symptoms, lower blood pressure (BP) to 140/90 mm Hg within 6 weeks, manage acute asthma flare-up without requiring hospitalization.

    (5) Examples of **long-term goals** include: prevent recurrence, maintain BP at less than 130/80 mm Hg, prevent progression of diabetic nerve disease.

  c. R = Resolution (including prevention): the intervention plan includes actual or proposed actions by the pharmacist or recommendations to other health-care professionals. The rationale for choosing a specific intervention should be stated. Intervention options may include:

    (1) Observing, reassessing, or following: no intervention necessary at this time. If no action was taken or recommended, the FARM note serves as a record of the event and should constitute part of the patient's pharmacy chart or database.

    (2) Counseling or educating the patient or caregiver

    (3) Making recommendations to the patient or caregiver

    (4) Informing the prescriber

    (5) Making recommendations to the prescriber

    (6) Withholding medication or advising against use

  d. M = Monitoring and follow-up: the parameters and timing of follow-up monitoring to assess the efficacy, safety, and outcome of the intervention. This portion of the FARM note should include:

    (1) The parameter to be followed (e.g., pain, depressed mood, serum potassium level)

    (2) The intent of the monitoring (e.g., efficacy, toxicity, adverse event)

    (3) How the parameter will be monitored (e.g., patient interview, serum drug level, physical examination)

    (4) Frequency of monitoring (e.g., weekly, monthly)

    (5) Duration of monitoring (e.g., until resolved, while on antibiotic, until resolved then monthly for 1 year)

    (6) Anticipated or desired finding (e.g., no pain, euglycemia, healing of lesion)

    (7) Decision point to alter therapy when or if outcome is not achieved (e.g., pain still present after 3 days, mild hypoglycemia more than two times a week)

Format of a SOAP note

The SOAP format is the one used most often by medical practitioners; however, when used within the pharmaceutical care context, the content of the sections must be revised to match the pharmacist's legal scope of practice.

a. S = Subjective Findings: the patient-specific *subjective* information that gives a basis for, or leads to, the recognition of a pharmacotherapy problem or indication for pharmacist intervention. Within the SOAP format, patient "findings" are delineated into subjective versus objective data.

  (1) Subjective data are open to individual interpretation, while objective data are easily duplicated or quantified. Examples of subjective findings include the patient's statement of complaint (the "cc:"), duration, or severity of symptoms.

  (2) Sometimes, the data to be noted are not clearly delineated as subjective or objective, or there may be a preponderance of one type of data. In these instances, the subjective and objective data may be combined as a single section, "S/O Findings."

b. O = Objective Findings: the patient-specific *objective* information that gives a basis for, or leads to, the recognition of a pharmacotherapy problem or indication for pharmacist intervention. Examples of objective information include lab data, weight, height, blood pressure, and pulse.

c. A = Assessment. In the medical model, the Assessment states the physician's working diagnosis and/or possible explanations for the patient's medical problem(s). In the pharmaceutical care model, however, diagnosis is not normally within the pharmacist's scope of practice. Instead, the Assessment section would include the pharmacist's evaluation of the subjective and objective findings in a manner similar to the description of the Assessment in the FARM format, above.

d. P = Plan. In the medical model, the Plan states the physician's intended drug regimen(s), surgical procedures, and/or diagnostic tests. In the pharmaceutical care model, pharmacists may not have the authority to initiate nor alter drug therapy regimens or order laboratory tests. Laboratory or prescriptive authority may be granted on a state-by-state basis, under collaborative protocol with specific physician(s), or within a specific health-care facility or system. Actions included within the Plan section should be identified as *recommended* actions when appropriate. In the pharmaceutical care model, the Plan is usually expanded to describe information included in the Monitoring/ Follow-up section in the FARM format, above.

V. FOCUSED AREAS OF PRACTICE. This phrase refers to areas of speciality practice in which pharmacists are increasingly being recognized for their therapeutic or management expertise. As such, pharmaceutical care provided by the pharmacist is augmented by activities not normally provided within the generalist pharmacist role. Categories of focused practice may best be described by the type and extent of specialty activities. *Activities for each descriptive level are additive to, or augment, the previous level.* That is, focused drug monitoring incorporates and expands the activities of pharmaceutical care; focused disease monitoring incorporates the activities of pharmaceutical care plus focused drug monitoring, etc.

A. Drug monitoring: specialized monitoring for a specific drug, or drug therapy for a specific disease state. Examples of activities would include, but not be limited to, the following:

1. Extensive patient education concerning the drug, the drug monitoring process, and the pharmacist's and patient's responsibilities for focused drug monitoring. It must be stressed to the patient that for the focused drug monitoring program to be effective, the pharmacist must have access to information concerning *all* the medications being taken by, or prescribed for, the patient.

2. Each time the patient returns for refill of the monitored medication (e.g., for hypertension, diabetes, hyperlipidemia, circulation, cardiovascular disease, glaucoma)

    a. Perform a compliance check (expected versus actual refill date), and determine *why* the needed medication or supplies are not being refilled. Physical, financial, intellectual, mental, or emotional issues may be involved, requiring referral to other health-care providers or requiring other innovative solutions. Take the responsibility and appropriate action to resolve these issues.

    b. Ask about the occurrence and frequency of side effects, especially those related to quality of life—such as orthostatic hypotension, changes in sexual function, energy level, exercise tolerance, hypoglycemia, hyperglycemia, and ability to concentrate. Counsel the patient about strategies to minimize these effects, or contact the prescriber to offer options to resolve the patient's reported problems.

3. With each new prescription or OTC medication added to the monitored drug regimen, observe and counsel the patient concerning the following:

    a. Drugs that may affect the efficacy of the monitored drug (drug–disease and drug–drug interactions). For example, for diabetes medications,

        (1) certain drugs may directly change blood glucose levels.

        (2) certain drugs may indirectly change blood glucose levels by interacting with the hypoglycemic agent.

    b. Drugs that may affect the course of the disease for the monitored drug. For example, certain drugs added to a diabetes regimen may affect the complications of diabetes by aggravating neuropathy and nephropathy, by causing decreased circulation, etc.

    c. Drugs that may affect comorbidity conditions of the disease for the monitored drug. For example, certain drugs added to a diabetes regimen may affect concurrent hypertension, lipid abnormalities, and other conditions that occur more frequently in the diabetic population.

4. Remind and encourage patients to adhere to schedules for recommended laboratory tests during the course of the drug therapy. Examples include prothrombin time tests, liver function tests, eye exams, and renal function tests. Adherence to such monitoring parameters will allow prevention or early detection and treatment of certain adverse drug effects.

B. Disease monitoring: specialized monitoring for a specific disease state. Disease monitoring activities are optimally performed at regular intervals (i.e., at set appointment times), but should at least be performed each time the patient returns for refill of a disease-related medication or supply.

A focused disease-monitoring program is extensive in time, effort, and patient education. At this level, however, the pharmacist does not initiate changes in pharmacological therapies.

Recommendations for changes are relayed to the medical provider, who then directs the pharmacist concerning specific regimen adjustments.

Examples of focused disease-monitoring activities would include, but not be limited to, the following:

1. Extensive patient education concerning the disease and its treatment, the disease-monitoring process, and the pharmacist's and patient's responsibilities for focused disease monitoring. Education will likely be needed initially and periodically during the monitoring program.

2. Focused monitoring of a *chronic* disease would include patient education to establish the patient's desired *targets or goals* and strategies to attain them.
   a. Encourage and assist patients to set long-term goals. Examples: lose 30 pounds, quit smoking.
   b. Encourage and assist patients to set short-term goals that are directed toward meeting the long-term goals. Examples: lose 1 pound in 1–2 weeks, decrease smoking by one cigarette per day.

3. Assessment for subjective evidence of *improvement or worsening of disease symptoms.*
   a. The frequent or consistent occurrence of certain symptoms (such as asthma attacks, hypoglycemia, chest pain, diarrhea from ulcerative colitis, etc) should be brought to the attention of the medical provider.
   b. Lack of subjective evidence of efficacy (failure of pain control, minimal or no improvement of nocturia, etc.) should also be reported to the prescriber.
   c. The patient's report of days of work or school missed, due to exacerbation of disease symptoms, is a valuable assessment of disease control or treatment.

4. Assessment for objective evidence or *certain indices of disease control or treatment.* For example, a pharmacist may review and guide a diabetic patient in interpretation of self-monitored blood glucose (SMBG) records. Using this data, the pharmacist can then advise the patient concerning the application of a prescribed insulin adjustment algorithm.
   a. Some data may be patient-derived, such as SMBG, weight, measurement of calf circumference, and readings from a peak-flow meter.
   b. Some data may be pharmacist-initiated, such as a pharmacy-based lipid monitoring program, blood glucose testing, blood pressure measurements, etc. It should be noted that a pharmacy may need to be CLIA-certified (Clinical Laboratories Improvement Act) before performing certain waived or moderately complex laboratory procedures.
   c. Some data may be obtained through the physician's office, with a copy being forwarded to the pharmacist or brought in by the patient.

C. **Drug/disease management by protocol.** The components of this focused practice include, but are not limited to, the following:

1. Disease and drug monitoring, including a significant component of patient education

2. Disease and quality-of-life outcomes identified and agreed upon by patient, medical provider, and pharmacist

3. Application of a drug-disease-management protocol, developed as a collaborative work relationship between pharmacist and medical provider, which elaborates specific authorizations or limitations for the pharmacist's activities. Components of a drug-disease-management protocol may include the following:
   a. Process by which the physician refers the patient to the pharmacist
   b. Drugs, devices, medical treatment, tests and procedures that may be prescribed, administered, or ordered, as appropriate for the treatment of the health problem addressed by the protocol
      (1) Drug initiation, dosage adjustment and/or discontinuation
      (2) Specific lab orders and interpretation
   c. Limited physical assessment
   d. Integration of the pharmaceutical care plan into the total medical care plan for the patient
   e. Predetermined plan for emergency services
   f. Written communication/documentation to/from medical provider (e.g., chart access and note entry)

VI. CLINICAL SKILLS AND PHARMACIST'S ROLES IN PHARMACEUTICAL CARE. The skills, activities, and services inherent in the provision of pharmaceutical care include, but are not limited to, the following:

A. Patient assessment

1. Physical assessment
2. Barriers to adherence
3. Psychosocial issues

B. Patient education and counseling

1. Interview skills
2. Communication skills (e.g., empathy, listening, speaking or writing at the patient's level of understanding)
3. Ability to motivate, inspire
4. Develop and implement a patient education plan based on an initial education assessment
5. Identification and resolution of compliance barriers

C. Patient-specific pharmacist care plans

1. Recognition, prevention, and management of drug interactions
2. Pharmacology and therapeutics (innovative and conventional)
3. Interpretation of laboratory tests
4. Knowledge of community resources, professional referrals
5. Communication and rapport with community medical providers

D. Drug treatment protocols

1. Develop and maintain (update) protocols.
2. Follow protocols as a pharmacist clinician.
3. Monitor aggregate adherence to treatment protocols [e.g., drug-utilization evaluations (DUE)], especially for a managed care or health system facility.

E. Dosage adjustment

1. Identify patients at risk for exaggerated or subtherapeutic response.
2. Apply pharmacokinetic principles to determine patient-specific dosing.
3. Order and interpret relevant tests at correct time intervals to assess dosage adjustment (e.g., plasma drug concentrations, blood glucose levels, blood pressure measurements).

F. Selection of therapeutic alternatives

1. Use drug information resources effectively.
2. Review and critique drug literature.
3. Construct comparative analyses to support therapeutic decisions.

G. Prescriptive authority in designated practice sites or positions

H. Preventive services

1. Immunizations
2. Screenings
3. Health and wellness education

I. **Managerial skills**

1. **Plan, direct,** and **implement** pharmaceutical care activities within various practice environments, such as community pharmacy, ambulatory care settings, managed or contractual care, home health services, long-term care facilities, inpatient hospital practice, and others.

2. **Allocate** resources.

VII. **PHARMACEUTICAL CARE AS THE MODEL FOR PHARMACY PRACTICE.** The concepts, activities, and services of pharmaceutical care form the basis for provision of clinical services directly to, and for the benefit of, patients in all pharmacy practice settings. These settings include home health, hospital, ambulatory care, primary care, consultation, long-term care, and community pharmacy practice. Work flow, staffing patterns, processes, and pharmacy programs might differ, but the core approach to patient care remains pharmaceutical care in all settings. Figures 20-1 and 20-2 illustrate pharmaceutical care models in the institutional and community pharmacy settings.

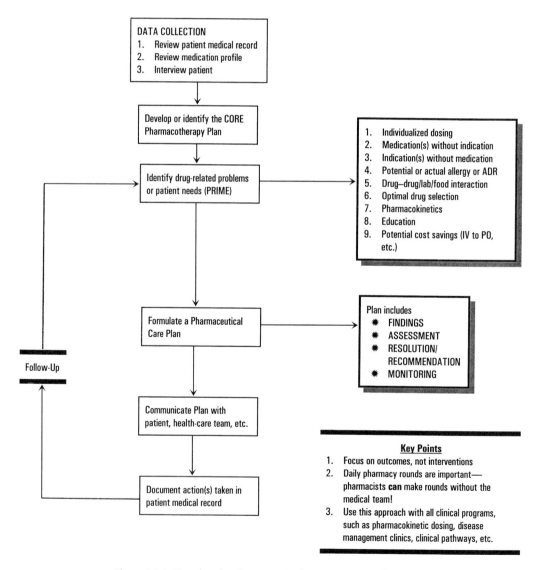

Figure 20-1. Template for pharmaceutical care: institutional practice.

Patient perceives problem or needs routine medical checkup

↓

1. Medical care provider
2. Diagnosis
3. Prescription/Treatment Plan

↓

Community Pharmacy

Pharmaceutical Care Component	Prescription Processing Component

1. Patient presents prescription to pharmacist or technician.

2. If new patient: fills out medical data information form.
   → 2a. Technician enters standard information into software.

3. Data collection: If new patient, pharmacist clarifies initial medical information (if needed) by interviewing patient. If established patient, pharmacist asks patient about
   a. recent changes in medical status
   b. recent OTC drug use
   c. drugs acquired at other facilities (e.g., physician samples; other pharmacies)
   d. drug concerns of patient or recent adverse effects

4. CORE Pharmacotherapy Plan: Pharmacist enters new data and prescription into software to integrate these with the existing CORE Plan.

5. PRIME pharmacotherapy problems: Pharmacist performs prospective drug utilization review (DUR), to identify problems or patient needs.
   → 5a. If no therapeutic concerns are raised, technician proceeds to fill prescription.

6. Pharmacist formulates FARM progress note to document care provided. Special attention should be given to
   a. RECOMMENDATIONS:
      1) If therapeutic concerns are raised, contact prescriber. Document resolution.
      → When therapeutic concerns are resolved, technician proceeds to fill prescription.
      2) If patient requires extensive counseling (e.g., beyond OBRA '90 requirements), document interventions provided. Example: instruction on use of insulin, actions of insulin, and recognition/prevention/treatment of hypoglycemia.
      → Technician processes claim form for submission to insurance company or prepares patient billing for expanded counseling.
      3) If patient is candidate for monitoring program or additional education services, recommend appropriate program and set up appointment for patient. Examples include: diabetes, hypertension, asthma, smoking-cessation monitoring and/or education sessions.
      → Technician maintains master schedule for pharmacist–patient appointments.
   b. MONITORING: see section 9 below.

7. Pharmacist counsels patient on prescription (or other interventions as determined in FARM note) while technician is completing dispensing process.

8. Prescription is checked by pharmacist when dispensing process is completed by technician.
   → Technician gives prescription to patient and concludes prescription processing by completing billing procedures (cash, charge, insurance billing, etc.).

9. MONITORING
   a. Follow-up with patient on new prescriptions: for example,
      1) call 2 days after dispensing of antibiotic to ascertain improvement of symptoms.
      2) call 7 days after antihypertensive prescription to determine if side effects are so bothersome that compliance may be affected.
   b. Relay follow-up findings to prescriber, when appropriate.
   c. Confirm follow-up appointment with patient who enrolled in a monitoring or education program.
   d. Document follow-up. New problems uncovered during follow-up become the FINDING of subsequent FARM note.

Figure 20-2. Template for pharmaceutical care: community practice.

VIII. DOCUMENTATION OF PHARMACEUTICAL CARE. "If it isn't documented, it isn't done!" Documentation of pharmaceutical care is integral to continuity of care, demonstration of clinician competence, communication among health-care providers, evidence of contributions to patient care, and reimbursement of professional services.

A. Pharmaceutical care, including the pharmaceutical care plan process (CORE, PRIME, FARM, or SOAP), is a systematic method for recording the pharmacist's examination of a patient's pharmacotherapy and subsequent identification of medication-related problems.

B. In most practice settings, **computer software programs** maintain patient data and drug-profile records. Thus, after documentation of the initial pharmaceutical care plan, patient data or drug regimens are included in subsequent FARM (or SOAP) notes only if a change occurs that is relevant to the therapeutic issue being addressed in the note.

C. Forms that summarize pharmacists' interventions using a **unified coding system** are useful for processing reimbursement or billing forms, but these forms are not adequate documentation of pharmaceutical care. These forms do not communicate to other health professionals the depth and quality of pharmacist interventions or the pharmacist's plan for ongoing pharmaceutical care.

IX. PHARMACEUTICAL CARE: AN ONGOING PROCESS. The **patient profile** (database) is revised and reassessed each time a new drug is added to or deleted from the medication regimen, a new disease or condition is diagnosed, or the patient undergoes other clinical intervention, such as surgery. When the patient returns to the pharmacy or is readmitted to the health system facility, the pharmacist uses the patient profile, PWDT, and FARM (or SOAP) notes (maintained in the patient pharmacy chart or in the medical chart) as the basis for ongoing pharmacist–patient interactions.

X. IMPORTANCE OF PHARMACEUTICAL CARE IN TODAY'S PHARMACY PRACTICE

A. The potential for **medication errors** is growing, and one professional group must assume a primary role in addressing this issue, rather than various groups or individuals making fragmented efforts. The pharmacist is trained specifically to address these therapeutic issues.

1. The use of prescription and nonprescription medications is growing and now constitutes the primary therapeutic modality available to health-care practitioners and patients.

2. The number, complexity, and potency of prescription and nonprescription drug products is increasing.

B. The need for pharmaceutical care secures an enduring role for the pharmacist in the U.S. health-care system. Every encounter with patients, regardless of practice setting, provides pharmaceutical care.

C. Pharmaceutical care activities integrate pharmacists into the health-care system of the future.

STUDY QUESTIONS

Directions: Each of the numbered items or incomplete statements in this section is followed by answers or by completions of the statement. Select the **one** lettered answer or completion that is **best** in each case.

1. Which of the following statements best describes FARM?

(A) Cultivation of a pharmacist's knowledge in order to better serve the public
(B) Findings, assessment, resolution, monitoring
(C) Findings, assessment, recognition, management
(D) The process by which an individual pharmacist interacts with a specific patient to attain pertinent medical information

2. An example of an expanded role of the pharmacist is

(A) community leader
(B) preparation of compounded prescriptions
(C) maintaining adequate inventory of orphan drugs
(D) triage of patients

3. What is the most important focus of pharmaceutical care?

(A) The pharmacist
(B) The patient
(C) The prescription
(D) The patient chart

4. Which of the following statements regarding pharmaceutical care is true? Pharmaceutical care

(A) usually does not overlap into other areas of heath care
(B) and clinical pharmacy are synonymous
(C) implies that the pharmacist is no longer responsible for dispensing functions
(D) is based on strategies to provide continuous patient care in order to attain desired outcomes

5. Essential components of pharmaceutical care include

(A) patient–pharmacist relationship, legible physician orders, and accurate data collection
(B) pharmacist–patient relationship and workup of drug therapy
(C) a software program that accesses medication history and prompts the pharmacist concerning questions to ask the patient
(D) maintenance of patient medication history for at least 2 years and a focus on acute illness

6. In the CORE pharmacotherapy plan, what does the "E" represent?

(A) Education of patient or caregiver
(B) Efficacy issues
(C) Elaboration
(D) Evaluation parameters

7. The most important reason for using the FARM note is to

(A) collect information for the physician
(B) document problem-solving and/or interventions performed by the pharmacist
(C) keep a log of all drug interactions
(D) create a uniform method of recording patient information

8. Which of the following topics would NOT be included in the assessment portion of the FARM note?

(A) Recommendations made to the patient or caregiver
(B) Severity, priority, or urgency of the problem
(C) Short-term and long-term goals of the intervention
(D) Additional information that is needed to best assess the problem

9. Immunizations, screenings, and wellness education are examples of which clinical skill?

(A) Community health overview
(B) Patient medication education and counseling
(C) Preventive services
(D) Managerial services

10. The pharmacist's role in the selection of therapeutic alternatives requires which of the following clinical skills?

(A) Review and critique drug literature
(B) Motivate and inspire patients
(C) Perform drug utilization evaluations (DUEs)
(D) Knowledge of community resources

ANSWERS AND EXPLANATIONS

1. The answer is B *[IV B 4]*.
A FARM progress note is used to describe and document the interventions intended or provided by the pharmacist. The acronym FARM means Findings, Assessment, Resolution, and Monitoring and follow-up.

2. The answer is D *[II A]*.
Pharmaceutical care has evolved from an emphasis on prevention of drug-related problems to the expanded roles of pharmacists in the triage of patients, treatment of routine acute illnesses, management of chronic diseases, and primary disease prevention.

3. The answer is B *[IV A]*.
Pharmaceutical care is based on a collaborative effort between pharmacist and patient.

4. The answer is D *[I B; IX]*.
The term pharmaceutical care describes specific activities and services through which an individual pharmacist cooperates with a patient and other professionals in designing, implementing, and monitoring a therapeutic plan that will produce specific therapeutic outcomes for the patient. The patient profile (database) is revised and the potential for drug-related problems reassessed each time a new drug is added to or deleted from the medication regimen, a new disease or condition is diagnosed, or the patient undergoes other clinical intervention (e.g., surgery).

5. The answer is B *[IV A, B]*.
The essential components of pharmaceutical care are the pharmacist–patient relationship and the pharmacist's workup of drug therapy.

6. The answer is D *[IV B 2]*.
The acronym CORE refers to the components of the pharmacotherapy plan, which is part of the pharmacist's workup of drug therapy. CORE stands for Condition or patient need, Outcome desired for that condition; Regimen selected to achieve that outcome, and Evaluation parameters to assess outcome achievement.

7. The answer is B *[IV C; VII]*.
The FARM note is the pharmacist's progress note, describing and documenting the interventions intended or provided by the pharmacist. This constitutes the progress note in the medical chart (in health system facilities) or in the pharmacy patient chart (in community pharmacy or sites without ready access to the medical chart).

8. The answer is A *[IV C]*.
The assessment portion of the FARM note states the pharmacist's evaluation of the findings. Recommendations are made to the patient or caregiver to resolve or prevent an actual or potential problem identified by the pharmacist. Thus, such recommendations would be included in the resolution portion of the FARM note.

9. The answer is C *[VI H]*.
Immunizations, screenings, and health and wellness education are examples of clinical skills used in a pharmacist's provision of preventive services.

10. The answer is A *[VI F]*.
For effective selection of therapeutic alternatives, a pharmacist would use certain clinical skills, including use of drug information resources, comparative analyses, and review and critique of drug literature.

21
Drug Information Resources

Paul F. Souney
Connie Lee Barnes

I. DEFINITION. Drug information is current, critically examined, relevant data about drugs and drug use in a given patient or situation.

   A. Current information uses the most recent, up-to-date sources possible.

   B. Critically examined information should meet the following criteria:

      1. More than one source should be used when appropriate.

      2. The extent of agreement of sources should be determined; if sources do not agree, good judgment should be used.

      3. The plausibility of information, based on clinical circumstances, should be determined.

   C. Relevant information must be presented in a manner that applies directly to the circumstances under consideration (e.g., patient parameters, therapeutic objectives, alternative approaches).

II. DRUG INFORMATION RESOURCES. There are three sources of drug information: journals (primary sources), indexing and abstracting services (secondary sources), and textbooks (tertiary sources).

   A. Primary sources

      1. Benefits. Journal articles provide the most current information about drugs and, ideally, should be the source for answering therapeutic questions. Journals enable pharmacists to:
        a. Keep abreast of professional news
        b. Learn how a second clinician handles a particular problem
        c. Keep up with new developments in pathophysiology, diagnostic agents, and therapeutic regimens
        d. Distinguish useful from useless or even harmful therapy
        e. Enhance communication with other health-care professionals and consumers
        f. Obtain continuing education credits
        g. Share opinions with other health-care professionals through letters-to-the-editor columns
        h. Prepare for the Board certification examination in pharmacotherapy, nutrition support, etc.

      2. Limitations. Although publication of an article in a well-known, respected journal enhances the credibility of information contained in an article, this does not guarantee that the article is accurate. Many articles possess inadequacies that become apparent as the ability to evaluate drug information improves.

   B. Secondary sources

      1. Benefits. Indexing and abstracting services (Table 21-1) are valuable tools for quick and selective screening of the primary literature for specific information, data, citation, and articles. In some cases, the sources provide sufficient information to serve as references for answering drug information requests.

      2. Limitations. Each indexing or abstracting service reviews a finite number of journals. Therefore, relying on only one service can greatly hinder the thoroughness of a literature search. Another important fact to remember is the substantial difference in lag time (i.e., the interval between publication of an article and citation of the article in an index) among various services. Several examples are given in Table 21-1.

Table 21-1. Examples of Abstracting/Indexing Services

Secondary References	Journals Indexed	Lag Time
CINAHL	1200	—
ClinAlert	150	1–6 weeks
Current Contents	1200	1–6 weeks
Drugdex	—	3–6 months
Medline/PubMed	4500	1 week
Inpharma	1800	3 weeks–6 months
International Pharmaceutical Abstracts	800	6–14 months
Iowa Drug Information System	200	3–12 months
Pharmaceutical News Index	—	2–8 weeks
Reactions	1800	3 weeks–6 months
Science Citation Index	3700	3–12 months

   a. Secondary sources usually **describe** only articles and clinical studies from journals. Frequently, readers respond to, criticize, and add new information to published articles and studies through letters. Services such as *Medline/PubMed* or the *Iowa Drug Information System* generally do include pertinent letters to the editor within the scope of coverage.
   b. Indexing and abstracting services are primarily used to **locate** journal articles. In general, abstracts should not be used as primary sources of information because they are generally interpretations of a study and may be a misinterpretation of important information. Pharmacists should obtain and evaluate the original article because abstracts might not tell the whole story.

C. Tertiary sources

   1. Benefits. General-reference textbooks can provide easy and convenient access to a broad spectrum of related topics. Background information on drugs and diseases is often available. Although a textbook might answer many drug-related questions, the limitations of these sources should not be overlooked.
   a. It could take several years to publish a text, so information available in textbooks might not include the most recent developments in the field. Other resources should be used to update or supplement information obtained from textbooks.
   b. The author of a textbook might not have done a thorough search of the literature, so pertinent data could have been omitted. An author also might have misinterpreted the primary or secondary literature. Reference citations should be available to verify the validity and accuracy of the data.

   2. General considerations when examining and using textbooks as sources of drug information include:
   a. The author, publisher, or both: What are the author's and publisher's track records?
   b. The year of publication (copyright date)
   c. The edition of the text: Is it the most current edition?
   d. The presence or absence of a bibliography: If a bibliography is included, are important statements accurately referenced? When were the references published?
   e. The scope of the textbook: How accessible is the information?
   f. Alternative resources that are available (e.g., primary and secondary sources, other relevant texts)

III. INTERNET

   A. Benefits. The Internet expands the ability to search therapies recently published or discussed in the media. An Internet search may be required for the following: company-specific information, issues currently in the news, alternative medicine, or U.S. government information. The most popular web browsers are Netscape Navigator/Communicator and Microsoft Internet Explorer. A variety of search engines have been developed to provide a

Table 21-2. Selected Web Sites

Site	Web URL
Agency for Healthcare Research and Quality	http://www.ahrq.gov
American Association of Colleges of Pharmacy	http://www.aacp.org
American Cancer Society	http.//www.cancer.org
American Diabetes Association	http://www.diabetes.org
American Heart Association	http://www.americanheart.org
American Society of Health-System Pharmacists	http://www.ashp.org
Centers for Disease Control and Prevention	http://www.cdc.gov
Department of Health and Human Services	http://www.os.dhhs.gov
DrugFacts	http://www.drugfacts.com
Drug Infonet	http://www.druginfonet.com
eMedicine	http://www.emedicine.com
Food and Drug Administration	http://www.fda.gov
Healthfinder	http://www.healthfinder.gov
Health On the Net Foundation	http://www.hon.ch
Mayo Clinic	http://www.mayo.edu
MD Consult	http://www.mdconsult.com
Medical Matrix	http://www.medmatrix.org
Medscape	http://www.medscape.com
MedWatch	http://www.fda.gov/medwatch
National Cancer Institute	http://www.cancer.gov
National Guideline Clearinghouse	http://www.guideline.gov
National Heart, Lung, and Blood Institute	http://www.nhlbi.nih.gov
National Institutes of Health	http://www.nih.gov
National Library of Medicine	http://www.nlm.nih.gov
Pharmaceutical Research and Manufacturers of America	http://www.phrma.org
PharmacyOneSource	http://www.pharmacyonesource.com
Pharmscope	http://www.pharmscope.com
RxList	http://www.rxlist.com
RxMed	http://www.rxmed.com
WebMD Corporation	http://www.webmd.com

method for searching the Internet. General search engines (AltaVista, Google, Overture, About, HotBot, Lycos) attempt to index as much of the Internet as possible. Also, medical search engines exist.

B. Limitations

1. Unlike information published in journals and textbooks, information obtained from the Internet may not be peer reviewed or edited prior to release.

2. Information received from the Internet may be only as reliable as the person who posted it and the users who read and comment on its content. A web site should be evaluated by its source (author) of information. The name, location, and sponsorship should be disclosed. Also, a reputable site will provide an ease of access to information and the ability to give feedback. Pharmacists should use traditional literature evaluation skills to determine whether the information is clear, concise, unbiased, relevant, and referenced.

C. Use. To obtain information from the Internet, the user must have an address [referred to as a URL (Uniform Resource Locator)] to insert in the browser, which will then find the site automatically. Many associations and organizations have web sites that are linked to other web pages. See Table 21-2 for selected web sites.

IV. STRATEGIES FOR EVALUATING INFORMATION REQUESTS. It is important to obtain as many clues as possible about drug information requests before beginning a literature search. Both time and money can be wasted doing a vast search. Below are important questions to ask the inquirer or evaluate before a manual or computerized search.

A. Talk with the inquirer. Before spending time searching for information, talk to the person who is requesting the information, and acquire any necessary additional information.

  1. Determine the reason for the inquiry. Find out where the inquirer heard or read about the drug. Is he or she taking the medication? If so, why? Because the search can be done by the drug or disease name, determine if the inquirer has a medical condition. Ascertaining the reason for the inquiry helps determine what additional information should be provided. For example, if the inquiry concerns a foreign drug, the inquirer might ask for a domestic equivalent.

  2. Clarify the drug's identification and availability. Make sure that the drug in question is available, and double-check information about the drug, such as:
    a. The **correct spelling** of the drug's name
    b. Whether it is a **generic** or **brand-name drug**
    c. What **pharmaceutical company** manufactures the drug and in what **country** the drug is manufactured
    d. Whether the drug is **prescription** or **nonprescription**
    e. Whether the drug is still **under investigation** and, if it is on the market, **the length of time on the market**
    f. The **dosage form** of the drug
    g. The **purpose** of the drug (i.e., what medical condition or symptom the drug is intended to alleviate; this information helps narrow the search if products with similar names are found)

B. To **identify** or **assess product availability,** consider using **these resources** (see Appendix E). Some of these resources are available as an electronic format or Internet/intranet version.

  1. For drugs manufactured in the **United States,** the following resources are available:
    a. *The American Drug Index,* which is updated annually
    b. *Drug Facts and Comparisons,* which is updated monthly and bound annually
    c. *Drug Topics Red Book,* which releases supplements and is updated annually
    d. The *Physician's Desk Reference (PDR),* which is updated annually
    e. The *American Hospital Formulary Service (AHFS) Drug Information,* which is supplemented quarterly and updated annually
    f. *Martindale: The Complete Drug Reference,* which is updated every 3 years

  2. For drugs manufactured in **foreign countries,** the following resources are available:
    a. *Martindale: The Complete Drug Reference*
    b. *Index Nominum*
    c. *United States Adopted Names (USAN)* and the *United States Pharmacopoeia (USP) Dictionary of Drug Names*

  3. For **investigational drugs,** the following resources are available:
    a. *Martindale: The Complete Drug Reference*
    b. *Drug Facts and Comparisons*
    c. *Unlisted Drugs*
    d. *The NDA Pipeline*

  4. For **orphan drugs** [i.e., drugs that are used to prevent or treat a rare disease (affects less than 200,000 people in the United States, so the cost of development is not likely to be offset by sales) and for which the United States Food and Drug Administration (FDA) offers assistance and financial incentives to sponsors undertaking the development of the drugs], the following resources are available:
    a. *Drug Facts and Comparisons*
    b. The *National Information Center for Orphan Drugs and Rare Diseases (NICODARD)*
    c. *Drugdex*

  5. For an **unknown drug** (i.e., one that is in hand but not identified), chemical analysis can be performed or the drug can be identified by physical characteristics, such as color, special markings, and shape. Consult the following sources for help:
    a. The *PDR, Drug Facts and Comparisons, Drug Topics Red Book, Ident-A-Drug Reference*
    b. *Identidex (Micromedex)*
    c. The manufacturer
    d. A laboratory
    e. *Lexi-Comp's Clinical Reference Library-Drug Identification*

V. SEARCH STRATEGIES. To develop an effective search strategy for locating drug information literature, the following tactics should be followed after determining whether primary or secondary sources are desired.

A. Determine whether the question at hand is **clinical** or **research-related. Define the question** as specifically as possible. Also, identify appropriate index terms (also called key words or descriptors) with which to search for the information.

B. Determine the **type of information** and **how much** is needed (i.e., only one fact, the most recent journal articles, review articles, or a comprehensive database search).

C. Ascertain as much information as possible about the drug being questioned and the **inquirer's association** with it. Remember that data on adverse drug effects or drug interactions are often fragmented and inadequately documented. See IV A 2 for the specific drug information that should be acquired, and also determine answers to the following questions:

  1. What is the indication for the prescribed drug?

  2. Is the drug's use approved or unapproved? This information can be found in the following resources (remember to check how often these resources are updated to ensure having the latest information).
   a. Approved uses of drugs can be checked in:
      (1) *AHFS Drug Information* for the current year and in the year's supplements
      (2) *Drug Facts and Comparisons*
      (3) The *PDR*
      (4) *USP DI*
      (5) *Drugdex (Micromedex)*
      (6) *Clinical Pharmacology*
      (7) *Drug Information Handbook*
   b. Unapproved uses of drugs can be found in:
      (1) *AHFS Drug Information*
      (2) *Drug Facts and Comparisons*
      (3) *Martindale: The Extra Pharmacopoeia*
      (4) Medline
      (5) *Drugdex*
      (6) *Inpharma*
      (7) *USP DI*

  3. What is the age, sex, and weight of the patient in question?

  4. Does the patient have any other medical conditions or renal or hepatic disease?

  5. Is the patient taking any other medications?

  6. What drugs has the patient taken during the past 6 months, and what were the dosages?

  7. Did the patient experience any signs or symptoms of a possible adverse drug reaction? If so:
   a. How severe was the reaction?
   b. When did the reaction appear?
   c. Has the patient (or any member of the patient's family) experienced any allergic or adverse reactions to medications in the past?
   d. Consult the following resources for more information:
      (1) Meyler's *Side Effects of Drugs* (SEDBASE online)
      (2) A general drug reference
      (3) *Reactions* (ADIS)
      (4) Medline
   e. Also, the manufacturer of the drug may be a useful source for missing information. In exchange for information, most companies expect to receive an adverse drug reaction form.

  8. Did the patient experience any signs or symptoms of a drug interaction? If so:
   a. What were the specific drugs in question?
   b. What were the respective dosages of the drugs?

    c. What was the duration of therapy?

    d. What was the length of the course of administration?

    e. What are the details of the events secondary to the suspected reaction?

    f. Consult the following resources for more information:

        (1) A drug interactions reference [e.g., *Drug Interaction Facts,* Hansten's *Drug Interaction Analysis and Management, Evaluations of Drug Interactions (EDI)*]

        (2) A general drug reference (e.g., *PDR*)

        (3) *Reactions*

        (4) Medline

  9. What is the patient's current medication status?

  10. Does the patient have any underlying diseases?

  11. How has the patient been managed so far?

  12. What is the stability of the drug, and how is compatibility of the drug with other drugs, the administration technique, and the equipment that holds it? Resources to check for this information include:

    a. Trissel's *Handbook on Injectable Drugs*

    b. King's *Guide to Parenteral Admixtures*

    c. Trissel's *Stability of Compounded Formulations*

D. Explore other possible information resources if necessary. For example, it may be useful to find background material in textbooks (tertiary references), and then go to the journal literature (primary references) for more current information.

VI. EVALUATING A CLINICAL STUDY.
Resource identification is followed by a critical assessment of the available information. This step is critical in developing an appropriate response for the inquirer.

  A. Evaluate the objective of the study. Determine the aim of the research that was performed.

    1. What did the researchers intend to examine?

    2. Is this goal stated clearly (i.e., is the objective specific)?

    3. Was the research limited to a single objective, or were there multiple drugs or effects being tested?

  B. Evaluate the subjects of the study. Determine the profile of the study population by looking for the following information:

    1. Were healthy subjects or affected patients used in the study?

    2. Were the subjects volunteers?

    3. What were the criteria for selecting the subjects?

    4. How many subjects were included, and what is the breakdown of age, sex, and race?

    5. If a disease was being treated, did any of the subjects have diseases other than that initially being treated? Were any additional treatments given? Were there any contraindications to the therapy?

    6. What was the patient selection method, and who was excluded from the study?

    7. A patient selection review should be done. You will find that most groups of subjects are homogeneous (i.e., they all have comparable characteristics). If a disease state is studied, patients should exhibit similar severity of symptoms. Researchers wish to eliminate interpatient variability. By selecting patients with similar characteristics, researchers can avoid results that are caused by individual differences among patients. Strong individual differences can obscure the results of the experiment. If studying a group of patients that exhibits significant interpatient variability is necessary, researchers may divide the patients into groups according to the variables likely to be associated with responsiveness to therapy. This is known as stratification.

C. Evaluate the administration of the drug treatment. For each drug being investigated, determine the following information:

1. **Details of treatment** with the agent being studied:
   a. Daily dose
   b. Frequency of administration
   c. Hours of day when administered
   d. Route of administration
   e. Source of drug (i.e., the supplier)
   f. Dosage form
   g. Timing of drug administration in relation to factors affecting drug absorption
   h. Methods of ensuring compliance
   i. Total duration of treatment

2. **Other therapeutic measures** in addition to the agent being studied

D. Evaluate the setting of the study. Try to determine the environment of the study and the dates on which the trial began and ended. Look for the following information:

1. People who made the observations; various professionals who offer different and unique perspectives based on their backgrounds and interests (Were the same people making observations throughout the study?)

2. Whether the study was done on an inpatient or outpatient basis

3. Description of physical setting (e.g., hospital, clinic, ward)

4. Length of the study (i.e., dates on which the trial began and ended)

E. Evaluate the methods and design of the study. The method section of the research paper explains how the research was conducted. The study design (i.e., retrospective, prospective, blind, crossover) and the methods used to complete the study are important in judging whether the study and the results are reliable and valid. From the study, try to determine answers to the following questions:

1. Are the methods of assessing the therapeutic effects clearly described?

2. Were the methods standardized?
   a. **Retrospective versus prospective**
      (1) **Retrospective** studies look at events that have already occurred to find some common link between them, require reliance on patient memories and accurate medical records, and are unable to show cause and effect. Retrospective studies are useful for studying rare diseases (or effects) and can help to decide if enough information exists to warrant prospective examination of a problem.
      (2) **Prospective** studies look forward in time at a question the study seeks to answer. They can be observational or experimental (i.e., clinical trials).
   b. **Treatment allocation**
      (1) **Parallel** study design is a protocol in which two or more patient groups are studied concurrently. The groups are treated identically except for one variable, such as a drug therapy (Figure 21-1).
      (2) **Crossover** design may be used as an additional control for interpatient and intrapatient variability (Figure 21-2). In this type of design, each patient group undergoes each type of treatment. However, the sequence in which the subjects undergo treatment is reversed for one group. Crossover design reduces the possibility that the results were strongly influenced by the order in which therapy was given. And because both groups of patients receive both types of treatment, any differences in responsiveness between the groups due to patient selection will be uncovered.

3. Were **control measures** used to reduce variation that might influence the results? Examples of such control methods include:
   a. Concurrent controls
   b. Stratification or matched subgroups
   c. A run-in period
   d. The patient as his or her own control (i.e., crossover design)
   e. Identical ancillary treatment

    4. Were controls used to reduce bias? Examples of such controls include:
      a. Blind assessment, which means that the people observing the patients do not know who is a subject and who is a control
      b. Blind patients, which means that the patients do not know whether they received the substance being studied or a placebo [**double-blind** combines points a and b] (Table 21-3)
      c. Random allocation, which means that patients involved in the study have an even chance of being assigned to either the group of subjects receiving the active drug or the group receiving a placebo
      d. Matching dummies, which are placebos that are physically identical to the active agent being studied
      e. Comparison of a placebo or a therapy to a recognized standard practice

F. Evaluate the analysis of the study. After looking at specific areas of the study separately, gather the information together to determine whether the trial is acceptable and the conclusions are justified by determining answers to the following questions (Figure 21-3):

    1. Were the subjects suitably selected in relation to the aim(s) of the study?

    2. Were the methods of measurement valid in relation to the aim(s) of the study?

    3. Were the methods adequately standardized?

    4. Were the methods sufficiently sensitive?

    5. Was the design appropriate?

    6. Were there enough subjects?

    7. Was the dosage appropriate?

Table 21-3. Types of Blind Studies

Types of Blinds	Patient Aware of Treatment	Physician Aware of Treatment
Open label (nonblind)	X	X
Single-blind	—	X
Double-blind	—	—

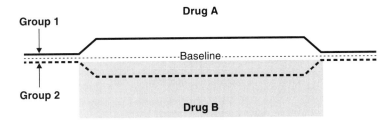

Figure 21-1. Parallel study design.

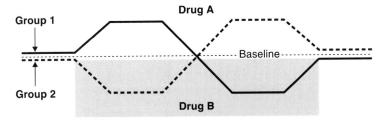

Figure 21-2. Crossover study design.

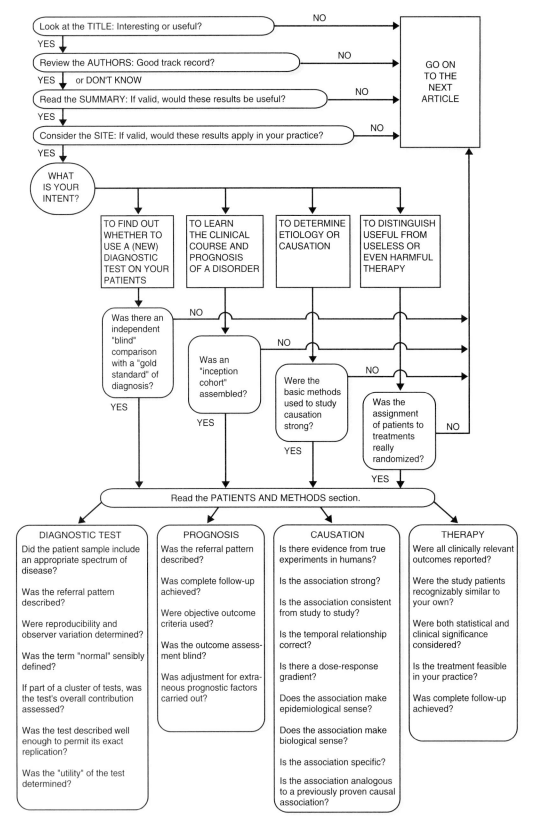

Figure 21-3. Evaluation of study analysis.

8. Was the duration of treatment adequate?

9. Were carryover effects avoided, or were compensations made for them?

10. If no controls were used, were they unnecessary or overlooked?

11. If controls were used, were they adequate?

12. Was the comparability of treatment groups examined?

13. Are the data adequate for assessment?

14. If statistical tests were not done, were they unnecessary or overlooked?

15. If statistical tests are reported, assess the following:
    a. Is it clear how the statistical tests were done?
    b. Were the tests appropriately used?
    c. If results show no significant difference between test groups, were there enough patients (i.e., statistical power)?

VII. GENERAL GUIDELINES FOR RESPONSES TO DRUG INFORMATION REQUESTS

A. Do not guess!

B. Responses to a member of the public must take several ethical issues into account.

1. Patient privacy must be protected.

2. Professional ethics must be maintained.

3. The patient–physician relationship cannot be breached.

4. Response is not necessary if the inquirer intends to misuse or abuse information that is provided. The inquirer often admits intent or offers clues to potential abuse, such as in the following examples:
   a. A patient asks how a certain drug is dosed (i.e., how much the drug can be increased, when it can be increased, what the maximum daily dose is). This kind of inquiry signals that the patient might be adjusting his or her own therapy.
   b. A patient asks a pharmacist to identify a tablet that is a prescription product known for a high rate of abuse.

C. Organize information before attempting to communicate the response to the inquirer. Anticipate additional questions.

D. Tailor the response to the inquirer's background. Also, consider the environment of the practice, institutional policy and procedure, and formulary.

E. Inform the inquirer where the information was found. Exercise caution with statements such as, "There are no reports in the literature."

F. Use **extreme** caution with statements such as, "I recommend ..." Do not hesitate to refer consumers to their physicians.

G. Use more than abstracts to answer drug information questions because they might be taken out of context and do not include all of the data available in the original article.

H. Alert the inquirer of a possible delay when it takes longer than anticipated to answer the question.

I. Ask if the information that is provided answers the inquirer's questions.

J. Ask if the inquirer wishes to have reprints of articles or a written response.

22
Adverse Drug Reaction Reporting

Barbara Szymusiak-Mutnick

I. **INTRODUCTION.** Adverse drug reactions (ADRs) are a cause of significant morbidity and mortality in patients in all arenas of health care today. There is wide variation in the current health-care literature, but it has been estimated that from one-third to as high as one-half of ADRs are believed to be preventable. The Institute of Medicine reported in January 2000 that an estimated 7000 deaths occur each year due to adverse drug events. Other studies estimate significantly higher numbers of deaths. The cost of morbidity and mortality due to drug-related events was recently estimated to be $136 billion annually. The suffering that patients experience because of drug-related events cannot be quantified.

II. **DEFINITIONS.** The terms adverse drug reaction, adverse drug event, untoward drug reaction, drug misadventure, side effect, or drug-related problem are many times used interchangeably but do not always describe the same situation.

   A. **Adverse drug reaction** is defined by the World Health Organization as "one which is noxious and unintended, and which occurs at doses normally used in man for the prophylaxis, diagnosis, or therapy of disease, or for the modification of physiological function."

   B. The United States Food and Drug Administration's (FDA) definition of **adverse drug event** is "any adverse event associated with the use of a drug in humans, whether or not considered drug related, including the following: an adverse event occurring in the course of the use of a drug in professional practice; an adverse event occurring from a drug overdose, whether accidental or intentional; an adverse event occurring from drug abuse; an adverse event occurring from drug withdrawal; and any significant failure of expected pharmacological action."

III. **TYPES**

   A. **Type A**

      1. Type A reactions are extensions of the drug's known pharmacology and are responsible for the majority of ADRs.

      2. Type A reactions are usually dose dependent and predictable but can be due to concomitant disease states, drug–drug interactions, or drug–food interactions.

      3. Ways to minimize type A reactions include understanding the pharmacology of the drug being prescribed, monitoring drugs with a narrow therapeutic window, and avoiding polypharmacy when possible.

   B. **Type B**

      1. Type B reactions include idiosyncratic reactions, immunological or allergic reactions, and carcinogenic/teratogenic reactions.

      2. Type B reactions are usually not due to a known pharmacology of the drug, but seem to be a function of patient susceptibility. They are rarely predictable, are usually not dose dependent, and seem to concentrate in certain body systems such as the liver, blood, skin, kidney, nervous system, and other body systems.

      3. Type B reactions are uncommon but are generally very serious and can be life-threatening.

      4. Except for immediate hypersensitivity reactions, type B reactions usually take 5 days before the patient demonstrates hypersensitivity to a drug. There is no maximum time for the occurrence of a reaction, but most occur within 12 weeks of initiation of therapy.

IV. RECOGNITION

A. Drugs must always be considered as a possible cause of disease or symptoms that are among a patient's list of complaints. Complete drug histories, including nonprescription drugs, must also be carried out.

B. Recognition is often subjective, and it is not always possible to demonstrate strong causality between the drug and the occurrence.

    1. Several factors may help in assessing the determination of causality.
      a. Did the patient actually ingest the drug in question?
      b. Did the onset of symptoms occur after the drug was taken?
      c. What is the time interval between taking the drug and the onset of symptoms?
      d. Did the symptoms resolve or improve after the drug was stopped or the dose decreased?
      e. Did the symptoms reoccur after the drug was reintroduced?
      f. Did drug–drug interactions contribute to the symptoms?
      g. Were the drugs measured in "toxic levels" in the patient's serum?
      h. Has this reaction been previously seen with use of the drug?
      i. What is the personal experience of the clinician with previous use of the drug and reactions secondary to the drug?

    2. Nomograms have been developed to aid in the assessment of causality.

V. SURVEILLANCE PROGRAMS.
Pharmacists, as well as all health-care professionals, should take an active role in monitoring, reporting, and trending ADR information. Some of the activities involved in a concurrent and ongoing ADR surveillance program at an institutional level include some of the following components:

A. Pharmacy departments should take the lead in the collection of information and should submit all reviews and reports to the Pharmacy and Therapeutics Committees for review and evaluation.

    1. Encourage all health-care professionals to be involved in reporting.

    2. Monitor patients using high-risk agents.

    3. Review patients who have received "antidote" type drugs.

    4. Notify prescribers of suspected ADRs, and encourage thorough documentation of the description of the reaction as well as the outcome in patients' medical records.

    5. Report appropriately identified ADRs to the FDA.

    6. Develop the use of pharmacy computer systems to track ADRs.

B. Evaluation of the causes of ADRs should be done. ADR report information should be used for educational purposes and identification of drug use and medication use processes to prevent further occurrences of ADRs. ADR reporting information should be incorporated into institutional Quality Improvement Programs.

VI. REPORTING TO THE FDA.
Three of the five major centers at the FDA are involved with evaluating the safety and efficacy of drugs. The largest center is the Center for Drug Evaluation and Research (CDER), which oversees both prescription and nonprescription [over-the-counter (OTC) drugs.] CDER established the Adverse Events Reporting System (AERS). Annually, the AERS receives about 250,000 reports of adverse experiences possibly associated with drugs. The Center for Biological Evaluation and Research (CBER) ensures the safety and efficacy of blood products, vaccines, allergenics, biological therapeutics, somatic cell therapy, gene therapy, and banked human tissue. The Center for Food Safety and Applied Nutrition (CFSAN) established the CFSAN Adverse Events Reporting Systems (CAERS) in 2002. The CAERS provides a monitoring system to identify potentially serious problems secondary to non–FDA-approved herbs, minerals, vitamins, dietary supplements, and other substances.

A. VAERS is the national Vaccine Adverse Event Reporting System coadministered by the Department of Health and Human Services (DHHS), the CBER of the FDA, and the Centers for Disease Control and Prevention (CDC). More than 10 million vaccines are given to children and many million more doses to adults each year. Although vaccines protect many people from dangerous diseases, they do have the potential to cause adverse effects.

1. The National Childhood Vaccine Injury Act (NCVIA) of 1989 requires health professionals and manufacturers of the vaccines to report to the DHHS adverse events following the administration of vaccines specified in the act, as described in the Table of Reportable Events Following Vaccination. In 1990, the VAERS was set up to receive all reports of suspected adverse events caused by any U.S. licensed vaccine (Figure 22-1).

2. The VAERS depends on voluntary reporting by health professionals to:
    a. Identify rare adverse reactions not detected in prelicensing studies
    b. Monitor for increases in already known reactions
    c. Identify risk factors or preexisting conditions that promote reactions
    d. Identify particular vaccine lots with unusually high rates or unusual types of events

B. MedWatch, the FDA's Medical Products Reporting Program, is a voluntary system for health-care providers (Figure 22-2) established in 1993. However, manufacturers and distributors of FDA-approved drugs, biologics, radiation-emitting devices, special nutritional products, dietary supplements, infant formulas, and devices are mandated to report problems to the FDA. The goals of the program are to increase awareness of reporting of medical-product–induced diseases and the importance of reporting, to clarify what should be reported, to make reporting as easy as possible, and to provide feedback to health professionals.

1. **Importance of reporting**
    a. The incidence of ADRs occurs at a high rate in health care today.
        (1) Generally, it is reported that 3%–11% of all hospital admissions can be attributable to ADRs, although some studies report the figure to be as high as 29%.
        (2) The likelihood that a patient will experience an ADR while hospitalized is reported in the literature to be in a range from 1%–44%.
    b. Prevention of ADRs is an important strategy in health care. It has been estimated that at least one-third of all ADRs may be preventable. It has been further noted that preventable ADRs tend to be the most costly to treat and cause the greatest degree of patient morbidity.
        (1) Future ADRs can be prevented in individual patients by careful and consistent documentation in patient records.
        (2) A program that tracks ADRs can help discover previously unidentified trends. These trends can be used within the institution to develop programs of prospective intervention to prevent reoccurrence of the reaction in the patient populations that are at similar risk.
    c. Recognition of previously undiscovered ADRs attributable to a drug is particularly true in the case of newly marketed products.
        (1) Although clinical trials are generally effective in assessing efficacy and risk–benefit ratio, inherent limitations exist in premarketing trials.
            (a) The trials are usually relatively short in duration and do not effectively mimic the exposure patients would experience if using the drug as a chronically administered agent.
            (b) Drug–drug interactions and use in patients with concomitant disease states may not be tested for in these trials.
            (c) The small size of the trials (usually 3000–4000 individuals) is insufficient to detect rarely occurring adverse reactions.
    d. Prompt recall in cases of product problems are accomplished when the MedWatch Program is used to report product problems or device defects.

2. **What should be reported?**
    a. ADRs that are serious, even if causality is not proven, including:
        (1) A patient's death that is suspected of being a direct outcome of an ADR
        (2) A life-threatening event
        (3) An initial or prolonged hospitalization
        (4) A significant, persistent, or permanent change or disability/incapacity
        (5) A congenital anomaly (including those occurring in a fetus)

VACCINE ADVERSE EVENT REPORTING SYSTEM
24 Hour Toll Free Information 1-800-822-7967
P.O. Box 1100, Rockville, MD 20849-1100
VAERS
PATIENT IDENTITY KEPT CONFIDENTIAL

For CDC/FDA Use Only

VAERS Number _____

Date Received _____

Patient Name:

Vaccine administered by (Name):

Form completed by (Name):

Last   First   M.I.

Responsible
Physician _____
Facility Name/Address

Relation   ☐ Vaccine Provider   ☐ Patient/Parent
to Patient ☐ Manufacturer   ☐ Other
Address *(if different from patient or provider)*

Address

City   State   Zip

City   State   Zip

City   State   Zip

Telephone no. (___) _____

Telephone no. (___) _____

Telephone no. (___) _____

| 1. State | 2. County where administered | 3. Date of birth ___/___/___ mm dd yy | 4. Patient age | 5. Sex ☐ M ☐ F | 6. Date form completed ___/___/___ mm dd yy |

7. Describe adverse events(s) (symptoms, signs, time course) and treatment, if any

8. Check all appropriate:
☐ Patient died   (date ___/___/___ mm dd yy)
☐ Life threatening illness
☐ Required emergency room/doctor visit
☐ Required hospitalization (_____days)
☐ Resulted in prolongation of hospitalization
☐ Resulted in permanent disability
☐ None of the above

9. Patient recovered   ☐ YES ☐ NO ☐ UNKNOWN

10. Date of vaccination ___/___/___ mm dd yy AM   Time _____ PM

11. Adverse event onset ___/___/___ mm dd yy AM   Time _____ PM

12. Relevant diagnostic tests/laboratory data

13. Enter all vaccines given on date listed in no. 10

	Vaccine (type)	Manufacturer	Lot number	Route/Site	No. Previous Doses
a.	_____	_____	_____	_____	_____
b.	_____	_____	_____	_____	_____
c.	_____	_____	_____	_____	_____
d.	_____	_____	_____	_____	_____

14. Any other vaccinations within 4 weeks prior to the date listed in no. 10

	Vaccine (type)	Manufacturer	Lot number	Route/Site	No. Previous doses	Date given
a.	_____	_____	_____	_____	_____	_____
b.	_____	_____	_____	_____	_____	_____

15. Vaccinated at:
☐ Private doctor's office/hospital   ☐ Military clinic/hospital
☐ Public health clinic/hospital   ☐ Other/unknown

16. Vaccine purchased with:
☐ Private funds   ☐ Military funds
☐ Public funds   ☐ Other/unknown

17. Other medications

18. Illness at time of vaccination (specify)

19. Pre-existing physician-diagnosed allergies, birth defects, medial conditions(specify)

20. Have you reported this adverse event previously?
☐ No   ☐ To health department
☐ To doctor ☐ To manufacturer

Only for children 5 and under

22. Birth weight _____ lb. _____ oz.

23. No. of brothers and sisters

21. Adverse event following prior vaccination (check all applicable, specify)

	Adverse Event	Onset Age	Type Vaccine	Dose no. in series
☐ In patient	_____	_____	_____	_____
☐ In brother or sister	_____	_____	_____	_____

Only for reports submitted by manufacturer/immunization project

24. Mfr./imm. proj. report no.

25. Date received by mfr./imm.proj.

26. 15 day report?
☐ Yes ☐ No

27. Report type
☐ Initial ☐ Follow-Up

Health care providers and manufacturers are required by law (42 USC 300aa-25) to report reactions to vaccines listed in the Table of Reportable Events Following Immunization. Reports for reactions to other vaccines are voluntary except when required as a condition of immunization grant awards.

Form VAERS-1(FDA)

Figure 22-1. VAERS form for reporting possible adverse drug reactions.

    (6) An important medical event based upon appropriate medical judgment that may jeopardize the patient and may require intensive intervention to prevent the outcomes listed above

  b. Malfunctioning devices such as heart valves, latex gloves, dialysis machines, and ventilators, and problems with nutritional products

Figure 22-2. Form for FDA Medical Products Reporting Program.

c. Product problems that can result in compromised safety or quality. This includes product contamination, mislabeling, unclear labeling, poor packaging, potency problems, and questionable stability.

3. **Confidentiality** of both the reporter and the patients whose cases are reported are substantially protected by the FDA.

4. Reporting of problems with OTC medications are required when the product has been marketed with a New Drug Application (NDA), including drugs formerly marketed as prescription-only drugs. OTC products marketed without an NDA do not require reporting, but it is strongly encouraged. Approval of the FDA is not required for the marketing of nonprescription herbs, minerals, vitamins, dietary supplements, and other substances. Because the FDA does not approve these substances, efficacy and safety do not have to be demonstrated, nor is it mandated to report problems to the FDA.
   a. Voluntary reporting of non–FDA-approved dietary supplements, herbs, and vitamins to the FDA occurs through the MedWatch system and is subsequently forwarded to the CAERS.
   b. Information about previously reported problems can be viewed at the web site http://vm.cfsan.fda.gov/~dms/aemsfull.html or obtained through the CFSAN.

5. Reporting to manufacturers is not described in the FDA's guidelines, although a section of the MedWatch form can be checked off to inform the FDA that a copy of the report has been forwarded to the manufacturer by the reporter.

VII. **AMERICAN SOCIETY OF HEALTH-SYSTEMS PHARMACISTS (ASHP) GUIDELINES** define criteria for classifying an ADR as significant. They encourage reporting of serious or unexpected ADRs to the FDA, the manufacturer, or both.

VIII. **JOINT COMMISSION ON ACCREDITATION OF HEALTHCARE ORGANIZATIONS (JCAHO)** requirements for accreditation describe the need for each health-care organization to monitor for adverse events involving drugs and devices in a continual, collaborative fashion.

Information about the MedWatch Program can be obtained by phone at 1-800-FDA-1088.
Information about the VAERS can be obtained by phone at 1-800-822-7967.
Further information about the FDA's reporting systems and programs, such as the CDER, can be found on the FDA's web site (www.fda.gov).

STUDY QUESTIONS

Directions: Each of the numbered items or incomplete statements in this section is followed by answers or by completions of the statement. Select the **one** lettered answer or completion that is **best** in each case.

1. The following definition, "one which is noxious and unintended, and which occurs at doses normally used in man for the prophylaxis, diagnosis, or therapy of disease, or for the modification of physiological function," describes

(A) a side effect
(B) an adverse drug reaction
(C) an adverse drug event

2. Type A reactions are characterized by which of the following?

(A) Idiosyncratic reactions
(B) A function of patient susceptibility
(C) Caused by drug–drug interactions
(D) All of the above
(E) None of the above

3. The MedWatch form is NOT the appropriate form to report which of the following events?

(A) A vaccine event described in the VAERS Reportable Events table
(B) An event caused by a drug that required an intervention to prevent permanent damage
(C) A malfunctioning ventilator
(D) A drug that is contained in a package with unclear labeling
(E) None of the above

4. Preventable ADRs

(A) generally display mild symptoms
(B) are always easily recognized
(C) are problems that are easily medically managed
(D) All of the above
(E) None of the above

5. Reporting problems with vitamins to the FDA is required by law in which of the following situations?

(A) When the product has been marketed with a New Drug Application (NDA)
(B) When the problem is discovered by the consumer
(C) When safety and efficacy has been proven by manufacturers to the FDA
(D) When a health-care professional discovers the problem
(E) None of the above

ANSWERS AND EXPLANATIONS

1. The answer is B *[II A].*
This is the definition by the World Health Organization.

2. The answer is C *[III A 2].*
Type A reactions can be caused by drug–drug interactions. Idiosyncratic reactions and reactions caused by patient susceptibility are generally in the classification of Type B reactions.

3. The answer is A *[VI A].*
All the others are reportable on the MedWatch form. The National Childhood Vaccine Injury Act of 1989 requires the use of a VAERS form to report vaccine-related injuries.

4. The answer is E *[VI B].*
Preventable ADRs can be the cause of serious medical problems that require intensive medical care. Although some preventable ADRs may appear obvious on review of a patient's medication history, this is not always the case.

5. The answer is E *[VI B 4].*
Marketing of these products does not depend on the manufacturers proving efficacy and safety of the products. No law requires reporting of subsequent problems. These products do not require an NDA. Although it is not required for health-care professionals to report problems, it is essential that voluntary reporting takes place.

23
Clinical Toxicology
John J. Ponzillo

I. OVERVIEW

A. This chapter is intended to provide the reader with an overview of the management of various toxic exposures. Emergency medical services (EMS) should be immediately contacted to provide advanced life support for patients with unstable vital signs resulting from a poisoning exposure. Additionally, these patients should be referred to a hospital for follow-up. As of September 2001, a nationwide toll-free poison center number became available. This number, (800) 222-1222, which is available 24 hours a day, should be used by health-care professionals and the general public when dealing with exposures to potentially toxic substances.

B. Definitions

1. **Clinical toxicology**—focuses on the effects of substances in patients caused by accidental poisonings or intentional overdoses of medications, drugs of abuse, household products, or various other chemicals

2. **Intoxication**—toxicity associated with any chemical substance

3. **Poisoning**—a clinical toxicity secondary to accidental exposure

4. **Overdose**—an intentional exposure with the intent of causing self-injury or death

C. Epidemiology. In 2000, more than 2 million accidental and intentional poisonings were reported to the American Association of Poison Control Centers (AAPCC). The majority of poison exposures (86.2%) were accidental. However, 920 of these exposures resulted in death. More information can be found at the AAPCC web site at http:www.aapcc.org.

D. Information resources

1. **Computerized databases**
   a. **Poisindex** is a computerized CD-ROM database that is updated quarterly and is a primary resource for poison control centers.
   b. **TOMES** (Toxicologic, Occupational Medicine and Environmental Series) provides information on industrial chemicals.

2. **Printed publications.** Textbooks and manuals provide useful information regarding the assessment and treatment of patients exposed to various substances, although their usefulness is limited by the lag time of information published in the primary literature reaching updated editions.
   a. Anderson IB, Benowitz NL, Blanc PD, Clark RF, et al. *Poisoning and Drug Overdose.* 3rd ed. Stamford, CT: Appleton and Lange, 1999.
   b. Ellenhorn MJ, ed. *Medical Toxicology: Diagnosis and Treatment of Human Poisonings.* 2nd ed. New York: Elsevier Science Publishing Co., 1997.
   c. Fraunfelder FT, Fraunfelder FW. *Drug-Induced Ocular Side Effects.* 5th ed. Butterworth-Heinemann, 2001.
   d. Goldfrank L, ed. *Toxicologic Emergencies.* 7th ed. Norwalk, CT: Appleton and Lange, 2002.
   e. Grant WM. *Toxicology of the Eye.* 4th ed. Springfield, IL: Charles C Thomas, 1995.
   f. Haddad LM, Shannon MW, Winchester JF, eds. *Clinical Management of Poisoning and Drug Overdose.* 3rd ed. Philadelphia: WB Saunders, 1998.
   g. Leikin JB, Paloucek FP. *Poisoning and Toxicology Compendium.* 3rd ed. Hudson, OH: Lexi-Comp, 2002.

3. **Internet**
   a. Centers for Disease Control and Prevention: www.cdc.gov
   b. FDA: www.fda.gov
   c. National Library of Medicine: www.nlm.nih.gov

      d. National Institute for Occupational Safety and Health (NIOSH): www.cdc.gov/niosh

      e. American Society of Health-System Pharmacists: www.ashp.org

    4. Poison control centers accredited by the AAPCC provide information to the general public and health-care providers. These centers are the most reliable and up-to-date sources of information, and as such, their phone numbers should be readily available.

II. GENERAL MANAGEMENT

  A. Supportive care and "ABCs." Evaluating and supporting vital functions (**a**irway, **b**reathing, and **c**irculation) are the mandatory first steps in the initial management of drug ingestions. After the patient is stabilized, the specific issue(s) of poison management should be addressed.[2]

  B. Treatment for patients with depressed mental status includes:

    1. To rule out or treat hypoglycemia, 50 mL of 50% dextrose in adults and 1 mL/kg in children, intravenously (IV)

    2. Thiamine 100 mg IV push (Glucose can precipitate the Wernicke-Korsakoff syndrome in thiamine-deficient patients.)

    3. Naloxone 0.4–2 mg IV push, if opiate ingestion is suspected

  C. Obtaining a history of exposure

    1. Identify the substance(s) ingested, the route of exposure, the quantity ingested, the amount of time since ingestion, signs and symptoms of overdose, and any associated illness or injury. **Corroborate** history and other physical evidence (e.g., pill containers) from prehospital providers.

    2. Neurological examination evaluates any seizures, alterations in consciousness, confusion, ataxia, slurred speech, tremor, headache, or syncope.

    3. Cardiopulmonary examination evaluates any syncope, palpitations, cough, chest pain, shortness of breath, or burning or irritation of the upper airway.

    4. Gastrointestinal (GI) examination evaluates any abdominal pain, nausea, vomiting, diarrhea, or difficulty in swallowing.

    5. Past medical history should include:
      a. Medications, including nonprescription substances
      b. Use of herbal medications
      c. Alcohol or drug abuse
      d. Psychiatric history
      e. Allergies
      f. Occupational or hobby exposures
      g. Travel
      h. Prior ingestions
      i. Social history with potential for domestic violence or neglect
      j. Last normal menstrual period or pregnancy

  D. Routine laboratory assessment

    1. Complete blood cell (CBC) count

    2. Serum electrolytes

    3. Blood urea nitrogen (BUN); serum creatinine (SCr)

---

[1]Note: Since the events of September 11, 2001, there has been an increased awareness regarding bioterrorism. While this chapter is not intended to review the management of biological or chemical warfare, the above-mentioned Web sites contain specific and updated links regarding the treatment of these exposures. The reader is encouraged to review this information.

[2]American College of Emergency Physicians. Clinical Policy for the Initial Approach to Patients Presenting with Altered Mental Status. *Ann Emerg Med* 1999;33:251–281.

4. Blood glucose

5. Urinalysis

6. Electrocardiogram (ECG)

7. Chest roentgenogram and/or **KUB**

E. Toxicology laboratory tests

1. **Advantages**
   a. Confirm or **determine** the presence of a particular agent
   b. **Predict** the anticipated toxic effects or severity of exposure to some poisons
   c. Confirm or **distinguish** differential or contributing diagnosis
   d. Occasionally help **guide therapy**

2. **Disadvantages**
   a. These tests cannot provide a specific diagnosis for all patients.
   b. All possible intoxicating agents cannot be screened.
   c. In critically ill patients, supportive treatment is needed before laboratory results of the toxicology screen are available.
   d. Laboratory drug-detection abilities differ.
   e. In general, only a **qualitative determination** of a substance or substances is necessary; however, **quantitative levels** of the following drugs are necessary to guide therapy:
      (1) Acetaminophen
      (2) Arsenic
      (3) Carbamazepine
      (4) Carboxyhemoglobin
      (5) Digoxin
      (6) Ethanol
      (7) Ethylene glycol
      (8) Iron
      (9) Lead
      (10) Lithium
      (11) Mercury
      (12) Methanol
      (13) Methemoglobin
      (14) Phenobarbital
      (15) Phenytoin
      (16) Salicylates
      (17) Theophylline
      (18) Valproic acid

F. Skin decontamination should be performed when percutaneous absorption of a substance may result in systemic toxicity or when the contaminating substance may produce local toxic effects (e.g., acid burns). The patient's clothing is removed, and the areas are irrigated with copious quantities of water. **Neutralization should not be attempted.** For example, neutralizing acid burns with sodium bicarbonate will produce an exothermic chemical reaction, thereby exacerbating the patient's condition.

G. Gastric decontamination may be attempted when supportive care is begun. GI decontamination involves removal of the ingestant with emesis or lavage, the use of activated charcoal potentially to bind any ingestants, and the use of cathartics to hasten excretion and thereby limit absorption.

1. **Emesis**
   a. **Contraindications**
      (1) Children younger than 6 months of age
      (2) Patients with central nervous system (CNS) depression or seizures
      (3) Patients who have ingested a strong acid, alkali, or a sharp object
      (4) Patients with compromised airway protective reflexes (including coma and convulsions)
      (5) Patients who have ingested some types of hydrocarbons or petroleum distillates
      (6) Patients who have ingested substances with an extremely rapid onset of action

(7) Patients with emesis following the ingestion
    b. Syrup of ipecac. Effects diminish with time. Data suggest that there are **NO** benefits following delayed administration. Consider ipecac if it can be administered within 60 minutes of the ingestion ***and only on the advice of a poison control center.***[3] Note: The use of ipecac has been declining due to concerns of safety and efficacy. The FDA is currently reviewing the role of ipecac in gastrointestinal decontamination. www.fda.gov accessed 12 June 2003.
        (1) Mechanism of action. The onset of emesis usually occurs within 30 minutes after syrup of ipecac. The effects last for approximately 2 hours and produce approximately three episodes of emesis in 60 minutes.
        (2) Dosages. Patients 6–12 months of age, 5–10 mL; patients 1–12 years of age, 15 mL; patients older than age 12 years, 30 mL. Each dose of syrup of ipecac should be followed with 120–240 mL of water. The patient should be upright to avoid accidental aspiration and should be supervised.
        (3) Adverse effects. Diarrhea, lethargy/drowsiness, and prolonged (>1 hour) emesis

  2. Gastric lavage
    a. Use. Gastric lavage is used in patients who are not alert or have a diminished gag reflex. This procedure should also be considered in patients who are seen early following massive ingestions. This procedure is ***contraindicated* in patients who have ingested acids, alkalis, or hydrocarbons. Additionally, patients should not receive gastric lavage if they are at risk for GI perforation or if they are combative.**
    b. Procedure. Patients are placed in the left lateral decubitus position. Lavage is performed after a cuffed endotracheal tube is in place to protect the airway. After aspiration of the gastric contents, 250–300 mL of tap water or saline is instilled and then aspirated. The sequence should be repeated until the return is continuously clear for at least 2 L.

  3. Activated charcoal adsorbs almost all commonly ingested drugs and chemicals and usually is administered to most overdose patients as quickly as possible. Commonly ingested substances not adsorbed include **ethanol, iron, lithium, cyanide, ethylene glycol, lead, mercury, methanol, organic solvents, potassium, strong acids,** and **strong alkalis.**
    a. Dosage. Activated charcoal is available as a colloidal dispersion with water or sorbitol. In **adults,** the dose of activated charcoal is 25–100 g; the dose in **children** 1–12 years of age is 25–50 g; the dose in children up to 1 year of age is 1 g/kg. Constipation has not been observed after the administration of a single dose of activated charcoal. **Multiple doses** of any cathartics should be avoided because they can cause electrolyte imbalances and/or dehydration. Toxic ingestions with drugs having an enterohepatic circulation (e.g., carbamazepine, theophylline, phenobarbital, tricyclic antidepressants, phenothiazines, digitalis) generally require that the charcoal be readministered every 6 hours to prevent reabsorption during recirculation.
    b. Adverse effects. Charcoal aspiration and empyema have been reported in the literature. As such, charcoal should be withheld if patients are vomiting. Bowel obstruction may occur with multiple doses of activated charcoal and/or patients who are receiving concomitant therapy with neuromuscular-blocking drugs.[4]

H. Whole-bowel irrigation has been shown to be effective under certain conditions, particularly when activated charcoal lacks efficacy. An isosmotic cathartic solution such as polyethylene glycol (Golytely, Colyte) is used. The dosage is 1–2 L/hr given orally or by nasogastric tube until the rectal effluent is clear.

I. Forced diuresis and **urinary pH manipulation** may be used to enhance the elimination of substances, whose elimination is primarily renal, if the substance has a relatively small volume of distribution with little protein binding. However, the use of these methods is associated with fluid and electrolyte disturbances.

  —**Alkaline diuresis** promotes the ionization of weak acids, thereby preventing their reabsorption by the kidney, which facilitates the excretion of these weak acids. This procedure has been

---

[3]American Academy of Clinical Toxicology; European Association of Poisons Centres and Clinical Toxicologists. Position Statement: Syrup of Ipecac. *Clin Toxicol* 1997;35:699–709.

[4]American Academy of Clinical Toxicology; European Association of Poisons Centres and Clinical Toxicologists. Position Statement: Single-Dose Activated Charcoal. *Clin Toxicol* 1997;35:721–741.

used in the management of patients who have ingested long-acting barbiturates such as phenobarbital or salicylic acid. Patients are given 50–100 mEq of sodium bicarbonate IV push, followed by a continuous infusion of 50–100 mEq of sodium bicarbonate in 1 L of 0.25%–0.45% normal saline, maintaining a urine pH of 7.3–8.5. Urine output should be 5–7 mL/kg/hr. **Complications** include metabolic alkalosis, hypernatremia, hyperosmolarity, and fluid overload.

J. Dialysis. In patients who fail to respond to the above measures of decontamination, hemodialysis, and to a lesser extent peritoneal dialysis, may enhance drug elimination. Substances that are removed by hemodialysis generally are water soluble, have a small volume of distribution (<0.5 L/kg), have a low molecular weight (<500 daltons), and are not significantly bound to plasma proteins. Hemodialysis usually is indicated for life-threatening ingestions of ethylene glycol, methanol, or paraquat. This technique also has been used to enhance the elimination of ethanol, theophylline, lithium, salicylates, and long-acting barbiturates.

K. Hemoperfusion is a technique in which anticoagulated blood is passed through (perfused) a column containing activated charcoal or resin particles. This method of elimination clears substances from the blood more rapidly than hemodialysis, but it does not correct fluid and electrolyte abnormalities, as does hemodialysis. Hemoperfusion, while more effective in removing phenobarbital, phenytoin, carbamazepine, methotrexate, and theophylline than hemodialysis, is less effective in removing ethanol or methanol. **Complications** of hemoperfusion include thrombocytopenia, leukopenia, hypocalcemia, hypoglycemia, and hypotension.

III. MANAGEMENT OF SPECIFIC INGESTIONS

A. Acetaminophen is an antipyretic–analgesic that can produce fatal hepatotoxicity in untreated patients through the generation of a toxic metabolite.

1. Available dosage forms. Acetaminophen is available in a variety of over-the-counter (OTC) and prescription drug products.

2. Toxicokinetics. Acetaminophen is well absorbed from the GI tract, has a half-life between 2 and 3 hours, and has less than 5% excreted unchanged in the urine, with the remainder metabolized in the liver by the cytochrome P450 system.

3. Clinical presentation
   a. Phase I (12–24 hours postingestion)—nausea, vomiting, anorexia, and diaphoresis
   b. Phase II (1–4 days postingestion)—asymptomatic
   c. Phase III (2–3 days in untreated patients)—nausea, abdominal pain, progressive evidence of hepatic failure, coma, and death

4. Laboratory data
   a. Serum acetaminophen levels. Patients with levels greater than 150, 70, or 40 mg/mL at 4, 8, or 12 hours after ingestion require antidotal therapy with *N*-acetylcysteine (NAC) according to the Rumack-Matthews nomogram.
   b. Baseline liver function tests should be done in all patients.
   c. Renal function tests, including a BUN and SCr, should be done.
   d. Coagulation studies include prothrombin time (PT), partial thromboplastin time (PTT), and bleeding time.

5. Treatment
   a. Adult patients who have ingested more than 7 grams or children who have ingested more than 100 mg/kg require treatment. Elderly or alcoholic patients have an increased susceptibility to acetaminophen hepatotoxicity.
   b. The recommended treatment is GI decontamination with syrup of ipecac or gastric lavage for patients presenting within 2 hours of ingestion.
   c. Antidotal therapy with NAC is indicated for patients with toxic blood levels of acetaminophen.
   (1) NAC dosage is 140 mg/kg as a loading dose followed by 70 mg/kg every 4 hours for a total of 17 doses. NAC is administered either orally or via a nasogastric tube. NAC (Mucomyst) 20% contains 200 mg/mL. Each dose must be diluted 1:3 in either cola or fruit juice to mask the unpleasant taste and smell. The dose of NAC should be repeated if the patient vomits within one half-hour of administration. Patients with severe nausea secondary to NAC may be pretreated with IV metoclo-

pramide 10 mg every 6 hours. Metoclopramide acts as an antiemetic while increasing the rate of NAC absorption.

(2) **IV NAC** is currently investigational for patients who are intolerant to oral NAC. Despite a shorter treatment period, IV NAC has produced a higher incidence of anaphylactoid reactions.

B. Alcohols

1. Ethylene glycol
  a. Available forms. Ethylene glycol commonly is used in antifreeze and windshield deicing solutions. This form is sometimes colorless and has a sweet taste.

  b. Toxicokinetics. Ethylene glycol is hepatically metabolized by alcohol dehydrogenase to glycolaldehyde, which is metabolized by aldehyde dehydrogenase to glycolic acid. Glycolic acid is converted to glyoxylic acid, whose most toxic metabolite is oxalic acid.

  c. Clinical presentation
    (1) **Stage I** (0.5–12 hours postingestion)—ataxia, nystagmus, nausea and vomiting, decreased deep tendon reflexes, and severe acidosis (more severe overdoses—hypocalcemic tetany and seizures, cerebral edema, coma, and death)
    (2) **Stage II** (12–24 hours postingestion)—tachypnea, cyanosis, tachycardia, pulmonary edema, and pneumonitis
    (3) **Stage III** (24–72 hours postingestion)—flank pain and costovertebral angle tenderness; oliguric renal failure

  d. Laboratory data may reveal severe metabolic acidosis, hypocalcemia, and calcium oxalate crystals in the urinalysis.

  e. Treatment
    (1) **Gastric lavage** is performed within 30 minutes of ingestion.
    (2) **IV ethanol (EtOH)**
      (a) **Indications** include an ethylene glycol level greater than 20 mg/dl, suspicion of ingestion pending level, or an anion gap metabolic acidosis with a history of ingestion, regardless of the level.
      (b) **EtOH dosage.** An EtOH level of at least 100 mg/dl should be maintained. Loading dose is 7.5–10 mL/kg of a 10% ethanol in dextrose 5% in water (d5w) over 1 hour followed by a maintenance infusion of 1.4 mL/kg/hr. Infusion rates may need to be increased in patients receiving hemodialysis.
    (3) **Fomepizole (Antizol)** is a potent inhibitor of alcohol dehydrogenase that can prevent the formation of the toxic metabolites of either methanol or ethylene glycol. Administer a **loading dose** of 15 mg/kg (up to 1 gram) in 100 mL of d5w or 0.9% NaCl infused over 30 minutes. **Maintenance doses:** 10 mg/kg every 14 hours for 4 doses, then increase to 15 mg/kg (to offset autoinduction phenomenon) until methanol or ethylene glycol levels are less than 20 mg/dl.
    (4) **Pyridoxine** (100 mg IV every day) and **thiamine** (100 mg IV every day) are cofactors that may convert glyoxylic acid to nonoxalate metabolites.
    (5) **Sodium bicarbonate** is used as needed to correct the acidosis.
    (6) **Hemodialysis.** EtOH infusion must be continued, and the rate of administration may need to be increased. **Indications** include ethylene glycol level more than 50 mg/dl, congestive heart failure, renal failure, or severe acidosis.

2. Methanol
  a. Available forms include gas-line antifreeze, windshield washer, and some sterno.

  b. Toxicokinetics. Alcohol dehydrogenase converts methanol to formaldehyde, which is then converted to formic acid.

  c. Clinical presentation
    (1) **Stage I**—euphoria, gregariousness, and muscle weakness for 6–36 hours, depending on the rate of formation of formic acid
    (2) **Stage II**—vomiting, upper abdominal pain, diarrhea, dizziness, headache, restlessness, dyspnea, blurred vision, photophobia, blindness, coma, cerebral edema, cardiac and respiratory depression, seizures, and death

  d. Laboratory data include severe metabolic acidosis, hyperglycemia, and hyperamylasemia.

  e. Treatment
    (1) **Gastric lavage.** Charcoal has not been shown to absorb alcohols.
    (2) **IV EtOH**

        (a) Indications include any peak methanol level greater than 20 mg/dl, a suspicious ingestion with a positive history, or any symptomatic patient with an anion gap acidosis.

        (b) Administration is the same as per ethylene glycol (see III B 1).

    (3) Folic acid administered at 1 mg/kg (maximum 50 mg) IV every 4 hours for 6 doses increases the metabolism of formate.

    (4) Fomepizole (Antizol) [see III B 1 e (3)]

    (5) Sodium bicarbonate is used for severe acidosis.

    (6) Hemodialysis is used for methanol levels greater than 50 mg/dl, severe and resistant acidosis, renal failure, or visual symptoms.

C. Anticoagulants[5,6,7]

  1. Heparin

    a. Available dosage forms include parenteral dosage forms for IV and subcutaneous administration.

    b. Toxicokinetics. Heparin has a half-life of 1–1.5 hours and is primarily metabolized in the liver.

    c. Clinical presentation. Look for any signs or symptoms of bleeding or bruising.

    d. Laboratory data. Obtain PTT, bleeding time, and platelet counts.

    e. Treatment

      (1) Stopping heparin administration for 1–2 hours and restarting therapy at a reduced dose can reverse mild over-anticoagulation.

      (2) Severe overdoses may require the administration of **protamine.** Protamine combines with heparin and neutralizes it. **One milligram of protamine neutralizes 100 units of heparin.** Protamine should be administered slowly, intravenously over 10 minutes. The maximum dose of protamine is 50 mg in any 10-minute period.

  2. Warfarin

    a. Available dosage forms include oral tablets and a solution for parenteral administration.

    b. Toxicokinetics. Warfarin is well absorbed following oral administration. Its mean half-life is 35 hours; protein binding is 99%, with a 5-day duration of activity. Vitamin K–dependent clotting factors begin to decline 6 hours after administration, but therapeutic anticoagulation may require several days.

    c. Clinical presentation includes minor bleeding, bruising, hematuria, epistaxis, and conjunctival hemorrhage. More serious bleeding includes GI, intracranial, retroperitoneal, and wound site.

    d. Laboratory data include PT, international normalized ratio (INR), and bleeding time.

    e. Treatment

      (1) If **PT** or **INR** is **slightly elevated,** withhold warfarin for 24–48 hours; then reinstitute therapy with a reduced dosage.

      (2) If **PT** or **INR** is **elevated** and **bleeding,** administer 10 mg of phytonadione (vitamin K) over 30 minutes. Patients who are bleeding may require the administration of blood products that contain clotting factors.

      (3) For mild over-anticoagulation, follow ACCP guidelines.

D. Antidepressants

  1. Tricyclic antidepressants (TCAs)

    a. Available forms include amitriptyline, nortriptyline, imipramine, desipramine, doxepin, protriptyline, and clomipramine.

    b. Toxicokinetics. The compounds are hepatically metabolized, undergo enterohepatic recirculation, are highly bound to plasma proteins, and have an elimination half-life of approximately 24 hours.

    c. Clinical presentation. Anticholinergic effects include mydriasis, ileus, urinary retention, and hyperpyrexia. **Cardiopulmonary toxicity** exhibits tachycardias, conduction blocks,

[5]Hirsh J, Dalen JE, Anderson DR, et al. Oral Anticoagulants: Mechanism of Action, Clinical Effectiveness, and Optimal Therapeutic Range. *Chest* 2001;119:8s–21s.

[6]Hirsh J, Warkentin TE, Shaughnessy SG, et al. Heparin and Low-Molecular-Weight Heparin: Mechanisms of Action, Pharmacokinetics, Dosing Considerations, Monitoring, Efficacy, and Safety. *Chest* 2001;119:64s–94s.

[7]Levine MN, Raskob G, Landefeld S, et al. Hemorrhagic Complications of Anticoagulant Treatment. *Chest* 2001;119:108s–121s.

hypotension, and pulmonary edema. **CNS manifestations** range from agitation and confusion to hallucinations, seizures, and coma.

    d. Laboratory data. Blood-level monitoring does not correlate well with clinical signs and symptoms of toxicity. Some authors suggest that electrocardiographic monitoring is a better guide to assessing the severity of ingestion.

    e. Treatment

        (1) GI decontamination. Syrup of ipecac is not recommended because patients may quickly become comatose and increase the risk of aspiration. **Activated charcoal** is given every 6 hours.

        (2) Alkalinization with sodium bicarbonate 1–2 mEq/kg to maintain an arterial pH of 7.45–7.55 decreases the free fraction of the absorbed toxins, while reversing some of the cardiac abnormalities.

        (3) Phenytoin and/or **benzodiazepines** may be required to control seizures. Phenytoin must be administered at a rate not exceeding 25 mg/min due to hypotensive side effects. (**Fosphenytoin** may be used because it has a lower incidence of hypotension than phenytoin.)

        (4) Physostigmine 2 mg IV over 1 minute may be used to reverse **severe** anticholinergic toxicity due to these drugs. **Because this antidote may cause asystole, the use of this antidote for TCA overdoses is declining.**

  2. Selective serotonin reuptake inhibitors (SSRIs)

    a. Available forms (nontricyclic agents) include fluoxetine, sertraline, and paroxetine.

    b. Toxicokinetics. SSRIs are well absorbed following oral administration. Peak levels occur within 2–6 hours. SSRIs are hepatically metabolized with a half-life between 8 and 30 hours.

    c. Clinical presentation includes mild symptomatology. Patients may become agitated, drowsy, or confused. Seizures and cardiovascular toxicity are rare.

    d. Laboratory data. ECG monitoring is recommended. Blood-level monitoring is not recommended.

    e. Treatment includes gastric lavage and supportive treatment.

E. Benzodiazepines

  1. Available forms include chlordiazepoxide, diazepam, flurazepam, midazolam, lorazepam, alprazolam, and triazolam.

  2. Toxicokinetics. These drugs are hepatically metabolized.

  3. Clinical presentation includes drowsiness, ataxia, and confusion. Fatalities are rare.

  4. Laboratory data. Drug-level monitoring is not indicated.

  5. Treatment

    a. Supportive treatment includes gastric emptying, activated charcoal, and a cathartic.

    b. Flumazenil is given 0.2 mg IV over 30 seconds; repeat doses of 0.5 mg over 30 seconds at 1-minute intervals for a maximum cumulative dose of 5 mg.

        (1) Flumazenil has a short elimination half-life.

        (2) Careful observation for **resedation** is necessary, especially for ingestions of long-acting benzodiazepines.

        (3) Flumazenil *is contraindicated in mixed overdose patients (particularly involving tricyclic antidepressants) in whom seizures are likely.*

F. β-adrenergic antagonists

  1. Available dosage forms. Class examples include propranolol, metoprolol, and atenolol. Oral and parenteral dosage forms are available.

  2. Toxicokinetics. All of the members within this class differ with regard to renal versus hepatic elimination, lipid solubility, and protein binding. Patients may become toxic due to changes in organ function.

  3. Clinical presentation includes hypotension, bradycardia, and atrioventricular block. Bronchospasm may occur, particularly with noncardioselective agents.

  4. Laboratory data include serum electrolytes and blood glucose (patients may become hypoglycemic).

5. Treatment
a. GI decontamination includes gastric lavage and activated charcoal.
b. Glucagon is given 50–150 μg/kg as a loading dose over 1 minute, followed by a continuous infusion of 1–5 mg/hr.
c. Epinephrine should be used cautiously in β-blocker overdoses. Unopposed α-receptor stimulation in the face of complete β-receptor block may lead to profound hypertension.

G. Calcium channel antagonists

1. **Available forms** include verapamil, diltiazem, and the dihydropyridine class (nifedipine derivatives).

2. **Toxicokinetics.** Onset of action is approximately 30 minutes, whereas the duration is 6–8 hours. Several compounds are available as sustained-release dosage forms, which may contribute to prolonged toxicity.

3. **Clinical presentation.** Hypotension is common to all classes. Bradycardia and atrioventricular block are more commonly seen with ingestions of verapamil or diltiazem. Pulmonary edema and seizures (verapamil) have been reported.

4. **Laboratory data** include ECG and serum electrolytes.

5. **Treatment**
   a. GI decontamination includes gastric lavage, activated charcoal, and whole-bowel irrigation (especially for ingestions with sustained-release products).
   b. Calcium. Calcium chloride 10% (10–20 mL) IV push is given for the management of hypotension, bradycardia, or heart block.
   c. Glucagon dosage is the same as for β-blocker overdose.

H. Cocaine

1. **Available forms** include alkaloid obtained from *Erythroxylon coca*.

2. **Toxicokinetics.** Cocaine is well absorbed following oral, inhalational, intranasal, and IV administration. Cocaine is metabolized in the liver and excreted in the urine.

3. **Clinical presentation** includes CNS and sympathetic stimulation (e.g., hypertension, tachypnea, tachycardia, nausea, vomiting, seizures). Death may result from respiratory failure, myocardial infarction, or cardiac arrest.

4. **Laboratory data** include cocaine and cocaine metabolite urine screens.

5. **Treatment** is **supportive:** benzodiazepines for seizures, labetalol for hypertension, and neuroleptics for psychosis.

I. Corrosives

1. **Available forms** include strong acids or alkalis.

2. **Toxicokinetics.** Corrosives are well absorbed following oral and inhalational administration.

3. **Clinical presentation.** These compounds produce burns on contact.

4. **Laboratory data.** Arterial blood gases (ABGs), chest radiographs, and at least 6 hours of observation are required for inhalation exposure.

5. **Treatment** is **decontamination.** Exposed skin must be irrigated with water. **Neutralization** should be **avoided** because these reactions are exothermic and will produce further tissue damage.

J. Cyanide

1. **Available forms** include industrial chemicals and some nail-polish removers.

2. **Toxicokinetics.** The drug is rapidly absorbed following oral or inhalation exposure.

3. **Clinical presentation** includes headache, dyspnea, nausea, vomiting, ataxia, coma, seizures, and death.

4. Laboratory data include cyanide levels, ABGs, electrolytes, and an ECG.

5. Treatment. A cyanide antidote kit is used. It contains the following:
   a. Amyl nitrite—pearls are crushed and held under the patient's nostrils
   b. Sodium nitrite 10 mL IV push—converts hemoglobin to methemoglobin, which binds the cyanide ion
   c. Sodium thiosulfate 50 mL of a 25% solution IV push—may be repeated if there is no response
   d. Oxygen
   e. Sodium bicarbonate—as needed for severe acidosis
   f. Hyperbaric oxygen—for patients not responding to above

K. Digoxin

1. Available dosage forms include oral and parenteral.

2. Toxicokinetics. Digoxin is well absorbed, is primarily renally eliminated, and has a half-life of 36–48 hours. Its volume of distribution is 7–10 L/kg. Equilibration between serum level and myocardial binding requires approximately 6–8 hours.

3. Clinical presentation includes confusion, anorexia, nausea, and vomiting in mild cases. In more severe cases, cardiac dysrhythmias are seen.

4. Laboratory data include serum digoxin levels, electrolytes, particularly serum potassium levels, and an ECG.

5. Treatment
   a. Decontamination by syrup of ipecac or activated charcoal is recommended.
   b. Supportive therapy includes managing hyper- or hypokalemia and inotropic support as needed.
   c. Digoxin-specific Fab antibodies. To determine the dosage, use the formula: Dose (vials) = [ingested digoxin (mg) $\times$ 0.8]/0.6. Each vial contains 40 mg of digoxin antibodies (Digibind) and should be reconstituted with 4 mL of sterile water.

L. Electrolytes

1. Magnesium
   a. Available dosage forms include oral, rectal, and parenteral. Magnesium-containing cathartics (e.g., magnesium citrate) have been reported to produce hypermagnesemia in patients receiving repetitive doses with activated charcoal.
   b. Toxicokinetics. Magnesium is found intracellularly and is renally eliminated.
   c. Clinical presentation
      (1) Mild—deep tendon reflexes may be depressed; lethargy and weakness
      (2) Severe—respiratory paralysis and heart block; prolonged PR, QRS, and QT intervals
   d. Laboratory data
      (1) Mild—more than 4 mEq/L
      (2) Severe—more than 10 mEq/L
   e. Treatment is **10% calcium chloride** 10–20 mL to temporarily antagonize the cardiac effects of magnesium. In severe cases, **hemodialysis** may be required.

2. Potassium
   a. Available dosage forms are oral and parenteral.
   b. Toxicokinetics. Potassium is primarily an intracellular cation. Changes in acid–base balance produce shifts in serum potassium values (e.g., a 0.1-unit increase in serum pH produces a 0.1–0.7 mEq/L decrease in serum potassium values).
   c. Clinical presentation includes cardiac irritability and peripheral weakness with minor increases. Cardiac dysrhythmias, including bradycardia, may progress to asystole.
   d. Laboratory data. ECG data include **peaked T waves** and prolongation of the QRS complex.
   e. Treatment
      (1) Calcium. Administer calcium chloride 10% 10–20 mL to antagonize the cardiac effects of hyperkalemia.
      (2) Sodium bicarbonate. 1–2 mEq/kg IV increases serum pH and causes an intracellular shift of potassium.

(3) Glucose and insulin. 50 mL of 50% dextrose and 5–10 units of regular insulin are administered via IV push to shift potassium from the extracellular fluid into the cells.

(4) Cation exchange resins bind potassium in exchange for another cation (sodium). **Sodium polystyrene sulfonate** (Kayexalate) is given 15 g/60 mL with 23.5% sorbitol in doses 15–30 g by mouth every 3–4 hours as needed until the hyperkalemia resolves. Alternatively, 50 g of sodium polystyrene sulfonate can be given rectally in 200 mL of sodium chloride as a retention enema.

(5) Hemodialysis is reserved for life-threatening hyperkalemia that does not respond to the above measures.

M. Iron (Fe)

1. **Available dosage forms.** Numerous OTC products are available. Toxicity is based on the amount of elemental iron ingested: sulfate salt 20% elemental Fe; fumarate salt 33% elemental Fe; and gluconate salt 12% elemental Fe.

2. **Toxicokinetics.** Iron is absorbed in the duodenum and jejunum.

3. **Clinical presentation**
   a. **Phase I**—nausea, vomiting, diarrhea, GI bleeding, hypotension
   b. **Phase II**—clinical improvement seen 6–24 hours postingestion
   c. **Phase III**—metabolic acidosis, renal and hepatic failure, sepsis, pulmonary edema, and death

4. **Laboratory data** include serum Fe levels, total iron-binding capacity (TIBC) **[is controversial],** ABGs, liver function tests (LFTs), hemoglobin, and hematocrit. Radiological evaluation of the abdomen notes the presence of radiopaque pills.

5. **Treatment**
   a. **Decontamination.** For ingestions greater than 30 mg/kg, ipecac emesis may be used if administered within a few minutes of exposure. Gastric lavage using sodium bicarbonate is of questionable efficacy. Whole-bowel irrigation is used for large ingestions.
   b. **Supportive treatment**
   c. **Deferoxime** is used to chelate iron. Administer 25–50 mg/kg up to a dose of 1 g, and observe for a red color in the urine. Then administer at a rate of 15 mg/kg/hr up to a maximum dose of 6 g/day. Continue until serum iron is within the therapeutic range.

N. Isoniazid (INH)

1. **Available dosage forms** include oral and parenteral.

2. **Toxicokinetics.** INH is well absorbed orally. Peak levels are within 1–2 hours postingestion. Isoniazid is hepatically metabolized.

3. **Clinical presentation** includes nausea, vomiting, slurred speech, ataxia, generalized tonic–clonic seizures, and coma.

4. **Laboratory data** include severe lactic acidosis, hypoglycemia, mild hyperkalemia, and leukocytosis.

5. **Treatment**
   a. **Decontamination.** Avoid emesis because patients are at high risk for developing seizures; for severe ingestions use activated charcoal gastric lavage.
   b. **Pyridoxine,** which reverses INH-induced seizures, is given in gram doses equivalent to the amount of isoniazid ingested. Pyridoxine is mixed as a 10% solution in D5W and infused over 30–60 minutes.
   c. **Sodium bicarbonate** corrects the acidosis.

O. Lead

1. **Available forms** include lead-containing paint or gasoline fume inhalation.

2. **Toxicokinetics.** Lead has slow distribution, with a half-life of approximately 2 months.

3. **Clinical presentation** includes nausea, vomiting, abdominal pain, peripheral neuropathies, convulsions, and coma.

4. **Laboratory data** include anemia and an elevated blood-lead level.

5. Treatment
   a. **Edetate Calcium Disodium** is given 50–75 mg/kg/day intramuscularly (IM) or slow IV in 4 divided doses.
   b. **Dimercaprol** is given 4 mg/kg IM every 4 hours for 3–5 days.

P. Lithium

1. **Available dosage forms** include liquid, capsules, and tablets (immediate- and sustained-release).

2. **Toxicokinetics.** Lithium is well absorbed following oral administration. It is not appreciably bound to plasma proteins and has a small volume of distribution (V_d) [0.5 L/kg]. Elimination is renal, with a half-life of 14–24 hours.

3. **Clinical presentation**
   a. **Mild intoxication:** polyuria, blurred vision, weakness, slurred speech, ataxia tremor, and myoclonic jerks
   b. **Severe intoxication:** delirium, coma, seizures, and hyperthermia

4. **Laboratory data**
   a. Therapeutic range: 0.6–1.2 mEq/L
   b. Mild toxicity: 1.5–2.5 mEq/L
   c. Moderate toxicity: 2.5–3 mEq/L
   d. Severe toxicity: more than 3 mEq/L

5. **Treatment**
   a. **Supportive** care, including basic life support and fluid and electrolyte replacement
   b. **Decontamination**
      (1) **Syrup of ipecac** only if administered within a few minutes after exposure
      (2) **Activated charcoal** ineffective
      (3) **Sodium polystyrene sulfonate** has been effective in experimental models. Need to monitor potassium levels.
      (4) **Whole-bowel irrigation** for large ingestions, especially those involving sustained-release products
      (5) **Hemodialysis** for severely symptomatic patients with acute exposure levels greater than 2.5 mEq/L or chronic levels greater than 1.5 mEq/L. **Note:** Lithium levels may rise after dialysis due to a rebound effect.

Q. Opiates

1. **Available dosage forms** include oral immediate-release and sustained-release preparations as well as parenteral agents.

2. **Toxicokinetics.** Some agents have prolonged elimination half-lives (e.g., heroin, methadone).

3. **Clinical presentation** includes respiratory depression and a decreased level of consciousness. Rare effects include hypotension, bradycardia, and pulmonary edema. Seizures have been reported in patients with renal dysfunction who are receiving meperidine due to the accumulation of the metabolite normeperidine.

4. **Laboratory data** include baseline ABGs and toxicology screens.

5. **Treatment**
   a. **Naloxone** is given 0.4–2 mg every 5 minutes up to 10 mg and 0.03–0.1 mg/kg in pediatric patients. Naloxone has a very short half-life, and resedation is a concern in patients overdosing on long-acting opioids or sustained-release dosage forms.
   b. **Nalmefene** has a half-life of approximately 4–8 hours. Initial dosages are 0.5 mg/70 kg. A follow-up dose 2–5 minutes later is 1 mg/70 kg.

R. Organophosphates

1. **There are a variety of available forms;** they are usually pesticides or chemical warfare agents.

2. **Toxicokinetics.** Organophosphates are absorbed through the lungs, skin, GI tract, and conjunctiva.

3. **Clinical presentation** includes excessive cholinergic stimulation.

4. **Laboratory data** include red blood cell acetylcholinesterase activity.

5. **Treatment**
   a. **Decontamination**
   b. **Atropine** is given 0.5–2 mg IV to reverse the peripheral muscarinic effects.
   c. **Pralidoxime (2-PAM)** is given 1 g IV over 2 minutes and repeated in 20 minutes as needed.

S. Salicylates

1. **Available dosage forms** include a variety of OTC products: oral, rectal, and topical.

2. **Toxicokinetics.** Salicylates are well absorbed following oral administration. The half-life is 6–12 hours at lower doses. In overdose situations, the half-life may be prolonged to more than 20 hours.

3. **Clinical presentation** includes nausea, vomiting, tinnitus, and malaise (mild toxicity). Lethargy, convulsions, coma, and metabolic acidosis appear in more severe overdoses. Potential **complications** from therapeutic and toxic doses include GI bleeding, increased PT, hepatic toxicity, pancreatitis, and proteinuria.

4. **Laboratory data** for the following 6-hour postingestion levels are:
   a. 40–60 mg/dl—tinnitus
   b. 60–95 mg/dl—moderate toxicity
   c. More than 95 mg/dl—severe toxicity
   d. With the presence of acidemia and aciduria, evaluate ABGs
   e. Additionally, laboratory evaluation may show leukocytosis, thrombocytopenia, increased or decreased serum glucose and sodium, hypokalemia, and increased serum BUN, creatinine, and ketones.

5. **Treatment**
   a. **Decontamination** includes emesis with syrup of ipecac if administered within 30 minutes of exposure at home. Repetitive doses of activated charcoal every 6 hours with 1 dose of cathartic for patients ingesting greater than 150 mg/kg. Whole-bowel irrigation for large ingestions.
   b. **Alkaline diuresis** is given as above to enhance salicylate excretion. This is indicated for levels greater than 40 mg/dl.
   c. **Hemodialysis** is used for severe intoxications when serum levels are greater than 100 mg/dl. This method of decontamination is much better than repetitive doses of activated charcoal.
   d. **Fluid** and **electrolyte** replacement is administered as needed.
   e. **Vitamin K** and **fresh frozen plasma** are used to correct any coagulopathy.

T. Snake bites

1. **Types.** There are numerous species of snakes found worldwide. The venomous snakes found in North America include the following: rattlesnake, cottonmouth, copperhead, and coral. While patients may be exposed to more exotic snakes, a herpetologist should be consulted for a more definitive identification.

2. **Toxicokinetics.** Onset of symptomatology depends on the species of snake and the patient's underlying medical condition.

3. **Clinical presentation** includes nausea, vomiting, diarrhea, syncope, tachycardia, and cold, clammy skin. Local findings include pain, edema, and erythema. More severe envenomations can lead to severe tissue injury, compartment syndrome, and shock.

4. **Laboratory data**
   a. CBC and platelet count
   b. Coagulation profile
   c. Fibrin degradation products
   d. Electrolytes
   e. BUN, SCr, and urinalysis

5. Treatment

a. Supportive. Move the patient away from striking distance of the snake. Ideally, the patient should be transported to a medical facility as soon as possible. Constrictive clothing, rings, watches, etc. should be removed. Tetanus immunization should be assessed, and surgical intervention may be necessary for severe cases.

b. Antivenoms

(1) Antivenin (Crotalidae) polyvalent is a horse-derived product that has been reported to produce allergic reactions. For mild bites, the recommended dose is 5–10 vials; moderate, 10–20; and severe envenomations may require 20 or more vials.

(2) Crotalidae polyvalent immune Fab is a polyvalent antivenin made from sheep sources. The initial dose is 4–6 vials diluted in 250 mL of 0.9% NS administered over 1 hour. Additional doses may be required for severe envenomations.

U. Theophylline

1. **Available dosage forms** include liquid, sustained-release tablets and capsules, as well as parenteral forms.

2. **Toxicokinetics.** Well absorbed orally with a V_d of approximately 0.5 L/kg. Theophylline is hepatically metabolized and has a half-life of approximately 4–8 hours. Theophylline clearance is highly dependent on age, concomitant disease states, and interacting drugs.

3. **Clinical presentation** includes nausea, vomiting, seizures, and cardiac dysrhythmias. Chronic toxicity carries a poorer prognosis than acute toxicity.

4. **Laboratory data.** Therapeutic theophylline levels are 5–20 μg/mL. Hyperglycemia and hypokalemia are seen with acute ingestions. Other useful laboratory tests include serum electrolytes, BUN, creatinine, hepatic function, and ECG monitoring.

5. **Treatment**

a. Supportive therapy includes maintaining an airway and treating seizures and dysrhythmias as they occur.

b. Decontamination. Syrup of ipecac only if administered within a few minutes of the ingestion. **Activated charcoal** (repetitive doses) to enhance elimination. **Whole-bowel irrigation** for massive ingestions (especially with sustained-release products). **Charcoal hemoperfusion** is utilized in unstable patients who are in status epilepticus. **Hemodialysis** is used when hemoperfusion is unavailable.

c. β-adrenergic antagonists (e.g., esmolol) are used to treat the hypotension, tachycardia, and dysrhythmias caused by elevated cyclic adenosine monophosphate levels.

IV. References

A. American Academy of Clinical Toxicology; European Association of Poisons Centres and Clinical Toxicologists. Position Statement: Single-Dose Activated Charcoal. *Clin Toxicol* 1997;35: 721–741.

B. American Academy of Clinical Toxicology; European Association of Poisons Centres and Clinical Toxicologists. Position Statement: Syrup of Ipecac. *Clin Toxicol* 1997;35:699–709.

C. American College of Emergency Physicians. Clinical Policy for the Initial Approach to Patients Presenting with Acute Toxic Ingestion or Dermal or Inhalation Exposure. *Ann Emerg Med* 1999;33:735–762.

D. American College of Emergency Physicians. Clinical Policy for the Initial Approach to Patients Presenting with Altered Mental Status. *Ann Emerg Med* 1999;33:251–281.

E. Bond RC. The Role of Activated Charcoal and Gastric Emptying in Gastrointestinal Decontamination: A State-of-the-Art Review. *Ann Emerg Med* 2002;39:273–285.

F. Gold BS, et al. Bites of Venomous Snakes. *New Engl Med* 2002;347:347–356.

G. Hirsh J, Dalen JE, Anderson DR, et al. Oral Anticoagulants: Mechanism of Action, Clinical Effectiveness, and Optimal Therapeutic Range. *Chest* 2001;119:8s–21s.

H. Hirsh J, Warkentin TE, Shaughnessy SG, et al. Heparin and Low-Molecular-Weight Heparin: Mechanisms of Action, Pharmacokinetics, Dosing Considerations, Monitoring, Efficacy, and Safety. *Chest* 2001;119:64s–94s.

I. Levine MN, Raskob G, Landefeld S, et al. Hemorrhagic Complications of Anticoagulant Treatment. *Chest* 2001;119:108s–121s.

J. Litovitz TL, Klein-Schwartz, Rodgers GC, et al. 2001 Annual Report of the American Association of Poison Control Centers Toxic Exposure Surveillance System. *Am J Emerg Med* 2002;20:1–62.

K. Mokhlesi B, Leiken JB, Murray P, et al. Adult Toxicology in Critical Care Part 1: General Approach to the Intoxicated Patient. *Chest* 2003;123:577–592.

L. Mokhlesi B, Leiken JB, Murray P, et al. Adult Toxicology in Critical Care Part 2: General Approach to the Intoxicated Patient. *Chest* 2003;123:897–922.

M. Paloucek F. Antidotal flumazenil use—the protamine of the 90s. *Crit Care Med* 1999; 27:10–11.

STUDY QUESTIONS

Directions: Each of the numbered items or incomplete statements in this section is followed by answers or by completions of the statement. Select the **one** lettered answer or completion that is **best** in each case.

1. A physician receives a call from the parent of a 2-year-old child who has ingested an unknown quantity of morphine controlled-release tablets and is now unconscious. The physician's initial recommendation is

(A) To call EMS and have the child taken to the hospital emergency department
(B) Administer 1 g/kg of activated charcoal with sorbitol
(C) Administer syrup of ipecac 15 mL by mouth to induce vomiting
(D) Suggest that the child receive emergency hemodialysis
(E) Suggest that the child receive acid diuresis with ammonium chloride

2. A 3-year-old child ingests an unknown quantity of Draino, which is a liquid caustic. The patient's parents question the physician as to whether to administer syrup of ipecac. The physician should recommend which of the following treatments?

(A) Administer 15 mL of syrup of ipecac.
(B) Give the child some water or juice to drink.
(C) Administer thiamine 100 mg IV push.

3. An unconscious patient is brought into the emergency department. The patient is given 50 mL of 50% dextrose in water, thiamine 100 mg IV, followed by naloxone 1 mg, at which point he awakens. This patient most likely has overdosed on which of the following substances?

(A) Methanol
(B) Amitriptyline
(C) Cocaine
(D) Haloperidol
(E) Heroin

4. Contraindications to the administration of syrup of ipecac include which of the following?

(A) An unconscious patient
(B) A patient who is experiencing a generalized tonic–clonic seizure
(C) A patient who has ingested a caustic substance
(D) All of the above
(E) None of the above

5. An unconscious patient is brought to the emergency department with a history of an unknown drug overdose. Which of the following actions should the physician perform?

(A) Administer 50 mL of 50% dextrose, thiamine 100 mg IV push, and naloxone 0.8 mg IV push
(B) Protect the patient's airway and ensure that vital signs are stable
(C) Order the following laboratory tests: CBC, electrolytes, and a toxicology screen
(D) All of the above

6. A patient who overdoses on acetaminophen is admitted to the hospital for antidotal therapy with *N*-acetylcysteine. The patient has the following medication orders: *N*-acetylcysteine 140 mg/kg loading dose followed by 70 mg/kg for a total of 17 doses, ranitidine 50 mg IV every 8 hours, prochlorperazine 10 mg IM every 6 hours as needed for nausea, thiamine 100 mg IV every day for 3 doses, and Darvocet N-100 1–2 tablets every 4 hours as needed for headache. What is the best course of action?

(A) Call the physician to increase the dosage of ranitidine to 50 mg IV every 6 hours.
(B) Call the physician to have the Darvocet N-100 discontinued.
(C) Call the physician to initiate hemodialysis therapy.
(D) Have the patient prophylactically intubated to protect the airway.
(E) Administer ethanol 10% at a loading dose of 7.5 mL/kg over 1 hour, followed by a continuous infusion of 1.4 mL/kg/hr for 48 hours.

7. Ethyl alcohol (EtOH) is administered to patients who have ingested either ethylene glycol or methanol because EtOH

(A) helps to sedate patients.
(B) increases the metabolism of ethylene glycol and methanol.
(C) blocks the formation of the toxic metabolites of ethylene glycol and methanol.
(D) increases the renal clearance of ethylene glycol and methanol.
(E) is not an antidote for ethylene glycol or methanol overdoses.

8. A patient with renal failure is inadvertently given 3 doses of potassium chloride 40 mEq IV in 100 mL of 0.9% sodium chloride over a 3-hour period. This error is immediately discovered and a STAT serum potassium level is 8.0 mEq/L. The patient is bradycardic with a markedly prolonged QRS complex. The patient should receive which of the following?

(A) Calcium chloride 10% 10 mL IV push
(B) Sodium bicarbonate 50 mEq IV push
(C) Insulin 10 units and 50% dextrose 50 mL IV push
(D) Sodium polystyrene sulfonate 30 g by mouth every 3 hours for 4 doses
(E) None of the above

9. Parenteral calcium is used as an antidote for which of the following situations?

(A) Verapamil overdoses
(B) Hyperkalemia
(C) Cocaine intoxication
(D) Verapamil overdoses and hyperkalemia

10. A 65-year-old woman with normal renal function is administered a 0.25 mg dose of digoxin IV push. A serum level obtained 1 hour after drug administration is 5 ng/mL. Your recommendation to the physician is which of the following?

(A) Administer 2 vials of digoxin immune antibodies STAT.
(B) Administer repetitive doses of activated charcoal.
(C) Call a nephrologist, and hemodialyze the patient.
(D) Repeat the serum digoxin level 6–8 hours after the dose, and reassess the patient.

11. A 16-year-old woman is reported to have overdosed on 40 sustained-release theophylline tablets. She is transported to the emergency department, where gastric lavage was performed and she was given one dose of activated charcoal. An initial theophylline level is 42 μg/mL, but a follow-up level in the intensive care unit (ICU) is 95 μg/mL. What is the most appropriate course of therapy?

(A) Charcoal hemoperfusion and multiple-dose activated charcoal
(B) Syrup of ipecac administration
(C) Forced alkaline diuresis
(D) Nasogastric administration of sodium-polystyrene sulfonate

12. A 23-year-old man is admitted to the ICU after ingesting 20 acetaminophen tablets 500 mg with a "six-pack" of beer. He was initially awake and alert in the emergency department and was given one dose of activated charcoal. His initial acetaminophen level taken approximately 2 hours after ingestion is 90 μg/mL. What would be the most appropriate course of action?

(A) Administer repeated doses of activated charcoal and sorbitol.
(B) Administer syrup of ipecac.
(C) Administer a loading dose of N-acetylcysteine, and repeat the acetaminophen level in 4 hours.
(D) Discharge the patient to home.

13. An overdose victim presents to the emergency department with an elevated heart rate, decreased blood pressure, dilated pupils, and lethargy. Upon arrival to the ICU, she has a generalized tonic–clonic seizure that is treated with IV diazepam and fosphenytoin. Which of the following is the most likely intoxicant?

(A) Ethyl alcohol
(B) Methanol
(C) Acetaminophen
(D) Oxycodone
(E) Amitriptyline

ANSWERS AND EXPLANATIONS

1. The answer is A *[I A].*
Patients with unstable vital signs should be taken to an emergency department for immediate treatment.

2. The answer is B *[II G 1 a].*
Vomiting should not be induced in patients who have ingested caustic substances because these chemicals can induce further burning when they come up in the emesis.

3. The answer is E *[III Q 5].*
Naloxone reverses the effects of opioid receptor agonists, such as heroin, morphine, and propoxyphene.

4. The answer is D *[II G 1].*
Contraindications to ipecac include "the three C's": caustics, conscious, convulsions.

5. The answer is D *[II].*
The management of unconscious overdose patients involves aggressive support of vital signs, the administration of empiric antidotal therapy, while obtaining various laboratory tests to determine the nature of the overdose.

6. The answer is B *[III A].*
Darvocet N-100 is an acetaminophen-containing product that should not be given to a patient with documented acetaminophen toxicity. Be aware particularly of OTC products containing acetaminophen.

7. The answer is C *[III B].*
Ethanol saturates alcohol dehydrogenase and prevents the formation of the toxic metabolites of either ethylene glycol or methanol.

8. The answer is A *[III L 2].*
All of the selections are used to manage hyperkalemia. Although, in an unstable patient, the cardiac effects of hyperkalemia must first be reversed with intravenous calcium.

9. The answer is D *[III G, L 2].*
Parenteral calcium is used to reverse the cardiac effects of calcium channel blocker overuse and hyperkalemia.

10. The answer is D *[III K].*
The plasma/tissue distribution phase for digoxin is 6–8 hours postadministration. Sampling digoxin levels sooner may give a falsely elevated level. Only symptomatic patients should receive digoxin immune antibodies. Hemodialysis is of no value in managing digoxin overdoses.

11. The answer is A *[III T].*
Large ingestions of sustained-release products may act as drug reservoirs, necessitating aggressive measures to remove the toxin.

12. The answer is C *[III A].*
Large acetaminophen ingestions (>140 mg/kg) may be fatal if unrecognized. The Rumack-Matthew nomogram requires a 4-hour level to accurately assess the potential for toxicity. If the 4-hour level is in the toxic range, the full course of *N*-acetylcysteine therapy should be administered.

13. The answer is E *[III D].*
Tricyclic antidepressant overdoses will produce seizures, hypotension, mydriasis, hypotension and ventricular dysrhythmias. The cardiac and CNS effects of tricyclic antidepressant toxicity will respond to bicarbonate therapy. Opiates such as oxycodone will produce miosis.

24
Federal Pharmacy Law

Robert C. Pavlan, Jr.

I. FEDERAL CONTROLLED SUBSTANCES ACT

A. Schedules of controlled substances. Certain drugs have a potential for abuse that leads to physical or psychological dependence. As a result, the U.S. federal government has placed these drugs into schedules (I, II, III, IV, and V) and refers to them as controlled substances. The Attorney General of the United States has the authority to add or remove a drug or substance from one of the federal schedules, or to transfer a drug from one federal schedule to another. The federal schedules are updated and published annually by the federal government.

1. Schedule I (CI; C-I) Schedule I drugs may not be kept in a pharmacy nor dispensed pursuant to a prescription (except for properly registered facilities for investigative or research purposes). A controlled substance analogue of a drug in any federal schedule, commonly referred to as a "designer drug," is considered a schedule I substance to the extent intended for human consumption. Required findings by the government for placement of a drug into schedule I include:
   a. The drug or other substance has a high potential for abuse.
   b. The drug or other substance has no currently accepted medical use in treatment in the United States.
   c. There is a lack of accepted safety for use of the drug or other substance under medical supervision.

2. Schedule II (CII; C-II). Required findings for placement of a drug into schedule II include:
   a. The drug or other substance has a high potential for abuse.
   b. The drug or other substance has a currently accepted medical use in treatment in the United States or a currently accepted medical use with severe restrictions.
   c. Abuse of the drug or other substance may lead to severe psychological or physical dependence.

3. Schedule III (CIII; C-III). Required findings for placement of a drug into schedule III include:
   a. The drug or other substance has a potential for abuse less than the drugs or other substances in schedules I and II.
   b. The drug or other substance has a currently accepted medical use in treatment in the United States.
   c. Abuse of the drug or other substance may lead to moderate or low physical dependence or high psychological dependence.

4. Schedule IV (CIV; C-IV). Required findings for placement of a drug into schedule IV include:
   a. The drug or other substance has a low potential for abuse relative to the drugs or other substances in schedule III.
   b. The drug or other substance has a currently accepted medical use in treatment in the United States.
   c. Abuse of the drug or other substance may lead to limited physical dependence or psychological dependence relative to the drugs or other substances in schedule III.

5. Schedule V (CV; C-V). Required findings for placement of a drug into schedule V include:
   a. The drug or other substance has a low potential for abuse relative to the drugs or other substances in schedule IV.
   b. The drug or other substance has a currently accepted medical use in treatment in the United States.
   c. Abuse of the drug or other substance may lead to limited physical dependence or psychological dependence relative to the drugs or other substances in schedule IV.

B. Registration requirements. This Act regulates the use of controlled substances by requiring all entities that lawfully handle them to register with the federal government, specifically, the Drug Enforcement Administration (DEA).

1. **Entities that must register**
    a. **Manufacturers** and **wholesalers** of controlled substances must register with the DEA initially and reregister every year thereafter.
    b. **Dispensers** (practitioners and pharmacies) of controlled substances must register with the DEA initially and reregister every 3 years thereafter. Pharmacists, pharmacy interns, pharmacy technicians, and all other employees or agents of a pharmacy do not have to register, providing the pharmacy is properly registered and the employee or agent is acting in the usual course of employment or business.
    c. All other entities that lawfully handle any controlled substance must register with the DEA, including researchers, clinics and laboratories, and teaching institutions.

2. **Separate registration for separate activities.** Every entity that engages in one of the following activities must register with the DEA. A separate registration is required for each activity, with certain exceptions (e.g., a manufacturer of a schedule of a controlled substance is allowed to distribute that schedule without being registered as a distributor).
    a. Manufacturing controlled substances
    b. Distributing controlled substances
    c. Dispensing controlled substances listed in schedules II–V (e.g., practitioners, pharmacies)
    d. Conducting research with controlled substances listed in schedules II–V
    e. Conducting instructional activities with controlled substances listed in schedules II–V
    f. Conducting a narcotic treatment program using any narcotic drug listed in schedules II, III, IV, or V
    g. Conducting research and instructional activities with controlled substances listed in schedule I
    h. Conducting chemical analysis with controlled substances listed in any schedule
    i. Importing controlled substances
    j. Exporting controlled substances
    k. Participating in maintenance or detoxification treatment and mixing, preparing, packaging, or changing the dosage form of a narcotic drug listed in schedules II, III, IV, or V for use in maintenance or detoxification treatment by another narcotic treatment program.

3. **Separate registrations for separate locations.** Each principal place of business of a registrant having more than one location must have its own registration certificate. Each pharmacy, chain pharmacy, and hospital that dispenses controlled substances must have its own registration certificate. Registration is not required for an office that is used by a registrant where controlled substances are neither stored nor dispensed.
    a. **Warehouses.** A warehouse where controlled substances are stored by or on behalf of a registrant is not required to register unless one of the following occurs:
        (1) Controlled substances are directly distributed from the warehouse to a registered location different than the location from which the substances were shipped.
        (2) Controlled substances are directly distributed from the warehouse to a person or entity not required to register under the Act.

4. **Registration procedure.** Applications to become registered must be submitted to the DEA on the appropriate form with the required fee, information, and signature of one of the following:
    a. The individual who owns and operates the entity, if doing business as an individual
    b. A partner of the applicant, if a partnership
    c. An officer of the applicant, if a corporation, corporate division, association, trust, or other entity
    d. One or more individuals who have been granted a power of attorney by an applicant. A **power of attorney** allows one to lawfully act in place of another. The power of attorney must be signed by one of the individuals listed above in a–c and by the individual receiving the power of attorney. The power of attorney remains valid until revoked by the applicant.

5. **Registration action by the DEA.** If an application is complete, it will be accepted for filing. If it is defective, the DEA will return the application with a statement indicating the reason for its nonacceptance. The application may be corrected and resubmitted at any time.
    a. **Issuance of certificate of registration.** A certificate of registration will be issued by the DEA when it determines that the registration is required by law in order to conduct such activity (e.g., manufacturing, distributing, or dispensing a controlled substance). The certificate must be conspicuously maintained and readily retrievable at the registered location.

b. Denial of registration. If the DEA determines that a registration is not required by law, it will issue an Order To Show Cause why the registration should not be denied. The applicant may request a hearing and explain why the certificate of registration should be issued. After the hearing, the DEA may deny the application or issue the certificate.

6. Modification of registration. A registrant may submit a letter of request to the DEA seeking to modify its registration. A modification may be sought when there is a change in the name or address that appears on the certificate, or when the pharmacy seeks DEA approval to dispense additional controlled substances [if initially authorized to only dispense a particular schedule(s) of controlled substances].

7. Transfer of registration. A registration to dispense controlled substances may not be transferred to any other person or entity except when the ownership of a pharmacy is being transferred from one entity to another. In such a case, controlled substances in schedules II–V must be properly disposed of or transferred to the new entity.

8. Suspension or revocation of registration. The DEA may suspend or revoke any registration. The DEA must first issue an Order To Show Cause (upon the registrant) why the registration should not be revoked or suspended. The registrant may request a hearing to explain why the registration should not be suspended or revoked. After a hearing, the DEA may suspend, revoke, or take no action on the registration.

  a. Order of suspension or revocation. After a registrant has received an order suspending or revoking its registration, it must take the following action:

    (1) Immediately deliver its certificate of registration and any DEA 222 order forms in its possession to the nearest office of the DEA

    (2) As instructed by the DEA, either:

      (a) deliver all controlled substances in its possession to the nearest office of the DEA or to authorized agents of the DEA or

      (b) place all controlled substances in its possession under seal.

  b. Imminent danger to public health or safety. The DEA may serve on a registrant an order of immediate suspension when it finds that there is an **imminent danger** to the **public health** or **safety.** The immediate suspension remains in effect until the conclusion of all proceedings, either administrative proceedings by the DEA or judicial proceedings. After receiving an order of immediate suspension, the registrant must take the same action as outlined above under I B 8 a.

9. Exemptions from registration. Certain individuals are exempt from registration under the Act. The following are exempt:

  a. Military officials. Military officials, including Public Health Service and Bureau of Prisons officials, who are authorized to prescribe, dispense, or administer, but not to procure or purchase, controlled substances in the course of their official duties, are exempt from registering with the DEA. The individual must, however, obtain a registration for such activities conducted during any separate private practice.

  b. Law-enforcement officials. Federal and state law-enforcement personnel acting in the course of enforcing any law relating to controlled substances are exempt from registration.

  c. Civil defense officials. Civil defense and disaster-relief organization officials are exempt from registration in order to maintain and dispense controlled substances during times of proclaimed emergencies or disasters.

  d. Agents and employees of registrants. Agents and employees, while acting lawfully in the usual course of their business or employment, are exempt from registration when the business or employment is conducted on behalf of a person (or business) who is registered under the Act. Delivery personnel (e.g., United Parcel Service, Federal Express) are therefore not required to register. Likewise, pharmacists working for a registered pharmacy are not required to register.

10. Termination of registration. The registration of any person or entity will terminate when the person dies, ceases legal existence (e.g., corporate dissolution, partnership dissolution), or discontinues business or professional practice. The DEA must be notified promptly when any of these occurs. In such a case, all controlled substances in schedules II–V must be properly disposed of.

C. Required inventories. The Act requires all pharmacies and hospitals (every separately registered location) to conduct an initial inventory and biennial inventory of all controlled substances in schedules II, III, IV, and V.

1. **Initial inventory.** The initial inventory must be taken on the date the entity commences business and begins dispensing controlled substances. If the entity has no controlled substances on hand, a record of this fact must be maintained as its initial inventory.

2. **Biennial inventory.** The biennial inventory must be taken at least every 2 years from the date of the initial inventory.
   a. **Biennial date.** The biennial date may be **any** date that is within 2 years of the previous biennial (or initial) date. This date does **not** have to be reported to the DEA if it is different than the biennial date that would otherwise apply (i.e., on the exact day 2 years after the previous inventory).

3. **Inventory procedures**
   a. All inventories must be maintained in a **written, typewritten,** or **printed form** and be conducted at either the opening of business or the close of business on the inventory date (which must be noted on the inventory).
   b. **Separate inventory record for schedule II controlled substances.** Because all records for schedule II controlled substances must be maintained separately from other records, schedule II inventories must be maintained separately from other controlled-substance inventories.

4. **Inventory content.** All inventory records must contain the following:
   a. Date the inventory is taken
   b. Each finished form of the substance (dosage form and strength)
   c. Number of units or volume of each finished form in each commercial container (e.g., 100-tablet bottle). For opened commercial containers, inventory must be taken as follows:
      (1) For schedule II controlled substances, an exact count or measure must be taken.
      (2) For schedule III, IV, and V controlled substances, an estimated count or measure may be taken, except that an exact count must be taken if the container holds more than 1000 tablets or capsules.
   d. For each controlled substance maintained for extemporaneous compounding, or for substances that are damaged, defective, or impure and awaiting disposal:
      (1) Name of the substance
      (2) Total quantity to the nearest metric unit weight or the total number of units of finished form
      (3) Reason the substance is being maintained and whether it is capable of use in the manufacture of any controlled substance in finished form

5. **Inventory record maintenance.** Every inventory record must be maintained at the registered location (e.g., pharmacy, hospital) for at least 2 years from the date of the inventory.
   a. Schedule II inventories must be maintained separately from all other records of the pharmacy.
   b. Schedule III–V inventory records must be maintained either separately from all other records of the pharmacy or in such a manner that the required information is readily retrievable from ordinary business records of the pharmacy. "Readily retrievable" means that the inventory records can be separated out from all other records in a reasonable time.

6. **Perpetual inventories.** The Act does not require a dispenser registrant (e.g., pharmacy, hospital) to maintain a perpetual inventory of any controlled substance.

7. **Newly controlled substances or changes in scheduling of a substance.** An inventory of a substance must be taken when, by order of the DEA, it becomes a newly controlled substance or it shifts into another schedule. The inventory of that particular controlled substance must be taken on the effective date of the change. A complete inventory of all controlled substances is not required, nor is an inventory required when a substance moves from a controlled-substance schedule to a nonfederal schedule.

8. **Transfer of business activity.** An inventory of controlled substances II–V must be taken at the time a pharmacy or hospital undergoes a change in ownership. The inventory must be taken on the date of transfer and serves as the final inventory of the transferor and the initial inventory of the transferee.

9. **Inventory record submission.** The Act does not require the submission of inventory records to anyone, including the DEA. The records must be maintained at the registered location for inspection and copying by authorized agents of the DEA.

D. Obtaining controlled substances. Schedule II controlled substances must be obtained from a supplier (wholesaler, manufacturer) by using DEA Form 222. The Act does not require the use of any special form to obtain controlled substances in schedules III–V.

1. DEA Form 222. Only entities that are registered to dispense or handle schedule II controlled substances may obtain Form 222. The forms are serially numbered and issued by the DEA with the name, address, registration number, authorized activity, and schedules of the registrant. Each form contains an original, duplicate, and triplicate copy (Copy 1, Copy 2, and Copy 3, respectively).

   a. Execution of Form 222. Form 222 may be executed only on behalf of the registrant named on the form and only if the registration has not expired nor been revoked or suspended. The form must be prepared in triplicate as provided by the DEA by use of a typewriter, pen, or indelible pencil in the following manner:

   (1) Only one item may be ordered on each of the 10 numbered lines on the form. The total number of items ordered must be noted on the form in the space provided.

   (2) One item may consist of one or more commercial or bulk containers of a product. A separate item must be made for different commercial or bulk containers of a product. For each item, the form must contain the following information:
   (a) Name of the article ordered
   (b) Finished or bulk form of the product (dosage form and strength)
   (c) Number of units or volume in each commercial or bulk container (e.g., 100-tablet bottle)
   (d) Number of commercial or bulk containers ordered
   (e) If the article is not in pure form, the name and quantity per unit of the controlled substances contained in the article.

   (3) The supplier's name and address must be included on the form. Only one supplier may be listed on any one form.

   (4) Each form must include the date of the order, and no form is valid more than 60 days after its execution by the purchaser.

   (5) The form must be signed either by the person who signed the most recent application for registration or reregistration, or by a person authorized to obtain and execute order forms by a **power of attorney.**
   (a) Any purchaser may authorize one or more individuals (does not have to be an attorney-at-law), whether or not located at the registered location, to obtain and execute 222 Forms by executing a power of attorney for the individual(s).
   (b) The power of attorney must be signed by the person who signed the most recent application for registration or reregistration and by the individual(s) receiving the power of attorney. This form must be similar or identical to the DEA's "Power of Attorney for DEA Order Forms."
   (c) Once properly executed, the individual receiving the power of attorney may obtain and sign DEA Form 222 to the same extent as the individual who signed the most recent application for registration or reregistration.
   (d) The power of attorney must be filed with the executed 222 Forms of the purchaser and be retained for the same period as any order form bearing the signature of the attorney [see I D 1 a (8)]. The power of attorney does not have to be submitted to the DEA.

   (6) Copies 1 and 2 must be submitted to the supplier. Copy 3 must be retained by the purchaser.

   (7) When the ordered schedule II controlled substances are received by the pharmacy, the following information must be recorded on the retained Copy 3:
   (a) Number of commercial or bulk containers furnished on each item (or line)
   (b) Date on which the containers are received by the pharmacy

   (8) DEA 222 Forms must be maintained at the registered location (pharmacy or hospital) for at least 2 years from their execution. The time of execution would be the date the last entry was made on Copy 3.

   b. Cancellation by purchaser. A purchaser may cancel all or part of an order by notifying the supplier in writing. The supplier must indicate the cancellation on Copies 1 and 2 by drawing a line through the canceled items and printing the word "canceled" in the space provided for number of items shipped. Likewise, a supplier may void all or part of an order by notifying the purchaser in writing and printing the word "canceled" in the space provided for number of items shipped.

c. **Maintenance of DEA Form 222.** Executed Copy 3 forms and Copies 1 and 2 of each un-accepted or defective form and the statement of refusal from the supplier must be main-tained by the purchaser. They must be kept separate from all other records and be avail-able for inspection for at least 2 years. All forms must be maintained at the registered location preprinted on the form, and not at a central location.

d. **Loss or theft of DEA Form 222.** Any used or unused form stolen from or lost by a pur-chaser or supplier must be reported immediately to the DEA. Such notification must in-clude the serial number of each form lost or stolen.

2. **Obtaining schedule III–V controlled substances.** There is no special form for obtaining schedule III–V controlled substances. Each registrant must, however, maintain a complete and accurate record of receipt for each such substance. The record must be maintained at either the registered location of the pharmacy or hospital, or at a central location, for 2 years. If a central location is used, the pharmacy must first notify the DEA, indicating its intention to keep central records. Central records may then be maintained unless the DEA denies the request to keep such records. An invoice or packing slip will suffice as a record of receipt, providing the following information is included:

a. Name of the controlled substance

b. Finished form of the substance (dosage form and strength)

c. Number of units or volume of the finished form in each commercial container (e.g., 100-tablet bottle)

d. Number of commercial containers of each such finished form received from other per-sons

e. Date of actual receipt of each commercial container

f. Name, address, and registration number of the person from whom the containers were received

E. **Storage of controlled substances.** All controlled substances in schedules II–V must be stored in one of the following ways:

1. In a securely locked, substantially constructed cabinet

2. Dispersed throughout the stock of unscheduled prescription medication to prevent any theft or diversion

F. **Theft or significant loss of schedule II–V controlled substances.** Every registrant must promptly notify the regional office of the DEA of the theft or significant loss of any controlled substance in schedules II–V. This report must be done using DEA **Form 106.**

G. **Disposal of controlled substances.** Every disposal of a controlled substance must be accom-plished by submitting DEA **Form 41** to the DEA (except for disposals pursuant to a valid pre-scription, discussed below). The form must list the controlled substances earmarked for dis-posal. The DEA will authorize the disposal and instruct the registrant to dispose of the controlled substances in one of the following ways:

1. By the transfer to a person or entity registered with the DEA and authorized to possess the substance. Schedule II controlled substances must be transferred by use of the transferee's (another pharmacy or hospital, or the wholesaler or manufacturer) DEA Form 222. A writ-ten record of the transfer of schedule III–V controlled substances must be kept for at least 2 years and include the following information:

a. Name of the controlled substance

b. Finished form of the substance (dosage form and strength)

c. Number of units or volume of the finished form in each commercial container (e.g., 100-tablet bottle)

d. Number of commercial containers of each finished form transferred

e. Date of the transfer

f. Name, address, and registration number of the transferee

2. By the delivery to an agent of the DEA or to the nearest office of the DEA

3. By the destruction in the presence of an agent of the DEA or other authorized person

4. By any other means that the DEA determines to ensure that the substance does not become available to unauthorized persons or entities

H. Regular disposals of controlled substances. If a registrant (usually a hospital) regularly disposes of controlled substances in schedules II–V the DEA may authorize disposals without prior approval in each instance. If the DEA grants this authority, the registrant must keep records of each disposal and file periodic reports to the regional office of the DEA summarizing the disposals. The DEA may place additional conditions on such disposal, including the method of disposal and the frequency and detail of reports.

I. Disposal of controlled substances pursuant to a valid prescription

1. **Persons who may issue prescriptions for controlled substances.** A controlled-substance prescription may be issued only by a practitioner who is granted such authority by the state in which that practitioner is licensed. Although the Act is federal legislation, each state determines who will be authorized to dispense controlled substances. Most states allow the following individuals to prescribe: physicians, dentists, podiatrists, and veterinarians. Some states allow the following individuals, referred to as midlevel practitioners, to prescribe (usually with certain restrictions): physician's assistants, nurse practitioners, certified nurse midwives, psychiatric nurses, mental health clinical specialists. All prescribers must be registered with the DEA or exempted from registration (see I B 9).

   a. **DEA numbers and authenticity.** After registering with the DEA, all registrants are assigned a DEA number by the DEA. A practitioner's DEA number consists of nine characters. The first two characters are letters. The first letter will be either A or B. The second letter will be the first letter of the practitioner's last name. The next six characters are randomly chosen numbers. The last character is a number often referred to as the "check digit." For example, Dr. Henry Jones may have a DEA number of AJ 4357782.

      (1) **Authentication of DEA number.** The DEA assigns DEA numbers with a quick method of verification built into the number. This allows a dispensing pharmacist to make a cursory review of the number for authenticity. For example, using the above DEA number, the practitioner's last name must start with a J. Also, the following quick calculation can be made to verify that the "check digit" is correct:

         (a) The digits in positions 1, 3, and 5 are added together to reach a number. In the above example, that would be $4 + 5 + 7 = 16$.

         (b) The digits in positions 2, 4, and 6 are added together, then multiplied by 2. In the above example, that would be $(3 + 7 + 8) \times 2 = 36$.

         (c) These numbers above are added together: $16 + 36 = 52$. The far-right digit becomes the check digit. The check digit must therefore be a 2. If the check digit is anything other than a 2, the number may not be a valid DEA number. In such a case, the DEA should be notified in order to verify the number.

      (2) **Midlevel practitioner DEA numbers.** Midlevel practitioner DEA numbers are similar to practitioner DEA numbers except for the first character. Instead of the letter A or B, midlevel practitioners have the letter M as the first character in their DEA number. The mathematical method for verifying the authenticity of the number is the same.

      (3) **DEA numbers for practitioners and midlevel practitioners who are employees of institutions.** Practitioners and midlevel practitioners who issue prescriptions in the course of their employment with an institution may issue prescriptions for all controlled substances under the institution's DEA registration. The practitioner's or midlevel practitioner's "DEA number" will be a specific internal code number issued by the institution. The code number must consist of numbers, letters, or a combination of numbers and letters and must be a suffix to the institution's DEA number, preceded by a hyphen (e.g., AP0123456-10 or AP0123456-A12).

2. **Purpose of issuance of controlled-substance prescriptions.** A controlled-substance prescription may be issued only in good faith for a legitimate medical purpose by a practitioner acting in the usual course of his or her professional practice. The practitioner and the dispensing pharmacist have the responsibility to ensure that a prescription is properly issued and dispensed (referred to as corresponding responsibility of the pharmacist).

   a. **Legitimate medical purpose.** Legitimate medical purpose and good faith are prerequisites for all controlled-substance prescriptions. With respect to a pharmacist, these requirements will be apparent from an objective point of view. As a general rule, if, from all the surrounding facts and circumstances, a reasonably prudent pharmacist would form the opinion that a prescription was issued for a legitimate medical purpose, then the pharmacist has fulfilled his or her responsibility under the Act, and the prescription may be legally dispensed.

    b. Usual course of professional practice. A **practitioner–patient relationship** for the purpose of treating and caring for the patient must be present. Usually, such a relationship includes the taking and recording of an appropriate medical history, and an appropriate physical exam. This limits a practitioner's ability to prescribe outside his or her course of professional practice (e.g., a veterinarian may not prescribe a controlled substance for a human). The notion of "usual course of practice" becomes more unclear with respect to medical doctors who specialize. Such specialists often issue prescriptions "outside" their specialty. Generally, all controlled-substance prescriptions from medical doctors are deemed to be "in the usual course of professional practice" as long as it is issued for a human, regardless of whether the problem being treated is within the doctor's specialty.

    c. Restrictions on issuance of a controlled-substance prescription

        (1) A prescription may not be issued by a practitioner in order for that practitioner to obtain controlled substances for the purpose of **general dispensing** to his or her patients.

        (2) A prescription may not be issued for the dispensing of controlled substances for **detoxification** or maintenance treatment. Administration and direct dispensing of controlled substances are allowed only when conducted in properly registered treatment programs. A prescription for **methadone** is valid only when issued as an analgesic in cases of severe pain. Methadone may be dispensed in a hospital to maintain a patient's addiction as long as the patient is admitted and being treated for some other medical condition and is not administered methadone solely for detoxification purposes.

3. Manner of issuance of a controlled-substance prescription. Schedule II controlled-substance prescriptions must be written with ink or indelible pencil or typewritten (except in cases of oral emergency schedule II prescriptions). Schedule III–V controlled-substance prescriptions may be orally ordered by the practitioner. Prescriptions may be prepared by either the practitioner or an agent of the practitioner, and communicated to the pharmacy by the practitioner or the agent. Authorization for the prescription (or refill) must, however, originate with the practitioner. Both the practitioner and dispensing pharmacist are responsible for the completeness of the prescription. All prescriptions for controlled substances must include the following information:

    a. Full name and address of the patient

    b. Date the prescription is issued and signed (one and the same)

    c. Drug name, dosage form and strength

    d. Quantity of drug prescribed

    e. Directions for use

    f. Name, address, and DEA registration number of the practitioner

    g. The signature of the practitioner (no preprinted or stamped signatures) as he or she would sign any legal document (all schedule II controlled-substance prescriptions must be manually signed by the practitioner)

4. Emergency dispensing of schedule II controlled substances

    a. An oral schedule II controlled-substance prescription may be received from a practitioner in an emergency situation. An emergency prescription must include all of the information required for any controlled-substance prescription. An emergency situation exists when **all three** of the following factors are present:

        (1) The immediate administration of the controlled substance is necessary for proper treatment of the patient.

        (2) No appropriate alternative treatment is available, including administration of a controlled substance that is not in schedule II.

        (3) It is not reasonably possible for the practitioner to provide a written prescription to be presented to the person dispensing the controlled substance before the dispensing.

    b. Proper dispensing. The quantity prescribed and dispensed must be limited to the amount necessary to adequately treat the patient during the emergency period. If the practitioner is not known to the pharmacist, the pharmacist must make a reasonable good-faith effort to determine that the oral authorization came from a registered practitioner.

        (1) Delivery of written prescription. The practitioner who authorizes the emergency prescription must, within 7 days of the oral authorization, deliver a written prescription to the dispensing pharmacist. The prescription must contain the information required of all controlled-substance prescriptions, have written on its face the words "Authorization for Emergency Dispensing," and the date of the oral authorization. The prescription may be delivered in person or by mail; if delivered by mail, it must be postmarked within the 7-day period. Upon receipt, the dispensing pharmacist must attach it to the oral emergency prescription, which was previously reduced to writing.

    (2) Failure to deliver a written prescription. If a practitioner fails to deliver the written prescription as required, the dispensing pharmacist must notify the regional office of the DEA. Failure by the pharmacist to notify the DEA serves to void the pharmacist's authority to dispense an oral emergency schedule II prescription. The pharmacist will be deemed to have unlawfully dispensed a schedule II controlled substance.

  5. Facsimile prescriptions. Prescriptions for controlled substances III, IV and V (and nonfederal controlled substances such as penicillin and furosemide) may be delivered to the dispensing pharmacy via facsimile machine. A facsimile prescription is deemed to be the written, signed prescription from the prescriber so long as it contains the information required of all prescriptions under federal law. The prescription must be sent directly from the prescriber or his authorized agent to the pharmacy.

    a. Schedule II controlled substances. Prescriptions for schedule II controlled substances may be sent via facsimile to a dispensing pharmacy to facilitate dispensing of the prescription. **No drug may be released** to the patient until the original, signed prescription is presented to the dispensing pharmacist. A schedule II controlled-substance facsimile prescription **will serve** as the original, signed prescription in the following situations:

      (1) Injectable home-health prescriptions. A facsimile schedule II narcotic prescription calling for the compounding of a solution for direct administration to a patient in a private residence, long-term–care facility, or hospice setting may serve as the original prescription. The exception applies so long as the solution will be administered by means of parenteral, intravenous, intramuscular, subcutaneous, or intraspinal infusion.

      (2) Long-term–care facility prescriptions. Any facsimile schedule II prescription issued for a resident of a long-term–care facility may serve as the original, signed prescription.

      (3) Hospice patient prescriptions. Any facsimile schedule II narcotic prescription issued for a patient enrolled in a hospice-care program certified and/or paid for by Medicare under Title XVIII or licensed by state law may serve as the original prescription. The prescriber, or his agent, **must** note on the prescription that the patient is a hospice patient.

  6. Electronic data transmission prescriptions. Prescription information that is transmitted directly from a practitioner to a pharmacy by electronic means such as the Internet is referred to as electronic data transmission prescriptions. Electronic signatures are recognized as legally acceptable signatures of practitioners and legend drugs, except for controlled substances, may be transmitted to pharmacies via the Internet if allowed by state law. A state may allow a practitioner and pharmacy to maintain the prescription information in electronic form without reducing it to writing, so long as they comply with state-mandated safeguards.

    a. Controlled-substance prescriptions. The DEA does not yet recognize electronic data transmission prescriptions as a means of communicating prescription information for any controlled substance. Therefore, prescription information for controlled substances may not be communicated from a practitioner to a pharmacy by electronic means.

  7. Persons who may dispense controlled-substance prescriptions. A **pharmacist** acting in the usual course of his or her professional practice in a DEA-registered pharmacy (or hospital or other registered facility) may dispense a controlled substance pursuant to a prescription. A **pharmacy intern** acting under the direct supervision of his preceptor in a DEA-registered facility may also dispense a controlled substance pursuant to a prescription.

  8. Dispensing procedures of controlled substances pursuant to a prescription. Once a controlled-substance prescription has been lawfully issued by a practitioner and presented to a pharmacist, it may be dispensed in accordance with the following:

    a. Presentation to the pharmacist. Schedules III and IV controlled-substance prescriptions are valid for 6 months from the date of issuance by the practitioner. Schedule II controlled-substance prescriptions have no time limit for presentation under the Act, although they are often recognized to be valid for up to 6 months. Schedule V controlled-substance prescriptions also have no set time limit for presentation under the Act. Regardless of which schedule of controlled substance is involved, the good-faith and "legitimate medical purpose" limitation will always apply and may serve to otherwise limit the validity of a prescription.

b. **Information that must be recorded on the prescription by the dispensing pharmacist.** Under the Act, a filled prescription is considered to be a lawful record of disposition for a controlled substance. As a result, every prescription for a controlled substance must contain certain information. Some of the information will already be contained in the prescription, although the dispensing pharmacist is responsible for ensuring that all of the following information is recorded (usually on the face of the prescription):

   (1) Name of the controlled substance

   (2) Finished form of the controlled substance (dosage form and strength)

   (3) Name and address of the person to whom it was dispensed

   (4) Date of dispensing

   (5) Number of units or volume dispensed (quantity)

   (6) Written or typewritten name or initials of the individual who dispensed the controlled substance

   (7) Serial number of the prescription

c. **Required information on prescription labels.** Every prescription label for a controlled substance must include the following information:

   (1) Name and address of the pharmacy

   (2) Serial number assigned to the prescription

   (3) Date of the initial filling of the prescription (for refills, the date originally filled)

   (4) Name of the patient

   (5) Name of the prescribing practitioner

   (6) Directions for use, and cautionary statements, if any

   (7) For schedule II, III, and IV controlled substances, the federal crime transfer warning must appear on the container: "Caution: Federal law prohibits the transfer of this drug to any person other than the patient for whom it was prescribed."

d. **Allowable quantities that may be dispensed.** The Act contains no limitation concerning the quantity of a controlled substance that may be dispensed pursuant to a prescription. All quantities are, of course, limited to the good-faith and "legitimate medical purpose" standards.

e. **Filing controlled substance prescriptions.** Written controlled-substance prescriptions must be maintained at the pharmacy for a period of 2 years from the date of the original dispensing or last refill, whichever is later. They must be available for inspection and copying by employees and agents of the DEA and be filed **segregated** from all other records in one of the following ways (state law usually dictates the method to be used):

   (1) Using **three separate files** as follows:

      (a) One file for schedule II controlled-substance prescriptions

      (b) One file for schedule III, IV, and V controlled-substance prescriptions

      (c) One file for unscheduled prescription drugs

   (2) Using **two separate files** as follows:

      (a) One file for all controlled-substance prescriptions (II–V), as long as schedule III, IV, and V prescriptions have the letter "C" stamped in red ink in the lower-right corner no less than 1 inch high

      (b) One file for unscheduled prescription drugs

   (3) Using **two separate files** as follows:

      (a) One file for schedule II controlled-substance prescriptions

      (b) One file for all other controlled substances (III–V) and unscheduled prescription drugs, as long as schedule III, IV, and V prescriptions have the letter "C" stamped in red ink in the lower-right corner no less than 1 inch high

   (4) In either **(2)** or **(3)** above, if a pharmacy utilizes an electronic record-keeping system for prescriptions (i.e., computerized records), which permits identification by prescription number and retrieval of original documents by prescriber's name, patient's name, drug dispensed, and date filled, then the requirement to mark the hard copy prescription with a red "C" is waived.

f. **Refill dispensing of controlled substances.** Prescriptions for schedule II controlled substances may not be refilled. Prescriptions for schedules III and IV controlled substances may be refilled up to five times within 6 months from the date of issue of the prescription.

Schedule V controlled-substance prescriptions have no limitations for refilling under the Act; however, once again, the good-faith and "legitimate medical purpose" limitations apply here, as well as to all controlled-substance refills.

(1) Refill information may be maintained either manually or by use of a computer. The Act requires that the information be maintained one way or the other, but not both ways. If **computerized refill records** are maintained, the system must have certain capabilities and the dispensing pharmacist must follow certain procedures.

(a) The computer must be able to provide on-line retrieval of the original prescription information, provide on-line retrieval of the refill history, a refill-by-refill audit trail, and an auxiliary procedure in those cases where the system experiences downtime.

(b) The system must also allow the pharmacist who refills a prescription to document that the information he or she entered into the computer is correct.

(2) When dispensing a refill, the pharmacist must record, on the back of the original prescription or by computer, the following information:

(a) Date of the refill

(b) Name or initials of the refilling pharmacist

(c) Amount of the medication dispensed (if the amount is omitted, the refill will be deemed to have been for the full face amount prescribed by the practitioner)

g. Partial dispensing of controlled substances. The Act does not prohibit the partial dispensing of controlled substances in schedules III and IV, provided that each partial filling is recorded in the same manner as refills, the total quantity dispensed in all partial fillings does not exceed the total quantity prescribed, and no partial filling occurs after 6 months from the date of issuance of the prescription. Likewise, all partial fillings of a schedule V prescription must not exceed the total quantity prescribed.

(1) Partial dispensing of a schedule II controlled substance. The partial dispensing of a schedule II prescription is allowed if the pharmacist is unable to supply the full quantity or the prescription is for a terminally ill patient or a patient in a long-term–care facility (LTCF). Under no other circumstance may a schedule II prescription be partially dispensed.

(a) Inadequate supply. In cases of an inadequate supply, the dispensing pharmacist must note on the face of the prescription the amount dispensed. The remaining balance of the schedule II prescription must be dispensed within 72 hours of the first partial filling. If, for any reason, the balance is not dispensed within the 72-hour period, the pharmacist must notify the prescribing practitioner of this fact. The pharmacist may not dispense any further amounts pursuant to this prescription beyond the 72-hour period.

(b) Terminally ill and patients in LTCFs. It is the pharmacist's responsibility to ensure that a patient has a medical diagnosis documenting a terminal illness or that the patient is in an LTCF. Before any partial dispensing, the pharmacist must record on the prescription whether the patient is "terminally ill" or an "LTCF patient." Any partial dispensing without one of these notations shall be deemed to be a dispensing in violation of the Act. The total amount of the schedule II substance dispensed in all partial fillings must not exceed the total quantity prescribed. Schedule II prescriptions for a terminally ill patient or a patient in an LTCF are valid up to 60 days from the date of issuance of the prescription by the practitioner. All of the following information must be recorded, either manually on the back of the prescription or via computer (with similar capabilities required for computerized refill record keeping), when partially dispensing a schedule II prescription for a terminally ill patient or a patient in an LTCF:

(i) Date of the partial filling

(ii) Quantity of drug dispensed

(iii) Remaining quantity authorized to be dispensed

(iv) Identification of the dispensing pharmacist

h. Transfer of refill information for a controlled-substance prescription. Refill information concerning schedules III, IV, and V controlled substances may be transferred to another pharmacy only once (if allowed by state law). Pharmacies electronically sharing a real-time, on-line database (such as chain pharmacies) may transfer refill information for these controlled substances up to the maximum number of refills permitted by law and the prescriber's authorization. The communication must be made directly between two licensed pharmacists. Both the original prescription and the transferred prescription must be maintained for 2 years from the date of the last refill. Certain information must be recorded as follows:

    (1) The **transferring pharmacist** must:

        (a) Write the word "void" on the face of the original prescription

        (b) On the back of the prescription, record the name, address, and DEA registration number of the pharmacy to which it was transferred and the name of the pharmacist receiving the information

        (c) Record the date of the transfer and the name of the transferring pharmacist

    (2) The **receiving pharmacist** must:

        (a) Write the word "transfer" on the face of the transferred prescription

        (b) Record all of the information required for any controlled-substance prescription (see I I 3), and include the following:

            (i) Date of issuance of the original prescription

            (ii) Original number of refills authorized on the original prescription

            (iii) Date the prescription was initially dispensed

            (iv) Number of valid refills remaining and the date of the last refill

            (v) Pharmacy's name, address, DEA registration number, and original prescription number from which the prescription information was transferred

            (vi) Name of the transferring pharmacist

J. Disposal of controlled substances to a patient without a prescription. Controlled substances that are not prescription (or legend) drugs under federal law may be dispensed to a patient at retail without a prescription. These drugs do not have on the manufacturer's label the federal statement: "Caution: Federal law prohibits dispensing without a prescription." The substances may be dispensed without a prescription in accordance with the following:

    1. The dispensing must be made only by a licensed pharmacist. The actual cash transfer or delivery may be made by a nonpharmacist.

    2. Not more than 8 oz of any substance containing opium, 4 oz of any other controlled substance, 48 dosage units of any substance containing opium, or 24 dosage units of any other controlled substance may be dispensed to the same purchaser in any 48-hour period.

    3. The purchaser is at least 18 years old.

    4. Any purchaser not known to the pharmacist must furnish suitable identification.

    5. A bound record book must be maintained for 2 years from the date of the last entry. The following information must be recorded for each purchase:

        a. Name and address of the purchaser

        b. Name and quantity of controlled substance purchased

        c. Date of each purchase

        d. Name or initials of the pharmacist who dispensed the substance to the purchaser

    6. All dispensing of a controlled substance without a prescription must be done in good faith and not to evade the provisions of the Act.

K. Security considerations

    1. Controlled-substance seals. Manufacturers must package certain controlled substances in a container with a securely affixed seal to reveal any tampering. Every bottle, multiple-dose vial, or other commercial container of any controlled substance listed in schedule II, or of any narcotic controlled substance listed in schedule III or IV, must be packaged with such a seal.

    2. Felony convictions. No DEA registrant may employ an individual who has access to controlled substances if that individual had previously been convicted of a felony offense related to controlled substances.

    3. Manufacturer's label. Every commercial container of a controlled substance must have on its label the symbol designating the schedule in which the controlled substance is listed. The symbol must appear in the upper-right corner of the label or be overprinted on the label.

L. Record maintenance. All records required to be maintained under the Act must be kept by the registrant for 2 years. The records may be maintained at a central location (e.g., at a chain pharmacy's regional office) after notifying the DEA. However, executed DEA 222 Forms (Copy 3), all controlled-substance prescriptions, and all inventories must be maintained at the pharmacy, not centrally. All schedule II controlled-substance records must be maintained separately and readily retrievable from all other records.

M. DEA inspections. Inspections by the DEA of any registered facility may be conducted only in a reasonable manner and during regular business hours. Inspection may be conducted after obtaining consent of the registrant or after the DEA has obtained an administrative warrant from a judge. An application for an administrative warrant must state with specificity the nature, extent, and authority to conduct the requested inspection. The scope of an administrative inspection extends to any records required under the Act, equipment and containers used in the handling of controlled substances, and the verification of compliance with any requirement of the Act. If records are removed from the registrant by the DEA, a receipt given to the registrant will list the items taken.

N. Long-term–care facilities (LTCFs). An LTCF is defined as a nursing home, retirement care, mental care, or other facility or institution that provides extended health care to resident patients. LTCFs are not normally registered with the DEA, although they often maintain controlled substances that are dispensed to a patient by prescription from a pharmacy. They are not required to be registered with the DEA because the controlled substance is dispensed to the ultimate user (the patient) and is not issued by or through the LTCF. When disposing of controlled substances, LTCFs must contact the nearest DEA Diversion Field Office for disposal instructions.

   1. Emergency kits for LTCFs. An LTCF may maintain controlled substances in emergency kits so long as state law specifically approves of such use and the state sets forth procedures that require the following:
      a. Source of supply: The LTCF must obtain controlled substances for the emergency kits from a DEA-registered hospital/clinic, pharmacy, or practitioner.
      b. Security safeguards: Access to each emergency kit in the LTCF must be restricted, and the type and quantity of controlled substances that may be placed in the emergency kit must be specifically limited.
      c. Proper control, accountability, and record keeping: The LTCF and the providing DEA-registered hospital/clinic, pharmacy, or practitioner must maintain complete and accurate records of the controlled substances placed in the emergency kit, including the disposition of these controlled substances, as well as take periodic physical inventories of the drugs.
      d. Administration of controlled substances. In emergency medical situations when medication is needed from the emergency kit, only LTCF personnel who are authorized by an individual practitioner can administer the controlled substances.
      e. Prohibited activities: Prohibited activities can result in the state revocation, denial, or suspension of having emergency kits containing controlled substances in an LTCF.

O. Violations under the Act. Penalties for violations of the Federal Controlled Substances Act depend on the schedule of controlled substance involved, the unlawful act, **and the knowledge and intent of the violator.** It will also depend on whether it is a first offense or a subsequent offense.

   1. Civil penalty. Generally, each violation of the Act may subject an individual to a civil penalty (fine) of up to $10,000. The government must prove that the violator was negligent with respect to compliance under the Act, as opposed to mere mistake or inadvertence.

   2. Imprisonment. If an individual knowingly and intentionally violates the Act, he or she may be sentenced to a term of years, in addition to a civil penalty.

II. FEDERAL FOOD, DRUG, AND COSMETIC ACT (FDCA). In 1937, sulfanilamide elixir containing deadly diethylene glycol (automobile antifreeze) was manufactured without any safety data. There were numerous deaths associated with its use, which prompted the federal government to pass the 1938 FDCA. The FDCA requires that all new drug products intended for use as labeled by the manufacturer in the United States must be proven to the federal government to be safe and effective. Such proof is submitted to the Food and Drug Administration (FDA) by use of a New Drug Application (NDA).

A. Definition. Under the FDCA, the term "drug" is defined as including all of the following:

1. Articles recognized in the official *United States Pharmacopeia (USP),* official *Homeopathic Pharmacopoeia of the United States,* or official *National Formulary,* or any supplement to these

2. Articles intended for use in the diagnosis, cure, mitigation, treatment, or prevention of disease in man or other animals

3. Articles (other than food) intended to affect the structure or any function of the body of man or other animals

4. Articles intended for use as a component of any article specified in 1, 2, or 3 above

B. Legend drugs. Legend drugs are those medications that have on their label from the manufacturer the following federally required statement: "**Rx** only." Such medications may be dispensed directly to the patient by means of a valid written or oral prescription from a practitioner or by a valid refill authorization of either. By law, these medications must bear a label with adequate directions for use, which can only be given by a licensed practitioner and, therefore, the requirement of a prescription. A drug, intended for use by humans, is considered a legend drug (and have the above caution on its label) if any of the following apply:

1. Because of the drug's toxicity or other potential for a harmful effect, or its method of use, or collateral measures necessary to its use, it is **not safe** for use **except under the supervision** of a practitioner licensed by law to administer such drug.

2. The drug is a **new drug** for which an approved NDA limits its use to the professional supervision of a practitioner licensed by law to administer such drug. A new drug is broadly defined as being one that generally is not recognized among experts as safe and effective for use under the conditions prescribed, recommended, or suggested in the labeling. It is also defined as being a drug that, as a result of investigations to determine its safety and effectiveness for use under such conditions, has become so recognized but that has not, other than in the investigations, been used to a material extent or for a material time under such conditions. Finally, a new drug may result from a change in the dosage form, labeling, indications, or any other change in a drug product that is already being marketed. The ultimate decision of whether a drug is a new drug lies with the FDA because of its expertise in resolving technical and scientific questions.

   a. **NDA.** Every new drug marketed in the United States must be safe and effective for its intended use as labeled by the manufacturer. Proof of safety and effectiveness must be submitted to the FDA by the manufacturer via the NDA. When a new chemical entity (NCE) is identified by a manufacturer, the manufacturer must obtain an Investigational New Drug Application (IND) before conducting preclinical animal tests and clinical human investigations.

   b. **IND.** Because an NCE has not yet been approved by the FDA as a safe and effective drug, a manufacturer is required to file an IND with the FDA. The IND allows a manufacturer to conduct research with the NCE and exempts the drug from certain prohibitions of the FDCA in order to facilitate clinical investigations; thus, INDs are sometimes referred to as an Investigational New Drug Exemption. Generally, clinical investigation of an NCE is divided into three phases, with each phase involving a greater number of human subjects.

      (1) **Phase 1.** A phase 1 investigation is the initial introduction of an investigational new drug into humans to determine the metabolism, pharmacology, side effects, mechanism of action, and early evidence on effectiveness.

      (2) **Phase 2.** A phase 2 investigation includes the well-controlled, closely monitored clinical studies in order to evaluate the effectiveness of the drug for a particular indication and to further determine side effects and risks.

      (3) **Phase 3.** A phase 3 investigation includes expanded clinical trials to gather additional information concerning safety, effectiveness, and the overall benefit–risk relationship associated with the drug's use. This phase also includes gathering information to provide an adequate basis for physician labeling.

   c. **Treatment INDs (or treatment protocols).** The FDA may allow a treatment IND, which allows a researcher (physician) to use an investigational drug as treatment in serious and life-threatening diseases where no comparable or satisfactory alternative drug or other therapy is available.

C. Over-the-counter (OTC) medications. Certain medications may be dispensed OTC at retail distributors without a prescription. The federal government has determined that these medications may be safely and properly self-administered without the supervision of a practitioner licensed by law to administer (or prescribe) such a drug. Generally, these medications are not habit-forming and have a low toxicity or other potential for a harmful effect. These medications do not have the federal statement "**Rx** only" on their label (see II B).

1. OTC preparations must have **adequate directions** for use on their label, and the product must comply with the applicable FDA monograph. The FDCA requires all drugs marketed in the United States to be generally recognized as safe and effective. As a result, it convened review panels to review OTC drug effectiveness and create monographs for each therapeutic class of OTC drugs. This review is referred to as the Drug-Efficacy (or Effectiveness) Study Implementation (DESI). All OTC drugs must comply with the applicable drug monograph or be considered misbranded (see II I) and subject to FDA regulatory action.

2. OTC preparations must have the following information on its label:
   a. Identity, in bold face, of the OTC product on the principal display panel
   b. Adequate directions for use
   c. Ingredients (including inert or inactive ingredients) in the product
   d. Net quantity of contents
   e. Expiration date of the product
   f. Lot number of the product
   g. Name and place of business of the manufacturer, packer, or distributor
   h. Disclosure of certain contents and the declaration of certain warnings, including habit-forming ingredients and warnings, pregnancy/nursing warnings, and aspirin warnings

3. **Prescription drug conversion to OTC.** A legend drug will convert to an OTC drug when the FDA finds that the prescription-only limitation is not necessary for the protection of the public health by reason of the drug's toxicity or other potential for harmful effect, the method of its use, or the collateral measures necessary to its use. The FDA must also find that the drug is safe and effective for use in self-medication as directed in proposed labeling.

4. **Miscellaneous regulations for OTCs.**
   a. **Ipecac syrup.** Although ipecac syrup can only be dispensed pursuant to a prescription, the FDA believes that it should be readily available OTC as an emergency treatment emetic for use in poisonings. The FDA allows the OTC sale of ipecac syrup in 1 fluid ounce containers so that it will be readily available in the household for emergency treatment of poisonings, under medical supervision, and that the drug be appropriately packaged and labeled for this purpose.
   b. **Pregnancy-nursing warning.** All OTC drugs intended for systemic absorption must contain a warning that if the user is pregnant or nursing a baby, she should first seek the advice of a health professional before using the product. Exceptions to this labeling requirement exist when an OTC is intended to benefit the fetus or nursing infant, and for OTC drugs that are labeled exclusively for pediatric use.
   c. **Aspirin warnings.** All OTC aspirin containing preparations must have a warning to keep out of children's reach and to contact a physician immediately in case of accidental overdose. Oral or rectal OTC aspirin containing preparations must also have a warning concerning Reye's syndrome in children and teenagers.
   d. **Chemicals and precursors.** It was discovered that combination drug products containing ephedrine, pseudoephedrine, or phenylpropanolamine are the precursor materials used by illegal methamphetamine laboratories. The Comprehensive Methamphetamine Control Act of 1996 requires all retail distributors of these OTC products to fulfill certain obligations. A retail distributor includes a grocery store, general merchandise store, a pharmacy, or any other entity or person who sells these items to customers for personal use. For regulated transactions, a retailer must maintain a record of these transactions for a period of 2 years, must obtain proof of identity from customers, and must report suspicious regulated sales immediately to the DEA. The record must be maintained separately from other records of controlled substances, and the DEA suggests that the record be made in a bound log book similar to the record kept for the sale of OTC controlled substances (see IJ). The following single transactions of these products in the amounts stated are considered to be "regulated transactions."
      (1) **Phenylpropanolamine (PPA).** PPA is no longer in any OTC drug product.

(2) **Pseudoephedrine.** Sales of combination products containing more than 24 g of pseudoephedrine. Blister-pack sales of these products exceeding 24 g are **not** regulated sales.

(3) **Ephedrine.** Sales of combination products containing more than 24 g of ephedrine **and all** single-entity ephedrine products regardless of the amount of ephedrine (more than zero grams).

D. Generic drugs

1. **Definition.** The *generic name* of a drug has been defined as its chemical name, a common name, or an official name used in an official compendium. A manufacturer seeking approval from the FDA for a drug that has already been proven to be safe and effective may file an Abbreviated New Drug Application (ANDA).

2. **ANDA.** A filing of an ANDA allows the approval of a drug for which exhaustive safety and efficacy studies have already been performed. A drug is considered to be the same as an approved drug when the two are identical in active ingredient(s), dosage form, strength, route of administration, indications, and conditions of use. Rigorous animal and human data to determine safety and effectiveness are not required in the ANDA. However, information showing that the generic version of the drug is bioavailable and bioequivalent to the pioneer (original) drug is necessary. Such approved drugs are listed by the FDA in the "Approved Drug Products with Therapeutic Equivalence Evaluations," commonly referred to as the FDA Orange Book (because it comes from the FDA in an orange binder).

E. Proprietary drugs.
The *proprietary name* of a drug is the name given by the manufacturer to designate the drug's source of manufacture and to differentiate it from the same or chemically similar drugs from other manufacturers. Another name for the proprietary name of a drug is its trade name.

F. Established names for drugs.
The FDCA authorizes the Commissioner of the FDA to designate an official name for any drug if he determines that such action is necessary or desirable in the interest of usefulness and simplicity. The FDCA also requires that a drug's established name appear on the label and labeling of the drug. A drug's *established name* is defined as follows:

1. It may be an **official name** designated by the Commissioner of Food and Drugs. For NCEs, the name should be simple and useful. In this regard, the FDA recognizes the U.S. Adopted Names Council (USAN) in deriving names for NCEs. The USAN name is considered to be an official name recognized in an official compendium. The FDA may use another name if the USAN or common or usual name is unduly complex, misleading, or is not useful for any other reason.

2. If no official name has been designated for the drug and the drug is an article recognized in an official compendium, then the **official title** contained in the compendium may be the established name.

3. If neither of the above two apply, then the **common** or **usual name** of the drug may be its established name.

G. Dispensing a prescription drug.
A prescription drug may be dispensed only by a practitioner or by a pharmacist pursuant to a written or oral prescription of a practitioner, or a refill of either. The prescription label on the container dispensed to the patient must contain certain information, or it will be considered misbranded and dispensed in violation of the FDCA. This information is minimal under the FDCA and is usually supplemented by state laws, which require more information. So long as this information is in English, the dispensing pharmacist will be in compliance with the FDCA. If any of the required information is in another language, then all of the required information must be in that language. The prescription must also be packaged in a child-resistant container as required under the Poison Prevention Packaging Act (see III). The following information must appear on every prescription label:

1. Name and address of the pharmacy

2. Serial number of the prescription

3. Date the prescription is filled or the date of the prescription

4. Name of the prescriber

5. Name of the patient (if stated in the prescription)

6. Directions for use and any cautionary statements contained in the prescription

H. Drug recall. The FDCA allows the FDA to initiate regulatory actions to ensure that unsafe, unfit, or ineffective products do not reach the market, or to promptly remove those products that do reach the marketplace. The enforcement actions that may be initiated include the release of information to the general public and/or professional groups; administrative actions and inspections; the institution of recall; or seizure, injunction, or criminal prosecution.

1. **Voluntary action of the manufacturer.** After several unsuccessful attempts by the FDA to receive court-ordered recalls, the FDA recognizes that recalls are voluntary actions of the manufacturers and distributors. As a result, a recall may be undertaken at any time, or upon request of the FDA. If the FDA is unsuccessful in persuading a company to recall a product, or when the FDA determines that a recall is or will be ineffective, it may seek a court order condemning the product and allowing the product's seizure.

2. **Drug recall classification.** After the FDA has evaluated the problem(s) associated with the product and after the degree of health hazard has been determined, the FDA will assign the recall one of the following classifications:
   a. **Class I**—a situation in which there is a reasonable probability that the use of or exposure to a violative product will cause serious adverse health consequences or death
   b. **Class II**—a situation in which use of or exposure to a violative product may cause temporary or medically reversible adverse health consequences or where the probability of serious health consequences is remote
   c. **Class III**—a situation in which use of or exposure to a violative product is not likely to cause adverse health consequences

3. **Recall procedure.** A recall strategy will be developed that will consider the depth of the recall (consumer level, retail level, wholesale level), the need for public warnings, and the extent of effectiveness checks for the recall. Every recalling company is responsible for notifying each of its affected direct accounts by first-class mail, mailgram, or telegram. Public notification is made by the FDA via the weekly *FDA Enforcement Report,* which publishes each recall according to its classification.

I. Adulteration and misbranding. A misbranding or adulteration of a drug is prohibited by the FDCA. Although the misbranding and adulteration provisions are mainly concerned with the manufacturing of a drug, a pharmacist may also misbrand or adulterate a drug. The purpose of the misbranding and adulteration statutes is to protect the public health of consumers who are largely unable to protect themselves where drugs are involved. The adulteration and misbranding statutes are criminal in nature and may subject a pharmacist to criminal proceedings in federal court, in addition to administrative proceedings.

1. **Adulteration.** In general, the term *adulteration* refers to a change or variation from official formulary standards or from the manufacturer's standards. A drug is considered adulterated if any of the following conditions occur:
   a. If the drug consists in whole or in part of any filthy, putrid, or decomposed substance
   b. If the drug has been prepared, packed, or held under unsanitary conditions where it may have been contaminated with filth or rendered injurious to health
   c. If the drug's container is composed, in whole or in part, of any poisonous or deleterious substance that may render the contents injurious to health
   d. If the drug contains, for purposes of coloring only, a color additive that is unsafe within the meaning of the FDCA
   e. If the drug is a new animal drug, or an animal feed containing a new animal drug, that is unsafe within the meaning of the FDCA
   f. If the drug is purported to be a drug that is recognized in an official compendium, and its strength differs from, or its quality or purity falls below, the standard set forth in the compendium, unless the deviation is plainly and specifically stated on its label
   g. If the drug is not a compound recognized by name in an official compendium; if its strength differs from, or its purity or quality falls below, that which it purports or is represented to possess
   h. If the drug has been mixed or packed with another substance so as to reduce the drug's quality or strength
   i. If the drug has been substituted, wholly or partially, with another substance

    j. If the drug is an OTC drug and it is not packaged in the required tamper-resistant packaging or properly labeled in conformity with the tamper-resistant regulations (see IV)

    k. If the drug (or medical device) is an ophthalmic preparation offered or intended for ophthalmic use that is not sterile

2. Misbranding. In general, the term *misbranding* means that a drug is sold or dispensed with a label or labeling that is in violation of the FDCA. *Label* is defined as being a display of written, printed, or graphic matter upon the immediate container of any article (or drug). *Labeling* is more broadly defined to include the label as well as other written, printed, or graphic matter upon any article or any of its containers or wrappers, or accompanying the article (or drug). A drug is considered misbranded if any of the following conditions occur:

    a. If the labeling is false or misleading in any particular

    b. If the drug is an imitation of another drug, or if it is offered for sale under the name of another drug

    c. If the drug is composed wholly or partly of insulin and it is not properly batch certified under the FDCA

    d. If the drug is composed wholly or partly of an antibiotic and it is not properly batch certified under the FDCA

    e. If the drug is dispensed by a name that is recognized in an official compendium and it is either not packaged or not labeled in conformity with the official compendium

    f. If the drug is determined by the federal government to be liable to deterioration and it is not packaged in a proper form and manner, and the label fails to bear a statement of proper precautions

    g. If the drug is dispensed in a non–child-resistant container, when a child-resistant container is otherwise required (see III)

    h. If the manufacturer fails to place on the label any of the following:

        (1) Fact that certain drugs may be habit forming

        (2) Name of each active ingredient

        (3) Name and place of business of the manufacturer, packer, or distributor

    i. If a pharmacist fails to place on a prescription container label any of the following:

        (1) Name and address of the pharmacy

        (2) Serial number of the prescription

        (3) Date of filling the prescription or the date of the prescription

        (4) Name of the prescriber

        (5) Name of the patient

        (6) Directions for use and any cautionary statements contained in the prescription

    j. If an oral contraceptive is dispensed without the required patient package insert

    k. If an intrauterine device that must be dispensed with a patient package insert is dispensed without the insert

    l. If an estrogen product is dispensed without the required patient package insert

    m. If a progestogen-containing product is dispensed without the required patient package insert

    n. If a legend drug is dispensed (or refilled) without a prescription (or refill authorization) of a licensed practitioner, it is deemed to be misbranded by the dispensing pharmacist.

    o. If the drug is an OTC drug and it is not packaged in tamper-resistant packaging or properly labeled in conformity with the tamper-resistant regulations (see IV)

    p. If the drug is an OTC drug and it is not properly labeled in conformity with the labeling requirements of the FDCA

    q. If the drug (or medical device) is an ophthalmic preparation offered or intended for ophthalmic use that is not sterile

3. Violations under the Act. Any misbranding or adulteration of a drug may subject the individual (e.g., a pharmacist) to imprisonment, a fine, or both. A pharmacy and pharmacist will be exempt from criminal sanctions in either of the following cases:

    a. Certain cases of good faith. When adulterated or misbranded products are received from a manufacturer or wholesaler in good faith by the pharmacy, the pharmacy may not be held responsible in certain situations. This exemption applies only if it is a first violation and, if requested, the pharmacy or pharmacist furnishes to the government the name and address of the person from whom the drug was received and copies of all documents pertaining to its delivery.

    b. Receipt of drug with a signed, written guaranty. A pharmacy and pharmacist will be exempt from misbranding and adulteration violations when a signed, written guaranty is received from the wholesaler or manufacturer. The guaranty must contain the name and address of the person residing in the United States from whom the drug was received in good faith and a statement that the drug is not adulterated or misbranded.

4. **Seizures.** Any adulterated or misbranded drug will be subject to condemnation and seizure by the U.S. government after a hearing in any district court of the United States (or territory) with proper jurisdiction. A seizure may be done without a hearing if the federal government has probable cause to believe that the violation would be dangerous to health or that the labeling of the misbranded article is fraudulent or would be materially misleading to the injury or damage of the purchaser or consumer.

5. **Investigations and inspections**
   a. The U.S. Secretary of Health and Human Services has the authority to conduct examinations and inspections through federal employees and by officers and employees of any state, territory, or political subdivision duly commissioned by the U.S. Secretary of Health and Human Services as an officer of the U.S. Department of Health and Human Services.
   b. **Scope of investigation.** An investigator may enter a pharmacy or other establishment where adulterated or misbranded drugs are held and inspect all drugs, materials, containers, and labeling. The inspection does not extend to financial data, sales data other than shipment data, pricing data, personnel data, and other records that have no bearing on adulteration and misbranding. The investigator must present appropriate credentials and a written notice to the owner, operator, or agent in charge that he or she is authorized to conduct an investigation. The inspection must be done at reasonable times, within reasonable limits, and in a reasonable manner.

6. **Current Good Manufacturing Practice (cGMP).** Under the FDCA, a drug is considered adulterated if it is not manufactured "in conformity with current Good Manufacturing Practice." FDA regulations state with particularity the minimum cGMPs for methods to be used in, and the facilities or controls to be used for, the manufacture, processing, packing, or holding of a drug. The cGMPs ensure that a drug meets the requirements of the FDCA as to safety and has the identity and strength and meets the quality and purity characteristics that it purports.

J. Registration of producers of drugs

1. Manufacturers and businesses that distribute a drug manufactured by another but sold under their own label or trade name must register their establishment with the FDA. They also must submit a list of every drug (prescription and OTC) in commercial distribution, with updates every June and December.

2. Pharmacies properly licensed by state law that do not manufacture or possess drugs for sale other than in the regular course of the practice of pharmacy are not required to register with the FDA. A pharmacy engaged in manufacturing or processing activities that are considered beyond the normal practice of pharmacy must register with the FDA and supply a list of every drug in commercial distribution.
   a. **Scope of pharmacy practice.** A pharmacy or pharmacist may not manufacture drug products. They may only compound drug preparations pursuant to a valid prescription of a practitioner for a particular patient. Large-scale manufacturing of drug products by a pharmacy or pharmacist is outside the scope of pharmacy practice and requires proper registration with the FDA and compliance with cGMPs.

K. Package inserts. The federal government has determined that prescription medication information needs to be disseminated to health professionals and, in the case of certain drugs, to the patient.

1. **Manufacturer's insert.** An amendment to the FDCA required that all manufacturers provide "full disclosure" concerning prescription medication that they market. Full disclosure is accomplished by means of a package insert that is enclosed with every commercial container of a drug product. The insert should contain essential scientific information needed for the safe and effective use of the drug and should be informative and accurate. It must not be promotional in tone, false, or misleading.

2. **Patient package insert.** The FDA has determined that, because of certain side effects associated with the use of particular drug products, patient package inserts must be dispensed to the patient at the time of dispensing the medications. The following products must be dispensed with a patient package insert, which is supplied with the product from the manufacturer:

   a. **Oral contraceptives.** Hospital inpatients or LTCF patients may receive the insert before administration of the first oral contraceptive and every 30 days thereafter, as long as the therapy continues.

   b. **Intrauterine devices** for human use in contraception. Every practitioner dispensing such a device must provide the patient with an informative insert.

   c. **Estrogen and estrogen-containing products.** Hospital inpatients or LTCF patients may receive the insert before administration of the first estrogen dose and every 30 days thereafter, as long as the therapy continues.

   d. **Progestational drug products.** Hospital inpatients or LTCF patients may receive the insert before administration of the first progestational drug product and every 30 days thereafter, as long as the therapy continues.

   e. **Isoproterenol inhalation products** require the following warning statement on the immediate container label of such a product: "Warning: Do not exceed the dose prescribed by your physician. If difficulty persists, contact your physician immediately."

   f. **Miscellaneous drug products.** Certain drug products were approved by the FDA with the provision that they must be dispensed along with a patient package insert that includes a particular warning or statement of benefits and risks associated with the use of the drug. For example, isotretinoin was approved for dispensing with an insert warning about serious fetal harm when administered to pregnant women.

L. **Prescription drug samples**

   1. An **amendment** to the FDCA (Prescription Drug Marketing Act) severely restricted the distribution of drug samples by manufacturers. Under the FDCA, no person may sell, purchase, or trade, or offer to sell, purchase, or trade any drug sample. Samples may only be distributed upon written request of a practitioner. Manufacturers must maintain records of every sample distribution for a period of three years. Pharmacies may not receive samples from a manufacturer except in certain situations in which a practitioner requests storage of his or her samples in the pharmacy.

   2. **Importation under the FDCA.** The Prescription Drug Marketing Act prohibits the import of prescription drugs once exported. Importation is allowed after notification and approval of the FDA and in cases of an emergency.

M. **Medical devices.** An amendment to the FDCA in 1976 (Medical Device Amendments) required a device manufacturer to provide reasonable assurance of the safety and effectiveness of the device. The amendment required the FDA to categorize each device on the market in 1976 into one of three classes: Class I, Class II, or Class III, depending on each device's safety and effectiveness. Generally, **Class I** devices are those that have a reasonable assurance of safety and effectiveness. **Class II** devices are those that do not have the reasonable assurance of safety and effectiveness, but there is sufficient information about the device to establish special controls to ensure its safety and effectiveness (and may be marketed with such controls). **Class III** devices are those for which information is not sufficient to provide reasonable assurance of their safety and effectiveness. Class III devices may be marketed only if they are proven to be substantially equivalent to a device on the market before 1976, by approval of a premarket application, or by reclassification into Class I or II.

   1. **Medical device tracking.** Manufacturers of medical devices whose failure would be reasonably likely to have a serious adverse health consequence must track the device down the chain of distribution to the patient. Such tracking allows the manufacturer to take appropriate action with respect to recalls, defects, or other relevant information concerning the device. Every final distributor such as a pharmacy, hospital, or home health-care company must report certain information to the manufacturer. Tracking information must be maintained by the manufacturer and distributor for the useful life of the device and be available for inspection by FDA personnel.

   2. **Manufacturer's reports.** Every device manufacturer must report to the FDA information, when received or made aware of, that reasonably suggests that one of its marketed devices may have caused or contributed to a death or serious injury. Likewise, hospitals and other

medical service facilities must provide reports on adverse reactions to, or malfunctioning of, medical devices.

3. **Adulteration and misbranding.** Medical devices may be adulterated or misbranded in the same way that drugs are adulterated or misbranded (see II I).

III. POISON PREVENTION PACKAGING ACT (PPPA).

The PPPA of 1970 requires that drugs for human use in an oral dosage form must be packaged for the consumer in special packaging. All such federal controlled substances and drugs dispensed pursuant to a prescription must be dispensed to the consumer in special packaging. *Special packaging,* referred to as **child-resistant** containers, is defined as a container that is designed to be significantly difficult for children under 5 years of age to gain access to within a reasonable time. The container must not be too difficult for normal adults (ones with no overt physical or mental handicaps) to use properly and does not include packaging that all such children cannot gain access within a reasonable time. The Consumer Products Safety Commission is responsible for interpreting, establishing rules and regulations for, and enforcing the provisions of the PPPA.

A. **Exceptions.** The following medications are exempt from the special packaging requirements:

1. Sublingual dosage forms of nitroglycerin; other dosage forms intended for oral administration, such as nitroglycerin sustained-release preparations, must be packaged in child-resistant containers

2. Sublingual and chewable forms of isosorbide dinitrate in dosage strengths of 10 mg or less

3. Erythromycin ethylsuccinate granules for oral suspension and oral suspensions in packages containing not more than 8 g of the equivalent of erythromycin

4. Cyclically administered oral contraceptives in manufacturers' mnemonic (memory-aid) dispenser packages that rely solely on the activity of one or more progestogen or estrogen substances

5. Anhydrous cholestyramine in powder form

6. All unit-dose forms of potassium supplements, including individually wrapped effervescent tablets, unit-dose vials of liquid potassium, and powdered potassium in unit-dose packages, containing not more than 50 mEq of potassium per unit dose

7. Sodium fluoride drug preparations, including liquid and tablet forms, containing no more than 264 mg of sodium fluoride per package and containing no other prescription medication

8. Betamethasone tablets packaged in manufacturers' dispenser packages, containing no more than 12.6 mg betamethasone

9. Pancrelipase preparations in tablet, capsule, or powder form and containing no other prescription medication

10. Prednisone in tablet form, when dispensed in packages containing no more than 105 mg of the drug, and containing no other prescription medication

11. Mebendazole in tablet form in packages containing not more than 600 mg of the drug and no other prescription medication

12. Methylprednisolone in tablet form in packages containing not more than 84 mg of the drug and no other prescription medication

13. Colestipol in powder form in packages containing not more than 5 g of the drug and no other prescription medication

14. Erythromycin ethylsuccinate tablets in packages containing no more than the equivalent of 16 g erythromycin

15. Conjugated estrogen tablets USP, when dispensed in mnemonic packages containing not more than 32 mg of the drug and no other prescription medication

16. Norethindrone acetate tablets USP, when dispensed in mnemonic packages containing not more than 50 mg of the drug and no other prescription medication

17. Medroxyprogesterone acetate tablets

B. **Requests for a non–child-resistant container.** A prescribing practitioner may make a request in the prescription that the medication be dispensed in a non–child-resistant container. A practitioner may not, however, make a blanket request that all prescriptions issued by him or her be dispensed in non–child-resistant containers. The purchaser, or patient, may also make a request that the medication be dispensed in a non–child-resistant container. The request of the purchaser, or patient, does not (under the PPPA) have to be in writing. The purchaser, or patient, may make a blanket request that none of his or her medications be dispensed in a child-resistant container. A dispensing pharmacist may never make the decision to use non–child-resistant containers.

C. **Reuse of child-resistant containers.** Reuse of child-resistant containers are prohibited by regulation of the federal Consumer Products Safety Commission. However, the Commission has indicated that glass containers may be reused as long as a new safety closure is used.

D. **Manufacturer's packaging.** Packaging from the manufacturer that is intended to be dispensed directly to the patient must be in child-resistant packaging. Bulk packaging intended to be repackaged by the pharmacist for each prescription does not have to be in special packaging from the manufacturer. Unit packaging from the manufacturer that will be dispensed directly to the consumer, or patient, must comply with the child-resistant requirements of the PPPA (unless specifically exempted; see III A).

E. **Exemptions for easy access.** Special packaging is not required in cases where OTC medication needs to be readily available to the elderly or handicapped persons. A manufacturer may supply a single size of a drug product in non–child-resistant packaging, as long as it also supplies the medication in packages that use the special packaging. Additionally, the package must be conspicuously labeled with the statement: "This package for households without young children." For those packages too small for this statement, the statement "Package not child-resistant" may be used.

F. **Hospitals and institutions.** The special packaging requirements of the PPPA apply to household substances. *Household substance* is defined as "any substance which is customarily produced or distributed for sale for consumption or use, or customarily stored, by individuals in or about the household. . . ." As long as the medication is administered by institutional personnel and is not directly dispensed to the consumer (patient), child-resistant containers are not required.

G. **Miscellaneous products requiring special packaging.** The PPPA requires that certain household substances be distributed to the consumer in special packaging. Examples of these substances include furniture polish containing petroleum distillates, drain pipe cleaners, turpentine, paint solvents, and lighter fluid.

IV. **ANTI-TAMPERING ACT.** The U.S. Congress passed the Anti-Tampering Act in 1984 due to a number of deaths that occurred in the early 1980s from OTC medication capsules contaminated with cyanide.

A. **Violations.** Unlawful acts involving a consumer product can be broken down into one of the following listed violations. The term *consumer product* includes any food, drug, device, or cosmetic, as well as any article, product, or commodity that is customarily used by individuals for purposes of personal care or to perform services ordinarily done within a household.

1. **Tampering.** Any individual who tampers or attempts to tamper with any consumer product that affects interstate or foreign commerce, or its labeling or container, may be in violation of the statute. A violation occurs when the individual acts (or threatens to act) with reckless disregard for the risk that another person will be placed in danger of death or bodily injury. Any individual who taints any consumer product or causes its labeling or container to be materially false or misleading is in violation of the statute if done with intent to cause serious injury to the business of another.

2. **False communications.** Knowingly communicating false information that a consumer product has been tainted may be a violation. If such tainting, had it occurred, would create a risk of death or bodily injury to another person, then the false communication is deemed a violation.

3. **Conspiracy.** An agreement between two or more persons to do (or further) either of the above acts is considered a violation.

B. OTC tamper-resistant packaging. Certain OTC products must be packaged, by FDA regulation, in tamper-resistant packaging. Examples include contact lens solutions and other ophthalmic solutions. A **tamper-resistant package** is one having one or more indicators or barriers to entry that, if breached or missing, can reasonably be expected to provide visible evidence to consumers that tampering has occurred. To reduce tampering, the package must have **one** of the following characteristics:

1. Be distinctive by design so that the product cannot be duplicated by commonly available materials or processes or

2. Use one or more indicators or barriers to entry that employ an identifying characteristic

C. OTC tamper-resistant labeling. The OTC product must be labeled with a prominently placed statement alerting consumers to the specific tamper-resistant feature of the package. The statement must be placed so that it will be unaffected if the tamper-resistant feature is breached or missing.

D. Medical devices and cosmetics. Certain medical devices and cosmetics must be packaged in tamper-resistant packaging. The packaging requirements are similar to the requirements outlined above for OTC drug products.

V. MAILING PRESCRIPTION MEDICATION

A. All prescription medication, including controlled substances and narcotics in schedules II–V, may be mailed from a physician, or pharmacist pursuant to a prescription, to the patient. Flammable substances (e.g., acetone) and alcoholic beverages may not be sent to a patient through the U.S. mail.

B. The medication must be placed in a plain outer container or be securely overwrapped in plain paper. There must be no markings of any kind on the outside wrapper or container that would indicate the nature of the contents.

VI. OMNIBUS BUDGET RECONCILIATION ACT OF 1990 (OBRA '90). Under the Constitution of the United States, the federal government has no power or authority to directly regulate the practice of pharmacy. Such power rests with each state. The federal government can, however, indirectly regulate, or affect, the practice of pharmacy by attaching conditions of participation and reimbursement for federally funded programs.

A. Medicaid prescriptions. With respect to prescriptions dispensed to Medicaid patients (paid in part by the federal government along with the state government), the federal government has attached certain conditions for reimbursement. Such conditions were deemed necessary to stem the always increasing cost of the Medicaid programs. It was believed that improved medication compliance by Medicaid recipients would, in the long run, reduce the cost of the programs by reducing subsequent hospitalizations and other subsequent utilization of health care. As a result, pharmacists are required to do the following in the course of dispensing a Medicaid prescription:

1. Make a reasonable good-faith effort to obtain and maintain a history of the patient, including a medication history

2. Conduct a review of every prescription for appropriateness and to screen for potential drug therapy problems

3. Make an offer to counsel each Medicaid recipient concerning the drug (if the offer is accepted, the counseling must include the drug's proper administration, common adverse or severe side effects, techniques for self-monitoring, and proper storage)

B. Manufacturer's best price. OBRA '90 requires manufacturers that wish to participate in the Medicaid program to offer the federal government their best price for prescription drugs. *Best price* is defined as the lowest price at which any purchaser is purchasing that drug product.

VII. HEALTH INSURANCE PORTABILITY AND ACCOUNTABILITY ACT OF 1996 (HIPAA).

HIPAA is federal legislation that requires all health-care providers, including pharmacies, to protect patient information from unauthorized use and disclosures. This is referred to as the Privacy Rule and was established as a result of the government's recognition that individually identifiable health information is readily available due to health-care plans, health-care clearinghouses, third-party billing practices, clinical research trials, and the transmission of health information in electronic form. Protected health information (PHI) must be confidentially maintained by a health-care provider to prevent any unauthorized use or disclosure. Other covered entities, such as Organized Health Care Arrangements, HMO's and insurance plans, must also follow the Privacy Rule.

A. Definitions. Under the Privacy Rule, certain terms have specific meanings.

1. **"Covered entity"** means:
    a. a health plan (e.g., group health insurance, Medicaid, Medicare).
    b. a health-care clearinghouse (e.g., billing service companies and companies that process health information received from another entity).
    c. a health-care provider who transmits any health information in electronic form in connection with a transaction covered by HIPAA. "Health care" is defined as including the sale or dispensing of a drug, device, equipment, or other item in accordance with a prescription.

2. **"Individually identifiable health information"** is information created or received by a covered entity that relates to the past, present, or future physical or mental health or condition of an individual; the provision of health care to an individual; or any payment for any provision of any health care, **and** that identifies the individual **or** that provides a reasonable basis to identify the individual. The items listed below are deemed sufficient to identify an individual:
    a. Name
    b. Address, including all geographic subdivisions smaller than a state (e.g., street address, city, county, zip code)
    c. Dates (except year), including birth dates, admission dates, discharge dates, dates of death
    d. Telephone numbers
    e. Fax numbers
    f. E-mail addresses
    g. Social Security numbers
    h. Medical record numbers
    i. Health plan beneficiary numbers
    j. Account numbers
    k. Certificate/license numbers
    l. Vehicle identifiers and serial numbers, including license plate numbers
    m. Device identifiers
    n. Web universal resource locaters (URLs)
    o. Internet protocol (IP) address numbers
    p. Biometric identifiers, including fingerprints and voice prints
    q. Full face photographic images and any comparable images
    r. Any other unique identifying number, charactistic, or code, except for codes assigned to reidentify information that has been de-identified
    s. Names of any relative, employer, or household member of the individual

3. **"Protected health information"** (PHI) is all individually identifiable health information that is transmitted or maintained in **any** form or medium, electronically or otherwise.

4. **"Notice of privacy practices for protected health information."** An individual has the right to adequate notice of the uses and disclosures of PHI that may be made by the covered entity, and of the individual's rights and the covered entity's legal duties with respect to PHI. Generally, the notice must contain information describing the individual's rights under the Privacy Rule and the covered entity's responsibilities.
    a. **Header.** Every notice must contain the following statement as a header or be otherwise prominently displayed: "THIS NOTICE DESCRIBES HOW MEDICAL INFORMATION ABOUT YOU MAY BE USED AND DISCLOSED AND HOW YOU CAN GET ACCESS TO THIS INFORMATION. PLEASE REVIEW IT CAREFULLY."

b. Individual's rights. An individual has the right to request restrictions on certain uses and disclosures of PHI, the right to receive confidential communications of PHI by alternative means or at alternative locations, the right to inspect and copy his PHI, the right to amend his PHI, the right to receive an accounting of disclosures of PHI, and the right to obtain a paper copy of the notice from the covered entity.

c. Covered entity's responsibilities. The notice must include a statement that the covered entity is required by law to maintain the privacy of PHI, a statement of its legal duties and privacy practices with respect to PHI, a statement that it must abide by the notice currently in effect, and a statement that it reserves the right to change the terms of its notice and how it will provide individuals with a revised notice.

d. Miscellaneous contents of notice. The notice must contain a statement that individuals may complain to the covered entity and to the U.S. Department of Health and Human Services if they believe their privacy rights have been violated. The notice must state a date on which it becomes effective. The effective date must be no later than the date of the first service delivery.

e. Posting of notice. A pharmacy must post the notice in a clear and prominent location where it is reasonable to expect individuals to be able to read the notice.

f. Written acknowledgment of notice. Every covered entity must obtain a written acknowledgment of receipt of the notice by the individual. If one is not obtained, the covered entity must document its good-faith efforts to obtain the acknowledgment and the reason why it was not obtained.

g. Exceptions for inmates. A person incarcerated in or otherwise confined to a correctional institution does not have a right to notice under the Privacy Rule, and the notice requirements do not apply to a correctional institution that is a covered entity.

5. **"Authorization"** for a covered entity to use or disclose PHI: a patient must give written authorization before a covered entity, including pharmacies and pharmacists, may use or disclose PHI. **No patient consent or authorization** is necessary when PHI use and disclosure is for **treatment, payment, or health-care operations.** This allows a health-care provider to consult with other covered entities (i.e., other health-care providers) to provide proper patient care without being unduly hindered by the Privacy Rule. For uses and disclosures that require an authorization, the **written authorization** must be written in plain language, and a **signed copy** must be provided to the individual. The signed authorization must be maintained by the covered entity for **6 years** from the date of its creation or the date when it was last in effect, whichever is later. The written authorization must at least contain the following core elements and statements:

a. A description of the information to be used or disclosed that identifies the information in a specific and meaningful fashion.

b. The name or other specific identification of the person(s), or class of persons, authorized to make the requested use or disclosure.

c. The name or other specific identification of the person(s), or class of persons, to whom the covered entity may make the requested use or disclosure.

d. A description of each purpose of the requested use or disclosure.

e. An expiration date or an expiration event that relates to the individual or the purpose of the use or disclosure.

f. Signature of the individual and date. If signed by a personal representative, it must also include a description of such representative's authority to act for the individual.

g. The written authorization must contain the following statements:

(1) The individual's right to revoke the authorization in writing along with the exceptions to the right to revoke and a description of how the individual may revoke the authorization.

(2) The ability or inability to condition treatment, payment, enrollment, or eligibility for benefits on the authorization, by stating either that the covered entity cannot require authorization, or that if the covered entity can require authorization, the consequences to the individual of his or her refusal to sign the authorization.

(3) The potential for the disclosed information to be redisclosed by the recipient and no longer be protected by the Privacy Rule.

6. **"Minimum necessary."** When using or disclosing PHI or when requesting PHI from another covered entity, a covered entity must make reasonable efforts to limit PHI to the **minimum necessary** to accomplish the intended purpose of the use, disclosure, or request. The minimum necessary rule **does not apply** to disclosures or requests by a health-care

provider for treatment, uses or disclosures made pursuant to an authorization, and uses or disclosures that are required by law. "Required by law" means a mandate in a law that compels an entity to make a use or disclosure of PHI. It includes a covered entity's compliance with state and federal laws and regulations that require the production of information; court orders and court-ordered warrants, subpoenas or summons issued by a court, a governmental or tribal inspector general, or an administrative body authorized to require the production of information and Medicare conditions of participation with respect to health-care providers participating in the program.

7. **"Business associates."** A business associate of a covered entity is a person or business that performs a function or activity on behalf of the covered entity, such as claims processing, billing, utilization review, quality assurance, etc., **and** that requires the use or disclosure of individually identifiable health information. A business associate would also include persons who provide services to the covered entity, **and** the service involves disclosure of individually identifiable health information, such as legal, actuarial, accounting, consulting, data aggregation, management, administrative, accreditation, or financial services. **Excluded** from the definition of business associates are members of the workforce of the covered entity, and functions or services that do not require disclosure of individually identifiable health information.

   a. **Business associate contracts.** Every business associate must enter into an agreement with the covered entity to ensure compliance with the Privacy Rule. Generally, the agreement must establish the required uses and disclosures of PHI by the business associate and require the return or destruction of PHI at termination of the contract.

B. **Additional responsibilities of covered entities.** Every covered entity must create policies and procedures for compliance with the Privacy Rule, must designate a privacy official responsible for creating such policies and procedures, must designate a contact person or office that is responsible for receiving complaints and that is able to provide further information about matters covered by the notice, and must train all members of its workforce with respect to the Privacy Rule. Every designation must be maintained by the covered entity for 6 years from the date it last was in effect. Lastly, every covered entity must have and apply appropriate sanctions against members of its workforce who fail to comply with the Privacy Rule.

C. **State law privacy rules.** The federal Privacy Rule is intended as the minimum requirement for privacy standards. If a state law is more stringent, then a covered entity must follow that state's privacy standards. If a state privacy law is not as stringent, the federal Privacy Rule preempts any contrary state law and a covered entity must abide by the federal Privacy Rule.

D. **Penalties for violation of the Privacy Rule.** Any person who violates the Privacy Rule may not be fined more than $100 for each violation up to a total of $25,000 per calendar year for all violations of an identical requirement. Additional penalties may be imposed for the following **wrongful disclosure** of individually identifiable health information:

   1. Wrongful obtainment or disclosure of PHI: fined not more than $50,000, imprisoned not more than 1 year, or both.

   2. Wrongful obtainment or disclosure of PHI under false pretenses: fined not more than $100,000, imprisoned not more than 5 years, or both.

   3. Wrongful obtainment or disclosure of PHI committed with intent to sell, transfer, or use same for commercial advantage, personal gain, or malicious harm: fined not more than $250,000, imprisoned not more than 10 years, or both.

VIII. **NARCOTIC TREATMENT PROGRAMS.** Methadone use is currently allowed as part of a total treatment program for narcotic addiction. Regulations concerning methadone treatment programs have been jointly established by the DEA and FDA. Narcotic-dependent individuals are those who physiologically need heroin or a morphine-like drug to prevent the onset of signs of withdrawal.

A. **Definition.** A narcotic treatment program is an organization that administers or dispenses a narcotic drug to a narcotic addict for maintenance or detoxification treatment, and provides, when appropriate or necessary, a comprehensive range of medical and rehabilitative services. The program must be:

1. Approved by the FDA

2. Approved by the appropriate state agency, usually the state's Department of Public Health or equivalent

3. Registered under the Federal Controlled Substances Act with the DEA to use a narcotic drug for the treatment of narcotic addiction

B. **Detoxification treatment** is defined as dispensing of narcotic drugs in decreasing doses to an individual to alleviate adverse physiological or psychological effects incident to withdrawal of narcotic drug use. Detoxification is for a period not in excess of 180 days.

C. **Maintenance treatment** is the dispensing of a narcotic drug, at relatively stable dosage levels, in the treatment of an individual for dependence on heroin or other morphine-like drug.

D. **Requirements to admit patients into a program.** In general, for a patient to be admitted into a comprehensive maintenance program, the following requirements must be met:

1. A program physician must determine that the person is currently physiologically dependent on a narcotic drug and became physiologically dependent at least 1 year before admission to the program.

2. The patient must have voluntarily chosen to participate in the program and must sign a "Consent to Methadone Treatment" (provided by the FDA) after being clearly and adequately informed about the use of methadone.

E. **Take-home methadone.** Take-home methadone may be given only to patients who, in the clinical judgment of the program physician, are responsible in handling narcotic drugs. The patient must come to the clinic for observation daily or at least 6 days a week. Over time, the program physician may reduce clinical observations to once weekly. Methadone for take-home use must be dispensed similarly to the dispensing of any schedule II controlled substance and include the treatment center's name, address, and telephone number on its label.

STUDY QUESTIONS

Directions: Each of the numbered items or incomplete statements in this section is followed by answers or by completions of the statement. Select the **one** lettered answer or completion that is **best** in each case.

1. All of the following prescription medications may be delivered by mail to the patient via the U.S. Postal Service EXCEPT

(A) procainamide
(B) ampicillin
(C) hydromorphone
(D) diazepam
(E) all of the above may be delivered by mail

2. Which of the following narcotic drugs has been approved by the FDA for use in the treatment of narcotic addiction?

(A) Morphine
(B) Codeine
(C) Methadone
(D) Hydrocodone
(E) None of the above

3. For the U.S. government to place a drug into schedule III, which of the following findings must be made concerning the drug?

(A) The drug or other substance has a high potential for abuse.
(B) Abuse of the drug or other substance may lead to limited physical dependence or psychological dependence relative to the drugs or other substances in schedule IV.
(C) The drug or other substance has no currently accepted medical use in treatment in the United States.
(D) Abuse of the drug or other substance may lead to moderate or low physical dependence or high psychological dependence.
(E) There is a lack of accepted safety for use of the drug or other substance under medical supervision.

4. Under the Federal Controlled Substances Act, all of the following items must appear on a controlled-substance prescription label EXCEPT the

(A) name, address, and DEA number of the pharmacy
(B) name of the patient
(C) name of the prescribing practitioner
(D) serial number assigned to the prescription
(E) date of the initial filling of the prescription

5. Under the Federal Controlled Substances Act, all of the following entities must register with the DEA EXCEPT

(A) prescribers of controlled substances
(B) pharmacists who dispense controlled substances
(C) distributors of controlled substances
(D) importers of controlled substances
(E) universities conducting instructional activities with controlled substances listed in schedules II–V

6. Under the Federal Controlled Substances Act, which of the following statements concerning the emergency dispensing of a schedule II controlled substance is true?

(A) The practitioner who authorizes the oral prescription must, within 7 days, deliver a written prescription to the dispensing pharmacist.
(B) The quantity prescribed and dispensed must be limited to the amount necessary to adequately treat the patient during the emergency period.
(C) It is not reasonably possible for the practitioner to provide a written prescription to be presented to the person dispensing the controlled substance before the dispensing.
(D) No appropriate alternative treatment is available, including administration of a controlled substance that is not in schedule II.
(E) All of the above statements are true.

7. Under the Federal Controlled Substances Act, the crime transfer warning, "Caution: Federal law prohibits the transfer of this drug to any person other than the patient for whom it was prescribed," must appear on the prescription container label of all controlled substances EXCEPT

(A) schedule II controlled substances
(B) schedule III controlled substances
(C) schedule IV controlled substances
(D) schedule V controlled substances

8. Which of the following statements concerning drug recall classification is true?

(A) A Class I recall is a situation in which use of, or exposure to, a violative product is not likely to cause adverse health consequences.

(B) A Class I recall is a situation in which use of, or exposure to, a violative product may cause temporary or medically reversible adverse health consequences or in which the probability of serious health consequences is remote.

(C) A Class I recall is a situation in which there is a reasonable probability that the use of, or exposure to, a violative product will cause serious adverse health consequences or death.

(D) A Class II recall is a situation in which use of, or exposure to, a violative product is not likely to cause adverse health consequences.

(E) A Class III recall is a situation in which there is a reasonable probability that the use of, or exposure to, a violative product will cause serious adverse health consequences or death.

9. Under the Federal Food, Drug, and Cosmetic Act, all of the following statements are considered a misbranding of a drug EXCEPT if

(A) the labeling is false or misleading in any particular.

(B) an oral contraceptive is dispensed without the required patient package insert.

(C) the drug is an imitation of another drug, or if it is offered for sale under the name of another drug.

(D) the drug consists in whole or in part of any filthy, putrid, or decomposed substance.

10. All of the following oral medications are exempt from child-resistant packaging EXCEPT

(A) anhydrous cholestyramine in powder form

(B) nitroglycerin preparations in sustained release form

(C) cyclically administered oral contraceptives in manufacturers' mnemonic (memory-aid) dispenser packages that rely solely upon the activity of one or more progestogen or estrogen substances

(D) pancrelipase preparations in tablet, capsule, or powder form that contain no other prescription medication

ANSWERS AND EXPLANATIONS

1. The answer is E *[V]*.
Narcotics and controlled substances in schedules II–V may be delivered to the patient by mail. The U.S. Postal Service no longer prohibits the mailing of narcotics by a physician or pharmacist (pursuant to a prescription) to the patient.

2. The answer is C *[VIII, VIII A, I I 2 c (2)]*.
Methadone is approved by the FDA for use in the treatment of narcotic addiction. Only a properly registered narcotic treatment program may dispense methadone for maintenance or detoxification treatment. Pharmacies that are not so registered may only dispense methadone for severe pain.

3. The answer is D *[I A 3]*.
To place a drug into schedule III, the U.S. government must make the following findings concerning the drug: (1) it has a potential for abuse less than the drugs or other substances in schedules I and II; (2) it has a currently accepted medical use in treatment in the United States; and (3) abuse of the drug may lead to moderate or low physical dependence or high psychological dependence.

4. The answer is A *[I I 8 c (1)–(7)]*.
A pharmacy's DEA number is not required to appear on the medication container label dispensed to the patient.

5. The answer is B *[I B 2 a–k, I B 9 d]*.
Agents and employees of DEA registrants, such as pharmacists, are exempt from registering with the DEA. Pharmacies, not the individual pharmacists, must register with the DEA.

6. The answer is E *[I I 4 a, b]*.
Emergency dispensing of an oral schedule II controlled-substance prescription must be done in strict compliance with the law. Before dispensing such a prescription, the pharmacist must make the threshold determination that ALL three factors that define an emergency situation (see I I 4 a) are present. If any one of the three factors is absent, the prescription is not for an emergency situation, and a written prescription must be presented to the pharmacist.

7. The answer is D *[I I 8 c (7)]*.
The federal crime transfer warning label is not required to appear on the prescription container label of schedule V controlled substances.

8. The answer is C *[II H 2 a–c]*.
A Class I recall is a situation in which there is a reasonable probability that the use of, or exposure to, a violative product will cause serious adverse health consequences or death.

9. The answer is D *[II I 1, 2]*.
The Federal Food, Drug, and Cosmetic Act states that a drug is considered adulterated if it consists in whole or in part of any filthy, putrid, or decomposed substance. The terms "misbranding" and "adulteration" are often referred to in literature and case law as being the same or similar violations under the law. However, the Act sets forth specific instances of adulteration and specific instances of misbranding.

10. The answer is B *[III A 1]*.
Only sublingual dosage forms of nitroglycerin are exempt from child-resistant packaging.

25
Reviewing and Dispensing Prescription and Medication Orders

Todd A. Brown

I. DEFINITIONS

A. Prescriptions are orders for medications, nondrug products, and services that are written by a licensed practitioner or midlevel practitioner who is authorized by state law to prescribe (see Appendix A). Pharmacists are increasingly being given prescribing privileges by enactment of state **collaborative drug therapy management** (CDTM) legislation. This allows pharmacists to order new medication or change the dose of existing medications under established protocols or guidelines agreed upon by the pharmacist and physician. Practitioners may only prescribe medications that are within their scope of practice. Prescriptions may be written, presented orally (by telephone), or presented electronically (i.e., via fax or computer network) to the pharmacist. The requirements of the prescription form may vary with state regulations. The prescription serves as a vehicle for communication from the prescriber to the pharmacist about the needs of the patient. The following information should be included on a prescription:

1. **Patient information,** including full name and address

2. **Date** on which the prescription was issued

3. **Name and dosage form of the product.** The name can be any of the following:
   a. Proprietary (brand)
   b. Nonproprietary (generic)
   c. Chemical

4. **Product strength.** The strength of the product is not required if only one strength is commercially available or if the product contains a combination of active ingredients. It is advisable to include the strength to reduce the chance of misinterpreting the prescription. If the dose is to be calculated by the pharmacist, then the pharmacist can decide the strength of the product dispensed after calculating the patient's dose.

5. **Quantity to be dispensed.** This should include the amount and the units of measure (e.g., grams, ounces, tablets). If the amount is not specified, the directions should specify the dose to be taken and the duration of therapy so that the pharmacist can calculate the quantity required for the patient.

6. **Directions for the pharmacist.** Directions may be required for:
   a. Preparation (e.g., compounding)
   b. Labeling (i.e., information to be put on the prescription label)

7. **Directions for the patient.** These should include explicit instructions on the quantity, schedule, and duration for proper use. "As Directed" should be avoided. If the directions vary, a minimum and maximum dose can be used.

8. **Refill information.** If refill information is not supplied, it is generally assumed that no refills are authorized. "As needed" [pro re nata (prn)] refills are usually interpreted as allowing for refills for 1 year.

9. **Prescriber information.** This should include the name, office address, signature of the prescriber, and the Drug Enforcement Administration (DEA) number (for controlled substances only). In some circumstances, prescriptions may be written by a midlevel practitioner (not licensed to prescribe alone) under the supervision of a licensed prescriber. In these cases, both the midlevel practitioner writing the prescription and the supervising licensed prescriber's name should be included.

B. Medication orders are orders for medications by an individual authorized to prescribe and are intended for use by patients while in an institutional setting. They may be written, presented orally (by telephone), or presented electronically (i.e., via fax or computer network) to the pharmacist. The medication order generally includes:

1. **Patient information** (e.g., full name, identification number)

2. **Date and time** the order was written

3. **Name of the product.** The name can be any of the following:
   a. Proprietary (brand)
   b. Nonproprietary (generic)
   c. Chemical

4. **Product strength, dosage, and route of administration.** The strength of the product is not required if only one strength is commercially available or if the product contains a combination of active ingredients. It is advisable to include the strength to reduce the chance of misinterpreting the order. The pharmacist may decide the strength of the product dispensed after calculating the patient's dose. The dosage and route of administration should be included to reduce the chance of misinterpreting the order and to allow for correct administration to the patient.

5. **Prescriber's signature.** If the order was taken verbally, the name of the person transcribing the order should be included.

6. **Directions for the pharmacist.** These can be used for:
   a. Preparation (e.g., compounding)
   b. Labeling (i.e., information to be put on the label)

7. **Instructions for administration,** including quantity, route of administration, schedule, and duration of use

II. UNDERSTANDING THE PRESCRIPTION OR MEDICATION ORDER AND EVALUATING ITS APPROPRIATENESS

A. Understanding the order. A complete understanding of all information contained in a prescription or medication order is required. Each piece of information should be appropriate and consistent with the remaining information (i.e., the instructions for use should be appropriate for the medication being ordered). The pharmacist should read the entire prescription or medication order carefully to determine the prescriber's intent by interpreting the following information:

1. The name and address of both the patient and the prescriber

2. The patient's disease or condition requiring treatment

3. The reason the order is indicated, relative to the medical need of the patient (e.g., an antibacterial for an infection)

4. The name of the product, the quantity prescribed, and instructions for use

5. All terminology, including units of measure (apothecary, metric, or English) and Latin abbreviations (see Appendix A)

B. Evaluating the appropriateness. Complete information is required on the prescription or medication order to provide the necessary information to allow the pharmacist to evaluate the appropriateness of the order. When the order is incomplete, the pharmacist must obtain the required information from either the patient or the prescriber. The following should be considered during an evaluation:

1. The patient's disease or condition requiring treatment

2. The patient's allergies or hypersensitivities

3. The pharmacological or biological action of the prescribed product

4. The prescribed route of administration

5. Whether the prescribed product might result in a drug–drug, drug–disease, or drug–food interaction

6. Whether the dose, dosage form, and dosage regimen are safe and likely to meet the needs of the patient

7. Whether the patient will have any difficulties adhering to the regimen and the potential impact on the therapeutic outcome desired

8. Whether the total quantity of medication prescribed is sufficient to allow proper completion of a course of therapy

9. Whether a physical or chemical incompatibility might result (i.e., if the product requires extemporaneous compounding)

10. Whether a licensed practitioner, acting in the course and scope of practice, issued the prescription in good faith, for a legitimate medical purpose

C. **Discovering inappropriate prescriptions or medication orders.** Pharmacists are required to review medication profiles to ensure the appropriateness of prescriptions or medication orders. This is commonly called **drug utilization review** (DUR). Pharmacists should not fill prescriptions or medication orders that they have concerns with or that are considered inappropriate, but rather, should contact the prescriber. The process of calling a prescriber to discuss concerns identified during a DUR is commonly called **therapeutic intervention.**

1. When performing a therapeutic intervention, the following information should be provided:
   a. A brief description of the problem
   b. A reference source that documents the problem
   c. A description of the clinical significance of the problem
   d. A suggestion of a solution to the problem

2. The following resolutions are possible to solve the problem or concern:
   a. The prescription or medication order will be dispensed as written.
   b. The prescription or medication order will not be dispensed.
   c. The prescription or medication order will be altered and dispensed.

3. Documentation of the results of a therapeutic intervention are required if the prescription or medication order is changed. The name of the prescriber, date of communication, issues discussed, and resolution should be included in the documentation. This information should be kept for the same time period as the prescription or medication order.

4. If the pharmacist feels that, in his or her professional judgment, an order is inappropriate and could harm the patient, the pharmacist should not process the order. The pharmacist may also be required to explain the situation to the patient. If, after a therapeutic intervention, the pharmacist believes the order is still inappropriate, the guidelines of the institution and professional judgment should be followed.

III. **PROCESSING PRESCRIPTIONS AND MEDICATION ORDERS** requires that the pharmacist follow appropriate guidelines. An environment that limits distractions and disruptions during these activities will assist in increasing the accuracy of this process. Automation and the use of pharmacy technicians allow the pharmacist to oversee these functions but spend less time performing these activities. The time saved allows the pharmacist greater time for patient-focused activities, such as counseling and patient education.

A. The following **information should be recorded on the prescription:**

1. The prescription number (for initial filling)

2. The original date of filling

3. The product and quantity dispensed

4. The pharmacist's initials

B. **Product selection.** Generic substitution statutes, as well as formulary and therapeutic substitution policies, might provide direction in product selection.

C. Product preparation for use by the patient. The following might be necessary for preparation:

1. Obtaining the proper amount of medication to be dispensed

2. Reconstitution (the addition of liquid to make a solution or suspension)

3. Extemporaneous compounding (see Chapter 5)

4. Assembly of the medication delivery unit

D. Selection of the proper package or container is required to ensure product stability, to promote patient compliance, and to comply with legal requirements. This information is commonly found in the *United States Pharmacopeia.*

E. Labeling the prescribed product

1. The **prescription label** must contain the following information:
   a. Name and address of the pharmacy
   b. Patient's name
   c. Original date of filling
   d. Prescription number
   e. Directions for use
   f. Product's brand name or generic name and manufacturer
   g. Product strength (if available in more than one strength)
   h. Quantity of medication dispensed
   i. Prescriber's name
   j. Expiration date of the medication
   k. Pharmacist's initials

2. **Unit-dose packages** contain one dose or one unit of medication. For a medication order that is dispensed in **unit-dose packages,** the label should identify the product's brand or generic name, strength, lot number, and expiration date.

3. **Auxiliary and cautionary labels.** To ensure proper medication use, storage, and compliance with applicable statutes, and to reinforce information provided during counseling, auxiliary and/or cautionary labels should be affixed when appropriate (see Appendix A).

4. For medication in schedules II–IV (see Chapter 24), a federal transfer warning is required.

F. Record keeping and confidentiality. The pharmacist is required to maintain **prescription files** and **records** in accordance with standards of sound practice and statutory requirements. The implementation of the **Healthcare Insurance Portability and Accountability Act of 1996** (HIPAA) has put additional requirements on all health professionals who have access to health information (see Chapter 24). The records should include a **patient profile system,** containing patient demographic information and a complete chronological record of all medication use and services provided in the delivery of pharmaceutical care.

1. The patient profile should contain the following **patient information:**
   a. Patient's name
   b. Patient's address (or room number in institutional settings)
   c. Any known allergies, sensitivities, or history of idiosyncratic reactions to previous medications
   d. Birth date (i.e., to assess the appropriateness of the dose)
   e. Clinical condition(s) [i.e., to help assess the appropriateness of the medication and to prevent drug–disease interactions]
   f. Weight (i.e., to assess the appropriateness of the dose)
   g. Occupation (i.e., to detect conditions associated with a particular occupation and to help determine if the patient will be able to comply with the regimen)
   h. Nonprescription medication use (i.e., to prevent drug–drug and drug–disease interactions, to assess medication effectiveness, and to detect possible adverse effects)

2. In addition, the patient profile should contain the following information from each prescription or medication order:
   a. Name of the medication
   b. Medication strength
   c. Dosage form

    d. Quantity dispensed
    e. Directions for use
    f. Prescription number
    g. Dispensing date
    h. Number of refills authorized and remaining
    i. Prescriber's name
    j. Pharmacist's initials

IV. DISPENSING MEDICATION AND COUNSELING.
The dispensing of medication requires that the pharmacist verify that patients have the necessary knowledge and ability to adhere to the prescribed treatment. This will increase the likelihood of obtaining the desired outcomes.

A. Counseling patients. The pharmacist should evaluate the patient's understanding of each medication and supply additional information when the patient's information is incorrect or insufficient. The pharmacist might need to advise patients regarding the proper dosage, appearance, and name of the medication. Information about the route of administration, instructions for use, duration of use, and the reason the product was prescribed may also be needed. In addition, the following topics might also be appropriate during the counseling session:

1. **Special procedures.** As appropriate, the pharmacist should advise patients on how to take the medication (e.g., on an empty stomach, with plenty of water) and instruct them on foods to avoid while taking the medication (e.g., alcoholic beverages, dairy products).

2. **Potential adverse effects.** The pharmacist should ensure that patients are aware of the possible adverse effects associated with the medication. Patients should understand:
    a. The **frequency** of an adverse effect. This will help patients recognize common adverse effects and not be overly concerned with those that are rare.
    b. The **severity** of an adverse effect. This will help patients focus on those adverse effects that are severe and not those that are inconsequential.
    c. What action should be taken to **manage** or **minimize** the adverse effect. This will help patients deal with possible adverse effects in the appropriate manner.

3. **Proper storage.** The pharmacist should counsel patients on how to store medications properly to ensure stability and potency.

4. **Over-the-counter (OTC) products.** The pharmacist should instruct patients about the use of OTC products that might or might not be appropriate when taking a prescribed product.

B. Counseling health professionals. Health professionals (i.e., in an institutional setting) may administer medications to patients. In these cases, the pharmacist should ensure that the health professional has sufficient knowledge to administer the product. Information that health professionals would need to administer medications safely and effectively include:

1. The choice of a particular product

2. The proper dosage, dosage regimen, and route of administration

3. The cost of the prescribed product and the costs associated with its use (i.e., administration costs and costs of treating possible adverse effects)

4. The availability of commercially made products

5. Potential adverse effects

6. Drug interactions

7. Physical incompatibilities

8. Safe handling and disposal procedures

9. Nutritional interactions or requirements

10. Drug interference with laboratory tests

V. PATIENT MONITORING.
The provision of pharmaceutical care requires a **pharmaceutical care plan** (see Chapter 20). Monitoring the impact of drug therapy should be performed on a reg-

ular basis. A pharmaceutical care plan maximizes the benefits of the prescribed therapy by increasing desired outcomes and decreasing undesired outcomes. Undesired outcomes associated with drug therapy are frequently called **drug-related problems.**

A. Pharmaceutical care plan. To increase the frequency and benefits of desired outcomes, a pharmaceutical care plan should include the following:

    1. Assessment—a review of the medical conditions and symptoms to determine the need for drug therapy

    2. Plan—a decision of an appropriate drug therapy based on the assessment of the patient

    3. Monitoring—a review of the outcomes of drug therapy (i.e., goals and end points) to determine if the patient is obtaining the desired outcomes

B. Drug-related problems are evidence of less-than-optimal drug therapy. Detection of drug-related problems requires an assessment of the need for a change in drug therapy. Possible problems include:

    1. Unnecessary drug therapy—medication that cannot be associated with a medical condition or the presence of a condition in which nondrug therapy is more appropriate.

    2. Wrong drug—The drug is not indicated for the condition or is not delivering the desired outcomes, or a more effective drug is available.

    3. Dose too low—incorrect dose, frequency, administration, or duration of therapy resulting in an insufficient dose of drug to the patient.

    4. Adverse drug reaction—allergic reaction, drug interaction, or an undesirable effect from a medication.

    5. Dose too high—incorrect dose, frequency, or duration, resulting in more medication than is required.

    6. Inappropriate compliance—the patient is not taking the optimal amount of medication due to cost, administration difficulties, alternative health beliefs, or a lack of understanding of the need for the medication.

    7. Need additional drug therapy—due to an undertreated condition, synergism with concurrent drug therapy, or prophylactic therapy required.

STUDY QUESTIONS

Directions: Each of the numbered items or incomplete statements in this section is followed by answers or by completions of the statement. Select the **one** lettered answer or completion that is **best** in each case.

1. Medication orders differ from prescriptions in which of the following ways? They

(A) are intended for ambulatory use.
(B) contain only the generic name of the medication.
(C) are intended for institutional use.
(D) may be transmitted electronically.
(E) contain the quantity of medication to be dispensed.

2. If a therapeutic intervention is necessary, all of the following information should be communicated to the prescriber EXCEPT

(A) a declaration that "a mistake was made."
(B) a brief description of the problem.
(C) a reference source that documents the problem.
(D) an alternative or suggestion to resolve the problem.
(E) a description of the clinical significance of the problem.

3. The following information should be recorded on a prescription EXCEPT the

(A) prescription number
(B) date of filling
(C) expiration date
(D) product and quantity dispensed
(E) pharmacist's initials

4. A prescription label should contain all of the following EXCEPT the

(A) quantity dispensed
(B) lot number
(C) patient's diagnosis
(D) expiration date
(E) prescriber's name

5. Auxiliary and cautionary labels should be utilized for all of the following purposes EXCEPT to

(A) substitute for verbal consultation.
(B) ensure proper usage.
(C) inform of storage requirements.
(D) comply with regulatory requirements.
(E) warn against the concomitant use of certain drugs or foods.

6. The following items are essential for a patient profile system EXCEPT

(A) the patient's name
(B) the prescriber's DEA registration number
(C) the patient's allergies
(D) the patient's birth date
(E) instructions for medication use

7. The following are drug-related problems EXCEPT

(A) an adverse effect from a medication
(B) symptoms due to undertreatment
(C) a drug–drug interaction
(D) an undiagnosed condition
(E) an allergic reaction to a medication

ANSWERS AND EXPLANATIONS

1. The answer is C *[I B]*.
Medication orders are written for the care of inpatients. Both medication orders and prescriptions may contain the brand or generic name of the drug and may be transmitted electronically. Only prescriptions contain the quantity of medication to be dispensed.

2. The answer is A *[II C 1]*.
Information provided to the prescriber during a therapeutic intervention should include a description of the problem, reference source, description of the clinical significance, and an alternative. Informing the prescriber that a mistake was made does not encourage cooperation and resolution of the problem.

3. The answer is C *[III A]*.
The prescription number, date of filling, product and quantity dispensed, and pharmacist's initials should be recorded on the prescription. The expiration date of the product being dispensed is not required.

4. The answer is C *[III E 1]*.
The quantity of medication dispensed, lot number, expiration date of the product, and prescriber's name should be included on the label. The patient's diagnosis, although listed in the patient's profile, is not included on the prescription label.

5. The answer is A *[III E 3; IV A 1]*.
Auxiliary and cautionary labels are an adjunct to, not a replacement for, verbal consultation. Appropriate uses for such labels include ensuring proper use, storage requirements, and compliance with statutory requirements, and warning against food and drug interactions.

6. The answer is B *[III F 1–2]*.
The patient's name is required to identify each patient. Often, the address or room number is required to identify patients with similar names. The patient's allergies, birth date, and instructions for use are required to prevent drug allergies and to assess the appropriateness of the prescription or medication order.

7. The answer is D *[V B]*.
Adverse effects, undertreated conditions, allergic reactions, and drug–drug interaction are all drug-related problems. An undiagnosed condition may lead to a drug-related problem once diagnosed; however, diagnosis is required before the need for medication can be assessed.

26
Sterile Products
John Fanikos

I. INTRODUCTION

A. Sterility, an absolute term, means the absence of living microorganisms.

1. **Sterile products** are pharmaceutical dosage forms that are sterile. This includes products like parenteral preparations, irrigating solutions, and ophthalmic preparations (see Chapter 29).

2. **Aseptic technique** refers to the procedures used during preparation that maintain the sterility of pharmaceutical dosage forms.

3. **Parenteral preparations** are pharmaceutical dosage forms that are injected through one or more layers of skin. Because the parenteral route bypasses the protective barriers of the body, parenteral preparations must be sterile. The pH of a solution may markedly influence the stability and compatibility of parenteral preparations (see V B).

4. **Pyrogens** are metabolic by-products of live or dead microorganisms that cause a pyretic response (i.e., a fever) upon injection.

5. **Tonicity** refers to the tone of a solution and is directly related to the osmotic pressure exerted by the solute.
   a. **Hypotonic solutions** have a lower osmotic pressure than blood or 0.9% sodium chloride solution. Because these solutions cause cells to expand, administration can lead to pain and hemolysis.
   b. **Isotonic solutions** exert the same osmotic pressure as blood or 0.9% sodium chloride solution.
   c. **Hypertonic solutions** have a greater osmotic pressure than blood or 0.9% sodium chloride solution. These solutions are administered through a large vein, either the subclavian or internal jugular vein to avoid phlebitis and ensure rapid dilution.

B. Design and function of sterile product areas

1. **Clean rooms.** These areas are specially constructed and maintained to reduce the probability of environmental contamination of sterile products during the manufacturing process. Clean rooms must meet several requirements:
   a. **High-efficiency particulate-air (HEPA) filters** are used to cleanse the air entering the room. These filters remove all airborne particles 0.3 mm or larger, with an efficiency of 99.97%. In addition, HEPA-filtered rooms generally are classified as Federal Class 10,000, which means that they contain no more than 10,000 particles 0.5 mm or larger per cubic foot of air.
   b. **Positive-pressure airflow** is used to prevent contaminated air from flowing into the clean room. In order to achieve this, the air pressure inside the clean room must be greater than the pressure outside the room, so that when a door to the clean room is opened, the airflow is outward.
   c. **Counters** in the clean room are made of stainless steel or other nonporous, easily cleaned material.
   d. **Walls** and **floors** do not have cracks or crevices and have rounded corners. Walls and floors should also be nonporous and washable to enable regular disinfection. If walls or floors are painted, an epoxy paint is used.
   e. **Airflow.** As with the HEPA filters used in clean rooms, the airflow moves with a uniform velocity along parallel lines. The velocity of the airflow is 90 feet per minute.

2. **Laminar flow hoods.** These clean-air work benches are specially designed, like clean rooms, to create an aseptic environment for the preparation of sterile products. A Class 100 environment exists inside a certified horizontal or vertical laminar airflow hood. Laminar flow hoods generally are used in conjunction with clean rooms. However, not all phar-

macies involved in preparing sterile products have clean rooms; in these instances, laminar flow hoods are vital to ensure aseptic preparation.

a. HEPA filter requirement. Like clean rooms, laminar flow hoods use HEPA filters, but the hoods use a higher-efficiency air filter than do clean rooms. Laminar flow hoods are classified as Federal Class 100, meaning that they contain no more than 100 particles 0.3 mm or larger per cubic foot of air and have an efficiency of 99.99%.

b. Types of laminar flow hoods

   (1) Horizontal laminar flow hoods (Figure 26-1) were the first hoods used in pharmacies for the preparation of sterile products. Airflow in horizontal hoods moves across the surface of the work area, flowing first through a prefilter and then through the HEPA filter. The major **disadvantage** of the horizontal hood is that it offers no protection to the operator, which is especially significant when antineoplastic agents are being prepared (see V D 2).

   (2) Vertical laminar flow hoods (Figure 26-2) provide **two major advantages** over horizontal flow hoods.

      (a) The airflow is vertical, flowing down on the work space. This airflow pattern protects the operator against potential hazards from the products being prepared.

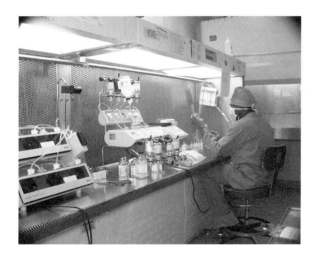

Figure 26-1. Horizontal laminar flow hood (photo taken by William Salkin).

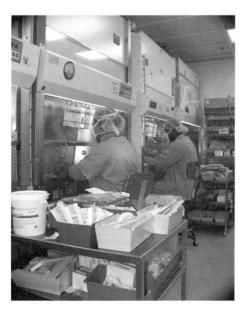

Figure 26-2. Vertical laminar flow hood (photo taken by William Salkin).

(b) A portion of the HEPA-filtered air is recirculated a second time through the HEPA filter. The remainder of the filtered air is removed through an exhaust filter, which may be vented to the outside to protect the operator from chronic, concentrated exposure to hazardous materials.

3. **Inspection and certification.** Clean rooms and laminar flow hoods are inspected and certified when they are first installed, at least every 6–12 months thereafter, and, in the case of hoods, when moved to a new location.
   a. **Inspections** are conducted by companies with the sensitive equipment needed for testing procedures and with personnel who are specially trained in these procedures.
   b. The **dioctyl phthalate (DOP) smoke test** ensures that no particle larger than 0.3 mm passes through the HEPA filter. In addition, an anemometer is used to determine airflow velocity, and a particle counter is used to determine the particle count.

II. STERILIZATION METHODS AND EQUIPMENT.
Sterilization is performed to destroy or remove all microorganisms in or on a product. Sterilization can be achieved through thermal, chemical, radioactive, or mechanical methods.

A. **Thermal sterilization** involves the use of either moist or dry heat.

1. **Moist-heat sterilization** is the **most widely used** and reliable sterilization method.
   a. Microorganisms are destroyed by **cellular protein coagulation.**
   b. The objects to be sterilized are exposed to saturated steam under pressure at a minimum temperature of **121°C** for at least **15 minutes.**
   c. An **autoclave** is commonly used for moist-heat sterilization.
   d. Because it does not require as high a temperature, moist-heat sterilization causes **less product and equipment damage** compared to dry-heat sterilization.

2. **Dry-heat sterilization** is appropriate for materials that cannot withstand moist-heat sterilization. Objects are subjected to a temperature of at least **160°C** for **120 minutes** (if higher temperatures can be used, less exposure time is required).

B. **Chemical (gas) sterilization** is used to sterilize surfaces and porous materials (e.g., surgical dressings) that other sterilization methods may damage.

1. In this method, **ethylene oxide** is used generally in combination with heat and moisture.

2. **Residual gas** must be allowed to dissipate after sterilization and before use of the sterile product.

C. **Radioactive sterilization** is suitable for the industrial sterilization of contents in sealed packages that cannot be exposed to heat (e.g., prepackaged surgical components, some ophthalmic ointments).

1. This technique involves either **electromagnetic** or **particulate radiation.**

2. Accelerated drug decomposition sometimes results.

D. **Mechanical sterilization (filtration)** removes but does not destroy microorganisms and clarifies solutions by eliminating particulate matter. For solutions rendered unstable by thermal, chemical, or radiation sterilization, filtration is the preferred method. A depth filter or screen filter may be used.

1. **Depth filters** usually consist of fritted glass or unglazed porcelain (i.e., substances that trap particles in channels).

2. **Screen (membrane) filters** are films measuring 1–200 mm thick made of cellulose esters, microfilaments, polycarbonate, synthetic polymers, silver, or stainless steel.
   a. A **mesh** of millions of microcapillary pores of identical size filter the solution by a process of physical sieving.
   b. **Flow rate.** Because pores make up 70%–85% of the surface, screen filters have a higher flow rate than depth filters.
   c. **Types of screen filters**
      (1) Particulate filters remove particles of glass, plastic, rubber, and other contaminants.
         (a) Other uses. These filters also are used to reduce the risk of phlebitis associated with administration of reconstituted powders. Filtration removes any undissolved powder particles that may cause venous inflammation.

    (b) The **pore size** of standard particulate filters ranges from 0.45–5 mm. Special particulate filters are required to filter blood, emulsions (e.g., fat emulsions), or colloidal dispersions or suspensions because these preparations have a larger particle size.

  (2) Microbial filters, with a pore size of 0.22 mm or smaller, ensure complete microbial removal and sterilization. This is referred to as cold sterilization.

  (3) Final filters, which may be either particulate or microbial, are often included as part of the tubing used in drug administration. They are referred to as in-line filters and are used to remove particulates or microorganisms from an intravenous (IV) solution during infusion.

III. PACKAGING OF PARENTERAL PRODUCTS. Parenteral preparations and other sterile products must be packaged in a way that maintains product sterility until the time of use and prevents contamination of contents during opening.

A. Types of containers

  1. Ampules, the oldest type of parenteral product containers, are made entirely of **glass.**

    a. Intended for **single use only,** ampules are opened by breaking the glass at a score line on the neck.

    b. Disadvantages. Because glass particles may become dislodged during ampule opening, the product must be filtered before it is administered. Their unsuitability for multiple-dose use, the need to filter solutions before use, and other safety considerations have markedly reduced the ampule as a package form.

  2. Vials are glass or plastic containers closed with a rubber stopper and sealed with an aluminum crimp (Figure 26-3).

    a. Vials have several **advantages** over ampules.

      (1) Vials can be designed to hold multiple doses (if prepared with a bacteriostatic agent).

      (2) The drug product is easier to remove from vials than from ampules.

      (3) Vials eliminate the risk of glass particle contamination during opening.

    b. However, vials also have certain **disadvantages.**

      (1) The rubber stopper can become cored, causing a small bit of rubber to enter the solution.

      (2) Multiple withdrawals (as with multiple-dose vials) can result in microbial contamination.

    c. Some drugs that are unstable in solution are packaged in vials unreconstituted and must be **reconstituted** with a diluent before use. Sterile water or sterile sodium chloride for injection are the most commonly used drug diluents.

      (1) To accelerate the dissolution rate and permit rapid reconstitution, many powders are lyophilized (freeze dried).

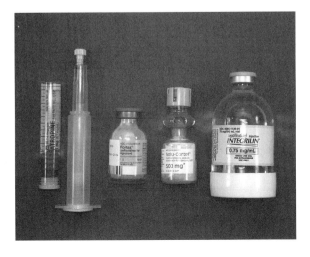

Figure 26-3. Syringes and vials (photo taken by William Salkin).

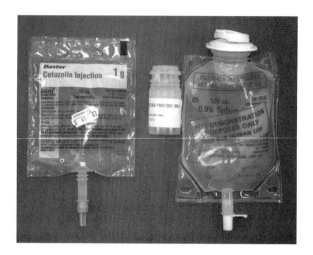

Figure 26-4. Left, prefilled antibiotic piggy-back dose; right, Abbott ADD-Vantage system (photo taken by William Salkin).

(2) Some of these drugs come in vials that contain a double chamber.
  (a) The top chamber, containing sterile water for injection, is separated from the unreconstituted drug by a rubber closure.
  (b) To dislodge the inner closure and mix the contents of the compartments, external pressure is applied to the outer rubber closure. This system eliminates the need to enter the vial twice, thereby reducing the risk of microbial contamination.

3. Some drugs come in vials that may be attached to an IV bag for reconstitution and administration (**ADD-Vantage** by Abbott) [Figure 26-4].
  a. The ADD-Vantage vial is screwed into the top of an ADD-Vantage IV bag, and the rubber diaphragm is dislodged from the vial, allowing the IV solution to dissolve the drug.
  b. The reconstituted ADD-Vantage vial and IV bag are ready for administration when hung.

4. Prefilled syringes and **cartridges** are designed for maximum convenience (see Figure 26-3).
  a. Prefilled syringes. Drugs administered in an emergency (e.g., atropine, epinephrine) are available for immediate injection when packaged in prefilled syringes.
  b. Prefilled cartridges are ready-to-use parenteral packages that offer improved sterility and accuracy. They consist of a plastic cartridge holder and a prefilled medication cartridge with a needle attached. The medication is premixed and premeasured. Narcotics (e.g., morphine, meperidine) are commonly available in prefilled cartridges.

5. Infusion solutions are divided into two categories: **small-volume parenterals** (SVPs), those having a volume less than 100 mL; and **large-volume parenterals** (LVPs), those having a volume of 100 mL or greater. Infusion solutions are used for the intermittent or continuous infusion of fluids or drugs (see VIII B).

B. Packaging materials. Materials used to package parenteral products include glass and plastic polymers.

  1. Glass, the original parenteral packaging material, has superior clarity, facilitating inspection for particulate matter. Compared to plastic, glass less frequently interacts with the preparation it contains.

  2. Plastic polymers used for parenteral packaging include polyvinylchloride (PVC) and polyolefin.
    a. PVC is flexible and nonrigid.
    b. Polyolefin is semirigid; unlike PVC, it can be stored upright.
    c. Both types of plastic offer several **advantages** over glass, including durability, easier storage and disposal, reduced weight, and improved safety.

IV. PARENTERAL ADMINISTRATION ROUTES. Parenteral preparations may be given by a variety of administration routes.

A. **Subcutaneous** administration refers to injection into the subcutaneous tissue beneath the skin layers, usually of the abdomen, arm, or thigh. Insulin is an example of a subcutaneously administered drug.

B. **Intramuscular** administration means injection into a muscle mass. The mid-deltoid area and gluteus medius are common injection sites.

1. No more than 5 mL of a solution should be injected by this route.

2. Drugs intended for prolonged or delayed absorption (e.g., methylprednisolone) commonly are administered intramuscularly.

C. **IV** administration is the most important and most common parenteral administration route. It allows an immediate therapeutic effect by delivering the drug directly into the circulation. However, this route precludes recall of an inadvertent drug overdose. Antibiotics, cardiac medications, and many other drugs are given intravenously.

D. **Intradermal** administration involves injection into the most superficial skin layer. Because this route can deliver only a limited drug volume, its use generally is restricted to skin tests and certain vaccines.

E. **Intra-arterial** administration is injection directly into an artery. It delivers a high drug concentration to the target site with little dilution by the circulation. Generally, this route is used only for radiopaque materials, thrombolytic agents, and some antineoplastic agents.

F. **Intracardiac** administration is injection of a drug directly into the heart.

G. **Hypodermoclysis** refers to injection of large volumes of a solution into subcutaneous tissue to provide a continuous, abundant drug supply. This route occasionally is used for antibiotic administration in children.

H. **Intraspinal** administration refers to injection into the spinal column. Local anesthetics (e.g., lidocaine, bupivacaine) are frequently administered via this route during surgical procedures.

I. **Intra-articular** administration means injection into a joint space. Corticosteroids (e.g., methylprednisolone, hydrocortisone) use this route for the treatment of arthritis.

J. **Intrasynovial administration** refers to injection into the joint fluid.

K. **Intrathecal administration** is injection into the spinal fluid; it sometimes is used for antibiotics and cancer chemotherapy.

L. **Epidural administration** refers to the injection of medications, usually local anesthetics and/or narcotics near or outside the dura mater of the central nervous system. This route is frequently used during childbirth.

V. PARENTERAL PREPARATIONS

A. **IV admixtures.** These preparations consist of one or more sterile drug products added to an IV fluid, generally dextrose or sodium chloride solution alone or in combination. IV admixtures are used for drugs intended for continuous infusion. Drugs that may cause irritation or toxicity when given as a rapid direct IV injection are also prepared as IV admixtures.

B. **IV fluids and electrolytes**

1. **Fluids** used in the preparation and administration of parenteral products include sterile water and sodium chloride, dextrose, and Ringer's solutions, all of which have multiple uses. These fluids serve as vehicles in IV admixtures, providing a means for reconstituting sterile powders. They serve as the basis for correcting body fluid and electrolyte disturbances and provide a caloric source in parenteral nutrition.

   a. **Dextrose (D-glucose) solutions** are the most frequently used glucose solutions in parenteral preparations.

      (1) **Uses.** Generally, a solution of dextrose 5% in water (d5w) is used as a vehicle in IV admixtures. D5W may also serve as a hydrating solution. In higher concentrations (e.g., a 10% solution in water), dextrose provides a source of carbohydrates in parenteral nutrition solutions.

      (2) Considerations. Because the pH of D5W ranges from 3.5–6.5, instability may result if it is combined with an acid-sensitive drug.

        (a) Dextrose concentrations greater than 15% must be administered through a central vein.

        (b) Dextrose solutions should be used cautiously in patients with diabetes mellitus.

  b. Sodium chloride usually is given as a 0.9% solution. Because it is isotonic with blood, this solution is called normal saline solution (NSS). A solution of 0.45% sodium chloride is termed half-normal saline. A solution of 0.225% sodium chloride is termed quarter-normal saline.

      (1) Sodium chloride for injection, which is a solution of 0.9% sodium chloride, is used as a vehicle in IV admixtures and for fluid and electrolyte replacement. In smaller volumes, it is suitable for the reconstitution of various medications.

      (2) Bacteriostatic sodium chloride for injection, which is also a 0.9% solution, is intended solely for multiple reconstitutions. It contains an agent that inhibits bacterial growth (e.g., benzyl alcohol, propylparaben, methylparaben), which allows for its use in multiple-dose preparations.

  c. Waters are used for reconstitution and for dilution of such IV solutions as dextrose and sodium chloride. Waters suitable for parenteral preparations include sterile water for injection and bacteriostatic water for injection.

  d. Ringer's solutions, which are appropriate for fluid and electrolyte replacement, commonly are administered to postsurgical patients.

      (1) Lactated Ringer's injection (i.e., Hartmann's solution, Ringer's lactate solution) contains sodium lactate, sodium chloride, potassium chloride, and calcium chloride. Frequently, it is combined with dextrose (e.g., as 5% dextrose in lactated Ringer's injection).

      (2) Ringer's injection differs from lactated Ringer's injection in that it does not contain sodium lactate and has slightly different concentrations of sodium chloride and calcium chloride. Like lactated Ringer's injection, it may be combined in solution with dextrose.

2. Electrolyte preparations. With ions present in both intracellular and extracellular fluid, electrolytes are crucial for various biological processes. Surgical and medical patients who cannot take food by mouth or who need nutritional supplementation require the addition of electrolytes in hydrating solutions or parenteral nutrition solutions.

  a. Cations are positively charged electrolytes.

      (1) Sodium is the chief extracellular cation.

        (a) Importance. Sodium plays a key role in interstitial osmotic pressure, tissue hydration, acid–base balance, nerve-impulse transmission, and muscle contraction.

        (b) Parenteral sodium preparations include sodium chloride, sodium acetate, and sodium phosphate.

      (2) Potassium is the chief intracellular cation.

        (a) Importance. Potassium participates in carbohydrate metabolism, protein synthesis, muscle contraction (especially of cardiac muscle), and neuromuscular excitability.

        (b) Parenteral potassium preparations include potassium acetate, potassium chloride, and potassium phosphate.

      (3) Calcium

        (a) Importance. Calcium is essential to nerve-impulse transmission, muscle contraction, cardiac function, bone formation, and capillary and cell membrane permeability.

        (b) Parenteral calcium preparations include calcium chloride, calcium gluconate, and calcium gluceptate.

      (4) Magnesium

        (a) Importance. Magnesium plays a vital part in enzyme activities, neuromuscular transmission, and muscle excitability.

        (b) Parenteral preparation. Magnesium is given parenterally as magnesium sulfate.

  b. Anions are negatively charged electrolytes.

      (1) Chloride is the major extracellular anion.

        (a) Importance. Along with sodium, it regulates interstitial osmotic pressure and helps to control blood pH.

        (b) Parenteral chloride preparations include calcium chloride, potassium chloride, and sodium chloride.

   (2) Phosphate is the major intracellular anion.

        (a) Importance. Phosphate is critical to various enzyme activities. It also influences calcium levels and acts as a buffer to prevent marked changes in acid–base balance.

        (b) Parenteral phosphate preparations include potassium phosphate and sodium phosphate.

   (3) Acetate

        (a) Importance. Acetate is a bicarbonate precursor that may be used to provide alkali to assist in the preservation of plasma pH.

        (b) Parenteral acetate preparations include potassium acetate and sodium acetate.

C. Parenteral antibiotic preparations are available as sterile unreconstituted powders, which must be reconstituted with sterile water, normal saline, or d5w, or as a sterile, ready-to-use liquid parenteral.

   1. Administration methods. Parenteral antibiotics may be given intermittently by direct IV injection, short-term infusion, intramuscular injection, or intrathecal injection.

   2. Uses. Parenteral antibiotics are used to treat infections that are serious and require high antibiotic blood levels or when the gastrointestinal tract is contraindicated, such as in ileus.

   3. Dosing frequencies of parenteral antibiotics vary from once daily to as often as every 2 hours, depending on the kinetics of the drug, seriousness of the infection, the site of infection, and the patient's disease or organ status (e.g., renal disease).

D. Parenteral antineoplastic agents. Studies suggest that these medications may be toxic to the personnel who prepare and administer them. The evidence is not conclusive, which necessitates special precautions to ensure safety and minimize risks. In addition, patients receiving antineoplastics can experience various problems associated with drug delivery.

   1. Administration methods. Parenteral antineoplastics may be given by direct IV injection, short-term infusion, or long-term infusion. Some are administered by a non-IV route, such as the subcutaneous, intramuscular, intra-arterial, or intrathecal route.

   2. Safe antineoplastic handling guidelines. All pharmacy and nursing personnel who prepare or administer antineoplastics should receive special training in the following guidelines to reduce the risk of exposure to these drugs.

     a. A **vertical laminar flow hood** should be used during drug preparation, with exhaust directed to the outside.

     b. All syringes and IV tubing should have **Luer-Lok fittings** (see VII B 1, 4).

     c. Clothing. Personnel should wear closed-front cuffed surgical gowns and double-layered latex surgeon's gloves.

     d. Negative-pressure technique should be used during withdrawal of medication from vials. This will prevent pressure from building up inside the vial and causing the drug to spray around the needle.

     e. Final dosage adjustment should be made into the vial, ampule, or directly into an absorbent gauze pad.

     f. Priming equipment. Special care should be taken when IV administration sets are primed. The IV tubing should be primed before adding the drug, or the tubing can be primed with drug-free fluid before connecting it to the chemotherapy drug container. If these are not available, prime the tubing into sterile gauze in a sealable plastic bag.

     g. Proper procedures should be followed for **disposal** of materials used in the preparation and administration of antineoplastics.

        (1) Needles should not be clipped or recapped.

        (2) Preparations should be discarded in containers that are puncture-proof, leak-proof, and properly labeled.

        (3) Hazardous waste. There is no completely acceptable method for disposing of hazardous waste. High-temperature incineration may be the preferred method. These materials may also be buried in an EPA-licensed hazardous waste dump or chemically deactivated.

   h. After removal of gloves, personnel should **wash hands** thoroughly.
   i. Personnel and equipment involved in the preparation and administration of antineo-plastic agents should be **monitored** routinely.

   3. Patient problems. Infusion phlebitis and extravasation are the most serious problems that may occur during the administration of parenteral antineoplastics.
   a. Infusion phlebitis (inflammation of a vein) is characterized by pain, swelling, heat sensation, and redness at the infusion site. Drug dilution and filtration can eliminate or minimize the risk of phlebitis.
   b. Extravasation (infiltration of a drug into subcutaneous tissues surrounding the vein) is especially harmful when antineoplastics with vesicant properties are administered. Measures must be taken immediately if extravasation occurs.
      (1) Depending on the drug involved, emergency measures may include stopping the infusion, injecting hydrocortisone or another anti-inflammatory agent directly into the affected area, injecting an antidote (if available), and applying a cold compress (to facilitate a drug–antidote reaction).
      (2) A warm compress may then be applied to increase the flow of blood, and thus the vesicant, away from damaged tissue.

E. Parenteral biotechnology products are created by the application of biological processes to the generation of therapeutic agents, such as monoclonal antibodies, various vaccines, and colony-stimulating factors.

   1. Potential uses of these agents include cancer therapy, infections, transplant rejection and vaccines against cancer, HIV infection, hepatitis B, herpes, rheumatoid arthritis, inflammatory bowel disease, respiratory diseases, and malaria.

   2. Characteristics. Protein and peptide biotechnology drugs have a shorter half-life, often require special storage such as refrigeration or freezing, and must not be shaken vigorously to avoid destroying the protein molecules.

   3. Administration. Many biotechnology products require reconstitution with sterile water or normal saline and may be parenterally administered by direct IV injection or infusion, or by intramuscular or subcutaneous injection.

VI. IRRIGATING SOLUTIONS. Although these sterile products are manufactured by the same standards used to process IV preparations, they are **not intended for infusion into the venous system.** Labeling differences between irrigation solutions and injections are specified in the *United States Pharmacopeia* (USP) and reflect differences in acceptable particulate matter levels, volume of solution available for use, and the container design.

   A. Topical administration. Irrigating solutions for topical use are packaged in pour bottles so that they can be poured directly onto the desired area. These solutions are intended for such purposes as irrigating wounds, moistening dressings, and cleaning surgical instruments.

   B. Infusion of irrigating solutions. This procedure, using an administration set attached to a Foley catheter, is commonly used for many surgical patients. Surgeons performing urological procedures often use irrigating solutions to perfuse tissues in order to maintain the integrity of the surgical field, remove blood, and provide a clear field of view. To decrease the risk of infection, 1 mL of Neosporin G.U. Irrigant, an antibiotic preparation, often is added to these solutions.

   C. Dialysis. Dialysates are irrigating solutions used in the dialysis of patients with such disorders as renal failure, poisoning, and electrolyte disturbances. These products remove waste materials, serum electrolytes, and toxic products from the body.

   1. In **peritoneal dialysis,** a hypertonic dialysate is infused directly into the peritoneal cavity via a surgically implanted catheter. The dialysate, which contains dextrose and electrolytes, removes harmful substances by osmosis and diffusion. After a specified period of time, the solution is drained. Antibiotics and heparin may be added to the dialysate.

   2. In **hemodialysis,** the patient's blood is transfused through a dialyzing membrane unit that removes the harmful substances from the patient's vascular system. After passing through the dialyzer, the blood reenters the body through a vein.

VII. NEEDLES AND SYRINGES

A. **Hypodermic needles** are stainless-steel or aluminum devices that penetrate the skin for the purpose of administering or transferring a parenteral product.

1. **Needle gauge** is the outside diameter of the needle shaft; the larger the number, the smaller the diameter. Gauges in common use range from 13 (largest diameter) to 27. Subcutaneous injections usually require a 24-gauge or 25-gauge needle. Intramuscular injections require a needle with a gauge between 19 and 22. Needles between 18 gauge and 20 gauge are commonly used for compounding parenterals.

2. **Bevels** are slanting edges cut into needle tips to facilitate injection through tissue or rubber vial closures.
   a. **Regular-bevel needles** are the most commonly used type, and they are suitable for subcutaneous and intramuscular injections and hypodermoclysis.
   b. **Short-bevel needles** are used when only shallow penetration is required (as in IV injections).
   c. **Intradermal-bevel needles** are designed for intradermal injections and have the most beveled edges.

3. **Needle lengths** range from $1/4$ inch to 6 inches. Choice of needle length depends on the desired penetration.
   a. For **compounding parenteral preparations,** $1 1/2$-inch-long needles are commonly used.
   b. **Intradermal and subcutaneous injections** necessitate a short needle length, usually $1/4$ inch to $5/8$ inch.
   c. **Intracardiac injection** requires a needle length of $3 1/2$ inches.
   d. **IV infusion** requires needles that range in length from $1 1/4$ inches to $2 1/2$ inches.

B. **Syringes** are devices for injecting, withdrawing, or instilling fluids. Syringes consist of a glass or plastic barrel with a tight-fitting plunger at one end; a small opening at the other end accommodates the head of a needle.

1. The **Luer syringe,** the first syringe developed, has a universal needle attachment accommodating all needle sizes.

2. **Syringe volumes** range from 0.3 to 60 mL. Insulin syringes have unit gradations (100 units/mL) rather than volume gradations.

3. **Calibrations,** which may be in the metric or English system, vary in specificity depending on syringe size; the smaller the syringe, the smaller the measurement scale.

4. **Syringe tips** come in several types.
   a. **Luer-Lok tips** are threaded to ensure that the needle fits tightly in the syringe. Antineoplastic agents should be administered with syringes of this type (see V D 2).
   b. **Luer-Slip tips** are unthreaded so that the syringe and needle do not lock into place. Because of this, the needle may become dislodged.
   c. **Eccentric tips,** which are set off center, allow the needle to remain parallel to the injection site and minimize venous irritation.
   d. **Catheter tips** are used for wound irrigation and administration of enteral feedings. They are not intended for injections.

VIII. INTRAVENOUS DRUG DELIVERY

A. **Injection sites**

1. **Peripheral vein injection** is preferred for drugs that do not irritate the veins, administration of isotonic solutions, and patients who require only short-term IV therapy. Generally, the dorsal forearm surface is chosen for venipuncture.

2. **Central vein injection** is preferred for administration of irritating drugs or hypertonic solutions, patients requiring long-term IV therapy, and situations in which a peripheral line cannot be maintained. Large veins in the thoracic cavity, such as the subclavian vein, are used.

B. Infusion methods

1. **Continuous-drip infusion** is the slow, primary-line infusion of an IV preparation to maintain a therapeutic drug level or provide fluid and electrolyte replacement.
   a. **Flow rates** must be carefully monitored. Generally, these rates are expressed as volume per unit of time (e.g., mL/hr, drops/min) and sometimes as mg/min for certain drugs.
   b. **Administration.** Drugs with a narrow therapeutic index such as aminophylline, heparin, and pressor agents (epinephrine, norepinephrine, phenylephrine) typically are administered by this method.

2. **Intermittent infusion** allows drug administration at specific intervals (e.g., every 4 hours) and is most often used for antibiotics.
   a. **Three different techniques** may be used.
      (1) **Direct (bolus) injection** rapidly delivers small volumes of an undiluted drug. This method is used to:
         (a) Achieve an immediate effect (as in an emergency)
         (b) Administer drugs that cannot be diluted
         (c) Achieve a therapeutic serum drug level quickly
      (2) **Additive set infusion,** using a volume-control device, is appropriate for the intermittent delivery of small amounts of IV solutions or diluted medications. The fluid chamber is attached to an independent fluid supply or placed directly under the established primary IV line.
      (3) The **piggyback method** is used when a drug cannot be mixed with the primary solution. A special coupling for the primary IV tubing permits infusion of a supplementary secondary solution through the primary system.
         (a) This method eliminates the need for a second venipuncture or further dilution of the supplementary preparation.
         (b) **Admixtures** in which the vehicle is added to the drug are known as manufacturers' piggybacks. Admixtures in which a special drug vial is attached to a special IV bag are known as the ADD-Vantage system (see Figure 26-4).
   b. In some cases, **intermittent infusion injection devices** are used. Also called scalp-vein, heparin-lock, or butterfly infusion sets, these devices permit intermittent delivery while eliminating the need for multiple venipunctures or prolonged venous access with a continuous infusion. To prevent clotting in the cannula, dilute heparin solution or NSS may be added. Benefits of intermittent infusion injection devices include the following:
      (1) This method is especially suitable for patients who do not require, or would be jeopardized by, administration of large amounts of IV fluids (e.g., those with congestive heart failure).
      (2) Because intermittent infusion injection devices do not require continuous attachment to an IV bottle or bag and pole, they permit greater patient ambulation.

C. Pumps and controllers are the electronic devices used to administer parenteral infusions when the use of gravity flow alone might lead to inaccurate dosing or risk patient safety. Pumps and controllers are used to administer parenteral nutrition, chemotherapy, cardiac medications, and blood products.

1. **Pumps** are used to deliver IV infusions with accuracy and safety.
   a. Two **types of mechanisms** are used in infusion pumps.
      (1) **Piston-cylinder mechanisms** use a piston in a cylinder or a syringe-like apparatus to pump the desired volume of fluid.
      (2) **Linear peristaltic mechanisms** use external pressure to expel the fluid out of the pumping chamber.
   b. **Types of pumps**
      (1) **Volumetric pumps** are used for intermittent infusion of medications such as antibiotics. They are also used for continuous infusion of IV fluid, parenteral nutrition, anticoagulants, and anti-asthma medications.
      (2) **Syringe pumps** are used to administer intermittent or continuous infusions of medications (e.g., antibiotics, opiates) in concentrated form.
      (3) **Mobile infusion pumps** are small infusion devices designed for ambulatory and home patients and used for administering chemotherapy and opiate medications.

(4) **Implantable pumps** are infusion devices surgically placed under the skin to provide a continuous release of medication, typically an opiate. The reservoir in the pump is refilled by injecting the medication through a latex diaphragm in the pump.

(5) **Patient-controlled analgesic pumps** are used to administer narcotics intermittently or on demand by the patient within the patient-specific parameters, which are ordered by the physician and programmed into the pump.

c. **Benefits.** Despite their extra costs and the training required by personnel, pumps provide a number of important benefits. They maintain a constant, accurate flow rate and can detect infiltrations, occlusions, and air. Pumps also may decrease the amount of time a nurse spends dispensing medication.

2. **Controllers,** unlike pumps, exert no pumping pressure on the IV fluid. Rather, they rely on gravity and control the infusion by counting drops electronically, or they infuse the fluid mechanically and electronically (e.g., volumetric controllers). In **comparison to pumps,** the following are characteristics of controllers:

a. They are less complex and generally less expensive.

b. They achieve reasonable accuracy.

c. They are very useful for uncomplicated infusion therapy but cannot be used for arterial drug infusion or for infusion into small veins.

D. **IV incompatibilities.** When two or more drugs must be administered through a single IV line or given in a single solution, an undesirable reaction can occur. Although such incompatibilities are relatively rare, their consequences may be catastrophic. A patient who receives a preparation in which an incompatibility has occurred could experience toxicity or an incomplete therapeutic effect.

1. **Types of incompatibilities**

a. A **physical incompatibility** occurs when a drug combination produces a visible change in the appearance of a solution.

(1) An **example** of physical incompatibility is the evolution of carbon dioxide when sodium bicarbonate and hydrochloric acid are admixed.

(2) Various **types** of physical incompatibilities may occur:

(a) Visible color change or darkening

(b) Formation of precipitate, which may result from the combination of phosphate and calcium

b. A **chemical incompatibility** reflects the chemical degradation of one or more of the admixed drugs, resulting in toxicity or therapeutic inactivity.

(1) The degradation is not always visible. **Nonvisible chemical incompatibility** may be detected only by analytical methods.

(2) Chemical incompatibility occurs in several **varieties.**

(a) **Complexation** is a reaction between products that inactivates them. For example, the combination of calcium and tetracycline leads to formation of a complex that inactivates tetracycline.

(b) **Oxidation** occurs when one drug loses electrons to the other, resulting in a color change and therapeutic inactivity.

(c) **Reduction** takes place when one drug gains electrons from the other.

(d) **Photolysis** (chemical decomposition caused by light) can lead to hydrolysis or oxidation, with resulting discoloration.

c. A **therapeutic incompatibility** occurs when two or more drugs, IV fluids, or both are combined and the result is a response other than that intended. An example of a therapeutic incompatibility is the reduced bactericidal activity of penicillin G when given after tetracycline. Because tetracycline is a bacteriostatic agent, it slows bacterial growth; penicillin, on the other hand, is most effective against rapidly proliferating bacteria.

2. **Factors affecting IV compatibility**

a. **pH.** Incompatibility is more likely to occur when the components of an IV solution differ significantly in pH. This increased risk is explained by the chemical reaction between an acid and a base, which yields a salt and water; the salt may be an insoluble precipitate.

b. **Temperature.** Generally, increased storage temperature speeds drug degradation. To preserve drug stability, drugs should be stored in a refrigerator or freezer, as appropriate.

    c. Degree of dilution. Generally, the more diluted the drugs are in a solution, the less chance there is for an ion interaction leading to incompatibility.

    d. Length of time in solution. The chance for a reaction resulting in incompatibility increases with the length of time that drugs are in contact with each other.

    e. Order of mixing. Drugs that are incompatible in combination, such as calcium and phosphate, should not be added consecutively when an IV admixture is being prepared. This keeps these substances from pooling, or forming a layer on the top of the IV fluid, and, therefore, decreases the chance of an incompatibility. Thorough mixing after each addition is also essential.

3. Preventing or minimizing incompatibilities. To reduce the chance for an incompatibility, the following steps should be taken:

    a. Each drug should be mixed thoroughly after it is added to the preparation.

    b. Solutions should be administered promptly after they are mixed to minimize the time available for a potential reaction to occur.

    c. The number of drugs mixed together in an IV solution should be kept to a minimum.

    d. If a prescription calls for unfamiliar drugs or IV fluids, compatibility references should be consulted.

E. Hazards of parenteral drug therapy. A wide range of problems can occur with parenteral drug administration.

1. Physical hazards

    a. Phlebitis, which is generally a minor complication, may result from vein injury or irritation. Phlebitis can be minimized or prevented through proper IV insertion technique, dilution of irritating drugs, and a decreased infusion rate.

    b. Extravasation may occur with administration of drugs with vesicant properties (see V D 3 b).

    c. Irritation at the injection site can be reduced by varying the injection site and applying a moisturizing lotion to the area.

    d. Pain from infusion is most common with peripheral IV administration of a highly concentrated preparation. Switching to central vein infusion and/or diluting the drug might alleviate the problem.

    e. Air embolism, potentially fatal, can result from entry of air into the IV tubing.

    f. Infection, a particular danger with central IV lines, may stem from contamination during IV line insertion or tubing changes. Infection may be local or generalized (septicemia). The infection risk can be minimized by following established protocols for the care of central lines.

    g. Allergic reactions can result from hypersensitivity to an IV solution or additive.

    h. Central catheter misplacement may lead to air embolism or pneumothorax. To ensure that the catheter has passed into the subclavian vein and advanced to the level of the vena cava, the placement should always be verified radiologically.

    i. Hypothermia, possibly resulting in shock and cardiac arrest, might stem from administration of a cold IV solution. This problem can be prevented by allowing parenteral products to reach room temperature.

    j. Neurotoxicity may be a serious complication of intrathecal or intraspinal administration of drugs containing preservatives. Preservative-free drugs should be used in these circumstances.

2. Mechanical hazards

    a. Infusion pump or **controller failure** can lead to runaway infusion, fluid overload, or incorrect dosages.

    b. IV tubing can become kinked, split, or cracked. It also may produce particulates, allow contamination, or interfere with the infusion.

    c. Particulate matter may be present in a parenteral product and can cause embolism.

    d. Glass containers may break, causing injury.

    e. Rubber vial closures may interact with the enclosed product.

3. Therapeutic hazards

    a. Drug instability may lead to therapeutic ineffectiveness.

    b. Incompatibility may result in toxicity or reduced therapeutic effectiveness.

    c. Labeling errors can cause administration of an incorrect drug or improper dosage.

    d. Drug overdose can be caused by runaway IV infusion, failure of an infusion pump or controller, or nursing or pharmacy errors.

e. Preservative toxicity can be a serious complication, especially in children. For example, premature infants receiving parenteral products containing benzyl alcohol can develop a fatal acidotic toxic syndrome, which is referred to as the **gasping syndrome.**

IX. QUALITY CONTROL AND QUALITY ASSURANCE

A. Definitions

1. **Quality control** is the day-to-day assessment of all operations from the receipt of raw material to the distribution of the finished product, including analytic testing of the finished product.

2. **Quality assurance,** an oversight function, involves the auditing of quality control procedures and systems, with suggestions for changes as needed.

B. Testing procedures.
Various types of tests are used to ensure that all sterile products are free of microbial contamination, pyrogens, and particulate matter.

1. **Sterility testing** ensures that the process used to sterilize the product was successful.
   a. The **official** USP **standard** for sterility testing calls for the following:
      (1) A 10-test sample for batches of 20–200 units
      (2) A minimum of two test samples for batches of less than 20 units
   b. The **membrane sterilization method** is often used to conduct sterility testing. Test samples are passed through membrane filters, and a nutrient medium is then added to promote microbial growth. After an incubation period, microbial growth is determined.

2. **Pyrogen testing** can be accomplished by means of qualitative fever response testing in rabbits or by in vitro limulus lysate testing. Commercial laboratories are available to perform these tests. People handling sterile products can attempt to avoid problems with pyrogens by purchasing pyrogen-free water and sodium chloride for injection from reputable manufacturers and by using proper handling and storage procedures.

3. **Clarity testing** is used to check sterile products for particulate matter. Before dispensing a parenteral solution, pharmacy personnel should check it for particulates by swirling the solution and looking at it against both light and dark backgrounds, using a clarity testing lamp or other standard light source.

C. Practical quality assurance programs
for noncommercial sterile products include training, monitoring the manufacturing process, quality control check, and documentation.

1. **Training of pharmacists and technicians** in proper aseptic techniques and practices is the single most important aspect of an effective quality assurance program. Training should impart a thorough understanding of departmental policies and procedures.

2. By **monitoring the manufacturing process,** a supervisor can check adherence to established policies and procedures and take corrective action as necessary.

D. Process validation
provides a mechanism for ensuring processes consistently result in sterile products of acceptable quality. This should include a written procedure to follow as well as evaluation of aseptic technique through process simulation.

E. Process simulation testing
duplicates sterile product production except that an appropriate growth media is used in place of the drug products. After preparation and incubation of the final product, no growth indicates proper aseptic techniques were followed.

F. Quality control
checking includes monitoring the sterility of a sample of manufactured products. The membrane sterilization method is practically employed using a commercially available filter and trypticase soy broth media.

G. Documentation
of training procedures, quality control results, laminar flow hood certification, and production records are required by various agencies and organizations.

STUDY QUESTIONS

Directions: Each of the numbered items or incomplete statements in this section is followed by answers or by completions of the statement. Select the **one** lettered answer or completion that is **best** in each case.

1. Parenteral products with an osmotic pressure less than that of blood or 0.9% sodium chloride are referred to as

(A) isotonic solutions
(B) hypertonic solutions
(C) hypotonic solutions
(D) iso-osmotic solutions
(E) neutral solutions

2. Aseptic technique should be used in the preparation of all of the following medications with the exception of;

(A) neomycin irrigation solution
(B) ganciclovir intraocular injection
(C) phytonadione subcutaneous injection
(D) ampicillin IV admixture piggyback
(E) bacitracin ointment

3. Which needle has the smallest diameter?

(A) 25 gauge, $3\frac{3}{4}$ inches
(B) 24 gauge, $3\frac{1}{2}$ inches
(C) 22 gauge, $3\frac{1}{2}$ inches
(D) 20 gauge, $3\frac{3}{8}$ inches
(E) 26 gauge, $3\frac{5}{8}$ inches

4. Intra-articular injection refers to injection into the

(A) muscle mass
(B) subcutaneous tissue
(C) spinal fluid
(D) superficial skin layer
(E) joint space

5. Advantages of the intravenous route include

(A) ease of removal of the dose
(B) a depot effect
(C) low incidence of phlebitis
(D) rapid onset of action
(E) a localized effect

6. A central vein, either subclavian or internal jugular, may be considered a suitable route for IV administration in which of the following situations?

(A) When an irritating drug is given
(B) When hypertonic drugs are given
(C) For long-term therapy
(D) For administering dextrose 35% as parenteral nutrition
(E) All of the above

7. To prepare a total parenteral nutrition (TPN) that requires 10 mEq of calcium gluconate and 15 mM of potassium phosphate, the appropriate action to take would be which of the following?

(A) Add the calcium first, add the other additives, then add the phosphate last, thoroughly mixing the solution after addition.
(B) Add the calcium gluconate and potassium phosphate consecutively.
(C) Not combine the agents together but give them as a separate infusion.
(D) None of the above.

8. Which needle gauge would be most likely used as a subcutaneous injection of epoetin?

(A) 25 gauge, $\frac{5}{8}$ inch
(B) 16 gauge, 1 inch
(C) 18 gauge, $1\frac{1}{2}$ inches
(D) 22 gauge, $1\frac{1}{2}$ inches
(E) None of the above

9. Which of the following drugs should NOT be prepared in a horizontal laminar flow hood?

(A) Ampicillin
(B) Dopamine
(C) Cisplatin
(D) Nitroglycerin
(E) Bretylium tosylate

10. All of the following statements about d5w are true EXCEPT

(A) its pH range is 3.5–6.5.
(B) it is hypertonic.
(C) it is a 5% solution of D-glucose.
(D) it should be used with caution in diabetic patients.
(E) it is often used in IV admixtures.

11. All of the following are potential hazards of parenteral therapy EXCEPT

(A) hypothermia
(B) phlebitis
(C) extravasation
(D) allergic reactions
(E) ileus

12. Procedures for the safe handling of antineoplastic agents include all of the following EXCEPT

(A) use of Luer-Lok syringe fittings.
(B) wearing double-layered latex gloves.
(C) use of negative-pressure technique when medication is being withdrawn from vials.
(D) wearing closed-front, surgical-type gowns with cuffs.
(E) use of horizontal laminar flow hood.

13. In preparing an intraspinal dose of bupivacaine, the best pore size filter for cold sterilization would be

(A) 8-mm filter
(B) 5-μm filter
(C) 0.45-μm filter
(D) 0.22-μm filter
(E) None of the above

14. Process simulation

(A) is a method of quality assurance.
(B) evaluates the adequacy of a practitioner's aseptic technique.
(C) requires the use of a microbial growth medium.
(D) is carried out in a manner identical to normal sterile admixture production.
(E) All of the above.

ANSWERS AND EXPLANATIONS

1. The answer is C *[I A 5 a]*.
Hypotonic solutions have an osmotic pressure less than that of blood (or 0.9% saline), whereas hypertonic solutions have an osmotic pressure greater than that of blood, and isotonic or iso-osmotic solutions have an osmotic pressure equal to that of blood.

2. The answer is E *[I A 1, A 3)]*.
Irrigation solutions, ophthalmic preparations and parenteral products, and subcutaneous and IV medications should be prepared using aseptic technique. Since Bacitracin ointment is applied to the skin and does not bypass the body's protective barriers, its preparation would not be held to the same requirements.

3. The answer is E *[VII A 1]*.
The gauge size refers to the outer diameter of the needle. The lower the gauge size number, the larger the needle.

4. The answer is E *[IV I]*.
Intra-articular injection refers to an injection into the joint space. This administration route generally is used for certain types of corticosteroids to reduce inflammation associated with injury or rheumatoid arthritis.

5. The answer is D *[IV C]*.
The IV route of drug administration allows for rapid onset of action and, therefore, immediate therapeutic effect. There can be no recall of the administered dose, and phlebitis, or inflammation of a vein, can occur. In addition, a depot effect (i.e., accumulation and storage of the drug for distribution) cannot be achieved by administering a drug intravenously. Delivering a drug intravenously results in a systemic rather than a localized effect.

6. The answer is E *[V B 1 a]*.
Irritating drugs, hypertonic drugs, long-term therapy, and dextrose 35% are best given by central IV administration. Peripheral vein injection is used for postoperative hydration, administration of nonirritating drugs, or isotonic solutions and for short-term IV therapy.

7. The answer is A *[VIII D 2 e]*.
Physical incompatibilities occur when two or more products are combined and produce a change in the appearance of the solution, such as the formation of a precipitate. Calcium and phosphate solutions when directly combined or added consecutively to a solution will form a white precipitate. By altering the order of mixing, they can be safely added to TPN solutions.

8. The answer is A *[VII A1, VII A 3 b]*.
Since subcutaneous injection does not require penetration through several skin layers or muscle tissue, a short needle with a narrow diameter is used. A 16- or 18-gauge needle is most commonly used in the pharmacy for preparing parenteral solutions. A 22-gauge needle would be used for intramuscular injection.

9. The answer is C *[I B 2 b 1]*.
CisPlatin is an antineoplastic agent and, consequently, should be prepared only in a vertical laminar flow hood because of the potential hazard of these toxic agents to the operator.

10. The answer is B *[V B 1 a]*.
d5w (dextrose [D-glucose] 5% in water) is acidic, its pH ranges from 3.5–6.5, and it is isotonic. It is often used in IV admixtures and should be used with caution in diabetic patients.

11. The answer is E *[VIII E 1 i, E 1 a, E 1 b, E 1g]*.
Parenteral therapy is often a treatment for ileus. Hypothermia, phlebitis, extravasation, and allergic reactions can be hazards of parenteral therapy.

12. The answer is E *[V D 2].*

In order to prevent drug exposure, a vertical flow laminar hood (not horizontal) should be used when an antineoplastic agent is prepared. The other precautions mentioned in the question are important safety measures for handling parenteral antineoplastics. All pharmacy and nursing personnel who handle these toxic substances should receive special training.

13. The answer is D *[II D 2 C (1) (b)].*

Since intraspinal and epidural doses of bupivacaine are frequently prepared from nonsterile powders, cold sterilization, accomplished by filtration, is a simple method of ensuring complete microbial removal. The filters listed 8 mm to 0.45 μm will remove only particulate matter. A 0.22 μM filter ensures the removal of microorganisms.

14. The answer is E *[IX E]*

Process simulation is one part of an overall quality assurance program. It requires duplicating sterile product preparation using a growth medium in place of actual products. It serves to evaluate the aseptic technique of the individual performing all the necessary steps of sterile product preparation.

Parapharmaceuticals, Home Diagnostics, and Medical Devices

Todd A. Brown

I. AMBULATORY AIDS

A. Canes. These simple ambulatory aids provide balance and allow for the transfer of weight off a weakened limb.

1. **Use.** A cane is usually used held on the strong side of the body to allow for a shifting of weight from the weakened side. The height of the cane must be adjusted to the individual patient. A cane that is correctly fitted allows for maximum weight transfer without allowing the patient to lock the elbow. The correct height should provide a 25° angle at the elbow, or the top of the cane should come to the crease of the wrist while the patient is standing erect.

2. **Types of canes.** Canes may be made of wood or metal.
   a. **Wooden canes** come in varying thicknesses. The thicker ones are intended for males, and the thinner ones are for females. Canes must be cut to the correct height for the patient.
   b. **Metal canes** are usually adjustable to fit the individual patient.
   c. **Folding canes** will fold into three sections to allow for easy transport or storage when not in use.
   d. A **quad cane** is a metal cane that has a quadrangular base with four legs. This allows for greater weight transfer. The base of the quad cane comes in two sizes. The larger base provides greater stability but is more difficult to manipulate because of the size and weight.

B. Crutches may be used by patients with temporary disabilities (e.g., sprains, fractures) or by those with chronic conditions.

1. **Use.** Crutches are used to take all the weight off an injured or weakened leg. The crutches are used in place of the leg. Crutch sizes range from toddler to adult. Accessories that are used with a crutch include a tip to prevent slipping, handgrip cushion, and arm pad (for axillary crutch).

2. **Types of crutches**
   a. An **axillary crutch,** the **most commonly used** crutch, is typically used for temporary disabilities. The top of the crutch should be 2 inches below the axilla to prevent "crutch paralysis" (i.e., injury to the axillary nerves, blood vessels, and lymph nodes). The height of the handgrip should be set so that the elbow forms a 25° angle.
   b. A **forearm crutch** (also called a **Canadian** or **Lofstrand** crutch) supports the wrist and elbows, attaching to the forearm by a collar or cuff. It is commonly used by patients who need crutches on a long-term basis.
   c. A **quad crutch** is a forearm crutch with a quadrangular base that has four legs. The base is attached to the crutch with a flexible rubber mount. This allows for more stability and constant contact with the ground.
   d. A **platform crutch** contains a rectangular area in which to place the forearm. The crutch may be held by a handgrip or secured by a belt that wraps around the forearm. It is commonly used by patients who do not have enough hand strength and control for a forearm crutch.

C. Walkers are lightweight rectangular-shaped devices that are made of metal tubing and have four widely placed legs.

1. **Use.** Walkers are used by patients who need more **support** than a cane or crutch or who have trouble with balance during ambulation. The use requires reasonably good arm, hand, and wrist function. The patient holds onto the walker and takes a step, then moves the walker and takes another step.

    2. Types of walkers. Walkers come in two sizes: **adult** and **child.** Some walkers are adjustable in height. Some walkers will fold to make storage or transporting easier. Walkers can have wheels on the legs. This allows the user to move the walker by rolling it instead of having to pick it up. Patients with loss of arm, wrist, or hand function on one side might use a **hemiwalker** or a **side walker.**

        a. A **hemiwalker** is similar to a standard walker except that it has one handle in the center of the walker for manipulation.

        b. A **side walker** is placed to the side of the patient instead of in front of the patient.

        c. A **reciprocal walker** contains two hinges, one on each side of the walker. This allows the user to swing each side alternately during ambulation.

D. Wheelchairs. Many different types of wheelchairs are available. The patient's disabilities, size, weight, and activities are the main considerations in wheelchair selection. The following options should be considered when selecting a wheelchair.

    1. Seat size. The standard chair is 18 inches wide and 16 inches deep. A narrow wheelchair is 16 inches wide. Wheelchairs are available in widths up to 48 inches. The chair should be 2 inches wider than the widest part of the patient's body (usually around the buttocks or thighs).

    2. Arms can be fixed, detachable, half length, full length, adjustable, or tilt back. The armrest and padding must also be considered.

    3. Tires can be hard rubber or pneumatic (i.e., air filled).

    4. Wheels can be reinforced with spokes or can be composite based.

    5. Leg rests can be of different sizes and are available with padding.

    6. Footrests can be of different sizes and are available with or without heel loops.

    7. Casters (i.e., **front wheels**) can be hard rubber or pneumatic.

    8. Calf rests can be of different sizes and are available with padding.

    9. Seat upholstery can be made of mesh or vinyl.

    10. Back upholstery can be made of mesh or vinyl.

    11. Cross braces add stability and durability to the chair.

    12. Weight. Standard wheelchairs weigh 35–50 lbs. Lightweight wheelchairs (25–35 lbs) are available for those who are unable to manipulate a standard chair and for ease of transport.

E. Sports chairs are wheelchairs that are lightweight and durable. They are designed for people who are very active.

F. Powered wheelchairs are designed for people who cannot wheel themselves. This type of wheelchair is powered by a motor and battery.

II. BATHROOM EQUIPMENT. This equipment is used for patients who cannot get to the bathroom or to provide assistance to patients using the toilet or bathtub.

A. Elevated toilet seats are used to increase the height at which the patient sits over the toilet. This assists patients with limited mobility in getting on and off the toilet. Additional support can be provided with **toilet safety rails.** These rails allow the patient to transfer weight from the feet to the hands, and they help to prevent the patient from falling when getting on or off the toilet.

B. Commodes are portable toilets that are used by patients who cannot get to the bathroom. Commodes contain a frame (with or without a backrest), a seat, and a bucket. Some are adjustable in height and have arms that drop to facilitate transfer to and from the commode. Folding commodes are available to make storage easier.

C. Three-in-one commodes function as combination commode, elevated toilet seat, and toilet safety rails. These are beneficial for patients requiring varying assistance during recuperation.

D. Bath benches are seats with or without a back that fit in the bathtub and allow the patient to sit while taking a shower.

E. Transfer benches are placed over the outside of the bathtub. They are available with or without a back. A transfer bench assists the patient in getting into the bathtub and serves as a bath bench while the patient takes a shower.

III. BLOOD PRESSURE MONITORS.
Patients with hypertension use this equipment to monitor blood pressure so that appropriate therapeutic decisions can be made. The type of monitor that is recommended should be determined by the patient's ability to use the product correctly. Types of monitors include:

A. Mercury sphygmomanometer. This type of monitor is the **most accurate** and does not need calibration. It does require the use of a stethoscope, which is difficult for some patients. Mercury in a graduated column rises in response to pressure applied to the cuff. The blood pressure is determined by measuring the length of the mercury column while listening for the Korotkoff sounds in the stethoscope.

B. Aneroid sphygmomanometer. This is similar to a mercury sphygmomanometer, except that instead of a column of mercury, it has a dial to be read. Aneroid models have the advantage of being **less expensive** than mercury models; however, they do require regular calibration to ensure proper results.

C. Electronic or digital monitor. This type of monitor detects blood pressure by using a microphone or by oscillometric technology, which converts movement of vessels into blood pressure. This type is easier to use than a sphygmomanometer and does not require the use of a stethoscope. These models are more **expensive** and need to be calibrated on a regular basis, but they represent an alternative for those patients who cannot use a sphygmomanometer.

D. Finger monitors. These detect blood pressure by compressing the finger and converting blood vessel movement into blood pressure by oscillometric technology. Many environmental conditions and medications can interfere with the results of these monitors, which are the **least accurate.**

IV. HEAT AND COLD THERAPY.
For musculoskeletal disorders (e.g., sprains, strains, arthritis), treatment may include the application of heat or cold to specific areas of the body.

A. Heat can be applied in a dry or moist form. **Dry** heat is less effective than moist heat but is tolerated better and, thus, its clinical effectiveness is similar. **Moist** heat has an advantage of not causing as much perspiration and is often recommended. The application of heat produces vasodilation and muscle relaxation. This facilitates pain relief and healing. Products that can deliver heat include:

1. A **hot water bottle,** a rubber container, should be half-filled with hot water. The remaining air is squeezed out of the container, which is then capped. This results in a flexible container that can be shaped to the area of the body for which it is being used to provide dry heat.

2. A **heating pad** is an electrically powered pad that can produce moist or dry heat. Moist heat is supplied by inserting a wet sponge in a pocket that is next to the pad. Patients should be instructed to place the pad on top of the body instead of lying on the pad in order to prevent burning.

3. A **moist-heat pack** (also called a hydrocollator) contains silica beads, which absorb heat when placed in boiling water. The heated pack is wrapped in a towel and applied to the body to provide moist heat. A moist-heat pack must be kept moist to retain its absorbent properties. The pack should be wrapped in plastic and stored in the refrigerator if use is anticipated or in the freezer if long-term storage is required.

4. A **gel pack** provides dry heat after it is heated in boiling water or in the microwave. It is reusable by repeating the heating process.

5. **Chemical hot packs** provide dry heat by mixing chemicals from two compartments. The chemicals undergo an exothermic reaction. Some packs are reusable by reheating in boiling water or in the microwave.

6. **Paraffin baths** provide moist heat by covering the body with heated paraffin. Once the wax cools and hardens, it is removed. This method is commonly used for patients with arthritis in the hands and fingers.

B. **Cold** application is indicated mainly as acute therapy to decrease circulation to a local area and to provide pain relief. Cold is contraindicated in patients with circulatory stasis or lacerated tissue. Products that can deliver cold include:

1. An **ice bag** is a flexible plastic container designed to hold ice. The bag is then applied to the body.

2. A **gel pack** can be used to apply cold by freezing and then applying to the body.

3. **Chemical packs** can be used to apply cold. Chemicals from two compartments are mixed together, resulting in a chemical reaction that produces cold. These packs are used once and then disposed of.

V. HOME DIAGNOSTIC AIDS

A. **Self-care tests** or **kits** are used as screening tests or for monitoring. Many factors can affect the accuracy of the tests. The most common factor is the patient not following directions or having poor technique. Pharmacists should be prepared to counsel patients on the proper use and interpretation and to refer patients to the appropriate health-care provider if necessary.

B. **Types of self-care tests**

1. **Urine tests**
   a. The **urine glucose test** detects sugar in the urine. Patients with diabetes can use this to evaluate glucose control. Blood glucose testing is preferred, however, because it is more accurate and gives a better description of current glycemia.
   b. The **ketone test** detects the presence of ketones in the urine. This is used by patients with diabetes as an indicator of severely uncontrolled diabetes.
   c. **Ovulation prediction tests** predict when ovulation occurs to increase the chance of conception. These tests detect the presence of **luteinizing hormone (LH)** in the urine. Its presence means that ovulation should occur within 20–48 hours. The test is performed daily until a positive result is obtained. The time in which the patient begins testing is dependent on the length and regularity of the menstrual cycle. Patients with menstrual cycles of consistent length may only need to test for 4 days, while those with menstrual cycles that change in length may need to test for 8 or 9 days.
   d. **Pregnancy tests** detect pregnancy by the presence in the urine of **human chorionic gonadotropin (hCG),** which is secreted after fertilization. Many pregnancy test kits can detect hCG one day after missed menses. Patients taking hCG (e.g., as part of infertility therapy) could get false-positive results. Patients should be referred to the appropriate health-care provider if they receive a positive result or two negative results 7 days apart and have not had menses.
   e. The **urinary bacteria test** detects the presence of nitrite in the urine. The presence of nitrite is used as an indicator of a **urinary tract infection (UTI)** because the most common bacteria associated with UTIs are gram-negative bacteria, which convert nitrate to nitrite. Because this test is not specific for bacteria, false results can occur. This test is used by patients who have chronic UTIs, as one indicator of a possible infection.

2. **Blood tests**
   a. The **cholesterol test** determines a patient's total cholesterol. The patient supplies a large drop of blood, and the test separates the total cholesterol. The measurement of the amount of cholesterol is determined by a chart that is provided with the test. This test can be useful for patients who want to monitor therapy; it is also useful as a screening test. Patients with results that are borderline or higher should be referred to the appropriate health-care provider.
   b. The **blood glucose test** measures the concentration of glucose in the blood. Patients with diabetes use this information, along with diet, exercise, and medication, to keep glucose

levels within a target range. Some blood glucose tests can be read visually by comparing the color change to a chart provided with the test. Visually read tests give an approximation of the blood glucose. Other tests are designed to be used with **blood glucose meters,** which read the test and display the actual blood glucose value. Some blood glucose meters contain optical units that measure the color change caused by glucose, while others measure the electric charge produced by glucose. The result is then calibrated to provide whole blood or plasma glucose concentration. Whole blood is approximately 12% lower than plasma glucose, which is what is measured in the standard laboratory tests. Patients using blood glucose tests must perform the test properly and understand appropriate actions to take when values are outside the desired range.

3. **Fecal occult blood tests** detect the presence of blood in the stool as a screening test for colorectal cancer. Patients drop a pad into the toilet after defecation. The pad will change color if blood is present. Patients should eat high-fiber foods during the testing period and are instructed to test three consecutive stool samples. Patients with a positive result should be referred to the appropriate health-care provider. Certain conditions (gastrointestinal bleed, nosebleed, menstruation), foods (red meat), medications [nonsteroidal anti-inflammatory drugs (NSAIDs)], and toilet-bowl cleaners can produce false-positive results.

4. **Home specimen collection kits** allow for collection of a specimen at home, which is then sent to a laboratory for testing. Blood-collection devices are available so that patients can test themselves for the presence of the human immunodeficiency virus (HIV) and the concentration of glycosylated hemoglobin (for patients with diabetes). A screening test for illicit drug use is also available. These tests require a urine or hair sample for analysis. The HIV and illicit drug use tests allow the patient to test anonymously by using an identification number included with the kit. The results can be obtained by calling a toll-free telephone number. The results of the glycosylated hemoglobin test are mailed to the patient and physician if supplied.

VI. HOSPITAL BEDS AND ACCESSORIES.

Hospital beds are used by patients who are confined to bed for long periods of time or who require elevation of the head or feet as part of their treatment. Hospital beds may be manually or electrically operated.

A. Types of hospital beds

1. A **manual** hospital bed has no electrically powered motors; the head, foot, and bed height are adjusted manually.

2. A **semielectric** hospital bed contains two motors that raise the head and foot of the bed. The patient can usually adjust the bed's position with a handheld control. The height of the bed is adjusted manually. The semielectric bed can usually be adjusted manually in case of loss of electricity.

3. A **fully electric** hospital bed contains three motors that can change the height of the bed as well as raise the head and foot via electrically powered motors. The fully electric hospital bed can usually be adjusted manually in case of loss of electricity.

B. Accessories

1. **Bed rails** keep the patient in the bed and assist in position changes.

2. A **trapeze** is a triangular-shaped object that hangs above the patient and is used to change the patient's position.

3. **Alternating pressure pads** are used by patients to prevent decubitus ulcers (i.e., bed sores). As a preventive measure, these pads inflate and change the areas of the body that receive pressure.

VII. INCONTINENCE AND INCONTINENCE PRODUCTS

A. Urinary incontinence

is a condition in which involuntary urine loss is a social or hygienic problem and is objectively demonstrable. Incontinence is a common problem in the elderly. Types of incontinence include:

1. **Urge** incontinence, which is uncontrolled contractions of the bladder

2. **Stress** incontinence, a weakness of the sphincter that causes leakage when intra-abdominal pressure increases (i.e., while laughing, coughing, sneezing); common in pregnancy

3. **Overflow** incontinence, which is caused by obstruction of urine flow from the bladder; common in elderly men due to prostate enlargement

4. **Functional incontinence,** which is related to physical or psychological problems that impair the patient's ability to get to the bathroom

5. **Iatrogenic incontinence,** caused by drugs or surgery

6. **Mixed incontinence,** a combination of more than one type of incontinence

B. Incontinence products

1. **Shields** are disposable, absorbent pads that are placed in the underwear and held with an adhesive strip on the back of the pad. These pads are used for light incontinence problems.

2. **Undergarments** are disposable absorbent garments that are worn under the underwear and held in place with elastic straps that go around the hips. They are designed for moderate incontinence problems.

3. **Briefs** look like adult-sized diapers that are kept in place with adhesive strips. They are designed for heavy incontinence problems.

4. **Pull-up pants** are absorbant disposable garments that look like underwear and are used for heavy incontinence problems.

5. **Underpads** are absorbent pads to be placed on the bed underneath a patient with incontinence. These pads have a barrier to protect the bedding.

6. **Waterproof sheets** are plastic or vinyl sheets that protect the mattress. They may be lined with a soft material to prevent friction against the skin.

7. **Incontinence systems** are garments that look like underwear but have a pouch or pocket designed for a disposable or reusable pad.

VIII. ORTHOPEDIC BRACES AND SURGICAL FITTINGS. These products promote proper body alignment and support injured areas. Pharmacists should have additional training before attempting to fit an orthopedic device.

A. Abdominal supports are elastic and are used to support and hold surgical dressings in place. Abdominal supports come in different widths.

B. Arm slings are used to provide comfort and support during recuperation from fractures, sprains, and surgery. The elbow should form a 90° angle in an arm sling to allow for proper circulation.

C. Back supports are worn by patients to provide support or promote proper alignment. The support is named to describe the area of the spine in which it is worn.

1. A **sacral belt** (also called **sacral cinch** or **sacroiliac belt**) supports the lower back.

2. A **lumbosacral support** supports the lower and middle back.

3. A **thoracolumbar support** supports the middle and higher areas of the back.

D. Cervical collars support or limit the range of motion of the neck. Cervical collars should be of sufficient length so that the patient can adjust the degree of compression. The width of the cervical collar should be the measurement from the chin to the sternum when the patient is standing straight, looking ahead.

1. **Soft** or **foam** cervical collars provide mild support and remind the wearer to keep the neck straight.

2. **Hard** or **rigid** cervical collars provide more support and limit movement to a greater degree.

3. A **Philadelphia** or **extrication** collar is used to immobilize the neck and is commonly used in emergency situations.

E. Clavicle supports are used as aids for the reduction and stabilization of the clavicle (i.e., collar-bone). These supports are sometimes called **figure-eight straps** because of their appearance.

F. Knee braces (also called **knee cages**) are used to support the knee. Some braces have metal stays on the side to prevent the lateral movement of the knee. Those with metal stays may also have hinges to allow for movement of the knee. Some knee braces have a cut-out hole and padding around the patella (i.e., knee cap) to prevent its movement.

G. Knee immobilizers prevent any motion of the knee and are used for severe injuries and fractures. They are available in different lengths and are adjustable in size.

H. Shoulder immobilizers prevent movement of the shoulder and arm. The elbow should be at a 90° angle to allow for healing without affecting circulation.

I. Tennis elbow supports apply pressure to the forearm to provide pain relief and decrease inflammation from tennis elbow (i.e., epicondylitis).

J. Wrist braces prevent movement of the wrist to allow healing. The brace may be shaped to have the wrist flexed so that the tendons in the hand remain stretched during the period of inactivity.

IX. OSTOMY APPLIANCES AND ACCESSORIES

A. Definitions. An **ostomy** is a surgical procedure in which an artificial opening is created in the abdominal wall for the purpose of eliminating waste. The opening is called a **stoma.** Each procedure is named to describe the anatomical location involved.

1. In a **colostomy,** part of the colon is cut and attached to the abdominal wall. This procedure is done mainly in patients with colon or rectal cancer, lower-bowel obstruction, or diverticulitis. A colostomy may be temporary or permanent, the discharge may be liquid or semisolid (as with an **ascending** colostomy), or it may be solid (as with a **descending** or **sigmoid** colostomy). Patients with an ascending colostomy and some patients with a transverse colostomy have gastric enzymes present in the discharge. These patients must take extra care to ensure that the discharge does not come into contact with the skin.

2. In an **ileostomy,** the ileum is attached to the abdominal wall. This procedure is performed in patients with ulcerative colitis or Crohn's disease.

3. A **urostomy** is performed in patients with bladder cancer. In this procedure, an **ileal conduit** is created by attaching the ureters to the ileum and the distal end of the ileum to the abdominal wall.

B. Ostomy appliances. The ostomy appliance contains a **flange** that attaches to the skin around the stoma. The flange protects the skin and allows for the collection device or **pouch** to be worn on the body. The selection of an ostomy appliance depends on the type of discharge produced. In addition to size, color, and flexibility, appliances may have detachable pouches and be able to be drained by releasing a clip at the bottom of the appliance.

C. Ostomy accessories

1. **Washers, powder paste,** and **barriers** are designed to protect the skin around a stoma.

2. **Cement, elastic belts,** and **tape** are used to hold the appliance in place.

3. **Deodorizers** help control fecal odor. **External** deodorizers can be placed into the appliance; systemic deodorizers (e.g., bismuth subgallate, chlorophyll, charcoal) can be ingested as **internal** deodorizers.

4. **Moisturizers** and **disinfectants** can be used to treat the skin and prevent complications.

5. **Irrigation devices** are used by patients who have control over the elimination of waste to facilitate removal of the accumulated waste. The devices are used to instill water into the intestine, which produces peristalsis.

D. Special considerations for ostomy patients. Drug therapy can present unique problems for ostomates. Absorption of enteric-coated or sustained-release products may not be possible. Antibiotics, sulfa drugs, laxatives, and diuretics are some of the common problem medications in these patients.

X. RESPIRATORY EQUIPMENT

A. Continuous positive airway pressure (CPAP) is used in patients with sleep apnea. The pressure supplied from this machine keeps the airway open. It is typically worn while sleeping to allow the patient to sleep without disturbance.

B. A **humidifier** puts moisture into the air by breaking water into small particles and blowing them into the air to be evaporated. Humidifiers are sometimes called "cool mist vaporizers." An **ultrasonic humidifier** contains a transducer, which produces a finer mist. It is commonly used to promote expectoration in patients with upper-respiratory infections. Both types of humidifiers need to be cleaned regularly to prevent the growth of mold or bacteria.

C. A **nebulizer** is used to deliver medication to the mouth or throat. Patients with a sore throat may use a nebulizer to deliver a topical anesthetic to the throat. An **ultrasonic nebulizer** is used to deliver medication into the lungs. The medication is diluted with normal saline and then inhaled. An ultrasonic nebulizer is used by patients with respiratory infections, asthma, or chronic obstructive pulmonary disease (COPD).

D. Oxygen is administered for a variety of conditions. Oxygen can be stored as a gas or a liquid or can be extracted from the air via a **concentrator.** The amount of oxygen required by the patient is measured in liters per minute (L/min). A **registered respiratory therapist** can be consulted for information on the correct procedures, cautions, and laws regarding oxygen use.

E. A **peak flow meter** is used by patients with asthma to detect constriction of the airways before symptoms appear. Early detection of an upcoming attack allows for therapy designed to stop or minimize the severity of the disease. Patients exhale as much as possible into a peak flow meter to obtain the expiratory flow rate. If this rate is below a predetermined baseline, patients might be instructed to change therapy.

F. Vaporizers are similar to humidifiers because they are used to deliver moisture to the air. These devices produce moisture by heating water to produce steam. They are commonly used to promote expectoration in patients with upper-respiratory infections.

XI. THERMOMETERS. These instruments measure body temperature and are **most commonly used** to detect or evaluate the treatment of infections.

A. A **mercury fever thermometer** has a sealed glass constriction chamber that contains liquid mercury. Responding to temperature changes, the mercury expands or contracts. It remains at the maximum temperature registered until shaken back into the reservoir at the bottom. Mercury fever thermometers are graduated from 96°F to 106°F in two-tenths of a degree increments. Mercury thermometers should be cleaned and sterilized with alcohol after each use.

1. The **oral** thermometer has a long slender reservoir. It is placed under the tongue, and the lips are sealed around the thermometer for 3 minutes.

2. The **rectal** thermometer has a blunt, pear-shaped bulb to prevent breakage and aid in retention. It is inserted 1 inch into the rectum and left for at least 2 minutes. A lubricant should be used to aid insertion. Rectal temperature is 1° higher than oral temperature.

3. The **security** thermometer (also called a **stubby** thermometer) has a short, stubby bulb to prevent it from breaking. It can be used as an oral or rectal thermometer.

4. Any of the three types of mercury thermometers can be used to take the **axillary temperature** if an oral or rectal temperature cannot be taken. An axillary temperature is taken by holding the thermometer snugly under the arm for 3–4 minutes. Axillary temperature is 1° lower than oral temperature.

B. **The basal thermometer** is used to measure basal body temperature. The basal body temperature is used to predict ovulation to increase or decrease the chance of conception. Basal body temperature is usually taken orally, rectally, or vaginally, as long as the route is consistent.

C. **Electronic thermometers** register temperature quickly. Heat alters the current running through a resistor, and the temperature is displayed via a digital readout. The current is supplied by a battery, some of which are rechargeable. Electric thermometers can be used orally or rectally and generally require placing a plastic sheath over the tip of the thermometer before using.

D. **Tympanic thermometers** use infrared technology to detect the temperature of the tympanic membrane. The temperature is determined within seconds and is less invasive than other thermometers. These thermometers use disposable tips that are inserted into the ear.

E. **Liquid-crystal strips** are placed directly on the skin (usually the forehead) to calculate body temperature. This method is not as accurate as others and should be reserved for situations in which other methods are not possible.

XII. **URINARY CATHETERS.** These devices allow for the **collection** and **removal of urine** from the bladder.

A. **External** catheters are used for **heavy incontinence** problems or complete loss of urine control. They are attached to a stationary collection device or a leg bag to allow for ambulation. Types of external catheters include:

   1. The **male** external catheter, which is also called a **condom** catheter because of its appearance. Some have adhesive to assist in keeping the catheter secure.

   2. The **female** external catheter, which is a contoured device that fits snugly in the vagina. It is connected to a stationary collection device or a leg bag, as with the male external catheter.

B. **Internal** catheters are used during **surgery** or when external catheters are inappropriate. Internal catheters can be used at home, but the patient must be taught proper insertion techniques to prevent infection. The catheter is inserted through the urethra into the bladder and is attached to a stationary collection device or leg bag. Catheters are sized by the **French scale:** the larger the number, the larger the diameter of the catheter. Types of catheters include:

   1. The **straight** catheter, which is used for **intermittent catheterization** to drain the bladder. It consists of a rubber tube in which one end has a hole to allow the drainage of urine; the other end connects to the collection device.

   2. The **Foley** catheter, an indwelling catheter that can be used for **up to 30 days before changing.** The end that is inserted into the bladder contains a balloon that is inflated with sterile water or saline. The inflated balloon holds the catheter in place. The balloon is deflated before removal.

STUDY QUESTIONS

Directions: Each of the numbered items or incomplete statements in this section is followed by answers or by completions of the statement. Select the **one** lettered answer or completion that is **best** in each case.

1. When a patient is fitted with an axillary crutch, how far below the underarm should the top of the crutch rest?

(A) 0.5 inch
(B) 1 inch
(C) 2 inches
(D) 3 inches
(E) 4 inches

2. What angle should the elbow form when a cane is the correct height?

(A) 10°
(B) 25°
(C) 45°
(D) 60°
(E) 90°

3. A product that delivers moisture to the air by heating water to produce steam is called a

(A) nebulizer
(B) humidifier
(C) ventilator
(D) peak flow meter
(E) vaporizer

4. An absorbent product designed for patients with light incontinence problems is a

(A) brief
(B) shield
(C) undergarment
(D) underpad
(E) catheter

5. When an oral temperature is taken, the thermometer should be placed into the mouth for

(A) 1 minute
(B) 2 minutes
(C) 3 minutes
(D) 4 minutes
(E) 5 minutes

6. The diameter of urinary catheters is measured by which of the following scales?

(A) Leur
(B) English
(C) French
(D) Gauge
(E) Metric

7. A cervical collar that immobilizes the neck is called a

(A) soft cervical collar
(B) hard cervical collar
(C) foam cervical collar
(D) extrication collar
(E) rigid cervical collar

8. Incontinence that is caused by an obstruction of the bladder is called

(A) overflow incontinence
(B) urge incontinence
(C) stress incontinence
(D) functional incontinence
(E) iatrogenic incontinence

9. A colostomy or ileostomy could be performed for all of the following conditions EXCEPT

(A) lower bowel obstruction
(B) malignancy of the colon or rectum
(C) ulcerative colitis
(D) duodenal ulcer
(E) Crohn's disease

10. Pregnancy test kits are designed to detect which substance?

(A) Luteinizing hormone (LH)
(B) Progesterone
(C) Human chorionic gonadotropin (hCG)
(D) Estrogen
(E) Follicle-stimulating hormone

ANSWERS AND EXPLANATIONS

1. The answer is C *[I B 2 a].*
When a patient is fitted for an axillary crutch, the top of the crutch should be 2 inches below the ax-illa (underarm).

2. The answer is B *[I A 1].*
When a patient is properly fitted for a cane, the elbow should form a 25° angle. This allows for maxi-mum weight transfer.

3. The answer is E *[X F].*
A vaporizer produces moisture by heating water to produce steam. A humidifier also produces mois-ture; however, it works by mechanically creating small water particles. A nebulizer is used to deliver liquid to the mouth and throat. A ventilator is used to assist in breathing. A peak flow meter is used to detect airway constriction.

4. The answer is B *[VII B 1].*
Shields are pads that are placed in the underwear and held with adhesive strips. They are used for pa-tients with light incontinence problems.

5. The answer is C *[XI A 1].*
Oral temperature is taken by inserting the bulb of the thermometer under the tongue and sealing the lips around the thermometer for 3 minutes.

6. The answer is C *[XII B].*
The French scale is used to measure the diameter of a urinary catheter. The Leur scale is used to mea-sure syringe tip size. The gauge scale is used to measure needle diameter. The metric scale is a general system of measurement.

7. The answer is D *[VIII D 3].*
An extrication collar (also known as a Philadelphia collar) is used to immobilize the neck. It is com-monly used in emergency situations. Soft or foam cervical collars provide mild support and remind the patient to keep the neck straight. Hard or rigid cervical collars provide moderate support but allow some movement.

8. The answer is A *[VII A 3].*
Overflow incontinence is caused by obstruction of the bladder. Urge incontinence is caused by un-controlled bladder contractions. Stress incontinence is caused by increases in intra-abdominal pres-sure. Functional incontinence is related to physical or psychological problems. Iatrogenic incontinence is caused by drugs or surgery.

9. The answer is D *[IX A 1–2].*
Lower-bowel obstruction, malignancy of the colon or rectum, and diverticulitis may all require a colostomy. Ulcerative colitis and Crohn's disease may require an ileostomy. The treatment of a duode-nal ulcer would not include a colostomy or an ileostomy.

10. The answer is C *[V B 1 d].*
Pregnancy tests detect hCG in the urine. This is secreted after the embryo has implanted in the uterus. Ovulation prediction tests detect LH. Progesterone, estrogen, and follicle-stimulating hormone are all involved in controlling the menstrual cycle.

28

OTC Otic, Dental, and Ophthalmic Agents

Larry N. Swanson
Connie Lee Barnes
Tina M. Harrison

I. OTIC OVER-THE-COUNTER (OTC) PRODUCTS

A. The ear structure

1. The **external ear** consists of the **auricle (pinna),** which is the visible outer structure of the ear that serves to funnel sounds into the ear canal.

2. The **ear canal,** also known as the external auditory meatus, is a channel that is about 1 inch in length, points downward, and ends in a cul-de-sac at the **tympanic membrane (eardrum).**

   a. The **skin lining the ear canal** is very thin and tightly stretched. The slightest degree of inflammation elicits a significant amount of pain. This canal is also lined with glands that secrete substances that form **cerumen (earwax),** which lubricates the lining of the ear canal and aids the removal of organisms and other foreign debris.

   b. The **tympanic membrane** vibrates when hit by sound waves, and it transmits that sound into the middle ear.

3. The **middle ear** is a small chamber about the size of a pea and contains the three small bones known as the **ossicles,** which amplify and transmit the sound waves farther into the inner ear.

   a. The middle ear is normally filled with air. The **eustachian tubes,** which are about the size of a pencil lead, connect the middle ear with the nasopharynx and equilibrate air pressure between the middle ear and the outer atmosphere. The "popping" (or "clicking") sensation that is heard upon swallowing is the sound of air bubbles passing through these tubes, which then open.

   b. In the presence of a cold or allergy, these eustachian tube walls may swell, which prevents air from passing through. A pressure drop in the middle ear may create a vacuum, which draws fluid into the middle ear. Bacteria may then grow in this fluid and produce a condition known as **otitis media** (middle ear infection).

4. The **inner ear** consists of the **cochlea** (the organ of hearing) and the **vestibular apparatus,** which is involved with maintaining balance and equilibrium.

B. Common ear disorders.

Table 28-1 differentiates the symptoms of the common otic disorders encountered by pharmacists. There are three ear-related conditions for which pharmacists may recommend OTC medications: earwax softening, prevention of "blocked ears" due to altitude changes, and treatment of water-clogged ears.

1. **Excessive/impacted earwax**

   a. **Functions** of cerumen include:

      (1) Lubrication of the lining of the ear canal

      (2) Aiding in the removal of organisms and debris by its outward movement (ceruminokinesis), which is caused by movement of the jaw during chewing and talking. The healthy ear is "self-cleaning" through this process.

      (3) Helping to protect the ear canal through its bacteriostatic and possibly fungistatic properties

   b. There are primarily **four reasons why earwax accumulates:**

      (1) Overactive ceruminous glands, which are rare

      (2) An anatomically narrowed ear canal

      (3) A large amount of hair in the canal, which occurs often in the elderly

      (4) Inefficient or insufficient chewing or talking, which may also occur in the elderly

Table 28-1. Symptoms of Otic Disorders

	Boil	Bacterial External Otitis	Impacted Cerumen	Suppurative Otitis Media
Pain*	Often	Often	Rarely	Usually
Hearing deficit	Rarely	Possibly	Often	Possibly
Purulent discharge	Rarely	Often	Rarely	Occasionally, when present, it indicates perforation
Bilateral symptoms	Rarely	Possibly	Rarely	Occasionally
Appropriateness of self-medication	Auricle only	Never	Carbamide peroxide	Never

*Pain is increased with chewing, traction on the auricle, and medial pressure on the tragus, except in otitis media, where it is knife-like and steady.

    c. Improper removal methods. Attempts should not be made to remove earwax by using cotton-tipped applicators, match sticks, or hairpins, as this usually pushes the earwax down farther in the canal and makes it more difficult to remove and may also contribute to the development of infection. Hence, the old adage: "Never put anything in your ear smaller than your elbow."

    d. Earwax-softening agents include:

      (1) Carbamide peroxide [urea hydrogen peroxide (e.g., Debrox, Murine Ear)] is the only approved safe and effective agent for earwax removal.

        (a) Action. Carbamide peroxide releases oxygen and, via a mechanical action of effervescence, loosens the wax debris and aids in its removal.

        (b) To **prevent vertigo,** one should warm the vial of this medication in the hands and put 5–10 drops in the ear.

        (c) Use. Carbamide peroxide should be used twice a day for 4 days, and the ear canal may be irrigated with the use of an ear syringe.

        (d) Cautions

          (i) Do not use if ear drainage, discharge, pain, or irritation or rash occurs.

          (ii) Do not use if injury or perforation of the ear drum exists.

          (iii) If the patient feels pain or a severe fullness in the ear when instilling drops into the ear, this might indicate the presence of a ruptured tympanic membrane.

      (2) Other agents that have been used for earwax softening include olive oil (sweet oil), mineral oil, glycerin, diluted hydrogen peroxide solution, propylene glycol, and baking soda solution (½ teaspoonful baking soda in 2 ounces of warm water).

      (3) Ear candles have gained some popularity, but they are not recommended. This is a hollow fabric cone (no wick) impregnated with beeswax or paraffin and is about 1 foot long. Instructions for these have the patient lie on his or her side with one ear up, cover the face and hair with a towel or paper plate, and have a second person insert the candle into the ear and light it on the other end. Heat presumably melts the earwax and creates a vacuum that draws the earwax out of the ear into the cone. Limited clinical trials have not confirmed the efficacy of these, and there have been reports of ear injuries, burns, eardrum perforations, and temporary hearing loss.

      (4) Cerumenolytics such as triethanolamine polypeptide oleate (Cerumenex) may be used for severely **impacted earwax.** This is available by prescription and must be administered under the supervision of a physician. Physicians may also use various devices/irrigating systems to remove impacted cerumen.

  2. Altitude and ear pressure. During situations such as airplane descent when there are rapid changes in air pressure, the **eustachian tubes** may not function properly. Traveling from low atmospheric pressure to a higher air pressure causes a vacuum to form in the middle ear. As a result, the eardrum retracts and cannot vibrate, which creates a muffled sound and some pain. Patients with a cold or allergy might be more susceptible to this problem.

    a. The act of **swallowing** (induced by chewing gum or letting hard candy dissolve in the mouth), activates the muscles that pull open the eustachian tubes and helps to unblock

the ears. Giving a baby a bottle of milk or juice upon airplane descent helps prevent ear pain.
- **b. Yawning** is also effective in opening the eustachian tubes.
- **c.** Another effective method of unblocking the ears is pinching the nostrils and, using the cheek and throat muscles, **forcing air into the back of the nose** as if trying to blow off the thumb and fingers from the nostrils.
- **d.** The use of **decongestant** medication may be recommended, either in the form of an oral agent such as pseudoephedrine (e.g., Sudafed), which should be taken about an hour before descent, or a topical decongestant such as oxymetazoline (e.g., Afrin), which should be administered 10–15 minutes before descent. In contrast to the effectiveness in adults, a recent study in children, however, failed to show that oral pseudoephedrine reduces air travel–associated ear pain in children.

3. **Otitis externa** is an inflammation of the external ear canal. The most common form is acute diffuse otitis externa (also called **swimmer's ear** or **hot weather ear**), which usually occurs during the summer months.
- **a.** Pathophysiology
    - **(1)** Typically, this condition develops when water accumulates in the external ear canal after swimming. The combination of heat and humidity results in softening and swelling of the ear wax, which interferes with the normal protective function of the ear wax. The pH in this area then increases and sets the stage for bacterial invasion.
    - **(2)** The resulting itching makes affected patients scratch the area [with fingers or cotton-tipped applicators (Q-tips)], which further interferes with the integrity of the ear canal.
    - **(3)** In more than 50% of cases, the microorganism that is involved is *Pseudomonas aeruginosa.* Other common bacteria include *Staphylococcus, Bacillus,* and *Proteus* organisms.
    - **(4)** The infection is commonly unilateral.
- **b.** Symptoms
    - **(1)** Itching
    - **(2)** Pain that is accentuated by moving the ear (i.e., pulling upward on the auricle or pressing on the tragus)
    - **(3)** A fluid discharge from the canal (in severe cases)
    - **(4)** A decrease or loss of hearing (if the ear canal is completely blocked)
- **c.** Treatment
    - **(1)** There is **no OTC treatment** for this condition.
    - **(2)** Prescription treatment usually includes an antibiotic/steroid combination, such as neomycin, polymyxin, hydrocortisone (e.g., Cortisporin Otic), or newer agents ofloxacin (Floxin) otic solution or ciprofloxacin/hydrocortisone (Cipro HC) otic suspension or an acetic acid and hydrocortisone combination (e.g., VoSol-HC Otic)
- **d. Prevention**
    - **(1)** After swimming or showering, the head should be turned to the side to drain water out of the ear. If otitis externa is a frequent occurrence, moldable silicone ear plugs or rubber ear inserts, which are placed in the ear before swimming, may be recommended. Earplugs get mixed results; they can help keep out water, but they can also trap it and irritate the ear canal.
    - **(2)** To dry the ear after swimming, several drops of a **50/50 solution of isopropyl alcohol and white vinegar,** which contains acetic acid and restores the acid pH to the external auditory canal, can be instilled in the ear. OTC agents like Swim-Ear or Auro-Dri (95% isopropyl alcohol and 5% anhydrous glycerin) may be tried as "ear-drying aids" for water-clogged ears. The FDA now prohibits the labeling of these agents for actual prevention of otitis externa.

4. **Boils** (i.e., **furuncles**) are infected hair follicles in the ear canal that usually involve the organism *Staphylococcus aureus.* This condition is usually self-limiting and is best treated by the application of warm compresses, which brings the boil to a head.

5. **Otitis media (OM)** is an infection of the middle ear. There are four types: myringitis, acute otitis media (AOM), chronic suppurative OM, and OM with effusion. *S. pneumoniae, Haemophilus influenzae,* and *Moraxella catarrhalis* are the **most frequent** organisms encountered for AOM. With the exception of colds, this is the most common infection in young children.

a. The **symptoms** include pain in the ear, fever, fluid discharge from the ear, and possible decreased hearing.

b. The **treatment** involves the use of oral antibiotics, which are available on prescription.

c. **Bottle feeding infants in a supine position should be avoided** because this allows milk to drain down the eustachian tubes into the middle ear. Infants have relatively short eustachian tubes and a horizontal configuration. Occasionally, when an infant is bothered by middle ear infections, a physician may choose to insert tympanostomy tubes into the ear drum for drainage and pressure-equalization purposes.

C. Administration of ear medication

1. When administering ear drops, pull the earlobe up and back to straighten the canal for adults and down and back to straighten in children.

2. Avoid touching the ear dropper tip to the ear; this prevents recontamination of the external ear if treating otitis externa.

3. One should instruct patients using a bulb syringe for ear irrigation to direct the solution up against the upper portion of the ear canal and not directly against the tympanic membrane.

4. The adult ear canal can hold about 17 drops (~0.85 mL) of fluid.

5. Warm ear drops in the hands to body temperature for 1–2 minutes. Drops that are too warm or too cold may cause vertigo (dizziness).

6. Tilt the head sideways with the affected ear upward when applying the drops.

II. DENTAL OTC PRODUCTS

A. Dental anatomy. Anatomically, the teeth are divided into two parts: the **crown** (above the gingival line) and the root (below the gingival line).

1. **Enamel** is the crystalline calcium salts (hydroxyapatite) that cover the crown to protect the underlying tooth structure.

2. **Dentin** is the largest part of the tooth structure, located beneath the enamel. It protects the dental pulp.

3. **Cementum** is a bone-like structure that covers the root and provides the attachment of the tooth with the periodontal ligaments.

4. **Pulp** consists of free nerve endings.

B. Common dental problems and OTC products

1. **Dental caries** (i.e., **cavities**) are formed by the growth and implantation of cariogenic microorganisms.
   a. **Causes**
   (1) **Bacteria** (primarily *Streptococcus mutans* and *Lactobacillaceae*) produce acids (e.g., lactic acid) that demineralize enamel. Initially, demineralized enamel appears as a white, chalky area and becomes bluish-white and eventually brown or yellow.
   (2) **Diet** is another factor in the development of dental caries. Foods with a high concentration of refined sugar (i.e., sucrose) increase the risk of dental caries. Sucrose is converted by bacterial plaque into volatile acids that destroy the hydroxyapatite.
   (a) **Fructose** and **lactose** are less cariogenic than sucrose.
   (b) **Noncariogenic sugar substitutes** are xylitol, sorbitol, and aspartame.
   b. **OTC products** for dental caries include products that can alleviate the pain and sensitivity until the patient can get to the dentist. Examples of ingredients that are beneficial in this regard include lidocaine, benzocaine (e.g., Anbesol, Orajel), or an oral analgesic (e.g., aspirin, acetaminophen).

2. **Plaque and calculus**
   a. **Causes**
   (1) **Plaque** is a sticky substance formed by the attachment of bacteria to the pellicle, which is a thin, acellular, glycoprotein (a mucoprotein coating that adheres to the enamel within minutes after cleaning a tooth).

(2) Calculus (or **tartar**) is the substance formed when plaque is not removed within 24 hours. The plaque begins to calcify into calculus when calcium salt precipitates from the saliva. Calculus can be removed only by a professional dental cleaning.

b. OTC products

(1) Toothbrushes. Soft, rounded, nylon bristles are preferred by dentists because hard bristles can irritate the gingival margins and cause the gums to recede. Electric toothbrushes can benefit patients who require someone to clean their teeth for them or patients who have orthodontic appliances.

(2) Irrigating devices direct a high-pressure stream of water through a nozzle to the hard-to-clean areas by gently lifting the free gingiva to rinse out crevices. Two types are available: **pulsating** (i.e., intermittent low- and high-pressure water streams) and **steady** (i.e., constant and consistent water pressure), neither of which has shown superior irrigating ability.

(a) Irrigating devices should serve as adjuncts in maintaining oral hygiene.

(b) Examples include Interplak Water Jet, Hydro Pik, and the Water Pik Oral Irrigator.

c. Dental floss is available waxed, unwaxed, thick, thin, flavored, or unflavored. Some dental flosses are impregnated or coated with additives such as baking soda and fluoride. Also, several manufacturers are marketing floss made of materials with superior antishredding properties (e.g., Glide, Colgate Precision). There are no differences between dental flosses in terms of plaque removal and prevention of gingivitis. There is no evidence of a residual wax film with the use of waxed dental floss.

(1) The selection of dental floss depends upon characteristics of the patient, such as tooth roughness or tightness of tooth contacts (e.g., waxed floss is recommended for tight-fitting teeth because it can pass easily between the teeth without shredding).

(2) The American Dental Association (ADA) recognizes the following brands as safe and effective: Butler, Johnson & Johnson, and Oral-B.

d. Dentifrices are products that enhance the removal of stains and dental plaque by the toothbrush. These include toothpastes, antiplaque and anticalculous mouthwashes, cosmetic whiteners, desensitizing agents, disclosing agents, and dental gums.

(1) Toothpastes are beneficial in decreasing the incidence of dental caries, reducing mouth odors, and enhancing personal appearance. Some toothpastes may contain an antioxidant, CoQ10 (e.g., Q-Dent CoQ10). **Ingredients** include the following:

(a) Abrasives are responsible for physically removing plaque and debris. Examples include silicates, sodium bicarbonate, dicalcium phosphate, sodium metaphosphate, calcium pyrophosphate, calcium carbonate, magnesium carbonate, and aluminum oxides. Mentadent contains sodium bicarbonate, whereas PeroxiCare contains sodium bicarbonate and peroxide. High-abrasive formulations are not advised for long-term use or for use by patients with exposed root surfaces.

(b) Surfactants are foaming agents that are incorporated into most dentifrices because their detergent action aids in removing debris. The **most frequently used** surfactants are **sodium lauryl sulfate** and **sodium dodecyl benzenesulfonate.** Sodium lauryl sulfate–containing dentifrices have been associated with an increase in the occurrence of canker sores. Dentifrices such as Rembrandt Natural, Sensodyne, and Biotene do not contain sodium lauryl sulfate.

(c) Humectants prevent the preparation from drying. Examples include sorbitol, glycerin, and propylene glycol.

(d) Suspending agents add thickness to the product. Examples include methylcellulose, tragacanth, and karaya gum.

(e) Flavoring agents include sorbitol or saccharin.

(f) Pyrophosphates are found in tartar-control toothpastes. These products retard tartar formation; however, they form an alkaline solution that may irritate the skin. Some patients might experience a rash around the outside of the mouth. These patients should use regular toothpaste with only occasional uses of tartar-control toothpaste. Tartar-control toothpastes do not penetrate below the gum-Line, where tartar does the most damage.

(g) Fluoride is anticariogenic because it replaces the hydroxyl ion in hydroxyapatite with the fluoride ion to form fluorapatite on the outer surface of the enamel. Fluorapatite hardens the enamel and makes it more acid resistant. Fluoride also has demonstrated antibacterial activity.

(i) Fluoride is **most beneficial** if used from birth through **age 12 or 13** because unerupted permanent teeth are mineralizing during that time.

Whether or not a patient receives fluoride depends upon the concentration in their drinking water (Table 28-2).

(ii) **Common fluoride compounds** in toothpaste include 0.24% sodium fluoride and 0.76% or 0.80% sodium monofluorophosphate (e.g., Aim, Crest, Aquafresh, Colgate). Crest Gum Care contains a reformulated version of stannous fluoride (0.454%), which might reduce gingivitis and bleeding of the gums by an average of 20% and 33%. It can also stain teeth brown.

(iii) A fluoride warning label, which recommends contacting a poison control center or seeking professional assistance if more than a brushful of fluoride toothpaste is ingested, is required by the FDA on fluoride-containing dentifrices because the federal agency lists fluoride as a toxic substance.

(iv) The estimated toxic dose of fluoride is 5–10 mg/kg.

(v) Acute fluoride toxicity causes nausea, vomiting, and diarrhea. The ADA limits the maximum amount of fluoride in ADA-accepted toothpaste to 260 mg per container.

(2) Agents with **antiplaque** potential for inclusion in dentifrices include plant extracts (sanguinarine), metal salts (zinc and stannous), phenolic compounds (triclosan), and essential oils (thymol and eucalyptol).

(a) **Triclosan** is an antimicrobial agent that has been demonstrated clinically to help prevent gingivitis, plaque, cavities, and tartar.

(i) Colgate Total contains 0.24% sodium fluoride and 0.30% triclosan and is formulated with a polymer, **Gantrez,** which works to prolong the contact of triclosan with oral structures.

(ii) Therefore, Colgate Total continues to work in between brushings.

(b) Colgate Total has been accepted by the ADA as efficacious.

(3) **Anticalculous dentifrices** include zinc chloride, zinc citrate, and 33% pyrophosphate as ingredients to prevent calculus formation.

(a) The ADA does not evaluate anticalculous claims because the ADA regards the inhibition of supragingival calculus as a nontherapeutic use.

(b) The ADA has directed that the following statement appear on all package and container labeling for accepted fluoride dentifrice products with calculus-control activity: "[*Product name*] has been shown to reduce the formation of tartar above the gumline, but has not been shown to have a therapeutic effect on periodontal diseases."

(4) **Cosmetic whitening agents.** The **most common ingredient** in these products that is responsible for whitening the teeth is **10% carbamide peroxide** (i.e., in Gly-Oxide, Simply White, or Proxigel) and hydrogen peroxide (i.e., in Crest Whitestrips).

(a) Carbamide peroxide is a white crystal that reacts with water to release hydrogen peroxide, which in turn liberates free oxides.

(b) Some cosmetic whiteners may contain hydrogen peroxide or perhydrol urea in gel or liquid form.

(c) Products specifically marketed to dentists include Platinum Professional Tooth Whitening System and Rembrandt Lighten Gel.

(i) Patients should only perform tooth bleaching with a dentist's supervision.

Table 28-2. Daily Fluoride Supplement Requirements for Infants and Children Based on Concentration of Fluoride in Drinking Water

Water Concentration	Age	Fluoride Supplement Required
>0.6 ppm of fluoride	6 months to 3 years	0
	3–6 years	0
0.3–0.6 ppm of fluoride	6 months to 3 years	0
	3–6 years	0.25 mg per day
	6–16 years	0.50 mg per day
<0.3 ppm of fluoride	6 months to 3 years	0.25 mg per day
	3–6 years	0.50 mg per day
	6–16 years	1.00 mg per day

(ii) Crest Extra Whitening uses a patented soft-silica technology. Due to this technology, the product contains 50% more silica, which greatly enhances the removal of extrinsic stains without increasing abrasiveness.

(d) **Possible risks** associated with using whitening products include alteration of normal flora, tissue damage, teeth sensitivity, gingivitis, and potentiation of carcinogenic effects of other agents.

(e) **Antiseptics** have been used as whiteners (e.g., Gly-Oxide, Proxigel).

(5) **Desensitizing agents** reduce the pain in sensitive teeth caused by cold, heat, acids, sweets, or touch. These products should be nonabrasive and should not be used on a permanent basis unless directed by a dentist.

(a) Examples of **5% potassium nitrate compounds** include Colgate Sensitive, Sensodyne, Aquafresh Sensitive, and Crest Sensitivity.

(b) Dibasic sodium citrate in pluronic gel and 10% strontium chloride were classified as Class III pending further evidence of effectiveness.

(6) **Disclosing agents** aid in visualizing where dental plaque has formed. These products are for occasional use only and should not be swallowed. The FDA-approved product is a vegetable dye, FD&C red No 3. Following use, the consumer should rinse the mouth with water and expectorate.

(7) **Mouthwashes** may contain astringents, demulcents, detergents, flavors, germicidal agents, and fluoride. They can be used for cosmetic purposes, reducing plaque, or supplementing fluoride consumption.

(a) **Cosmetic mouthwashes** freshen the breath. They are nontherapeutic and are not effective as an antiseptic agent. These mouthwashes are classified by their active ingredients, alcohol content, and appearance. The most popular products are those that contain medicinal phenol and mint. The higher the percent of alcohol, the higher the impact of flavor within the mouth.

(b) **Antiplaque mouth rinses.** Mouth rinses claiming anticalculous or tartar-control activity contain the same active ingredients as anticalculus dentifrices. Cool Mint Listerine has received the ADA seal of approval.

(i) Cetylpyridinium chloride (CPC), a mouthwash ingredient, has been approved for Class I for plaque and gingivitis treatment. Examples of products in this class include Cepacol, Scope, and Oral-B Anti-Plaque Rinse.

(ii) Staining is associated with the overuse of CPC.

(c) **Fluoridated mouthwashes** are used after cleaning the teeth and should be expectorated. Nothing should be put into the mouth for 30 minutes after using these mouthwashes. The ADA has approved the following products: ACT Anti-Cavity Dental Rinse, ACT for Kids, Fluorigard Anti-Cavity Dental Rinse, and Reach Fluoride Dental Rinse, and Oral-B Rinse Therapy and Anti-Cavity Treatment.

(8) **Dental gums** are promoted to reduce plaque, whiten teeth, possibly reduce the risk of tooth decay, and freshen breath. Chewing gum is associated with increased salivary flow, which apparently produces a beneficial buffering effect against acids in the oral cavity.

(a) Some contain baking soda as a mild abrasive cleaner and to neutralize acid.

(b) Calcium may be added to help remineralize the teeth and prevent cavities.

(c) These gums also contain xylitol, a sweetener that is less likely to cause cavities than sugar or sorbitol. Examples are Trident Advantage, Arm & Hammer Dental Care, BreathAsure, Dental Care, Advance Breath Care, Aquafresh Whitening, and Biotene. BreathAsure Dental Gum contains an ingredient called PXT-20, which is an emulsion of polydimethylsiloxane and poloxamer 407. It forms a thin coating on the tooth that is supposed to reduce plaque buildup.

(d) These gums are not a substitute for good oral hygiene including brushing and flossing, but may be useful for people who are unable to brush after lunch.

(e) It is not known if these products have any advantage over regular sugarless gum.

3. **Gingivitis** is inflammation of the gingiva. The gingiva may appear larger in size with a bluish hue caused by engorged gingival capillaries and a slow venous return.

a. **Cause.** Gingivitis is caused by microorganisms that eventually damage cellular and intercellular tissues. **Chronic gingivitis** may be localized or generalized. The gums readily bleed when probed or brushed, and the patient should seek dental assistance.

b. OTC products include anesthetics containing eugenol or benzocaine (e.g., Orajel) to relieve the pain. Mouthwashes may freshen the breath; however, it is important to consider the potential of these products to disguise and delay treatment of pathological conditions (e.g., gingivitis) before use. Also, acetaminophen (Tylenol) can be recommended. The patient should seek the advice of a dentist.

4. Periodontal disease is the result of chronic gingivitis left untreated.
   a. The periodontal ligament attachment and alveolar bone support of the tooth deteriorate.
   b. Periodontitis may be treated with prescription products:
   (1) Periostat (doxycycline hyclate, 20-mg capsules)
   (2) Atridox (doxycycline hyclate 10%) in the Atrigel Delivery System.
      (a) Atridox provides local antibacterial effects.
      (b) Low-dose doxycycline inhibits collagenase, an enzyme that destroys connective tissue in the gums, leading to tooth loss.

5. Acute necrotizing ulcerative gingivitis (ANUG) is also called **trench mouth** and is characterized by necrosis and ulceration of the gingival surface with underlying inflammation. This condition is usually seen in teens and young adults.
   a. Signs and **symptoms** of ANUG include severe pain, halitosis, bleeding, foul taste, and increased salivation.
   b. The **cause** of ANUG is unknown. It is postulated that it might be associated with the overgrowth of spirochete and fusiform organisms.
   c. Risk factors include anxiety, stress, smoking, malnutrition, and poor oral hygiene.
   d. Treatment consists of local debridement. Also, penicillin VK (penicillin V is a derivative of penicillin G; however, it is more stable in an acidic medium and, therefore, is better absorbed from the gastrointestinal tract; K stands for potassium) or metronidazole may be used in certain cases (e.g., widespread lesions).
   e. OTC products include acetaminophen and products with benzocaine (not eugenol because it may cause soft-tissue damage). The patient should be advised to see a dentist. The use of salicylates is not recommended if the patient is predisposed to bleeding. Also, adequate nutrition, high fluid intake, and rest are essential. Rinsing the mouth with warm normal saline or 1.5% peroxide solution might be helpful for the first few days.

6. Temporomandibular joint (TMJ) syndrome is caused by an improper working relationship between the chewing muscles and the TMJ.
   a. Signs and **symptoms** include a dull, aching pain around the ear, headaches, neck aches, limited opening of the mouth, and a clicking or popping noise upon opening the mouth.
   b. Risk factors include bruxism (i.e., grinding the teeth) and occlusal (i.e., bite) abnormalities.
   c. Treatment consists of moist heat applied to the jaw, muscle relaxants, bite plates or occlusal splints, a diet of soft foods, correcting the occlusion, or surgery.
   d. OTC products that can help relieve the pain include oral analgesics (e.g., acetaminophen, ibuprofen).

7. Teething pain. The ADA has not accepted any product for teething pain. A **frozen teething ring** can provide symptomatic relief. Persisting pain may be treated with a local anesthetic such as benzocaine (found in Anbesol Baby and Orajel Baby). If a teething child presents with a fever, a physician should be contacted.

8. Xerostomia (i.e., dry mouth) is caused by improper functioning of the salivary glands (as in Sjögren's syndrome and diabetes mellitus). **Artificial saliva** is available as an OTC product. The ADA has approved the following artificial saliva products: Moi-Stir, Salivart, Xero-Lube, and Oralbalance Gel.

C. Common oral lesions and OTC products

1. Canker sores (also called **recurrent aphthous ulcers** or **recurrent aphthous stomatitis**)
   a. The **cause** of canker sores is unknown. Studies suggest that the cause may be due to hypersensitivity to bacteria found in the mouth or dysfunction of the immune system initiated by minor trauma or stress. This is why physicians or dentists may use prednisone or a topical steroid to reduce allergic reaction, or have the patient rinse with a tetracycline suspension. Peridex and Listerine appear to help decrease the bacteria in the mouth.
   b. Lesions can occur on any nonkeratinized mucosal surface in the mouth (i.e., tongue, lips) and usually appear gray to yellow with an erythematous halo of inflamed tissue surrounding the ulcer. Most lesions persist for 7–14 days and heal without scarring.

c. OTC products can control the pain of canker sores, shorten the duration of current lesions, and prevent new lesions. Products include **protectants, local anesthetics,** and **debriding and wound-cleansing agents.**

(1) Protectants include Orabase, denture adhesives (see II F 2), and benzoin tincture. Denture adhesives are not approved for this use by the FDA.

(2) Local anesthetics, such as benzocaine or butacaine, are the **most common anesthetics** found in these OTC products.

(a) The FDA has approved the following ingredients:
  (i) Benzocaine (5%–20%)
  (ii) Benzyl alcohol (0.05%–0.1%)
  (iii) Dyclonine (0.05%–0.1%)
  (iv) Hexylresorcinol (0.05%–0.1%)
  (v) Menthol (0.04%–2%)
  (vi) Phenol (0.5%–1.5%)
  (vii) Phenolate sodium (0.5%–1.5%)
  (viii) Salicyl alcohol (1%–6%)

(b) Examples of OTC local anesthetics for oral use include Anbesol, Blistex, Campho-Phenique, Orajel, Orajel CoverMed, Zilactin-B, Zilactin-L, Benzodent, and Rembrandt Canker Pain Relief Kit.

(c) The use of products containing substantial amounts of menthol, phenol, camphor, and eugenol should be discouraged due to their ability to irritate tissue.

(d) Aspirin should not be retained in the mouth or placed on an oral lesion in an attempt to provide relief.

(e) Prescription products. Amlexanox (Aphthasol) has been approved for the treatment of canker sores.
  (i) It is applied four times daily after meals and at bedtime.
  (ii) Advise patients to start using the product as soon as they notice symptoms and to continue until the ulcer is healed, approximately 10 days.

(f) Gelclair is indicated for local management and relief of oral pain associated with aphthous ulcers. It provides oral pain relief by acting as a protective adherent barrier over the surface of the mouth and throat.
  (i) Patient should use one packet at least three times a day or as needed.
  (ii) Advise patients to mix one packet with 3 tablespoons of water, swish for a minute, then expectorate. Do not eat or drink for approximately 1 hour after treatment.

(g) Investigational products: Thalidomide. Thalidomide is being studied for the treatment of AIDS-associated oral canker sores.

(3) Debriding and wound-cleansing agents include 10%–15% carbamide peroxide, 3% hydrogen peroxide, 1.2 g sodium perborate monohydrate, and sodium bicarbonate. The FDA considers these four active ingredients to be safe and effective for debriding or wound-cleansing agents for oral health care.

2. Cold sores/fever blisters (also called **herpes simplex labialis**) are caused primarily by the herpes simplex type I virus (HSV-1). HSV-1 is contagious and is thought to be transmitted by direct contact. An outbreak may be provoked by stress, minor infection, fever, or sunlight. Cold sores usually occur on the lips and are recurrent, often arising in the same location.

a. Presentation. An outbreak is preceded by burning, itching, or numbness. Red papules of fluid-containing vesicles then appear, and these eventually burst and form a crust. These sores are typically self-limited and heal in 10–14 days without scarring.

b. OTC products for cold sores include products that contain softening compounds (e.g., emollient creams, petrolatum, protectants), which keep the cold sore moist to prevent it from drying and fissuring. Local anesthetics in nondrying bases (e.g., Orabase, with benzocaine) decrease pain. Highly astringent bases should be avoided. The ADA contraindicates caustic agents (e.g., phenol, silver nitrate), camphor and other counterirritants, and hydrocortisone for the treatment of cold sores. Lesions should be kept clean by gently washing with mild soap.

(1) If a **secondary infection** develops, bacitracin or Neosporin antibiotic ointments should be recommended. If necessary, the patient should consult a physician for a systemic antibiotic prescription.

      (2) A lip **sunscreen** should be used for patients whose cold sores appear to be due to sun exposure.

      (3) The essential amino acid l-lysine has been used in oral doses of 300–1200 mg daily to accelerate recovery or suppress recurrence of cold sores. However, studies have produced conflicting data regarding l-lysine and its effect on the duration, severity, and recurrence rate of cold sores.

   c. Prescription products.

      (1) Docosanol 10% cream (Abreva) is indicated for the treatment of recurrent oral-facial herpes simplex. It blocks the virus from entering the cells. Patients should apply the cream five times a day until the lesion is healed.

      (2) Valacyclovir (Valtrex) is the first 1-day oral antiviral medication for the treatment of herpes labialis.

      (3) Acyclovir 400 mg orally twice a day has been studied for delaying recurrence and reducing the frequency of cold sores. Also, **acyclovir 5%** in a modified aqueous cream applied four times daily significantly reduced the healing time of cold sores and the number of recurrent sores.

      (4) Penciclovir (Denavir), an active metabolite of famciclovir (Famvir) has been approved for the treatment of recurrent herpes labialis in adults. Patients should apply Denavir every 2 hours while awake for 4 days beginning at the first sign of tingling or swelling.

      (5) Viractin 2% tetracaine cream and gel is used for the treatment of cold sores.

D. Common oral infections and OTC products

   1. Candidiasis (also called **thrush**) is caused by the fungus *Candida albicans,* which is the most common opportunistic pathogen associated with oral infections. Thrush has a milky curd appearance, and affected patients should contact a physician.

   2. Oral cancer. The most common oral cancer is **squamous cell carcinoma,** which can appear as red or white lesions, ulcerations, or tumors.

     a. Signs and **symptoms** include a color change in the tongue, a sore throat that does not heal, and persistent or unexplained bleeding. Patients with any of these signs should contact a physician or a dentist.

     b. Risk factors include smoked and smokeless tobacco as well as alcohol.

     c. Treatment consists of eliminating use of tobacco and alcohol in any form (e.g., alcoholic beverages, mouth rinses with alcohol). Also, treatment generally includes **wide local excision** for small lesions and **en bloc excisions** for larger lesions (in continuity with radical neck dissection if lymph nodes are involved). Radiation, alone or combined with surgery, may be appropriate. Chemotherapy may be used as palliation or as an adjunct to surgery and radiation.

     d. OTC medications should not be administered until after checking with a physician. For example, OTC medications used for inflammation can increase the effects of methotrexate. Chemotherapeutic agents can produce many possible side effects that require immediate medical attention (e.g., chest pain, inflammation, unusual bleeding). Some examples of side effects that usually do not require medical attention include nausea, vomiting, loss of appetite or hair, and trouble sleeping. OTC medications can be useful in these cases; however, nausea and vomiting are treated by prescription medications such as ondansetron or metoclopramide. Nonpharmacological measures, such as avoiding disturbing environmental odors and vestibular disturbances, might be helpful in minimizing nausea and vomiting.

E. Recommended standard prophylaxis for prevention of endocarditis

   1. Amoxicillin 2.0 g orally 1 hour before the procedure for adults, and 50 mg/kg orally for children, is the recommended standard prophylactic regimen for all dental, oral, upper-respiratory tract, and esophageal procedures.

   2. For patients who are **allergic to penicillin,** the recommended **alternative oral regimens** include:

     a. Clindamycin, 600 mg for adults; 20 mg/kg for children

     b. Cephalexin or **cefadroxil,** 2.0 g for adults; 50 mg/kg for children

     c. Azithromycin or **clarithromycin,** 500 mg for adults; 15 mg/kg for children, 1 hour prior to the procedure

F. OTC denture products

1. **Denture cleansers** are either **chemical** or **abrasive** in respect to their cleansing ability.
   a. **Chemical** denture cleansers include alkaline peroxide, alkaline hypochlorite, or dilute acids.
      (1) **Alkaline peroxide** is the **most commonly used** chemical denture cleanser and is available as tablets or powders. It causes oxygen to be released, which creates a cleansing effect. Alkaline peroxide does not damage the surface of acrylic resins; however, it may bleach them.
      (2) **Alkaline hypochlorite** (i.e., bleach) dissolves the matrix of plaque but has no effect on calculus. It is both bactericidal and fungicidal. A **disadvantage** of alkaline hypochlorite is that it **corrodes metal denture components.** It can also bleach acrylic resin. Therefore, it should not be used more than once a week.
   b. **Abrasive** denture cleansers are available as gel, paste, or powder (e.g., silicates, sodium bicarbonate, dicalcium phosphate, calcium carbonate).
      (1) Dentures should not be soaked in hot water because the heat could distort or warp the appliances.
      (2) The ADA accepts the following denture cleansers as safe and effective: Denture-Brite, Efferdent, and Polident.

2. **Denture adherents** contain materials (e.g., karaya gum, pectin, methylcellulose) that swell, gel, and become viscous in order to promote adhesion, which increases the denture attachment to underlying soft tissues.
   a. **Disadvantages.** As the use of denture adherents increases, the soft tissue deteriorates. Denture adherents can also provide a medium for bacterial and fungal growth. Daily use of denture adherents is not recommended.
   b. The ADA accepts the following denture adherents as safe and effective: Fixodent, Orafix, Sea-Bond, Super Poli-Grip, and Effergrip.

G. Pharmacists' responsibilities to the patient using OTC oral products

1. **Refer** a patient to a dentist if the oral complaint involves an abscess with fever, swelling, malaise, lymphadenopathy, or purulent exudate.

2. **Remind** patients that cold and canker sores, with appropriate treatment, are usually a self-limiting problem.

3. Patients should be informed about **how to use recommended products,** the duration of use, the expectations of using the product, and the procedure to follow if the product is ineffective.

4. If a nonprescription product does not improve a condition, or if the condition worsens, use of the product should be discontinued and a physician or dentist should be contacted.

III. OPHTHALMIC OTC PRODUCTS

A. Anatomy

1. **Eyelids** are folds of tissue that protect the eye and distribute tears.

2. The **external eye** is formed by the lacrimal apparatus and the conjunctival cul-de-sac.

3. **Internal eye**
   a. The **sclera** is the outer coating over the eyeball.
   b. The **iris** is the colored membrane that regulates the entrance of light through the pupil.
   c. **Aqueous humor** is the fluid derived from the blood by a process of secretion and ultrafiltration.
   d. The **lens,** which is a transparent refracting membrane, focuses rays to form an image on the retina.
   e. The **retina** receives the image formed by the lens.
   f. The **conjunctiva** is the mucous membrane that lines the eyelids.
   g. The **trabecular meshwork** and **Schlemm's canal** serve as exit pathways for aqueous humor.
   h. The **pupil** is the contractile opening at the center of the iris that responds to light and darkness.

B. Eye disorders

1. **Conditions affecting the eyelid** include irritation, inflammation, and infections [e.g., contusions (black eyes), styes].

   a. **Symptoms of a stye** include pain, tenderness, redness, and swelling. A stye is defined as a localized, purulent, inflammatory infection of one or more sebaceous glands of the eyelid. Styes cannot be treated with OTC medications. Often, hot compresses applied four times a day are helpful. However, some patients may require treatment with an antibiotic.

   b. **Inflammation of the eyelid** (blepharitis) can be detected by redness of the lids and burning, itching, and scaly skin. The underlying problem (e.g., seborrheic dermatitis, *S. aureus*) should be treated, which often requires an antibiotic.

   c. **Black eyes** may be treated with cold compresses for the first 24 hours, then with warm compresses. Damage to the eyelid itself should be referred to a physician.

2. **External ocular disorders** include chemical burns, conjunctivitis, and lacrimal system disorders.

   a. **Chemical burns** should not be self-treated with OTC products. Patients should be referred to a physician immediately.

   b. **Conjunctivitis** is caused either by viruses (most common), allergies, bacteria, or chlamydia.

   c. **Symptoms of conjunctivitis** include redness, itching, and discharge.

      (1) **Viral conjunctivitis,** or "pink eye," is a contagious form. Treatment is aimed at symptom relief. Artifical tears and topical decongestants can be used. Patients should be counseled to wash hands thoroughly, to not share towels with others, and to dispose of tissues properly.

      (2) **Allergic conjunctivitis** is commonly caused by animal dander, pollen, or topical eye preparations. Itching is considered the hallmark of this form of conjunctivitis. Removal or avoidance of the offending substances is recommended. However, cold compresses, oral or topical antihistamines or decongestants may be used.

      (3) **Bacterial and Chlamydial conjunctivitis** require treatment with prescription antibiotics.

   d. **Dacryoadenitis** (i.e., swelling of the lacrimal gland) should be referred to a physician. Symptoms include red, burning eyes and the sensation of a foreign body in the eye.

   e. **Corneal edema** is the result of an underlying cause (e.g., damage to the eye). Hypertonic solutions and decongestants can be helpful treatments. However, if edema persists for more than 24 hours, a physician should be contacted.

   f. **Insufficient tearing** can be a side effect of many medications, especially those with anticholinergic activity. Treatment for dry eyes should include an evaluation of the current medications and use of artificial tears. A chronic condition where insufficient tearing occurs (e.g., Sjögren's syndrome) is generally successfully treated with artificial tear products (see III D 5). The use of pilocarpine is also used to treat Sjögren's syndrome when artificial tears are ineffective.

3. **Internal ocular disorders** include glaucoma (i.e., an increase in intraocular pressure, optic neuropathy and visual field loss), cataracts (i.e., opacity of the crystalline lens of the eye or its capsule), and uveitis (i.e., inflammation of the uvea). These internal ailments should be diagnosed and treated by a physician.

C. Ophthalmic products. The following agents are included in ophthalmic products for the specific purposes listed below.

1. **Antioxidants** and **stabilizers** are used to delay or prevent deterioration of the drug. Examples include edetic acid, sodium bisulfite, sodium metabisulfite, sodium thiosulfate, and thiourea.

2. **Buffers** are designed to keep products within the appropriate pH range, which is 6.0–8.0 (tears are 7.4). Buffers include acetic acid, boric acid, hydrochloric acid, phosphoric acid, potassium bicarbonate, potassium borate, potassium citrate, the potassium phosphates, potassium tetraborate, sodium acetate, sodium bicarbonate, sodium biphosphate, sodium borate, sodium carbonate, sodium citrate, sodium hydroxide, and sodium phosphate.

3. **Clarifying or wetting** agents reduce surface tension of the lens. Examples include polysorbate 20, polysorbate 80, poloxamer 282, and tyloxapol.

4. **Preservatives** destroy or inhibit the development of microorganisms. Examples of these agents are benzalkonium chloride and benzethonium chloride.

5. **Tonicity adjusters** include dextrose, glycerine (1%), potassium chloride, propylene glycol (1%), and sodium chloride. Agents considered to be isotonic should equal 0.9%–60.2% sodium chloride. When applied to the eye, these agents pull water from the middle of the cornea. Nonisotonic agents used in the eye may produce excessive blinking or cause damage.

6. **Viscosity-increasing agents** are used to increase the retention time for ophthalmic medications. These agents include cellulose derivatives, dextran 70, gelatin (0.01%), and liquid polyols.

D. Medicinal agents. **There are no FDA-approved anti-infective products available for OTC ophthalmic use. The following compounds are medicinal agents used for ophthalmic therapy.**

1. **Astringents.** The only FDA-recommended astringent is zinc sulfate (0.25%). This agent is relatively mild but still provides some relief from eye irritation because it decreases inflammation. The recommended dose is 1–2 drops four times a day.

2. **Demulcents** are relatively free of side effects and are used to protect and lubricate the eye from dryness and irritation from sun exposure. Demulcents include carboxymethylcellulose sodium, dextran 70, gelatin, glycerin, hydroxyethyl cellulose, hydroxypropyl methylcellulose, methylcellulose, polyethylene glycol 300, polyethylene glycol 400, polysorbate 80, polyvinyl alcohol, povidone, and propylene glycol.

3. **Decongestants and vasoconstrictors**
   a. **Mechanism of action.** These agents work by producing a temporary constriction of the blood vessels located in the conjunctiva.
   b. **Products** include naphazoline hydrochloride (e.g., Clear Eyes), phenylephrine hydrochloride (e.g., Isopto Frin), tetrahydrozoline hydrochloride (e.g., Murine Plus), and oxymetazoline hydrochloride (OcuClear). Combination decongestant and antihistamine products include Naphazoline Plus Solution, Naphcon-A, and Opcon-A.
   c. **Rebound congestion** can occur with a long duration of use.
   d. **Contraindication.** The available OTC agents are useful in relieving eye redness and irritations and are contraindicated in angle-closure glaucoma patients.

4. **Hypertonic agents** (e.g., sodium chloride 2%–5%) are used for the relief of corneal swelling. Although they are available as nonprescription products, these products should be used under the supervision of a physician because of their concentration.

5. **Artificial tears** (combination of hypertonic agent, buffer, viscosity agent, and preservative) are used to lubricate the eye for relief of dry eyes or irritation. Preservative-free (PF) products are also available for single- or unit-dose use.

E. **Home remedies** (e.g., boric acid eyewash, chamomile tea compresses, internal echinacea) should be avoided. These homemade remedies have not been proven safe or effective. There are also risks due to nonsterilization of placing these products into one's eye.

F. **General patient information**

1. Patients should be counseled regarding appropriate administration of individual products. They also should be told to wash hands thoroughly before applying these products.

2. If a patient presents with a headache or vision abnormalities, has had symptoms persisting for more than 3 days, or if a recommended OTC product has not abated symptoms during this time, a physician should be contacted. In general, OTC ophthalmic products should not be used for more than 3 days without physician supervision.

3. Proper administration technique is important when using these agents. The tip of the container should never come in contact with the eye itself. Suspensions should be shaken before being administered. Any agent that has changed color should be discarded immediately.

4. Systemic absorption may occur; therefore, patients should be instructed to compress the lacrimal sac for 1–2 minutes during and following instillation of drops.

5. If more than one ophthalmic product is being used, an interval of at least 5 minutes should be allowed before administering the next product.

6. Ophthalmic ointments may blur vision during waking hours. Use with caution in conditions where visual clarity is critical.

G. Contact lenses. Wearing contact lenses successfully depends on adequate tear production.

1. General considerations

    a. Indications include keratoconus (protrusion of the central part of the cornea), aphakia (absence of lens), visual aberrations, myopia (nearsightedness), hyperopia (farsightedness), astigmatism (improper focus of light rays), presbyopia (diminution of the accommodation of the lens), and monovision.

    b. Contraindications include occupations with exposure to excessive dust, wind, or smoke; chronic conjunctivitis or blepharitis; and recurrent bacterial, fungal, or viral infections.

    c. Caution should be taken by patients suffering from diseases that can affect the normal eye (e.g., epilepsy, high blood pressure, heart disease, diabetes mellitus). Certain diseases and drugs may have direct effects on the eye. For example, high blood pressure can produce retinal hemorrhage; diabetes mellitus produces an outgrowth of vessels in the iris and anterior chamber of the eye; and oral contraceptives have numerous possible effects on the eye (e.g., increased corneal sensitivity, color changes, decreased visual acuity).

2. Types of contact lenses

    a. Daily-wear soft lenses are made of soft, flexible plastic that allows oxygen to pass through to the eyes. They are designed to be removed and cleaned nightly and often require once weekly enzymatic cleaning. Sleeping in these lenses is not recommended due to the possibility of serious eye damage. These lenses are usually replaced yearly.

    b. Daily-wear disposable soft lenses are like the daily-wear lenses; however, these are designed for single daily use and should be discarded and replaced daily with a brand-new pair. Virtually no lens care is required.

    c. Extended-wear soft lenses are designed to be worn continuously for up to 6 nights then replaced with new lenses.

    d. Frequent-replacement soft lenses are designed for daily use (but are removed at night) for a set period of time (e.g., 2 weeks, 1 month).

    e. Rigid gas permeable (RGP) lenses are made from a combination of the soft materials and a harder plastic, polymethylmethacrylate (PMMA). These are considered "hard" lenses if compared to the soft lenses, but these are not the same as the traditional "hard" lenses that were made solely from PMMA. The combination of materials allows oxygen to flow through to the eye, lessens discomfort, and allows for easier cleaning. The RGP lenses are available in daily- and extended-wear versions.

3. Solution ingredients

    a. Cleaning products generally contain nonionic or amphoteric surfactants, which dislodge mucus, lipids, and proteins from the lens. Contact lenses should be rinsed following the cleansing step to prevent eye irritation.

    b. Wetting solutions are applied directly to the lens before insertion into the eye. Wetting solutions are intended to lubricate, decrease lens surface tension, and change the lens surface from hydrophobic to hydrophilic.

    c. Soaking and **storage solutions** are used to provide an aseptic environment and to hydrate the lens.

    d. Preservatives used in these solutions include benzalkonium chloride, thimerosal, phenylmercuric nitrate, sorbic acid, and sodium edetate. Thimerosal causes a great deal of irritation to many soft contact lens wearers.

4. General patient information

    a. Never swap contact lenses with another person.

    b. Wash and rinse your hands before handling your lenses.

    c. Never use saliva on your lenses.

    d. Don't wear lenses longer than prescribed.

    e. If eyes become irritated, remove the lenses immediately and consult a physician.

    f. Throw away disposable lenses after the recommended wearing period.

    g. Visit a reputable eye care professional annually for a complete eye exam, or more frequently if needed.

STUDY QUESTIONS

Directions: Each of the numbered items or incomplete statements in this section is followed by answers or by completions of the statement. Select the **one** lettered answer or completion that is **best** in each case.

1. Ophthalmic agents contraindicated in glaucoma patients include which of the following substances?

(A) Antioxidants

(B) Antipruritics

(C) Decongestants

(D) Emollients

2. Which of the following is the only FDA-recommended astringent?

(A) Benzalkonium chloride

(B) Sodium chloride

(C) Zinc sulfate

(D) Edetic acid

3. Abrasives, ingredients in dentifrices, are noted for which of the following actions?

(A) Providing flavor

(B) Cleansing via a foaming detergent action

(C) Removing plaque and debris

(D) Preventing dental caries

(E) Adding thickness to the product

4. The appropriate pH range for ophthalmic products is

(A) 2.0–3.0

(B) 4.0–6.0

(C) 6.0–8.0

(D) 8.0–10.0

5. Which of the following lenses are designed to be worn continuously for up to 6 nights?

(A) RGP lenses

(B) Daily-wear soft lenses

(C) Daily-wear disposable soft lenses

(D) Extended-wear soft lenses

(E) Frequent-replacement soft lenses

6. All of the following statements concerning the use of alkaline peroxide as a denture cleanser are true EXCEPT

(A) it may bleach the denture

(B) it is available as tablets or powders

(C) it acts by releasing oxygen

(D) it is fungicidal and bactericidal

(E) it does not damage the surface of acrylic resins

7. All of the following statements concerning teeth-whitening products are true EXCEPT

(A) possible risks include tissue irritation and gingivitis

(B) most products contain 10% carbamide peroxide

(C) most products contain zinc to prevent calculus formation

(D) antiseptics (e.g., Proxigel) have been used as bleaching agents

(E) hydrogen peroxide–containing products are teeth-whitening agents

8. All of the following desensitizing agents are recommended for sensitive teeth EXCEPT

(A) 10% carbamide peroxide

(B) 5% potassium nitrate

(C) dibasic sodium citrate

(D) 10% strontium chloride

9. Which of the following statements is NOT correct?

(A) The "clicking" sound you hear when you swallow is caused by the air movement in the eustachian tubes.

(B) Giving a baby a bottle of milk can help prevent ear pain during aircraft descent.

(C) Chewing and talking actually aid in the natural outward movement of ear wax.

(D) The pain of otitis media is usually made worse by pressing on the tragus.

(E) The product Swim-Ear® could be recommended to treat water-clogged ears.

10. Carbamide peroxide appears to soften earwax by

(A) causing oxygen to be released, which loosens the wax
(B) stimulating fluid secretion in the ear canal
(C) actually dissolving the ear wax
(D) decreasing lipid content of the wax
(E) none of the above

11. All of the following statements are true regarding acute diffuse otitis externa EXCEPT:

(A) One of the other names for this condition is "swimmer's ear."
(B) Heat and humidity are considered contributing factors in the pathogenesis of this condition.
(C) Although there are no OTC agents available to treat this condition, Debrox is considered a useful preventive agent.
(D) This condition may require prescription topical antibiotic ear drops.
(E) The use of cotton-tipped applicators (e.g., Q-tips) in the ear canal may predispose a person to this condition.

12. A common oral problem caused by herpes simplex type I virus (HSV-1) is

(A) aphthous ulcers
(B) canker sores
(C) aphthous stomatitis
(D) fever blisters
(E) thrush

13. Mrs. Smith enters a pharmacy and says, "I think I've picked up one of my grandchildren's colds and have developed painful cold sores." The pharmacist would offer all of the following statements as advice for the treatment of cold sores EXCEPT:

(A) Lesions should be kept clean by gently washing them with mild soap solutions.
(B) Factors that delay healing (e.g., wind, sunlight, fatigue) should be avoided.
(C) Cold sores should be kept moist to prevent drying and fissuring by using Orabase cream.
(D) Hydrocortisone should be placed directly on the lesion.
(E) Application of a topical antibiotic (e.g., Neosporin) 3–4 times daily may be warranted if there are signs and symptoms of secondary bacterial infection.

14. The definition of a surfactant (an ingredient in toothpaste) can best be described by which of the following statements? Surfactant

(A) prevents drying of the preparation.
(B) removes debris by its detergent action and causes foaming, which is usually desired by the patient.
(C) physically removes plaque and debris.
(D) determines the texture, dispersiveness, and appearance of the product.
(E) adds flavor to the preparation, which makes it more appealing to the patient.

15. A 16-year-old girl stops by a pharmacy on her way home from school. She says to the pharmacist, "I have been using Proxigel daily to bleach my teeth in preparation for my spring formal. However, my teeth are becoming very sensitive." All of the following statements are advice that the pharmacist might suggest EXCEPT:

(A) There is a possibility that you may damage the gingival tissue and tooth pulp.
(B) Oxidizing agents may have the potential for mutating or enhancing the carcinogenic effects of other agents (e.g., tobacco).
(C) Bleaching teeth is best done under dental supervision.
(D) Proxigel is an antiseptic that contains zinc and should not be used for cosmetic whitening of the teeth.
(E) The most common ingredient in products responsible for teeth whitening is 10% carbamide peroxide, which can cause sensitivity.

16. All of the following products may be recommended by a pharmacist for the treatment of canker sores EXCEPT

(A) Benzocaine
(B) Zilactin-B
(C) Bayer aspirin placed directly on the oral lesion
(D) Anbesol
(E) Orajel

17. An FDA-approved ingredient for protection against painful sensitivity of the teeth due to cold, heat, acids, sweets, or contact is

(A) dicalcium phosphate
(B) sodium lauryl sulfate
(C) 5% potassium nitrate
(D) zinc chloride
(E) calcium carbonate

Directions: Each item below contains three suggested answers of which **one** or more is correct. Choose the answer

A	if **I only** is correct
B	if **III only** is correct
C	if **I and II** are correct
D	if **II and III** are correct
E	if **I, II, and III** are correct

18. Which of the following compounds are considered a suspending agent (an ingredient in dentifrices)?

I. Dicalcium phosphate
II. Karaya gum
III. Methylcellulose

19. Cold-sore treatment might include which of the following ingredients?

I. Benzocaine
II. Dyclonine
III. Camphor

20. Pharmacists can recommend OTC drug treatment for which of the following ear conditions?

I. Treatment of accumulated ear wax
II. Prevention of "blocked ears" due to altitude changes
III. Treatment of water-clogged ears

ANSWERS AND EXPLANATIONS

1. The answer is C *[III D 3]*.
Decongestants can cause a slight pupillary dilation. Although this is not significant in open-angle glaucoma, these agents should be avoided in angle-closure patients. In angle-closure glaucoma, the blockage to outflow is more severe and directly involves the anterior chamber.

2. The answer is C *[III D 1]*.
Zinc sulfate is the only ophthalmic astringent recommended by the FDA. Sodium chloride is a hypertonic agent. Benzalkonium chloride is a preservative used in contact lens solutions. Edetic acid is an antioxidant used to slow or prevent deterioration of ophthalmic drugs.

3. The answer is C *[II B 2 d (1) (a)]*.
Abrasives are components in dentifrices that are responsible for physically removing plaque. Patients should use the least abrasive dentifrice, unless directed otherwise by the dentist.

4. The answer is C *[III C 2]*.
The appropriate pH range for ophthalmic agents is 6.0–8.0, which is similar to the pH of tears (7.4).

5. The answer is D *[III G 2 c]*.
The extended-wear soft lenses may be worn for up to 6 nights before replacement is needed. They should not be worn for longer periods to avoid the possibility of serious eye damage.

6. The answer is D *[II F 1 a (1)]*.
The mechanism of action of alkaline peroxide is the release of oxygen for a mechanical cleaning effect. It can be used safely on acrylic appliances; however, it may bleach the appliance. It is available in tablet or powder form. Alkaline hypochlorite, not alkaline peroxide, is both bactericidal and fungicidal.

7. The answer is C *[II B 2 d (4)]*.
Teeth-whitening agents usually contain 10% carbamide peroxide, which is a white crystal that reacts with water to release hydrogen peroxide and, therefore, liberates free oxides. Cosmetic agents can alter the normal flora or cause tissue irritation, gingivitis, and teeth sensitivity. Antiseptics (e.g., Gly-Oxide, Proxigel) and hydrogen peroxide (e.g., Crest Whitestrips) have been used as teeth-whitening agents.

8. The answer is A *[II B 2 d (4)]*.
Desensitizing agents should not be abrasive or used on a chronic basis unless directed by a dentist. The products approved by the American Dental Association (ADA) include the ingredients 5% potassium nitrate, 10% strontium chloride, and dibasic sodium citrate 2% in pluronic gel. The ingredient 10% carbamide peroxide is a whitening agent that can cause teeth sensitivity and, therefore, should not be used by a patient with sensitive teeth.

9. The answer is D *[I B 3 b (2)]*.
The pain of acute diffuse otitis externa (not otitis media) is made worse by moving the ear (pulling upward on the auricle or pressing the tragus). Because otitis media involves the middle ear, this pain is not affected by movement of the external ear structure.

10. The answer is A *[I B 1 d (1) (a)]*.
Carbamide peroxide releases oxygen and, via a mechanical action of effervescence, loosens the wax debris and aids in its removal.

11. The answer is C *[I B 3 and 1B 1 d (1)]*.
Debrox, a trade name for carbamide peroxide, is used to soften ear wax, not as a preventive agent for otitis externa. The FDA does not allow any OTC agents to be labeled for the prevention of otitis externa, but the instillation of ear drops containing either a 50:50 solution of isopropyl alcohol and white vinegar, or an isopropyl alcohol/anhydrous glycerin solution, will treat water-clogged ears.

12. The answer is D *[II C 2]*.
Cold sores/fever blisters (also called herpes simplex labialis) are primarily caused by the herpes simplex type I virus.

13. The answer is D *[II C 2]*.

Stress, minor infection, fever, or sunlight may provoke and delay healing of cold sores. OTC products for the treatment of cold sores include products that contain softening compounds (e.g., emollient creams, petrolatum, protectants), which keep the cold sore moist to prevent it from drying and fissuring. If a secondary infection develops, bacitracin or neomycin ointments should be recommended.

14. The answer is B *[II B 2 d (1) (b)]*.

Sodium lauryl sulfate is used frequently as a surfactant in most dentifrices. Its detergent action aids in the removal of debris, and the foaming is usually desired by the patient. There is no evidence that surfactants possess anticaries activity or decrease periodontal disease. The FDA considers surfactants an inactive ingredient in dentifrices.

15. The answer is D *[II B 2 d (4)]*.

Teeth-whitening agents usually contain 10% carbamide peroxide, which is a white crystal that reacts with water to release hydrogen peroxide and, therefore, liberates free oxides. Cosmetic agents can alter the normal flora or cause tissue irritation, gingivitis, and teeth sensitivity. Antiseptics have been used as cosmetic whiteners (e.g., Gly-Oxide, Proxigel) along with calcium peroxide (e.g., calprox in EpiSmile). EpiSmile also contains sodium monofluorophosphate.

16. The answer is C *[II C 1 c (2)]*.

Local anesthetics can provide relief of canker sore pain. The most common local anesthetics found in OTC products include benzocaine and butacaine. Some examples are Anbesol, Zilactin-B, and Orajel. Aspirin should not be retained in the mouth before swallowing or placed in the area of the oral lesions because of the high risk for chemical burn with necrosis.

17. The answer is C *[II B 2 d (5)]*.

Desensitizing agents should not be abrasive or used on a chronic basis unless directed by a dentist. The products approved by the ADA include the ingredients 5% potassium nitrate, 10% strontium chloride, and dibasic sodium citrate 2% in pluronic gel.

18. The answer is D (II, III) *[II B 2 d (1) (d)]*.

Suspending agents are products that add thickness to the dentifrices. Examples are tragacanth, karaya gum, and methylcellulose. Dicalcium phosphate is categorized as an abrasive product.

19. The answer is C (I, II) *[II C 2 a, b]*.

Cold-sore treatment involves keeping the lesion moist with emollient creams, petrolatum, or protectants. In addition, local anesthetics (e.g., benzocaine, dyclonine, salicyl alcohol) may be used. Topical counterirritants (e.g., camphor) and caustics or escharotic agents (e.g., phenol, menthol, silver nitrate) are not recommended because they may further irritate the tissue. Cold sores are usually self-limiting and heal within 10–14 days without scarring.

20. The answer is E (all) *[I B]*.

OTC drug treatment can be recommended for all of these ear conditions.

29

OTC Dermatological Agents

Larry N. Swanson

I. PEDICULOSIS AND PEDICULICIDES

A. Introduction. Pediculosis is a skin infestation produced by blood-sucking lice. Lice are small, flat, wingless insects with stubby antennae and three pairs of legs that end in sharp, curved claws. Three **types of lice infest humans.**

1. *Pediculus humanus capitis* (i.e., the head louse)

2. *Pediculus humanus corporis* (i.e., the body louse)

3. *Phthirus pubis* (i.e., the pubic, or crab, louse)

B. Life cycles. The lice that infest humans pass through similar life cycles.

1. **Location.** All lice need human warmth to survive.
   a. Head and **pubic lice** spend their entire cycle on the skin of the human host.
   b. Body lice live in clothing, coming to the skin surface only to feed.

2. **Development**
   a. Each type of louse develops from **eggs (nits)** that incubate for about 1 week. When the small, gray-white, tear-shaped eggs hatch, the nymphs appear.
   b. In about 3 weeks, the **nymphs** mature; then, the females start to lay eggs.
   c. Each type of louse survives about 1 month as a **mature adult.** During this time, the female head louse can produce 3–6 eggs a day.

3. **Egg deposit**
   a. Body lice deposit their eggs on fibers of clothing, particularly in the seams. These lice can survive without food up to 10 days, and the eggs may remain viable for about 1 month.
   b. Head and **pubic lice** deposit their eggs on hair strands, about ¼ inch from the skin. Adult head lice can survive on inanimate objects for about 20 hours; head lice nits may survive up to 10 days off the body.

C. Incidence. The incidence of lice infestations increases each year.

1. More than 10 million cases of head lice occur each year in the United States.

2. The bulk of these cases occur between September and November, when students are back in school.

3. In outbreaks of head lice, 70% of cases occur in children younger than 12 years.

4. Infestations tend to be more common in girls, presumably because of their greater tendency to share grooming items.

5. Unlike the other two forms of lice, body lice are associated with improper hygiene and are often present in homeless people. This infestation is rare in the United States, especially when people follow proper hygiene routines.

D. Medical problems

1. Both adult and nymph lice are blood-sucking; they feed on humans by piercing the skin and introducing a small amount of saliva (which contains an **anticoagulant**) into the feeding area. All lice types feed on blood for about 30–45 minutes every 3–6 hours.
   a. The attachment of lice to the body causes an **erythematous papule,** which may **itch.**
   b. The female louse produces a sticky **cement-like secretion** that holds the eggs in place on the hair shaft so securely that ordinary shampooing does not remove it.

2. Neither head nor crab lice transmit infections, but body lice transmit **typhus, relapsing fever,** and **trench fever.**

3. Lice and humans have a true **parasitic relationship;** lice depend on the human host for shelter, food, and reproductive success. Once hatched, nymphs must have access to the human host within the first 12- to 24-hour period, if they are to survive.

E. Methods of transmission

1. **Head lice** are most commonly **spread by head-to-head contact** with an infested person through hats, caps, scarves, pillowcases, communal combs and brushes, or clothing that is hung close together (e.g., on a coat rack).

2. **Pubic lice** are **transmitted primarily through sexual contact,** but also through shared undergarments, towels, or toilet seats.
   a. The lice affect teens and young adults most often through sexual contact.
   b. Lice frequently coexist with other sexually transmitted diseases.
   c. Scratching in the genital areas may transmit pubic lice to other hairy regions, such as the eyelashes, eyebrows, sideburns, and mustaches.

F. Signs and symptoms

1. **Head lice**
   a. Most patients have fewer than 10 lice.
   b. The most common sign is **head scratching.**
   c. **Skin redness around the nape (i.e., back) of the neck** and above the ears is usually seen.
   d. The lice can be identified by direct examination using wooden applicator sticks or a comb to part the hair, then looking at the hair through a magnifying glass.
   e. The lice appear as tiny brownish-gray spots that are often difficult to see. The shiny, **whitish-silver eggs,** which appear almost as grains of sugar, are more likely to be seen than the lice. The nits are initially **deposited** about **one-quarter of an inch from the scalp** on the hair shaft, and they may be **confused with dandruff or hair spray droplets.** Usually, hair grows at a rate of about ½ inch per month, so the duration of infestation can be assessed based on this information.

2. **Pubic lice.** The primary symptom is scratching in the genital area.

3. **Body lice.** The most common symptoms are bites and itching, which are commonly seen as vertical excoriations on the trunk area.

G. Treatment

1. There are **three steps** in the treatment of lice.
   a. Treat the lice and nits with a pediculicide agent.
   b. Control the symptoms of itching in order to prevent secondary infection.
   c. Clean the environment of potential lice and nits.

2. **Itching.** Pharmacists should advise patients that even after the causative organism and nits have been killed, itching may persist for several days. This aspect is very important because patients may decide to use pediculicides excessively, thinking that they have been ineffective when the itching continues. **Excessive use of pediculicides may result in excessive drying, which can cause further itching.**

3. Home remedies. Because of the social stigma attached to lice infestation, some individuals may resort to harmful home remedies. Examples of such uncomfortable, ineffective, and potentially dangerous approaches that should not be used include:
   a. Shaving the head and pubic area
   b. Applying heat to the infested area with a hair dryer
   c. Soaking the head in hot water for several minutes
   d. Soaking the area of infestation with gasoline or kerosene

4. **Over-the-counter (OTC) pediculicide products** are considered first-line treatments and include:
   a. **Pyrethrins 0.17%–0.33% with piperonyl butoxide 2%–4%.** This product is safe and effective for the treatment of head and pubic lice. The combination of ingredients is an example of **pharmacological synergism.**
      (1) **Pyrethrins** kill by **disrupting ion-transport mechanisms at the nerve membranes.** These natural insecticides are derived from a mixture of substances obtained **from** the

flowers of the **chrysanthemum** plant. Because not all eggs may be killed (it takes about 4 days for the nervous system of the louse to develop) with a single application of this agent (~70%–80% ovicidal activity and no residual effect) or removed with a nit comb, it may be necessary to reapply the pyrethrin product within 7–10 days of the first application (because the usual hatching time of the eggs is 7–10 days).

  (2) **Piperonyl butoxide** enhances the pediculicide effect of pyrethrins by **suppressing the oxidative degradation mechanisms of the lice.** Therefore, the length of time that the pyrethrins contact the lice is increased.

  (3) **Side effects** from either agent are **uncommon.**

    (a) **Contact dermatitis** (see IV) is the most frequently reported side effect.

    (b) **Allergic reactions.** Because pyrethrins are derived from a plant (chrysanthemum), they may produce hay fever (i.e., allergic rhinitis) and asthma attacks in susceptible individuals. Thus, patients who have known allergies to ragweed or chrysanthemum plants should use this product with caution.

  (4) Common **trade names** for this product include A-200 Lice Killing Shampoo, R and C, and RID.

  (5) **Directions for use (shampoo)**

    (a) **Apply the product, undiluted,** to the dry hair until it is entirely wet.

    (b) Allow the product to **remain on the head for 10 minutes.**

    (c) **Rinse thoroughly** with warm water.

    (d) Dry the area, preferably with a disposable cloth.

    (e) **Comb hair** in the previously infested area **with a fine-toothed comb** to remove dead lice and eggs.

    (f) Do not exceed two applications within 24 hours. It may be necessary to reapply the shampoo in 7–10 days [see above in (1)].

b. Permethrin (Nix) is a pyrethroid (i.e., a synthetic version of a pyrethrin). It is safe and effective for the treatment of head lice only.

  (1) **Mechanism of action.** Permethrin has a **similar mechanism of action as the pyrethrins.**

  (2) **Application.** Permethrin comes in the form of a 1% **creme rinse** and should be applied like a conventional hair conditioner after the hair has been shampooed (use a shampoo with no conditioner), rinsed, and towel-dried. The hair should be thoroughly saturated with undiluted permethrin (about 25–30 ml), which should **remain on the hair for 10 minutes then rinsed.**

  (3) **Effectiveness.** A single application is generally quite effective in killing lice and has a 70%–80% ovicidal activity. Because the agent is retained on the hair shaft, the product provides **continuing activity for up to 14 days.** This 2-week therapeutic effect persists regardless of normal shampooing.

    (a) Even with the residual activity, there still may be the need for retreatment in 7–10 days.

    (b) **Comb hair** in the previously infested area **with a fine-toothed comb** to remove dead lice and eggs.

    (c) There is, at least theoretically, the speculation that because low-level residual amounts of this agent are retained on the hair, it may be possible that when suboptimal levels are present, some lice may survive and give rise to strains that are resistant.

c. OTC pediculicide treatment failure. The National Pediculosis Association (NPA) has received reports of treatment failure with the use of the preceding agents. Speculations as to the cause of this treatment failure include failure to follow product instructions, noncompliance with nit removal, and possible head-lice drug resistance. Studies support the theory that there are now "super lice" that have survived exposure to pyrethrins and permethrin.

  5. **Prescription products** are included here to put into perspective how the OTC agents fit into therapy.

    a. Malathion (Ovide) is an organophosphate cholinesterase inhibitor that has been widely used as a lawn and garden insecticide. It is indicated only for head lice. Malathion kills both lice and nits in vitro (95% ovicidal activity). It has been on and off the market over the past several years.

      (1) **Mechanism of action.** Sulfur atoms in the malathion bind with sulfur groups on the hair, giving a residual protective effect against reinfestation.

(2) Application. Malathion is prepared as a lotion in 78% alcohol; therefore, caution should be used near an open flame or a hair dryer. The product should be sprinkled on dry hair and left for 8–12 hours before rinsing. A fine-toothed comb should be used to remove the dead lice and eggs.

(3) No systemic **adverse effects** have been reported with topical use of this medication.

(a) The alcoholic vehicle may produce stinging and possible flammability.

(b) Although this agent is very effective, its unpleasant odor (due to sulfhydryl compounds), the required time of 8–12 hours on the scalp, and those points noted in (a) above represent the main drawbacks.

b. Lindane, or gamma-benzene hexachloride has fallen into disfavor because of the potential for toxicity and the fact that its efficacy is less than the other agents available (both prescription and OTC products) [45%–70% ovicidal activity]. It is available as a shampoo, cream, or lotion. It is indicated for head, pubic, and body lice.

(1) Mechanism of action. Lindane is neurotoxic to head lice and their eggs.

(2) Application. For head lice, the lindane shampoo should be applied to dry hair and thoroughly worked into the hair and scalp of the infested individual.

(a) The area should **be shampooed for 4 minutes,** then rinsed and towel dried.

(b) The nits should **be removed** with a fine-toothed comb designed for this purpose.

(3) It has **neurotoxicity potential** because of percutaneous absorption; therefore, its use should be avoided in infants, pregnant and nursing women, and anyone with a neurological disorder. Severe **central nervous system (CNS) toxicity** has occurred in infants, with seizures and deaths reported, particularly when the lotion is used or when the agent is ingested. Toxicity has been minimal when the shampoo is used properly to treat head lice.

6. Adjunctive therapy

a. Nit removal

(1) The pediculicide products mentioned vary in their ability to kill the lice nits. To ensure successful therapy, after pediculicide application, the nits should be removed with a **fine-toothed comb.** A sturdy **metal comb** (like the LiceMeister) is recommended by the NPA. Many schools have a **"no nit" policy;** that is, a child's hair and scalp must be free of nits before he or she is allowed to return to the classroom.

(2) Although various substances have been used in an effort to dislodge the nits from the hair shafts, most have been unsuccessful. A mixture of 50% vinegar and 50% water applied and left on the hair for 1 hour has been recommended. A lice egg remover containing various enzymes comes as part of a kit in the Clear 2 Step Total Lice Elimination System.

(3) Neon Nits is a topical aerosol spray to help locate nits. It dyes the nits bright pink to make them easier to see for subsequent removal. It does not kill or remove the nits by itself.

b. Treatment of other household members. Once a lice infestation has been identified in one member of the household, all other members should be examined carefully. Everyone who is infested should be treated at the same time.

c. Adjunctive methods for controlling lice infestations

(1) Washable material items such as linens, towels, hats, and clothing should be machine-washed in hot water and dried in a hot dryer to destroy lice and nits.

(2) Nonwashable material goods should be dry-cleaned or sealed in a plastic bag for 2 weeks.

(3) Personal items (e.g., comb, brushes) should be soaked in hot water (130°F) for at least 15 minutes.

(4) Furniture and household items (e.g., carpets, chairs, couches, pillows) should be vacuumed thoroughly. OTC spray products that contain pyrethrins are no more effective than vacuuming in terms of removing the risk of reinfestation.

d. Pediculicides should not be used around the eyes. For **eyelash pubic lice infestations, petrolatum** applied five times a day asphyxiates lice, or gentle removal with baby shampoo may be helpful.

H. Head lice myths are numerous. The following additional facts may reassure and inform patients and parents of patients.

1. No significant difference in incidence occurs among the various socioeconomic classes or races.

2. Hygiene and hair length are not contributing factors.

3. Head lice do not fly or jump from person to person.

4. Head lice do not carry other diseases.

5. Head lice cannot be contracted from animals, and pets are not susceptible to *Pediculus humanus capitis.*

6. The head does not have to be shaved to get rid of lice.

7. Washing hair with "brown" soap is not effective.

8. Head lice are unrelated to ticks.

9. Hair does not fall out as a consequence of infestation.

10. Head lice infestations can occur at any time of the year.

II. ACNE AND ITS TREATMENT

A. Overview

1. **Definition.** *Acne vulgaris* is a disorder of the pilosebaceous units, mainly of the face, chest, and back. The lesions usually start as open or closed comedones and evolve into inflammatory papules and pustules that either resolve as macules or become secondary pyoderma, which results in various sequelae.

2. **Incidence**
   a. Acne vulgaris is the **most common** skin disease of adolescence; it affects about 85% of all people between the ages of 12 and 24.
   b. It affects primarily adolescents in junior high and senior high, then decreases in adulthood.

3. **Importance**
   a. Acne vulgaris is usually **self-limiting.**
   b. However, the condition is significant to adolescents because of heightened self-consciousness about appearance.
   c. A great majority of people do not consult a physician for treatment of acne; therefore, a pharmacist can play a significant role.

B. Etiology and pathophysiology

1. The **pathogenesis** of acne vulgaris involves **three events.**
   a. **Increased sebum production**
      (1) Sebum secretion is regulated primarily by **androgens,** which are actively secreted in both sexes beginning at puberty.
      (2) One of these androgens, testosterone, is converted to **dihydrotestosterone (DHT).**
      (3) DHT levels induce the sebaceous glands to increase in size and activity, resulting in increased amounts of sebum.
   b. **Abnormal clumping of epithelial horny cells within the pilosebaceous unit**
      (1) Normally, keratinized horny cells are sloughed from the epithelial lining of the pilosebaceous duct in the hair follicles and are carried to the skin surface with a flow of sebum.
      (2) In the patient with acne, the keratinization process is abnormal, characterized by increased adherence and production of follicular epithelial cells. This process is called **retention hyperkeratosis,** and it results in obstruction of the outflow of the pilosebaceous unit.
   c. **Presence of *Propionibacterium acnes*** (a gram-positive anaerobe)
      (1) People with acne have skin colony counts of *P. acnes* that are significantly higher than the counts of those without acne.
      (2) *P. acnes* produces several enzymes, including lipases, that break down sebum triglycerides to short-chain free fatty acids (FFAs), which are irritating, cause comedones, and result in inflammation.

2. **Sequence of acne lesion development**
   a. Mechanical blockage of a pilosebaceous duct by clumped horny cells results in a closed comedo (i.e., a whitehead).

    b. When a closed comedo develops, it can form either a papule or an open comedo (i.e., a blackhead). The color is attributed to melanin or oxidized lipid, not to dirt.

    c. The lesion may enlarge and fill with pus, which is then termed a pustule.

    d. In more severe cases of acne, papules may develop into nodules or cysts.

    e. The term "pimple" nonspecifically refers to whiteheads, blackheads, papules, and pustules.

C. Clinical features

    1. Location. Acne vulgaris lesions usually occur on the face, neck, chest, upper back, and shoulders. Any or all types of lesions may be seen on a single patient.

    2. Symptoms. This condition is usually asymptomatic; however, some patients may have pruritus or pain if large, tender lesions are present.

    3. Classification. It is important to differentiate **noninflammatory** from **inflammatory** acne to determine the best treatment approach. There have been many rating or grading scales for acne severity (Table 29-1). **Cystic acne** is present when the follicular wall ruptures occur deeper in the dermis and nodules and cysts are seen. Because of the potential for scarring, cystic acne patients should be referred to a physician for treatment. Scarring occurs with hypertrophic ridges, keloids, or atrophic "ice pick" pits.

D. Complicating factors. Other factors have been implicated in the exacerbation of acne.

    1. Drugs and hormones

        a. Many topical and systemic medications (e.g., bromides, iodides, topical coal tar products, androgens, phenytoin, progestins, lithium, corticosteroids) can be comedogenic and can make acne worse or can induce acne-like eruptions (i.e., acneiform lesions).

        b. Acneiform eruptions differ from true acne lesions in that apparently no comedo forms, eruptions are usually acute, and the lesions usually are all in the same stage of development.

    2. Stress does not cause acne but may exacerbate it.

    3. Diet. There is very little evidence to support a relationship between diet and acne. Many different foods have been blamed for acne, from chocolates and sweets to shellfish to nuts and other fatty foods. Several studies have demonstrated that **chocolate does not affect acne.** The majority of dermatologists today make the following recommendations regarding diet.

        a. The patient should be eating a well-balanced diet. As with most other diseases, and as a matter of good health, excess fats and carbohydrates should be avoided.

        b. The patient who insists that certain foods cause exacerbation of acne should probably avoid those foods.

    4. Physical trauma or **irritation** can promote the rupture of plugged follicles, which can produce more inflammatory reactions. Scrubbing the face, wearing headbands, cradling the chin with the hand, and picking at the pimples can contribute to the primary inflammation process. **Gentle** regular **washing** with soap and water can be beneficial.

Table 29-1. Assessment of Acne Severity

Grade of Acne	Qualitative Description	Quantitative Description
I	Comedonal acne	Comedones only, <10 on face, none on trunk, no scars; noninflammatory lesions only
II	Papular acne	10–25 papules on face and trunk, mild scarring; inflammatory lesions <5 mm in diameter
III[a]	Pustular acne	More than 25 pustules, moderate scarring; size similar to papules but with visible, purulent core
IV[a]	Severe/persistent pustulocystic acne	Nodules or cysts, extensive scarring, inflammatory lesions >5 mm in diameter
—	Recalcitrant severe cystic acne	Extensive nodules/cysts

[a]Some overlap with previous grade of acne.
Adapted from *Handbook of Nonprescription Drugs: An Interactive Approach to Self-Care,* 13th ed. Washington, DC, American Pharmaceutical Association, 2002:780.

5. **Cosmetics.** Some cosmetic bases and certain cosmetic ingredients are comedogenic (e.g., lanolins, petroleum bases, cocoa butter). Preparations such as cleansing creams, suntan oils, and heavy foundations should be avoided.

6. **Menstrual cycle.** Some women may notice flare-ups of acne during the premenstrual part of the cycle. Fluctuations in the level of progesterone are the probable cause.

7. **Environmental factors.** Very humid environments or heavy sweating lead to keratin hydration, swelling, and a decrease in the size of the pilosebaceous follicle orifice, which results in duct obstruction. The sun, as well as artificial ultraviolet (UV) light, can help acne by drying and peeling the skin, but both also can aggravate acne.

E. **Treatment and care**

1. **General**
   a. Most patients can be treated successfully with either topically or systemically administered medications or both. Acne often improves when patients reach their early twenties.
   b. Even the most effective treatment programs may take several weeks to produce any clinical improvement. This aspect must be emphasized.
   c. People affected with acne should avoid anything that seems to worsen the condition (e.g., cosmetics, clothing, cradling the chin with the hand).
   d. The number and type of lesions should be roughly determined to assess further therapeutic responses.
   e. **Self treatment with OTC agents** is appropriate only for patients with **noninflammatory grade I acne** of mild to moderate severity.

2. **Cleansing recommendations**
   a. Because many acne patients have oily skin, **gentle cleansing** two to three times daily is recommended for removing excess oil.
   b. Acne lesions cannot be scrubbed away. Compulsive scrubbing may actually worsen the acne by disrupting the follicular walls and, thus, setting the stage for inflammation.
   c. Mild facial soaps, such as Dove, Neutrogena, and Purpose, should be used to cleanse the skin.
   d. Medicated soaps containing sulfur, resorcinol, or salicylic acid are of little value because the medication rinses away rather than penetrates the follicle.
   e. Patients with mild comedonal acne might find benefit from cleansers containing pumice, polyethylene, or aluminum oxide particles (e.g., Brasivol). However, patients with inflammatory acne or sensitive skin should avoid these products.

3. **Approaches** to treatment depend on the severity of the condition. Although acne cannot be cured, most cases can be managed successfully with topical treatment alone. Based on the pathogenesis of the condition, potential methods include:
   a. **Unblocking** the sebaceous duct so that the contents can be easily expelled
   b. **Decreasing** the amount of sebum that is secreted
   c. **Changing** the composition of the **sebum** to make it less irritating by decreasing the population of *P. acnes*

4. **Nonprescription topical medications**
   a. **Benzoyl peroxide** (e.g., Oxy, Exact) [Category III; 2.5%–10%] has traditionally been recognized as the most effective topical OTC agent for acne, and many OTC acne products contain it. However, the final monograph from the FDA changed the status of benzoyl peroxide from Category I (generally recognized as safe and effective) to Category III, indicating that more data are needed to prove its safety with regard to long-term photocarcinogenic effects.
      (1) **Effects.** Benzoyl peroxide has irritant, drying, peeling, comedolytic, and antibacterial effects. The clinical response shows only minimal differences among the 2.5%, 5%, and 10% concentrations. (Additional products are available in 4%, 5.5%, and 20% concentrations.)
         (a) A **beneficial effect** should be noticed within about 2 weeks, but the usual length of a therapeutic trial is 6–8 weeks.
         (b) As for **adverse effects,** benzoyl peroxide may cause a burning or stinging sensation, which gradually disappears. Most of the adverse effects from this agent relate to its therapeutic effect of irritating and drying the skin. For this reason, the lowest concentration available should be chosen initially. From 1%–3% of patients may be hypersensitive to benzoyl peroxide.

        (c) The vehicle for the benzoyl peroxide is also important in its overall activity. The alcohol gel vehicle tends to be more effective than the lotion or cream formulations.

        (d) Benzoyl peroxide can discolor certain types of fabric or clothing material and can also bleach hair.

    (2) Mechanism of action. Benzoyl peroxide has a dual mode of action, so it is effective against both inflammatory and noninflammatory acne.

        (a) Benzoyl peroxide decomposes to release oxygen, which is lethal to the *P. acnes* anaerobe.

        (b) As an irritant, it increases the turnover rate of epithelial cells, resulting in increased sloughing and promoting of resolution of comedones.

    (3) Application

        (a) The affected area should be washed with mild soap and water, then gently patted dry.

        (b) The product should be massaged gently into the skin, avoiding the eyes, mouth, lips, and inside of the nose.

        (c) The product can be applied at night, left on for 15 or 20 minutes to test sensitivity, then washed off.

        (d) If no excessive irritation develops, apply once daily for the first few days.

        (e) If drying, redness, or peeling does not occur in 3 days, increase application to twice daily.

        (f) If patients have to use benzoyl peroxide during the day, advise them to use a sunscreen and avoid unnecessary sun exposure.

  b. Salicylic acid (Category I; 0.5%–2%), an irritant keratolytic agent, results in increased turnover of the epithelial lining. Through this effect, salicylic acid probably promotes the penetration of other acne products.

  c. Sulfur (3%–8%), sulfur 3%–8% combined with resorcinol 2%, or **resorcinol monoacetate 3%** (Category I; Clearasil Adult Care, Acnomel)

    (1) Sulfur is a keratolytic agent and has antibacterial actions.

    (2) Sulfur traditionally has been recognized as a less desirable product because it may be acnegenic with continued use, and it has an offensive color and odor.

  d. Resorcinol (Category II; as a single agent) is a keratolytic agent that has been recognized as effective against acne when the agent is combined with sulfur.

F. Prescription medications, both topical and systemic, are included here to put into perspective how OTC agents fit into acne therapy.

  1. Topical prescription agents

    a. Tretinoin (vitamin A acid, retinoic acid, Retin-A) increases the turnover rate of nonadhering horny cells in the follicular canal, which results in comedo clearing and inhibits new comedo development.

      (1) Effectiveness. Tretinoin is probably the most effective topical agent for acne, especially acne characterized by comedones. It is best used for **noninflammatory** acne. Tretinoin also may be used in combination with antibiotics or benzoyl peroxide for management of severe inflammatory acne.

      (2) Side effects. Because of its irritant properties, tretinoin can cause **excessive irritation, erythema, peeling,** and increased risk for **severe sunburn.** There may be an initial exacerbation of the acne, and a total of 12 weeks may be necessary to fully assess treatment efficacy.

      (3) Application. The cream formulation of tretinoin, which is less irritating than the gel form (which in turn is less irritating than the solution form), should be used initially. Because of the irritant properties, tretinoin should be applied 30 minutes after washing. Initially, it should be applied every other day, then daily. Other irritating substances, such as strong abrasive cleaners and astringents, should be avoided during treatment with tretinoin. Newer reformulations of this agent (Retin-A Micro, Avita) are less irritating.

    b. Adapalene (Differin) is a topical retinoid-like compound that is dosed once daily.

      (1) Effectiveness. It appears to cause less irritation than tretinoin and to be more effective. Therapeutic results should be noticed in 8–12 weeks. It can be used as an alternative to tretinoin in individuals with mild to moderate acne.

      (2) Side effects. The same precautions that apply to tretinoin apply also for adapalene.

c. Tazarotene gel and cream (Tazorac) is a retinoid prodrug for mild to moderately severe facial acne that is applied once daily in the evening. It is used for psoriasis also. It has similar precautions as tretinoin, and the dose-related **adverse effects** include itching, burning, stinging, and erythema (redness). The gel form appears to be more irritating than tretinoin or adapalene.

d. Antibiotics: tetracycline (Topicycline), **meclocycline sulfosalicylate** (Meclan), **erythromycin** (T-Stat, Eryderm), **clindamycin** (Cleocin-T). Combination products containing benzoyl peroxide and erythromycin (Benzamycin) and benzoyl peroxide and clindamycin (BenzaClin) are also available.

   (1) Mechanism of action. The mechanism of action apparently involves suppression of the *P. acnes* organism, which in turn minimizes the inflammatory response due to the acne.

   (2) Application. These antibiotics are applied directly to acne sites, thus minimizing serious side effects from oral administration.

   (3) Side effects. There are **minimal** side effects to these topically applied antibiotics. **Mild burning** or **irritation** may occur. **Tetracycline** may **discolor the skin and fluoresce** in black light. **Clindamycin** can be absorbed to result in **pseudomembranous colitis.**

e. Azelaic acid 20% cream (Azelex) is a topical agent that appears to be **as effective** as benzoyl peroxide or tretinoin for the treatment of mild to moderate inflammatory acne. This agent has both antibacterial and antikeratinizing activity. It inhibits the growth of *P. acnes* and has an antiproliferative effect on keratinocytes. It seems to be less irritating than benzoyl peroxide or tretinoin. **Stinging, burning, tingling, pruritus,** and **erythema** have been reported in a low number of patients. It also decreases pigmentation in the areas of increased pigmentation but apparently does not affect freckles, nevi, or normal skin. Because of its dual action, it can be used as a single-product option in the treatment of mild to moderate acne.

2. Systemic prescription agents

a. Oral antibiotics/anti-infectives are the most effective against inflammatory lesions because they suppress *P. acnes*. Oral antibiotics have an onset of action of 3–4 weeks. Antibiotics do not affect existing lesions, but prevent future lesions through this effect. *P. acnes* resistance has been observed with erythromycin and tetracycline, but most strains remain sensitive.

   (1) Tetracycline is the **most frequently used** oral antibiotic for acne. It is preferred because of its effectiveness, low toxicity, and low cost.

      (a) Initial doses are 250 mg, two to four times daily, gradually reduced to a maintenance dose of about 250 mg per day.

      (b) Side effects. The more common adverse effects include upset stomach, vaginal moniliasis, and photosensitivity.

   (2) Erythromycin (E-Mycin) may be used as an alternative to tetracycline.

      (a) Initial doses range from 500–2000 mg per day in divided doses. A maintenance dose ranges from 250–500 mg per day.

      (b) Side effects. The primary side effect associated with erythromycin is gastrointestinal distress.

   (3) Clindamycin. Diarrhea and rare cases of pseudomembranous colitis limit the use of clindamycin.

   (4) Minocycline (Minocin) **or doxycycline** (Vibramycin). Either of these agents can be taken in doses of 50–200. Because of greater lipid solubility and enhanced penetration into sebaceous follicles, these agents are useful for refractory cases. Either can be taken if clinical resistance is suspected to erythromycin or if intolerable gastric irritation occurs after oral tetracycline. These two agents can be taken with food. Side effects to minocycline, including dizziness or vertigo and headache, discoloration of skin and visceral tissue, and drug-induced lupus erythematosus, limit the use of this agent.

   (5) Trimethoprim-sulfamethoxazole (Bactrim, Septra) has been used successfully in patients with acne resistant to erythromycin or tetracyclines. **Azithromycin** has also been used.

b. Isotretinoin (Accutane) is a vitamin A derivative indicated for **severe recalcitrant nodulocystic acne.** A single course of therapy can result in a complete and prolonged remission period.

(1) Mechanism of action. Although the exact mechanism is unknown, isotretinoin decreases sebum production and keratinization, and it reduces the population of *P. acnes.*

(2) Dosage. Doses range from 0.5–2 mg/kg/day given twice daily for 15–20 weeks.

(3) Side effects include:

    (a) Mucocutaneous dryness. Cheilitis (i.e., inflammation of the lips), dryness of the nasal mucosa, and facial dermatitis may occur with isotretinoin use. These effects can be treated with topical lubricants. Dryness of the eyes can also occur, so people using isotretinoin should not wear contact lenses.

    (b) Elevated serum levels. Isotretinoin may elevate serum triglycerides and cholesterol, as well as liver enzymes.

    (c) Birth defects. Isotretinoin is a **potent teratogen** and should not be given to pregnant women.

    (d) Depression. There have been reports of depression, psychosis, and rarely suicidal ideation, suicide attempts, and suicide. This must be taken in the context that teenagers with acne may often be depressed related to their appearance.

c. Antiandrogens and hormones

    (1) Estrogens can decrease sebum production through an antiandrogenic effect.

    (2) Some progestin agents in oral contraceptives (e.g., norethindrone, norgestrel) have androgenic activity that can stimulate sebum secretion resulting in acne. One of the progestins, **norgestimate,** is minimally androgenic, and when it is combined with **ethinyl estradiol** as a triphasic combination oral contraceptive agent (Ortho Tri-Cyclen), it is effective in the treatment of moderate acne in some women and is FDA approved for such. **Norethindrone acetate/ethinyl estradiol** (Estrostep) is also FDA approved for acne.

    (3) Corticosteroids. Although corticosteroids have been implicated as causing acne, they also can be used to treat severe acne. Intralesional injections of triamcinolone and systemic corticosteroids have been used for severe inflammatory acne and severe cystic acne, respectively. Prednisone (or its equivalent) in doses of 20 mg per day or higher may be used for a short period of time to quickly improve acne for important events like a wedding. Topical corticosteroids are not effective.

    (4) Spironolactone (Aldactone) is an androgen antagonist that may be used on a limited basis.

III. SUNLIGHT, SUNSCREENS, AND SUNTAN PRODUCTS

A. Introduction. Overexposure to sunlight damages skin. A suntan, which has traditionally been associated with health, is actually a response to injury. Of the three types of solar radiation, only the UV spectrum produces sunburn and suntan.

  1. The **UV spectrum** ranges from 200–400 nanometers (nm). Natural and artificial UV light is further subdivided into three bands.

    a. UVA (320–400 nm) can cause the skin to tan, and it tends to be weak in causing the skin to redden. UVA is about 1000 times less potent than a comparable dose of UVB in causing erythema, but it is only slightly blocked out by the ozone layer and reaches the earth's surface in 10–100 times the amount of UVB. Some have proposed that UVA be further subdivided into UVA I (340–400 nm) and UVA II (320–340 nm). UVA I is less erythrogenic and melanogenic than UVA II or UVB. UVA II is similar in effect to UVB.

    (1) Uses. UVA is often used in tanning booths and in psoralen plus UVA (PUVA) treatment of psoriasis.

    (2) Disadvantages. UVA is responsible for many **photosensitivity** reactions, **photoaging,** and **photodermatoses.** UVA rays can also **penetrate deeply into the dermis** and augment the cancerous effects of UVB rays.

    b. UVB (290–320 nm) **causes the usual sunburn reaction** and stimulates tanning. It has long been associated with sunlight skin damage, including the various skin cancers. It is the **most erythrogenic** and **melanogenic** of the three UV radiation bands. Small amounts of this radiation are required for normal **vitamin D synthesis** in the skin.

    c. UVC (200–290 nm) does not reach the earth's surface because most of it is absorbed by the ozone layer. Artificial UVC sources (e.g., germicidal and mercury arc lamps) can emit this radiation.

2. The **visible spectrum** (400–770 nm) produces the "brightness" of the sun.

3. The **infrared spectrum** (770–1800 nm) produces the "warmth" of the sun.

B. Sunburn and suntan

1. Sunburn is generally a **superficial burn involving the epidermis.** This layer is rapidly repaired while old cells are being sloughed off in a process called **peeling.** The newly formed skin is thicker and offers protection for the lower dermal layers.

    a. Normal sequence after mild to moderate sunlight UV radiation (UVR) exposure

        (1) Erythema occurs within 20–30 minutes as a result of oxidation of bleached melanin and dilation of dermal venules.

        (2) The initial erythema rapidly fades, and true sunburn erythema begins 2–8 hours after initial exposure to the sun.

        (3) Dilation of the arterioles results in increased vascular permeability, localized edema, and pain, which become maximal after 14–20 hours and last 24–72 hours.

    b. Manifestations range from mild (a slight reddening of the skin) to severe (formation of blisters and desquamation). If the effect is severe, the patient may experience pain, swelling, and blistering. Fever, chills, and nausea may also develop, as well as prostration, which is related to excessive synthesis and diffusion of prostaglandins.

2. Suntan is the result of two processes:

    a. Oxidation of melanin, which is already present in the epidermis

    b. Stimulation of melanocytes to produce additional melanin, which is subsequently oxidized upon further exposure to sunlight

        (1) With increased melanin production, the melanocytes introduce the pigment into keratin-producing cells, which gradually become darkened keratin and a full suntan in 2–10 days.

        (2) Tanning increases tolerance to additional sunlight and reduces the likelihood of subsequent burning. However, dark skin is not totally immune to sunburn.

C. Factors affecting exposure to UVR

1. Time of day and season. The greatest exposure to harmful UVB rays occurs between 10 A.M. and 2 P.M. in midsummer. UVA rays are fairly continuous throughout the day and season.

2. Altitude. Sunburn is more likely to occur at high altitudes. UVB intensity increases 4% with each 1000-foot increase in altitude.

3. Environmental factors. Atmospheric conditions (e.g., smog, haze, smoke) may affect (i.e., decrease) the amount of UVR reaching the skin. Although direct sunlight greatly reduces the amount of UV exposure needed to produce a burn, sunburn can occur without it. For example, a sunburn can also develop on a cloudy day due to the percentage of UVR penetration through cloud layers (60%–80%). However, the **reflection of light rays** (e.g., by snow, sand, water) greatly **increases** the amount of UV **exposure to sunlight.**

4. Predisposing factors. People with fair skin and light hair are at greater risk for developing sunburn and other UVR skin damage than their darker counterparts.

D. Other reactions to sunlight (UVR) exposure

1. Actinic keratosis is a precancerous condition and may occur after many years of excessive exposure to sunlight. Typically arising during middle age or later, this disorder manifests as a sharply demarcated, roughened, or hardened growth, which may be flat or raised, and it may progress to **squamous cell carcinoma.**

2. Skin cancer. Chronic overexposure to sunlight may lead to **squamous cell carcinoma, basal cell carcinoma,** or **malignant melanoma.**

    a. Squamous cell carcinoma. Lesions usually appear as thickened, rough, scaly patches, which can bleed, and most commonly develops from actinic keratosis. It accounts for about 15% of skin cancers.

    b. Basal cell carcinoma. This is the most common of all skin cancers and accounts for about 80% of skin cancers. It may appear as pearly or translucent bumps and originates in the basal cells.

c. Malignant melanoma. Malignant melanoma originates from melanocytes and is the deadliest form of skin cancer, and its incidence has been increasing. Moles should be watched for indications of malignancy—the ABCDs are **a**symmetrical shape, **b**order irregularity, nonuniform **c**olor, and **d**iameter greater than 6 mm. Malignant melanoma formation may be associated with intense, intermittent overexposure to the sun (sunburning).

3. Drug-induced photosensitivity reactions
   a. Types
      (1) Photoallergy reactions occur when light makes a drug become antigenic or act as a hapten (i.e., a photoallergen). These reactions also require previous contact with the offending drug. Photoallergy reactions are relatively **rare** and are associated more frequently with topically applied agents than with oral medications.
         (a) Occurrence of these reactions is not dose-related. The patient is usually cross-sensitive with chemically related compounds.
         (b) Rashes are most prominent on light-exposed sites (i.e., face, neck, forearms, back of hands), and they usually occur, after an incubation period of 24–48 hours of combined drug and sun exposure, as an intensely pruritic eczematous dermatitis (a severe rash).
      (2) Phototoxic reactions occur when light alters a drug to a toxic form, which results in tissue damage that is independent of an allergic response.
         (a) Occurrence. These reactions are usually dose-related, and the patient usually has no cross-sensitivity to other agents.
         (b) Rashes often appear as an exaggerated sunburn and are usually confined to areas of combined chemical and light exposure.
   b. Implicated drugs. Many drugs have been implicated in causing photoallergy and phototoxic reactions: thiazides, tetracyclines, phenothiazines, sulfonamides, and even sunscreens. Some drugs may produce both types of reactions.
   c. Prevention. Standard sunscreens do not always prevent photosensitivity reactions caused by drugs. UV light above 320 nm (i.e., UVA light) has been implicated in inducing photosensitivity reactions, so a chemical or physical sunscreen must cover this spectrum (see III E 2).

4. Photodermatoses are skin conditions that are triggered or worsened by light within specific wavelengths. These conditions include polymorphous light eruption (PMLE), lupus erythematosus, and solar urticaria.

5. Photoaging is a skin condition that is not merely an acceleration of normal aging. UVA radiation is thought to be involved. The skin appears dry, scaly, yellow, and deeply wrinkled; it is also thinner and more fragile.

E. Sunscreen agents. People can protect their skin from harmful UVR by avoiding exposure to sunlight and other sources of UVR, wearing protective clothing, and applying sunscreen.

   1. Application and general information. All exposed areas should be covered evenly and liberally (2 mg/cm^2, which requires about 1 ounce of sunscreen per one total body application for an average-size adult in a swimsuit) with sunscreen, optimally 30 minutes (2 hours for PABA and PABA esters) before sun exposure to allow for penetration and binding to the skin.
      a. Substantivity. Perspiration, swimming, sand, towels, and clothing tend to remove sunscreen and may increase the need for reapplication.
         (1) Substantivity is the ability of a sunscreen formulation to adhere to the skin while swimming or perspiring.
         (2) "**Water resistant**" labeling indicates that the formula retains SPF after 40 minutes of activity in the water, sweating, or perspiring.
         (3) Labeling a product as "**very water resistant**" indicates that the product retains SPF after 80 minutes of activity in the water, sweating, or perspiring.
      b. Protection. Sunscreen products vary widely in their ability to protect against sunburn; the SPF and UVA/UVB ray protection should be noted to determine the level of protection. Moreover, baby oil, mineral oil, olive oil, and cocoa butter are not sunscreens (but are often used to attain a tan).
         (1) SPF gives the consumer a guide for determining how the product will protect the skin from UV rays, principally UVB rays. An SPF of 30 blocks ~97% of the UVB rays. Scientific evidence shows a point of diminishing returns at levels more than

30; any benefits that might be derived from using sunscreens with SPFs more than 30 are negligible. The FDA's final monograph requires sunscreens with SPFs higher than 30 to use one collective term "SPF 30 Plus" or "30+". An SPF of at least 15 for most individuals is recommended by the Skin Cancer Foundation.

    (a) **Definitions. Minimal sun protection product**—SPF of 2 to under 12; **moderate sun protection product**—SPF of 12 to under 30; **high sun protection product**—SPF of 30 or above.

    (b) **Derivation.** SPF is defined as the **minimal erythema dose (MED)** of protected skin divided by the MED of unprotected skin. MED is the amount of solar radiation needed to produce minimal skin redness.

    (c) **Example.** A person who usually gets red after 20 minutes in the sun and wants to stay in the sun for 2 hours (120 minutes) should apply a sunscreen with an SPF of 6 (120 minutes divided by 20 minutes = SPF 6). An SPF 6 product should provide adequate coverage, provided it is not washed off (as from swimming) or dissolved by sweat. An SPF of 15 blocks ~93% of the UVB rays.

    (d) There is **no generally accepted comparable term that measures UVA protection,** although a few have been proposed. One major concern is that people may be staying out in the sun longer as they use sunscreen products that have high SPF values. If inadequate UVA protection is provided in that product, these individuals may be exposing themselves to very high amounts of UVA with the potential for significant overexposure to this form of UV radiation.

  (2) Skin cancer prevention. Sunscreen application has been shown to prevent squamous cell carcinoma, but it is not absolutely confirmed that their use prevents melanoma. In fact, some studies have found that individuals who regularly use sunscreen have a higher risk of this cancer (perhaps by allowing people to stay out in the sun longer before burning and thus giving them longer periods of sun exposure).

 c. Sensitivity. Some people may be hypersensitive to sunscreen agents. Discontinue use if signs of irritation or a rash occur. Contact dermatitis may occur with some of these agents. If sensitive to benzocaine, procaine, sulfonamides, or thiazides, avoid PABA or PABA esters.

 d. Specific information

  (1) Do not use these on infants younger than 6 months of age (there is concern about absorption of these agents).

  (2) Do not use a product with less than an SPF of 4 on children less than 2 years of age (there is concern that SPFs less than this will not provide adequate protection).

  (3) Recommend sunscreen products that are broad-spectrum sunscreens (i.e., that block both UVB and UVA).

2. The two basic **types of sunscreen agents** are physical sun blocks and chemical sunscreens (Table 29-2).

 a. Physical sun blocks are opaque formulations that reflect and scatter up to 99% of light in both the UV and visible spectrums (290–700 nm). Examples include titanium dioxide and zinc oxide. These sun blocks are less cosmetically acceptable than chemical sunscreens because they have a greasy appearance, but they may be useful for protecting small areas (e.g., the nose). These sun blocks are also useful for photosensitization protection. Newer, more dilute versions of titanium dioxide products and microfine, transparent forms of zinc oxide are more cosmetically appealing. Red petrolatum covers a lesser spectrum (290–365 nm).

 b. Chemical sunscreens act by absorbing a specific portion of the UV light spectrum to keep it from penetrating the skin. They can be categorized on the basis of their spectra of UVR blockage and basic chemical classification. Five main groups of chemical sunscreens are available.

  (1) PABA and **PABA esters** primarily absorb UVB rays. Examples are *p*-aminobenzoic acid, padimate O, and glyceryl PABA.

  (2) Cinnamates primarily absorb UVB rays. Examples are cinoxate and octyl methoxycinnamate.

  (3) Salicylates primarily absorb UVB rays. Examples are ethylhexyl salicylate and homosalate.

  (4) Benzophenones absorb UVB rays and sometimes extend into the UVA range. Examples are oxybenzone and dioxybenzone. Because of their extension into the UVA range, they are somewhat protective against photosensitivity reactions.

Table 29-2. Sunscreen Ingredients

Sunscreens		UV Spectrum (nm)	Concentrations (%)
Chemical	*Benzophenones*	UVA and UVB	
	Oxybenzone	270–350	2–6
	Dioxybenzone	260–380[1]	3
	PABA and PABA esters	UVB	
	P-aminobenzoic acid	260–313	5–15
	Ethyl dihydroxy propyl PABA	280–330	1–5
	Padimate O (octyl dimethyl PABA)	290–315	1.4–8
	Glyceryl PABA	264–315	2–3
	Cinnamates	UVB[2]	
	Cinoxate	270–328	1–3
	Ethylhexyl p-methoxycinnamate	290–320	2–7.5
	Octocrylene	250–360	7–10
	Octyl methoxycinnamate	290–320	—
	Salicylates	UVB[3]	
	Ethylhexyl salicylate	280–320	3–5
	Homosalate	295–315	4–15
	Octyl salicylate	280–320	3–5
	Miscellaneous	UVB	
	Menthyl anthranilate	260–380[4]	3.5–5
	Digalloyl trioleate	270–320	2–5
	Avobenzone (butyl methoxy-dibenzoylmethane; Parsol 1789)	UVA 320–400	3
Physical	Titanium dioxide	290–700	2–25
	Red petrolatum	290–365[5]	30–100
	Zinc oxide	290–700	—

[1]Values available when used in combination with other screens.
[2]Some UVA spectrum.
[3]Primarily UVB, but has about ⅓ the absorbency of PABA.
[4]Values are concentrations higher than normally found in nonprescription drugs.
[5]At 334 nm, 16% UV radiation is transmitted; at 365 nm, 58% is transmitted.
©Jan 2000 by Facts and Comparisons. Used with permission from *Drug Facts and Comparisons*. St. Louis: Facts and Comparisons: p 1715.

    (5) Miscellaneous. The newest agent, **avobenzone (Parsol 1789)** or butyl methoxydiben-zoylmethane, provides coverage over the entire UVA range although its absorbance decreases dramatically at 370 nm. Photosensitivity reactions from medications may not be completely prevented in the 370–400 nm range. In combination with oxybenzone and octyl methoxycinnamate, a product such as Shade UVA Guard offers the greatest protection in both the UVA and UVB ranges. There are a number of other sunscreen combination products that contain avobenzone (i.e., PreSun Ultra).

  c. OTC sunscreen products. Most sunscreen products on the market contain combinations of two or more of the classes of chemical sunscreen agents noted in the preceding paragraphs. To get adequate UVA protection, choose a product with avobenzone or a product with titanium dioxide or zinc oxide.

F. Special agents of interest

  1. Dihydroxyacetone (DHA) is a chemical agent that darkens the skin by interacting with keratin in the stratum corneum to produce an **artificial "suntan."** It provides **no protection against UV rays** and may not produce a natural-looking tan. DHA must be applied evenly. If an artificial suntan is achieved with this chemical, it wears off in a few days. In addition, it can discolor hair and clothing.

  2. Beta-carotene, a vitamin A precursor, may produce skin coloration when ingested orally. While beta-carotene is protective against some forms of abnormal photosensitivity (e.g., erythropoietic protoporphyria), it has not been shown to protect against sunburn in normal individuals.

3. **Canthaxanthine** is a carotenoid (provitamin A). It has been used as a food-coloring agent but has not been approved by the FDA for use as an oral tanning agent. It **does not produce a true suntan** but is deposited into fatty tissues under the skin. It probably does not protect the skin from sunburn.

4. **Tyrosine** has been promoted as a tan accelerator or **tan magnifier.** Because melanin pigment is eventually synthesized from tyrosine, the theory is that topically applied tyrosine will enhance the formation of melanin. However, **studies have not confirmed an enhanced tanning effect from this agent.**

IV. CONTACT DERMATITIS AND ITS TREATMENT

A. Introduction

1. **Types of contact dermatitis.** Contact dermatitis is one of the **most common** dermatological conditions encountered in clinical practice. It has traditionally been divided into **irritant contact dermatitis** and **allergic contact dermatitis** on the basis of the etiology and immunological mechanism.

a. **Irritant contact dermatitis** is caused by direct contact with a primary irritant. These irritants can be classified as absolute or relative primary irritants.

   (1) **Absolute primary irritants** are intrinsically damaging substances that injure, on first contact, any person's skin. Examples include strong acids, alkalis, and other industrial chemicals.

   (2) **Relative primary irritants** cause most cases of contact dermatitis seen in clinical practice. These irritants are less toxic than absolute primary irritants, and they require repeated or prolonged exposure to provoke a reaction. Examples of relative primary irritants include soaps, detergents, benzoyl peroxide, and certain plant and animal substances.

b. **Allergic contact dermatitis.** Many plants, and almost any chemical, can cause allergic contact dermatitis. Poison ivy is a classic example of allergic contact dermatitis, which is classified as a type IV hypersensitivity reaction. This type of allergic reaction is T–cell-mediated, and the following **sequence of events** must occur to provoke it:

   (1) The epidermis must come in **contact** with the hapten (i.e., the specific allergen).

   (2) The **hapten–epidermal protein complex** (i.e., the complete antigen) must form.

   (3) The antigen must **enter the lymphatic system.**

   (4) **Immunologically competent lymphoid cells,** which are selective against the antigen, must form.

   (5) On **reexposure** to the hapten, the typical, local delayed hypersensitivity reaction (i.e., contact dermatitis) occurs.

   (6) The **induction period,** during which sensitivity develops, usually requires 14–21 days but may take as few as 4 days or more than several weeks. **Once sensitivity is fully developed:**

   (a) Reexposure to even minute amounts of the same material elicits an eczematous response, typically with an onset of 12 hours and a peak of 48–72 hours after exposure.

   (b) Sensitivity usually persists for life.

      (i) Most contact allergens produce sensitization in only a small percentage of exposed persons.

      (ii) Allergens or substances such as poison ivy, however, produce sensitization in more than 70% of the population (50%–95% are sensitive to the poison ivy plant).

2. **General phases of contact dermatitis**

a. **Acute stage.** "Wet" lesions, such as blisters or denuded and weeping skin, are evident in well-outlined patches. Also evident are erythema, edema, vesicles, and oozing.

b. **Subacute stage.** In this phase, crusts or scabs form over the previously wet lesions. Allergic contact dermatitis and irritant contact dermatitis caused by absolute primary irritants produce both the acute and subacute stages.

c. **Chronic stage.** In this phase, the lesions become dry and thickened (i.e., lichenified). Initially, dryness and fissuring are the signs. Later, erythema, lichenification, and excoriations appear. The chronic phase of contact dermatitis usually occurs more often with irritant contact dermatitis caused by relative primary irritants.

B. **Toxic plants.** Poison ivy and poison oak are the **most common causes** of allergic contact dermatitis in North America. These plants were formerly known as the *Rhus* genus, but they are now properly referred to as the *Toxicodendron* genus.

   1. **Poison ivy** (*Toxicodendron radicans* and *T. rydbergii*) grows as a vine or as a bush. It is found in most parts of the United States, but is especially prevalent in the northeastern part of the country. Poison ivy is often identified by its characteristic growth pattern, described by the saying, "Leaves of three, let it be."

   2. **Poison oak** (*T. diversilobum*) is found in the western United States and Canada. It grows as an upright shrub or a woody vine. *T. toxicarium* is found in the eastern United States.

   3. **Poison sumac** (*T. vernix*) grows in woody or swampy areas as a coarse shrub or tree and is prevalent in the eastern United States and southeastern Canada.

C. **Toxicodendron dermatitis.** In order for dermatitis to develop, previous sensitization (a 5- to 21-day incubation period) caused by direct contact with a sensitizing agent is required (see IV A 1 b). An oleoresin, **urushiol oil,** which is a pentadecacatechol, is the active sensitizing agent in poison ivy, poison oak, and poison sumac. There are slight differences in the chemical structures of the sensitizing agent in each of these plants, but the three agents cross react.

   1. **Release of the urushiol oil.** The plants must be bruised or injured to release the oleoresin. It is **present in** the **roots, stems, leaves,** and **fruit.** The urushiol oil may remain active on tools, toys, clothes, pets, and under fingernails if those items have had contact with the broken plants.
      a. Urushiol oil does not volatilize, so one cannot get dermatitis from just being near a poison ivy plant; direct contact is necessary. **Burning plants,** however, can cause droplets of oil carried by smoke to enter the respiratory system, which can cause significant respiratory distress.
      b. A cut or damaged poison ivy, poison oak, or poison sumac plant yields a milky sap containing the oleoresin, which turns black within a few minutes. This change can be a means for confirming identification of these plants.
      c. Because the oleoresin can rapidly penetrate the skin, the affected **area must be washed with soap and water within 10 minutes** after exposure to prevent the dermatitis eruption. Washing up to 30 minutes after exposure is still useful in removing some of the oleoresin.

   2. If an individual has been **previously sensitized,** the lesions usually occur within 6–48 hours after contact with the allergen.

   3. Typically, the **initial eruption** exists as small patches of erythematous papules (usually streaks). **Pruritus (itching) is the primary symptom.**
      a. Papules may progress to vesicles, which may then ooze and bleed when they are scratched. Secondary infection may then develop. Often, the inflammation is severe, and a significant amount of edema occurs over the exposed area.
      b. The lesions may last from a few days to several weeks. Left untreated, the condition rarely persists longer than 2–3 weeks.

   4. **Poison ivy dermatitis does not spread.** New lesions, however, may continue to appear for several days despite lack of further contact with the plant. This reaction may be due to the following facts:
      a. Skin that has been minimally exposed to the antigen begins to react only as the person's sensitivity heightens.
      b. Antigen is absorbed at varying rates through the skin of different parts of the body.
      c. The person inadvertently touches contaminated objects or may have residual oleoresin underneath the fingernails, for instance.

   5. **Poison ivy is not contagious.** The serous fluid from the weeping vesicles are not antigenic. No one can "catch" poison ivy from another person.

D. Treatment. The treatment of irritant and allergic contact dermatitis focuses on therapy for the specific symptomatology.

1. A pharmacist should **refer a patient** with a poison ivy eruption to a physician if:
   a. The eruption involves more than 15% of the body.
   b. The eruption involves the eyes, genital area, mouth, or respiratory tract (some patients may experience respiratory difficulties if they inhale the smoke of burning poison ivy plants).

2. The **severity of the eruption** depends on:
   a. The quantity of allergen that the patient has been exposed to
   b. The individual patient's sensitivity to the allergen

3. **For severe eruptions,** a patient should consult a physician, who may prescribe **systemic corticosteroids.**
   a. Systemic corticosteroids are the cornerstone of therapy. One should use sufficiently high doses to suppress this inflammation. Generally, it is recommended that prednisone be given in a dose of 60 mg/day for 5 days, then reduced to 40 mg/day for 5 days, then 20 mg/day for 5 days, then discontinued.
   b. Some blisters may be drained at their base. The skin on top of the blister should be kept intact. Draining the blister allows more topical medication to penetrate for an antipruritic effect. Baths and soaks [see IV D 4 b (1) (b)] may be beneficial as well.

4. **For a less severe eruption,** the principal goals are to relieve the itching and inflammation and to protect the integrity of the skin.
   a. Several therapeutic classes of agents can be used **to relieve itching.**
      (1) The application of **local anesthetics** [e.g., benzocaine (5%–20%)] may relieve itching. Relief may be of short duration (30–45 minutes), but application of benzocaine may be especially useful at bedtime, when pruritus is most bothersome. There is some question about the frequency of the sensitizing ability of benzocaine (0.17%–5%). Certainly, treatment should be discontinued if the rash worsens.
      (2) **Oral antihistamines** may be helpful in alleviating pruritus mainly due to their sedating effect rather than a specific antipruritic effect. The principal concern with these agents involves the effect of CNS depression (drowsiness) and possible anticholinergic effects.
      (3) **Topical antihistamines** [e.g., diphenhydramine (Benadryl cream or spray)] provide relief of mild itching principally through a topical anesthetic effect rather than any antihistamine effect. The main concern with topical antihistamines is that they may also have a significant sensitizing potential, and in children with varicella infections (where the integrity of the skin is compromised), systemic absorption has occurred with symptoms of anticholinergic toxicity produced.
      (4) **Counterirritants** include camphor (0.1%–3%), phenol (0.5%–1.5%), and menthol (0.1%–1%). These agents have an analgesic effect due to depression of cutaneous receptors. The exact antipruritic mechanism is not fully known, but a placebo effect may result from the characteristic "medicinal" odors of these agents.
      (5) **Astringents** are mild protein precipitants that result in contraction of tissue, which in turn decreases the local edema and inflammation.
         (a) The principal agent used is **aluminum acetate** (Burow's solution).
         (b) **Calamine** (zinc oxide with ferric oxide [which provides the pink color]) is also used sometimes. Calamine contracts tissue and helps dry the area, but the formation of the thick dried paste may not be tolerated by some people.
      (6) **Topical hydrocortisone** (e.g., Cortaid), which is available in concentrations up to 1%, is useful for its antipruritic and anti-inflammatory effects.
   b. Basic treatment
      (1) Acute (weeping) lesions (see IV A 2 a)
         (a) **Wet dressings** work on the principle that water evaporating from the skin cools it and, thus, relieves itching. Wet dressings have an additional benefit of causing gentle debridement and cleansing of the skin.
         (b) **Burow's solution** (Domeboro) in concentrations of 1:20–1:40 as a wet dressing or a cool bath of 15–30 minutes three to six times per day provides a significant antipruritic effect.
         (c) **Colloidal oatmeal baths** (e.g., Aveeno) may also provide an antipruritic effect.
         (d) **Topical therapy that may hinder treatment**

        (i)   **Local anesthetics and topical antihistamines** may sensitize.

        (ii)   **Calamine** may "make a mess" without doing much good!

    (2) Subacute dermatitis (see IV A 2 b). A thin layer of hydrocortisone cream or lotion (0.5%–1%) may be applied three or four times a day to treat subacute dermatitis. Supplemental agents, such as oral antihistamines or topical anesthetics, may be used as well.

    (3) Chronic dermatitis (see IV A 2 c) is best treated with hydrocortisone ointment. This stage is observed more frequently in forms of contact dermatitis that involve continuous exposure to the irritant or allergen.

E. Prevention

    1. The best treatment for poison ivy contact dermatitis is to **prevent contact** with the offending cause. This approach involves avoiding the plant and wearing protective clothing.

    2. Barrier preparations. Bentoquatam (quaternium-18 bentonite) [Ivy Block], an organoclay, is the first poison ivy blocker proven safe and effective. It comes as a lotion that should be applied at least 15 minutes before contact with the plant and then every 4 hours for continued protection against urushiol. It should be applied to leave a smooth, wet, visible film on the skin. Ivy Block may be removed with soap and water. Because of its alcohol content, patients should be instructed to stay away from flame during application until the product has dried on the skin.

    3. Hyposensitization using plant extracts of poison ivy was used in the past with mixed success. Maximal hyposensitization requires 3–6 months to develop, and it diminishes rapidly when administration of the extract ceases. No products are currently available that can be recommended for this use.

STUDY QUESTIONS

Directions: Each of the numbered items or incomplete statements in this section is followed by answers or by completions of the statement. Select the **one** lettered answer or completion that is **best** in each case.

1. A woman, who has not been in the sun for 4 months, develops redness on her chest after lying in the sun for 20 minutes. The next day, she applies a suntan lotion and develops the same degree of redness on her back in 2 hours and 20 minutes. What is the sun protection factor (SPF) of the lotion she is using?

(A) 14
(B) 10
(C) 12
(D) 9
(E) 7

2. Which of the following cleansing products would a pharmacist recommend for a patient with inflammatory acne?

(A) An abrasive facial sponge and soap used four times daily
(B) Aluminum oxide particles used twice daily
(C) Sulfur 5% soap used twice daily
(D) Mild facial soap used twice daily

3. If a patient needs a second application of an over-the-counter (OTC) pyrethrin pediculicide shampoo, how many days after the first application should this be done?

(A) 4–5
(B) 6
(C) 7–10
(D) 14–21
(E) 15–17

4. All of the following treatments for personal articles infested with head lice would be effective EXCEPT

(A) placing woolen hats in a plastic bag for 2 weeks
(B) using an aerosol of pyrethrins with piperonyl butoxide sprayed in the air of all bathrooms
(C) machine-washing clothes in hot water and drying them using the hot setting on the dryer
(D) dry-cleaning woolen scarves
(E) soaking hair brushes in hot water for 15 minutes

5. All of the following sunscreen agents or combinations of agents would likely help prevent a drug-induced photosensitivity reaction EXCEPT

(A) titanium dioxide
(B) octyl methoxycinnamate plus homo-salate
(C) oxybenzone and padimate O
(D) zinc oxide
(E) padimate O plus avobenzone

6. All of the following would be appropriate recommendations for an adult patient in the acute stage (i.e., blistering, weeping) of poison ivy contact dermatitis EXCEPT

(A) two 25-mg capsules of diphenhydramine at night for itching
(B) 60 mg per day of prednisone initially, then tapered over 15 days
(C) Burow's solution; 1:20 wet dressing to area for 15–30 minutes, four times per day
(D) two soaks per day in Aveeno Bath Treatment
(E) two applications of Ivy Block

7. All of the following nonprescription agents have been classified by the United States Food and Drug Administration (FDA) as safe and effective (Category I) for acne EXCEPT

(A) sulfur
(B) salicylic acid
(C) sulfur-resorcinol combination
(D) benzoic acid

8. Pharmacists educating patients about acne should mention all of the following EXCEPT

(A) eliminating all chocolate and fried foods from the diet
(B) cleansing skin gently two to three times daily
(C) using water-based noncomedogenic cosmetics
(D) not squeezing acne lesions
(E) keeping in mind that acne usually resolves by one's early 20s

9. A 15-year-old male patient has been using benzoyl peroxide 5% cream faithfully every day for the past 2 months with no apparent side effects. All of the following can be said about this patient EXCEPT

(A) he has been using this product for a long enough time to determine if the dose and dosage form are going to have any benefit

(B) he should use this product no more frequently than every other day because of its irritating properties

(C) this starting dose and dosage form are useful, especially if he has dry skin or it is wintertime

(D) his scalp hair may look bleached if the product comes in contact with it

(E) the product would sting if it got into his eyes

10. All of the following descriptions match the therapeutic agent for poison ivy EXCEPT

(A) Calamine—phenolphthalein gives it the pink color

(B) Ivy Block—useful in preventing poison ivy dermatitis

(C) Benzocaine—data regarding incidence of hypersensitivity are conflicting

(D) hydrocortisone—useful for its antipruritic and anti-inflammatory effects

11. All of the following statements related to sun protection are true EXCEPT

(A) the sun's intensity increases 20% when going from sea level to an altitude of 5000 feet

(B) "water resistant" labeling on a sunscreen product indicates that it will retain its SPF after 40 minutes of activity in water, sweating, or perspiring

(C) baby oil is not a sunscreen, but its application to the skin after tanning causes melanin to rise to the surface

(D) per the FDA, a product with an SPF of 50 must now be labeled "SPF 30 plus"

(E) the SPF is really only a measure of ultraviolet B (UVB) protection

12. All of the following statements about sunscreens are correct EXCEPT

(A) malignant melanoma formation may be associated with intense, intermittent overexposure to the sun (sunburning)

(B) dihydroxyacetone (DHA) will not prevent sunburn

(C) sunscreens are best applied immediately before going out in the sun

(D) avobenzone provides sunscreen coverage for the UVA spectrum

(E) tyrosine has been marketed as a tan accelerator or tan magnifier

ANSWERS AND EXPLANATIONS

1. The answer is E *[III E 1].*
The sun protection factor (SPF) is the minimal erythema dose (MED) of protected skin divided by the MED of unprotected skin. Thus, 2 hours and 20 minutes (140 minutes) divided by 20 minutes equals an SPF of 7.

2. The answer is D *[II E 2].*
For patients with inflammatory acne, the best product is a mild facial soap used twice daily. The soap should be gently rubbed into the skin with only the fingertips. Cleansing products that irritate already inflamed skin should be avoided.

3. The answer is C *[I G 4 a (1)].*
Reapplication of pyrethrins with piperonyl butoxide should be within 7–10 days of the first application. Any lice nits that were not killed on the first application would have time to hatch and then be killed with the second application.

4. The answer is B *[I G 4 a, 6 c].*
Pyrethrins with piperonyl butoxide in an aerosol form can be sprayed directly on inanimate objects (e.g., chairs, headrests) to kill head lice, but the combination should not be sprayed in the air like an aerosol deodorizer. Moreover, vacuuming the furniture would probably be as effective as spraying it. The other selections are appropriate for personal articles infested with head lice.

5. The answer is B *[III E 2, III D 3 c].*
Octyl methoxycinnamate and homosalate protect against only ultraviolet B (UVB) exposure. Because photosensitivity reactions are often associated with UVA radiation exposure, people also need sunscreen protection for this portion of the UV radiation band. The other agents listed cover at least part of both UVA and UVB spectra.

6. The answer is E *[IV D 3, 4, IV E 2].*
Ivy Block is used as a barrier protectant for the prevention of poison ivy dermatitis, *not* for the treatment of an acute eruption. The other options are appropriate to recommend to someone suffering from the acute stage of poison ivy dermatitis.

7. The answer is D *[II E 4].*
Benzoic acid has not been shown to be effective for acne treatment. The other agents, sulfur, salicylic acid, and a sulfur-resorcinol combination, are all safe and effective products for treating acne.

8. The answer is A *[II D 3].*
Evidence does not show that acne worsens from any particular type of food, including chocolate or fried foods. The other choices are pieces of information that the pharmacist should convey to a patient with acne.

9. The answer is B *[II E 4 a].*
Although the irritating properties of benzoyl peroxide might dictate applying it only every other day upon initiating treatment, this patient has tolerated the agent on a daily basis for 2 months. Thus, there would be no need to decrease the application frequency. All of the other choices do apply to this patient's use of benzoyl peroxide.

10. The answer is A *[IV D 4 a].*
Ferric oxide provides the pink color of calamine. All of the other descriptions match their associated agents.

11. The answer is C *[III C 2, E 1 b, c, 2 b].*
Baby oil is not a sunscreen, and it has no effect on melanin. Sun protection factor (SPF) does measure ultraviolet B (UVB) protection, and an SPF higher than 30 must be labeled "SPF 30 Plus." "Water resistant" sunscreen products must retain their SPF value after 40 minutes of water activity. The intensity of the sun does increase by 4% with each 1000-foot elevation.

12. The answer is C *[III D 2, E 1, 2 b; F 1, 4].*
Optimally, sunscreens should be applied 1–2 hours before exposure to the sun. This allows time for the product to bind to the stratum corneum, which provides better protection. The other responses are correct.

30
OTC Weight-Control, Sleep, and Smoking-Cessation Aids

Larry N. Swanson
Tina M. Harrison

I. WEIGHT CONTROL

A. Obesity

1. **Definition.** In recent years, there has been a move to define "overweight" and "obese" individuals by making use of the **body mass index (BMI).** While being overweight can raise the risk of disease, especially cardiovascular disease, the risk is only partially determined by body weight. The **BMI** is used as a parameter to assess the overall risk of developing heart disease when patients are overweight.

$$BMI = \frac{Weight\ (kg)}{Height^2\ (meters)}\ or\ \frac{Weight\ (lb) \times 700}{Height\ (inches)}, \text{ then divide by the height again.}$$

   a. Normal weight is generally considered to be in a BMI range of 18.5 to 24.9. Overweight individuals have a BMI between 25.0 and 29.9. Class I obesity has a BMI range of 30.0 to 34.9; Class II obesity, 35.0 to 39.9; and Class III obesity, greater than 40.0 (Table 30-1).

   b. Some believe that a BMI of 27 or above is the cutoff for significant concern for the need for weight loss. A BMI of 27.8 for men and 27.3 for women corresponds roughly to 20% above the desirable weight (the midpoint of the desirable weight range for a medium-frame person in the 1983 Metropolitan Height and Weight tables).

2. **Types**
   a. Overweight people with large abdomens are generally in worse health than equally obese people who have fat distributed around their hips and limbs.
   b. Waist measurement to hip measurement ratios of greater than 0.95 for men and 0.80 for women are associated with higher death rates. A high-risk waist circumference for men has been determined to be greater than 40 inches; for women, this is greater than 35 inches (see Table 30-1).

3. **Cause.** Although many hypotheses, theories, and proposed mechanisms have been discussed, no uniform cause of obesity has been determined. Patients can become obese because they consistently ingest more calories than their body is able to metabolize. Observations about the cause of obesity include the following.

Table 30-1. Classification of Overweight and Obesity and Relative Disease Risk

	BMI (kg/m²)	Obesity Class	Disease Risk* Relative to Normal Waist Circumference	
			Men ≤40 inches Women ≤35 inches	>40 inches >35 inches
Underweight	<18.5		—	—
Normal**	18.5–24.9		—	—
Overweight	25.0–29.9		Increased	High
Obesity	30.0–34.9	I	High	Very high
	35.0—39.9	II	Very high	Very high
Extreme obesity	≥40	III	Extremely high	Extremely high

*Disease risk for non–insulin-dependent diabetes mellitus, hypertension, and cardiovascular disease.

**Increased waist circumference can also be a marker for increased risk even in persons of normal weight. Adapted from *Preventing and Managing the Global Epidemic of Obesity. Report of the World Health Organization Consultation of Obesity.* Geneva: WHO, June 1997.

    a. Patients may have an **elevated body weight "set point."** When these patients lose weight, compensatory adjustments in metabolism result in their regaining the weight, even with a decreased caloric intake.

    b. Heredity is accepted as an important factor in the etiology of obesity. Studies of identical twins raised apart show that each twin's weight does not vary significantly, which indicates that genetics has a more important role than environmental factors in determining obesity.

    c. Obese patients may be **more responsive to external food cues** (e.g., taste, smell, sight of food).

4. Statistics

    a. Obesity afflicts more people in the United States than does any disease. As much as **one-third of the United States population over 30 years of age** may be obese, and a recent study suggests that one in three adults in the United States is attempting to lose weight.

    b. Yearly, more than **30 billion dollars** is spent on the treatment of obesity, yet less is known about its cause than is known about the cause of most other medical conditions.

    c. The **medical management** of obesity is almost universally unsuccessful. An estimated 90% of all patients who lose more than 25 pounds in a diet program regain that weight within 3 years.

5. Medical consequences

    a. Numerous studies have shown that a significant number of patients with hypertension, non–insulin-dependent diabetes mellitus, and osteoarthritis can significantly control their conditions through weight loss. According to a recent study, it now appears that **even a modest weight gain as one ages** puts middle-aged women at **a higher risk of heart disease.** Women who gained 12–18 pounds after age 18 had a 25% greater chance of suffering a heart attack than their leaner counterparts.

    b. People who are 20% or more over their ideal body weight are more likely to suffer from the following diseases or disorders:

        (1) Amenorrhea

        (2) Cancer of the cervix, colon, endometrium, gallbladder, prostate, and uterus

        (3) Congestive heart failure

        (4) Coronary heart disease

        (5) Diabetes mellitus

        (6) Fatty liver

        (7) Gallbladder disease

        (8) Hirsutism

        (9) Hypertension

        (10) Dyslipidemia

        (11) Respiratory tract infections and other problems

        (12) Varicose veins

B. Management. Weight reduction involves an integrated program of diet, correct eating habits, exercise, patient follow-up, and, sometimes, medication. An approximate **weight-loss goal** should be set when the patient and physician are establishing ideal body weight. Realistic goals about the frequency of weight loss should be established.

    1. A weight loss goal of 1–2 pounds per week is appropriate.

    2. To lose 1 pound in a week, a person must expend 3500 calories through physical work or decrease caloric intake by 3500 calories during that week.

    3. For example, a patient who normally consumes 3000 calories per day must decrease that intake by 500 calories per day in order to lose 1 pound in 1 week (500×7 days = 3500 calories).

C. Diets are specific eating plans that provide a certain number of calories per day.

    1. Balanced diets with calories derived from protein, carbohydrate, and fat are optimal. The caloric intake of fat should be minimized (i.e., less than 30% of total calories, less than 10% saturated fat) for general health reasons (e.g., incidence of ischemic heart disease, certain types of cancer). Also, fat contains 9 calories per gram; carbohydrate or protein contains 4 calories per gram.

    2. Fad diets do not teach patients how to eat properly for long-range benefits. Weight maintenance is the key.

3. **Caloric restriction** is usually at two levels: low-calorie diets (LCDs) usually of 1000–1500 calories per day and very-low–calorie diets (VLCDs) of 800 calories or less. VLCDs need to be conducted under strict medical supervision and monitoring and are designed for severely overweight individuals. Formula diet programs (i.e., Optifast, Slim-Fast) use low-calorie, nutritionally balanced products (e.g., flavored drinks, nutritional bars) to control and limit caloric intake. One dieting approach might be to use the liquid Slim-Fast shakes (approximately 220 calories/can) for one or two meals and then eat regular food for the third meal.

4. **Food additives** like artificial sweeteners (e.g., saccharin, aspartame) can substitute for sugar and its 33 calories/teaspoonful. Fat substitutes (e.g., olestra) provide the taste and "feel" of fat, but with fewer calories. **Olestra** (Olean) is a nondigestible, noncaloric fat substitute for use in snack foods such as potato chips. Side effects such as loose stools, diarrhea, abdominal cramps, and nausea may occur in some patients. This agent may have some effect on the absorption of fat-soluble vitamins (A, D, E, and K) and beta-carotene.

D. **Eating habits.** Patients need to be trained in gaining self-control of their eating behavior if they are planning to lose weight and maintain the weight loss.

1. **Behavior modification programs,** which seek to eliminate improper eating behaviors (e.g., eating while watching television, eating too rapidly, eating when not hungry), may be beneficial.

2. **Self-help groups** (e.g., Weight Watchers, Nutri-System, Jenny Craig) use a program of diet, education, and positive emotional support to help patients lose weight.

E. **Exercise.** Because 3500 calories of work must be expended to lose 1 pound, exercise is clearly a difficult way to lose weight. However, an effective weight-loss program incorporates exercise.

1. **Benefits**
   a. Exercise burns calories [e.g., walking (2 mph) burns 200 calories per hour; running (5.3 mph) burns 570 calories per hour].
   b. Exercise raises body metabolism, which can have an extended effect on weight loss.
   c. Exercise can decrease appetite.
   d. Patients usually feel better (mentally and emotionally) when they exercise regularly.
   e. Exercise helps to prevent the loss of muscle mass.

2. **Effective exercise expends energy.** Vibrating belts, continuous passive motion machines, and similar products do not result in increased weight loss because using them does not expend energy.

F. **Prescription weight-loss products**

1. **Overview.** Despite the interest in pharmacotherapy, there had been no new drugs approved for weight control in the United States for more than 20 years until dexfenfluramine (Redux) came on the market in 1996. This has been due to a combination of factors, but an important one has been the manner in which the Drug Enforcement Agency (DEA) has classified these drugs.
   a. The initial drugs used for appetite suppression, **amphetamine, methamphetamine,** and **phenmetrazine** (Preludin) are classified as Schedule II because they have a high potential for abuse. These drugs are no longer used for weight control.
   b. Drugs that were marketed later, **phendimetrazine** (Plegine), **diethylpropion** (Tenuate), and **phentermine** (Ionamin), have shown little evidence of abuse potential but have still been classified as controlled substances and are only recommended for short-term use (usually no more than a few weeks). Because of the association of valvular heart disease with the combination of fenfluramine and phentermine ("fen-phen") and the increased risk of primary pulmonary hypertension and brain neurotoxicity associated with both fenfluramine and dexfenfluramine, these two agents were removed from the market in 1997. The other United States Food and Drug Administration (FDA)-approved prescription agents for short-term treatment of obesity are benzphetamine (Didrex) and mazindol (Sanorex).
   c. The newest agents available for weight loss are **sibutramine** (Meredia) and **orlistat** (Xenical). **Only these two agents have FDA approval for long-term use (greater than 3 months at a time).**
      (1) **Sibutramine** is usually given 10 mg daily, although the dose may be increased to 15 mg daily after 4 weeks if weight loss is inadequate. This agent has both sero-

tonin and norepinephrine reuptake effects, which affects satiety and hunger in the hypothalamus. In clinical trials, sibutramine showed a statistical improvement in amount of weight lost versus placebo. However, there was no statistical improvement in total cholesterol, high-density lipoprotein (HDL), or fasting blood glucose. This agent is contraindicated in patients with known seizure disorders, congestive heart failure (CHF), a history of myocardial infarction, and arrhythmias.

(2) **Orlistat** is a potent and irreversible inhibitor of gastric, pancreatic, and pancreatic carboxylester lipases. These enzymes are required for the hydrolysis of fat in the gastrointestinal (GI) tract to free fatty acids and monoacylglycerols, which are absorbable. Inhibition of these enzymes results in: (1) inhibition of the digestion of dietary triglycerides, (2) inhibition of the hydrolysis and absorption of dietary fat, and (3) decreased solubility and absorption of cholesterol.

   (a) Orlistat, like sibutramine, is indicated for the treatment of obesity in patients who have a BMI of more than 30 or a BMI more than 27 with at least one risk factor. This agent should be used in conjunction with diet and exercise.

   (b) The dose is 120 mg three times a day with each main meal. The most commonly reported **side effects** include fatty/oily stools, increased defecation, soft stool, and fecal urgency, and these side effects directly correlate to the amount of fat in the diet. The patient should be cautioned that the absorption of the fat-soluble vitamins (A, D, E, and K) may be decreased in patients who take orlistat.

2. **Indication.** Prescription weight-loss drugs have been justified for someone who has lost weight on a diet and then reaches a plateau or, more rarely, for someone who is beginning a diet. These agents traditionally have been used for short-term therapy (8–12 weeks), and their use results in small, but statistically significant weight loss (~0.5 lb per week more than with placebo). It is more widely accepted to use prescription weight-loss products when obese patients are at high risk for adverse health consequences. Sibutramine is specifically recommended for patients with a BMI ≥30 or a BMI ≥27 in the presence of other risk factors.

3. The **mechanism of action** apparently involves suppression of the satiety center in the hypothalamic ventromedial nucleus. Most suppressants augment brain catecholamine action with the exception of agents such as fenfluramine (removed from the market), which acts specifically on serotonin. Other mechanisms may be involved as well. Sibutramine inhibits the reuptake of serotonin, norepinephrine, and dopamine in the central nervous system (CNS). (See above for orlistat's mechanism of action.)

4. **Drug selection and side effects.** No superiority has been shown for the appetite suppressant effects of any of these agents. Patients often tolerate one agent better than another. Restlessness, insomnia, tremors, tachycardia, nausea, diarrhea, constipation, dry mouth, and mydriasis are commonly reported side effects. In susceptible patients, elevated blood pressure and cardiac arrhythmias may occur. There is the potential for dependence and abuse of all of these agents (except orlistat).

5. **Long-term use.** There is a growing interest in treating obesity as a **long-term chronic disease** in the same manner that we view hypertension and diabetes mellitus. Diet modification and exercise is the best known combination for maintenance of weight loss.

G. OTC weight-loss products

1. Two agents [**phenylpropanolamine** (PPA) and **benzocaine**] were originally considered by the FDA as generally recognized safe and effective (Category I) over-the-counter (OTC) weight-control drugs. However, safety (PPA) and efficacy (benzocaine) issues have removed these agents from the market. No OTC agents have proven efficacy as weight-loss drugs. In October 2000, the Non-Prescription Advisory Committee of the FDA recommended that PPA be classified as "unsafe" because research has shown that patients taking PPA are at higher risk of hemorrhagic stroke. In November 2000, the FDA took steps to remove PPA from all drug products and requested that all drug companies discontinue marketing products containing PPA. **Benzocaine** appears to act topically on nerve endings in the oral cavity to decrease the ability to detect different degrees of sweetness. Supposedly by this numbing effect using gum, candy, or lozenge dosage forms (3–15 mg per dose), the desire for food is decreased. Surprisingly, systemic benzocaine administered in the form of tablets or capsules also was included as Category I even though there is no lo-

cal effect. The FDA has advised manufacturers of benzocaine-containing products that there is **insufficient evidence of efficacy** for this agent and additional studies would need to be conducted to verify this agent's role in weight loss. The manufacturers responded by removing benzocaine from their products.

2. **Additional agents.** A number of other OTC agents have been proposed for the treatment of obesity, but support for their effectiveness is weak. For example, the bulk-producing laxatives have been proposed to create a feeling of fullness in the stomach. However, x-ray studies have shown that the bulk leaves the stomach within 30 minutes. No herbal products are considered safe and effective treatments for weight loss, and one agent (ma huang, a natural form of ephedrine) can have significant sympathomimetic and CNS side effects.

II. SLEEP AIDS

A. Normal sleep and sleep requirements

1. **Length.** Sleep time and quality of sleep vary widely among individuals. The usual range of sleep time per night is 5–10 hours, with an average of about 7½ hours.

2. **Sleep requirements** change as a person ages. Newborns may sleep up to 18 hours. Preteens usually fall asleep within 5 or 10 minutes, sleep for 9½ hours, and spend 95% of their time in bed in solid, continuous, deep sleep. By adulthood, 7 or 8 hours of sleep usually provides adequate rest. In old age, 6 hours may suffice.

3. **Polysomnography** uses electroencephalogram (EEG), electro-oculogram (EOG), and electromyogram (EMG) recordings to note changes that occur during sleep.
   a. **Stages.** Using polysomnography, researchers have discovered five stages of sleep.
      (1) **One rapid eye movement (REM) stage** occupies about 25% of normal total sleep time.
      (2) **Four non–rapid eye movement (NREM) stages** make up the remaining 75% of normal total sleep time. Stages three and four of NREM sleep are considered to be the deepest sleep and are often referred to collectively as **delta sleep** or **restorative sleep.**
   b. Most **dreaming** occurs during the REM stage of sleep, and the degree of "restfulness" of sleep is associated with the amount of REM sleep.
   c. Most of the **medications** used to treat insomnia, including the OTC agents, interfere with some component of the sleep stages, especially the REM sleep.

B. Insomnia

1. **Definition.** Insomnia is an interruption of the natural sleep cycle that results in impaired daytime performance. Insomnia must be defined not only in terms of the amount of sleep but also with attention to the perceived quality of sleep.

2. **Diagnosis.** Daytime performance deficits, not the number of hours slept, should be the primary determinant of an insomnia diagnosis.
   a. An occasional night of inadequate or no sleep is of little concern in healthy individuals. Apart from **extreme sleepiness** and the occurrence of **"microsleeps,"** remarkably **little pathology** is associated with extended sleeplessness.
   b. As long as patients awake each morning feeling fully refreshed and do not need an afternoon nap, they should be reassured that they do not have insomnia and that the full 8-hour sleep pattern at night is not absolutely necessary. Oftentimes, simple **reassurance** may be all that is needed to "cure" insomnia.

3. **Categories.** Insomnias can generally be divided into three categories.
   a. **Transient** insomnia, which accounts for approximately 15% of insomnia cases, generally lasts less than 7 days. Causes of transient insomnia include **jet lag, shift work,** or **acute anxiety.**
   b. **Short-term** insomnia lasts from 1–3 weeks. Causes of short-term insomnia include usually identifiable, often self-limiting problems, such as **grief, pain, noise,** or an **anxiety-provoking situation.**
   c. **Long-term** insomnia (or chronic insomnia) lasts longer than 3 weeks, indicates an underlying pathology, and requires a thorough assessment of the patient's physical and

emotional health. Long-term insomnia may stem from an underlying medical condition such as **hyperthyroidism** or **arthritis.** Often, treatment strategies that relieve the underlying physical disorder resolve the insomnia complaint.

4. **Causes.** Patients who experience insomnia have different causes for this condition.
   a. **Intrinsic sleep disorders**
      (1) **Psychophysiological insomnia** is a conditioned form of sleep loss in which the patient associates increased wakefulness with the bedroom and the bedtime routine.
      (2) **Restless legs syndrome** is characterized by extremely uncomfortable sensations in leg muscles at rest, which are relieved only by getting up and moving around.
      (3) **Sleep apnea** can be obstructive or centrally mediated. The hallmark is breathing that stops for short periods during sleep. Patients with sleep apnea should not use hypnotics or OTC sleep aids.
      (4) **Sleep-related myoclonus** is the periodic, rhythmic curling or jumping of the feet during sleep.
   b. **Extrinsic sleep disorders**
      (1) **Adjustment sleep disorder** is prompted by a stressful life change.
      (2) **Inadequate sleep hygiene** is caused by a lifestyle that reduces the amount of quality sleep.
      (3) **Hypnotic-, stimulant-,** or **alcohol-dependent** sleep disorder is caused by dependence, tolerance, or overreliance on a given agent.
   c. **Circadian sleep disorders**
      (1) **Delayed sleep phase syndrome** occurs in people whose natural sleep times are altered due to work. For instance, a person who must be at work at 8 A.M., but naturally gets tired after 2 A.M. and wakes after 10 A.M., would be affected by this type of disorder.
      (2) **Jet lag** is primarily a problem for people who travel across several time zones.
   d. **Psychiatric disorders,** such as **major depressive disorder,** result in poor sleep that usually improves with specific antidepressant medication.

5. **Treatment** of insomnia is highly dependent on the type of insomnia. It is very important to distinguish among transient insomnia, short-term insomnia, and long-term insomnia (see II B 3).
   a. **Nondrug intervention** and **sleep-hygiene measures** include the following lifestyle and environmental recommendations:
      (1) Establishing a regular bedtime
      (2) Going to bed when tired and ready to sleep
      (3) If unable to sleep, getting out of bed
      (4) Shortly before bedtime, engaging in a relaxing activity, such as taking a warm bath, eating a light snack, or doing relaxation exercises
      (5) Avoiding strenuous exercise or other stimulating activity for several hours before bedtime
      (6) Avoiding alcohol because it could produce fragmented sleep
      (7) Making sure that the bedroom and the bed are comfortable for sleeping
      (8) Avoiding stimulants (e.g., caffeine, nicotine, PPA, pseudoephedrine) late in the day
      (9) Avoiding naps during the day
   b. **Drug treatment of transient and short-term insomnia.** Wakefulness and sleep are antagonistic states competing for control of brain activity. Several neurotransmitters play a role in arousal. Their actions help explain why medications that mimic or counteract their effects can influence sleep. **Serotonin** and **γ-aminobutyric acid (GABA)** are believed to promote slow-wave sleep. **Acetylcholine** regulates REM sleep. **Norepinephrine, epinephrine,** and **dopamine** stimulate wakefulness. Individuals vary greatly in their natural levels of neurotransmitters and their sensitivity to these chemicals. Hypnotics exert their effects by modulating brain neurotransmitters and neuropeptides such as serotonin, norepinephrine, acetylcholine, histamine, adenosine, and GABA.
      (1) The **goal of therapy** for transient and short-term insomnia is:
          (a) Restoring daytime functioning
          (b) Avoiding the self-reinforcing pattern that may develop into chronic insomnia
      (2) **Therapeutic contract.** A wise strategy for using hypnotics is to enter into a therapeutic contract with patients, limiting hypnotic use to no more than two or three nights in succession, followed by one or more medicine-free nights. In this way, hypnotics can serve as a safety net, and patients can be assured that they will have no more than one night of sleeplessness without obtaining relief.

Table 30-2. Examples of Short-, Intermediate-, and Long-Acting Benzodiazepines

Agent	Rate of Elimination	Onset of Action (minutes)	Usual Adult Dose (mg)
Triazolam (Halcion)	Rapid	15–30	0.125–0.25
Estazolam (ProSom)	Intermediate	15–30	1–2
Temazepam (Restoril)	Intermediate	45–60	15–30
Flurazepam HCl (Dalmane)	Slow	15–30	15–30
Quazepam (Doral)	Slow	15–30	7.5–15

(3) Prescription hypnotic agents are reserved primarily for this type of insomnia. Sedative hypnotic agents should be used only as part of a plan that makes use of good sleep-hygiene techniques.

    (a) Benzodiazepines have been considered to be the drugs of choice for symptomatic relief of insomnia.

        (i) Mechanism of action. The benzodiazepines work by enhancing the activity of the inhibitory neurotransmitter GABA, which calms brain activity.

        (ii) Selection of a benzodiazepine is based on the specific pharmacokinetic profile that matches the particular sleep problem (Table 30-2).

        (iii) Adverse effects of these hypnotics include daytime sedation and mental cloudiness. Triazolam has been associated with anterograde amnesia and rebound insomnia.

    (b) Zolpidem (Ambien) is unique because it is a nonbenzodiazepine with the structure of an imidazopyridine. It acts on the benzodiazepine receptor (v-1 subtype) in the CNS. It has a minimal effect on sleep stages and, therefore, is reported to promote a more natural sleep.

        (i) Advantages over the benzodiazepines include lack of withdrawal effects, no rebound insomnia, and little or no tolerance demonstrated. It has a rapid onset of action and is useful for both initiating and maintaining sleep.

        (ii) Adverse effects of zolpidem include nightmares, agitation, headaches, GI upset, dizziness, and daytime drowsiness.

    (c) Zaleplon (Sonata) was approved by the FDA in August 1999. Like zolpidem, this agent is a pyrazolopyrimidine derivative that binds selectively to BNZ_1 receptors. Because of its very short half-life (0.9–1 hour), it is particularly useful **for patients with difficulty falling asleep** as the major sleep complaint. Also, again because of its very short half-life, patients with insomnia during the night can take zaleplon if they **have at least 4 or more hours in bed.**

    (d) Older prescription drugs. The **barbiturates** are prescribed less commonly for management of insomnia because of the risk of excessive CNS depression. The **early nonbarbiturate nonbenzodiazepine** sedative hypnotics were originally thought to be superior to the barbiturates, but they were found to share many disadvantages in addition to having disadvantages of their own. **Chloral hydrate** might be considered an exception, but it still has some issues of concern (e.g., displaces some highly protein-bound drugs, some GI irritation).

    (e) Antidepressants with sedative side effects (e.g., amitriptyline, doxepin, and trazodone) have been used in lower doses than those used in depression to treat insomnia.

(4) OTC drug therapy

    (a) The FDA has deemed two antihistamines, **diphenhydramine** (e.g., Nytol, Sominex, Compoz Nighttime Sleep Aid, Unisom Sleepgels) and **doxylamine** (e.g., Unisom Nighttime Sleep-Aid), safe and effective sleep aids. They are both ethanolamine antihistamines, which possess the highest sedative effects and the lowest GI side effects of the various antihistamines.

        (i) The **therapeutic use** of these agents capitalizes on the drowsiness side effect.

        (ii) Indications. These OTC products are indicated for mild situational insomnia.

        (iii) The usual **dose** for adults is 25 mg for doxylamine and 50 mg for diphenhydramine. Increasing the dose of diphenhydramine does not produce a linear increase in hypnotic effect. However, it does produce greater anticholinergic side effects, particularly in elderly people.

(iv) The most common **side effects** include dizziness, dry mouth, blurred vision, and upset stomach. Both doxylamine and diphenhydramine cause REM suppression and, therefore, some REM rebound after discontinuation. Anticholinergic effects include constipation and urinary retention. Central anticholinergic effects that also affect the elderly include confusion, disorientation, impaired short-term memory, and, at times, visual and tactile hallucinations.

(v) **Contraindications.** These agents should not be used by individuals under age 12 and should not be taken for longer than 2 weeks. In addition, they should be used cautiously by patients who have asthma, narrow-angle glaucoma, and prostate enlargement.

(vi) **Efficacy.** Diphenhydramine and doxylamine are considered to be roughly equivalent in efficacy.

(b) **Melatonin** (e.g., Melatonex) has been prominently featured in the media because of various therapeutic claims. Among these has been the recommendation to use this agent to treat insomnia and jet lag. It has **not** been approved by the FDA for this use. This hormone is produced in a predictable daily rhythm by the pineal gland, which is located deep in the brain between the two hemispheres. Levels of melatonin climb after dark and ebb after dawn. Older people, who often suffer from insomnia, have lower serum concentrations of melatonin. There is evidence to support the contention that melatonin has a hypnotic effect in humans (especially in jet lag); however, large controlled trials have not been done. The purity of the products sold in health food stores and the adverse effects of taking the hormone are unknown.

(c) The effectiveness of the herbal product **valerian** as a hypnotic is questionable, and it has a delayed onset of effect; therefore, it is not recommended for acute management of insomnia.

III. SMOKING CESSATION

A. Introduction. Nicotine, the physically addictive component of tobacco, is readily absorbed in the lungs from inhaled smoke. Nicotine from smokeless tobacco products, such as chewing tobacco and snuff, is absorbed from the oral mucosa. Despite reports of an increased incidence of lung disease, heart disease, and cancer, many Americans continue to use tobacco products. The economic impact of these smoking-related illnesses exceeds $97 billion annually in direct costs for medical care and loss of wages.

B. Physiological effects of nicotine involve primarily the CNS (e.g., enhanced relaxation, improved attention) and cardiovascular system (e.g., elevated blood pressure, tachycardia, peripheral vasoconstriction). Reports of weight loss, early menopause, and osteoporosis are also found with nicotine use.

C. Benefits of smoking cessation include a longer life and better health. Smokers who are motivated to quit for health reasons have a higher success rate. Studies have shown that success rates have been associated with a desire to protect future health, a sense of personal vulnerability to smoking health risks, and a desire for greater self-mastery, self-confidence, or self-esteem. Helpful social support, smokers who use low-nicotine-content cigarettes, and those with a lower smoking rate are also the most successful with smoking cessation.

D. Smoking-cessation strategies have been developed by the Agency for Healthcare Research and Quality (AHRQ). The panel recommends that clinicians use the following five strategies:

1. **Ask** patients about their use of tobacco products.
2. **Advise** all users to quit.
3. **Identify** smokers willing to attempt to quit.
4. **Assist** the patient in quitting.
5. **Arrange** for follow-up contact.

Table 30-3. Transdermal Patches Available for Nicotine-Replacement Therapy

Product Name	Nicotine Delivery (mg/24 hr)	Duration of Therapy (weeks)
Nicoderm CQ	21, 14, 7	6–8
Nicotrol	15	6
Habitrol[§]	21, 14, 7	6–8
Prostep[§]	22, 11	8

§ = available only with a prescription.

E. **Interventions** with a counselor or group have provided the greatest success rate for persons desiring to quit smoking. Patients need to be instructed about the possible **nicotine-withdrawal symptoms,** which can include anxiety, depression, difficulty concentrating, headache, restlessness, insomnia, and increased appetite.

F. **Nicotine-replacement therapy** reduces the withdrawal symptoms associated with smoking cessation. Four nicotine dosage forms—polacrilex (chewing gum, lozenge), transdermal systems (patches), oral inhaler, and nasal spray—are approved by the FDA for smoking cessation. Product selection is based primarily on patient preference. The oral and nasal spray (e.g., Nicotrol NS, Nicotrol Inhaler) are available only by prescription. Buproprion (e.g., Zyban) is also available by prescription only. The suggested dose of buproprion for smoking cessation is 150 mg every day for 3 days, increased to 150 mg twice daily for 7–12 weeks.

1. **Nicotine gum** (e.g., Nicorette) is available in 2- and 4-mg dosage forms. Nicotine gum is most effective when given to patients along with some behavioral intervention. The 4-mg strength works best in highly dependent smokers. The most common adverse effects are sore jaw and mouth, mouth ulcers, and indigestion. It is recommended not to exceed 30 pieces of gum in 24 hours. Most people find that 10–12 pieces a day will control their urge to smoke.

2. A **nicotine lozenge** (i.e., Commit) was approved in late 2002 for OTC marketing. It contains the same active ingredient as the nicotine gum. It also comes in 2-mg and 4-mg strengths and is sugar free. The dosage strength is based on the amount of time it takes for the smoker to crave tobacco after awakening. People who feel an urge to smoke within 30 minutes of waking should use the 4-mg lozenge. The recommended dosing interval is 1–2 hours during the first 6 weeks of treatment, 2–4 hours for the next 3 weeks, and 4–8 hours during the final 3 weeks of the recommended 12-week program. The product should be sucked until dissolved (not chewed or swallowed). No more than 20 lozenges should be taken in a day.

3. **Transdermal nicotine** (e.g., Nicoderm CQ, Nicotrol) is sometimes preferred over the gum because of the avoidance of bad taste, GI complications, and the likelihood of enhanced compliance. The patches also allow for more steady nicotine serum concentrations. The most distinguishing characteristics of the nicotine patches are nicotine content, dosage, and release rate. Heavy smokers (>10 cigarettes per day) should be instructed to begin with the higher-dosed patch. The most commonly reported side effect is local skin irritation. Table 30-3 illustrates the transdermal products available.

G. **Other treatment options** have included agents such as benzodiazepines, antidepressants (e.g., doxepin, fluoxetine), propranolol, and clonidine. Due to the lack of clinical trials for these agents in smoking cessation, they are not routinely recommended.

H. **Patient counseling** should include information on avoidance of the concomitant use of tobacco. Patients using the patch should be told to apply it on a relatively hairless area between the neck and waist as soon as they awaken.

STUDY QUESTIONS

Directions: Each of the numbered items or incomplete statements in this section is followed by answers or by completions of the statement. Select the **one** lettered answer or completion that is **best** in each case.

1. Based on the calorie decrease necessary to lose 1 pound of body fat, how many pounds will a woman likely lose in 20 days if she cuts her caloric intake from 2200 per day to 1600 per day but does not increase her physical activity?

(A) 10 pounds
(B) Approximately 5 pounds
(C) Approximately 3.5 pounds
(D) Slightly less than 2 pounds
(E) Not enough data to calculate

2. All of the following statements about diphenhydramine are true EXCEPT

(A) a 50-mg dose that is ineffective should be doubled for the elderly patient
(B) it suppresses rapid eye movement (REM) sleep
(C) it should not be taken with alcohol
(D) it is similar in efficacy to doxylamine as a sleep aid

3. All of the following statements about sleep stages are true EXCEPT

(A) a normal, young, healthy adult spends about 20%–25% of total sleep time in rapid eye movement (REM) sleep
(B) the degree of restfulness of sleep is associated with the amount of REM sleep
(C) dreaming appears to occur most often in the first stage of non–rapid eye movement (NREM) sleep
(D) stages three and four of NREM sleep are often referred to as delta sleep

4. All of the following would be useful sleep-hygiene measures EXCEPT

(A) exercising intensely just before bedtime
(B) taking a warm bath just before bedtime
(C) reading until drowsy
(D) keeping the bedroom somewhat cool
(E) establishing a regular bedtime

5. All of the following statements about obesity are true EXCEPT

(A) obesity is now defined as a person who has surplus body fat and a BMI ≥ 30.0
(B) phenylpropanolamine was removed from the market because of safety concerns
(C) fad diets do not teach patients how to eat for long-term maintenance of the decreased weight
(D) a bulk laxative such as Metamucil has been proven to be an effective weight-loss agent

6. Which of the following is NOT a motivational factor associated with successful quitting of smoking?

(A) Previous history of depression
(B) Desire to protect future health and overcome minor smoking-related symptoms
(C) Desire for greater self-mastery, self-control, or self-esteem
(D) Confidence in ability to quit

7. All of the following statements about patient counseling for smoking cessation are true EXCEPT

(A) adverse effects associated with the nicotine gum include bad taste, mouth sores, and sore throat
(B) physical withdrawal symptoms are not likely with smoking cessation
(C) concomitant use of other nicotine-containing products (e.g., cigarettes) should not be used with smoking-cessation products
(D) certain medications (e.g., theophylline) may require dosage adjustment when you stop smoking

8. Which of the following are associated with the LEAST effective means of smoking cessation?

(A) Group counseling used with the nicotine gum
(B) Transdermal nicotine
(C) Self-controlled abstinence with no pharmacological/psychological intervention
(D) Group counseling with no pharmacological intervention

9. All of the following statements are TRUE about nicotine replacement therapy EXCEPT

(A) the transdermal patches are usually preferred over the gum because of the gum's side effects
(B) the transdermal patches provide more consistent serum levels over 24 hours than the gum
(C) the transdermal patches generally allow for dosage titration
(D) addiction to the nicotine-replacement therapy will not occur

ANSWERS AND EXPLANATIONS

1. The answer is C *[I B]*.
The woman would lose about 3.5 pounds. To lose 1 pound of fat, caloric intake must decrease by 3,500 calories. This woman decreased her caloric intake from 2,200 calories per day to 1,600 calories per day, a decrease of 600 calories. Six hundred calories multiplied by 20 days equals a decrease of 12,000 calories. Twelve thousand divided by 3,500 equals 3.43 pounds, or approximately 3.5 pounds.

2. The answer is A *[II B 5 b (4) (a)]*.
Increasing the dose of diphenhydramine does not automatically bring a linear increase in hypnotic effect. However, it does produce greater anticholinergic side effects, which are particularly troublesome in the elderly. Diphenhydramine, which suppresses rapid eye movement (REM) sleep, produces a sedation more unpleasant than that of alcohol or benzodiazepines. Diphenhydramine should not be taken with alcohol. As a sleep aid, it is similar in efficacy to doxylamine.

3. The answer is C *[II A 3]*.
Most dreaming appears to occur during rapid eye movement (REM) rather than non-REM (NREM) sleep. The average, young, healthy adult spends about one-quarter of the time sleeping in REM sleep. The amount of REM sleep is associated with the degree of restfulness. Delta sleep consists of stages three and four of NREM sleep.

4. The answer is A *[II B 5 a]*.
Exercising intensely just before going to bed will usually have a stimulating effect. Taking a warm bath shortly before bedtime, reading until drowsy, keeping the bedroom cool, and establishing a regular bedtime are considered appropriate sleep-hygiene measures.

5. The answer is D *[I A 1, C 1–3]*.
Bulk laxatives produce a feeling of fullness, but x-ray studies show that the bulk leaves the stomach within 30 minutes. They may decrease appetite somewhat, but the effectiveness of bulk laxatives as a weight-loss agent is weak. Obese people are those who have surplus body fat and have a BMI ≥30. Hemorrhagic stroke was reported in association with phenylpropanolamine use. Fad diets do not teach people how to eat to maintain any achieved weight loss. Consequently, many people who follow fad diets regain weight.

6. The answer is A *[III C]*.
Smokers with no past history of depression and who have psychosocial assets (e.g., self-esteem, self-management skills, manageable life stress, freedom from other chemical dependencies) are more likely to be successful with smoking cessation.

7. The answer is B *[III E, F 3, H]*.
Smoking cessation may precipitate both physical and psychological withdrawal symptoms.

8. The answer is C *[III E]*.
Successful smoking cessation has been achieved with and without pharmacological intervention; however, psychological support is the cornerstone of treatment. Lack of psychosocial support and not using some nicotine-delivery system has shown to have the lowest cessation success rate.

9. The answer is D *[III F]*.
Addiction to the nicotine found in the replacement products has been noted; however, there are fewer adverse effects on the lungs with the use of these products.

31
OTC Agents for Fever, Pain, Cough, Cold, and Allergic Rhinitis

Gerald E. Schumacher
Larry N. Swanson

I. ANALGESIC, ANTI-INFLAMMATORY, AND ANTIPYRETIC AGENTS. Over-the-counter (OTC) analgesics and antipyretics relieve mild-to-moderate pain and reduce inflammation and fever. These agents are effective for somatic pain (e.g., musculoskeletal pain in the joints; pain from headache, myalgia, and dysmenorrhea; discomfort resulting from generalized inflammation), but they are not effective in reducing discomfort from the visceral organs (e.g., stomach, lungs, heart). Salicylates and nonsteroidal anti-inflammatory drugs (NSAIDs) reduce pain, inflammation, and fever, but acetaminophen generally is effective for only pain and fever.*

A. Pathogenesis of pain. Intense stimulus (e.g., tissue injury) releases substances that sensitize pain receptors to mechanical, thermal, and chemical stimulation. This triggers pain receptors to send pain impulses over afferent nerve fibers to the central nervous system (CNS).

1. **Awareness** of pain occurs in the thalamus.

2. Pain **recognition** and **localization** occur in the cortex.

3. **Mechanism of analgesic, anti-inflammatory, and antipyretic action.** These agents inhibit (centrally, peripherally, or both) the biosynthesis of various **prostaglandins,** substances involved in the development of pain and inflammation as well as in the regulation of body temperature.

B. Salicylates

1. **Therapeutic uses.** Salicylates are used to relieve mild-to-moderate pain and reduce inflammation and fever. Aspirin (acetylsalicylic acid), specifically, is also used to reduce the incidence of:
   a. **Strokes** in men at risk. Present evidence does not support the value of using aspirin in women. There is no evidence that aspirin is useful after strokes are complete for men or women.
   b. **Transient ischemic attacks (TIAs)** in men with recurrent attacks. There is no evidence that aspirin is useful in women.
   c. **Myocardial infarction** in men and women who have had a previous infarction, stable and unstable angina pectoris, or coronary artery bypass surgery.

2. **Mechanism of action**
   a. **Analgesic and anti-inflammatory actions.** The action of aspirin results from both the acetyl and the salicylate portions of the drug. Actions of other salicylates (e.g., sodium salicylate, salicylsalicylic acid, choline salicylate) result only from the salicylate portion of the agents.
      (1) These drugs **inhibit cyclooxygenase,** the enzyme that is responsible for the formation of precursors of prostaglandins and thromboxanes from arachidonic acid (Figure 31-1).
      (2) Analgesia is produced mainly by **blocking the peripheral generation of pain impulses** mediated by prostaglandins and other chemicals. Analgesia probably secondarily involves a reduction in the awareness of pain in the CNS.

---

*In some instances, aspirin is considered to be a nonsteroidal anti-inflammatory drug (NSAID), whereas in other instances it is not. For the purpose of demonstrating different information, aspirin and NSAIDs are discussed separately in this chapter.

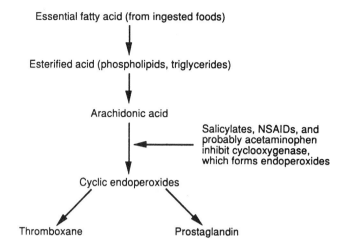

Essential fatty acid (from ingested foods)

Esterified acid (phospholipids, triglycerides)

Arachidonic acid

Salicylates, NSAIDs, and probably acetaminophen inhibit cyclooxygenase, which forms endoperoxides

Cyclic endoperoxides

Thromboxane   Prostaglandin

Figure 31-1. Inhibition of prostaglandin formation by aspirin, NSAIDs, and acetaminophen.

    b. Antipyretic action. The principal antipyretic action occurs in the CNS. Salicylates act on the hypothalamic heat-regulating center to produce peripheral vasodilation, which results from the inhibition of prostaglandin synthesis.

    c. Antiplatelet and antithrombotic actions

        (1) Antiplatelet. Aspirin (but not other salicylates, acetaminophen, or NSAIDs) **irreversibly inhibits cyclooxygenase in platelets,** which prevents the formation of the aggregating agent thromboxane A_2.

        (2) Antithrombotic. At low doses, aspirin inhibits thromboxane A_2 formation but has a relatively small effect on prostacyclin. This results in blocking the platelet aggregant thromboxane A_2, while preserving the action of the aggregation inhibitor, prostacyclin [prostaglandin I_2 (PGI_2)].

3. Administration and dosage

    a. For **analgesia** or **antipyresis in adults,** 325–650 mg every 4 hours or 650–1000 mg every 6 hours should be administered as needed. The maximum daily dose is 4000 mg for no longer than 10 days for pain or 3 days for fever, without consulting a physician.

    b. Child dosage depends on age. The dosages are 160 mg every 4 hours for children 2–4 years of age and 400–480 mg every 4 hours for children 9–12 years of age. Salicylates should be given for no longer than 5 days for pain, 3 days for fever, and 2 days for sore throat, without consulting a physician.

    c. The **antirheumatic dosage for adults** is 3600–4500 mg daily in divided doses.

    d. For patients with **ischemic heart disease,** a 325-mg dose is given daily. Every other day is recommended for individuals with stable angina, unstable angina, and evolving myocardial infarction. For patients without clinically apparent ischemic heart disease, the hemorrhagic complications associated with routine aspirin use may outweigh its benefit, unless subjects have established risk factors for atherosclerotic disease.

    e. Anti-inflammatory dosages. Although antipyretic and analgesic effects should appear within the first few doses, the anti-inflammatory effect may take 2 or more weeks to appear, even at high doses. The usual anti-inflammatory dosage of aspirin is 4000–6000 mg per day. The usual anti-inflammatory dosage of ibuprofen is 1200–3200 mg per day.

4. Precautions

    a. Hypersensitivity to aspirin occurs in up to 0.5% of the population.

        (1) Allergic reactions resulting in bronchoconstriction occur most frequently in people with **nasal polyps.**

        (2) Cross-reactivity with other NSAIDs occurs in more than 90% of people. Cross-reactivity with acetaminophen occurs in 5% of people.

    b. Contraindications. Aspirin is contraindicated in patients with bleeding disorders or peptic ulcers. Also, aspirin should not be given to children or teenagers with a viral illness, because Reye's syndrome (i.e., fatty liver degeneration accompanied by encephalopathy) may occur.

    c. Pregnancy. Salicylates in chronic high doses are recommended with extreme caution during the last trimester of pregnancy because of:

        (1) Potential bleeding problems in the mother, fetus, or neonate

        (2) Prolonging or complicating delivery

    d. Gastrointestinal (GI) disturbances resulting from the inhibition of the gastric prostaglandins occur in 10%–20% of people at analgesic and antipyretic dosages. Anti-inflammatory regimens affect up to 40% of people. These percentages decrease by using enteric-coated dosage forms and taking salicylates with food or large doses of antacids. Buffered aspirin products contain insufficient "buffers" to counteract the adverse GI effects of aspirin.

    e. CNS disturbances such as tinnitus, dizziness, or headache may occur at anti-inflammatory doses in some patients.

    f. Salicylism (salicylate toxicity) may occur at anti-inflammatory doses. In addition to the CNS disturbances above, respiratory alkalosis, nausea, hyperthermia, confusion, and convulsions may occur.

5. Significant interactions

    a. Salicylates potentiate the effect of **anticoagulants** and **thrombolytic agents.**

    b. Salicylates potentiate (at anti-inflammatory doses) the effect of **hypoglycemics.**

    c. Salicylates potentiate the adverse gastrointestinal reaction resulting from chronic **alcohol** or **NSAID** use.

    d. Aspirin may competitively inhibit the metabolism of **zidovudine,** resulting in potentiation of zidovudine or aspirin toxicity.

    e. Caffeine taken in conjunction with salicylates appears to enhance the analgesic effect.

C. Acetaminophen

1. Therapeutic uses. Acetaminophen is used to relieve mild-to-moderate pain and reduce fever. Guidelines from the American College of Rheumatology now recommend it as first-line therapy for osteoarthritis of the knee and hip. Because it has minimal anti-inflammatory activity, it cannot be used to treat the swelling or stiffness resulting from rheumatoid arthritis.

2. Mechanism of action. The analgesic and antipyretic actions of acetaminophen are the same as those for aspirin (see I B 2 a–b).

3. Administration and dosage. Available dosage forms are 325 mg and 500 mg. A prolonged-dosage-form caplet of 650 mg is also available.

    a. For **analgesia** or **antipyresis in adults,** the dosage is 500–1000 mg three times daily as needed. The maximum daily dose is 4000 mg for no longer than 10 days for pain or 3 days for fever, without consulting a physician. For osteoarthritis, 1000 mg four times daily is recommended.

    b. For **children age 6 years or older,** 325 mg is administered every 4–6 hours as needed. The maximum daily dose is 1600 mg for no longer than 5 days for pain, 3 days for fever, or 2 days for sore throat, without consulting a physician.

    c. Routine use. Acetaminophen is routinely used in patients who are:

        (1) Sensitive to the GI disturbances caused by salicylates and NSAIDs

        (2) Prone to bleeding disorders

        (3) Hypersensitive to salicylates

4. Precautions. Patients with active alcoholism, hepatic disease, or viral hepatitis are at risk from chronic administration of acetaminophen. Toxicity is rare, but chronic daily ingestion of 5 g or more for longer than 1 month is likely to result in liver damage. Acute doses of 10 g or more are hepatotoxic.

5. Significant interactions. Acetaminophen may competitively inhibit the metabolism of **zidovudine,** resulting in potentiation of zidovudine or acetaminophen toxicity.

D. NSAIDs. Currently, **ibuprofen, naproxen,** and **ketoprofen** are the only NSAIDs available without a prescription.

1. Therapeutic uses. NSAIDs are used to relieve mild-to-moderate pain and reduce inflammation and fever. OTC drug use largely focuses on the analgesic and antipyretic indications of these agents. Maximum OTC drug dosage is generally recommended for osteoarthritis.

2. Mechanism of action

    a. Analgesic and anti-inflammatory actions. NSAIDs inhibit prostaglandin synthesis both peripherally and centrally. Like salicylates, these drugs inhibit cyclooxygenase (see Figure 31-1). NSAIDs produce analgesia mainly by blocking the peripheral generation of pain impulses that are mediated by prostaglandins and other chemicals. Secondarily, analgesia probably involves a reduction in the awareness of pain in the CNS.

    b. Antipyretic action. The principal antipyretic action is central. NSAIDs act on the hypothalamic heat-regulating center to produce peripheral vasodilation, which results from the inhibition of prostaglandin synthesis.

3. Administration and dosage. The available OTC dosage forms of ibuprofen are a 200-mg tablet and a 100-mg per 5-mL oral suspension. Naproxen sodium OTC is available as a 220-mg (200 mg of naproxen) tablet. Ketoprofen OTC is a 12.5-mg tablet.

    a. For **analgesia** or **antipyresis in adults,** the dosage of **ibuprofen** is 200–400 mg every 4–6 hours as needed. The maximum daily dose is 1200 mg for no longer than 10 days for pain or 3 days for fever, without consulting a physician. For **naproxen sodium,** the recommended dose is 220 mg every 8–12 hours as needed. The maximum daily dose is 660 mg. **Ketoprofen** is recommended as 12.5 mg every 4–6 hours as needed, with a maximum daily dose of 75 mg. Both naproxen and ketoprofen caution about the same limitations on the duration of treatment without consulting a physician as recommended for ibuprofen.

    b. For **rheumatoid arthritis dosage in adults, ibuprofen** is recommended to a maximum daily dosage of 3200 mg (administered on a 4–6-hour basis), **naproxen sodium** to a daily maximum of 1100 mg (divided in doses every 8–12 hours), and **ketoprofen** to a maximum of 300 mg per day (administered every 4–6 hours).

    c. Naproxen sodium and **ketoprofen** are not recommended for children under 12 years of age. **Ibuprofen** is available as a suspension for children 2–11 years of age.

4. Precautions

    a. NSAIDs are contraindicated in patients with **bleeding disorders** or **peptic ulcers.**

    b. NSAIDs are recommended with extreme caution during the last trimester of **pregnancy** because of:

        (1) Potential adverse effects on fetal blood flow

        (2) The possibility of prolonging pregnancy

    c. GI disturbances resulting from the inhibition of the gastric prostaglandins occur in 5%–10% of people at analgesic and antipyretic doses. Anti-inflammatory regimens (i.e., higher doses) affect up to 20% of people. These percentages decrease by taking NSAIDs with food or large doses of antacids. Ibuprofen is often preferred to aspirin by patients because ibuprofen causes fewer GI disturbances and bleeding events.

    d. Renal toxicity during chronic administration is a significant concern and may occur in the form of nephrotic syndrome, hyperkalemia, or interstitial nephritis.

5. Significant interactions

    a. NSAIDs potentiate the effect of **anticoagulants** and **thrombolytic agents.**

    b. NSAIDs potentiate (at anti-inflammatory doses) the effect of **hypoglycemics.**

    c. NSAIDs potentiate the adverse GI reactions resulting from chronic **alcohol** or **salicylate** use.

    d. Caffeine taken in conjunction with ibuprofen appears to enhance the analgesic effect.

    e. Hypersensitivity to **aspirin** can occur with NSAID use.

    f. OTC labeling for these agents cautions against use of an NSAID with other NSAIDs.

II. THE COMMON COLD

A. General

1. The common cold has been described as the **most expensive illness** in the United States. It is estimated that **30 million days** are lost from work or school each year due to the common cold.

2. In the United States, **100 million cases** are reported annually. Generally, adults will have 2–4 colds per year; children (preschoolers) will have 6–10 colds per year.

3. There is probably no other category of self-medication that requires more of the pharmacist in terms of time, advice, and patient counseling.

4. Although certain single OTC medications and combinations have been shown to reduce cold symptoms in adults and adolescents, there is very limited demonstrated effectiveness data for these agents in preschool children.

B. Etiology

1. There are **about 200 identified viral strains** that invade the nasal and bronchial epithelial cells to cause the common cold.

2. The viruses **most commonly responsible** for the common cold are the **rhinoviruses** (about 50% of cases) followed by the **coronaviruses.**

3. In order to produce infection, a rhinovirus must penetrate the protective mucous blanket that covers the nasal epithelium.

4. Mucus in the nasal passages traps and removes most contaminants, but the rhinovirus remains attached to the **nasal mucous membranes** via a specific receptor.

5. Rhinovirus infection leads to the release of various **inflammatory mediators.** Mediators like **prostaglandins, leukotrienes,** and **kinins** are involved in symptoms such as nasal congestion, runny nose, and sore throat.

6. Histamine is not involved in the inflammation associated with rhinovirus infection, but it is associated with the immediate phase of allergic response (sneezing and itching). Now that the importance of chemical mediators in the common cold is understood, new therapies can be developed to relieve symptoms. Because inflammation plays a dominant role, anti-inflammatory therapy may emerge as an appropriate course of action (Figure 31-2).

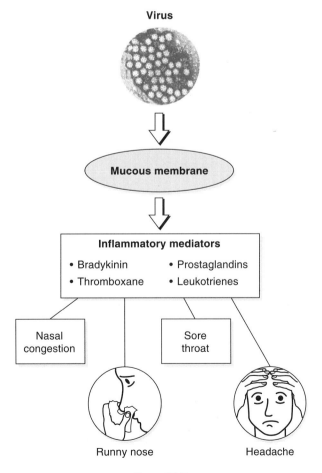

Figure 31-2.

7. Scientists believe that the common cold is actually **200 different infections** caused by 200 viruses. Each infection may result in lifetime immunity or at least long-term immunity so that each cold endured means one less virus to worry about. Indeed, people generally get fewer colds as they get older. Immunity is partly responsible, but less contact with children as people age may be an even more important factor.

C. Pathogenesis

1. Experts disagree on how colds are transmitted. Some say through the air (i.e., in the mist created by a sneeze). Evidence favors **direct contact,** such as shaking hands with a cold sufferer who has just blown his nose, as the main route of transmission.

2. On the skin, certain fabrics, and hard nonporous materials, such as stainless steel and wood, self-inoculation occurs readily. These **viruses can survive up to 3 hours outside the body.** For example, a susceptible person picks up the virus from a **contaminated surface** and then, when **fingers rub the nose or eyes, transfers** the **virus** to the **nasal mucous membranes** (a favorite nesting spot of the cold virus).

3. Shaking hands, opening a door, picking up a toy, and rubbing noses are **more frequent infection routes** than sneezing, coughing, and even kissing. It is probably easier to catch a cold by shaking hands than by kissing. Cold viruses are present in very low amounts in saliva. Studies of kissing couples (one with a cold, one without) found that kissing seldom led to inoculation.

4. "Catching" a cold occurs most probably by having contact with the hands of an infected person as well as objects that the infected person has touched.

5. To **avoid infection,** experts advise:
   a. Washing hands frequently with soap and hot water *(this is probably the simplest and most effective way to keep from getting colds or spreading them)*
   b. Keeping **hands away from the eyes and nose**
   c. Washing contaminated objects or surfaces
   d. Using disposable tissues instead of a handkerchief
   e. Covering a cough or a sneeze

6. Getting chilled or wet will not cause a cold. Viruses, not weather, cause colds. Studies have shown that people exposed to bone-chilling temperatures, icy baths, and drafts with or without wet feet or hair do not catch colds unless they are exposed to viruses. Colds are more common in winter because: (a) humidity is low (cold viruses survive better in low humidity); (b) cold weather dries the lining of the nasal passages, making them more vulnerable; and (c) people (especially kids in school) spend more time indoors and thus are exposed to more viruses.

7. Several factors affecting susceptibility and transmission of viruses have been identified. **Poor nutritional state, fatigue,** and **emotional stress** are all associated with decreased resistance to viral infection.

8. Children's noses have been called "the chief reservoirs for infectious rhinoviruses." Preschoolers have the most colds (between 6 and 10 per year), and young parents (especially mothers) often catch the virus from their children.

D. Symptoms

1. The **common cold** is usually **benign** and **self-limiting.** Typically, cold symptoms begin slowly, 18–48 hours after exposure to a virus.

2. The **first symptoms** are usually a **scratchy, sore throat** followed by a **runny nose, watery–itchy eyes, sneezing,** and a general feeling of **fatigue.** Patients note an increase in the secretions found in the nose, throat, and bronchial tubes, and a cough may develop.

3. With time, the **watery discharge** is transformed to a **thick, tenacious consistency.** Generally, the most annoying and troublesome symptoms of the **cold last approximately 4–5 days,** with symptoms gradually diminishing and disappearing **completely after 10 days** or so.

4. There are **five symptom areas** where a pharmacist can recommend treatment: **stuffy or runny nose, sore or scratchy throat, cough, headache,** and a general feeling of **malaise.**

E. Treatment

 1. **Decongestants. Nasal** decongestants are **sympathomimetic amines.** They stimulate the α-adrenergic receptors of vascular smooth muscle, which constrict dilated arterioles. Vessels that are located within the nasal mucosa become smaller and less engorged with blood. This decreases edema and, thus, increases nasal ventilation and drainage. Headache caused by congested sinuses may also be relieved. **Excessive nose blowing,** which irritates the nostrils and mucous membranes, is decreased with the use of decongestants. Too much nose blowing can further spread the virus and cause discomfort to the patient due to the possibility of pushing infected fluids into nasal sinuses or into the eustachian tubes. Decongestants may be applied to the nasal mucosa or taken orally.

   a. **Intranasal decongestants**

      (1) Intranasal decongestants induce **prompt and profound vasoconstriction** with relief of congestion.

      (2) The **major disadvantage** for **intranasal decongestants** is the potential to develop a **rebound congestion** (rhinitis medicamentosa). Rebound congestion may be expected whenever topical decongestants are **used longer than 3–5 days.** This effect is more common with the short-acting agents.

         (a) The **mechanism** for rebound congestion is not completely known. If the patient truly has a cold, a duration of 3–5 days for the use of topical decongestants is all that will usually be necessary.

         (b) **Treatment** of rebound congestion

            (i) The simplest but least comfortable therapy for rebound congestion is to **completely withdraw** the topical vasoconstrictor.

            (ii) As this action above promptly results in bilateral vasodilation with total nasal obstruction, a more acceptable method is to **initially discontinue the medication in only one nostril.** When the rebound condition subsides in the drug-free nostril (normally 1–2 weeks), a total withdrawal from the other side is undertaken.

            (iii) An alternative approach is to discontinue the topical decongestant and **give an oral decongestant.**

            (iv) The patient can use **saline drops or spray** (i.e., Ocean, Ayr, NaSal). A saline product has the dual function of keeping the nasal mucosa moist while providing psychological assistance to the individual. ("We're doing something for the nose.")

      (3) These topical agents have varying durations of action. Selection of these agents can be administered in a convenient every 12-hour dosage form [e.g., oxymetazoline (Afrin)].

      (4) These topical agents usually are not absorbed to any significant extent to cause problems with the patient who has high blood pressure. Because of the short duration of any blood pressure–elevating effect, the short-acting agents should be used if a topical decongestant is needed in a hypertensive patient. Some of these products may not be used in young children (e.g., topical naphazoline has resulted in CNS depression in young children).

      (5) These agents are similarly effective in equipotent doses with duration of action varying. The addition of aromatic vapors (e.g., menthol, camphor, eucalyptol) does not add any therapeutic benefit.

      (6) **Topical saline nasal products** are recommended for children less than age 2 years (unless directed by a physician) and pregnant women (because of concern of possible harm to the fetus by sympathomimetic agents). Because infants less than 6 months of age are obligate nose breathers, saline should be used because the sympathomimetic decongestants could cause rebound congestion and apnea in these patients.

      (7) These are the intranasal decongestants approved by the Food and Drug Administration (FDA):

         (a) Ephedrine (topical) 0.5% (q 4–6h)—**not less than (NLT) age 6 years**

         (b) Naphazoline (topical) 0.025%–0.05% (Privine) [q 4–6h]—**NLT age 12 years**

         (c) Phenylephrine (topical) 0.125%–1% (Neo-Synephrine, Nostril) [q 4–6h]

         (d) Propylhexedrine (inhaled) [Benzedrex] (q 2h)—**NLT age 6 years**

         (e) 1-Desoxyephedrine (inhaled) [Vicks Inhaler] (q 2h)—**NLT age 6 years**

         (f) Xylometazoline (topical) 0.05%–0.1% (Otrivin) [q 8–10h]

         (g) Oxymetazoline (topical) 0.025%–0.05% (Afrin, Neo-Synephrine 12 Hour, Nostrilla) [q 12h]

      (8) See Table 31-1 for patient counseling information.

Table 31-1. Patient Counseling Information on Nasal Decongestants

Drops	Spray (Atomizer)	Inhalers	Metered-Dose Pump (Spray)
• Blow your nose. • Squeeze rubber bulb on dropper and withdraw medication from bottle. • Recline on a bed and hang head over the side (preferred) OR tilt head back while standing or sitting. • Place drops into each nostril and gently tilt the head from side to side to distribute the drug. • Keep head tilted back for several minutes after instilling the drops. • Rinse the dropper with hot water.	• Blow your nose. • Remove cap from spray container. • For best results, do not shake the squeeze bottle. • Administer one spray with head in upright position. • Sniff deeply while squeezing the bottle. • Wait 3–5 minutes and blow nose. • Administer another spray if necessary. • Rinse the spray tip with hot water taking care not to allow water to enter the bottle. • Replace cap.	• Blow your nose. • Warm inhaler in your hand to increase volatility of the medication. • Remove the protective cap. • Inhale medicated vapor in one nostril while closing off the other nostril; repeat in other nostril. • Wipe the inhaler clean after each use. • Replace cap immediately. • Note: Inhaler loses its potency after 2–3 months even though the aroma may linger.	• Blow your nose. • Remove the protective cap. • Prime the metered pump by depressing several times (for first use), pointing away from the face. • Hold the bottle with the thumb at the base and nozzle between first and second fingers. • Insert pump gently into the nose with the head upright. • Depress pump completely, and sniff deeply. • Wait 3–5 minutes, and then blow nose. • Administer another spray if necessary. • Rinse the spray tip with hot water, taking care not to allow water to enter the bottle. • Replace cap.

b. Oral decongestants

(1) An oral decongestant may be useful in reaching deep into the **nasopharyngeal** and **sinus passages** where topical solutions may not be accessible. Because oral agents induce less intense vasoconstriction locally, they have not been associated with rebound congestion.

(2) Oral agents also may be favored for use in **small children** when topical application of a sympathomimetic amine may sometimes prove difficult.

(3) Because these agents are administered orally, potential systemic **side effects** may be more likely. CNS stimulation is the most common.

(4) Oral decongestants should be **avoided (or used cautiously)** in patients with problems such as **heart disease, hypertension, diabetes, hyperthyroidism, benign prostatic hypertrophy,** and **narrow angle glaucoma.** (Pseudoephedrine may have the least effect on blood pressure in the controlled hypertensive population.)

(5) Decongestants are **contraindicated** in patients taking monoamine oxidase (**MAO) inhibitors.**

(6) FDA-approved oral decongestants include:[*]
   (a) Phenylephrine 10 mg q 4h
   (b) Pseudoephedrine 60 mg q 6h (Sudafed)

(7) General **guidelines** for dosages for **children** regarding decongestants (Note: This also applies to antihistamines, guaifenesin, and antitussives.)
   (a) Ages 6–12 years—$1/2$ the adult dose
   (b) Ages 2–6 years—$1/4$ the adult dose
   (c) Under age 2 years—not specified

---

*Note–Phenylpropanolamine was removed from the market in late 2000 because of its association with hemorrhagic stroke in some patients.

    c. Nasal strips (e.g., Breathe Right). This is an adhesive bandage device (looks like a Band-Aid) that pulls open the nostrils and might relieve nasal congestion and decrease snoring. This device might be useful in persons who need to avoid the sympathomimetic agents (e.g., pregnant women). Even though these products are used by athletes and might improve breathing, there is no evidence that their use results in improved athletic performance.

2. Antihistamines

    a. Overview. A common cold is an infection caused by a virus that results in the release of chemicals called **kinins.** Kinins cause inflammation in the lining of the nose. This inflammation results in sneezing, runny nose, and stuffiness.

    b. Use. Although antihistamines have been prescribed by physicians for colds for decades (presumably because the symptoms are similar to those caused by allergies), scientific studies have conclusively demonstrated that these symptoms are **not** caused by **histamine.** Therefore, it is generally viewed that there is **questionable rationale for the use of antihistamines** to treat the common cold (may **rely on the anticholinergic effect** of these agents). The use of antihistamines to treat the common cold is **controversial.** Some studies show no effect, whereas others have shown **a decrease in sneezing and nasal secretions (runny nose)** with specific antihistamines (e.g., chlorpheniramine, doxylamine, clemastine). These studies' results should not be extrapolated to all of the available antihistamines, although the FDA announced in summer 2000 that it intends to allow the indications for sneezing and runny nose caused by the common cold to be part of the first-generation antihistamine final monograph.

    c. Classes of first-generation antihistamines

        (1) Alkylamines

            (a) Brompheniramine—4 mg q 4–6h (Dimetane)

            (b) Dexbrompheniramine—6 mg q 12h (time-release in Drixoral)

            (c) Chlorpheniramine—4 mg q 4–6h (Chlor-Trimeton, Teldrin)

            (d) Pheniramine—12.5–25 mg q 4–6h

            (e) Triprolidine—2.5 mg q 6–8h (in Actifed)

        (2) Ethylenediamines

            (a) Pyrilamine—25–50 mg q 6–8h

            (b) Thonzylamine—50–100 mg q 6–8h

        (3) Ethanolamines

            (a) Diphenhydramine—25–50 mg q 4–6h (Benadryl)

            (b) Doxylamine—7.5 mg q 4–6h

            (c) Clemastine—1.34 mg q 12h (in Tavist)

        (4) Piperidines (e.g., Phenindamine—25 mg q 4–6h)

    d. Side effects

        (1) Because of their anticholinergic properties, first-generation antihistamines may cause **dry mouth ("cotton mouth"), blurred vision, difficulty in urination, constipation, irritability,** and **dizziness** (see III B 1).

        (2) Patients with **narrow angle glaucoma** and **benign prostatic hypertrophy** should **avoid first-generation antihistamines** because the anticholinergic activities may exacerbate their condition.

        (3) It has long been thought that asthma sufferers should not take first-generation antihistamines because their anticholinergic properties would exacerbate asthma; however, the FDA found no evidence that the mucus-drying action is harmful in asthmatic patients.

        (4) Other side effects of first-generation antihistamines include nausea, vomiting, and **GI upset.** GI upset is more common with the ethylenediamines.

        (5) OTC antihistamines vary in the degree of drowsiness produced. All OTC first-generation antihistamines have sedative effects, but **ethanolamines** cause the **most sedation.** Among the most potent H_1-antagonists is the chemical class of alkylamines, which include chlorpheniramine (Chlor-Trimeton) and brompheniramine (Dimetane). These agents **(alkylamines) have a lower incidence of drowsiness** and may cause **CNS stimulation** (usually in children; caution should be noted in hyperactive children receiving antihistamines).

        (6) The newer, **second-generation antihistamines,** which are currently available by prescription (with the exception of Loratadine) have difficulty crossing the blood–brain barrier. Consequently, they tend to cause fewer unwanted CNS sedative effects. None of these agents has significant anticholinergic effects.

3. **Expectorants and antitussives.** Cough is a physiological protective reflex that assists in clearing the respiratory tract of mucus, inhaled irritants, and other foreign debris. Coughing from the common cold usually is caused by stimulation of cough receptors located within the **epithelial lining** of the **tracheobronchial tree.** The **cough center** in the **medulla** coordinates a series of events that leads to the cough response. A cough may be nonproductive or productive. **Nonproductive** coughs can be suppressed with **antitussives. Productive** coughs respond best to increased fluid intake and an OTC **expectorant.** Productive coughs generally should not be suppressed because they are essential to the removal of accumulated debris.

a. **Antitussives**
   (1) Patients with **dry, nonproductive coughs** are candidates for therapeutic cough suppression. Such coughs, if persistent, bothersome, or sleep disrupting, may be suppressed with an **antitussive.**
   (2) The nonproductive cough, if not treated, may become self-perpetuating as rapid air expulsion via the cough (up to 75 mph) may cause further irritation of the tracheal and pharyngeal mucosa.
   (3) Antitussives inhibit or suppress coughing. Most act centrally to depress the medullary cough center and thus elevate the threshold for incoming cough impulses. Examples include **narcotics,** such as **codeine,** and the nonnarcotic antitussive **dextromethorphan.**
   (4) Antitussives may act peripherally on sensory nerve receptors within the respiratory tract. These agents are exemplified by the volatile agents such as **camphor** and **menthol** (e.g., Vicks Vaporub).
   (5) There are limited data that support the efficacy of these agents for cough due to colds.
   (6) **Demulcents,** such as hard candy or cough drops, soothe an irritated throat and bronchial passageway and may produce an antitussive action.
   (7) **FDA-approved OTC antitussives** include the following:
      (a) **Codeine** and its salts are widely used cough suppressants and the standard against which all other antitussives are measured (dose = 10–20 mg q 4–6h).
         (i) The potential for codeine **abuse** is negligible but has been observed.
         (ii) Because codeine in this dosage form is schedule C-V, its OTC sale in cough syrups may be restricted in some states.
         (iii) **Adverse effects** include drowsiness, lightheadedness, excitement, loss of appetite, nausea and vomiting, headache, abdominal discomfort, and constipation.
         (iv) **Children** under 6 years of age are most vulnerable to serious adverse effects of codeine.
         (v) **Respiratory depression** usually occurs with prescription analgesic doses of this drug. Respiratory arrest, coma, and death have been reported in the less than 6 years of age group following single doses of 5–12 mg/kg.
      (b) **Dextromethorphan** is a synthetic nonnarcotic agent, having no analgesic or addictive properties (dose = 10–20 mg q 4h or 30 mg q 6–8h).
         (i) As a cough suppressant, it is as effective as codeine on a milligram-to-milligram basis.
         (ii) Dextromethorphan may be indicated in persons for whom adverse effects of codeine are particularly bothersome.
         (iii) Usual therapeutic doses do not cause a significant effect on either respiratory or cardiovascular functions.
         (iv) Adverse effects include drowsiness, GI upset, nausea, and dizziness.
         (v) Pharmacists should be aware of reports of high-dose recreational abuse of this agent.
      (c) **Diphenhydramine** is an antihistamine and antitussive agent. Its antitussive effects are due to its central-acting mechanism through the medullary cough center (dose = 25 mg q 4h).
         (i) Diphenhydramine **acts centrally** on the cough center similarly to codeine, rather than by generalized depression of the CNS.
         (ii) Part of diphenhydramine's antitussive action may be mediated through **anticholinergic activity.**
         (iii) As an ethanolamine antihistamine, this agent may produce **sedation** and symptoms of anticholinergic action (e.g., dry mouth, blurred vision, urinary retention).

(d) Camphor and menthol. A 4.7%–5.3% camphor and a 2.6%–2.8% menthol concentration in petrolatum (e.g., Vick's Vaporub) rubbed on the chest or neck effectively reduces coughing. Likewise, **camphor** and **menthol used in a hot steam vaporizer** at a concentration of 6.2% camphor or 3.2% menthol in water are safe and effective antitussives. **Menthol,** in doses of 5–10 mg in a **lozenge** (e.g., Hall's Mentho-Lyptus) or a compressed tablet dissolved in the mouth, is safe and effective as an antitussive.

(i) These agents produce a sensation of coolness on the respiratory tract, presumably by stimulating cold sensory receptors. This engenders a **local anesthetic effect** on respiratory passageways, which produces an antitussive effect.

b. Expectorants

(1) Expectorants purportedly **facilitate removal of mucus** and other irritants from the respiratory tract. This supposedly produces formation of less tenacious secretions and/or **decreases the viscosity of thickened secretions.** Some clinicians believe that an **expectorant action is best obtained by pushing fluids (i.e., 8–10 glasses of water per day).**

(2) Their major pharmacological action is to irritate receptors in the gastric mucosa. This promotes increased output from secretory glands of the GI system and reflexively increases flow of fluids from glands lining the respiratory tract. The outcome is increased volume and decreased viscosity of bronchial secretions.

(3) Guaifenesin (e.g., Robitussin) is the **only expectorant** that has demonstrated safety and efficacy for self-administration per the FDA. There is still controversy as to whether this agent is truly effective (dose = 200–400 mg q 4h).

(a) Guaifenesin occasionally causes gastric disturbance, nausea, and vomiting. Taking it with a full glass of water may reduce gastric irritation.

(b) Because of the conflicting therapeutic end points, some clinicians **question the rationale for combined use** in the same product of an **antitussive** and an **expectorant** (e.g., Robitussin DM).

4. Demulcents are used to relieve dry or sore throat. Sucking on hard candy works by promoting salivary flow, which is soothing. Often, **lozenges** and **gargles** containing analgesics may help soothe a sore throat, though relief is only short term because the antiseptics and topical anesthetics found in these products are not powerful enough to fight off a virus. If demulcents or gargles do not relieve discomfort to a tolerable level, local **anesthetic sprays** (e.g., Chloraseptic) or lozenges such as benzocaine may be administered to provide short-term comfort. These remedies should be given every 3–4 hours.

5. Analgesics. Early symptoms of the common cold include **mild malaise** and **headaches.** OTC products available to relieve these symptoms include aspirin, acetaminophen, ibuprofen, naproxen sodium, and ketoprofen.

6. Combination products

a. It is best to treat a specific symptom that is causing the patient most difficulty, as opposed to recommending a "shotgun" product with a large number of ingredients that may not be necessary. Such a product may expose the patient to the possibility of side effects for medications that are not needed (e.g., Nyquil).

b. There are a large number of combination cough and cold products on the market. Certain product name designations help to identify the ingredients (Table 31-2).

(1) "Nighttime" or **"PM"** usually signifies that the product contains **diphenhydramine** or, more rarely, **doxylamine.**

(2) "Sinus" usually signifies a **decongestant** (e.g., pseudoephedrine) and/or an **analgesic** (e.g., acetaminophen).

(3) "Cough" usually signifies that the product contains **dextromethorphan.**

(4) "No drowsiness" or **"daytime"** on the label usually indicates that the product contains a **decongestant** (e.g., pseudoephedrine) and does not contain an antihistamine.

(5) "Allergy" signifies that it contains an **antihistamine.**

(6) "AM" indicates that it contains a decongestant (i.e., no antihistamine).

(7) "Cold" or **"flu"** usually signifies that it contains a **decongestant** or **decongestant and antihistamine.**

7. Zinc. A well-publicized study in 1996 suggested that zinc administration **could speed the recovery from a cold**—coughing, headaches, hoarseness, congestion, runny noses, and

Table 31-2. Tylenol Products (January, 2003)

	Trade Name		Antihistamine	Decongestant	Cough Agents	Diuretic
				Active Ingredients		
1	Tylenol Extra Strength	Acetaminophen				
2	Tylenol Regular Strength	Acetaminophen				
3	Tylenol Arthritis Pain Extended Relief	Acetaminophen				
4	Tylenol Sore Throat Liquid	Acetaminophen				
5	Infant's Tylenol Concentrated Drops	Acetaminophen				
6	Children's Tylenol Chewable Tablets	Acetaminophen				
7	Junior Strength Tylenol Chewable Tablets	Acetaminophen				
8	Children's Tylenol Suspension Liquid	Acetaminophen				
9	Tylenol PM	Acetaminophen	Diphenhydramine			
10	Women's Tylenol Menstrual Relief	Acetaminophen				Pamabrom
11	Tylenol Sinus Day Non-Drowsy	Acetaminophen		Pseudoephedrine		
12	Children's Tylenol Sinus Chewable Tablets	Acetaminophen		Pseudoephedrine		
13	Infant's Tylenol Cold Concentrated Drops	Acetaminophen		Pseudoephedrine		
14	Tylenol Severe Allergy	Acetaminophen	Diphenhydramine			
15	Children's Tylenol Sinus Liquid Suspension	Acetaminophen		Pseudoephedrine		
16	Tylenol Sinus **Day**/Night Convenience Pack	Acetaminophen		Pseudoephedrine		
17	**Night**	Acetaminophen	Doxylamine	Pseudoephedrine		
18	Tylenol Cold Day Non-Drowsy	Acetaminophen		Pseudoephedrine	Dextromethorphan	
19	Children's Tylenol Cold Liquid	Acetaminophen	Chlorpheniramine	Pseudoephedrine		
20	Children's Tylenol Cold Chewable Tablets	Acetaminophen	Chlorpheniramine	Pseudoephedrine		
21	Tylenol Flu Day Non-Drowsy	Acetaminophen		Pseudoephedrine	Dextromethorphan	
22	Tylenol Flu Night Time	Acetaminophen	Diphenhydramine	Pseudoephedrine		
23	Tylenol Sinus Night Time	Acetaminophen	Doxylamine	Pseudoephedrine		
24	Tylenol Allergy Sinus Day Time	Acetaminophen	Chlorpheniramine	Pseudoephedrine		
25	Tylenol Allergy Sinus Night Time	Acetaminophen	Diphenhydramine	Pseudoephedrine		
26	Infant's Tylenol Cold Plus Cough Concentrated Drops	Acetaminophen		Pseudoephedrine	Dextromethorphan	
27	Children's Tylenol Allergy-D Liquid	Acetaminophen	Diphenhydramine	Pseudoephedrine		
28	Tylenol Cold **Day**/Night Convenience Pack	Acetaminophen		Pseudoephedrine		
29	**Night**	Acetaminophen	Chlorpheniramine	Pseudoephedrine		
30	Tylenol Cold Night Time Complete Formula	Acetaminophen	Chlorpheniramine	Pseudoephedrine	Dextromethorphan	
31	Tylenol Cold Severe Congestion Non-Drowsy	Acetaminophen		Pseudoephedrine	Dextromethorphan & guaifenesin	
32	Children's Tylenol Flu Suspension Liquid	Acetaminophen	Chlorpheniramine	Pseudoephedrine	Dextromethorphan	
33	Children's Tylenol Cold Plus Cough Liquid	Acetaminophen	Chlorpheniramine	Pseudoephedrine	Dextromethorphan	
34	Children's Tylenol Cold Plus Cough Chewable Tablets	Acetaminophen	Chlorpheniramine	Pseudoephedrine	Dextromethorphan	

sore throats disappeared in fewer days (4.4 days versus 7.6 days on placebo); subsequent studies have not been able to confirm this benefit. Because a large percentage of the zinc group (80% versus 30% in the placebo group) reported a bad taste in their mouths, there were questions regarding bias in this study because patients may have known they were on zinc, perhaps leading them to believe that they would recover faster.

8. **Echinacea** (see Chapter 34). Trials in Germany have suggested that extracts of this agent can reduce the severity and duration of cold symptoms. Echinacea is thought to stimulate the immune system by **increasing the number of white blood cells.** There are numerous kinds of echinacea and dosage forms, which makes interpretation of study results difficult. Because of its potential to stimulate immune cells, patients with autoimmune disorders, such as rheumatoid arthritis and lupus, should avoid this agent.

9. **Vitamin C.** Several controlled studies have failed to validate earlier reports that high-dose vitamin C is effective in preventing the common cold. A few studies have suggested that this agent may slightly reduce the severity of cold symptoms, but **most of the research shows no benefit.**

F. Patients with the following signs or symptoms should be referred for medical follow-up because these may indicate the presence of **strep throat, bacterial pneumonia,** or **other** more **serious** infections.

1. A **fever** greater than 101°F (38.3°C) accompanied by shaking chills, and coughing up thick phlegm (especially if greenish or foul smelling)

2. Sharp chest pain when taking a deep breath

3. Cold-like symptoms that do not improve after 7 days

4. Any fever greater than 103°F or 39.4°C

5. Coughing up blood

6. Any significant throat pain in a child

7. A painful throat in addition to any of the following:
   a. Pus (yellowish-white spots) on the tonsils or throat
   b. Fever greater than 101°F or 38.3°C
   c. Swollen or tender glands or bumps in the front of the neck
   d. Exposure to someone who has a documented case of strep throat
   e. A rash that appears during or after a sore throat
   f. A history of rheumatic fever, rheumatic heart disease, kidney disease, or chronic lung disease, such as emphysema or chronic bronchitis

III. ALLERGIC RHINITIS (Table 31-3)

A. **Introduction.** Approximately 20% of Americans suffer symptoms of allergic rhinitis, which can be seasonal or perennial. **Seasonal** outbreaks are cyclic and associated with pollination patterns of offending allergens. Although seasonal rhinitis is commonly called **"hay fever,"** the term is inappropriate. Hay is not a causative agent, and fever is not a symptom. **Perennial** rhinitis is chronic and is caused by antigens, such as house dust or animal protein, that are not linked to the changing seasons.

1. There are **three separate allergy seasons.**
   a. Spring (trees)
   b. Late spring–early summer (grasses)
   c. Late summer to the first killing frost (weeds, most commonly **ragweed**)

2. **Symptoms** include **sneezing** episodes, **nasal pruritus** with **congestion, clear rhinorrhea, itching** of the **palate, conjunctival erythema** and **itching,** and **ear fullness** with popping and pressure on the cheeks and forehead. Constitutional feelings of weakness, malaise, and fatigue may also be seen.
   a. Symptoms are similar and overlap with those of the common cold. For this reason, consumers often refer to allergic rhinitis as a **"summer cold."**
   b. The symptoms associated with allergic rhinitis are due to an **immunoglobulin E** (IgE)-mediated immunological reaction.

Table 31-3. How Do the Common Cold and Allergic Rhinitis Differ?

Sign	Common Cold	Allergic Rhinitis
Sneezing	Occurs	Common
Nasal discharge	Mucopurulent; occurs especially during days 1–3	Watery; common, occurs anytime
Itchy nose and eyes	Occurs	Common
Watering and redness of eyes	Common	Common
Nasal congestion	Common	Common
Cough	Common, especially in later phase	Uncommon
Fever	Rare	Absent
Pruritus	Uncommon	Common
Inciting cause	Virus	Allergen
Occurrence	Anytime	Seasonal (seasonal type); anytime (perennial type)

3. **Pathophysiology.** The **allergic response** is divided into **several phases:** sensitization, early phase, cellular recruitment, and late phase. Inhaled allergens interact with T- and B-cell lymphocytes to produce IgE antibodies, which become attached to mast cells and basophils (sensitization). On subsequent reexposure to the allergen, degranulation of the mast cells and basophils occurs, causing the release of histamine, leukotrienes, prostaglandin, and bradykinin. Rhinorrhea, sneezing, itching, and discomfort occur within minutes as part of the **early-phase** response. A **late-phase** inflammatory response occurs 4–24 hours later, with migration and activation of eosinophils, neutrophils, basophils, macrophages, and monocytes in the nasal mucosa. Renewed allergic symptoms of increasing nasal secretions and nasal congestion occur without additional allergen exposure.

B. **Treatment.** The **best treatment** for allergic rhinitis, although not always practical, is to **avoid the allergen or allergens** that trigger the allergic symptoms. For example, if a patient is allergic to ragweed, counsel him or her to stay in an air-conditioned environment as much as possible. Air conditioning, with frequent filter changes, helps reduce the pollen count in the room. If the patient is allergic to dust mites, removing rugs, furniture, or mattresses that harbor dust mites is helpful. Encasing items such as mattresses in airtight plastic can also decrease the number of mites.

1. **Antihistamines**
   a. There are two types of H_1-receptor–blocking antihistamines: **first generation** (sedating, nonselective) and **second generation** (nonsedating, selective) agents. Most of the OTC agents are first-generation antihistamines, but as of December 2002, **loratadine** (Claritin, others) a second-generation agent, was approved for OTC marketing.
   b. The **first-generation** antihistamines cross the blood–brain barrier. **Drowsiness, sedation, dizziness, confusion,** and **slowed reaction time** are side effects. Drowsiness may be transient and tolerance may occur in some patients after 5–7 days of therapy. These agents also produce anticholinergic action, with **dry mouth, urinary retention, blurred vision,** and **constipation** as additional side effects. Also, these agents have been associated with decreased work and academic performance and higher accident (automobile and occupational) risks. Performance impairment may "spill over" into the next day after a nighttime dose.
   c. The **second-generation** antihistamines do not cross the blood–brain barrier and do not have anticholinergic actions, so sedation (rare) and anticholinergic side effects are not associated with these agents. They have a more favorable safety and side-effect profile.
   d. The **primary nonprescription medication** used to treat allergic rhinitis is an oral antihistamine. Antihistamines cause competitive blockade of the actions of histamine at H_1-receptor sites.
   e. If possible, antihistamine therapy should be started 1–2 weeks before a known allergy season or several hours before exposure to a known allergen. **Regular, rather than as needed, dosing** of antihistamines is more effective.

f. Whereas there are variations in potency, duration of action, and extent of adverse effects, there are no major therapeutic differences in the various OTC antihistamines.

g. Antihistamines **should be taken uninterrupted throughout the pollen season.** To be effective, they must combine with the specific histamine receptor and block histamine binding. This is a dynamic competition between the antihistamine and histamine.

h. Antihistamines are **useful for** treating the **sneezing, rhinorrhea, pruritus, lacrimation,** and **irritated itchy eyes** (early-phase symptoms). They do not work to correct nasal congestion (late-phase symptom).

i. The **first-generation** and **second-generation** antihistamines are **roughly of equal efficacy** in their ability to relieve symptoms of histamine release.

2. Decongestants

a. Antihistamines are less effective in reversing nasal and ocular congestion. Decongestants **counter congestion** and **help reverse drowsiness** associated with **first-generation antihistamines.**

b. Systemic decongestants are preferred when a decongestant action is required for longer than 3–5 days, because of the rebound congestion that occurs with intranasal decongestants.

c. If the patient does not respond fully to antihistamines alone (i.e., **continues to have nasal congestion)** the next step would be to **add an oral decongestant.**

d. See II E I for decongestant use and side effects.

3. Cromolyn sodium (Nasalcrom)

a. The proposed mechanism of action is **stabilization of mast cells,** interfering with calcium transport and induction of degranulation.

b. This agent is **more effective in treating seasonal** versus perennial allergic rhinitis.

c. It reduces rhinorrhea, congestion, and sneezing by the mechanism noted above.

d. To be maximumly effective, it must be **started 2–4 weeks before the exposure** of the offending allergens and continued throughout the contact period.

e. Dosed 4–6 times per day in each nostril initially, administration frequency may be decreased when the symptoms are under control.

f. To be effective, it **must be used on a regular basis.**

4. Prescription treatment

a. Corticosteroids

(1) Intranasal steroids have emerged as the most effective treatment of allergic rhinitis, relieving sneezing, nasal pruritus, congestion, and rhinorrhea associated with the inflammation.

(2) Intranasal steroids are ineffective in the treatment of ocular tearing or ocular pruritus.

(3) Symptom relief is thought to be related to the ability of steroids to inhibit the activity of multiple cell types (e.g., mast cells, basophils, eosinophils, neutrophils, macrophages, lymphocytes) and mediators of the inflammatory response.

(4) Decreased capillary permeability and decreased nasal mucous secretion also contribute to the effectiveness achieved by intranasal steroids.

(5) The more recently developed formulations of beclomethasone (Vancenase, Beconase), budesonide (Rhinocort), flunisolide (Nasalide), fluticasone (Flonase), and triamcinolone (Nasacort) avoid the adrenal suppression at recommended doses.

(6) Major **adverse effects** of intranasal steroids are local dryness or irritation as evidenced by stinging, irritation, nose bleeds, sore throat, or burning and irritation.

(7) It may take up to 3 weeks for the peak effects of clinical improvement to occur.

(8) Treatment with these medications should start at the first signs of clinical symptoms and is usually continued throughout the allergen season.

b. Ipratropium bromide (Atrovent) nasal spray **reduces rhinorrhea** via an anticholinergic effect in patients with allergic or nonallergic perennial rhinitis or the common cold. **It is not recommended for general use in allergic rhinitis** because it does not prevent itching or sneezing nor much improvement in nasal congestion. Forty percent of each dose is absorbed systemically, and drowsiness occurs in about 10% of patients.

c. Azelastine (Astelin) antihistamine nasal spray is approved for the treatment of seasonal allergic rhinitis symptoms. This agent appears **comparable in efficacy to oral antihistamines** and may be more tolerable than first-generation drugs. About 20% of patients note a bitter taste, and systemic absorption results in the potential for drowsiness (11%).

d. Montelukast (Singulair), the leukotriene inhibitor that has been used for asthma, has now been approved for the relief of symptoms of seasonal allergic rhinitis in patients over the age of 2. The dose is once daily, the same as for asthma.

e. Immunotherapy

(1) Immunotherapy is usually begun only when the patient does not show a response to environmental modification and pharmacotherapy or cannot tolerate the medications.

(2) Routine injections of the diluted antigen are administered initially, with the concentration of the antigen increasing over time.

(3) Although the precise mechanism is not known, serum IgE levels specific to the antigens given tend to decrease during the course of immunotherapy. Conversely, there is an increase in serum IgG levels. A blocking antibody is thought to compete with mast cell-bound IgE for antigen binding.

(4) Because of the **time** and the **expense** involved, immunotherapy is usually reserved for **moderate to severe cases** of chronic allergic rhinitis.

STUDY QUESTIONS

Directions: Each of the numbered items or incomplete statements in this section is followed by answers or by completions of the statement. Select the **one** lettered answer or completion that is **best** in each case.

1. Which statement concerning the use of OTC analgesic agents is true?

(A) Aspirin is indicated for mild to moderate analgesia, inflammatory diseases, antipyresis, and prophylaxis for patients with ischemic heart disease.

(B) Ibuprofen is indicated for mild to moderate analgesia, reduction of fever, and prophylaxis for patients with ischemic heart disease, but not for inflammatory disorders.

(C) Acetaminophen is indicated for mild to moderate analgesia but not for reduction of fever and arthritis.

(D) Naproxen sodium is indicated for mild to moderate analgesia, antipyresis, and prophylaxis for patients with ischemic heart disease.

2. Which statement concerning drug interactions with OTC analgesic agents is true?

(A) Aspirin potentiates the effects of antihypertensives, cardiac glycosides, and anticoagulants.

(B) Ibuprofen potentiates the effect of zidovudine, hypoglycemics, and aminoglycosides.

(C) Acetaminophen potentiates the effect of zidovudine.

(D) For naproxen sodium, the OTC dosage recommendations are similar to the prescription dosage.

3. All of the following statements concerning contraindications with **chronic** use of OTC analgesic agents are correct EXCEPT

(A) aspirin, ibuprofen, naproxen sodium, and ketoprofen are contraindicated in patients with bleeding disorders, peptic ulcer, and the third trimester of pregnancy

(B) aspirin, acetaminophen, and ibuprofen are implicated in Reye's syndrome

(C) acetaminophen is contraindicated in patients with active alcoholism, hepatic disease, or viral hepatitis

4. Which statement concerning dosage recommendations for OTC analgesic agents is true?

(A) Aspirin for analgesia or antipyresis in adults is 325–650 mg every 4 hours or 650–1000 mg every 6 hours, with a maximum daily dose of 4000 mg for no longer than 10 days for pain or 3 days for fever, without consulting a physician; the antirheumatic dosage for adults is 3600–4500 mg daily in divided doses; and patients with ischemic heart disease take 325 mg daily or every other day.

(B) Ibuprofen for analgesia or antipyresis in adults is 300–600 mg every 6–8 hours, with a maximum daily dose of 1800 mg for no longer than 10 days for pain or 3 days for fever, without consulting a physician; and the anti-inflammatory dosage for adults is 1800–3600 mg daily in divided doses.

(C) Acetaminophen for analgesia or antipyresis in adults is 325 mg every 8–12 hours, with a maximum daily dose of 2000 mg for no longer than 10 days for pain and 3 days for fever, without consulting a physician; and patients with ischemic heart disease take 325 mg daily or every other day.

5. A 57-year-old male with hypertension has a dry, irritating, nonproductive cough due to a "cold." He is feeling better on the fifth day of having common cold symptoms, and the cough is the only current problem. Of the following choices, the best recommendation for this patient would be

(A) a product that contains pseudoephedrine and chlorpheniramine

(B) a product that preferably contains only guaifenesin

(C) a product that contains dextromethorphan to be given at bedtime

(D) Nyquil (dextromethorphan, acetaminophen, doxylamine, pseudoephedrine)

(E) Sudafed (pseudoephedrine) long-acting tablets to be taken twice daily

6. A 32-year-old woman with perennial allergic rhinitis asks a pharmacist's advice for the treatment of her symptoms. She has never used any product for this condition and informs the pharmacist that she is hyperthyroid. Which of the following medicines would be the best recommendation?

(A) Sudafed 30-mg tablets—usual dose and frequency per directions on package
(B) Afrin nasal spray—2 sprays in each nostril bid
(C) Drixoral tablets (pseudoephedrine and dexbrompheniramine)—per directions on the package
(D) Chlor-Trimeton 12-mg sustained-action tablets—1 tablet p.o. q 12h
(E) Neo-synephrine nasal spray—2 sprays q 6h

7. A patient with seasonal allergic rhinitis comes into a pharmacy and asks the pharmacist to recommend a product for him. He has been taking Chlor-Trimeton 12-mg tablets bid with some significant relief, but he is still complaining of some nasal congestion. What would be the best recommendation for this patient?

(A) Switch to another antihistamine
(B) Afrin nasal spray—2 sprays in each nostril bid for 10 days
(C) Neo-Synephrine nasal spray—2 sprays in each nostril q 4h until congestion goes away
(D) Add an oral decongestant to the Chlor-Trimeton regimen
(E) Ocean nasal spray as required for nasal stuffiness

8. All of the following statements regarding the common cold are true EXCEPT

(A) about 75% of common colds are caused by rhinoviruses
(B) histamine is not involved in the inflammation associated with the common cold
(C) there is no vaccine available to prevent the common cold because there are so many viral strains involved in causing this condition
(D) when you are infected with a particular cold virus strain, lifetime or long-term immunity develops to that specific virus
(E) the incidence of colds is highest in children, followed next by mothers of young children

9. All of the following statements about intranasal decongestants are true EXCEPT

(A) the menthol present in some of these products results in an antitussive action in addition to the decongestant effect
(B) the metered-dose pump dosage form prevents "back flow" of nasal secretions that may occur with the atomizer-spray dosage form
(C) after it is opened, the inhaler dosage form loses its potency after 2–3 months
(D) ideally, one should restrict the use of a topical decongestant spray to one individual in the family to prevent spread of the cold virus from person to person
(E) a second administration of the nasal decongestant metered-dose pump can be given about 3–5 minutes after the first dose—the patient should blow his or her nose prior to this second administration

10. All of the following statements regarding Breathe-Right nasal strips are true EXCEPT they

(A) might relieve nasal congestion
(B) might decrease snoring
(C) might be useful for pregnant women where there is concern about the use of sympathomimetic decongestants
(D) have been proven to increase athletic performance
(E) look like a Band-Aid that is worn across the nose

11. All of the following measures would be useful in preventing the spread of the cold virus EXCEPT

(A) cover a cough or sneeze
(B) keep hands away from your eyes and nose
(C) make sure that a person with a cold is kept warm
(D) use disposable tissues rather than a cloth handkerchief
(E) wash hands frequently with soap and water

ANSWERS AND EXPLANATIONS

1. The answer is A *[I B].*
Aspirin is the only analgesic agent with an approved labeling for analgesia, antipyresis, inflammation, and prophylaxis for ischemic heart disease.

2. The answer is C *[I C].*
Acetaminophen may competitively inhibit the metabolism of zidovudine, resulting in potentiation of zidovudine or acetaminophen toxicity. As for the other choices, OTC dosage levels are generally one-half the prescription dosage; aspirin is not commonly recognized to interact with antihypertensives or cardiac glycosides; nor is acetaminophen expected to interact with aminoglycosides.

3. The answer is B *[I B 4 b].*
Aspirin is the only analgesic agent associated with the development of Reye's syndrome.

4. The answer is A *[I B 3, C 3, D 3].*
The aspirin dosage OTC recommendations are correct; the levels for acetaminophen are too low, and for ibuprofen, too high. In addition, acetaminophen does not carry an ischemic heart disease prophylaxis recommendation.

5. The answer is C *[II E 3 a].*
It appears that this patient's cold is resolving. The only bothersome symptom is a nonproductive cough. An antitussive should be given at bedtime to permit the patient to get some sleep. A product containing the safe and effective dextromethorphan is indicated. The patient has hypertension and usually should not take an oral decongestant. A single-ingredient product aimed at the specific symptom is best.

6. The answer is D *[III A, B].*
The patient should try to identify the cause of her allergic rhinitis and avoid the allergen if possible. Perennial allergic rhinitis is caused by things like animal dander and house dust mites. Keeping a pet outdoors, encasing pillows, etc. might be useful. Pharmacological treatment is usually begun with an antihistamine. The patient does not have any contraindications to this agent. Oral decongestants should usually be avoided when hyperthyroidism is present. Because of rebound congestion, topical agents are not indicated for long-term use in allergic rhinitis.

7. The answer is D *[III B 1, 2].*
The first line of pharmacological therapy is the antihistamines. These agents will correct most of the symptoms but may not completely alleviate the symptoms of nasal congestion. The addition of an oral decongestant would be the next therapeutic intervention. Tolerance to the therapeutic benefit may develop to the antihistamines with continued use, but in this patient, significant relief has been obtained; only the congestion remains. Topical decongestants can only be used for a few days, so they have limited value in allergic rhinitis.

8. The answer is A *[II B C 8].*
Approximately 50% of colds are caused by rhinoviruses. Histamine is not believed to be a chemical mediator that is released in response to viral invasion. There are up to 200 different viral strains that have been identified as causing the common cold; it is, therefore, virtually impossible to develop a vaccine that would be able to cover such a large spectrum of viruses. Immunity (oftentimes, lifetime) does develop to the specific strain that infects a person. Colds are most common in children because they have not had time to develop immunity to many of these agents. Women in their 20s and 30s are the next most commonly infected group because many of these women are mothers of the children who become infected with the cold virus and then end up having the virus transmitted to them.

9. The answer is A *[II E 3 a (7) (d) and Table 31-1].*
In the appropriate concentration as a lozenge, compressed tablet, or topical ointment, menthol is an effective antitussive. Small amounts of aromatic vapors (i.e., menthol, camphor, eucalyptol) do not add any therapeutic benefit to the topical sympathomimetic decongestants. The metered-dose pump dosage form does prevent "back flow" of nasal secretions. The inhaler dosage form does lose its potency after 2–3 months after it is opened, and it is appropriate to administer a second dose of decongestant after 3–5 minutes and after blowing the nose to ensure the appropriate spread of the medication into the nasal passages.

10. The answer is D *[II E 1 c].*
Nasal strips have been used by professional athletes with the thought that this might improve athletic performance because the nostrils are more "open" and, therefore, able to take in more oxygen. There is no proof of this, however. The United States Food and Drug Administration (FDA) approved the use of this agent for nasal congestion and snoring. It may be especially useful in patients who should not use topical or oral sympathomimetic amines (i.e., the pregnant patient).

11. The answer is C *[II C].*
The most likely route of transmission of the cold virus from one patient to the next is via nasal secretions from the infected person to the hands of the noninfected person, who then puts his or her fingers in the eye or nose. The virus is also spread via sneezing and coughing. Efforts should, therefore, be directed toward measures to break these transmission pathways. Covering a cough or sneeze, washing the hands frequently, using disposable tissues versus a handkerchief, and keeping one's fingers away from the eyes or nose are all appropriate methods to decrease transmission. Patients do not "catch a cold" simply by being exposed to a chilly or drafty environment; the cold virus must be present. Thus, keeping a patient warm has no bearing on the transmission of the common cold.

32
OTC Agents for Constipation, Diarrhea, Hemorrhoids, and Heartburn

Stephen H. Fuller
Michelle A. Long
Steven M. Davis

I. CONSTIPATION

A. General information

1. **Definition.** Constipation is the difficult or infrequent passage of stool. Normal stool frequency ranges from two to three times daily to two to three times per week. Patients may experience abdominal bloating, headaches, or a sense of rectal fullness from incomplete evacuation of feces.

2. **Causes.** Constipation can be caused by many factors, including:
   a. **Insufficient dietary fiber**
   b. **Lack of exercise**
   c. **Poor bowel habits,** such as failure to respond to the defecatory urge or hurried bowels (i.e., incomplete evacuation)
   d. **Medications,** such as narcotics, antacids, or anticholinergics (e.g., antidepressants, antihypertensives, antihistamines, phenothiazines, antispasmodics)
   e. **Organic problems,** such as intestinal obstruction, tumor, inflammatory bowel disease, diverticulitis, hypothyroidism, hyperglycemia, irritable bowel syndrome, cerebrovascular disease, or Parkinson's disease

3. **Practitioners should question the patient about the following:**
   a. Normal stool frequency
   b. Duration of the constipation
   c. Frequency of constipation episodes
   d. Exercise routine
   e. Amount of dietary fiber consumed
   f. Presence of other symptoms
   g. Medications used currently
   h. Medications used to relieve constipation and their effectiveness

B. Treatment

1. **Nonpharmacological**
   a. Increase intake of fluids and fiber (e.g., whole-grain breads and cereals, beans, prunes, raisins, peas, carrots, corn)
   b. Increase exercise to increase and maintain bowel tone
   c. Bowel training to increase regularity

2. **Pharmacological.** Therapeutic agents are classified according to their mechanism of action. Laxatives should not be taken if nausea, vomiting, or abdominal pain is present.
   a. **Bulk-forming laxatives.** These medications are natural or synthetic polysaccharide derivatives that adsorb water to soften the stool and increase bulk, which stimulates peristalsis. Bulk-forming laxatives work in both the small and large intestines. The onset of action of these agents is slow (12–24 hours and up to 72 hours), which is why they are best used to prevent constipation rather than to treat severe acute constipation. There are both natural and synthetic products. All bulk-forming agents must be given with at least 8 oz of water to minimize the possible constipation experienced by some patients. Some bulk-forming medications may contain sugar, so diabetics should use sugar-free products. Bulk-forming agents should not be used if patients have an obstructing bowel le-

sion, intestinal strictures, or Crohn's disease because they can make this situation worse and possibly result in bowel perforation.

(1) Natural bulk-forming laxatives

 (a) Psyllium (e.g., Metamucil, Konsyl-D, Fiberall, Perdium Fiber Granules). An **adult dosage** is 1 rounded teaspoon (3.5 g) in 8 oz of water one to three times per day. A **child's dosage** is half the adult dosage one to three times per day.

 (b) Malt soup extract (e.g., Maltsupex). An **adult dosage** is 8–16 g (1–2 scoops) two to four times per day. A **child's dosage** is 16 g one to two times per day.

(2) Synthetic bulk-forming laxatives

 (a) Methylcellulose (e.g., Citrucel). An **adult dosage** is 1–2 g (1 tablespoon) one to three times per day. A **child's dosage** is 0.5 g one to three times per day.

 (b) Polycarbophil (e.g., Konsyl Fiber, Fiber Con, Mitrolan). An **adult dosage** is 1 g (2 tablets) one to four times per day. A **child's dosage** is 0.5 g one to three times per day. Calcium polycarbophil may impair the absorption of tetracyclines if the drugs are taken concurrently.

b. Saline and **osmotic laxatives** work by creating an osmotic gradient to pull water into the small and large intestines. This increased volume results in distention of the intestinal lumen, causing increased peristalsis and bowel motility. These laxatives also increase the activity of cholecystokinin-pancreozymin, which is an enzyme that increases the secretion of fluids into the gastrointestinal (GI) tract. The **onset of action varies** depending on the ingredient and dosage form. Rectal formulations (e.g., enemas, suppositories) have an onset of action of 5–30 minutes, whereas oral preparations work within 3–6 hours.

(1) Saline laxatives include sodium and magnesium salts. As much as 20% of magnesium may be absorbed from these products, which may lead to hypermagnesemia in patients with preexisting renal impairment. Patients with hypertension or congestive heart failure should not receive saline laxatives on a prolonged basis due to fluid retention from sodium absorption. Products include:

 (a) Magnesium citrate (e.g., Magnesia Citrate): Adults, $\frac{1}{2}$ of bottle; children (6–12 yr), $\frac{1}{3}$ of bottle

 (b) Magnesium hydroxide (e.g., Phillips' Milk of Magnesia): Adults, 30 mL; children (6–12 yr), 15 mL; children (2–5 yr) 5–15 mL

 (c) Magnesium sulfate (e.g., Epsom salt): Adults, 5–10 mL in 8 oz of water; children (6–12 yr), 2.5–5 mL

 (d) Sodium phosphate (e.g., Fleet Phospho-Soda): Adults, 20–45 mL; children (6–12 yr), 5–20 mL

(2) Osmotic laxatives

 (a) Glycerin is available in rectal products in suppository or liquid form (e.g., Fleet Babylax). Rectal burning may occur with glycerin products. In addition to the osmotic effect, sodium stearate in these products can produce a local irritant effect. An **adult dose** is 3 g in suppository form or 5–15 mL as an enema. A **child's dose** is 1.5 g in suppository form or 2–5 mL as an enema.

 (b) Lactulose (e.g., Chronulac, Enulose) is available only by prescription and is used to decrease blood ammonia levels in hepatic encephalopathy. It may cause flatulence and cramping and should be taken with fruit juice, water, or milk to increase the palatability. An **adult dosage** is 15–30 mL one to two times daily. A **child's dosage** is 2.5–5 mL two to three times daily.

 (c) Sorbitol, a nonabsorbable sugar, is similar in efficacy to lactulose, which can be administered orally (70% solution) or rectally (25% solution). The **adverse effects** are the same and include flatulence, cramping, and abdominal pain over the first few days. An **adult dose** is 15 mL orally (70% solution) or 120 mL rectally (25% solution). A **child's dose** is 15 mL orally (70% solution) or 30–60 mL of a rectal solution (25%).

 (d) Polyethylene glycol 3350 (Miralax) is available only by prescription and can be used for bowel evacuation if other products have not worked. It has been shown to be more effective than lactulose in short-term trials with less abdominal cramping. An **adult dose** is 1 cap dissolved in 8 oz of clear fluid once daily for up to 2 weeks. A **child's dose** is 0.8 g/kg/day.

c. Stimulant laxatives. These medications work in the small and large intestines to stimulate bowel motility and increase the secretion of fluids into the bowel. All stimulant laxatives can cause abdominal cramping. The oral preparations usually have an onset of action within 6–10 hours. Rectal preparations usually have an onset of action within

30–60 minutes. Stimulant laxatives are effective as initial drug therapy to treat constipation but should not be used for more than 1 week. Chronic use of stimulant laxatives can lead to **cathartic colon,** which results in a poorly functioning colon and resembles the symptoms of ulcerative colitis. However, most cases of cathartic colon were published before 1960, when more toxic ingredients (e.g., podophyllin) were used in laxative products. Another issue surrounds the possible carcinogenicity of stimulant laxatives. Phenolphthalein was removed from the market as suggested by the FDA when data reported carcinogenic tumors and genetic damage in rats. Subsequently, senna and the structurally similar products aloe and cascara sagrada are now considered category III, with more data needed to assess their safety.

   (1) Anthraquinone laxatives include senna, cascara sagrada, and casanthranol. **Melanosis coli,** which is a dark pigmentation of the colonic mucosa, can result with long-term use of anthraquinone laxatives. This usually disappears 6–12 months after discontinuing the medication. In addition, there is no indication that melanosis results in adverse consequences. Discoloration (pink/red, yellow, or brown) of the urine may occur. Cascara sagrada is excreted into breast milk. Anthraquinone products include:

   (a) Sennosides (e.g., Senokot, Ex-Lax, Fletcher's Castoria) is considered to be more potent than cascara products; however, senna causes more abdominal cramping. An **adult dosage** of sennosides is 12–50 mg twice daily. A **child's dosage** is 6–25 mg twice daily.

   (b) Cascara sagrada. Liquid preparations of cascara are more reliable than solid dosage forms. An **adult dosage** is 300–1000 mg/day (or 200–400 mg of cascara extract, or 0.5–1.5 mL of fluid extract) once daily. Children should receive 50% of the adult dose.

   (c) Casanthranol is considered to be a mild stimulant laxative and is present in Peri-Colace, which also contains docusate. An **adult dose** is 30–90 mg once daily.

   (2) Bisacodyl (e.g., Dulcolax) is a **diphenylmethane derivative.** The tablet formulations of bisacodyl are enteric coated, so they should not be crushed or chewed. Also, bisacodyl-containing products should not be taken within 1 hour of ingesting antacids or milk. An **adult** oral dose is 5–15 mg daily, with children receiving 5 mg daily. The rectal dose is 10 mg (1 suppository) for adults and 5 mg ($\frac{1}{2}$ suppository) for children.

   (3) Castor oil (e.g., Purge) has an onset of action within 2–6 hours. Castor oil works primarily at the small intestine, which can result in strong cathartic effects (e.g., excessive fluid and electrolyte loss). These cathartic effects can lead to dehydration. Castor oil should not be used in pregnant patients because it may induce premature labor. An **adult dose** is 15–60 mL; a **child's dose** is 5–15 mL.

d. Emollient laxatives act as surfactants by allowing absorption of water into the stool, which makes the softened stool easier to pass. These medications are particularly useful in patients who must avoid straining to pass hard stools, such as those who recently had a myocardial infarction or rectal surgery. However, clinical trials evaluating emollient "stool-softening" laxatives show that these products, when compared to placebo, do not affect the weight or water content of the stool or the frequency of stool passing. Emollient laxatives have a **slow onset of action** (24–72 hours), which is why they are not considered the drug of choice for severe acute constipation, and they are more useful for preventing constipation.

   (1) Products. Emollient laxatives are salts of the surfactant **docusate.** These products contain insignificant amounts of calcium, sodium, or potassium, and there are no specific guidelines for the selection of any one product. The products include:

   (a) Docusate sodium (Colace, Exlax stool softener)

   (b) Docusate calcium (Surfak)

   (c) Docusate potassium (Kasof)

   (2) Dosage information. The **adult dosage** is 50–300 mg per day. A **child's dosage** is 50–150 mg per day. Each dose must be taken with at least 8 oz of water. Liquid preparations should be taken in fruit juice or infant formula to increase palatability. Docusate products may facilitate the systemic absorption of mineral oil, so these agents should not be used concurrently.

e. Lubricant laxative (mineral oil). Mineral oil works at the colon to increase water retention in the stool to soften the stool. It has an **onset of action** of 6–8 hours.

   (1) Dosage information. An **adult dosage** is 15–45 mL per day. A **child's dosage** is 5–15 mL per day.

(2) Warnings

(a) Mineral oil can **decrease absorption of fat-soluble vitamins** (i.e., vitamins A, D, E, and K), so it should not be used on a chronic basis.

(b) Elderly, young, debilitated, and dysphagic patients are at the greatest risk of **lipid pneumonitis** from mineral oil aspiration.

(c) Emollients (e.g., docusate) may increase the systemic absorption of mineral oil, which can lead to **hepatotoxicity.**

(d) Mineral oil products may cause anal seepage, which results in itching (i.e., pruritus ani) and perianal discomfort. Mineral oil should be taken on an empty stomach.

(e) Mineral oil should not be given to patients with rectal bleeding or appendicitis.

(f) Mineral oil should not be given to children less than 6 years of age.

C. Special patient issues

1. Pediatric patients. The bowel patterns of pediatric patients vary. During the first weeks of life, infants pass approximately four stools per day. As children get older, approximately one to three stools are passed per day. Constipation should be expected if there is a drastic change from a child's baseline bowel function.

a. Nonpharmacological methods, such as increasing the amount of fluid or sugar in a child's formula in younger children or increasing the bulk content of the child's diet (fruit, fiber cereals, vegetables), should be tried before medications are used.

b. If nonpharmacological methods do not work, rectal stimulation may be useful. Pharmacological agents that can be used for acute relief include glycerin suppositories and magnesium laxatives. Stimulant laxatives should be administered as a last resort, but enemas should not be used in children less than 2 years of age and with extreme caution in children 2–5 years of age (see I C 4). Bulk-forming agents and stool softeners can be used if the constipation does not need immediate relief.

2. Pregnant patients. Constipation in pregnancy is common and is often due to compression of the colon by the enlarged uterus. Pregnant patients should avoid any preparation that may be absorbed systemically (e.g., stimulant laxatives), any preparation that can interfere with vitamin absorption (e.g., mineral oil), or any preparation that can induce premature labor (e.g., castor oil). Pregnant patients should use bulk-forming agents or stool softeners.

3. Geriatric patients tend to be at risk for constipation due to insufficient dietary (fiber) and fluid ingestion, failure to establish a regular bowel time habit, and abuse of stimulant laxatives resulting in a loss of smooth muscle tone in the bowel that promotes constipation (see I C 5). These causes should be investigated in addition to primary disease states (e.g., hypothyroidism) and medications (e.g., opiates, anticholinergics) that may lead to constipation in elderly patients. A **major concern** with geriatric patients is the possible loss of fluid that can be induced by aggressive laxative treatment (e.g., enemas, high-dose saline laxatives). Geriatric patients should not use stimulant laxatives on a chronic basis, and patients with renal impairment should not use magnesium products. Glycerin suppositories or orally administered lactulose may be useful for initial treatment of constipation and bulk-forming agents used to prevent constipation.

4. Use of enemas. Enemas are useful for evacuation of the bowel before surgery, childbirth, and for the treatment of acute constipation that has not responded to other medications (e.g., bisacodyl suppositories). An enema is the dosage route with the enema fluid determining the mechanism of evacuation (e.g., stimulant, osmotic). When administered correctly, an enema evacuates only the distal colon similar to a normal bowel movement. This is accomplished by having the patient lie on his or her side with the knees tucked toward the chest. While in this position, 1 pint (500 mL) of enema solution should be slowly squeezed into the rectum. This should be retained up to 1 hour or until definite lower abdominal cramping is felt. At this point, the bowel movement is ready for expulsion. Although all enemas cause abdominal cramping, some may have more serious **adverse effects** than others. Soap sud enemas can cause much rectal irritation and have been reported to cause anaphylaxis and rectal gangrene. The popular sodium phosphate enemas (e.g., Fleet) are very effective but have resulted in hyperphosphatasemia, hypocalcemia (tetany), hypokalemia, metabolic acidosis, and cardiac death usually due to conduction abnormalities in very small children. This has mainly occurred in children less than 2 years of age or from 2–5 years of age with predisposing factors. These factors include chronic renal disease, anorectal malformations, and/or Hirschsprung's disease, which allow phosphate blood concentrations to become abnormally high and potassium and calcium to become low, predisposing these patients to cardiac arrhythmias and potentially death. Therefore, the use of enemas is highly discouraged in children under 5 years of age.

5. **Laxative abuse** is a term to describe the routine, chronic use of laxatives on a daily basis (e.g., elderly patients) to the administration of high doses several times daily by patients with anorexia nervosa or bulimia for weight control. Excessive use of laxatives can lead to excessive diarrhea and vomiting, resulting in fluid and electrolyte abnormalities. In addition to the risks to patients from hypokalemia (e.g., metabolic alkalosis, cardiac conduction problems), patients can also develop osteomalacia, liver disease, and cathartic colon. Cathartic colon results from superficial ulcerations in the colon as well as damage to the muscularis mucosa and submucosa. This results in a loss of tone of the smooth and striated muscle and causes poor bowel function.

II. **DIARRHEA** is an abnormal increase in the frequency and looseness of stools. The overall weight and volume of the stool is increased (more than 200 g or mL/day), and the water content is increased to 60%–90%. In general, diarrhea results when some factor impairs the ability of the intestine to absorb water from the stool, which causes excess water in the stool. **Antidiarrheals** may serve to prevent an attack of diarrhea or to relieve existing symptoms.

A. **Classification.** Diarrhea can be classified based on mechanisms or etiology.

1. **Classification by mechanism**
   a. **Osmotic diarrhea** occurs when a nonabsorbable solute pulls excess water into the intestinal tract.
      (1) Ingestion of large meals or certain osmotic substances (e.g., sorbitol, glycerin) can lead to diarrhea.
      (2) Disaccharidase deficiency, which is a lack of enzymes needed to break down disaccharides in the gut for absorption (e.g., lactase deficiency), results in an increase in osmotic sugars (i.e., lactose, sucrose) in the intestinal tract.
      (3) Medications that can induce osmotic diarrhea include lactulose and magnesium-containing antacids and laxatives.
   b. **Secretory diarrhea** occurs when the intestinal wall is damaged, resulting in an increased secretion rather than absorption of electrolytes into the intestinal tract. Common sources include:
      (1) **Bacterial endotoxins** (e.g., *Escherichia coli, Vibrio cholerae, Shigella, Staphylococcus aureus*)
      (2) **Bacterial infections** (e.g., *Shigella, Salmonella*)
      (3) **Viral infections** (e.g., rotavirus, Norwalk virus)
      (4) **Protozoal infections** (e.g., *Giardia lamblia, Entamoeba histolytica*)
      (5) **Miscellaneous causes**—inflammatory bowel disease and medications (e.g., prostaglandins, antibiotics, colchicine, chemotherapeutic agents)
   c. **Motility disorders.** Diarrhea induced by motility disorders results from decreased contact time of the fecal mass with the intestinal wall, so less water is absorbed from the feces.
      (1) **Motility disorders** include irritable bowel syndrome, scleroderma, diabetic neuropathy, gastric/intestinal resection, and vagotomy.
      (2) **Medications** that can induce motility disorders include parasympathomimetic agents that enhance the effects of acetylcholine (e.g., metoclopramide, bethanechol), digitalis, quinidine, and antibiotics.
         (a) Antibiotics cause diarrhea by causing intestinal irritation, increased bowel motility, and altered bowel microbial flora.
         (b) Most antibiotic-induced diarrhea can be minimized by taking the agent with food.

2. **Classification by etiology**
   a. **Acute diarrhea** (usually self-limiting for 2–3 days but may last up to 2 weeks)
      (1) **Infection. Most common** sources include viral and bacterial, but protozoal diarrhea also occurs. Organisms include:
         (a) **Viruses** that commonly cause diarrhea include rotaviruses and the Norwalk virus.

(i) **Rotaviruses** usually affect children under 2 years of age. The virus has an onset of 1–2 days and lasts 5–8 days. Patients usually have vomiting, a mild fever, and may experience severe dehydration. There is usually no blood or pus in the stool.

(ii) The **Norwalk virus** affects older children and adults. It has an onset of 1–2 days and lasts 24–48 hours (the "24-hour bug"). As with rotaviruses, there is mild fever but no blood or pus in the stool.

(b) **Bacteria.** Most bacterial diarrhea results from consumption of contaminated water or food, with an onset of diarrhea in 8 hours to several days. Diarrhea due to consumption of contaminated food or water that occurs in a foreign country (e.g., Mexico, third-world countries) is referred to as traveler's diarrhea.

(i) **Toxigenic bacteria.** Diarrhea caused by toxigenic *E. coli, S. aureus, V. cholerae,* and *Shigella* results from the secretory effects of enterotoxins released by these organisms in the small intestine. Patients usually experience large-volume stools that are watery or greasy.

(ii) **Invasive bacteria.** Diarrhea caused by invasive *E. coli, Shigella, Salmonella, Campylobacter,* and *Clostridium difficile* results from mucosal invasion of the colon. This results in a dysentery-like diarrhea, which is characterized by an extreme urgency to defecate, abdominal cramping, tenesmus, fever, chills, and small-volume stools that contain blood or pus.

(c) **Protozoa.** *G. lamblia, E. histolytica,* and *Cryptosporidium* cause explosive, foul-smelling, large-volume, watery stools. This is thought to be caused by invasion of the small intestine, which causes damage to the microvilli and, therefore, decreases absorption of fluids. This type of diarrhea can result in large fluid losses, and patients are at risk for dehydration. Although protozoan-induced diarrhea is self-limiting, it may persist for several months, so therapy should be considered to eradicate the organism.

(2) **Diet-induced diarrhea.** Diarrhea induced by foods results from food allergies, high-fiber diets, fatty or spicy foods, large amounts of caffeine, or milk intolerance. The best treatment is prevention, by avoiding troublesome foods.

(3) **Drug-induced diarrhea** (see II A 1 a–c)

b. **Chronic diarrhea** (lasts longer than 2 weeks). If a patient suffers from diarrhea for long periods of time, or from recurrent episodes of diarrhea, the following causes must be considered: protozoal organisms, food-induced diarrhea (e.g., lactose intolerance), irritable bowel syndrome, malabsorption syndromes (e.g., celiac sprue, diverticulosis, short bowel syndrome), inflammatory bowel disease, pancreatic disease, and hyperthyroidism.

B. Patient evaluation

1. Pharmacists who are consulted by patients should ask the patient for the following information before recommending a therapy:

   a. **Age** of the patient
   b. **Onset and duration** of the diarrhea
   c. **Description of stool** (i.e., frequency, volume, blood, pus, watery)
   d. **Other symptoms** (e.g., abdominal cramping, fever, nausea, vomiting, weight loss)
   e. **Medications** recently started or medications used to relieve the diarrhea
   f. **Recent travel** (where and how long ago)
   g. **Medical history** (history of GI disorders)

2. **Referrals to a physician** should be made by the pharmacist who encounters a patient with diarrhea that meets the following criteria:

   a. **Younger than 3 years** of age or **older than 60 years** of age (with multiple medical problems), pregnant patients, and patients with HIV.
   b. **Bloody stools**
   c. **High fever** (greater than 101°F or 38°C)
   d. **Dehydration or weight loss** greater than 5% of total body weight; signs of dehydration—dry mouth, sunken eyes, crying without tears, dry skin that is not elastic like normal skin
   e. **Duration of diarrhea longer than 5 days**
   f. **Vomiting**

C. Treatment

1. Nonpharmacological

a. Food/breast feeding. In the past, there was much controversy regarding the decision "to feed" or "not to feed" children during acute episodes of diarrhea. Originally, parents were told that children should not receive food, milk products, or breast–feed for 6–48 hours after the onset of diarrhea. Parents were also told that if children did receive food, they should receive the "BRAT" diet, which consists of bananas, rice, applesauce, and toast. This diet does not work and is deficient in calories, protein, and fat. All patients should receive their normal diet or breast–feeding during bouts of diarrhea because these do not make the diarrhea worse and may actually improve the diarrhea.

b. Fluids. The most important part of treating acute diarrhea is the replacement of lost fluids. If patients experience mild to moderate fluid loss, fluid replacement can be achieved with oral-rehydration solutions (ORS). If fluid loss is severe (more than 10% loss of body weight) and/or severe vomiting persists, then patients may need intravenous rehydration before oral maintenance fluids can be administered. ORSs can be easily made at home (Table 32-1) or purchased ready-to-use (e.g., Pedialyte, Rehydralyte). All of these solutions are considered equally safe and effective but have no effect on the duration of the diarrhea. The secretory and absorptive mechanisms of the bowel function separately, and this allows these ORS to be absorbed during acute episodes of diarrhea, preventing severe dehydration and complications. Not every patient needs ORS. For a child without evidence of dehydration (see II B 2 d), administer 10 mL/kg or ½–1 cup of ORS for each loose stool. If a child is vomiting, administer smaller amounts (1–2 teaspoonful) every 2–5 minutes as tolerated.

(1) Fluid and electrolyte replacement. Fluid and electrolyte therapy is aimed at replacing what the body has lost. During this situation, the patient's fluid input and output as well as weight should be monitored. The World Health Organization has established guidelines for oral-replacement therapy (see Table 32-1). Recommended doses are given in Table 32-2.

(2) Fluids to be avoided include hypertonic fruit juices and drinks (e.g., apple juice, powdered drink mixes, gelatin water), carbonated beverages, and caffeine-containing beverages, which can make diarrhea worse and do not contain needed electrolytes (i.e., Na^+, K^+). Gatorade diluted in water (1:1) is adequate and provides the necessary combination of glucose, sodium, and potassium.

Table 32-1. Guidelines for Oral-Replacement Therapy Established by the World Health Organization (WHO)

Ingredients	Dose
Sodium chloride (table salt)	90 mEq (½ teaspoon)
Potassium chloride (potassium salt)	20 mEq (¼ teaspoon)
Sodium bicarbonate (baking soda)	30 mEq (½ teaspoon)
Glucose (sugar)	20 g (2 teaspoons)
Water	Enough to make 1 L of solution

Table 32-2. Guidelines for Fluid- and Electrolyte-Replacement Therapy

Age Group	Dose	
	Mild (2–3 stools/day)	**Moderate (4–5 stools/day)**
Adults (>5 years of age)	2 L/first 4 hours, then replace ongoing losses	2–4 L/first 4 hours, then replace ongoing losses
Children (<5 years of age)	50 mL/kg/first 4 hours, then 10 mL/kg or ½–1 cup per stool	100 mL/kg/4 hours, then 10 mL/kg or ½–1 cup per stool

2. **Pharmacologic.** Based on the Food and Drug Administration (FDA) review of the various antidiarrheal products, three agents have been identified as Category I (i.e., safe and effective) ingredients: **kaolin, bismuth subsalicylate,** and **loperamide.** In April 2003, the FDA reclassified attapulgite and polycarbophil products from category I to category III due to insufficient effectiveness data. Antidiarrheal agents are classified in different categories on the basis of their chemical class or pharmacologic mechanism of action.
   a. **Antiperistaltic drugs**
      (1) **Mechanism of action.** Antiperistaltic drugs act by stimulating mu opioid receptors on the circular and longitudinal musculature of the small and large intestines to normalize peristaltic intestinal movements. They slow intestinal motility and affect water and electrolyte movement through the bowel. Loperamide is considered more potent than diphenoxylate and morphine in its ability to slow GI motility. Loperamide is effective in nonspecific diarrhea and traveler's diarrhea. The frequency of bowel movements is decreased, and the consistency of stools is increased. However, replacement of fluids (through ORS) is still the main focus of therapy for diarrhea.
      (2) **Contraindication.** Antiperistaltic medications have always been restricted in patients with acute bacterial diarrhea associated with fecal leukocytes, high fever, or blood/mucus in the stool because of the potential for these drugs to decrease clearance of the organism and enhance systemic invasion of the organism. Most information shows that this is not significant and probably will cause no harm. However, these medications should not be used in patients with colitis (potential for the development of toxic megacolon) or in children less than 2 years of age.
      (3) **Prescription agents** in this class include the opiate-related agent diphenoxylate/atropine (e.g., Lomotil).
      (4) **Nonprescription agents. Loperamide** (e.g., Imodium A-D, Maalox Anti-Diarrheal, Pepto Diarrhea Control) provides effective control of diarrhea as quickly as 1 hour after administration. Antiperistaltic drugs should not be used for more than 48 hours in acute diarrhea.
         (a) **Dosage information.** An **adult dosage** is 4 mg followed by 2 mg after each unformed stool, not to exceed 16 mg/day. A **child's dosage** is 1–2 mg up to three times per day, depending on weight and age.
         (b) **Side effects.** At recommended doses, loperamide is generally well tolerated. Side effects are infrequent and consist primarily of abdominal pain, distention, or discomfort; drowsiness; dizziness; and dry mouth.
   b. **Adsorbents.** These medications adsorb toxins, bacteria, gases, and fluids. They are not absorbed systemically, so they produce **few adverse effects.** There are several products available; some are more effective than others, but none are very effective for severe acute diarrhea. These products are given for symptomatic relief and are usually administered in large doses immediately following a loose stool.
      (1) **Kaolin**
         (a) **Dosage information.** Adults and children 12 years of age and older: oral dosage is 26.2 g after each loose stool. Continue to take every 6 hours until stool is firm but not for more than 2 days. Do not exceed 262 g in 24 hours.
         (b) **Side effects.** Because activated kaolin is inert and is not absorbed systemically, **side effects** are minor with few patients experiencing constipation. It is recommended that this product not be given within two hours of other medications since it may decrease the absorption of other orally administered medications.
   c. **Miscellaneous agents**
      (1) **Bismuth subsalicylate** (e.g., Pepto-Bismol). Bismuth salts work as adsorbents but also are believed to decrease secretion of water into the bowel. Bismuth preparations have moderate effectiveness against the prevention and treatment of traveler's diarrhea and nonspecific diarrhea, but doses required for relief are large and must be administered frequently, so these preparations may be inconvenient.
         (a) **Dosage information.** An **adult dosage** is 2 tablets or 30–60 mL (524 mg) every hour as needed to a maximum of 8 doses in a 24-hour period. A **child's dosage** is ⅓ to ½ the adult dose. Bismuth subsalicylate can prevent traveler's diarrhea when 2 tablets are taken four times per day.
         (b) **Side effects** may include harmless grayish-charcoal coloring of stools or tongue. Ringing in the ears can occur with high doses especially if the patient is simultaneously taking other salicylate products. However, patients with black or bloody stools should not use this product.

Table 32-3. Drugs and Doses Used to Treat Infectious Diarrhea

Antibacterials	Antiprotozoals	Dose[+]
Azithromycin	N/A	500 mg, then 250 mg daily
Ciprofloxacin	N/A	500 mg twice daily
Doxycycline	N/A	100 mg twice daily
Metronidazole♦	—	250–750 mg three times daily
Norfloxacin	N/A	400 mg twice daily
Ofloxacin	N/A	300 mg twice daily
Quinacrine	—	100 mg three times daily
Trimethoprim/Sulfamethoxazole DS*	N/A	1 tablet twice daily
Vancomycin♦	N/A	125 mg QID

+Antibiotics are used for 3–5 days for bacterial- and protozoal-induced diarrhea.

♦Metronidazole and vancomycin are used for 10–14 days for clostridial diarrhea.

*Trimethoprim/sulfamethoxazole is not considered first line because of resistance problems.

    (c) Contraindication. Bismuth subsalicylate should not be given to children or teenagers during or after recovery from chicken pox or flu because of the possible association of salicylates with Reye's syndrome. Patients with documented allergies to salicylates should not take this product. Patients on anticoagulants should be monitored closely if taking these products.

  (2) Lactobacillus (e.g., Bacid, Lactinex) products are intended to replace the normal bacterial flora that is lost during the administration of oral antibiotics. However, there is little information to show that these products are useful for antibiotic-induced diarrhea, so most clinicians do not recommend their use.

  (3) Lactase (e.g., LactAid, Lactrase, Dairy Ease) is indicated for individuals who have insufficient amounts of lactase in the small intestine. Lactose (a disaccharide present in dairy products) must be broken down to glucose and galactose to be fully digested. If it is not, lactose draws water into the GI tract, and diarrhea results. Lactase is the enzyme responsible for digesting lactose. The dose is 1–2 capsules taken with milk or dairy products or added to milk before drinking. Titration of doses to higher levels may be required in some cases.

  (4) Anti-infectives. Depending on the suspected etiology of the infectious diarrhea, prescription antibiotics and antiprotozoal medications can be used to eradicate the organisms and decrease the duration of symptoms (Table 32-3). If antibiotics are used to prevent traveler's diarrhea, therapy should be started 1 day before arrival in high-incidence regions and continued until 2 days after departure. If diarrhea has occurred, antibiotic treatment should last for 3–5 days.

  (5) Anticholinergics (e.g., atropine, hyoscyamine) decrease bowel motility, which results in an increase of fluid absorption from the intestinal tract and a decrease in abdominal cramping. These products are found in combination with adsorbents or opiates. However, the amount of anticholinergic found in most products is not considered to be enough to alter the course of severe acute diarrhea. **Adverse effects** include dry mouth, blurred vision, and tachycardia. These products should not be used in patients with narrow angle glaucoma.

III. HEMORRHOIDS (also known as piles) are defined as clusters of dilated blood vessels in the lower rectum (internal hemorrhoids) or anus (external hemorrhoids). Simply, hemorrhoids represent downward displacement of anal cushions that contain arteriovenous anastomoses. Hemorrhoids are common, with approximately 10%–25% of the U.S. population afflicted. The risk of developing hemorrhoids increases with advancing age and peaks in individuals 45–65 years of age. Although they are considered a minor medical problem, they may cause considerable discomfort and anxiety. A proper diagnosis is important, because there are a number of conditions that may produce symptoms that mimic those of hemorrhoids (see III D). For example, colorectal cancer may cause bleeding, which is a common symptom of hemorrhoids. Fortunately, patient reassurance and the proper administration of a few simple treatments usually improve the condition.

A. Types of hemorrhoids are determined by their anatomical position and vascular origin.

1. An **internal** hemorrhoid is an exaggerated vascular cushion with an engorged internal hemorrhoidal plexus located above the dentate line and covered with a mucous membrane.

2. An **external** hemorrhoid is a dilated vein of the inferior hemorrhoidal plexus located below the dentate line and covered with squamous epithelium.

3. A **mixed** hemorrhoid appears as a baggy swelling and exhibits simultaneous characteristics of internal and external hemorrhoids.

B. Etiology. Although heredity may predispose a person to hemorrhoids, the exact cause is probably related to acquired factors.

1. Situations that result in **increased venous pressure** in the hemorrhoidal plexus (e.g., chronic straining during defecation; small, hard stools; prolonged sitting on the toilet; occupations that routinely require heavy lifting; pelvic tumors; pregnancy) can transform an asymptomatic hemorrhoid into a problem. Pregnancy is the most frequent cause of hemorrhoids in women of childbearing age.

2. The hemorrhoidal veins are pushed downward during defecation or straining, and, with increased venous pressure, they **dilate** and **become engorged.** Over time, the **fibers** that anchor the hemorrhoidal veins to their underlying muscular coats **stretch,** which results in **prolapse.**

C. Signs/symptoms

1. The **most common** sign/symptom of hemorrhoids is **painless bleeding** occurring during a bowel movement. The blood is usually bright red and may be visible on the stool, on the toilet tissue, or coloring the water in the toilet.

2. **Prolapse** is the **second most common** sign/symptom of hemorrhoids. A temporary protrusion may occur during defection, and it may need to be replaced manually. A permanently prolapsed hemorrhoid may give rise to chronic, moist soiling of the underwear. These patients may complain of a dull, aching feeling.

3. **Pain** is unusual unless **thrombosis** involving external tissue is present, and then the pain can be excruciating.

4. **Discomfort, soreness, pruritus, swelling, burning,** and **seepage** may also occur with hemorrhoids.

D. Other conditions that may **mimic** hemorrhoids include the following, which usually require a physician's intervention:

1. An **anal abscess,** usually a *Staphylococcus* infection

2. **Cryptitis,** which is inflammation of the crypts (small indentations at the mucocutaneous junction)

3. An **anal fissure,** which is a small tear in the lining of the anus

4. An **anal fistula,** which is an abnormal communication between the mucosa of the rectum and the skin adjacent to the anus

5. **Inflammatory bowel diseases**

6. A **polyp,** which is a tumor of the large intestine

7. **Colorectal cancer**

E. Internal hemorrhoids are graded and classified into one of four groups.

1. A **first-degree** hemorrhoid (grade 1) does not descend nor prolapse during straining upon defecation.

2. A **second-degree** hemorrhoid (grade 2) descends but returns spontaneously with relaxation.

3. A **third-degree** hemorrhoid (grade 3) requires manual replacement into the rectum after prolapse.

4. A **fourth-degree** hemorrhoid (grade 4) is permanently prolapsed and cannot be manipulated manually.

F. **Treatment.** The symptoms of hemorrhoids are produced by a cycle of events: the protrusion of the vascular submucosal cushion through a tight anal canal, which becomes further congested and hypertrophic, which causes the cushion to protrude further. All treatments of hemorrhoids aim to break this cycle, and they fall into a number of broad groups.

1. For **first-** and **second-degree internal** hemorrhoids that bleed minimally, a conservative approach can usually be taken.
    a. To **reduce straining** and **downward pressure** on the hemorrhoids, patients should avoid straining when defecating and avoid sitting on the toilet longer than necessary.
    b. **Correction of constipation is of paramount importance.** This can be accomplished by eating a high-fiber diet and increasing water intake and physical activity. Bulk-forming laxatives, such as psyllium, and stool softeners, such as docusate, may be helpful.
    c. **Sitz baths** for 15 minutes, three to four times a day, can soothe the anal mucosa. Tepid water should be used, and prolonged bathing should be avoided. Epsom salts (magnesium sulfate) added to the bath or the application of an ice pack can help reduce the swelling of an edematous or clotted hemorrhoid.
    d. **OTC hemorrhoidal ointments, creams, foams,** and **suppositories** may also help relieve symptoms (see III G).

2. **Higher-grade internal hemorrhoids** usually require physician expertise and specialized procedures for treatment.
    a. Symptomatic grades 2 or 3 hemorrhoids are often best treated with **hemorrhoid banding** (rubber band ligation). This procedure is performed through an anoscope; a rubber band ligature is placed on the rectal mucosa above the hemorrhoid, well above the dentate line to avoid excessive discomfort. The ligated area sloughs off in a few days.
    b. **Infrared photocoagulation** can be used for grade 2 hemorrhoids; it is less effective than banding with large hemorrhoids. Infrared light is focused at the base of the hemorrhoid, thereby destroying the varicosity secondary to the formation of a white coagulum.
    c. **Sclerotherapy** (injection of a sclerosing agent into the hemorrhoid) or cryotherapy ("freezing" the hemorrhoid) are older therapies that have been used.
    d. **Surgical hemorrhoidectomy** should be undertaken only for grades 3 or 4 hemorrhoids. Whether the procedure is done traditionally or with a laser, most patients have significant discomfort and a period of postoperative disability.

3. An **external, thrombosed hemorrhoid** can be completely excised in an office setting, clinic, or operating room.

G. **Nonprescription medication for hemorrhoidal and other anorectal diseases (Table 32-4).** The FDA has identified several ingredients as safe and effective to alleviate burning, discomfort, inflammation, irritation, itching, pain, and swelling. These products are simply palliative; they are not meant to cure hemorrhoids or other anorectal disease. If these products do not improve symptoms within 7 days, a physician should be consulted. A physician should also

Table 32-4. Guide to Hemorrhoidal Therapy Based on Approved Indication for OTC Anorectal Drug Products

	Burning	Discomfort	Irritation	Itching	Pain	Soreness	Swelling
Analgesic, Anesthetic, Antipruritic	Yes	Yes		Yes	Yes	Yes	
Astringent	Yes	Yes	Yes	Yes			
Keratolytic		Yes		Yes			
Local anesthetic	Yes	Yes		Yes	Yes	Yes	
Protectant	Yes	Yes	Yes	Yes			
Vasoconstrictor		Yes	Yes	Yes			Yes
Hydrocortisone		Yes		Yes			Yes

be consulted if bleeding, prolapse, seepage of feces or mucus, thrombosis, or severe pain occurs. Patients younger than 12 years of age should not rely upon self-treatment but should seek medical attention immediately.

1. **Ointments versus suppositories.**Generally, the ointment or cream dosage form is believed to be superior to a suppository, which may bypass the affected area. Patients should wash the anorectal area with mild soap and warm water and pat (not wipe) the area dry before applying a product. Alternatively, patients can use an OTC anal-cleansing pad (e.g., Tucks). Some ointments come with rectal pipes (pile pipes) that allow the patient to insert and apply the medication directly in the rectum. The openings in the rectal pipe allow the ointment to cover large areas of the rectal mucosa unreachable with the finger. The rectal pipe should be lubricated by spreading ointment around the tip of the pipe before insertion. Some clinicians advise against the use of the rectal pipe because the anal canal could be traumatized if the pipe is not inserted properly.

2. **Local anesthetics** block nerve-impulse transmission. They should be used for symptoms of pain, itching, burning, discomfort, and irritation in the perianal region or lower anal canal (not in the rectum). The rectum contains no sensory pain receptors.
    a. **Agents** deemed safe and effective include benzocaine 5%–20% (e.g., Lanacane), pramoxine 1% (e.g., ProctoFoam), benzyl alcohol 1%–4% (e.g., Tucks Clear Gel), dibucaine 0.25%–1% (e.g., Nupercainal), dyclonine 0.5%–1% (e.g., Dyclone), lidocaine 2%–5% (e.g., Xylocaine), and tetracaine 0.5%–1% (e.g., Pontocaine).
    b. **Adverse effects.** These agents may produce a hypersensitivity reaction with burning and itching similar to that of anorectal disease. Systemic absorption is minimal unless the perianal skin is abraded. As a result of its unique chemical structure, pramoxine exhibits little cross-sensitivity when compared to the other local anesthetics.

3. **Vasoconstrictors** decrease mucosal perfusion by causing arteriole constriction in the anorectal area after topical application. However, because bleeding in this area may be a sign of more serious disease, vasoconstrictors are not approved for control of minor bleeding. For temporary relief of itching and swelling, these agents have a local anesthetic effect of unknown mechanism.
    a. **Agents** deemed safe and effective include ephedrine sulfate 0.1%–1.25% in aqueous solution, epinephrine HCl 0.005%–0.01% in aqueous solution, and phenylephrine HCl 0.25% in aqueous solution. These agents are present in various ointments (e.g., Pazo) and suppositories (e.g., Preparation H).
    b. **Contraindications** apply to people with cardiovascular disease, high blood pressure, hyperthyroidism, diabetes, and prostate enlargement because of the possibility of systemic absorption.

4. Protectants provide a **physical barrier,** forming a protective coating over skin or mucous membranes, for temporary relief of itching, irritation, discomfort, and burning. They prevent irritation of anorectal tissue and prevent water loss from the stratum corneum. Protectants are often the bases or vehicles for other agents used for anorectal disease. Products include aluminum hydroxide gel, cocoa butter, kaolin, lanolin, hard fat, mineral oil, white petrolatum, petrolatum, glycerin (external use only), topical starch, cod liver oil, shark liver oil, and zinc oxide. When protectants are incorporated into the formulation of an OTC product, they should make up at least 50% of the dosage unit. If two to four protectants are used, their total concentration should represent at least 50% of the whole product. Lanolin, a derivative of wool alcohol, may be allergenic to susceptible individuals.
    a. **Absorbents** take up fluids that are on or secreted by skin or mucous membranes.
    b. **Adsorbents** attach to substances secreted by skin or mucous membranes.
    c. **Demulcents** combine with water to form a colloidal solution, which protects the skin in a way similar to mucus.
    d. **Emollients,** which are derived from animal or vegetable fats or petroleum products, soften or protect internal or external body surfaces.

5. **Astringents** lessen mucus and other secretions and protect underlying tissue through a local and limited protein coagulant effect. Action is limited to surface cells, but astringents provide temporary relief of itching, discomfort, irritation, and burning. Products considered to be safe and effective include calamine 5%–25%, witch hazel 10%–50% (external use only), and zinc oxide 5%–25%.

6. **Keratolytics** cause desquamation and debridement of the surface cells of the epidermis and provide temporary relief of discomfort and itching. Theoretically, keratolytics expose underlying tissue to other therapeutic agents. Products considered to be safe and effective include aluminum chlorhydroxyallantoinate (alcloxa) 0.2%–2.0% and resorcinol 1%–3%. Resorcinol should not be used on an open wound due to the potential for a serious hypersensitivity reaction. Keratolytics are reserved for external use only.

7. **Analgesics, anesthetics,** and **antipruritics** provide temporary relief of burning, discomfort, itching, pain, and soreness. The FDA has redesignated several ingredients into this category that were formerly classified as **counterirritants.** Ingredients considered to be safe and effective for external use in the anorectal area include menthol (0.1%–1%), juniper tar (1%–5%), and camphor (0.1%–3%). These agents should not be used to treat internal hemorrhoids.

8. **Wound-healing agents.** Live yeast cell derivative (LYCD) [skin-respiratory factor], which is a water-soluble extract of brewer's yeast, was present in Preparation H in the past. LYCD was removed from the list of **"safe and effective"** active ingredients by the FDA, as it determined that this agent was not proven effective as per the studies submitted to it. Preparation H products have been reformulated without LYCD. Preparation H Ointment now contains protectants (petrolatum, mineral oil, shark liver oil, lanolin, and glycerin) and the vasoconstrictor phenylephrine.

9. **Hydrocortisone (0.25%–1%)** causes vasoconstriction, stabilization of lysosomal membranes, and antimitotic activity. These agents have the potential to reduce itching, inflammation, and discomfort in the anorectal area. Until recently, hydrocortisone-containing hemorrhoidal products were available by prescription only. As with any steroid cogener, hydrocortisone may mask the symptoms of bacterial or fungal infections. Hydrocortisone concentrations greater than 1% are available by prescription only.

IV. GASTROESOPHAGEAL REFLUX DISEASE (HEARTBURN)

A. General information

1. **Definition.** The reflux of gastric contents into the esophagus, or gastroesophageal reflux, is generally a benign physiological process that occurs in normal individuals multiple times throughout the day. However, patients with gastroesophageal reflux disease (GERD) may experience esophageal tissue damage (reflux esophagitis) and/or symptoms of heartburn when the acidic gastric contents stay in prolonged contact with the esophagus.

2. **Symptoms.** Heartburn (pyrosis) typically is described as a burning sensation or pain located in the lower chest. Because the pain may radiate up into the chest, heartburn may be confused with pain associated with myocardial infarction. Symptoms usually occur soon after meals and when lying down at bedtime. Pain on swallowing (odynophagia) may suggest severe mucosal damage in the esophagus.

3. **Complications.** Patients with severe, uncontrolled GERD may suffer bleeding from esophageal ulcers and pulmonary complications resulting from the aspiration of refluxed material into the upper airways and lungs. Patients who describe difficulty swallowing (i.e., dysphagia) may have an esophageal stricture, cancer, or a motility disorder.

4. **Causes.** There is an imbalance of aggressive and protective forces. Aggressive forces include acid and pepsin. The most important protective force is probably the lower esophageal sphincter (LES). Many patients with GERD have a weak lower esophageal sphincter. As a result, the high pressure in the stomach creates enough force to overcome the weak squeeze of the LES and allows reflux to occur. Other protective forces include esophageal clearance, gastric emptying rate, and esophageal mucosal defense. Drugs that reduce LES tone include:
   a. Calcium channel antagonists (e.g., nifedipine, verapamil, diltiazem)
   b. Nitrates
   c. Anticholinergic agents (e.g., tricyclic antidepressants, antihistamines)
   d. Oral contraceptives and estrogen

5. Pharmacists who are consulted by patients should ask for the following information before recommending a therapy.
   a. Duration and frequency of symptoms
   b. Severity of the pain and symptoms

  c. Timing of the symptoms (especially in relation to meals and at bedtime)
  d. Presence of other symptoms (nausea, vomiting, bloody stools, weight loss)
  e. Use of alcohol or tobacco
  f. Amount of high-fat foods, caffeine-containing products, chocolate, and tomato-based foods consumed
  g. Medications used currently, including nonprescription medications
  h. Medications used to relieve heartburn and their effectiveness

6. Patients with the following symptoms or conditions should be referred to a physician for evaluation rather than treated with nonprescription agents.
  a. Severe abdominal or back pain
  b. Unexplained weight loss
  c. Chest pain that is indistinguishable from ischemic pain
  d. Difficulty or pain on swallowing
  e. Presence or history of vomiting blood
  f. Black tarry bowel movements (if not taking iron or bismuth subsalicylate)
  g. Children younger than 12 years of age
  h. Possibility of being pregnant
  i. Symptoms not responding to antacids or nonprescription histamine$_2$-receptor antagonists (H$_2$RAs) within 2 weeks or recurring soon after stopping

B. Treatment

1. **Nonpharmacological** interventions for GERD attempt to reduce or eliminate dietary and lifestyle factors that promote reflux. Specific recommendations include:
  a. Elevate the head of the bed about 6 inches with blocks. This position improves esophageal clearance and reduces the duration of reflux. Try to avoid just propping a patient's head up with pillows because this may worsen symptoms by increasing abdominal pressure.
  b. Eat evening meals at least 3 hours before going to bed to allow adequate time for gastric emptying.
  c. Avoid foods that reduce LES tone.
     (1) Chocolate
     (2) Mints
     (3) High-fat foods
  d. Avoid foods that irritate the esophagus.
     (1) Tomato-based products
     (2) Coffee
     (3) Citrus juices
  e. Reduce the size of meals.
  f. Avoid lying down after meals.
  g. Stop smoking.
  h. Limit alcohol intake.
  i. Limit caffeine-containing beverages.
  j. Lose weight if appropriate.
  k. Avoid wearing tight-fitting clothing.

2. **Pharmacological.** The management of GERD may be viewed as a stepped-care approach, with antacids, nonprescription H$_2$RAs, and nondrug measures forming the basis for the first step (Figure 32-1). These measures may help to alleviate symptoms in patients with mild to moderate GERD but cannot be expected to heal damaged esophageal mucosa or prevent complications. Steps 2 and higher utilize prescription-strength H$_2$RAs and other prescription medications.
  a. **Antacids.** Antacids neutralize gastric acid, which increases the pH of refluxed gastric contents. As a result, the refluxed contents are not as damaging to the esophageal mucosa. Antacids generally relieve heartburn within 5–15 minutes of administration. Antacid suspensions generally dissolve more easily in gastric acid and thereby work quicker. The duration of relief ranges from 1–3 hours. Because of their short duration, patients may need to take 4–5 doses throughout the day for adequate symptom relief. Antacids will not provide sustained neutralization of acid throughout the night. An **adult dose** is 40–80 mEq acid-neutralizing capacity (ANC) taken as needed for symptoms. If

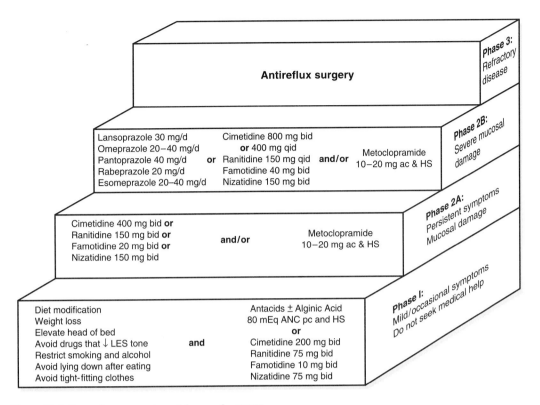

Figure 32-1. Step-wise progression of therapy for GERD.
ac = before meals; HS = bedtime; bid = twice daily; qid = four times daily; ANC = acid-neutralizing capacity.

necessary, these doses may be titrated to a scheduled regimen, such as 40–80 mEq after meals and at bedtime.

(1) **Sodium bicarbonate** (e.g., Alka-Seltzer, Bromo-Seltzer) should be used only for short-term relief of symptoms. Because each gram of sodium bicarbonate contains 12 mEq of sodium, it is contraindicated in patients with edema, congestive heart failure, renal failure, cirrhosis, and patients on low-salt diets. It is the only systemic antacid available and can thus alter systemic pH.

(2) **Calcium carbonate** (e.g., Tums) is useful for GERD but may cause constipation or, less likely, diarrhea. It is a good source of elemental calcium.

(3) **Aluminum hydroxide** (e.g., Amphojel, Alternagel) often causes constipation and should be avoided in patients with hemorrhoids or constipation, which is common in the elderly. Aluminum accumulation can be a problem in patients with chronic renal insufficiency.

(4) **Magnesium hydroxide** (e.g., Milk of Magnesia) rarely is used alone for heartburn because it frequently causes diarrhea.

(5) **Magnesium–aluminum** combination antacids (e.g., Maalox, Mylanta) provide the highest ANC per volume of antacid and are used most frequently. The predominant adverse effect of these combinations is diarrhea.

(6) **Patient information**
  (a) Patients with renal failure should avoid the use of all antacids. Potassium and magnesium content of antacids should be considered for patients with cardiac disease.
  (b) Patients should not take more than 500–600 mEq ANC of antacid per day.

(7) Antacids can interfere with the absorption of many drugs. In general, antacids should be spaced at least 2 hours apart from the administration of interacting drugs.

This is often quite difficult to accomplish. Important clinical interactions with antacids may occur with the following drugs:

- **(a)** Tetracycline antibiotics
- **(b)** Quinolone antibiotics (e.g., ciprofloxacin, levofloxacin)
- **(c)** Iron supplements
- **(d)** Digoxin

b. Alginic acid

(1) Mechanism of action. Alginic acid works by reacting with sodium bicarbonate and saliva to form a viscous solution of **sodium alginate.** This viscous solution floats on the surface of gastric contents so that, when reflux occurs, sodium alginate rather than acid is refluxed, and irritation is minimized.

(2) Patient information

- **(a)** Alginic-acid tablets must be chewed to be effective and should be followed by a full glass of water so that the viscous foam can float on it in the stomach.
- **(b)** Alginic-acid products work best when patients are in the upright position. Thus, these products should not be taken at bedtime or just before lying down.

c. Nonprescription H_2RAs. These medications inhibit gastric acid secretion by competitively blocking H_2-receptors on the parietal cell. By decreasing gastric acid secretion, the refluxed material is less damaging to the esophagus. The onset of symptom relief with H_2RAs is approximately 1–2 hours, which is considerably longer than antacids; however, the duration of action can last up to 10 hours.

(1) Cimetidine (Tagamet-HB)

- **(a)** The **adult dosage** of nonprescription cimetidine is 200 mg as needed for symptoms, up to twice daily. Cimetidine 200 mg suppresses gastric acid for approximately 6 hours.
- **(b)** Nonprescription doses of cimetidine may **impair** the **hepatic metabolism** and thus increase serum concentrations and the pharmacological effects of the following drugs:
    - **(i)** Warfarin
    - **(ii)** Phenytoin
    - **(iii)** Theophylline

(2) Famotidine (Pepcid-AC). The **adult dosage** of nonprescription famotidine is 10 mg as needed for symptoms, up to twice daily. Patients who anticipate heartburn or indigestion may take one famotidine 10-mg tablet 1 hour before eating, with a maximum of two tablets within a 24-hour period. Famotidine 10 mg suppresses acid secretion for 8–10 hours. Unlike cimetidine, famotidine rarely impairs hepatic metabolism of other drugs.

- **(a)** Famotidine/calcium carbonate/magnesium hydroxide (Pepcid Complete)
    - **(i)** A chewable combination of an H_2RA and an antacid.

(3) Ranitidine (Zantac75). The **adult dosage** of nonprescription ranitidine is 75 mg as needed for symptoms, up to twice daily. Ranitidine inhibits hepatic metabolism 5–10 times less than cimetidine; therefore, the potential for drug interactions is very small.

(4) Nizatidine (Axid-AR). The **adult dosage** of nizatidine is 75 mg as needed for symptoms, up to twice daily. Nizatidine rarely impairs hepatic metabolism of other drugs.

(5) Adverse effects. These agents are extremely well tolerated. The **most common** adverse effects reported with nonprescription doses are headache, diarrhea, dizziness, and nausea.

d. Prescription H_2RAs. Patients with moderate to severe symptoms and/or esophageal mucosal lesions require higher doses of H_2RAs than are available over the counter. Unlike patients with peptic ulcer disease, patients with GERD respond best to multiple daily doses of H_2RAs rather than to single bedtime doses.

e. Prokinetic agents. Patients with moderate to severe GERD may benefit from the addition of these medications, which stimulate esophageal motility and increase LES tone. Prokinetic agents are available only by prescription.

(1) Metoclopramide (Reglan, generic). Adverse effects limit the usefulness of this agent for many patients. Such effects include sedation, depression, and extrapyramidal effects.

(2) Cisapride (Propulsid). The numerous drug interactions with this product have caused the manufacturer to voluntarily remove it from the market. Propulsid may still be obtained through an investigational limited-access program.

    f. Proton pump inhibitors. These prescription-only agents (except omeprazole) provide complete acid suppression by inhibiting the hydrogen-potassium ATPase pump on the surface of the parietal cell. The duration of acid suppression with these agents is about 3 days. Proton pump inhibitors are the most potent and effective agents available for relieving severe GERD symptoms and healing esophageal lesions. In June, 2003, the FDA switched omeprazole to OTC status for the prevention of symptoms of frequent heartburn. OTC drugs should be used for no more than 14 days every 4 months, unless directed by a physician.

      (1) Omeprazole (Prilosec)

        (a) This drug may inhibit hepatic metabolism and thus increase serum concentration/pharmacologic effects of the following drugs: phenytoin, warfarin, and diazepam.

        (b) Adverse effects. Although rare, these may include headache, diarrhea, constipation or dizziness.

      (2) Lansoprazole (Prevacid) has no clinically significant drug interactions.

      (3) Pantoprazole (Protonix) is the only proton pump inhibitor with an oral and intravenous formulation.

      (4) Rabeprazole (Aciphex)

      (5) Esomeprazole (Nexium)

C. Special patient populations

    1. Pediatric patients. Gastroesophageal reflux occurs commonly in infants and children. Signs and symptoms in pediatric patients include vomiting, chest pain, irritability, feeding refusal, belching, and apnea. Serious complications (e.g., failure to thrive, esophageal strictures) can occur in infants and children.

      a. Antacids, with or without alginic acid, have been widely used in infants and children, but their safety has not been clearly established.

      b. H$_2$RAs have been used safely in children under the supervision of health-care providers. However, the nonprescription H$_2$RAs are not approved for use in children younger than 12 years of age unless directed by a physician.

    2. Pregnant patients. Heartburn occurs commonly during pregnancy because of increased abdominal pressure due to the expanding uterus, as well as reduced LES pressure resulting from high concentrations of estrogen and progesterone. Nearly half of pregnant women experience GERD, especially during the third trimester.

      a. Antacids are generally considered safe in pregnancy as long as chronic high doses are avoided. It is best to avoid sodium bicarbonate because of the risks of systemic alkalosis and the sodium load leading to edema and weight gain.

      b. Data regarding the **safety** of **alginic acid** during pregnancy are not available.

      c. Controlled data regarding the safety of **H$_2$RAs** in pregnancy are limited. Pregnant women seeking a nonprescription H$_2$RA for GERD should be directed to use antacids, unless a physician has instructed her otherwise.

    3. Elderly patients. Antacids and nonprescription H$_2$RAs may be safely used in elderly patients without any dosage adjustments.

      a. Dosage reduction of prescription H$_2$RAs may be necessary in elderly patients with reduced renal function.

      b. Elderly patients are more likely to be taking drugs that interact with antacids, H$_2$RAs, omeprazole, and/or cisapride.

      c. Elderly patients are also more likely to have symptoms or conditions that require referral to a physician before beginning nonprescription therapy.

STUDY QUESTIONS

Directions: Each of the numbered items or incomplete statements in this section is followed by answers or by completions of the statement. Select the **one** lettered answer or completion that is **best** in each case.

1. Which laxative should NOT be used to treat acute constipation because of its slow onset of action?

(A) Glycerin
(B) Bisacodyl suppository
(C) Psyllium
(D) Milk of Magnesia

2. Which is NOT a risk factor for hyperphosphatemia and death from sodium phosphate enemas when used in children?

(A) Renal insufficiency
(B) Hirschsprung's disease
(C) Anorectal malformations
(D) Children 6–12 years of age

3. All of the following statements about emollient "stool softener" laxatives are true EXCEPT

(A) they are not good for acute constipation
(B) they are good for patients who should not strain by passing a hard stool (e.g., post-surgical patients)
(C) they never have been found to be better than placebo for long-term use
(D) they are more effective than placebo for long term use

4. Which of the following statements adequately describes bulk-forming laxatives?

(A) Can cause diarrhea if not taken with water
(B) Are derived from polysaccharides and resemble fiber (bran) in mechanism of action
(C) Onset of action is in 4–8 hours
(D) Produce much more complete evacuation of constipation than stimulant products

5. Which of the following statements about non-drug therapies for acute diarrhea is NOT correct?

(A) Breast feeding should be continued as normal.
(B) Even if the patient is not vomiting, food should be withheld for 6–12 hours.
(C) Fluids can be given to patients who experience vomiting, but small amounts of fluid should be used.
(D) Replacement fluids mainly consist of water, sugar, potassium, sodium, and bicarbonate.

6. Which of the following products should NOT be used to replenish lost fluids from acute diarrhea?

(A) Pedialyte solution
(B) Kool-Aid
(C) Gatorade (half-strength diluted with water)
(D) The World Health Organization (WHO) solution

7. Which of the following statements about adsorbent drugs used for diarrhea is true?

(A) Useful for treatment of severe diarrhea
(B) Very unsafe because not absorbed systemically
(C) In general, small doses are needed to relieve diarrhea.
(D) Kaolin is now generally recognized as a safe and effective OTC antidiarrheal agent.

8. Which of the following statements concerning traveler's diarrhea (TD) is true?

(A) TD can usually be avoided by not eating raw vegetables, seafood, or eggs when traveling to third-world countries.
(B) TD can be prevented by taking one dose of antibiotic 1 day before a trip.
(C) A specie of *Helicobacter pylori* is the primary pathogen responsible for TD.
(D) Phillip's Milk of Magnesia is used to prevent/treat TD.

9. All of the following agents are considered close to ideal laxatives EXCEPT

(A) emollient laxatives
(B) bulk-forming laxatives
(C) fiber
(D) stimulant laxatives

10. All of the following statements about stool softeners are true EXCEPT

(A) there is minimal systemic absorption
(B) the onset of action is usually 1–2 days
(C) they are useful in patients with constipation who have experienced an acute myocardial infarction
(D) they can be taken with little or no water

11. All of the following statements adequately describe bulk-forming laxatives EXCEPT

(A) they produce a much more complete evacuation of constipation than stimulant products
(B) they can cause constipation if not taken with water
(C) they are derived from polysaccharides and resemble fiber (bran) in the mechanism of action
(D) the onset of action is 24–72 hours

12. A patient suffering from acute infectious diarrhea caused by *Shigella* can be managed in all of the following ways EXCEPT

(A) no treatment because signs and symptoms usually resolve in 48 hours
(B) use of glucose solutions (e.g., soda, apple juice) to settle the stomach and decrease the number of stools
(C) avoiding food for at least 6 hours, then slowly increasing fluid intake
(D) using antibiotics (e.g., Bactrim, doxycycline) for 7 days

13. Which local anesthetic should be used to treat symptoms of pain, itching, burning, and discomfort in patients with an established lidocaine allergy?

(A) Tetracaine
(B) Dibucaine
(C) Pramoxine
(D) Benzocaine

14. All of the following items are part of a standard conservative approach to the treatment of first- or second-degree hemorrhoids EXCEPT

(A) topical anesthetic (hemorrhoidal ointment)
(B) stool softener
(C) sitz baths
(D) rubber band ligation

15. What is the most common sign/symptom of hemorrhoids?

(A) Bleeding
(B) Pain
(C) Seepage
(D) Pruritus

16. Which of the following agents is designated as a safe and effective analgesic, anesthetic, and antipruritic by the Food and Drug Administration?

(A) Witch hazel
(B) Juniper tar
(C) Hydrocortisone
(D) Phenylephrine

17. All of the following vasoconstrictors are deemed safe and effective for the temporary relief of itching and swelling EXCEPT

(A) ephedrine 0.1%–1.25%
(B) epinephrine 0.005%–0.01%
(C) phenylpropanolamine 1%–10%
(D) phenylephrine 0.25%

18. All of the following symptoms associated with gastroesophageal reflux disease (GERD) may be treated with nonprescription agents EXCEPT

(A) burning sensation located in the lower chest
(B) pain that is worse after meals
(C) pain or difficulty when swallowing
(D) pain that is worse upon lying down at bedtime

19. Which of the following is an appropriate nonpharmacological recommendation for patients with gastroesophageal reflux disease (GERD)?

(A) Eat larger but fewer meals
(B) Avoid meals high in protein
(C) Eat evening meals at least 3 hours before bed
(D) Prop a patient's head up with two pillows at night

20. All of the following statements regarding antacid use in gastroesophageal reflux disease (GERD) are correct EXCEPT

(A) the onset of symptom relief with antacids is 1–2 hours
(B) antacids will relieve symptoms for 1–3 hours
(C) sodium bicarbonate should not be used in patients with edema, congestive heart failure, or those on low-salt diets
(D) the most frequent side effect of aluminum-magnesium combination antacids is diarrhea

21. All of the following statements regarding use of nonprescription H₂RAs in gastroesophageal reflux disease (GERD) are correct EXCEPT

(A) the most common adverse effects of nonprescription H₂RAs are headache, diarrhea, dizziness, and nausea
(B) cimetidine may increase serum concentrations of warfarin, theophylline, and phenytoin
(C) the onset of symptom relief with these agents is 1–2 hours
(D) nonprescription H₂RAs will heal severely damaged esophageal mucosa

22. All of the following statements regarding use of nonprescription products for gastroesophageal reflux disease (GERD) in special populations are correct EXCEPT

(A) nonprescription H₂RAs are not approved for use in children younger than 12 years of age
(B) antacids may be safely used in pregnant patients as long as chronic high doses are avoided
(C) sodium bicarbonate is the preferred antacid in pregnant patients
(D) doses of nonprescription H₂RAs do not need to be reduced in elderly patients

Directions: Each item below contains three suggested answers, of which **one or more** is correct. Choose the answer

A	if **I only** is correct
B	if **III only** is correct
C	if **I and II** are correct
D	if **II and III** are correct
E	if **I, II, and III** are correct

23. Which of the following drugs most commonly causes constipation?

I. Ampicillin
II. Narcotic analgesics
III. Drugs possessing anticholinergic properties

24. Which of the following statements about stimulant laxatives is correct?

I. They produce a stool quicker than any other type of laxative.
II. They are associated with more adverse effects than any other type of laxative.
III. They work by irritating the lining of the colon wall to increase peristalsis and produce a stool.

25. When should a patient experiencing diarrhea be referred to a physician by a pharmacist?

I. If the patient has pus or blood in the stool.
II. If the patient also suffers from vomiting.
III. If the patient has a fever.

ANSWERS AND EXPLANATIONS

1. The answer is C *[1 B]*.
Glycerin and the bisacodyl suppository all produce stools in one-half hour to a few hours, whereas psyllium, a bulk-forming laxative, produces stool in 24–72 hours in the same manner as a normal bolus of food or fiber.

2. The answer is D *[1 C 4]*.
The popular sodium phosphate enemas (e.g., Fleet) are very effective but have resulted in hyperphosphatemia, hypocalcemia (tetany), hypokalemia, metabolic acidosis, and cardiac death usually due to conduction abnormalities in very small children. This has mainly occurred in children younger than 2 years of age or between 2 and 5 years of age with predisposing factors. These factors include chronic renal disease, anorectal malformations, and/or Hirschsprung's disease, which allow phosphate blood concentrations to become abnormally high and potassium and calcium to become low. These conditions predispose these patients to cardiac arrhythmias and potentially death. Therefore, the use of enemas is highly discouraged in children under 5 years of age.

3. The answer is D *[I B 2 d]*.
These agents have a long onset of action (24–48 hours); thus, they should never be used for acute constipation but should be used mainly for patients who should not strain to pass hard stools (e.g., pregnant patients, postsurgical patients, post–myocardial infarction). However, they have never been found to be more effective than placebo in long-term use.

4. The answer is B *[I B 2 a, c]*.
Stimulant products result in a quicker, more complete, and often more violent evacuation of the bowel than do the bulk-forming agents. Bulk-forming agents are developed from complex sugars, similar to fiber, that provide bulk to increase gastrointestinal motility and water absorption into the bowel. However, patients must drink plenty of water to facilitate the absorption of water into the bowel, or they may become more constipated.

5. The answer is B *[II C 1]*.
The most important part of treating acute diarrhea is the replacement of lost fluids. If patients experience mild to moderate fluid loss, replacement can be done with oral-rehydration solutions. If fluid loss is severe (more than 10% loss of body weight) and/or severe vomiting, then patients may need intravenous rehydration before oral-maintenance fluids can be administered. Oral-rehydration solutions can be easily made at home (see Table 32-1) or purchased ready to use (e.g., Pedialyte, Infalyte, Rehydralyte, Resol). Because the secretory and absorptive mechanisms of the bowel function separately, this allows these oral-rehydration solutions to be absorbed during acute episodes of diarrhea, preventing severe dehydration and complications. There has been much controversy regarding the decision to feed or not feed children during acute episodes of diarrhea. Originally, parents were told that children should not receive food, milk-products, or breast milk for 6–48 hours after the onset of diarrhea. Recent information shows that children should remain on their normal diet or breast feeding during episodes of diarrhea because these do not make the diarrhea worse and may actually improve the diarrhea.

6. The answer is B *[II C 1 b]*.
Replacement fluids for diarrhea should contain the appropriate amount of electrolytes (K^+, Na^+, Cl^-, citrate) and glucose per specified amount of water, as found in commercially available oral-rehydration solutions such as Pedialyte and Rehydralyte. The World Health Organization (WHO) solution can be made easily at home to provide the necessary ingredients. In addition, one-half–strength Gatorade will provide the necessary electrolytes and glucose to replenish lost fluids. Kool-Aid does not contain potassium. Carbonated beverages are low in potassium, and some are too high in glucose.

7. The answer is D *[II C 2 b]*.
Adsorbents are not effective for severe diarrhea because they simply cannot adsorb enough water and do not reverse the cause of the diarrhea. Large doses may decrease symptoms. Of all the adsorbents, kaolin is the most effective and is now recognized by the FDA as safe and effective. All adsorbents are safe because they are not adsorbed systemically.

8. The answer is A *[II A 2 a (1) (b)]*.
Traveler's diarrhea (TD) primarily is caused by bacteria (mainly enterotoxin *Escherichia coli*). Prophylaxis and treatment regimens include oral antibiotics (fluoroquinolones, sulfonamides, doxycycline) and bismuth subsalicylate (Pepto-Bismol). *Helicobacter pylori* is the organism shown to contribute to refractory peptic ulcer disease.

9. The answer is D *[I B 2]*.
The ideal laxative is natural (i.e., similar to food) and produces stool on a regular basis. The product produces stool quickly (i.e., in several hours) without adverse effects such as abdominal cramping or the formation of a hard stool, which may be difficult to pass. Products such as fiber or bulk-forming agents produce a stool similar to a bolus of food, without adverse effects. Emollient laxatives (i.e., stool softeners) produce soft stools without difficult defecation. Stimulants produce a stool quickly, but patients often experience severe abdominal cramping and hard stools.

10. The answer is D *[I B 2 d]*.
Stool softeners are safe and do not produce any adverse systemic effects. Because stool softeners work as surfactants, they allow absorption of water into the stool, which makes the stool softer and easier to pass. These products are useful in patients who should avoid straining to pass hard stools (e.g., post-myocardial infarction patients) because straining may be stressful to the patient. Each dose must be taken with 8 oz of water.

11. The answer is A *[I B 2 a, c]*.
Stimulant products result in a quicker, more complete, and often more violent evacuation of the bowel than do the bulk-forming agents. Bulk-forming agents are developed from complex sugars, similar to fiber, that provide bulk to increase gastrointestinal motility and increase water absorption into the bowel. However, patients must drink plenty of water to facilitate the absorption of water into the bowel, or they may become more constipated.

12. The answer is B *[II C; Table 32-3]*.
Giving highly osmotic solutions of glucose (e.g., soda, fruit juice) can result in more water absorbed into the intestinal tract and, thus, further diarrhea. Many cases of diarrhea resolve within 48 hours without treatment. People with diarrhea can avoid food for at least 6 hours, then increase their fluid intake slowly. Severe cases of infectious diarrhea can be treated with antibiotics or antiprotozoals, depending on the organism that caused the episode.

13. The answer is C *[III G 2 b]*.
Due to its chemically distinct structure, pramoxine exhibits less cross-sensitivity when compared to the other anesthetics and should be used in patients with a lidocaine allergy.

14. The answer is D *[III F 1]*.
A conservative approach to treatment includes sitz baths, the use of stool softeners to prevent straining when passing a stool, and the use of an anesthetic hemorrhoidal preparation. If improvement is not seen, more aggressive therapy may be pursued (e.g., rubber band ligation).

15. The answer is A *[III C 1]*.
The most common sign/symptom of hemorrhoids is painless bleeding occurring during a bowel movement.

16. The answer is B *[III G 7]*.
Juniper tar, menthol, and camphor are the only three agents deemed safe and effective as analgesics, anesthetics, and antipruritics by the FDA. These agents were formerly classified as counterirritants.

17. The answer is C *[III G 3 a]*.
Vasoconstrictors deemed safe and effective by the FDA are ephedrine HCl 0.1%–1.25%, epinephrine HCl 0.005%–0.01%, and phenylephrine HCl 0.25%.

18. The answer is C *[IV A 2–3, 6]*.
Pain on swallowing often suggests severe esophageal mucosal damage, which would require prescription medications for healing. Difficulty on swallowing may indicate an esophageal stricture, cancer, or motor disorder. All of these conditions require diagnosis and treatment by a health-care provider.

19. The answer is C *[IV B 1 a–k].*
Patients should be instructed to eat evening meals at least 3 hours before going to bed. This allows sufficient time for gastric emptying, so that the volume of refluxed material will be smaller and less irritating to the esophagus.

20. The answer is A *[IV B 2 a].*
One of the major advantages of antacid use in heartburn is its quick onset of action. Most patients with mild gastroesophageal reflux disease (GERD) will experience relief from antacids within 5–15 minutes of administration.

21. The answer is D *[IV B 2 c–d].*
Nonprescription doses of H_2RAs are too low to heal esophageal damage. Esophageal mucosal damage is very difficult to heal and requires very high doses of H_2RAs that are available only by prescription. Alternatively, proton pump inhibitors, which completely suppress acid secretion, may be used to heal esophageal mucosal damage.

22. The answer is C *[IV C 2].*
Sodium bicarbonate should be avoided in pregnant patients because the high sodium load may cause systemic alkalosis, edema, and/or weight gain.

23. The answer is D (II, III) *[I A 2 d].*
Opiate analgesics (e.g., narcotics) and drugs with anticholinergic properties decrease bowel motility, which results in increased water absorption from the intestinal tract. This can cause a harder, drier stool, which results in constipation. Ampicillin is often poorly absorbed from the intestinal tract and can alter the flora of the intestinal bowel. This destruction of bowel organisms causes increased secretions into the bowel, which results in diarrhea.

24. The answer is D (II, III) *[I B 2 c].*
Stimulant laxatives do have a quick onset of action but not any quicker than the saline laxatives, which usually work in 4–6 hours. The mechanism of action for stimulant laxatives is that they irritate the lining of the colon wall, which increases peristalsis and produces a stool. These laxatives are associated with more adverse effects than other laxatives.

25. The answer is E (all) *[II B 2].*
Patients with pus or blood in the stool, vomiting, or fever may be suffering from severe bacterial diarrhea and may lose large amounts of fluid, which could result in severe dehydration.

33

OTC Menstrual, Vaginal, and Contraceptive Agents

Tina M. Harrison
Mollie A. Scott
Larry N. Swanson

I. MENSTRUATION AND MENSTRUAL PRODUCTS

A. Introduction. Menstruation is a cyclic, physiological discharge of blood and mucus through the vagina of a nonpregnant woman. The menstrual cycle eliminates a mature, unfertilized egg and prepares the endometrium for the possible implantation of a fertilized egg the following month. The **average** duration of the menstrual cycle is 28 days. The duration of menstrual flow is 3–7 days.

B. Menstrual abnormalities

1. **Dysmenorrhea** is painful menstruation.
   a. **Types**
      (1) **Primary dysmenorrhea** is pain associated with menstruation with the absence of identifiable pelvic disease. It is prompted by increased levels of prostaglandins in the menstrual fluids.
      (2) **Secondary dysmenorrhea** is associated with an underlying pelvic disorder. Possible causes include endometriosis, pelvic inflammatory disease (PID), and ovarian cysts.
   b. **Symptoms** of dysmenorrhea often include nausea, vomiting, diarrhea, headache, dizziness, and lower abdominal cramping.
   c. **Treatment**
      (1) **Recommendation of therapy** should be based on the patient's assessment of the degree of pain. Pain associated with dysmenorrhea generally tapers within 2 days. Prolonged pain may be associated with an underlying problem, and patients should be referred to a physician.
      (2) **Agents** for the relief of dysmenorrhea include:
         (a) **Analgesics** are used as primary treatment of dysmenorrhea and for relief of cramping associated with premenstrual syndrome (PMS) [see I B 4]. Analgesic treatment with aspirin or acetaminophen may begin at the onset of the menstrual period or 2–3 days before menses and continue throughout the menstrual flow. Nonsteroidal anti-inflammatory drugs (NSAIDs) also are approved for treatment. The dosage of ibuprofen (e.g., Advil, Midol IB, Nuprin) is 200 mg every 4–6 hours with the maximum not exceeding 1200 mg per day. Other NSAIDs include ketoprofen (e.g., Orudis-KT, Actron) 12.5 mg every 4–6 hours, not to exceed 25 mg in a 4–6-hour period or 75 mg in 24 hours, and naproxen (Aleve) 200 mg every 8–12 hours, not to exceed 600 mg per day. For women who do not receive relief from over-the-counter (OTC) analgesics, prescription NSAIDs may prove more useful.
         (b) **Diuretics** are **recommended** by the Food and Drug Administration (FDA) for use in eliminating water during premenstrual and menstrual periods. When administered approximately 5 days before menses, diuretics help relieve bloating, excess water, cramps, and tension. Included in this category are ammonium chloride, caffeine, and pamabrom.
            (i) **Ammonium chloride** (NH_4Cl) is an acid-forming salt often used in combination with caffeine. Up to 3 grams of NH_4Cl per day can be administered in three divided doses per day. Larger doses are often associated with gastrointestinal (GI) symptoms. OTC products include Aqua Ban and Aqua Ban Plus, which contains NH_4Cl and caffeine.
            (ii) **Caffeine,** a xanthine derivative, promotes diuresis by inhibiting tubular reabsorption of sodium and chloride. The **recommended dosage** is 100–200

mg every 3–4 hours. **Side effects** associated with caffeine use are GI disturbances and CNS stimulation.

    (iii) Pamabrom (Midol PMS, Pamprin) is a theophylline derivative often used in combination with analgesics and antihistamines. Dosages should not exceed 200 mg per day.

2. Amenorrhea is an absence of menstruation. The development of primary or secondary amenorrhea requires physician evaluation.

3. Intermenstrual pain and **bleeding** generally occur at midcycle and may last from several hours to days. Pain is often associated with ovulation (mittelschmerz). Therapy consists of nonprescription analgesics. Patients with pain lasting longer than 2 days should be referred to a physician.

4. PMS
    a. Symptoms (e.g., marked mood swings, fatigue, appetite changes, bloating) begin 1–7 days before the onset of menses.
    b. Nonpharmacological therapy includes regular exercise and reduction of stress factors. Patients experiencing symptoms abnormal to their cycle should be referred to a physician.
    c. Pharmacological treatment. The efficacy and safety of pharmacological treatment of PMS are aimed at the proposed etiologies (e.g., a drop in progesterone concentrations, high levels of prolactin, elevated estrogen concentrations, deficiencies of vitamins A or B_6, or an underlying disorder) and are not well studied. Although clinical trials do not support the efficacy of vitamins A or B_6, both have been used for the treatment of PMS. Nonprescription diuretics are commonly used to reduce fluid accumulation associated with PMS. Prescription drug products that have been studied in the management of PMS include benzodiazepines, monoamine oxidase inhibitors, tricyclic antidepressants, and serotonin reuptake inhibitors. Fluoxetine (under the brand name Sarafem) has recently been approved for the treatment of premenstrual dysphoric disorder.

5. Menorrhagia is excessive menstrual blood loss. Low hematocrit, low hemoglobin, and low serum iron levels may occur. Treatment for menorrhagia is usually an estrogen-progestin combination (i.e., oral contraceptive).

C. Toxic shock syndrome (TSS) is a rare but sometimes fatal disease often associated with menstruation.

    1. TSS can be categorized either as menstrual or nonmenstrual, with approximately two-thirds of cases associated with menstruation. TSS is known to occur in both men and women.

    2. This condition usually affects women under 30 years of age who use tampons. Women between the ages of 15 and 19 years are at the highest risk.

    3. TSS is characterized by an abrupt onset (8–12 hours) of flu-like symptoms (e.g., high fever, myalgia, vomiting, diarrhea).

    4. TSS results from an exotoxin produced by *Staphylococcus aureus.*

    5. The **primary risk factor** for TSS is the **use of tampons.** Additional risk factors include barrier contraceptives (e.g., diaphragms, cervical sponges).

    6. When TSS is suspected, patients should be hospitalized immediately. To lower the risk of TSS, women should use lower-absorbency tampons and alternate the use of tampons with feminine pads.

D. Menstrual products like feminine pads and tampons are used to absorb menstrual and other vaginal discharges. **Feminine pads** are available in a wide variety of sizes and absorbencies. "Super" or "maxi" pads may be used for the heaviest menstrual flow (usually occurring on day 2 of the cycle). "Mini" or "light" pads and "junior" or "teen" pads are designed for the smaller anatomy and lighter flow. Frequent changing of sanitary pads minimizes the occurrence of unpleasant odors, and it helps to minimize irritation and chafing. **Tampons** are intravaginal inserts designed to absorb vaginal discharge. Many women prefer tampons because they are worn internally, which lessens chafing, odor, bulkiness, and irritation. "Super" tampons are designed for heavier flow. "Junior" or "regular" tampons are designed for moderate to light menstrual flow. Frequent changing of tampons will minimize the risks associated with TSS.

II. VAGINAL PRODUCTS

A. Vaginal yeast infections

1. General considerations

a. Occurrence. Approximately 75% of all women will experience a yeast infection at least once, and 50% will have a second episode during their lifetime. Only 5% of women experience recurrent infections.

b. Cause. *Candida albicans* is responsible for up to 92% of infections. Infections due to *Candida glabrata* are increasing.

c. Predisposing factors. Antibiotics, oral contraceptives containing high-dose estrogen, pregnancy, diabetes, and immunosuppression increase the risk for infection.

d. Symptoms. Can include a thick, white, "cottage cheese"–like nonmalodorous vaginal discharge, dysuria, vaginal burning, and pruritus.

2. Patient assessment

a. Patients should be questioned about presence of symptoms, medication use, medical conditions, and history of vaginal yeast infections.

b. The following patients should be referred to their primary care provider for diagnosis and treatment:

   (1) First episode of symptoms
   (2) Pregnant
   (3) Less than 12 years of age
   (4) Systemic symptoms such as fever
   (5) History of recurrent vaginal yeast infections
   (6) Patients who complain of a "fishy" odor to their discharge (indicative of bacterial vaginosis most often caused by anaerobic bacteria) or a thin, malodorous purulent discharge (indicative of *Trichomonas* infection)

3. Pharmacological treatment

a. Nonprescription agents are recommended only for patients who have had a prior yeast infection and who can potentially recognize the infection and self-medicate.

b. The choice of nonprescription therapy is based on patient preference.

c. Available formulations include intravaginal creams, suppositories, and ointments.

d. External vaginal creams can be used in combination with intravaginal products to treat vulvar symptoms of pruritus.

e. Intravaginal products are used at bedtime, whereas the external creams can be used any time of day.

f. Available nonprescription therapies include the antifungal agents Gyne Lotrimin (clotrimazole), Monistat 3 and Monistat 7 (miconazole), Femstat 3 (butoconazole), and Monistat 1 and Vagistat 1 (tioconazole).

   (1) Gyne Lotrimin and Monistat 7 are used for 7 consecutive days; Monistat 3 and Femstat 3 are used for 3 consecutive days; Monistat 1 and Vagistat 1 are used for 1 day.
   (2) Efficacy rates approach 80%–90%.

4. Patient counseling

a. Nonpharmacological

   (1) Dry vaginal area well after bathing with a towel or a hairdryer on a low setting.
   (2) Avoid tight or damp clothing.
   (3) Wear cotton underwear.
   (4) Use unscented soap to avoid irritation.
   (5) Avoid douching.

b. Pharmacological

   (1) Complete course of therapy even if symptoms improve.
   (2) Wash vaginal area with mild soap prior to application.
   (3) Avoid sexual intercourse during therapy.
   (4) Avoid condoms or diaphragm use for 72 hours after therapy is completed.
   (5) Continue use during menstrual period.
   (6) Avoid tampons during use.
   (7) Sanitary pads can be used for leakage of intravaginal products.
   (8) Side effects can include burning or irritation.

B. Feminine hygiene products. There are a variety of feminine hygiene products available for cleansing and controlling odor associated with normal vaginal discharge. These products are not used to treat vaginal infections.

1. Vaginal douches such as Summers Eve irrigate the vagina and can be used for cleansing, soothing, as an astringent, or to produce a mucolytic effect.

2. Vaginal suppositories such as Betadine medicated suppositories are used for soothing, to relieve minor irritations, and to reduce the number of pathogenic microorganisms.

III. OTC CONTRACEPTIVES

A. Introduction. The **efficacy** and **pregnancy rates** for various means of contraception depend greatly on the **degree of compliance.** Table 33-1 gives ranges of pregnancy rates reported for various means of contraception.

B. Methods of contraception that may make use of nonprescription products or devices include:

1. **Fertility awareness methods** make use of information concerning the menstrual cycle to determine the days when intercourse is most likely to result in a pregnancy. **Periodic abstinence** is also referred to as the **rhythm method, natural family planning,** or **ovulation detection method.** The various natural family planning methods allow the patient to monitor the natural physiological signs that can in many women predict the fertile period (periovulatory phase of the menstrual cycle), enabling the couple to avoid coital exposure at that time. These methods are based on reproductive anatomy and physiology and are applied according to the signs and symptoms naturally occurring in the menstrual cycle. Calculations of the period of fertility take into account the **sperm viability** in the female reproductive tract, which is estimated to average **2–3 days** (up to 5 days), and the **fertile**

Table 33-1. Pregnancy Rates for Various Means of Contraception (%)[1]

Method of contraception	Typical[2]	Lowest[3]
Oral Contraceptives		
Combination (estrogen/progestin)	0.1–0.34	0.1
Progestin-only	0.5–1.5	0.5
Mechanical/Chemical		
Cervical cap[4]		
Multiparous	40	26
Nulliparous	20	9
Male condom without spermicide	12–14	3
Male condom with spermicide	4–6	1.8
Diaphragm[4]	20	6
Female condom	21	5
IUD	≤1–2	≤1–1.5
Levonorgestrel implants	≤1	≤1
Medroxyprogesterone injection	≤1	≤1
Spermicide alone	20–22	6
Rhythm (all types)	25	1–9
Vasectomy/Tubal Ligation	≤1	≤1
Withdrawal	40–50	30
No contraception	85	85

[1]During first year of continuous use.

[2]A typical couple who initiated a method that was either not always used correctly or was not used with every act of sexual intercourse, and who experienced an accidental pregnancy.

[3]The method of birth control was always used correctly with every act of sexual intercourse but the couple still experienced an accidental pregnancy.

[4]Used with spermicide.

Adapted from *Nonprescription Drug Therapy Guiding Patient Self Care, Facts and Comparisons,* St. Louis, 2002, p 1155.

period of the ovum, which is estimated to be **24 hours.** Recent studies indicate that conception is most likely to occur when couples have intercourse during a 6-day period ending on the day of ovulation. **Conception is highly unlikely if sexual intercourse occurs 6 or more days <u>prior</u> to ovulation or the day <u>after</u> ovulation. Disadvantages** to the rhythm method (but necessary to ensure efficacy) include both the **long periods of abstinence** and the **charting of menses** that are required. Methods of natural family planning and periodic abstinence include temperature method, calendar method, Billings method, and sympto-thermal method.

a. **Temperature method.** Basal body temperature (**BBT**) determination makes use of a **basal thermometer,** which can be purchased without a prescription. The thermometer covers the range of temperature from 96°F–100°F, with 0.1°F gradations.
   (1) The significance of basal temperature determination lies in the fact that within 24 hours preceding ovulation, there is a **moderate drop in the basal temperature** followed by a **noticeable rise in the body temperature,** usually about 24 hours after ovulation. This rise is usually maintained for the remainder of the cycle and is thought to be due to the thermogenic properties of **progesterone,** the hormone indicative of the transition from the ovulatory phase to the luteal phase. Therefore, ovulation is represented by the transition of the falling temperature to the rising temperature.
   (2) For many women, **abstinence** should be practiced from approximately **5 days after the onset of menses until 3 days after the transition in temperature.**
   (3) Because the basal temperature reflects the amount of heat radiation when the body is at its metabolic low, the temperature should be taken first thing in the morning (i.e., before any activity). The thermometer may be placed under the tongue, in the rectum, or in the vagina (the temperature should always be taken from the same place) and should be left undisturbed for at least 5 minutes (mercury thermometer). Electronic digital thermometers are also available that have shorter recording times (45–90 seconds). Infection, tension, a restless night, or any type of excessive movement can cause variations nonreflective of the basal temperature.
b. The **calendar method** estimates the possible day of ovulation. **Abstinence** should be practiced during the period around ovulation when there may be a fertilizable egg present. Whereas the calendar rhythm method was used for several decades, it has not been promoted as a method of natural family planning for many years. Although women who have regular menstrual cycles are able to use the calendar rhythm method successfully, women with irregular cycles, women who are breast feeding, or women with postponed ovulation cannot depend on the calendar rhythm method.
   (1) For a span of **approximately 1 year,** the patient records her menstruation dates on a calendar.
   (2) Calendar charting allows women to calculate the onset and duration of their fertile period—the time during which a viable egg is available for fertilization by sperm. Calculation of the fertile period rests on three assumptions.
      (a) **Ovulation** occurs on day **14 (plus or minus 2 days) before the onset of the next menses.**
      (b) **Sperm remain viable for 2–3 days.**
      (c) **The ovum survives for 24 hours.**
   (3) The calendar is then reviewed to determine the length of her shortest and longest cycle.
      (a) Eighteen days should be subtracted from the number of days of the shortest cycle. This number should correspond with the first possible fertile day in any given cycle: 14 + 2 = 16 days; 16 + 2 = 18 days (viability of sperm) [see III B 1 b].
      (b) Eleven days should be subtracted from the number of days of the longest cycle. This number should correspond with the last possible fertile day in any given cycle: 14 – 2 = 12 days; 12 – 1 = 11 days (viability of ova) [see III B 1 b].
   (4) **Abstinence** should be practiced from the first possible fertile day through the last possible fertile day.
   (5) **Example.** Assume the shortest number of days between two consecutive menses is 25 and the longest number of days between two consecutive menses is 32. Eighteen days subtracted from 25 days (the shortest cycle) equals 7 (or day 7). Eleven days subtracted from 32 days (the longest cycle) equals 21 (or day 21). Therefore, abstinence should be practiced from day 7 through and including day 21 of each cycle.

    c. The **cervical mucus (Billings or cervical secretions)** method of rhythm is based on the principle that the normal, thick, creamy white vaginal mucus becomes clear and tenacious around the time of ovulation (much like a raw egg white).

        (1) The woman should watch for this change in mucus consistency and practice abstinence around the time of ovulation.

        (2) The woman should consider herself fertile for 3–4 days after the peak change.

    d. The **symptothermal** method, rather than relying on a single physiological index, uses several indices to determine the fertile period.

        (1) The **most common** calendar calculations and **changes in the cervical mucus** are used to estimate the **onset of the fertile period.**

        (2) Changes in the mucus or basal temperature are used to estimate the end of the fertile period.

        (3) Because several indices need to be monitored, this method is more difficult to learn than the single-index method, but it is more effective than the cervical mucus method (i.e., Billings method) alone.

2. Spermicidal agents are composed of an **active spermicidal chemical,** which immobilizes or kills sperm, and an **inert base** (e.g., foam, cream, jelly, gel, tablet, or suppository), which localizes the spermicidal chemical in proximity to the cervical os.

    a. Mode of action. These agents work by disrupting the sperm membrane and by decreasing the ability of sperm to metabolize fructose.

    b. Active ingredients include **nonoxynol-9** or rarely **octoxynol-9.**

        (1) Both are considered safe and effective by the FDA.

        (2) Side effects [e.g., sensation of warmth, rare allergic reactions **(contact dermatitis with rash, stinging, itching, and swelling)**] are minimal. If a suspected reaction occurs, one should be instructed to use another product as the issue might be the concentration of the spermicide or an additive specific to a given brand.

        (3) There are no significant differences in birth-defect rates between users and nonusers.

    c. Effects against sexually transmitted diseases (STDs). Nonoxynol-9 is lethal to selected microbes in the laboratory setting and may help to inhibit a variety of sexually transmissible organisms, including those responsible for gonorrhea, chlamydial infection, candidiasis, genital herpes, syphilis, trichomoniasis, and acquired immune deficiency syndrome (AIDS). There have been inconsistent results in human studies, however. One concern relates to the fact that frequent use of spermicides can cause vulvovaginal epithelial disruption, which may increase susceptibility to human immunodeficiency virus (HIV). In addition, **spermicides** may alter the vaginal flora and, therefore, **should not be relied upon alone for STD prevention.**

    d. Dosage forms. Contraceptive spermicides offer the greatest variety within one specific method of contraception, being available in various forms, including the following (Table 33-2).

        (1) Creams, jellies, and gels are used with a diaphragm. The concentration of spermicide is less than the necessary 8% to be employed as a single contraceptive method.

        (2) Foams disperse better into the vagina and over the cervical opening. They usually contain a higher concentration of spermicide (i.e., **the optimal concentration of 8% or higher**). Volume differences among brands may require various dosage amounts. If vaginal or penile irritation develops, another brand should be tried.

            (a) The can should be shaken vigorously 20 times before use.

            (b) The foam should be inserted intravaginally about two-thirds the length of the applicator, and the contents should be discharged.

            (c) Foam should be reapplied during prolonged intercourse (e.g., that lasting longer than 1 hour) and before every subsequent act of intercourse.

            (d) In order to ensure efficacy, at least 8 hours should pass before douching because this may dilute the spermicide effect or even "force" sperm into the cervix.

        (3) Suppositories and foaming tablets. These agents are both small and convenient. Although solid at room temperature, suppositories melt at body temperature, whereas foaming tablets effervesce.

            (a) The tablets should be wetted before insertion, which may create a sensation of warmth.

            (b) The tablet or suppository should be inserted high into the vagina, and approximately 10–15 minutes should pass before intercourse.

            (c) Intercourse must occur within 1 hour, or the dose must be repeated.

Table 33-2. Spermicides

Representative Products (Brand Names)	Spermicidal Agent	Comments
Film		
VCF (Vaginal Contraceptive Film)	Nonoxynol-9	Contraceptive protection begins in 5–15 minutes after insertion; remains effective no more than 1 hour
Foam		
Ortho Options Delfen, Koromex	Nonoxynol-9	Contraceptive protection is immediate; remains effective no more than 1 hour
Jellies, creams, gels		
K-Y Plus Lubricating, Koromex, Ortho Options Gynol II, Ortho Options Conceptrol	Nonoxynol-9	Contraceptive protection is immediate; used alone remains effective no more than 1 hour; when used with diaphragm or cap, keep diaphragm or cap in place for at least 6 hours after last intercourse
Ortho Options Ortho-Gynol	Octoxynol-9	Contraceptive protection is immediate; than 1 hour; when used with diaphragm than 1 hour; when used with diaphragm or cap, keep diaphragm or cap in place for at least 6 hours after last intercourse
Suppositories and tablets		
Encare, Semicid inserts	Nonoxynol-9	Contraceptive protection begins in 10–15 minutes after insertion; remains effective no more than 1 hour

Adapted from Hatcher RA. *Contraceptive Technology 1994–1996,* 16th ed. NY, Irvington Publishers, 1994, p. 180.

        (d) Another tablet or suppository should be inserted before each repeated act of intercourse.

        (e) In order to ensure efficacy, 6–8 hours after the last act of intercourse should pass before douching.

    (4) Film comes as small paper-thin sheets (e.g., VCF). It is inserted on the tip of the finger into the vagina and placed at the cervical opening; 5–15 minutes must pass before intercourse.

    (5) Sponge. This was a fairly popular product that was removed from the market in the mid-90s because of cost issues related to its manufacture. The new owner of the Today™ sponge (Allendale Pharmaceuticals) is planning to remarket this product. It is a doughnut-shaped polyurethane device containing the spermicide, nonoxynol-9, which is inserted into the vagina before sexual intercourse. Efficacy is approximately comparable to that of a cervical cap. It is believed to act as a contraceptive in three ways: (1) mechanically blocking the cervical entrance, (2) absorbing semen, and (3) providing a spermicide. It can remain in place for 24 hours. Concerns are a higher risk for TSS and a higher pregnancy rate for women who have never given birth (nulliparous women).

  3. Condoms are used to prevent transmission of sperm into the vagina.

    a. Types. They are made of latex rubber, processed collagenous lamb caecum sheaths (lambskin), or polyurethane.

        (1) Latex condoms may help prevent the transmission of many STDs. They are usually packaged with the following label "when used properly, the latex condom may prevent the transmission of many STDs such as syphilis, gonorrhea, chlamydia infections, genital herpes, and AIDS."

            (a) Latex affords greater elasticity than lambskin, and latex condoms are more likely to remain in place on the penis.

(b) Various types are available (e.g., lubricated, ribbed, colored), including some with spermicide (concentration much less than that of a vaginal spermicide product). It is doubtful that spermicide-lubricated condoms offer any better protection than plain latex condoms and they have a shorter shelf life. There is a standard size, but recently smaller and larger versions were put on the market.

    (i) Latex condoms are available with a plain end or with a reservoir tip (sometimes designated as "enz"). The reservoir tip provides room for the ejaculate; however, a space may be left when using the plain-end condom, which accommodates the fluid just as effectively.

    (ii) The **prelubricated condom** helps prevent dyspareunia in a couple with insufficient natural lubrication. Prelubrication decreases the risk of tearing the condom. However, the extra lubrication may be excessive, to the extent of lessening sexual fulfillment in a couple who have adequate natural lubrication or when contraceptive foam is also used.

    (iii) Latex rubber may cause an allergic reaction. An estimated 1%–2% of the population is sensitized to natural rubber latex, with higher percentages likely for those frequently exposed to latex (e.g., health-care workers). The most common symptoms are genital inflammation with redness, itching, and burning. Sometimes, antioxidants or accelerators used during the manufacturing process may be the cause of the allergy.

(2) **Lambskin** condoms are **not** considered as effective as latex condoms (and cannot be labeled as such) in preventing the transmission of STDs, including AIDS. The lambskin condoms are structured to consist of membranes that reveal layers of fibers crisscrossing in various patterns. This gives the lambskin strength, but also allows for an occasional pore. Therefore, lambskin may allow HIV and hepatitis B virus, which are smaller than a sperm, to pass through.

    (a) Lambskin has less elasticity than latex, and lambskin condoms may slip off the penis.

    (b) Lambskin affords **greater sensitivity** than latex.

    (c) Lambskin condoms are more expensive than latex condoms.

(3) A **polyurethane condom** (e.g., Avanti, Trojan Supra) is available for men and is marketed for individuals who are allergic to latex. Some evidence exists that slippage and breakage rates may be higher than for latex condoms. In contrast to the latex condom, petroleum-based products will not degrade the polyurethane.

b. Advantages and disadvantages. The relative accessibility, ease of transport, and low cost make condoms an attractive method of contraception. However, the coital act must be interrupted to apply the condom, and often one or both partners complain of a partial or complete decrease in sensation.

c. Use

    (1) The female external genitalia should not be touched with the exposed penis, and the vagina should not be penetrated, until the condom is unrolled onto the erect penis.

    (2) The condom should be unrolled onto the penis as far as it will go. With the plain-end condom, a space between the tip of the penis and the tip of the condom should be left to catch the ejaculate.

    (3) With either reservoir-tip or plain-end condoms, the tip of the condom must be held between the thumb and index finger to avoid trapping air while unrolling the condom onto the penis. (The space will decrease the likelihood of both rupture secondary to pressure and regurgitation of the ejaculate onto the external genitalia.)

    (4) Proper lubrication to minimize the possibility of tearing can be ensured by using either a lubricated condom or by applying K-Y jelly, spermicidal cream, or jelly to either the condom or the woman's genitalia. [Petroleum jelly (Vaseline) should never be used because it causes deterioration of the rubber (latex) and is a poor lubricant.] Spermicidal foam, cream, or jelly is an excellent adjunctive contraceptive.

    (5) **Before the penis becomes flaccid,** it must be withdrawn from the vagina and the condom eased off. The **condom** should be handled with special care so as not to lose it into the vagina or spill any of the ejaculatory fluid onto the external genitalia.

    (6) A condom should never be reused.

    (7) Condoms should not be stored near excessive heat.

    (8) If the condom should break or leak, spermicide foam should be immediately inserted vaginally.

(9) Do not buy or use condoms that have passed their expiration date.

(10) Be sure to store condoms in a cool, dry place, out of direct sunlight. The glove compartment of a car is not a good place to store condoms. Do not store condoms in pockets, purses, or wallets for more than a few hours.

4. The **female condom** (Reality) is a **disposable polyurethane sheath** that fits into the vagina and **provides protection from pregnancy and STDs.** The sheath resembles a plastic vaginal pouch and consists of an **inner ring,** which is inserted into the vagina near the cervix much like a diaphragm, whereas the **outer ring** remains outside the vagina, covering the labia. The condom is prelubricated, and additional lubricant is provided for use if needed. The polyurethane sheath is **stronger** and probably **less likely to tear or break** than the latex sheath of male condoms. It should be removed immediately after intercourse (before the woman stands up). It may be inserted up to 8 hours before intercourse. If it is used properly, it provides the woman with a method to prevent the transmission of sexually transmitted disease. However, with the noted pregnancy failure rate (see Table 33-1), it is certainly not that reliable for disease transmission. It has not been very popular; some women complain that it interferes with sensation and that it makes unpleasant noises during use.

5. **The diaphragm** is a contraceptive device that is self-inserted into the vagina to block access of sperm to the cervix. It requires a prescription but must be used in conjunction with a nonprescription spermicide to seal off crevices between the vaginal wall and the device.

   a. The diaphragm is held in place by the spring tension of a wire rim encased by rubber. When positioned properly, the diaphragm forms a flexible dome to cover the cervix, the sides pressing against the vaginal muscle wall and the pubic bone.

   b. There are **four types** of diaphragms, including the **coil spring,** the **flat spring,** the **arcing spring,** and a **wide-seal rim.** The tone of vaginal muscles as well as the position of the uterus and adjacent organs usually determine the type of diaphragm necessary.

   c. Sizes of the diaphragm range from 50–95 mm in diameter, in 5-mm gradations.

   d. Use

   (1) The diaphragm plus spermicide can be inserted as long as 6 hours before coitus. The device should be left in place for at least 6 hours after intercourse, but no longer than 24 hours. Additional spermicide is required for repeated intercourse.

   (2) Before inserting the diaphragm, 1 teaspoonful (2–3-inch ribbon) of spermicidal cream or jelly should be spread over the inside of the rubber dome.

   (3) Also, spermicide should be spread around the rim to permit a good seal between the diaphragm and the vaginal wall. (For added protection, it is applied outside the dome.)

   (4) To ensure efficacy, the diaphragm should not be removed for 6–8 hours after intercourse.

   e. Proper care

   (1) The diaphragm should be washed with soap and water, rinsed thoroughly, and dried with a towel.

   (2) It should be dusted with cornstarch and kept in its original container (away from heat).

6. The **cervical cap** is a prescription rubber device smaller than a diaphragm that fits over the cervix like a thimble. It is more difficult to fit than the diaphragm.

   a. It remains effective for more than one episode of intercourse, without adding more spermicide.

   b. The cap should be filled one-third full of spermicide cream or jelly; the spermicide is then applied to the rim.

   c. The cervical cap may be left in place for a maximum of 48 hours and should be left in place for at least 8 hours after intercourse.

STUDY QUESTIONS

Directions: Each of the numbered items or incomplete statements in this section is followed by answers or by completions of the statement. Select the **one** lettered answer or completion that is **best** in each case.

1. The most common cause of vaginal yeast infections is

(A) *Candida albicans*
(B) *Candida glabrata*
(C) *Trichomonas*
(D) anaerobic bacteria

2. The efficacy rate for nonprescription antifungal agents for vaginal yeast infections is

(A) 50%
(B) 60%
(C) 70%
(D) 80%

3. Which of the following statements about nonprescription antifungal agents for vaginal yeast infections is INCORRECT?

(A) Femstat 3 should be applied intravaginally for 3 consecutive nights.
(B) Antifungal agents should be continued during menstruation.
(C) Monistat 1 contains miconazole.
(D) The choice of formulation is based on patient preference.

4. The best product to treat vulvar pruritus in a woman with a vaginal yeast infection is

(A) external miconazole (Monistat)
(B) external miconazole and intravaginal miconazole (Monistat 7 combination pack)
(C) intravaginal tioconazole (Vagistat 1)
(D) intravaginal butoconazole (Femstat 3)

5. Which of the following patients complaining of vaginal yeast infection symptoms should be referred to a physician?

(A) If there is a history of recurrent vaginal yeast infection
(B) If she is pregnant
(C) If she is less than 12 years of age
(D) All of the above

6. All of the following statements regarding contraceptives are correct EXCEPT

(A) using the basal temperature method, intercourse should be avoided for a full 6 days after the noted temperature transition
(B) if a condom should break or leak, one could recommend immediate insertion of a vaginal spermicide foam
(C) vaginal spermicides may kill many of the causative agents of sexually transmitted diseases (STDs), but they should not be relied upon alone for STD prevention
(D) latex condoms are the type that can be labeled for the prevention of human immunodeficiency virus (HIV) transmission
(E) nonoxynol-9 and octoxynol-9 are the two safe and effective United States–marketed vaginal spermicides

7. All of the following statements concerning the vaginal spermicides are correct EXCEPT

(A) used without a condom or diaphragm, it is recommended that the nonoxynol-9 concentration should be at least 8%
(B) foams probably disperse the spermicide throughout the vaginal canal better than cream or jelly forms
(C) douching should not occur for 6–8 hours after the last intercourse since this may dilute the spermicide effect or even "force" sperm into the cervix
(D) evidence to date shows no definite link between these agents and birth defects
(E) none; all of the above statements are correct

8. All of the following statements concerning contraception or contraceptive agents are correct EXCEPT

(A) progesterone is apparently responsible for the increase in basal temperature after ovulation
(B) Vaseline should not be used as a lubricant with latex condoms
(C) using a condom alone is more effective as a contraceptive than taking a combination oral contraceptive
(D) according to the Billings method, vaginal mucus appears like raw egg white at around the time of ovulation
(E) sperm may be viable for up to 5 days in the female reproductive tract with the right conditions

Directions: The group of items in this section consists of lettered options followed by a set of numbered items. For each item, select the **one** lettered option that is most closely associated with it. Each lettered option may be selected once, more than once, or not at all.

Questions 9–10

Match the following primary nonprescription treatments with the correct drug.

(A) Diuretics
(B) Salicylates
(C) Nonsteroidal anti-inflammatory drugs (NSAIDs)
(D) Narcotic analgesics

9. The primary nonprescription pharmacological treatment for pain associated with dysmenorrhea

10. Recommended by the Food and Drug Administration (FDA) for elimination of water before and during menstruation

ANSWERS AND EXPLANATIONS

1. The answer is A *[II A 1 b]*.
Candida albicans remains the most common cause. Infections caused by *Candida glabrata* are increasing. *Trichomonas* and anaerobic bacteria cause other types of vaginal infections.

2. The answer is D *[II A 3 f (2)]*.
Nonprescription antifungal agents' efficacy rates approach 80%–90%.

3. The answer is C *[II A 3 f]*.
Monistat 1 contains tioconazole, a long-acting ointment.

4. The answer is B *[II A 3 d]*.
External creams can be helpful to treat external itching. The vaginal yeast infection still must be treated with an intravaginal cream.

5. The answer is D *[II A 2 b]*.
All of these patients should be referred for diagnosis and treatment.

6. The answer is A *[III B 1 a (2)]*.
Intercourse should be avoided for a full 3 days after the noted temperature transition. All of the other statements (B–D) are correct.

7. The answer is E *[III B 2]*.
Statements A–D are correct.

8. The answer is C *[Table 33-1]*.
The most effective contraceptive product available today is the combination oral contraceptive. All of the other statements (A, B, D, and E) are correct.

9–10. The answers are: 9-C *[I B 1 c (2) (a)]*, **10-A** *[I B 1 c (2) (b)]*.
Nonsteroidal anti-inflammatory drugs (NSAIDs) are approved by the Food and Drug Administration (FDA) for the treatment of primary dysmenorrhea. For premenstrual and menstrual relief of water retention, bloating, and tension, the FDA has approved over-the-counter (OTC) diuretics.

34
Herbal Medicines and Nutritional Supplements

Teresa Klepser

I. **INTRODUCTION.** Many of the drugs available on the market are derived from plants. Some of those include aspirin, atropine, belladonna, capsaicin, cascara, colchicine, digoxin, ephedrine, ergotamine, ipecac, opium, physostigmine, pilocarpine, podophyllum, psyllium, quinidine, reserpine, scopolamine, senna, taxol, tubocurarine, vinblastine, and vincristine. Herbs are also derived from plants; however, herbs are not considered drugs by the Food and Drug Administration (FDA).

A. **Regulations**

1. **The Federal Food, Drug and Cosmetic Act of 1938** mandated pharmaceutical companies to test drugs for safety before marketing.

2. **The Kefauver-Harris Drug Amendments of 1962** mandated pharmaceutical companies to test drugs for efficacy before marketing.

3. **Dietary Supplement Health and Education Act of 1994**
   a. Dietary supplements are not drugs or food. They are intended to supplement the diet.
   b. Herbs are considered dietary supplements.
   c. Dietary supplements do not have to be standardized.
   d. The Secretary of Health and Human Services may remove a supplement from the market only when it has been shown to be hazardous to health.
   e. Dietary supplements may only make claims regarding the effects on structure or function of the body. No claims regarding a particular disease or condition can be made.
   f. This statement is required on the product label: "This product has not been evaluated by the FDA. It is not intended to diagnose, treat, cure, or prevent."

4. **German Federal Health Agency**
   a. In 1978, the German Federal Health Agency established the Commission E.
   b. The Commission E evaluates the safety and efficacy of herbs through clinical trials and cases that are published in scientific literature.
   c. There are more than 300 published monographs on herbs.

B. **Herbs considered unsafe for human consumption**

1. Carcinogenic herbs include borage, calamus, coltsfoot, comfrey, life root, and sassafras.

2. Hepatotoxic herbs include chaparral, germander, kava, and life root.

3. High doses of licorice for long periods may cause pseudoaldosteronism, a condition that may include headache, lethargy, sodium and water retention, hypokalemia, high blood pressure, heart failure, and cardiac arrest.

4. Ma huang is considered unsafe for patients with hypertension, diabetes, or thyroid disease.

5. Pokeroot may be fatal in children.

6. FDA unsafe herbs. The FDA's Center for Food Safety and Applied Nutrition had published the Special Nutritional Adverse Event Monitoring System website for dietary supplements. Unfortunately, the website had not been added to or updated since 1999, and the website has now been removed. Prior to removal, the following dietary supplements were considered unsafe by the FDA.
   Arnica → muscle paralysis, death
   American and European mistletoe → seizures, coma
   Bittersweet and deadly nightshade → cardiac toxicity
   Bloodroot → hypotension, coma
   Broom → dehydration

Comfrey → cancer
Dutch and English tonka bean → hepatotoxicity
Heliotrope → hepatotoxicity
Horse chestnut → bleeding
Jimson weed → anticholinergic, hallucinations
Kava → hepatotoxicity
Lily of the valley → cardiac toxicity
Lobelia (nicotine) → coma, death
Mandrake/Mayapple → severe gastrointestinal symptoms
Morning glory → psychosis
Periwinkle → renal and hepatotoxicity
Snakeroot → reserpine derivative
Spindle tree → seizures
St. John's wort → drug interactions
Sweet flag → hallucinations, liver cancer
True jalap → purgative cathartic
Wahoo → seizures
Wormwood → seizures, paralysis
Yohimbe → renal failure, hypertension

II. COMMONLY USED HERBS

A. Black cohosh *(Cimicifuga racemosa)*

1. **German Commission E indications.** Premenstrual symptoms, painful or difficult menstruation, and neurovegetative symptoms (hot flashes) caused by menopause

2. **Mechanism of action**
   a. Animal studies do not show estrogenic effects.
   b. Mechanism of action is unknown.

3. **Efficacy.** There are four clinical trials that are open-controls and one double-blind, randomized, placebo-controlled trial that compare black cohosh to hormone therapy in peri- and postmenopausal women with neurovegetative menopausal symptoms of varying degrees of severity. The Kupperman Menopause Index and psychiatric clinical and self-evaluation scales were significantly reduced after 3 months of treatment with black cohosh. Vaginal-cytological parameters also improved in regard to estrogen stimulation. Black cohosh was shown to be superior to placebo and comparable to estriol, conjugated estrogens, and estrogen–progesterone therapy.

4. **Contraindications/precautions**
   a. Pregnancy
   b. Unknown if suitable in cases where hormone-replacement therapy is contraindicated, such as estrogen-receptor–positive breast cancer
   c. German Commission E recommends that length of use should not exceed 6 months.

5. **Drug interactions.** None known

6. **Side effects**
   a. Occasional intestinal problems may occur, and weight gain is possible.
   b. Large doses of black cohosh may cause dizziness, nausea, severe headaches, stiffness, and trembling limbs.

7. **Dosage.** Remifemin™ is a standardized product that contains 20 mg of black cohosh to be taken twice daily. It is standardized to 1 mg of 27-deoxyactein per tablet.

B. Chaste tree berry *(Vitex agnus castus)*

1. **German Commission E indications.** Disorders of menstrual cycle, breast swelling, and premenstrual symptoms

2. **Mechanism of action.** Chaste tree berry binds to dopamine receptors and inhibits prolactin secretion. It also increases the pituitary gland's production of luteinizing hormone and inhibits follicle-stimulating hormone (FSH).

3. **Efficacy.** Schellenberg et al. performed a randomized, double-blind, placebo-controlled, parallel group study that included 170 women with premenstrual syndrome. Vitex was given 20 mg QD × 3 cycles. Self-assessment and clinical global impression significantly improved.

4. **Contraindications/precautions.** Pregnancy and women receiving hormone-replacement therapy

5. **Drug interactions.** None known

6. **Side effects.** Mild gastrointestinal upset, skin rash, increased menstrual flow

7. **Dosage.** Recommended dose of chaste tree berry is the liquid extract 40 drops daily.

C. **Cranberry** *(Vaccinium macrocarpon)*

1. **German Commission E indications.** Recurrent urinary tract infections

2. **Mechanism of action**
   a. Urinary acidification
   b. Benzoic and quinic acids break down and form hippuric acid (bacteriostatic)
   c. Inhibition of *Escherichia coli* adherence to epithelial cells of urinary tract

3. **Efficacy.** Avorn et al. performed a quasi-randomized, double-blind, placebo-controlled study including 153 women who received 300 mL of cranberry juice daily for 6 months. Bacteriuria with pyuria occurred less often in the cranberry group (15%) versus placebo (28%).

4. **Contraindications.** Benign prostatic hyperplasia, urinary obstruction, and nephrolithiasis

5. **Drug interactions**
   a. Vitamin B_{12} absorption ($\uparrow$)
   b. Potential to enhance elimination of renally excreted drugs by changing urine pH

6. **Side effects**
   a. Nausea, vomiting, diarrhea
   b. Nephrolithiasis

7. **Dosage.** Recommended dose of cranberry is 300–400 mg twice daily using a standardized product to include 11%–12% quinic acid per dose. Patients may also take 8–16 oz of 100% cranberry juice daily. Drinking lots of fluids is recommended.

D. **Dong quai** *(Angelica senensis)*

1. **Traditional Chinese medicine indications.** Menstrual disorders, anemia, constipation, insomnia, rheumatism, neuralgia, and hypertension

2. **Mechanism of action**
   a. Dong quai contains 1/400th estrogen. However, it does not appear to produce any changes to the ovaries or vaginal tissue.
   b. It contains seven different coumarin derivatives, including oxypeucedanin, osthol, psoralen, and bergapten. Many coumarins have been shown to have vasodilatory and antispasmodic effects. One of the coumarins (osthol) is a central nervous system stimulant.
   c. It inhibits experimentally induced IgE titers, suggesting that components of the plant may have immunosuppressive activity.
   d. It inhibits prostaglandin E_2 release and, therefore, possesses analgesic, antipyrexic, and anti-inflammatory actions.
   e. It has a quinidine-type effect, so it may control tachycardia.
   f. It normalizes uterine contractions.
   g. It has antibiotic activity against gram-negative bacteria *(Bacillus dysenteriae, Bacillus typhi, Bacillus comma, Bacillus paratyphi,* and *E. coli)* and against gram-positive bacteria (hemolytic *Streptococcus* type A and B, *Corynebacterium diphtheriae).*

3. **Efficacy.** Hirata et al. performed a randomized, double-blind, placebo-controlled trial that included 71 postmenopausal women (mean age 52.4 years) who had FSH less than 30 mIU/mL with hot flashes. Women received 3 capsules of dong quai three times daily (equivalent to 4.5 grams of dong quai root daily) or placebo for 24 weeks. Dong quai

did not produce estrogen-like responses in endometrial thickness or in vaginal maturation or relieve menopausal symptoms. The study is criticized for using dong quai alone, because in Traditional Chinese medicine, dong quai is used along with four or more other herbs.

4. **Contraindications/precautions**
   a. Pregnancy (uterine stimulant) and lactation
   b. Diarrhea
   c. Hemorrhagic disease
   d. Hypermenorrhea
   e. During colds or flus
   f. Allergy to parsley

5. **Drug interactions**
   a. Dong quai interacts with anticoagulants such as warfarin
   b. Unknown if it interacts with other cardiovascular drugs such as procainamide

6. **Side effects**
   a. Photodermatitis may occur in persons collecting the plant
   b. Burping, flatulence, and headache
   c. Safrole, found in the oil of dong quai, is carcinogenic and not recommended for ingestion

7. **Dosage.** A variety of doses are suggested. No standardized product is available.

E. **Echinacea** *(Echinacea purpurea, Echinacea angustifolia)*

1. **German Commission E indications**
   a. Internal use: supportive therapy for infections of the upper respiratory tract (colds) and lower urinary tract
   b. External use: local application for the treatment of hard-to-heal superficial wounds and ulcers

2. **Mechanism of action.** Echinacea increases the body's resistance to bacteria by:
   a. Caffeic acid derivatives, which include cichoric acid, chlorogenic acid, and cynarin, increase phagocytosis and stimulate the production of immune-potentiating substances such as interferon, interleukins, and tumor necrosis factor.
   b. Polysaccharides, such as inulin, stimulate macrophages and inhibit hyaluronidase activity to decrease inflammation.
   c. Alkylamides, such as echinacein, have a local anesthetic effect and inhibit hyaluronidase activity to decrease inflammation.
   d. Echinacea has little or no direct bactericidal or bacteriostatic properties.

3. **Efficacy.** Melchart et al. reviewed 26 controlled clinical trials evaluating echinacea's ability to strengthen the body's own defense mechanisms. Thirty of 34 echinacea therapies were more effective compared to controls.

4. **Contraindications/precautions**
   a. Echinacea is contraindicated in infectious and autoimmune diseases such as tuberculosis, leukosis, collagenosis, multiple sclerosis, acquired immune deficiency syndrome (AIDS), human immunodeficiency virus (HIV) infections, and lupus.
   b. Caution should be used in patients who are allergic to members of the ragweed family.
   c. The effects of echinacea in pregnancy, lactation, and children are unknown.
   d. Therapy should not exceed 8 weeks. Theoretically, prolonged use of echinacea may depress the immune system possibly through overstimulation.

5. **Drug interactions.** Unknown if Echinacea interacts with immunosuppressants

6. **Side effects.** Nausea, vomiting, allergic reactions, and anaphylaxis. May interfere with male fertility.

7. **Dosage.** There are a variety of doses recommended. The most common dose is as the dried powder, 1 gram or two 500-mg capsules orally three times daily. Recommended to use only for 2 weeks during a cold.

F. **Feverfew** *(Tanacetum parthenium)*

1. **German Commission E indication.** Prophylaxis of migraine headaches

2. Mechanism of action

    a. Feverfew inhibits the release of 5-hydroxytryptamine (serotonin) from platelets, which may be the same mechanism as methysergide maleate (Sansert).

    b. It irreversibly inhibits prostaglandin synthesis through a different mechanism than the salicylates. It inhibits phospholipase A_2 by α-methylene butyrolactones (parthenolide and epoxyartemorin).

    c. It inhibits polymorphonuclear leukocyte (PMN) degranulation, which reduces PMN-induced damage to the rheumatoid synovium.

    d. It inhibits phagocytosis of human neutrophils, which may reduce tissue damage from oxygen radicals.

    e. It inhibits mast cell release of histamine.

    f. It may have cytotoxic activity against human tumor cells.

    g. There is an antithrombotic potential due to a phospholipase inhibition that prevents the release of arachidonic acid.

    h. It may possess antimicrobial activity.

3. Efficacy. A randomized, double-blind, placebo-controlled study included 60 patients who received one feverfew capsule (70–114 mg/capsule) daily for 4 months. The prevention of migraines occurred in 59% of patients treated with feverfew as compared to 24% with placebo. The number and severity of migraine attacks and the degree of vomiting were reduced with feverfew. The duration of attacks was unaltered.

4. Contraindications/precautions. Feverfew should be avoided in pregnancy, lactation, and children under 2 years of age.

5. Drug interactions. Feverfew may interact with anticoagulants, increasing the risk of bleeding.

6. Side effects

    a. Gastric discomfort on oral consumption

    b. Minor ulcerations of oral mucosa, irritation of tongue, and swelling of lips may occur when fresh leaves are chewed.

    c. Heart rate increased by 26 beats/minute in two patients.

    d. Because there is a lack of precise information regarding potential long-term toxicity, the Canadian Health Protection Branch advises consumers not to take feverfew continuously for more than 4 months without medical advice.

    e. Discontinuation of feverfew may produce muscle/joint stiffness and a cluster of nervous system reactions (rebound of migraines, anxiety, and poor sleep patterns).

7. Dosage. The usual dose of feverfew is 125 mg daily. A product containing at least 0.2% parthenolide is recommended.

G. Garlic *(Allium sativum)*

1. German Commission E indications. Support dietary measures for the treatment of hyperlipoproteinemia and to prevent age-related changes in the blood vessels (arteriosclerosis)

2. Mechanism of action

    a. Garlic inhibits platelet function by interfering with thromboxane synthesis.

    b. It increases the levels of two antioxidant enzymes in the blood: catylase and glutathione peroxidase.

    c. Organic disulfides found in garlic oil inactivate the thiol enzymes such as coenzyme A (CoA) and hydroxymethyl glutaryl (HMG) CoA reductase.

3. Efficacy

    a. Silagy et al. performed a meta-analysis of eight studies evaluating the effect on blood pressure. The overall pooled difference in change of systolic blood pressure was 7.7 mm Hg lower with garlic than placebo; diastolic blood pressure was 5.0 mm Hg lower with garlic.

    b. Warshafsky et al. performed a meta-analysis of five studies evaluating the effect on total serum cholesterol. Patients were excluded if they were receiving lipid-lowering drugs. Overall pooled total cholesterol difference between garlic and placebo was -23 mg/dl (-29 to -17).

4. Contraindications/precautions

    a. Caution in diabetics

    b. Caution in pregnancy (emmenagogue and abortifacient)

    c. Caution in lactation

    d. Peptic ulcer disease and gastroesophageal reflux

    e. Discontinue 2 weeks prior to surgery

  5. **Drug interactions**

    a. Anticoagulants (increased bleeding)

    b. Protease inhibitors (decreased efficacy)

    c. Increases amphotericin B activity against *Cryptococcus neoformans*

    d. Antihypertensives

    e. Diabetic agents

  6. **Side effects.** Gastrointestinal discomfort (heartburn, flatulence), sweating, light-headedness, allergic reactions, and menorrhagia

  7. **Dosage.** 0.6–1.2 grams of dried powder (2–5 mg of allicin) daily or 2–4 grams of the fresh garlic

  8. **Comments.** Alliinase (enzyme that converts alliin to allicin) is inactivated by acids. Enteric-coated tablets or capsules allow more absorption because they pass through the stomach and release their contents in the alkaline medium of the small intestine.

H. Ginger *(Zingiber officinale)*

  1. **German Commission E indications.** Dyspepsia and prophylaxis of symptoms of travel sickness

  2. **Mechanism of action**

    a. Ginger promotes saliva and gastric juice secretion, which increases peristalsis and the tone of the intestinal muscle.

    b. It has no central nervous system effects.

    c. It has positive inotropic activity.

    d. It inhibits thromboxane synthesis as a prostacyclin agonist.

  3. **Efficacy.** A double-blind study included 36 blindfolded subjects with high susceptibility to motion sickness who were given ginger 940 mg, dimenhydrinate 100 mg, or placebo for the prevention of motion sickness induced by a tilted rotating chair. Ginger subjects remained in the chair an average of 5.5 minutes, dimenhydrinate 3.5 minutes, and placebo 1.5 minutes. The ginger group took longer to feel sick, but once sick, the sensations of nausea and vomiting progressed at the same rate in all groups.

  4. **Contraindications/precautions**

    a. It is suggested to avoid the use of ginger for the treatment of postoperative nausea because it may prolong bleeding time and delay immunological changes.

    b. It is contraindicated for gallstone pain.

    c. It is recommended for use in pregnancy only on the advice of a physician [uterine relaxant (low doses); uterine stimulant (high doses)].

  5. **Drug interactions.** Ginger interacts with antiplatelets and anticoagulants.

  6. **Side effects.** None reported

  7. **Dosage (for travel sickness).** Daily dose is 2–4 grams. Two 500-mg capsules taken 30 minutes prior to travel, then 1–2 more capsule(s) every 4 hours as needed.

I. Ginkgo *(Ginkgo biloba)*

  1. **German Commission E indications**

    a. Treatment for cerebral circulatory disturbances resulting in reduced functional capacity and vigilance (vertigo, tinnitus, weakened memory, and mood swings accompanied by anxiety)

    b. Treatment of peripheral arterial circulatory disturbance such as intermittent claudication

  2. **Mechanism of action**

    a. Ginkgo contains flavonoids (quercetin, kaempferol, and isorhamnetin) and terpenoids (ginkgolides A, B, C, and bilobalide).

    b. Flavonoids provide the antioxidant activity, reduce capillary fragility, and increase the threshold of blood loss from capillaries.

    c. Ginkgolides antagonize platelet-activating factor (PAF). PAF induces platelet aggregation, the degranulation of neutrophils, and the production of oxygen radicals.

    d. Bilobalide protects nerve cells.

3. Efficacy

    a. Kleijnen reviewed the clinical and pharmacological studies on ginkgo and cerebral insufficiency. Eight were of good quality. Seven of the trials showed positive effects of ginkgo compared to placebo. Symptoms of cerebral insufficiency that were evaluated were difficulties of concentration and memory, absentmindedness, confusion, lack of energy, tiredness, decreased physical performance, depression, anxiety, dizziness, tinnitus, and headaches.

    b. For intermittent claudication, there were 15 controlled trials, two of acceptable quality. Bauer et al. showed an increase in walking distance (ginkgo 112–222 m; placebo 145–176 m). Saudreau et al. showed amelioration of pain at rest; ginkgo showed a decrease on a 100-mm visual analogue scale for pain from 61 to 30 mm; placebo 51 to 39 mm.

    c. A randomized, double-blind, placebo-controlled study included 202 patients with either Alzheimer's or multi-infarct dementia. These patients were given ginkgo 40 mg three times daily or placebo for 1 year. Ginkgo had a statistically significant improvement by at least two points or better on the Alzheimer's Disease Assessment Scale–Cognitive 70-point subscale compared to placebo (50% versus 29%). Ginkgo showed statistically significant improvement on the Geriatric Evaluation by Relative's Rating Instrument (37% versus 23%). There was no difference between ginkgo and placebo on the Clinical Global Impression of Change.

4. Contraindications/precautions. None known

5. Drug interactions

    a. Ginkgo may potentiate the bleeding properties of antiplatelets—there is a case report of spontaneous hyphema (bleeding from the iris into the anterior chamber) from ginkgo and aspirin.

    b. Aminoglycosides (increased ototoxicity)

    c. Thiazide (increases blood pressure)

    d. Trazodone (coma)

6. Side effects

    a. Gastric disturbances, headache, dizziness, and vertigo

    b. Toxic ingestion may produce tonic–clonic seizures and loss of consciousness

7. Dosage. Recommended dose is 40 mg three times daily with meals for at least 4–6 weeks. Standardized preparations that contain 6% terpene lactones and 24% ginkgo flavone glycosides are recommended.

J. Asian ginseng *(Panax ginseng, Panax quinquefolius)*

1. German Commission E indications. Tonic to combat feelings of lassitude and debility, lack of energy, and ability to concentrate, and during convalescence

2. Mechanism of action

    a. At least 28 active ingredients known as ginsenosides have been isolated.

    b. Ginseng effects vary with extract derivative, drying method, dose, duration of treatment, and animal species that was studied. Each ginsenoside produces different pharmacological effects on the central nervous system, cardiovascular system, and other body systems. Different ginsenosides are capable of producing biological effects in direct opposition with those produced by others. For example, the ginsenoside Rb_1 has been shown to have a suppressive effect on the central nervous system; whereas Rg_1 produces a stimulatory effect.

3. Efficacy

    a. A randomized, double-blind, placebo-controlled, crossover study included 50 male sports teachers who performed a treadmill exercise test. Volunteers received 2 ginseng capsules (Geriatric Pharmaton™) daily for 6 weeks or placebo. Volunteers used energy more efficiently and had greater endurance while taking ginseng.

b. A case-controlled study including 1987 pairs evaluated ginseng's effect on various human cancers. Ginseng had a significant decreased risk for cancer compared with nonintakers. There may be a dose-response relationship; as the frequency and duration of ginseng use increased, the risk of cancer decreased. According to cancer site, ginseng significantly reduced the risk of cancer of the lip, oral cavity, and pharynx; esophagus; stomach; colon and rectum; liver; pancreas; lung; and ovaries. There was no risk reduction for cancers of the female breast, uterine cervix, urinary bladder, and thyroid gland.

4. Contraindications/precautions
  a. Pregnancy
  b. Children
  c. Avoid in patients with hypertension, emotional/psychological imbalances, headaches, heart palpitations, insomnia, asthma, inflammation, or infections with high fever.
  d. Caution should be used in patients with a history of bleeding.
  e. Discontinue 2 weeks before surgery
  f. Caution should be used in patients with a history of breast cancer. Ginseng may stimulate breast cancer cells.

5. Drug interactions
  a. Ginseng may interact with phenelzine, producing hallucinations and psychosis.
  b. Ginseng may decrease the International Normalized Ratio (INR) of warfarin.
  c. Ginseng may interact with stimulants, including caffeine.
  d. Ginseng may interact with hypoglycemics, causing hypoglycemia.
  e. It is unknown whether ginseng interacts with hormonal therapy, antihypertensives, or cardiac medications.

6. Side effects
  a. Nervousness and excitation for the first 4 days
  b. Inability to concentrate with long-term use
  c. Diffuse mammary nodularity and vaginal bleeding may be due to ginseng having an estrogen-like effect in women.
  d. Hypertension, euphoria, restlessness, nervousness, insomnia, skin eruptions, edema, and diarrhea have been reported with long-term ginseng use with an average dose of 3 grams of ginseng root daily.

7. Dosage. 1–2 grams of crude herb daily or 100–300 mg of ginseng extract three times daily. Standardized products that contain at least 4%–5% ginsenosides are recommended.

K. Siberian ginseng *(Eleutherococcus senticosus)*

  1. German Commission E indications. Tonic for fatigue, convalescence, decreased work capacity, or difficulty in concentration

  2. Mechanism of action. Animal research suggests that Siberian ginseng may stimulate the hypothalamic-pituitary-adrenal cortex. It may bind to progestin, mineralocorticoid, and glucocorticoid receptors.

  3. Efficacy. A randomized, double-blind, placebo-controlled study evaluated 20 highly trained distance runners who received *E. senticosus* extract 60 drops daily for 6 weeks or placebo. Subjects underwent a maximal treadmill test and a 10K race. No significant difference was observed between treatment and placebo for heart rate, oxygen consumption, expired minute volume, ventilatory equivalent for oxygen, or respiratory exchange ratio.

  4. Contraindications/precautions
    a. Avoid in hypertension
    b. Not recommended in patients with febrile states, hypertonic crisis, or myocardial infarction
    c. Caution should be used in diabetics and active bleeding.

  5. Drug interactions
    a. Serum levels of digoxin may increase when taken with Siberian ginseng.
    b. Hexobarbital and Siberian ginseng increase sleep latency and duration.
    c. Siberian ginseng may increase the risk of hypoglycemia with diabetic agents.
    d. Siberian ginseng may interact with anticoagulants.
    e. It is unknown whether Siberian ginseng interacts with stimulants, such as caffeine.
    f. It is unknown whether Siberian ginseng interacts with antihypertensives.

6. Side effects
   a. Mild, transient diarrhea, and insomnia
   b. Siberian ginseng may lower blood glucose.

7. Dosage. Two capsules (each capsule containing 400–500 mg of powdered root) three times daily; total of 2–3 grams daily. Solid concentrated extract standardized on eleuthero-sides B and E 300–400 mg daily are recommended. Recommended not to use longer than 3 weeks.

L. Kava *(Piper methysticum)*

1. German Commission E indications. Insomnia and nervousness

2. Mechanism of action
   a. The active components of kava are known as kavapyrones or kavalactones.
   b. The kavapyrones, especially dihydromethysticin, have a central depressant action similar to pentobarbital.
   c. Some of the kavapyrones have varying effects in regard to dopamine concentration levels. Low doses of DL-kawain decreased dopamine levels, whereas higher doses increased or did not change dopamine levels. Yangonin decreased dopamine levels and desmethoxyyangonin increased dopamine levels.
   d. DL-kawain has been shown to cause a decrease in serotonin levels.
   e. Some of the kavapyrones, especially desmethoxyyangonin and methysticin, inhibit monoamine oxidase B (MAO-B).
   f. Kava resin and pyrones exert some weak binding on γ-aminobutyric acid A (GABA-A) binding sites.

3. Efficacy. A randomized, placebo-controlled, multicenter trial evaluated 101 patients with one of the following diagnoses: agoraphobia, specific phobia, social phobia, generalized anxiety disorder, or adjustment disorder with anxiety. Patients either received 100 mg of kava (standardized to 70% kava lactones) TID for 25 weeks or placebo. Hamilton Anxiety Scale improved with either kava (30.7 to 9.7) or placebo (31.4 to 15.2), but it was statistically significant between the two groups. The Clinical Global Impression change of "very much improved" was statistically significant between two groups: kava—20% to 53.1%; placebo—10.5% to 30.2%.

4. Contraindications/precautions
   a. Avoid in depression because there is an increased risk of suicide.
   b. Caution should be used when operating machinery or motor vehicles.
   c. Kava should not be taken longer than 3 months without a doctor's supervision.
   d. Avoid during pregnancy/lactation.
   e. Avoid use in children.

5. Drug interactions
   a. Kava may potentiate the sedative effect of barbiturates, benzodiazepines, opiates, antidepressants, anxiolytics, or alcohol.
   b. Kava may potentiate the effects of MAO inhibitors.
   c. Kava may potentiate the effects of antiplatelets, increasing the risk of bleeding.
   d. Kava may reduce the efficacy of levodopa by decreasing the levels of dopamine.

6. Side effects
   a. Hepatotoxicity (considered to be an unsafe herb because of this)
   b. Yellowing skin, nails, and hair
   c. Allergic skin reactions
   d. "Kava dermopathy" (dry, scaly skin rash on palms of hands, soles of feet, forearms, back, and shins; swollen face; bloodshot eyes)
   e. Gastrointestinal complaints
   f. Visual disturbances (pupil dilation and disorders of oculomotor equilibrium)
   g. Morning fatigue
   h. Neurological (choreoathetosis, dystonic reactions, dyskinesia)
   i. Tolerance: not reported
   j. Toxicity may include ataxia, muscle weakness, and ascending paralysis without loss of consciousness.

7. **Dosage.** 200–250 mg of kavalactones or kavapyrones divided into two or three divided doses.

M. **Milk thistle** *(Silybum marianum)*

1. **German Commission E indications.** Chronic inflammatory liver conditions and cirrhosis

2. **Mechanism of action**
   a. Milk thistle produces antioxidants.
   b. Milk thistle stimulates the activity of RNA polymerase A.
   c. Milk thistle alters the outer liver membrane cell structure.

3. **Efficacy.** Saller et al. reviewed 36 studies with milk thistle. In acute viral hepatitis, no formally valid conclusion could be drawn. In alcoholic liver disease, prothrombin times and liver function tests improved. Milk thistle was shown to reduce liver-related mortality (OR = 0.54).

4. **Contraindications/precautions.** Avoid in pregnancy

5. **Drug interactions.** Unknown

6. **Side effects.** Diarrhea and rash

7. **Dosage.** Recommended dose of milk thistle is 200–400 mg/day divided into three doses using a standardized product that includes 70%–80% silymarin.

N. **Saw palmetto** *(Serenoa repens)*

1. **German Commission E indications.** Treatment of micturition difficulties associated with benign prostatic hyperplasia

2. **Mechanism of action**
   a. Saw palmetto inhibits dihydrotestosterone to androgen receptors in prostate cells.
   b. It may inhibit testosterone-5-alpha-reductase, the enzyme responsible for the conversion of testosterone to dihydrotestosterone.

3. **Efficacy.** A randomized, multicenter study evaluated 1069 men with moderate benign prostatic hyperplasia who received saw palmetto 160 mg twice daily or finasteride 5 mg daily for 6 months. There was no significant difference between saw palmetto and finasteride for the patient self-rated quality-of-life score and the International Prostate Symptom Score.

4. **Contraindications/precautions**
   a. Avoid in pregnancy
   b. Avoid in children

5. **Drug interactions.** It is unknown whether saw palmetto interacts with anticoagulants.

6. **Side effects**
   a. Intraoperative hemorrhage
   b. Headache
   c. Stomach upset

7. **Dosage.** 1–2 grams of saw palmetto or 320 mg of lipophilic extract daily, usually given 160 mg twice daily and taken with food. Products standardized to contain 90% free and 7% esterified fatty acids are recommended.

O. **St. John's wort** *(Hypericum perforatum)*

1. **German Commission E indications.** In supportive treatment for anxiety and depression

2. **Mechanism of action**
   a. Active ingredients include hypericin, pseudohypericin, quercetin, quercitrin, isoquercitrin, hyperoside, rutin, amentoflavone, hyperin, hyperforin, adhyperforin, and xanthones.
   b. Hypericin, flavonoids, and xanthones show in vitro irreversible MAO inhibitors type A and B activity.
   c. St. John's wort may inhibit serotonin reuptake.
   d. St. John's wort may inhibit synaptic GABA uptake and GABA-receptor binding.
   e. It may reduce cytokine expression, such as interleukin-6. This may be helpful in depression because interleukins may induce depression.

3. Efficacy
   a. A meta-analysis of 23 randomized trials (15 placebo controlled; 8 other antidepressants) was performed. St. John's wort extract given 350–1000 mg/day (hypericin 0.48–2.7 mg/day) for 4–8 weeks to patients with mild to moderate depression had significantly more "treatment responders" than placebo (55% versus 22%). St. John's wort 500–900 mg/day (hypericin 0.4–2.7 mg/day) given 4–6 weeks compared to other antidepressants (maprotiline 75 mg/day, imipramine 50–75 mg/day, and amitriptyline 30 mg/day) had similar "treatment responders" (St. John's wort 64%; other antidepressants 58.5%).
   b. St. John's wort may not be effective for major depression.

4. Contraindications/precautions
   a. Caution in fair-skinned persons when exposed to bright sunlight
   b. Caution in pregnancy (emmenagogue and abortifacient)
   c. No negative influence on general performance or the ability to drive a car or operate heavy machinery has been reported.

5. Drug interactions
   a. St. John's wort may interact with other drugs metabolized through the cytochrome P450 system isoenzymes 1A2, 2C9, and 3A4.
   b. Antidepressants such as paroxetine, sertraline, and nefazodone have been reported to cause serotonin syndrome when taken with St. John's wort.
   c. St. John's wort may decrease the INR of warfarin.
   d. Antiretroviral levels may decrease.
   e. Cyclosporine levels may decrease.
   f. Digoxin levels may decrease.
   g. Theophylline levels may decrease.
   h. Oral contraceptives may have a decreased effect.
   i. Irinotecan levels may decrease.

6. Food interactions
   a. Older studies suggested that St. John's wort was an MAO inhibitor.
   b. Newer studies suggest St. John's wort no longer acts like an MAO inhibitor (*Pharmacopsychiatry* 1997;30:102–107).
   c. No case reports published of MAO-type food interactions such as tyramine-containing foods: cheeses, beer, wine, herring, and yeast.

7. Side effects
   a. Photodermatitis
   b. Gastrointestinal irritations
   c. Allergic reactions
   d. Tiredness
   e. Restlessness

8. Dosage. 2–4 grams daily. Standardized products containing 0.4–2.7 mg hypericin/ day or 0.3% hypericin are recommended.

P. Valerian *(Valeriana officinalis)*

1. German Commission E indications. Restlessness and nervous disturbance of sleep

2. Mechanism of action
   a. Several active compounds have been isolated from valerian and grouped into three categories: volatile oil, valepotriates, and alkaloids. It is believed that the sedative activity of valerian is secondary to the valepotriates.
   b. Valepotriates, valeranone 6, kessane derivatives 3a–f, valerenic acid 5a, and valerenal 5b have been reported to prolong barbiturate-induced sleeping time.
   c. Valerenic acid 5a has been shown to possess pentobarbital-like central depressant activity rather than muscle relaxant or neuroleptic effects.
   d. Valerenic acid 5a has also been shown to inhibit the enzyme that triggers the breakdown of GABA.
   e. Valtrate and isovaltrate have exhibited antidepressant properties; didrovaltrate possesses a tranquilizing ability similar to the benzodiazepines.

3. Efficacy. A double-blind, randomized study included eight volunteers suffering from mild insomnia who received valerian aqueous extract 450 mg or 900 mg or placebo at bedtime.

Valerian 450 mg significantly improved sleep quality, sleep latency, and sleep depth compared to placebo. The 900-mg dose offered no advantage over the 450-mg dose.

4. **Contraindications/precautions.** Caution while driving or performing other tasks requiring alertness and coordination is recommended.

5. **Drug interactions.** Valerian may potentiate the sedative effect of barbiturates, benzodiazepines, opiates, alcohol, or other sedatives.

6. **Side effects**
   a. Headaches, hangover, excitability, insomnia, uneasiness, and cardiac disturbances
   b. Toxicity includes ataxia, decreased sensibility, hypothermia, hallucinations, and increased muscle relaxation

7. **Dosage** (dried root) 2–3 grams daily, up to three times daily. Standardized to contain 0.8%–1% valeremic acids/dose extract 400–900 mg 30–60 minutes before bedtime.

III. OTHER DIETARY SUPPLEMENTS THAT ARE POTENTIALLY SAFE

A. Chondroitin

1. **Nonapproved indications.** Viscoelastic agent in opthalmic procedures and the treatment of osteoarthritis

2. **Mechanism of action**
   a. It concentrates in cartilage, where it can be used in the synthesis of new cartilagenous matrix.
   b. It increases the ribonucleic acid (RNA) synthesis of chondrocytes that may increase the synthesis of proteoglycans and collagens.
   c. It may inhibit leukocyte elastase activity. Leukocyte elastase is found in high concentrations in the blood and synovial fluid of patients with rheumatic diseases.

3. **Efficacy.** Morreale et al. performed a 6-month randomized, parallel study that included 146 patients with knee osteoarthritis. Patients received either chondroitin sulfate 400 mg three times daily or diclofenac 50 mg three times daily for 3 months. Chondroitin was as effective for relieving symptoms associated with osteoarthritis, but the onset of action was much slower than diclofenac.

4. **Contraindications/precautions**
   a. Previous hypersensitivity to chrondroitin sulfate
   b. Bleeding disorders
   c. Use caution because chondroitin is usually produced from bovine cartilage (possible transmission of mad cow disease)

5. **Drug interactions.** May interact with heparin

6. **Side effects.** Nausea, epigastric pain, and headache

7. **Dosage.** 400 mg three times daily

B. Coenzyme Q_{10} (ubiquinone or ubidecarenone)

1. **Nonapproved indications.** Congestive heart failure (CHF), hypertension, stable angina, ventricular arrhythmias, cancer, heart surgery, and periodontal disease

2. **Mechanism of action**
   a. It is a naturally occurring coenzyme that has a predominant role in oxidative phosphorylation and synthesis of adenosine triphosphate (ATP), which is needed for muscle contraction and relaxation.
   b. It may have antioxidant properties.
   c. It has been shown to reduce myocardial injury from ischemia and to reduce toxic myocardial damage from anthracyclines such as doxorubicin.

3. **Efficacy**
   a. **CHF.** Morisco et al. performed a randomized, double-blind, placebo-controlled, multicenter study that included 641 patients with chronic CHF New York Heart Association Class III and IV receiving conventional treatment such as digoxin, diuretics, angiotensin-

converting enzyme (ACE) inhibitors, and calcium-channel blockers. Patients received coenzyme Q_{10} 2 mg/kg/day for 1 year or placebo. The number of patients requiring hospitalization secondary to CHF was less in the coenzyme Q_{10} group (n = 73) versus placebo (n = 118, p <0.001). Episodes of pulmonary edema and cardiac asthma were reduced with coenzyme Q_{10} (p <0.001).

    b. Adjuvant to HMG CoA reductase inhibitors. Hanaki et al. performed a study that evaluated the plasma levels of coenzyme Q_{10} in 245 normal subjects, 104 patients with coronary artery disease, and 29 patients with coronary artery disease taking pravastatin. In the normal subjects, coenzyme Q_{10} did not vary with age. In the coronary artery disease patient groups with and without pravastatin, coenzyme Q_{10} levels were lower than in the normal subjects. The authors concluded that a deficiency of coenzyme Q_{10} may increase the symptoms of atherosclerosis and that HMG CoA reductase inhibitors do not increase coenzyme Q_{10}. Therefore, patients taking HMG CoA reductase inhibitors should receive coenzyme Q_{10} supplementation.

4. Contraindications/precautions
    a. Biliary obstruction
    b. Diabetes mellitus (hypoglycemia)
    c. Hepatic insufficiency
    d. Renal insufficiency

5. Drug interactions
    a. Hypolipidemic agents lower plasma concentrations of coenzyme Q_{10}.
    b. Oral hypoglycemic agents potentially inhibit effects of exogenous administration.

6. Side effects
    a. Rash and gastrointestinal disturbances such as nausea, anorexia, epigastric pain, and diarrhea
    b. Elevations of serum aminotransferases have occurred with relatively high oral doses.

7. Dosage. 100 mg daily, up to 600 mg daily

C. Glucosamine

1. Nonapproved indication. Osteoarthritis

2. Mechanism of action
    a. Glucosamine enhances cartilage proteoglycan synthesis.
    b. It inhibits the deterioration of cartilage secondary to osteoarthritis.
    c. It maintains an equilibrium between cartilage catabolic and anabolic processes.
    d. It may have an anti-inflammatory action unlike cyclooxygenase.

3. Efficacy. A double-blind trial included 40 patients with unilateral osteoarthritis of the knee. Patients were given glucosamine 500 mg three times daily or ibuprofen 400 mg three times daily for 8 weeks. Pain scores decreased faster during the first 2 weeks in the ibuprofen group than in the glucosamine group. No significant difference in swelling was observed between the two groups.

4. Contraindications/precautions
    a. Hypersensitivity to glucosamine or shellfish
    b. Diabetics may have impaired insulin secretion.

5. Drug interactions
    a. Fluoxetine may increase glucosamine serum concentrations.
    b. Glucosamine may interact with diabetic agents.

6. Side effects
    a. Gastrointestinal side effects such as epigastric pain and tenderness, heartburn, diarrhea, and nausea
    b. Central nervous system side effects such as drowsiness, headache, and insomnia
    c. Long-term side effects are unknown.

7. Dosage. 500 mg three times daily

D. Melatonin

1. Orphan drug status. Treatment of circadian rhythm sleep disorders in blind people with no light perception

2. **Nonapproved indications.** Jet lag, insomnia, depression, and cancer

3. **Mechanism of action**
   a. It is a hormone made from serotonin and secreted by the pineal gland. Melatonin controls the periods of sleepiness and wakefulness.
   b. It may possess antioxidant properties.

4. **Efficacy**
   a. **Jet lag.** A randomized, placebo-controlled trial evaluated the effect of melatonin in 52 aircraft personnel. Melatonin was given either 5 mg daily 3 days before departure until 5 days after arrival (early group) or 5 mg daily upon arrival and for 3 additional days (late group). The late group had significantly less jet lag, fewer overall sleep disturbances, and a faster recovery of energy compared to the placebo group and the early group.
   b. **Insomnia.** A randomized, double-blind, placebo-controlled trial evaluated the effect of melatonin in 10 patients with persistent complaints of insomnia. Patients were given 1 week of placebo or melatonin 1 mg or 5 mg 15 minutes before the onset of sleep. Melatonin was comparable to placebo. Authors concluded that patients who may benefit from melatonin have a deficiency of melatonin.

5. **Contraindications/precautions**
   a. Avoid in pregnancy
   b. Melatonin may aggravate depressive symptoms.
   c. Melatonin may increase the incidence of seizures.

6. **Drug interactions**
   a. Vitamin B_{12} influences melatonin secretion. Low levels of vitamin B_{12} will produce low levels of melatonin.
   b. MAO inhibitors may increase melatonin serum concentrations.
   c. Selective serotonin reuptake inhibitors may increase melatonin serum concentrations.
   d. β-Blockers may decrease nocturnal secretion of melatonin.
   e. Other sedatives may exacerbate the sedative effects of melatonin.
   f. Melatonin may interact with immunosuppressants.

7. **Side effects**
   a. Side effects include drowsiness, daytime fatigue, headache, and transient depression.
   b. Long-term side effects are unknown.

8. **Dosage.** 0.3–5 mg at bedtime

STUDY QUESTIONS

Directions: Each of the numbered items or incomplete statements in this section is followed by answers or by completions of the statement. Select the **one** lettered answer or completion that is **best** in each case.

1. Which of the following herbs is known to cause cancer?

(A) Chaparral
(B) Comfrey
(C) Ma huang
(D) Licorice
(E) St. John's wort

2. Which of the following is a correct statement?

(A) Dietary supplements must be proven safe and effective before marketing in the United States.
(B) The following statement is optional for labeling of herbal products: "This product has not been evaluated by the FDA. It is not intended to diagnose, treat, cure, or prevent."
(C) Herbs must be standardized in order to be considered dietary supplements.
(D) Dietary supplement manufacturers may claim that their products affect the structure and function of the human body.

3. Which of the following herbs should be used with caution while driving or performing other tasks that require alertness and coordination?

(A) Kava
(B) Echinacea
(C) Dong quai
(D) Feverfew
(E) Saw palmetto

4. Tom would like to try Echinacea to prevent colds and flus during the winter months. Which of the following statements is true about Echinacea?

(A) It is contraindicated in patients allergic to parsley.
(B) It should only be taken continuously for 3 months.
(C) It is contraindicated in patients with lupus and leukosis.
(D) Prolonged use of Echinacea will upregulate the immune system.
(E) Side effects include headache, rash, and dizziness.

5. Mary has a family history of heart disease and wonders if garlic would be beneficial to her. Which of the following statements is correct about garlic?

(A) Enteric-coated tablets release their contents in the stomach.
(B) Side effects include heartburn, flatulence, and sweating.
(C) The safety of garlic in pregnancy is unknown.
(D) Garlic does not interact with warfarin.

6. An 80-year-old man takes warfarin for his mechanical heart valve. He would also like to take the following herbs: Asian ginseng, feverfew, Siberian ginseng, and garlic. Which of the following may decrease the effectiveness of warfarin?

(A) Asian ginseng
(B) Feverfew
(C) Siberian ginseng
(D) Garlic

7. A 30-year-old female is 10 weeks pregnant with her second child. During her first pregnancy, she became depressed and was started on Prozac 20 mg every day. She is already beginning to notice early symptoms of depression during her second pregnancy. She would like to try St. John's wort for her depression. Which of the following statements is correct regarding St. John's wort?

(A) The safety of St. John's wort in pregnancy is unknown.
(B) St. John's wort is not helpful in treating mild depression.
(C) St. John's wort may interact with serotonin reuptake inhibitors.
(D) St. John's wort may interact with dairy products like milk and eggs.

8. A 65-year-old is interested in taking ginkgo. Which of the following statements is correct regarding ginkgo?

(A) Ginkgo is contraindicated in diabetes and pregnancy.
(B) There is a drug–herb interaction between ginkgo and aspirin.
(C) Toxic effects include hypertension and cardiac arrest.
(D) There is a drug–herb interaction between ginkgo and phenelzine.
(E) Ginkgo is contraindicated in patients with gallstone pain.

9. A 20-year-old athletic man would like to take Asian and Siberian ginseng to increase his physical stamina. His girlfriend suggested that he ask a pharmacist about the safety of Asian and Siberian ginseng. Which of the following statements is correct?

(A) Asian ginseng may interact with phenelzine, warfarin, and digoxin.
(B) Asian ginseng is potentially harmful in patients with autoimmune diseases.
(C) Asian and Siberian ginseng are the same ginseng but are grown in different countries.
(D) Asian and Siberian ginseng should be avoided in patients with hypertension.
(E) Asian and Siberian ginseng have an estrogen-like effect in women.

ANSWERS AND EXPLANATIONS

1. The answer is B *[I B 1].*
Carcinogenic herbs include borage, calamus, coltsfoot, comfrey, life root, and sassafras. Hepatotoxic herbs include chaparal, germander, and life root. High doses of licorice for long periods may cause pseudoaldosteronism, a condition that may include headache, lethargy, sodium and water retention, hypokalemia, high blood pressure, heart failure, and cardiac arrest. Ma huang is considered unsafe for patients with hypertension, diabetes, or thyroid disease.

2. The answer is D *[I A 3].*
The Dietary Supplement Health and Education Act of 1994 states that dietary supplements are not considered drugs or food. Since dietary supplements are not regulated as drugs, their safety and efficacy are not mandated by the United States Food and Drug Administration (FDA). Dietary supplements are intended to supplement the diet. Dietary supplements do not have to be standardized. Dietary supplements may only make claims regarding the effects on structure or function of the body. No claims regarding a particular disease or condition can be made. This statement is required on the product label: "This product has not been evaluated by the FDA. It is not intended to diagnose, treat, cure, or prevent."

3. The answer is A *[II L 4].*
Caution while driving or performing other tasks requiring alertness and coordination is recommended with kava. Kava may potentiate the sedative effect of barbiturates, benzodiazepines, opiates, or alcohol. Kava is considered to be unsafe because of hepatotoxicity.

4. The answer is C *[II E 4].*
Echinacea is contraindicated in infectious and autoimmune diseases such as tuberculosis, leukosis, collagenosis, multiple sclerosis, acquired immune deficiency syndrome (AIDS), human immunodeficiency virus (HIV) infections, and lupus. Caution should be used in patients who are allergic to members of the ragweed family. The effects of Echinacea in pregnancy, lactation, and children are unknown. Therapy should not exceed 8 weeks. Theoretically, prolonged use of Echinacea may depress the immune system possibly through overstimulation. There are no known drug interactions with Echinacea. Side effects include nausea, vomiting, allergic reactions, anaphylaxis, and interference with male fertility.

5. The answer is B *[II G 4].*
Caution should be used in diabetics when taking garlic. Garlic should be avoided in pregnancy because it is an emmenagogue (stimulates uterine bleeding) and abortifacient. Garlic may interact with anticoagulants and increase the risk of bleeding. Side effects include gastrointestinal discomfort (e.g., heartburn, flatulence), sweating, light-headedness, allergic reactions, and menorrhagia. Enteric-coated tablets or capsules allow more absorption because they pass through the stomach and release their contents in the alkaline medium of the small intestine.

6. The answer is A *[II J 5].*
Asian ginseng may decrease the International Normalized Ratio (INR) of warfarin. Feverfew and garlic may increase the INR of warfarin. Siberian ginseng may increase serum levels of digoxin and potentiate hexobarbital's effects. St. John's wort may also decrease the INR of warfarin.

7. The answer is C *[II O 4].*
St. John's wort is indicated in Germany for depression and anxiety. Caution should be used in fair-skinned persons when exposed to bright sunlight. St. John's wort should be avoided in pregnancy because it is an emmenagogue (stimulates uterine bleeding) and abortifacient. No negative influence on general performance or the ability to drive a car or operate heavy machinery has been reported. St. John's wort may interact with other drugs metabolized through the cytochrome P450 system isoenzymes 1A2, 2C9, and 3A4. Antidepressants such as paroxetine, sertraline, and nefazodone have been reported to cause serotonin syndrome when taken with St. John's wort. Antiretroviral levels may decrease. Cyclosporine levels may decrease. Digoxin levels may decrease. Theophylline levels may decrease. Oral contraceptives may have a decreased effect. Irinotecan levels may decrease. Food interactions may be similar to those of the MAO inhibitors (tyramine-containing foods: cheese, beer, wine, herring, and yeast).

Herbal Medicines and Nutritional Supplements* **659**

8. The answer is B *[II I 5].*
There are no known contraindications for ginkgo. Ginkgo may potentiate the bleeding properties of antiplatelets. Side effects include gastric disturbances, headache, dizziness, and vertigo. Toxic ingestion may produce tonic–clonic seizures and loss of consciousness.

9. The answer is D *[II J 4, K 4].*
Asian ginseng's contraindications include pregnancy, children, and patients with hypertension, emotional/psychological imbalances, headaches, heart palpitations, insomnia, asthma, inflammation, or infections with high fever. Asian ginseng may interact with phenelzine, producing hallucinations and psychosis. Asian ginseng may decrease the INR of warfarin. Asian ginseng's side effects include nervousness and excitation for the first 4 days, inability to concentrate with long-term use, diffuse mammary nodularity, and vaginal bleeding. Siberian ginseng's contraindications/precautions include hypertension and patients with febrile states, hypertonic crisis, or myocardial infarction. Siberian ginseng may increase serum levels of digoxin and potentiate hexobarbital's effects. Siberian ginseng's side effects include mild, transient diarrhea, and insomnia. Siberian ginseng may also lower blood glucose.

35
Clinical Pharmacokinetics and Therapeutic Drug Monitoring

Gerald E. Schumacher

I. INTRODUCTION

A. Objectives

1. **Therapeutic drug monitoring** (TDM) in a general sense is about using serum drug concentrations (SDCs), pharmacokinetics, and pharmacodynamics to individualize and optimize patient responses to drug therapy.

2. **TDM** aims to promote optimum drug treatment by maintaining SDC within a **therapeutic range,** above which drug-induced toxicity occurs too often and below which the drug is too often ineffective.

B. Definitions

1. Specifically, **TDM** is a practice applied to a small group of drugs in which there is a direct relation between SDCs and pharmacological response, as well as a narrow range of concentrations that are effective and safe and for which SDCs are used in conjunction with other measures of clinical observation to assess patient status.

2. **Clinical pharmacokinetics,** a term often used interchangeably with TDM, is more generally the application of pharmacokinetic principles for the rational design of an individualized dosage regimen.

3. For definitions of the terms used and the concepts applicable in basic and clinical pharmacokinetics, see Chapter 6 on pharmacokinetics.

C. Rationale and reasons

1. **The rationale** for TDM makes three assumptions.
   a. Measuring patient SDC provides an opportunity to adjust for variations in patient pharmacokinetics by individualizing drug dosage.
   b. The SDC is a better predictor of patient response than is dose.
   c. There is a good relation between SDCs and pharmacological response.

2. **Reasons for measuring SDC**
   a. Drug levels are used in conjunction with other clinical data to assist practitioners in determining how a patient is responding.
   b. Drug levels provide a basis for **individualizing** patient dosage regimens.
   c. Drug levels assist in determining if a change in **patient-specific** pharmacokinetics has occurred during a course of treatment, either as a result of a change in physiological state, a change in diet, or addition of other drugs.
   d. Assuring **drug compliance** is often cited as a reason for measuring SDC, but it is unreliable for this purpose. In truth, a noncompliant patient may outwit practitioners by manipulating preappointment behavior to induce an SDC that is nonreflective of the patient's drug-taking behavior.

II. APPLYING CLINICAL PHARMACOKINETICS IN TDM

A. What the practitioner controls and does not control in TDM

1. Figure 35-1 shows the relation between dose rate of drug administered, pharmacokinetic variables, SDC, and pharmacological response.

2. Note that the only variables that the practitioner controls are the amount of drug administered and how often it is given. These variables may be manipulated to compensate for the

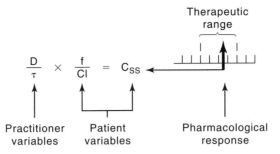

Figure 35-1. Pharmacokinetic factors influencing serum drug concentration and pharmacological response. Bioavailability is f, clearance is Cl, steady-state serum drug concentration is C_{ss}, D is dose, and τ is frequency of administration of dose.

patient's pharmacokinetic and pharmacodynamic variables (i.e., bioavailability, clearance, steady-state SDC, pharmacological response), which the practitioner does not control, to achieve some designated SDC that yields a pharmacological response usually observed within the drug's commonly accepted therapeutic SDC range.

B. The concept of therapeutic range

1. For many drugs, a specific serum concentration range can be designated for each drug that maximizes effectiveness and minimizes toxicity. The range of SDC is called the **therapeutic range** for the drug.

2. The notion of a therapeutic range is more a **probabilistic concept** than an absolute entity. It is probable that the majority of patients will show effective and safe responses within the therapeutic range. However, a minority of patients will need SDC above or below the upper or lower limits, respectively, of the therapeutic range to achieve an effective response. Similarly, a minority of patients will not show toxicity at SDC modestly above the therapeutic range, whereas others will show toxicity below the therapeutic range.

3. Therefore, TDM is about **individualizing** patient dosage regimens to achieve SDC within patient-specific therapeutic ranges for a drug. More often than not, a patient-specific range will fall within the generally stated therapeutic range.

C. The concept of population pharmacokinetic values

1. **A population pharmacokinetic value or parameter** refers to the mean (average) value noted for a given cohort of people (e.g., adults 20–60 years of age, patients with a defined range of renal impairment). Usually, this population value is normalized on a weight basis (e.g., theophylline volume of distribution in adult normals of 0.5 L/kg). When a population parameter is stated without defining the target population, it usually refers to adults; further, when the value also is not normalized (e.g., volume of distribution of theophylline of 35 L), it usually refers to adults of average weight (approximately 60–80 kg).

2. Hardly anyone is average. Individual values of the population studied are summed to determine a mean value that is then reported as the **population value.** Individualizing patient dosage regimens takes this into account by adjusting observed patient-specific values and responses to expected population measures.

3. So the practitioner starts the determination of a patient-specific dosage regimen by assuming that the patient behaves like the average member of his or her population with respect to pharmacokinetics, serum level, and expected response, and uses population pharmacokinetic parameters to calculate the dosage regimen needed to meet the desired SDC objective.

4. If after administering the dosage regimen until steady state is reached, based on using population values, the patient is responding appropriately, then no adjustment in regimen is necessary.

5. If, however, the starting assumption of using average values turns out to be incorrect, because the patient's response is either subtherapeutic or toxic due to patient-specific pharmacokinetic and/or pharmacodynamic values that are atypical for the population, the practitioner's only option (except for changing the drug) is to manipulate the practitioner-

controlled input variables, **dose and frequency,** to bring the pharmacological response within the desired range.

D. Timing of SDC measurements

1. SDCs are sometimes measured **early in a course of therapy,** before steady state is reached, to determine patient-specific pharmacokinetic parameters, rather than relying on population values.

2. More commonly, SDCs are measured **during a steady-state dosage interval** (τ_{ss}), because the objective is to determine if the SDC is within a desired therapeutic range, a range that has previously been determined almost invariably during τ_{ss}.

3. Because SDCs are most commonly measured at steady state and referenced to values obtained at steady state, it is necessary to wait after starting drug administration until at least three to four assumed half-life ($t_{1/2}$) values (88%–94% of reaching full steady state) so that SDC will be measured during a period when steady state may be assumed, for clinical purposes, to have been reached or approximated (e.g., approximately 90% of steady state or greater; so for an assumed $t_{1/2}$ of 6 hours, wait 18–24 hours after initiating drug treatment to measure SDC)

4. If there are no changes in patient response, there is usually **no need to take subsequent daily SDC measurements,** once an appropriate SDC has been achieved. Only if something occurs that may be expected to alter the patient's pharmacokinetic values (e.g., co-administration of another potentially modifying drug, change in physiological state), are frequent measurements necessary.

5. If a steady-state SDC (**C_{ss}**) is used appropriately to relate a patient's C_{ss} to a population or patient-specific therapeutic range, then it is important to note when during the steady-state dosage interval (τ_{ss}) the C_{ss} was measured in studies determining the therapeutic range. In other words, is the therapeutic range the practitioner is using as a basis for individualizing regimens based on C_{ss} measured **early** (apparent **$C_{max,ss}$**), near the **midpoint** (apparent **$C_{avg,ss}$**), or near the end (apparent **$C_{min,ss}$**) of τ_{ss}?

6. **Errors** in interpretation occur when C_{ss} for a patient is measured at a time during τ_{ss} that is markedly different than the time used for establishing the therapeutic range [e.g., measuring C_{ss} in a patient 1 hour after giving a dose on a q12h regimen when the C_{ss} for the referenced therapeutic range was actually taken at the end of τ_{ss} (**$C_{min,ss}$**)].

7. Errors in timing of C_{ss} are of greater concern for drugs with a short $t_{1/2}$ than for drugs with a long $t_{1/2}$. C_{ss} fluctuation during τ_{ss} is much greater in the former than the latter case.

III. TDM DRUGS AND COMMON CHARACTERISTICS

A. TDM drugs

1. Drugs for which TDM is commonly used are noted in Table 35-1, along with the population therapeutic range.

2. Drugs for which TDM is infrequently used in general situations, but perhaps commonly used by specialty practitioners or clinics, are noted in Table 35-2.

B. Common characteristics of TDM drugs. Drugs that qualify for TDM have, as a minimum, the following characteristics in common.

1. SDC is the most practical intermediate end point to be used when there is no clearly observable therapeutic or toxic end point.

2. SDC is a reasonable proxy for drug concentration at the site of action.

3. The range of therapeutic and safe serum concentrations is narrow.

4. There is no predictable dose-response relation.

5. The pharmacological effect observed persists for a relatively long time. Acute, short, or intermittent effects are not well regulated by using serum drug levels.

6. A drug assay is available that is accurate, precise, specific, rapid, and relatively inexpensive.

Table 35-1. Drugs Often Monitored Using Serum Drug Concentrations

Drug	Therapeutic Range for C_{ss}
Amikacin	$C_{max,ss}$ = 20–30 mcg/mL; $C_{min,ss}$ <10 mcg/mL
Cyclosporine	50–125 ng/mL
Digoxin	0.8–2* ng/mL
Gentamicin	$C_{max,ss}$ = 5–10 mcg/mL; $C_{min,ss}$ <2 mcg/mL
Phenytoin	10–20 mcg/mL
Theophylline	5–20 mcg/mL
Tobramycin	$C_{max,ss}$ = 5–10 mcg/mL; $C_{min,ss}$ <2 mcg/mL
Vancomycin	$C_{max,ss}$ = 30–50 mcg/mL; $C_{min,ss}$ = 5–10 mcg/mL

*Levels for atrial fibrillation often exceed 2 ng/mL.

Table 35-2. Drugs Monitored Using Serum Drug Concentrations in Specialty Situations

Amitriptyline
Carbamazepine
Imipramine
Lidocaine
Lithium
Methotrexate
Nortriptyline
Salicylates
Valproic acid

IV. EQUATIONS FREQUENTLY USED IN TDM

A. Linear pharmacokinetic drug clearance—normal renal function. Linear clearance assumes that a **proportional** change in dose leads to the same **proportional** change in SDC. It also assumes that $t_{1/2}$ and drug clearance remain **constant** as the dose changes. See IV D for an example of using some of the following equations.

1. **Estimating drug clearance (Cl):**

$$Cl = \frac{V}{1.4t_{1/2}} \tag{1}$$

where V is the apparent volume of distribution of drug.

2. **Maximum concentration ($C_{max,ss}$)** during τ_{ss}, when absorption is assumed to be much faster than elimination:

$$C_{max,ss} = \frac{(S)(f)(dose/V)}{1 - 10^{-0.3(\tau/t_{1/2})}} \tag{2}$$

where S is the fraction of the dosage form that is the active moiety and f is the bioavailability.

3. **Minimum concentration ($C_{min,ss}$)** during τ_{ss}, when absorption is assumed to be much faster than elimination:

$$C_{min,ss} = (C_{max,ss}) \, [10^{-0.3(\tau/t_{1/2})}] \tag{3}$$

4. **Average concentration resulting from intermittent administration ($C_{avg,ss}$)** during τ_{ss}:

$$C_{avg,ss} = \frac{(S)(f)(dose/\tau)}{Cl} \tag{4}$$

where dose/τ is the amount of drug administered during each selected unit of time (e.g., hours, minutes).

5. **Steady-state concentration resulting from continuous administration ($C_{inf,ss}$).** For the same dose rate (dose/τ), ($C_{avg,ss}$) for intermittent administration **is the same as** ($C_{inf,ss}$) for continuous administration:

$$C_{inf,ss} = \frac{(S)(f)(dose/t_{inf})}{Cl} \qquad (5)$$

B. Linear pharmacokinetic drug clearance—impaired renal function

1. **Estimating creatinine clearance from serum creatinine** when serum creatinine is assumed to be stable, not changing daily, and weight is expressed by the patient's total weight, unless total weight is equal to or more than 20% of ideal (lean) body weight, in which case ideal weight should be used in the calculation:

$$Cl_{cr} \text{ (mL/min, males)} = \frac{(140 - age)(weight)}{(Cr_s)(72)} \qquad (6)$$

where Cr_s denotes serum creatinine in mg/dl. The female value is 85% of the estimated male value in (6).

2. **Estimating prolonged drug $t_{1/2}$ or reduced drug Cl associated with reduced Cl_{cr}:**

$$\frac{(Cl)_{ri}}{(Cl)_n} = \frac{(t_{1/2})_n}{(t_{1/2})_{ri}} = 1 - F + F [(Cl_{cr})_{ri}/(Cl_{cr})_n] \qquad (7)$$

where ri and n denote the renal impaired and normal conditions, respectively; F is the fraction of drug administered that is eliminated unchanged (unmetabolized); and Cl_{cr} represents creatinine clearance in mL/min. Important F values for some common TDM drugs are: aminoglycosides = 0.98, digoxin = 0.98, and vancomycin = 0.95.

3. **Using $C_{avg,ss}$ as a target** so that $C_{avg,ss}$ in the renal impaired patient is maintained the same as $C_{avg,ss}$ in normals:

$$\frac{(dose/\tau)_{ri}}{(dose/\tau)_n} = \frac{dose_{ri} \times \tau_n}{dose_n \times \tau_{ri}} = 1 - F + F [(Cl_{cr})_{ri}/(Cl_{cr})_n] \qquad (8)$$

4. **Using $C_{max,ss}$ as a target** so that $C_{max,ss}$ in the renal impaired is maintained the same as $C_{max,ss}$ in normals:

$$\text{dose per } \tau_{ri} = (dose_L) [1 - 10^{-0.3(\tau_{ri}/t_{1/2ri})}] \qquad (9)$$

where $dose_L$ is a loading dose intended to achieve the same $C_{max,ss}$ in the renal impaired as in the normal patient.

C. Nonlinear pharmacokinetic drug clearance—normal renal function. Nonlinear clearance assumes that a proportional change in dose leads to a **disproportional** change in SDC. It also assumes that $t_{1/2}$ and Cl **change** as the dose changes and also as the amount of drug in the body from a given dose changes. Drugs exhibiting nonlinear clearance present a much greater challenge than linear clearance drugs because the assumptions in the latter case of proportional changes in dose yielding same proportional changes in C_{ss} and constant Cl and $t_{1/2}$ do not apply for nonlinear drugs. For nonlinear drugs, increases in dose lead to increases in $t_{1/2}$, decreases in Cl, and changes in C_{ss} that are excessive compared to the proportionate change in dose.

1. **Estimating drug clearance:**

$$Cl = \frac{V_{max}}{K_m + C_{avg,ss}} \qquad (10)$$

where V_{max} is the maximum amount of drug that can be eliminated per unit of time (e.g., day) and K_m is the drug serum concentration at which the rate of elimination is 50% of V_{max}.

2. **Estimating $C_{avg,ss}$ resulting from a given dose/τ:**

$$C_{avg,ss} = \frac{(K_m)(S)(f)(dose/t)}{V_{max} - (S)(f)(dose)/\tau} \qquad (11)$$

3. **Estimating dose/τ needed for a desired $C_{avg,ss}$:**

$$dose/\tau = \frac{(V_{max})(C_{avg,ss})}{(K_m + C_{avg,ss})(S)(f)} \qquad (12)$$

D. An example of applying some of the above equations to developing and modifying dosage regimens

1. A common dosage regimen for intravenous (IV) gentamicin is 1.7 mg/kg q8h (as a 30-minute infusion). Regimens are usually adjusted to achieve $C_{max,ss}$ and $C_{min,ss}$ within 5–10 mcg/mL and less than 2 mcg/mL, respectively. Does the above regimen meet the target concentration objectives in normal patients? Assume the following population parameters in normals: $Cl = 0.09$ L/kg/hr, $t_{1/2} = 2.5$ hr, $V = 0.25$ L/kg. For IV administration, $f = 1$, and $S = 1$ for the dosage form (label amount represents the actual amount of gentamicin).

2. **In normals,** using equations (2) and (3):

$$C_{max,ss} = \frac{(1)(1)(1.7 \text{ mg/kg})/(0.25 \text{ L/kg})}{1 - 10^{-0.3\,(8\text{ hr}/2.5\text{ hr})}} = 7.6 \text{ mcg/mL}$$

$$C_{min,ss} = 7.6 \text{ mcg/mL} \times 10^{-0.3\,(8\text{ hr}/2.5\text{ hr})} = 0.8 \text{ mcg/mL}$$

These values fall within the target concentration ranges for the average patient with normal renal function.

3. **In the renal impaired,** what should be done to modify the above regimen for a patient who is 60 years old, 70 kg, male, with a Cr_s of 2.5 mg/dl? In this patient, if the above regimen were used, the prolonged $t_{1/2}$ would yield $C_{max,ss} = 15.2$ mcg/mL and $C_{min,ss} = 8.4$ mcg/mL, values clearly above the target concentration ranges.

   a. Using equation (6) for estimating Cl_{cr} in this patient:

$$Cl_{cr} = \frac{(140 - 60 \text{ yr})(70 \text{ kg})}{(2.5 \text{ mg/dl})(72)} = 31 \text{ mL/min}$$

   b. Then using equation (7) for estimating $t_{1/2}$ in this patient, assuming $F = 0.98$ and $(Cl_{cr})_n = 120$ mL/min:

$$\frac{(2.5 \text{ hr})}{(t_{1/2})_{ri}} = 1 - 0.98 + 0.98(31/120) = 0.27$$

$$(t_{1/2})_{ri} = 9.3 \text{ hr}$$

   c. Then using equation (9), first determine a loading dose (D_L) to achieve the same $C_{max,ss}$ of approximately 8 mcg/mL as estimated in IV D 2 for a patient with normal renal function:

$$D_L = (C_{max,ss})(V)/(S)/(f)$$

$$D_L = (8 \text{ mcg/mL})(0.25 \text{ L/kg})/(1)(1) = 2 \text{ mg/kg}$$

   Next, determine fraction of drug lost during τ, assuming a τ_{ri} of 24 hours, and using the $(t_{1/2})_{ri}$ of 9.3 hours estimated in IV D 3 b:

$$\text{Fraction lost} = 1 - 10^{-0.3(\tau/t_{1/2})} = 1 - 10^{-0.3(24/9.3)} = 0.84$$

   Lastly, calculate D per τ_{ri}:

$$D \text{ per } \tau_{ri} = (D_L)[1 - 10^{-0.3(\tau/t_{1/2})}]$$
$$= (2 \text{ mg/kg})(0.84) = 1.7 \text{ mg/kg}$$

   Thus, a D_L of 2 mg/kg followed by 1.7 mg/kg q24h is expected to maintain levels in this patient similar to that in normals.

V. EFFECT OF PHYSIOLOGICAL ALTERATIONS ON PHARMACOKINETIC VARIABLES

   A. General considerations. It is apparent from Figure 35-1 and the equations in Section IV, that any changes in pharmacokinetic variables result in changes in C_{ss} and perhaps pharmacodynamic outcomes. This may necessitate changes in D/τ compared to normals. For renal impairment, **quantitative** estimates of resulting changes in Cl and $t_{1/2}$, compared to normal values, are available using the equations in Section IV. For hepatic, cardiac, pulmonary, and other impairments potentially inducing changes in normal pharmacokinetic variables, only **qualitative** estimates are possible.

B. Renal impairment, when marked, reduces drug clearance for drugs primarily dependent on the kidney for elimination. As noted in the equations in Section IV B, physiological markers like serum creatinine and creatinine clearance are used to estimate the changes in Cl and $t_{1/2}$ resulting from reductions in Cr_s and Cl_{cr}.

C. Hepatic impairment exerts a complex influence on drug pharmacokinetics. Two processes may be altered, blood flow rate in delivering drug to the liver and the capacity of enzymes to metabolize the drug. In general terms, moderate to severe hepatic impairment is expected to slow overall Cl and prolong $t_{1/2}$ for drugs highly dependent on the liver for elimination.

D. Cardiac impairment, when substantial, decreases hepatic and renal clearances, reduces volume of distribution, and may slow absorption for some drugs. The effect of compromised perfusion is most critical for drugs that are both highly dependent on the liver for clearance and efficiently metabolized by the liver in normal patients.

E. Aging results in reductions in renal (consistently) and hepatic (inconsistently) clearances. The clearance of drugs primarily dependent on the kidney declines by nearly 50% and the half-life nearly doubles over a 40–50-year period from young adulthood. On the other hand, some drugs primarily dependent on the liver for clearance show no age-related changes, while others do. Changes with age in absorption, volume of distribution, and serum protein binding of drugs show no consistent pattern.

F. From a clinical viewpoint, serum **protein binding** of drugs becomes an important issue in TDM for drugs bound more than 80% to serum proteins. Because hepatic and renal clearances, volume of distribution, and pharmacological response are mediated by the free (unbound) form of the drug in serum, interpatient variations in protein binding not only result in variations in pharmacokinetics in normals, but also loss of serum proteins during renal and hepatic impairments may result in modified drug clearance and pharmacological response.

VI. THE TOTAL TESTING PROCESS APPLIED TO TDM

A. Defining the total testing process (TTP)

1. TDM involves both the laboratory for analysis and clinicians for interpretation of SDC. TTP refers to all aspects of the steps of laboratory testing beginning with a clinical question that is prompted by the patient–clinician encounter and concluding with the impact of the test result on patient care.

2. TTP emphasizes that TDM is a process involving a series of steps and interrelated activities and should not be viewed simply as a numerical value for an SDC.

3. TTP focuses on identifying all steps of the TDM testing process, highlighting where variations and errors can occur, interpreting SDC results in light of the steps involved, and improving the contribution of testing to achieving desired patient outcomes.

B. Components and steps in TTP. There are 4 components and 11 steps in TTP.

1. **The preanalytical component** consists of four steps:

   (1) clinical question, (2) test selected, (3) test ordered, and (4) specimen collection.

2. **The analytical component** then follows with three steps:

   (5) sample prepared, (6) analysis performed, and (7) result verified.

3. **The postanalytical component** then concludes with four steps: (8) result reported, (9) clinical answer, (10) action taken, and (11) effect on patient care.

4. The three components are affected by the fourth component, the **regulatory environment** within which TDM is performed.

C. Contributions of TDM to TTP

1. TDM has the potential to improve many of the steps in TTP: providing education, drug information, interpretation of TDM results, assessing the appropriateness of the TDM order,

scheduling specimen collection, developing drug dosage guidelines, and providing written and oral consultation concerning TDM results.

2. The pharmacist's greatest involvement in TTP is in steps (2) assessing the appropriateness of TDM for a given situation, (4) timing of specimen collection, and (9) clinical interpretation of TDM results.

VII. USING TEST PERFORMANCE CHARACTERISTICS IN TDM

A. Rationale and reasons

1. In TDM, the SDC functions like a diagnostic test to assist in classifying patient status.

2. On the one hand, the patient's SDC may be used, in conjunction with a population SDC cutoff value measure for the drug, which acts as a separator, to classify the patient as a member of either drug-induced toxic (patient SDC > upper cutoff value) or therapeutic (within therapeutic range) subpopulations.

3. Alternately, the patient's SDC may classify the patient as part of the therapeutic or subtherapeutic (SDC < lower cutoff value) subpopulations.

4. Although classifying patients in subpopulations is the most common use of SDC in TDM, a more informed application of SDC is to use the result to modify the clinician's probability of patient status. This is the use of SDC as part of a Bayesian approach to diagnostic test interpretation.

B. Test performance characteristics.
Test performance indices are not perfect classifiers of patient status and should never be used as the sole measure for determining how the patient is reacting to the drug. A number of test performance indices characterize the accuracy of a diagnostic test to accurately classify patients as toxic, therapeutic, or subtherapeutic. Four of these indices are most useful in interpreting SDC.

1. **Positive predictive value (PPV)**
   a. **Comparing drug-induced toxic versus nontoxic patients (using upper SDC cutoff level).** PPV denotes the proportion of patients with a **positive test** (patient SDC > upper cutoff SDC) who are in a drug-induced **toxic** condition. So, the value of PPV represents the probability of a positive test being accurate in classifying the patient as toxic.
   b. **Comparing therapeutic versus subtherapeutic patients (using lower SDC cutoff level).** PPV denotes the proportion of patients with a **positive test** (patient SDC > lower cutoff SDC) who are **responding appropriately.** So, the value of PPV in this case represents the probability of a positive test being accurate in classifying the patient as therapeutic.

2. **Negative predictive value (NPV)**
   a. **Comparing drug-induced toxic versus nontoxic patients (using upper SDC cutoff level).** NPV denotes the proportion of patients with a **negative test** (patient SDC < upper cutoff SDC) who are **not** manifesting drug-induced **toxicity.** So, the value of NPV represents the probability of a negative test being accurate in classifying the patient as nontoxic.
   b. **Comparing therapeutic versus subtherapeutic patients (using lower SDC cutoff level).** NPV denotes the proportion of patients with a **negative test** (patient SDC < lower cutoff SDC) who are **subtherapeutic.** So, the value of NPV in this case represents the probability of a negative test being accurate in classifying the patient as subtherapeutic.

3. **Positive likelihood ratio (PLR).** In defining conditions as + or − (as in + = toxic and − = negative, or + = therapeutic and − = subtherapeutic), **PLR** is the probability that a **+ patient** has a **+ test** divided by the probability that a **− patient** has a **+ test** (e.g., the probability that a **toxic** patient has an SDC > cutoff divided by the probability that a **nontoxic** patient has an SDC > cutoff). The **higher** the **PLR,** the **more** discriminating the test.

4. **Negative likelihood ratio (NLR).** NLR is the probability that a **+ patient** has a **− test** divided by the probability that a **− patient** has a **− test.** The **lower** the **NLR,** the **more** discriminating the test.

5. **Illustrating the use of PPV, NPV, PLR, and NLR.** For theophylline, using a test upper cutoff of 20 mcg/mL, PPV is 0.5, NPV is 0.95, PLR is 6, and NLR is 0.4.

    a. For PPV, this means that the proportion of patients with a positive test result (SDC > upper cutoff) who truly have theophylline-induced toxicity is 50%. For an individual patient with SDC > cutoff, the probability of toxicity is 0.5.

    b. For NPV, this means that the proportion of patients with a negative test result (SDC < upper cutoff) who truly are nontoxic is 95%. For an individual patient with SDC < cutoff, the probability of nontoxicity is 0.95.

    c. For PLR, toxic patients will have a positive test result six times more often than do nontoxic patients.

    d. For NLR, toxic patients will have a negative test result 40% as often as will nontoxic patients.

    e. These results suggest that a negative theophylline test result rules out toxicity (0.95) about twice as effectively as a positive test rules in toxicity (0.5). A positive test appears to be unreliable as an indicator of toxicity, but a negative test appears to be highly predictive of nontoxicity. Furthermore, the PLR suggests that a positive SDC test is six times more likely to come from a toxic than a nontoxic patient. On the other hand, the NLR implies that it is considerably less than one-half as likely (0.4) that a negative test comes from a toxic compared to a nontoxic patient.

    f. Knowledge of test performance characteristics of SDC measures provides the practitioner with an index of the usefulness of the SDC in categorizing patients.

C. Using a Bayesian approach. Using SDC in conjunction with likelihood ratio information enhances the application of the SDC in decision making. A Bayesian approach to probability revision allows the practitioner to make a pretest assessment of patient status, order a diagnostic test, and use the probability information contained in the test result to revise the assessment of status.

    1. The relation between pretest, test, and posttest assessment is shown in the following equation:

$$\text{(pretest odds)(likelihood ratio)} = \text{(posttest odds)} \qquad \textbf{(13)}$$

    where pretest refers to the pretest odds of the condition being present prior to obtaining the patient's SDC and posttest refers to the posttest odds of the condition being present after learning the SDC.

    2. Odds are defined as + results divided by − results (+/−). **Probability** is defined as + results divided by total results (+/total, where total is the sum of + and − results).

    3. Odds are converted to probability as follows:

    Probability = odds/(1 + odds) $\qquad \textbf{(14)}$

    4. Probability is converted to odds as follows:

    Odds = probability/(1 − probability) $\qquad \textbf{(15)}$

    5. An example of applying a Bayesian approach to modifying the probability of patient status. Using the theophylline test performance characteristics noted in VII B 5:

    a. Assume that a practitioner assesses by visual inspection that the probability of theophylline-induced toxicity in a patient is 0.25 (the pretest probability). She orders a serum theophylline concentration (STC), and uses the measurement to revise her assessment of toxicity in the patient (the posttest probability).

    b. Further assume that the test performance characteristics for the STC are: PLR = 6 and NLR = 0.4.

    c. Using equations (13), (14), and (15), a pretest probability of 0.25 is the same as pretest odds of toxicity of 1/3 [0.25/(1 − 0.25)], using equation (15).

    d. If the STC test for the patient comes back positive (STC > 20 mcg/mL), then PLR = 6 is used to revise the odds of toxicity. If the STC test is negative (STC ≤ 20 mcg/mL), then NLR = 0.4 is used.

    e. Assume the patient's **STC = 22 mcg/mL,** then using equation (13) yields (1/3)(6) = 2. So, the posttest odds of toxicity are 2/1. Converting these odds to probability using equation (14): [2/(1 + 2)] = 0.67. The **posttest probability of toxicity is 0.67.** The pretest probability of 0.25 has nearly tripled using the STC as feedback.

    f. Assume instead that the patient's **STC = 14 mcg/mL;** then using equation (13) yields (1/3)(0.4) = 0.13. So, the posttest odds of toxicity are 0.13/1. Converting these odds to probability using equation (14): $[0.13/(1 + 0.13)] = 0.12$. **The posttest probability of toxicity is 0.12.**

g. While a positive STC test nearly tripled the probability of toxicity above, a negative test cuts the probability in half. This demonstrates the usefulness of using SDC in combination with practitioner assessment as a guide to quantifying the probability of patient status.

VIII. SUMMARY

A. TDM applies to a small number of drugs with a narrow range of effective and safe SDC wherein optimum drug treatment is promoted by maintaining SDC within a population or patient-specific therapeutic range, above which drug-induced toxicity occurs too often and below which the drug is too often ineffective.

B. A practitioner initiates drug treatment using a dose rate that assumes that the patient shows mean population values for the pharmacokinetic variables, even though it is expected that few patients will ever possess the mean value being used. If the resulting C_{ss} and/or pharmacological response is other than expected and the patient becomes at risk for subtherapeutic or drug-induced toxicity, it is likely due to the interpatient variability in pharmacokinetic values and pharmacodynamic response that characterizes the need for TDM; therefore, the dose rate is modified to produce a patient-specific C_{ss} that represents the best tradeoff of effectiveness and toxicity.

C. Timing of sampling of SDC is critical to reduce errors in interpretation of the measurement. SDC should be sampled at steady state, after postabsorption and postdistribution equilibrium is achieved, and a time during τ_{ss} that matches the time at which the therapeutic range was established.

D. The choice of $C_{max,ss}$, $C_{min,ss}$, $C_{avg,ss}$, or $C_{inf,ss}$ to estimate dosage regimens depends on the therapeutic range objective and, in the latter case, intravenous rather than intermittent administration.

E. For the renal-impaired patient, the dosage reduction factor is calculated to achieve, depending on the therapeutic range objective, a $C_{max,ss}$ or $C_{avg,ss}$ in the renal-impaired patient that is similar to that desired if the patient had normal renal function.

F. The TTP is the systematic sequence of events in which TDM is practiced from identification of the need for an SDC measurement, to proper timing of sample collection, laboratory analysis, interpretation of results, and dosage regimen modification, if indicated.

G. The SDC measure is more than a number used to relate the patient's value to a population therapeutic range. The SDC is a form of diagnostic test used (1) to assist in classifying patient status and (2) as feedback to revise practitioner estimates of patient status. Therefore, it is important to know the predictive values and likelihood ratios of SDC tests.

STUDY QUESTIONS

Directions: Each of the numbered items or incomplete statements in this section is followed by answers or by completions of the statement. Select the **one** lettered answer or completion that is **best** in each case.

1. Define therapeutic drug monitoring. What is meant by the term TDM?

(A) The use of drug serum concentration measurements, for drugs in which there is (1) a correlation between serum concentration and response, as well as (2) a narrow range of effective and safe concentrations, to assess patient status as an adjunct to clinical observation

(B) The use of drug serum concentration measurements to determine population values for a drug's half-life value

(C) The use of drug serum concentration measurements to assess the accuracy of the drug concentration assay

(D) Observing the effects of drugs in man

(E) Using drug serum concentration measurements to differentiate effective from ineffective drugs

2. The therapeutic range for theophylline is often stated as 10–20 mcg/mL. What does this mean?

(A) Fifty percent of people taking theophylline show a safe and effective response when the serum drug concentration is between 10–20 mcg/mL.

(B) Most people achieve the desired response to theophylline, with minimum adverse effects when the serum theophylline concentration is maintained between 10–20 mcg/mL. Fewer patients are managed effectively at <10 mcg/mL, but some may respond quite appropriately at lower levels. The frequency of adverse effects increases as the level increases above the upper limit of the therapeutic range, but a few patients are managed effectively, without adversity, above the range.

(C) Twenty-five percent of people show an effective response to theophylline at 10 mcg/mL, and 75% show an effective response at 20 mcg/mL.

(D) Twice daily administration of theophylline, but not three times daily, requires that serum drug concentrations stay within 10–20 mcg/mL.

(E) Theophylline serum drug concentrations outside of the 10–20 mcg/mL range are ineffective and/or unsafe.

3. Assume that for a digoxin, the therapeutic range is cited as $C_{avg,ss}$ = 0.8–2 ng/mL. If the patient is assumed to have an estimated digoxin $t_{1/2}$ of 48 hours, how long would you wait to take a serum digoxin concentration measurement, and when during τ would you schedule it?

(A) 28 days, then 3–4 hours after the dose is administered

(B) 14 days, then 6–8 hours after the dose is administered

(C) 7 days, then 10–14 hours after the dose is administered

(D) 3 days, then 1–2 hours after the dose is administered

(E) 1 day, then 18–22 hours after the dose is administered

4. Differentiate linear from nonlinear drug clearance. What is the effect on TDM?

(A) Linear drug clearance is first order, the Cl and $t_{1/2}$ are independent of drug dosage, and proportional changes in dose result in the same proportional changes in C_{ss}. Nonlinear drug clearance is zero order, Cl and $t_{1/2}$ change as dose changes (or as the amount of drug in the body changes), and proportional changes in dose yield disproportionate changes in C_{ss}.

(B) Linear drug clearance presents fewer serum concentration peaks and troughs during the dosage interval than does nonlinear drug clearance.

(C) Linear drug clearance is zero order, the Cl and $t_{1/2}$ are dependent on drug dosage, and proportional changes in dose do not result in the same proportional changes in C_{ss}. Nonlinear drug clearance is first order, and equations are not available to predict drug serum concentration from the dose rate.

(D) Drugs with linear clearance have shorter $t_{1/2}$ values than drugs with nonlinear clearance.

(E) Drugs with linear clearance are administered less often than drugs with nonlinear clearance.

5. What is the positive predictive value of a diagnostic test?

(A) The fraction of patients with a positive outcome who have a positive test result

(B) Being more than 50% correct in predicting success or failure upon using a drug regimen

(C) The fraction of patients who achieve a successful response in using a drug

(D) The fraction of patients with a positive test result who turn out to have a positive outcome

(E) The probability that knowledge of a drug serum concentration results in a successful response to treatment

6. A 70-year-old, 80-kg male, with serum creatinine of 3 mg/dL, is scheduled to start tobramycin therapy. What regimen is recommended to achieve $C_{max,ss}$ within 5–10 mcg/mL (use the midpoint of 7.5 mcg/mL for the calculation) and $C_{min,ss}$ <2 mcg/mL. Try a q24h regimen to start and, if unsuccessful in achieving the target concentration goals, alter τ and recalculate. Assume in normals the following values: $t_{1/2}$ = 2.5 hr, V = 0.25 L/kg, F = 0.98, S = 1, f = 1, Cl_{cr} = 120 mg/dL.

(A) A loading dose of 1.8–2.0 mg/kg followed by 1.0 mg/kg qd

(B) A loading dose of 1.8–2.0 mg/kg followed by 1.5 mg/kg qd

(C) 2.0 mg/kg qd

(D) 1.0 mg/kg qd

(E) 0.5 mg/kg qd

ANSWERS AND EXPLANATIONS

1. The answer is A *[1 B].*

2. The answer is B *[II B].*

3. The answer is C *[II D 3].*
If the patient's estimated $t_{1/2}$ is 48 hours, 90% of steady state is expected to be achieved between 3–4 $t_{1/2}$ intervals or 6–8 days in this case. For clinical purposes, we choose 90% attainment of steady state as the minimum time to estimate drug accumulation. A level drawn at 7 days seems reasonable. Once a τ_{ss} has been selected, the time for scheduling a level should correspond with the reference time for the therapeutic range. In this case, $C_{avg,ss}$ was cited as the reference time, so a measurement scheduled for sometime near the midpoint of τ_{ss} (around 12 hours) is reasonable.

4. The answer is A *[IV A, C].*
This presents challenges in TDM, because for linear drugs the clinician can expect a change in C_{ss} proportional to a change in dose, but for nonlinear drugs this is not true.

5. The answer is D *[VII B 1].*
The positive predictive value of a diagnostic test is an index of how effective the test is in classifying patients correctly. For example, using a C_{ss} measure for a given drug, knowing that the positive predictive value is 0.8, given a group of patients with a C_{ss} above the test cutoff value, 80% of the patients will be accurately classified as having a positive outcome. If the test is being used to classify toxic versus nontoxic patients, 80% of the patients with C_{ss} above the test cutoff will experience drug-induced toxicity. If, instead, the test is being used to classify effective versus subeffective response in patients, 80% of the patients with C_{ss} above the test cutoff will experience effective response.

6. The answer is B *[IV D 3].*
Using the equation for estimating Cl_{cr} in this patient from IV B 1:

$$Cl_{cr} = \frac{(140 - 70 \text{ yr})(80 \text{ kg})}{(3 \text{ mg/dL})(72)} = 26 \text{ mL/min}$$

Then, using the equation for estimating $t_{1/2}$ in this patient from IV B 2:

$$\frac{(2.5 \text{ hr})}{(t_{1/2})_{ri}} = 1 - 0.98 + 0.98 \, (26/120) = 0.23$$

$$(t_{1/2})_{ri} = 10.9 \text{ hr}$$

Then, using equation [IV D 3 b], first determine a loading dose: (D_L) to achieve the desired $C_{max,ss}$ of 7.5 mcg/mL:

$$D_L = (C_{max,ss})(V)/(S)(f)$$

$$D_L = (7.5 \text{ mcg/mL})(0.25 \text{ L/kg})/(1)(1) = 1.9 \text{ mg/kg}$$

Then, determine fraction of drug lost during τ, assuming a τ_{ri} of 24 hr, and using the $(t_{1/2})_{ri}$ of 10.9 hr estimated above using the equation in IV D 3 c:

$$\text{fraction lost} = 1 - 10^{-0.3(24/10.9)} = 0.78$$

Lastly, calculate D per τ_{ri}:

$$D \text{ per } \tau_{ri} = (D_L)(\text{fraction lost per } \tau_{ri})$$

$$= (1.9 \text{ mg/kg})(0.78) = 1.5 \text{ mg/kg}$$

Thus, a D_L of 1.9 mg/kg followed by 1.5 mg/kg q24h is expected to attain the desired $C_{max,ss}$ and $C_{min,ss}$ levels in this patient. Of course, many estimates were made along the way (Cl_{cr}, $t_{1/2}$, V), so if the patient's $C_{max,ss}$ and $C_{min,ss}$ vary from what has been expected from the calculations, it is likely due to the estimates being at variance with the actual value(s) in the patient.

36
Drug Use in Special Patient Populations: Pediatric, Pregnant, Geriatric

Mark K. Sorenson
Beth Bryles Phillips
Alan H. Mutnick

I. DRUG THERAPY IN PEDIATRIC PATIENTS

A. General considerations

1. Pediatric drug therapy challenges the pharmacist, because children are uniquely different from adults. Many of the assumptions made in adult drug therapy do not apply to children. For example, in contrast to the relatively stable pharmacokinetic profile that characterizes most of the adult years, **pharmacokinetic parameters in children change as they mature from birth to adolescence.** Complex processes relating to drug absorption, distribution, metabolism, and elimination are not fully developed at birth and mature at varying rates throughout childhood.

2. Drug selection, doses, and dosage intervals change throughout childhood, making **drug therapy monitoring** essential. The outline below describes pharmacokinetic differences in childhood that influence drug therapy. A discussion of problems inherent to pediatric drug monitoring follows, as well as some brief comments on adverse drug reactions. Finally, some cautions are suggested concerning drug dosing in children.

B. Pharmacokinetic considerations

1. **Gastrointestinal absorption.** Oral drug absorption is a complex and variable process. Many drug- and patient-related factors influence absorption, although drug-related factors are generally constant and patient-related factors change. These include underlying disease states and patient-related factors that change with advancing age: gastric pH, gastric emptying time, an underlying disease state, bile salt production, and pancreatic enzyme function.

   a. **Gastric pH.** Neonates are relatively achlorhydric. Increases in acid production correlate with starting enteral feedings. Acid production rises steadily in the first month of life but is variable. Relative achlorhydria (i.e., gastric pH >4) is present in approximately 20% of neonates at 1 week of age, 15% at 2 weeks, and 8% at 3 weeks. By 6 weeks of age, gastric acid production is comparable to that in older infants and reaches adult values at 2 years of age. Relative achlorhydria may explain the increased bioavailability of basic drugs and the unpredictable, slower absorption of acidic agents. Additionally, drugs normally degraded by gastric acid, such as penicillins, may have an increased bioavailability.

   b. **Gastric emptying.** The rate of gastric emptying is important in determining the rate and extent of drug absorption. Gastric emptying is highly variable in neonates and is affected by gestational and postnatal ages and the type of feeding administered. At 6–8 months of age, infants acquire the same rate of gastric emptying as adults.

      (1) Because most drugs are absorbed in the small intestine, a **reduced rate of emptying** slows the rate of absorption, which can reduce peak drug concentrations. **Prematurity** slows gastric emptying from an already reduced rate in term neonates [typical half-life ($t_{1/2}$) of gastric emptying is 90 minutes but may be as long as 6–8 hours] as compared with adults ($t_{1/2}$ is 65 minutes).

      (2) An **increased rate of emptying** may reduce the extent of absorption, because contact time with absorptive surfaces in the small intestine is reduced.

      (3) **Breast-fed infants** empty their stomachs approximately twice as fast as formula-fed infants. The increased caloric density of formula feedings delays gastric emptying.

c. Underlying disease state
    (1) Disease states that can significantly **prolong gastric emptying** include pyloric stenosis, gastroesophageal reflux, respiratory distress syndrome, and congenital heart disease.
    (2) Short-bowel syndrome greatly **reduces the total surface area available for drug absorption.**
    (3) Cholestatic liver disease, biliary obstruction, and distal ileum resection can **interfere with bile acid excretion or reabsorption and reduce the absorption of lipid-soluble substances,** including vitamins A, D, and E.
d. Bile salt production. The bile salt pool and the rate of bile salt synthesis are reduced approximately 50% in premature and young term infants as compared with adults. Decreased fat absorption from enteral feedings, as well as decreased drug absorption, can occur. For example, when vitamin D (i.e., calcifediol, also called 25-hydroxycholecalciferol) is administered to neonates, absorption is only 30% as compared with 70% in adults.
e. Pancreatic enzyme function. The absorption of lipid-soluble drugs is also affected by gastrointestinal concentrations of pancreatic enzymes. Neonates have low levels of lipases, and, when combined with reduced bile acid production, lipid-soluble drugs may be left insoluble and thus unabsorbed in the intestine. Oral suspensions, such as chloramphenicol palmitate, which require intraluminal hydrolysis by pancreatic lipases before being absorbed, have been associated with unreliable absorption of the active moiety in premature and term infants.

2. Percutaneous absorption. The skin is made up of three layers: the epidermis, dermis, and subcutaneous tissue. The stratum corneum, the outer layer of the epidermis, provides the main barrier function of the skin. Factors responsible for changing percutaneous absorption include the degree of skin hydration and the stratum corneum maturity.
  a. Skin hydration is increased in neonates and premature neonates.
  b. Stratum corneum maturity. Full-term neonates have an intact epidermal layer including a mature stratum corneum, unlike premature neonates who have an immature stratum corneum. Maturation of the premature skin is related to postnatal age, with the attainment of epidermal barrier properties similar to the full-term neonate within 3 weeks of life.
  c. Clinical significance. Due to the immature epidermal barrier and increased skin hydration, premature neonates have increased insensible fluid loss via transepidermal water loss and increased drug absorption compared to full-term neonates. The skin of a full-term neonate has barrier properties to drug absorption similar to adult skin.

3. Intramuscular (IM) absorption. The surface area available for absorption, blood flow to the injection site, and muscle activity are physiological factors that influence absorption of drugs administered by IM injection. Preterm neonates demonstrate erratic drug absorption following IM administration because of their small muscle mass, weak muscle contraction ability, and hemodynamic instability. IM therapy is generally well absorbed in infants and older children but is often discouraged secondary to the pain associated with this route of administration.

4. Distribution. How a drug distributes in the body is important in both the selection and dosage of a drug. Volume of distribution is affected by many age-dependent factors, including the degree of protein binding, the sizes of various body compartments, and the presence of various endogenous substances.
  a. Protein binding. Acidic drugs bind to **albumin,** while basic substances bind primarily to **alpha$_1$-acid glycoprotein (AGP).** Both of these proteins are reduced in neonates, which allows greater amounts of free drug in the serum and tissues. In addition to reduced amounts, these proteins are also less efficient at binding drugs in neonates. This has been demonstrated for phenytoin, phenobarbital, chloramphenicol, penicillin, propranolol, lidocaine, and several other substances. The increase in the free fraction of certain drugs in neonates and infants may result in enhanced pharmacological activity for a given dose and challenges the reliability of serum concentration monitoring, which generally uses parameters derived from adult populations. Adult levels for albumin and AGP occur at approximately 10–12 months of age.
  b. Size of body compartments. At birth, extracellular fluid volume constitutes approximately 40% of total body weight, decreasing to 25% by 6 months, and 20% by 12 years. For polar compounds, such as the aminoglycosides that distribute into extracel-

lular spaces, **larger mg/kg doses** are required in neonates to achieve therapeutic concentrations. The dosage interval will likely be greater (e.g., q12–24 hours) in neonates compared to older infants and children, however, due to decreased drug elimination. Changes in the percent of total body fat with age can also alter drug distribution. A 29-week neonate is comprised of only 1% body adipose tissue compared to a full-term newborn with 12%–16% body fat. This increases to between 20%–25% body fat at 1 year of age and then falls slightly between 1 and 2 years of age. The decreased percent of body fat in the premature neonate and newborn results in a smaller volume of distribution for fat-soluble or lipophilic drugs. For example, the volume of distribution of diazepam in a neonate is 1.4–1.8 L/kg compared to 2.2–2.6 L/kg in adults. Smaller mg/kg doses of diazepam are required in neonates to achieve a therapeutic effect.

c. **Endogenous substances.** In neonates, various endogenous substances can bind to plasma proteins and reduce the degree of drug-protein binding. The two most important substances are **free fatty acids** and **unconjugated bilirubin,** which, when present in high concentrations, can increase the unbound to bound drug ratio in the plasma.

(1) The serum concentration of these two substances normalizes in early infancy.

(2) Caution is urged, however, in evaluating bilirubin- or free fatty acid–induced drug-displacement reactions, because significant increases in the plasma concentrations of the drug occur only when the displaced drug is more than 90% bound and its metabolism is rate-limited.

(3) Usually, increases in unbound concentrations are only transient, because hepatic metabolism for most drugs is not rate-limited.

d. Because **bilirubin** competes with certain drugs for albumin-binding sites, it can be displaced, which presents a **theoretical** concern for the development of **drug-induced kernicterus** in neonates. **Hyperbilirubinemia** develops because heme catabolism is accelerated and the conjugating ability of the liver is reduced due to prematurity.

(1) Unconjugated bilirubin normally binds noncovalently to plasma albumin, but the binding affinity is reduced in neonates, not approaching **adult values** until 6 months of age. Thus, it can potentially be displaced when certain highly bound acidic compounds are administered.

(2) The concern for drug-induced bilirubin displacement is theoretical, because it is derived from in vitro studies. It may be that drug-induced displacement of bilirubin and the development of clinical kernicterus are unlikely because the affinity of bilirubin for albumin greatly exceeds that of most drugs. This remains controversial, however, and requires further study.

5. **Metabolism.** Drug metabolism occurs primarily in the liver, with additional biotransformation occurring in the intestine, lung, adrenal gland, and skin. In the liver, metabolism involves a series of **phase I and phase II reactions,** both of which are susceptible to enzyme-inducing (e.g., phenytoin, phenobarbital, carbamazepine, rifampin) and enzyme-inhibiting (e.g., cimetidine, erythromycin) agents.

a. **Phase I reactions** are nonsynthetic reactions (i.e., oxidation, reduction, hydrolysis, and hydroxylation) that result either in inactive compounds or in metabolites with equal, lesser, or, rarely, greater pharmacological action.

(1) The major **enzymes** responsible for phase I oxidation reactions are those in the cytochrome P450 monooxygenase system, which at birth are at approximately 50% of the activity of adult levels.

(2) Consequently, the **metabolism of many drugs** (e.g., phenobarbital) **is reduced** and **drug serum half-lives are prolonged** correspondingly.

(a) The **ability to oxidize** drugs increases with increasing postnatal age so that by several weeks of postnatal life, metabolic rates generally are equal to or greater than adult rates.

(b) **Metabolic rates** remain high for 1–5 years and gradually decline to adult levels at puberty.

b. **Phase II reactions** are synthetic reactions (i.e., conjugation with glycine, glucuronide, or sulfate) that result in polar, water-soluble, inactive compounds for renal and biliary elimination.

(1) The underlying **enzyme systems** are unevenly depressed at birth and mature at varying rates.

(2) For example, the **ability to conjugate drugs with glucuronide** (e.g., chloramphenicol) is greatly reduced at birth and does not reach adult values until 3–4 years of age.

(3) Also, the **acetylation of sulfonamides** is significantly reduced at birth.

(4) However, the **ability to conjugate sulfate groups** (e.g., acetaminophen) is well developed at birth.

(5) The **ability to conjugate carboxyl groups with glycine** apparently is only slightly reduced at birth, and adult levels are achieved by about 6 months of age.

6. **Elimination.** The kidney is the major route of drug elimination for both water-soluble drugs and water-soluble metabolites of lipid-soluble drugs. Three basic processes contribute to renal elimination: glomerular filtration, tubular secretion, and tubular reabsorption. Both glomerular filtration and secretion promote the renal elimination of drugs, whereas reabsorption reduces it. All three processes display age-dependent changes in maturity.

    a. At birth, **glomerular filtration in full-term neonates** is 30%–50% of the adult value and matures quickly, approaching 85% of adult values by 3–5 months of age. **Premature infants** (i.e., less than 34 weeks' gestational age) at birth have glomerular filtration rates that are further reduced due to incomplete nephrogenesis and do not obtain rates comparable to those of full-term infants until 4–6 weeks of age.

    b. Tubular function

        (1) Tubular secretion is an active process, using separate protein carriers for acids and bases. In contrast to glomerular filtration, secretion matures at a slower rate. At birth, **full-term infants** have secretory rates of approximately 20% of adult values and do not achieve adult rates until 6–7 months of age. Before secretion is fully mature, some drugs (e.g., penicillin) may stimulate their own secretion, leading to decreased efficacy unless the dosage is increased.

        (2) Tubular reabsorption can be an active or passive process. It increases with postconceptional age and is reduced in neonates. Unlike tubular secretion, its development remains poorly understood.

    c. Two other considerations in renal elimination include renal blood flow and drug-protein binding.

        (1) Renal blood flow is the driving force underlying glomerular filtration. As cardiac output increases and renal vascular resistance decreases, renal blood flow increases, and adult values are attained by 6–12 months of age.

        (2) Protein binding significantly affects glomerular filtration because only unbound drug is filtered.

C. **Problems in pediatric drug monitoring.** Several problems are inherent in pediatric pharmacotherapy, and lack of recognition or concern for them may lead to greater morbidity or drug-related toxicity.

1. As previously discussed, children display unique **age-dependent changes** in pharmacokinetic parameters. Absorption, distribution, metabolism, and elimination of a drug can vary greatly between different age groups. Lack of proper clinical monitoring can lead to underdosage, overdosage, therapeutic failure, or drug-related toxicity.

2. **Therapeutic drug monitoring** assumes a correlation exists between serum drug concentrations and therapeutic effects (see Chapter 35). Many of these correlations have been displayed in adult patients but not in children. Extrapolating target serum drug concentrations, which are derived from adults, to children may not always be appropriate. Multiple factors, including drug-protein binding differences, different metabolite patterns, and altered body composition with changes in volume of distribution, can change the amount of free drug availability at the receptor site and alter the therapeutic effects of a drug.

    a. A potential complication in interpreting serum drug levels is the **presence of endogenous substances,** which may cross-react with analytical drug assays. This has been demonstrated for digoxin in neonates and infants, and it may be applicable to other drugs.

    b. Drug levels are not constant (except when administered by continuous infusion) in the serum and may fluctuate greatly during dosage intervals. Accurate timing of drawing blood for therapeutic monitoring is essential to correctly interpret drug concentrations.

3. **Technical problems** may interfere with proper drug delivery. Pediatric drug doses often are in small fluid volumes, which may greatly prolong drug delivery when given through typical intravenous (IV) administration sets, which may contain 20–30 mL of fluid dead space. The use of microbore tubing and syringe infusion pumps can help prevent this problem. Enteral feeding tubes present similar problems.

D. Adverse drug reactions are not uncommon in children. Antibiotics (especially vancomycin, cephalosporins, and penicillins), anticonvulsants, narcotics, antiemetics, and contrast agents are leading causes of adverse drug reactions in children. The majority of these are mild (e.g., red-man syndrome with IV vancomycin) and are managed relatively simply.

 1. However, approximately **3 out of every 10 reactions prolong or require hospitalization** [e.g., syndrome of inappropriate antidiuretic hormone (SIADH) with carbamazepine], and approximately 1 out of 10 is considered severe (i.e., the reaction is life-threatening or fatal, requires a prolonged recovery time, or is permanently disabling).

 2. Examples of severe reactions include anaphylaxis after administering a cephalosporin, or respiratory arrest following the combined IV use of a benzodiazepine and a narcotic.

E. Dosing considerations in pediatric patients. Paracelsus's (1493–1541) statement concerning drug dosages is applicable to children: "All substances are poisons; there is none which is not a poison. The right dose differentiates a poison from a remedy."

 1. **Drug dosages** for adults cannot be extrapolated to children. This is especially true in neonates and infants and for drugs with a narrow therapeutic index. As previously reviewed, children differ considerably pharmacokinetically from adults, and various rules for dosing children based on age or weight are unreliable and are not recommended. Pediatric dosages should be verified whenever possible using a reference specific to pediatric patients. Pediatric references provide dosing information based most commonly on a patient's weight or body surface area (BSA). If a pediatric dosage needs to be calculated based on BSA, it can be determined by using a BSA nomogram or the following equation:

$$\text{BSA (in } m^2) = \sqrt{\frac{\text{height (cm)} \times \text{weight (kg)}}{3600}}$$

 2. Pediatric drug dosages for many commonly used drugs can be obtained from standard **pediatric references,** such as the *Harriet Lane Handbook* (Mosby), *The Pediatric Drug Handbook* (Mosby), or the *Pediatric Dosage Handbook* (Lexi-Comp). It should be noted that for many drugs (especially antibiotics), varying dosage ranges may exist in different reference sources.

 3. **Dosing intervals** are often different for children. For example, because of reduced renal and hepatic function, neonates generally require a longer dosing interval compared to children and adults. Older infants and children may require a shorter interval because of their enhanced elimination of drugs.

 4. **Underlying disease states** may also affect pediatric doses and dosage intervals. For example, patients with cystic fibrosis and cancer often require larger doses and shorter dosing intervals for aminoglycoside antibiotics due to enhanced drug clearance.

 5. **Errors in dosage calculations or drug preparation** are more likely to occur in pediatric patients than in adults. Common errors made include decimal point errors (resulting in 10 to 100 to 1000-fold errors), dosing on a mg/kg/day versus mg/kg/dose basis, dosing on a mg/kg versus mg/m² BSA basis, and confusing kg with pounds in dosage calculations. Arithmetic errors are prone to occur when extemporaneously preparing pediatric dosage forms or when calculating dosages.

II. DRUG USE IN PREGNANT PATIENTS. Pregnant women may require drug therapy for preexisting medical conditions or for problems associated with their pregnancy. This patient population may be exposed to drugs or environmental agents that have adverse effects on the unborn. Clinical situations also exist where the fetus may be pharmacologically treated when the mother takes medication. It is important to understand the principles of drug use in these patients because any drug administered to a pregnant woman may directly harm the developing fetus or adversely influence her pregnancy. Furthermore, pharmacotherapy in such a patient population requires knowledge of drug clearance as well as latent effects that are unique in pregnancy.

A. Fetal development. The effects of drug therapy in pregnancy depend largely on the **stage of fetal development** during which exposure occurs. Limited information exists regarding the effects of drugs in the period of conception and implantation. However, it is suggested that women who are at risk of conceiving or who wish to become pregnant should withdraw all unnecessary medication 3–6 months before conception.

1. **Blastogenesis.** During this stage (the first 15–21 days after fertilization), cleavage and germ layer formation occur. The embryonic cells are in a relatively undifferentiated state.

2. **Organogenesis** (14–56 days). All major organs start to develop during this period. Exposing the embryo to certain drugs at this time may cause major congenital malformations. Organogenesis is the most critical period of development.

3. **Fetal period** (ninth week to birth). At the ninth week, the embryo is referred to as a fetus. Development during this time is primarily maturation and growth. Exposure to a drug during this period is generally not associated with major congenital malformations. However, the developing fetus may be at risk from exposure to the pharmacological effects of a variety of fetotoxic drugs and microorganisms.

B. **Placental transfer of drugs.** The placenta, a product of conception, is the functional unit between the fetal body and the maternal blood.

1. The **functions** of the placenta include nutrition, respiration, metabolism, excretion, and endocrine activity to maintain fetal and maternal well-being. In conjunction with the fetus, the placenta produces a number of pregnancy-related hormones that are mainly secreted into the maternal circulation. In order for a drug to cause a teratogenic or pharmacological effect in the embryo or fetus, it must cross from the maternal circulation to the fetal circulation or tissues. Generally, this passage occurs via the placenta.

2. The **placenta is not a protective barrier.** Previously, the placenta was considered to be a protective barrier that isolated the fetus from drugs and toxins present in the maternal circulation. However, the protective characteristics of the placenta are, in fact, limited. The concept that a placental barrier exists should be disregarded. The transfer of most nutrients, oxygen, waste products, drugs, and other substances occurs via **passive diffusion** primarily driven by the concentration gradient. A few compounds, however, are actively transported across the placental membranes.

3. **Factors affecting placental drug transfer.** Generally, the principles that apply to drug transfer across any lipid membrane can be applied to placental transfer of a drug. Most substances administered for therapeutic purposes have, by design, the ability to cross the placenta to the fetus. The critical factor is whether the rate and extent of transfer are sufficient to cause significant drug concentrations in the fetus. There are many factors that affect the rate and extent of placental drug transfer.
   a. **Molecular weight.** Low–molecular-weight drugs [i.e., less than 500 daltons (d)] diffuse freely across the placenta. Drugs of a higher molecular weight (500–1000 d) cross less easily. Drugs comprised of very large molecules (e.g., heparin) do not cross the placental membranes.
   b. **pH.** The pH gradient between the maternal and fetal circulation and the pH of the drug itself affect the degree of placental transfer. Weakly acidic and weakly basic drugs tend to rapidly diffuse across the placental membranes.
   c. **Lipid solubility.** Moderately lipid-soluble drugs easily diffuse across the placental membranes. It is important to note that many drugs that have been formulated for oral administration, and hence gastrointestinal absorption, are designed for optimal lipid membrane transfer. Generally, these drugs can cross the placenta.
   d. **Drug absorption.** During pregnancy, gastric tone and motility are decreased, which results in delayed gastrointestinal emptying time. This may affect oral drug absorption. Nausea and vomiting, which are most common in the first trimester but may continue throughout pregnancy, may also affect oral drug administration and absorption.
   e. **Drug distribution.** The volume of distribution increases significantly during pregnancy and increases with advancing gestational age. The alteration in volume of distribution is the result of a combination of changes associated with pregnancy, including increased plasma volume and increased cardiac output secondary to an increase in stroke volume and heart rate. Total body fluid (i.e., both intravascular and extravascular volume) increases, as does fat content.
   f. **Plasma protein binding.** Placental transfer of plasma protein-bound drug is unlikely, because only the free unbound drug crosses the placenta. During pregnancy, a reduction in the levels of two major drug-binding proteins is observed, namely albumin and AGP.

(1) The reduction of these two important proteins potentially alters the free fraction of a drug.

(2) When these plasma protein concentrations are decreased, there are fewer binding sites available for acidic drugs, and an increase in free drug concentration may result.

(3) However, concomitant increases in drug catabolism in the liver, renal clearance, increased tissue uptake, and altered receptor activity may counteract the effect of changes in plasma protein binding.

g. **Physical characteristics of the placenta.** As pregnancy progresses, the placental membranes become progressively thinner, resulting in a decrease in diffusion distance.

h. **The pharmacological activities of the drug.** Drugs with vasoactive properties may affect maternal and placental blood flow, and therefore influence the amount of drug reaching the fetus.

i. **Coexistent disease states.** Maternal hypertension or diabetes may reduce or enhance placental drug transfer, as a result of alterations in placenta permeability.

j. **Rate of maternal and placental blood flow.** Factors that influence maternal blood flow (e.g., exercise, meals, vasoactive medications) may affect drug absorption, maternal drug concentration deliverable to the placenta, and ultimately the fetus.

4. **Embryotoxic drugs** are drugs that harm the developing embryo, resulting in termination of pregnancy or shortening of gestational length.

a. Many drugs [e.g., hormones, antidepressants, angiotensin-converting enzyme (ACE) inhibitors, and certain antibiotics] administered in early pregnancy may be embryotoxic.

b. Because the placenta has not quite fully formed by organogenesis (see II A 2), the embryo risks damage from a variety of compounds.

c. Some drugs may result in miscarriage by causing a severe chemical insult to the products of conception.

5. **Teratogenic drugs** cause physical defects in a developing fetus. This risk of teratogenesis is highest during the first trimester.

a. Teratogenesis may lead to physical malformation and/or mental abnormalities that may affect the long-term viability of the developing fetus.

b. Because fetal organ systems develop at different times, specific teratogenic effects depend mainly on the point of gestation when the drug was ingested.

c. The Food and Drug Administration has developed a **classification system** that groups drugs according to the degree of their potential risk during pregnancy [*Fed Regis* 1979 Jun 26, 44(124): 37434–37467].

(1) **Category A.** Adequate, well-controlled studies in pregnant women have not shown an increased risk of fetal abnormalities.

(2) **Category B.** Animal studies have revealed no evidence of harm to the fetus; however, there are no adequate and well-controlled studies in pregnant women; **or** Animal studies have shown an adverse effect, but adequate and well-controlled studies in pregnant women have failed to demonstrate a risk to the fetus.

(3) **Category C.** Animal studies have shown an adverse effect and there are no adequate and well-controlled studies in pregnant women; **or** No animal studies have been conducted, and there are no adequate and well-controlled studies in pregnant women.

(4) **Category D.** Studies, adequate well-controlled or observational, in pregnant women have demonstrated a risk to the fetus. However, the benefits of therapy may outweigh the potential risk.

(5) **Category X.** Studies, adequate well-controlled or observational, in animals or pregnant women have demonstrated positive evidence of fetal abnormalities. The use of the product is contraindicated in women who are or may become pregnant.

d. **Examples** of teratogenic and potentially toxic drugs include the following:

(1) **Vitamin A derivatives.** The drugs in this group—which includes vitamin A, isotretinoin, and etretinate—are potent animal teratogens. Using these agents shortly before or during pregnancy may result in severe human deformities.

(2) **ACE inhibitors.** It remains unclear if this class of antihypertensive drugs produces structural abnormalities in the developing human fetus. These drugs may, however, compromise the fetal renal system and result in severe renal failure and possibly fetal death.

(3) **Warfarin and warfarin derivatives.** The use of warfarin during the first trimester has been associated with a pattern of defects that commonly include nasal hypoplasia and a depressed nasal bridge. The characteristic defects are collectively referred to as fetal warfarin syndrome (FWS). Warfarin use during the second and third

trimesters is associated with increased risk of fetal central nervous system (CNS) malformations. Heparin, which is poorly transferred across the placenta, may be substituted for warfarin when anticoagulant therapy is necessary.

(4) Estrogen and androgens. These category X drugs may cause serious genital tract malformations.

(5) Other hormonal agents. Drugs such as thyroid preparations and cortisone may affect the development of fetal endocrine glands. Methimazole and carbimazole have been associated with malformations in newborns exposed in utero. Propylthiouracil (PTU) is the drug of choice in pregnancy and lactation for antithyroid therapy.

(6) Ethanol. Alcohol consumed in large amounts or for prolonged periods during pregnancy has been associated with a pattern of defects collectively referred to as fetal alcohol syndrome (FAS). Features of FAS include abnormalities in growth and in cardiac, skeletal, craniofacial, muscular, genitourinary, cutaneous, and CNS development.

(7) Antibiotics

    (a) Mottling of the teeth may occur when **tetracycline** is taken by the mother after week 18 of pregnancy. This teratogenic effect does not become evident until later in childhood when the teeth erupt.

    (b) Metronidazole is mutagenic in animals and is contraindicated for treating trichomoniasis during the first trimester. Use for other indications must be carefully evaluated, especially in the first trimester.

    (c) Quinolone antibiotics are not recommended for use during pregnancy because of arthropathies observed in immature animals.

(8) Anticonvulsants such as phenytoin, trimethadione, valproic acid, and sodium valproate have been associated with malformations when used during the first trimester.

(9) Lithium. Congenital malformations, primarily in the cardiovascular system, have been associated with first trimester administration of lithium. Ebstein's anomaly (i.e., tricuspid valve malformation) has been reported in a significant number of fetuses exposed to the drug during this period. Exposure to the drug near term has resulted in neonatal lithium toxicity, which is generally reversible.

(10) Antineoplastics. Many agents belonging to this class of drugs have been associated with fetal malformations following first-trimester exposures. Examples include busulfan, chlorambucil, cyclophosphamide, and methotrexate.

(11) Finasteride may cause abnormal development of the genitalia of male fetuses exposed to the drug in utero. Pregnant women should avoid handling crushed tablets of the drug and should avoid contact with the semen of men who are taking this medication.

6. Fetotoxic drug effects are the result of pharmacological activity of a drug that may physiologically affect the developing fetus.

  a. During the **fetal period,** these effects are more likely to occur than are teratogenic effects.

  b. Clinically significant fetotoxic effects include the following:

    (1) CNS depression may occur with barbiturates, tranquilizers, antidepressants, and narcotics. Also, analgesics and anesthetics commonly given during labor may cause significant CNS and respiratory depression in newborns.

    (2) Neonatal bleeding. Maternal ingestion of agents such as nonsteroidal anti-inflammatory drugs (NSAIDs) and anticoagulants at therapeutic doses near term may cause bleeding problems in the newborn. NSAIDs may prolong gestation and interfere with the progress of labor. Acetaminophen is a safe and effective analgesic for use in pregnancy.

    (3) Drug withdrawal. Habitual maternal use of barbiturates, narcotics, benzodiazepines, alcohol, and other substances of abuse may lead to withdrawal symptoms in newborns.

    (4) Reduced birth weight. Pregnant women who smoke cigarettes, consume large amounts of alcohol, or abuse drugs have an increased risk of delivering a low–birth-weight infant.

    (5) Constriction of the ductus arteriosus. Maternal use of NSAIDs in the third trimester may cause the ductus arteriosus to close prematurely and may result in pulmonary hypertension in the newborn.

C. Drug excretion in breast milk. Recent appreciation of the benefits of breast-feeding for the infant and mother has become evident. Today, more than 60% of women choose to breast-feed their infants. Of these women, 90%–95% receive a medication during the first postpartum week. It is important to understand the principles of drug excretion in breast milk and specific information on the various medications in order to minimize risks from drug effects in the nursing infant.

1. **Transfer of drugs from plasma to breast milk** is governed by many of the same principles that influence human membrane drug transfer.
   a. Many drugs cross the mammary epithelium via **passive diffusion** along a concentration gradient formed by the un-ionized drug content on each side of the membrane.
   b. This membrane is a **semipermeable lipid barrier** like other human membranes.
   c. The membrane also consists of **small pores** that allow for direct passage of low–molecular-weight substances (i.e., less than 200 d).
      (1) **Larger drug molecules,** which are unable to pass through the pores, must dissolve in the lipid part of the membrane in order to pass through to the breast milk.
      (2) **Active transport mechanisms** are described for some substances; however, there are no drugs known to use this process.

2. **Physiochemical characteristics of the drug** and its environment that **influence the rate and extent** of drug passage into the breast milk include:
   a. **Molecular weight of the drug** (see II C 1 c)
   b. The **pit gradient between the breast milk and plasma.** Human milk tends to be more acidic than plasma.
      (1) Therefore, weak acids may diffuse across the membrane and remain un-ionized, allowing for passage back into the plasma.
      (2) Weak bases may diffuse into the breast milk and ionize, which causes drug trapping (i.e., a clinically significant increase in the concentration of weak bases in the breast milk).
   c. **Degree of drug ionization.** Only the ionized form of a drug is able to pass through the lipid membrane. Drugs that exist un-ionized in large concentrations in the plasma would not be available to diffuse across the lipid membrane.
   d. **Plasma protein binding.** Only the unbound portion of a drug is available to pass into the breast milk. In general, drugs with high plasma protein binding properties tend to remain in the plasma and pass into the breast milk in low concentrations. While milk proteins exist and drug binding to these proteins may occur, the clinical relevance is limited.
   e. **Lipid solubility of the drug.** Lipid solubility is necessary for a drug to pass into the breast milk. Highly lipid-soluble drugs (e.g., diazepam) may pass into the breast milk in relatively high amounts and therefore may present a significant dose of drug to the nursing infant.

3. **After a drug is administered to a nursing mother,** the drug may be partially activated or inactivated in the maternal liver. The drug may be metabolized to active or inactive metabolites.
   a. **Maternal pharmacology** plays a significant role in the rate and extent of drug passage into breast milk. The extent of plasma protein binding, as well as changes in the mother's ability to metabolize or eliminate the drug, influence the amount of drug in the plasma that is available to pass into the breast milk.
   b. Equally important in affecting drug concentrations in breast milk are the **maternal dose of the drug,** the **dosing schedule or frequency,** and the **route of administration.**

4. **Drugs affecting hormonal influence of breast milk production.** The primary hormone responsible for controlling breast milk production is **prolactin.**
   a. **Following delivery,** serum prolactin levels increase to promote the production and secretion of breast milk. Prolactin continues to be released in response to infant feeding.
   b. However, infant feeding is not the only influence on serum prolactin levels. There are frequently prescribed **medications that may alter serum prolactin levels** and therefore the amount of breast milk produced.
      (1) A decrease in milk production may result in diminished weight gain in the nursing infant, the need for supplementation, or premature cessation of breast-feeding.
      (2) **Drugs that decrease serum prolactin levels.** Drugs such as **bromocriptine** have been used to suppress lactation in women who choose not to breast-feed. Other drugs include:
         (a) Ergot alkaloids
         (b) L-dopa

(3) Drugs that increase serum prolactin levels. Metoclopramide and sulpiride have been useful therapeutically to enhance milk production. The following drugs are known to increase serum prolactin levels, but they have not been used therapeutically.

(a) Methyldopa
(b) Amphetamines
(c) Haloperidol
(d) Phenothiazines
(e) Theophylline

5. **Factors to assess the risk of toxicity to the infant** include:
   a. Inherent toxicity of the drug
   b. Amount of drug ingested
   c. Degree of prematurity
   d. Nursing pattern of the infant

6. **Factors to minimize drug exposure to the infant.** One of the goals when using medications in the breast-feeding mother is to maintain a natural, uninterrupted pattern of nursing. In many instances, it may be possible to withhold a drug when it is not essential or delay therapy until after weaning. Other factors include:
   a. Product selection. When a specific product is being selected from a class of drugs, it is important to choose the product that is distributed into the milk the least.
      (1) Other desirable characteristics include a short half-life, inactive metabolites, and no accumulation in breast milk.
      (2) Additionally, it is desirable to select a particular route of administration associated with a lower concentration of the drug in breast milk.
   b. Maternal dose relative to infant feeding. One of the goals of drug dosing in lactating women is minimal infant exposure to the drug. In drugs taken on a scheduled basis, it is desirable to adjust the dosing and nursing schedules so that a drug dose is administered immediately before the infant's feeding.

7. **Examples of drugs that readily enter breast milk** and should be used with caution in nursing mothers include the following:
   a. Narcotics, barbiturates, and benzodiazepines, such as diazepam, may have a hypnotic effect on the nursing infant. These effects are related to the maternal dose. Alcohol consumption may have a similar effect.
   b. Antidepressants and antipsychotics. These classes of drugs appear to pass into the breast milk; however, no serious adverse effects are reported. The long-term behavioral effects of chronic exposure to these drugs on developing newborns are unknown.
   c. Metoclopramide. This antiemetic passes readily into the breast milk and may accumulate as a result of ion trapping. Its use may be of concern because of its potential strong CNS effects. However, there are no published reports involving serious effects associated with using this drug in lactating women.
   d. Anticholinergic compounds. These drugs may result in adverse CNS effects in the infant and may reduce lactation in the mother. Dicyclomine is contraindicated in nursing mothers because it may result in neonatal apnea.

III. DRUG USE IN GERIATRIC PATIENTS.

III. DRUG USE IN GERIATRIC PATIENTS. More than 12% of the American population is over 65 years of age, representing more than 34 million Americans. It is estimated that three out of every four elderly people are taking prescription medications. Overall, these drugs account for one-third of all prescription medications in the United States. Estimated total drug usage, including nonprescription medications, increases this estimate to 50% of all drugs used in the United States.

A. Elderly patients are at increased risk for drug-induced adverse effects. Incidence of **adverse drug reactions** (ADRs) in patients over the age of 65 is two to three times greater compared to younger patients. One in five of all geriatric patients experiences an ADR. In some patients, ADRs are overlooked because they mimic the characteristics of other diseases.

B. Factors that are responsible for the higher prevalence of ADRs in the geriatric population include polypharmacy, multiple disease states, increasing severity of illness, reduced drug elimination, and increased sensitivity to drug effects.

1. Studies have shown that more than 35% of geriatric patients living in the community use six or more medications; approximately one-half of patients residing in long-term–care facilities use five or more medications.

2. Patients taking multiple medications have a greater chance of experiencing ADRs due to drug–drug interactions and the potential for overlap or synergy between adverse effect profiles.

3. Patients with multiple disease states are at higher risk of having a drug–disease state interaction.

4. In addition to the aforementioned risk factors for developing an ADR, it is difficult to predict how geriatric patients will respond to any given medication due to altered pharmacokinetic and pharmacodynamic profiles.

5. Another issue complicating geriatric drug therapy is adherence. Factors that have been shown to increase nonadherence include female gender, lower socioeconomic status, living alone, polypharmacy, complicated drug regimens, and multiple diseases. As many as 60% of geriatric patients do not take their medications as prescribed and may self-medicate as often as once a week.

6. Elderly patients can have diseases that make adhering to drug therapy difficult. Conditions that affect vision, such as macular degeneration or cataract formation, can make reading prescription labels and medication instructions troublesome. Hearing loss can prevent patients from understanding and health-care professionals from effectively communicating medication information and patient instructions. Arthritis can add to the difficulty of opening medication bottles. In these instances, providing patients with medication or "pill" boxes and written medication lists may limit potential barriers to patient adherence. Recognizing these factors, pharmacists can increase adherence in elderly patients.

7. Pharmacists can provide recommendations to eliminate unnecessary drug therapy and monitor medication profiles to avoid potential drug–drug or drug–disease state interactions that may prove harmful. Efforts to optimize drug therapy, including simplifying and employing more cost-effective regimens, may ultimately afford better patient adherence.

C. **Pharmacokinetics.** Pharmacokinetic parameters may be altered in the elderly due to age-related physiological changes. Specific age-related physiological changes affecting drug therapy are depicted in Table 36-1.

Table 36-1. Age-Related Physiological Changes Affecting Drug Therapy

Pharmacokinetic Factor	Change	Clinical Significance
Gastrointestinal motility	↓	May affect the rate but not the extent of drug absorption
Gastric pH	↑	No significant change in drug absorption
Renal function	↓	Reduced elimination of renally excreted drugs
Serum albumin	↓	Decreased protein binding leading to an increased free fraction of drug
Phase I hepatic metabolism	↓	Potential accumulation of drugs metabolized by oxidation, reduction, or hydrolysis reactions
Body fat/lean muscle mass ratio	↑	Increased volume of distribution of fat-soluble drugs
Total body water	↓	Decreased volume of distribution of water-soluble drugs
Pharmacodynamic Factor	**Change**	**Clinical Significance**
Beta-receptor sensitivity	↓	Potential diminished response to beta-blockers
Baroreceptor sensitivity	↓	Greater risk of orthostatic hypotension
Response to benzodiazepines and opioid analgesics	↑	Increased risk of adverse effects with typical doses

1. **Absorption.** Physiological changes that can alter absorption in the elderly include delayed gastric emptying, decreased splanchnic blood flow, elevated gastric pH, and impaired intestinal motility. Although the rate of drug absorption may be altered in some patients, the extent of absorption is rarely affected.

2. **Distribution.** Several age-related physiological changes may affect drug distribution.
   a. Elderly patients have a decrease in total body water, causing water-soluble drugs (e.g., acetaminophen) to have a smaller volume of distribution.
   b. The volume of distribution of lipid-soluble drugs (e.g., diazepam, propranolol) is increased because elderly patients tend to have a greater ratio of adipose tissue to lean muscle mass.
   c. These age-related changes impacting drug distribution may lead to increases in ADRs.
   d. Aging may also affect the pharmacokinetics of drugs that are highly protein bound. For example, drugs that are highly bound to albumin (e.g., warfarin, phenytoin) may have a greater free concentration because albumin can be decreased in the elderly.
   e. Although AGP concentrations tend to increase with age, the increase in the concentrations of basic drugs (e.g., lidocaine, propranolol) that bind to AGP are usually clinically meaningful only in acutely ill patients.

3. **Renal excretion.** Perhaps the best documented age-related physiological change is the decline in renal function, specifically glomerular filtration rate and the tubular secretion rate.
   a. In patients without renal dysfunction, it is estimated that there is a 50% decline in renal function by age 70.
   b. Serum creatinine may not be a good predictor of renal function, as creatinine production also declines with age.
   c. Drugs primarily eliminated by the kidneys can result in increased concentrations and subsequent adverse effects. All renally eliminated drugs used in geriatric patients should be monitored for possible dosage reduction and potential toxicity.
   d. Certain drugs, such as digoxin, procainamide, H_2-receptor antagonists, lithium, and aminoglycosides, have been shown to cause serious or pronounced ADRs when doses are not adjusted for renal function.

4. **Hepatic metabolism.** Age-related changes affecting the liver include a reduction in hepatic blood flow and a decline in hepatic metabolism.
   a. Phase II reactions (glucuronidation, acetylation, and sulfation) are relatively unchanged in the elderly.
   b. A reduction in phase I reactions (oxidation, reduction, and hydrolysis), however, can occur. Benzodiazepines and certain analgesics, dependent on phase I reactions for metabolism, represent situations where changes in hepatic metabolism may be important. The elimination half-lives of these agents are prolonged and may result in drug accumulation and possible adverse effects.

D. **Pharmacodynamics**

1. Elderly patients can be more or less responsive, compared to younger patients, to certain drugs. One reason is due to altered receptor sensitivity in the elderly. Studies have shown that elderly patients may show a diminished response to beta-blockers.

2. In contrast, elderly patients seem to have an exaggerated response to analgesics, benzodiazepines, and warfarin. Elderly patients should be monitored carefully when taking these medications. Low doses of benzodiazepines should be used in these patients, if at all. When initiating warfarin therapy, lower doses (e.g., 2.5 mg every day) should also be used. One important rule of thumb to follow when initiating drug therapy in the elderly population is to "start low and titrate slow."

E. **Drug therapy considerations**

1. Drug therapy in geriatric patients is involved and can be very complex because of age-related changes in pharmacokinetics and pharmacodynamics.

2. A lack of clinical trials designed to evaluate the safety and efficacy of drug therapy in the elderly population increases the problem.

3. The higher incidence of adverse effects in geriatric patients may be due in part to the complexity of drug therapy and the relative lack of clinical trials in this population. Table 36-2

Table 36-2. Target Drugs and Doses to Avoid in Geriatric Patients

Drug	Comment
Analgesics	
Pentazocine	Avoid due to safer and more effective alternatives
Propoxyphene	Avoid due to lack of efficacy and potential for accumulation and adverse effects
Antibiotics	
Oral antibiotics	Therapy >4 weeks should be avoided except when treating osteomyelitis, prostatitis, tuberculosis, or endocarditis
Antidepressants	
Amitriptyline	Avoid due to anticholinergic adverse effects and increased risk of falls; use nortriptyline or desipramine as alternatives
Amitriptyline/perphenazine	Avoid; use separate antidepressant and antipsychotic agents in appropriate geriatric doses as necessary
Antiemetics	
Trimethobenzamide	Avoid; more effective alternatives available
Antihypertensives	
Hydrochlorothiazide	Doses >50 mg/day should be avoided
Methyldopa	Avoid due to safer alternatives
Propranolol	Lipophilic nonselective beta-blocker with increased potential for adverse effects; avoid (unless indicated for controlling violent behaviors)
Reserpine	Avoid due to risk of adverse effects (e.g., sedation, depression)
Antipsychotics	
Haloperidol	Avoid doses >3 mg/day unless indicated for psychotic disorder
Thioridazine	Avoid doses >30 mg/day unless indicated for psychotic disorder
Antispasmodics	
Belladonna	Avoid long-term use due to anticholinergic adverse effects
Clidinium	
Dicyclomine	
Hyoscyamine	
Decongestants	
Oxymetazoline	Daily use for >2 weeks should be avoided
Phenylephrine	
Pseudoephedrine	
Dementia Treatments	
Isoxsuprine	Avoid due to lack of efficacy
H$_2$-Antagonists	
Cimetidine	Avoid doses >900 mg/day and therapy longer than 12 weeks
Rantidine	Avoid doses >300 mg/day and therapy longer than 12 weeks
Hypoglycemic Agents	
Chlorpropamide	Avoid; long $t_{1/2}$ can cause prolonged hypoglycemic episodes and can induce SIADH
Muscle Relaxants	
Carisoprodol	Risk of adverse events greater than potential benefits; all use should be avoided
Cyclobenzaprine	
Methocarbamol	
Orphenadrine	
NSAIDs	
Indomethacin	Avoid due to CNS adverse effects; use alternative NSAID
Phenylbutazone	Avoid due to hemotological adverse effects; use alternative NSAID
Platelet Inhibitors	
Dipyridamole	Avoid due to lack of efficacy and adverse effects (orthostatic hypotension) at high doses; aspirin is safer and more effective

(Continued on next page)

Table 36-2. *Continued*

Drug	Comment
Sedative-Hypnotics	

Long-acting benzodiazepines
  Chlordiazepoxide
  Diazepam
  Flurazepam
	Avoid due to accumulation and increased risk of falls

Short-acting Benzodiazepines
  Alprazolam
  Oxazepam
  Triazolam
	Nightly use for >4 weeks should be avoided due to potential for addiction; avoid oxazepam doses >30 mg/day

Meprobamate	All use should be avoided

Short-duration barbiturates
  Pentobarbital
  Secobarbital
	All use should be avoided because safer alternatives exist

Adapted from references: Beers MH, Ouslander JH, Rollingher I, et al. Explicit criteria for determining inappropriate medication use in nursing home residents. *Arch Intern Med* 1991;151:1825–1832; Stuck AE, Beer MH, Steiner A, et al. Inappropriate medication use in community-residing older persons. *Arch Intern Med* 1994; 154:2195–2200.

lists several drugs and doses that should be avoided in the elderly due to higher risks of adverse effects and/or lack of efficacy.

4. Due to alterations in gait, balance, and mobility, falls and consequent adverse events are frequent occurrences in geriatric patients.
   a. The prevalence of osteoporosis in the elderly results in a higher incidence of fractures. Complications associated with fractures, particularly hip fractures, are significant causes of increased morbidity and mortality.
   b. It is important to consider medications that can place elderly patients at risk for falls.
   c. Medications causing orthostatic hypotension, drowsiness, dizziness, blurred vision, or confusion have the potential to cause or worsen postural instability and increase falls in the elderly.
   d. It is established that many psychoactive agents, especially long-acting benzodiazepines, are associated with an increased risk of falls in the elderly. To minimize this likelihood, long-acting benzodiazepines should never be used in these patients. If a benzodiazepine must be prescribed, lorazepam or oxazepam are optimal choices due to a lack of active metabolites and because are metabolized by pathways dependent on phase I hepatic reactions.

5. Geriatric patients tend to be sensitive to medications that possess anticholinergic effects. Dry mouth, urinary retention, blurry vision, constipation, tachycardia, memory impairment, and confusion are typical anticholinergic adverse effects associated with several classes of drugs (Table 36-3).
   a. When possible, drugs with anticholinergic effects should be avoided in the elderly. In those instances when this is not an option, the least anticholinergic agent should be chosen and initiated at the lowest effective dose. One example is the tricyclic antidepressants. When a tricyclic antidepressant is needed, desipramine and nortriptyline possess less anticholinergic activity than amitriptyline and imipramine and therefore would be better initial therapeutic options.
   b. Frequent monitoring for and patient education on signs and symptoms of possible anticholinergic adverse effects is always warranted when these drugs are prescribed in the elderly.

F. **General principles.** To aid clinicians in providing appropriate geriatric drug therapy, some general principles have been developed.

1. Start with a low dose, and titrate the medication dose slowly.

2. Due to reduced renal and hepatic function, the half-lives of many drugs are prolonged in the elderly.

Table 36-3. Drugs and Drug Classes Possessing Anticholinergic Effects

Antidiarrheal agents
    Diphenoxylate/atropine

Antiemetics/antivertigo agents
    Dimenhydrinate
    Meclizine
    Scopolamine
    Trimethobenzamide

Antihistamines

Antipsychotic agents

Antispasmodics
    Belladonna alkaloids
    Clidinium bromide
    Hyoscyamine
    Propantheline
    Oxybutynin

Class Ia antiarrhythmic agents
    Disopyramide
    Procainamide
    Quinidine

Parkinson's agents
    Benztropine
    Procyclidine
    Trihexyphenidyl

Skeletal muscle relaxants
    Cyclobenzaprine
    Orphenadrine

Tricyclic antidepressants

3. Rapid dose escalations prevent attainment of the optimal therapeutic response because a steady-state concentration of the drug is not reached and increases the risks for developing an ADR.

4. The fewest number of drugs should always be used to treat patients.

5. Always evaluate possible drug toxicity. Geriatric patients can have atypical presentations of ADRs, which may manifest as CNS changes (e.g., altered mental status).

STUDY QUESTIONS

Directions: Each of the numbered items or incomplete statements in this section is followed by answers or by completions of the statement. Select the **one** lettered answer or completion that is **best** in each case.

1. All of the following medications should not be used routinely in pregnant patients during the third trimester EXCEPT

(A) acetaminophen
(B) nonsteroidal anti-inflammatory drugs
(C) warfarin
(D) lithium
(E) aspirin

2. Which of the following medications may have the potential to cause falls in a geriatric patient?

(A) Amitriptyline
(B) Trazodone
(C) Acetaminophen with codeine
(D) Diazepam
(E) All of the above

3. Placental transfer of a drug is affected by all of the following characteristics EXCEPT

(A) molecular weight
(B) fetal gender
(C) gestational age
(D) lipid solubility of the drug
(E) plasma protein binding

4. All of the following are taken into account when calculating dosage for children EXCEPT

(A) height
(B) weight
(C) hepatic and renal function
(D) age
(E) body surface area

5. When selecting a benzodiazepine product for a woman who has chronic panic disorder, all of the following drug properties are desirable for breast-feeding her 8-month-old infant who was born at term EXCEPT

(A) hepatic metabolism to inactive metabolites
(B) a short half-life
(C) a rapid onset of action
(D) a tendency to bind to milk proteins

6. All of the following drugs may enhance breast milk production by increasing prolactin levels EXCEPT

(A) haloperidol
(B) methyldopa
(C) metoclopramide
(D) bromocriptine
(E) theophylline

7. Which of the following drugs is expected to cause anticholinergic adverse effects in the elderly?

(A) Propoxyphene
(B) Ciprofloxacin
(C) Amitriptyline
(D) Propranolol
(E) Cimetidine

8. Which of the following antihypertensive agents should be avoided in elderly patients?

(A) Amlodipine 5 mg every day
(B) Atenolol 25 mg every day
(C) Benazepril 10 mg every day
(D) Hydrochlorothiazide 25 mg every day
(E) Methyldopa 250 mg three times a day

9. Which of the following benzodiazepines is expected to cause the LEAST amount of adverse effects in the elderly?

(A) Chlordiazepoxide
(B) Diazepam
(C) Flurazepam
(D) Oxazepam
(E) Temazepam

10. Which of the following factors is associated with an increased risk of noncompliance in the elderly?

(A) Polypharmacy
(B) Hypertension
(C) Male gender
(D) Living with a spouse in an isolated environment
(E) Expensive medications

Directions: The question below contains three suggested answers, of which **one or more** is correct. Choose the answer

A	if **I only** is correct
B	if **III only** is correct
C	if **I and II** are correct
D	if **II and III** are correct
E	if **I, II, and III** are correct

11. According to the principles of drug excretion into the breast milk, which combination of the following properties would result in the HIGHEST drug concentration in breast milk?

 I. Low molecular weight, moderately lipophilic
 II. Low plasma protein bound, weakly basic
III. Highly plasma protein bound, weakly acidic

ANSWERS AND EXPLANATIONS

1. The answer is A *[II B 5 d (3), (9), 6 b (2)].*
Acetaminophen is a safe and effective analgesic that can be used in therapeutic doses during pregnancy. Nonsteroidal anti-inflammatory drugs (NSAIDs) may interfere with the onset or progress of labor when used in the third trimester. NSAIDs and warfarin, when used near delivery, may cause bleeding problems in the newborn infant. Additionally, warfarin use in the third trimester may be associated with fetal central nervous system (CNS) abnormalities. Lithium use in the third trimester may cause neonatal lithium toxicity.

2. The answer is E *[III E 4 c].*
Medications that can cause orthostatic hypotension, drowsiness, dizziness, blurred vision, or confusion have the potential to cause falls in geriatric patients. Thus, all of the medications listed may put the patient at a fall risk.

3. The answer is B *[II B 3].*
Fetal gender does not affect placental transfer of a drug. The molecular weight and the lipid solubility of a drug greatly influence its ability to cross the placental membranes. Plasma protein binding affects the amount of free drug available to cross the placenta. Gestational age influences the volume of distribution of the drug as well as the thickness of the placental membranes.

4. The answer is D *[I E].*
When calculating dosage for children, the child's height, weight, body surface area, and renal and hepatic function must be taken into account. Age, although sometimes used, may result in improper dosing because of the variations in body size and level of development found in children of the same age.

5. The answer is D *[II C 6 a (1)].*
When any drug is used by a nursing mother, it is desirable to have the least amount of active drug available in the maternal circulation to diffuse into the breast milk. A rapidly acting (for maternal onset of action), rapidly eliminated (i.e., short half-life) drug with inactive metabolites is optimal. If the drug binds in high quantities to milk proteins, it may tend to remain or accumulate in the breast milk.

6. The answer is D *[II C 4 b (2) (3)].*
Bromocriptine effectively decreases serum prolactin levels and has been used therapeutically to suppress lactation. Haloperidol, methyldopa, metoclopramide, and theophylline may increase serum prolactin levels. Of these drugs, only metoclopramide (as well as sulpiride) has been useful therapeutically to enhance milk production.

7. The answer is C *[III E 5; Table 36-3].*
Tricyclic antidepressants are an established cause of anticholinergic adverse effects in the elderly. When these agents are indicated, nortriptyline and desipramine are associated with a lower incidence of anticholinergic adverse drug reactions (ADRs) and are more desirable alternatives.

8. The answer is E *[III; Table 36-2].*
The use of methyldopa should be avoided in elderly patients due to risk of central nervous system adverse effects and hypotension.

9. The answer is D *[III; Table 36-2].*
Chlordiazepoxide, diazepam, and flurazepam should be avoided in elderly patients due to active metabolites and long-elimination half-lives. Oxazepam represents the safest alternative because of a relatively short half-life, absence of active metabolites, and it is devoid of phase I hepatic metabolism.

10. The answer is A *[III B].*
Female gender, lower socioeconomic status, living alone, polypharmacy, complicated drug regimens, and multiple disease states are all risk factors for noncompliance in the geriatric population.

11. The answer is C (I, II) *[II C 1–3].*
High–molecular-weight substances are less likely to pass into breast milk because of their size. Drugs that are highly plasma protein bound may only reach the breast milk in small amounts, because a large portion of the drug is bound to the maternal plasma proteins, and therefore only a small amount is free to diffuse into breast milk. A low–molecular-weight, moderately lipophilic drug passes easily into breast milk. A drug that has a low degree of plasma protein binding has a significant amount of drug free to diffuse into breast milk. A weakly basic drug may ionize after reaching the breast milk and therefore remain trapped in the milk.

37
Clinical Laboratory Tests

D. Byron May
Larry N. Swanson

I. GENERAL PRINCIPLES

A. Monitoring drug therapy

1. **Laboratory test results** are used to investigate potential problems with a patient's anatomy or physiology. Pharmacists usually monitor laboratory tests to:
   a. **Assess the therapeutic and adverse effects of a drug** (e.g., monitoring the serum uric acid level after allopurinol is administered, checking for increased liver function test values after administration of isoniazid)
   b. **Determine the proper drug dose** (e.g., assessment of the serum creatinine or creatinine clearance value before use of a renally excreted drug)
   c. **Assess the need for additional or alternate drug therapy** [e.g., assessment of white blood cell (WBC) count after an antibiotic is administered]
   d. **Prevent test misinterpretation resulting from drug interference** (e.g., determination of a false positive for a urine glucose test after cephalosporin administration)

2. These tests can be **very expensive,** and requests for them must be balanced against potential benefits for patients and how the laboratory test will affect your decision regarding therapy. Generally, lab tests should only be ordered if the results will affect the decisions about the management of the patient.

B. Definition of normal values

1. **Normal laboratory test results** fall within a predetermined range of values, and **abnormal values** fall outside that range. The normal range of a laboratory test is usually determined by applying statistical methods to results from a representative sample of the general population. Usually, the mean ± 2 standard deviations is taken as the normal range.
   a. **Normal limits may be defined somewhat arbitrarily;** thus, values outside the normal range may not necessarily indicate disease or the need for treatment (e.g., asymptomatic hyperuricemia).
   b. Many factors (e.g., age, sex, time since last meal) must be taken into account when evaluating test results.
   c. **Normal values also vary among institutions** and may depend on the method used to perform the test.
   d. The goal is NOT to make all lab values normal; resist urges to do something in a clinically stable patient.
   e. Attempts have been made in recent years to standardize the presentation of laboratory data by using the International System of Units (SI units). Controversy surrounds this issue in the United States, and resistance to adopt this system continues. The SI unit of measure is a method of reporting clinical laboratory data in a standard metric format. The basic unit of mass for the SI is the mole. The mole is not influenced by the addition of excess weight of salt or ester formulations. Technically and pharmacologically, the mole is more meaningful than the gram because each physiological reaction occurs on a molecular level.

      Efforts to implement the SI system began in the 1970s, resulting in the adoption of full SI-transition policies by a few major medical and pharmaceutical journals in the 1980s. Reluctance to use this system by many clinicians in the United States has forced changes in the policies by some journals to report both conventional and SI units or to report the conversion factor between the two systems. It is still controversial which method should be used to report clinical laboratory values. There are arguments for and against the universal conversion to the SI system. Readers should be aware that some journals report SI and/or conventional units in their text. Particular attention should be paid to the units associated with a reported laboratory value, and access to a conversion table may be necessary to avoid confusion in the interpretation of the data. When appropriate, both conventional and SI units will be reported in this chapter.

2. **Laboratory error** must always be considered when **test results do not correlate with expected results for a given patient.** If necessary, the test should be repeated. Common sources of laboratory error include spoiled specimens, incomplete specimens, specimens taken at the wrong time, faulty reagents, technical errors, incorrect procedures, and failure to take diet or medication into account.

3. During hospital admission or routine physical examination, a **battery of tests** is usually given to augment the history and physical examination. Basic tests may include an electrocardiogram (ECG), a chest x-ray, a sequential multiple analyzer **(SMA) profile, electrolyte tests, a complete blood count (CBC),** and **urinalysis.**

C. **Quantitative tests, qualitative tests, and analytical performance**

1. Tests with normal values reported in ranges (i.e., 3.5–5.0 mEq/L) are called *quantitative.*

2. Tests with positive (+) or negative (–) outcomes are called *qualitative.*

3. Those with varying degrees of positivity (e.g., 1+, 2+, 3+ glucose in the urine) are termed *semiquantitative.*

4. The quality of a quantitative assay is measured in terms of *accuracy* (accuracy is defined as the extent to which mean measurement is close to the true value). *Precision* refers to the reproducibility of the assay.

II. **HEMATOLOGICAL TESTS.** Blood contains three types of formed elements: red blood cells (RBCs), WBCs, and platelets (Figure 37-1). A CBC includes hemoglobin (Hb), hematocrit (Hct), total WBCs, total RBCs, mean cell volume (MCV), and platelet count.

A. **RBCs (erythrocytes)**

1. The **RBC count,** which reports the number of RBCs found in a cubic millimeter (mm³) of whole blood, provides an indirect estimate of the blood's Hb content. **Normal values** are:
   a. 4.3–5.9 million/mm³ of blood for men ($\times 10^{12}$/L)
   b. 3.5–5.0 million/mm³ of blood for women ($\times 10^{12}$/L)

2. The **Hct or packed cell volume (PCV)** measures the percentage by volume of packed RBCs in a whole blood sample after centrifugation. The Hct value is usually three times the Hb value (see II A 3) and is given as a percent or fraction of 1 (42%–52% or 0.42–0.52 for men; 37%–47% or 0.37–0.47 for women).
   a. Low Hct values indicate such conditions as anemia, overhydration, or blood loss.
   b. High Hct values indicate such conditions as polycythemia vera or dehydration.

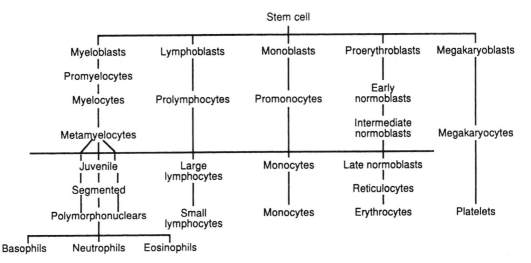

Figure 37-1. Derivation of blood elements from stem cells. Cells located below the *horizontal line* are found in normal peripheral blood, with the exception of the late normoblasts.

3. The **Hb test** measures the grams of Hb contained in 100 mL (1 dl) or 1 L of whole blood and provides an estimate of the oxygen-carrying capacity of the RBCs. The Hb value depends on the **number of RBCs** and the **amount of Hb in each RBC.**
   a. **Normal values** are 14–18 g/dl for men and 12–16 g/dl for women.
   b. **Low Hb** values indicate anemia.

4. **RBC indices** (also known as **Wintrobe indices**) provide important information regarding RBC size, Hb concentration, and Hb weight. They are used primarily to categorize anemias, although they may be affected by average cell measurements. A peripheral blood smear can provide most of the information obtained through RBC indices. Observations of a smear may show variation in RBC shape **(poikilocytosis),** as might occur in sickle-cell anemia, or it may show a variation in RBC size **(anisocytosis),** as might occur in a mixed anemia (folic acid and iron deficiency).
   a. **MCV** is the ratio of the Hct to the RBC count. It essentially assesses average RBC size and reflects any anisocytosis.

   $$\frac{\text{Hct (\%)} \times 10}{\text{RBC count (in millions)}} = \text{MCV}$$

      (1) **Low MCV** indicates **microcytic** (undersized) **RBCs,** as occurs in iron deficiency.
      (2) **High MCV** indicates **macrocytic** (oversized) **RBCs,** as occurs in a vitamin B_{12} or folic acid deficiency.
      (3) **Normal range for MCV** is 90 ±10.
   b. **Mean cell Hb (MCH)** assesses the amount of Hb in an average RBC.
      (1) MCH is defined as:

   $$\frac{\text{Hb} \times 10}{\text{RBC count (in millions)}} = \text{MCH}$$

      (2) **Normal range for MCH** is 30 ±4.
   c. **Mean cell Hb concentration (MCHC)** represents the average concentration of Hb in an average RBC, defined as:

   $$\frac{\text{Hb} \times 100}{\text{Hct}} = \text{MCHC}$$

      (1) **Normal range for MCHC** is 34 ±3.
      (2) **Low MCHC** indicates **hypochromia** (pale RBCs resulting from decreased Hb content), as occurs in iron deficiency.
   d. **RBC distribution width (RDW)** is a relatively new index of RBCs. Normally, most RBCs are approximately equal in size, so that only one bell-shaped histogram peak is generated. Disease may change the size of some RBCs—for example, the gradual change in size of newly produced RBCs in folic acid or iron deficiency. The difference in size between the abnormal and less abnormal RBCs produces either more than one histogram peak or a broadening of the normal peak. This value is used primarily with other tests to diagnose iron-deficiency anemia.
      (1) **An increased RDW** is found in factor-deficiency anemia (e.g., iron, folate, vitamin B_{12}).
      (2) **A normal RDW** is found in such conditions as anemia of chronic disease.
      (3) The **RDW index** is never decreased.

5. The **reticulocyte count** provides a measure of immature RBCs (reticulocytes), which contain remnants of nuclear material (reticulum). Normal RBCs circulate in the blood for about 1–2 days in this form. Hence, this test provides an index of bone marrow production of mature RBCs.
   a. Reticulocytes normally comprise 0.1%–2.4% of the total RBC count.
   b. **Increased reticulocyte count** occurs with such conditions as hemolytic anemia, acute blood loss, and response to the treatment of a factor deficiency (e.g., an iron, vitamin B_{12}, or folate deficiency). **Polychromasia** (the tendency to stain with acidic or basic dyes) noted on a peripheral smear laboratory report usually indicates increased reticulocytes.
   c. **Decreased reticulocyte count** occurs with such conditions as drug-induced aplastic anemia.

6. The **erythrocyte sedimentation rate (ESR)** measures the rate of RBC settling of whole, uncoagulated blood over time, and it primarily reflects plasma composition. Most of the sedimentation effect results from alterations in plasma proteins.

a. Normal ESR rates range from 0–20 mm/hr for males and from 0–30 mm/hr for females.
b. ESR values increase with acute or chronic infection, tissue necrosis or infarction, well-established malignancy, and rheumatoid collagen diseases.
c. ESR values are used to:
  (1) Follow the clinical course of a disease
  (2) Demonstrate the presence of occult organic disease
  (3) Differentiate conditions with similar symptomatology [e.g., angina pectoris (no change in ESR value) as opposed to a myocardial infarction (increase in ESR value)]

B. WBCs (leukocytes)

  1. The **WBC count** reports the number of WBCs in a cubic millimeter of whole blood.
    a. Normal values range from 4,000–11,000 WBC/mm³.
    b. Increased WBC count (leukocytosis) usually signals infection; it may also result from leukemia or tissue necrosis. It is most often found with **bacterial infection.**
    c. Decreased WBC count (leukopenia) indicates bone marrow depression, which may result from metastatic carcinoma, lymphoma, or toxic reactions to substances such as antineoplastic agents.

  2. The **WBC differential** evaluates the distribution and morphology of the five major types of WBCs—the **granulocytes** (i.e., **neutrophils, basophils, eosinophils**) and the **nongranulocytes** (i.e., **lymphocytes, monocytes**). A certain percentage of each type comprises the total WBC count (Table 37-1).
    a. Neutrophils may be mature (**polymorphonuclear leukocytes,** also known as PMNs, "polys," segmented neutrophils, or "segs") or immature ("**bands**" or "stabs").
      (1) Chemotaxis. Neutrophils that **phagocytize and degrade many types of particles** serve as the body's first line of defense when tissue is damaged or foreign material gains entry. They congregate at sites in response to a specific stimulus, through a process known as chemotaxis.
      (2) Neutrophilic leukocytosis. This describes a response to an appropriate stimulus in which the total neutrophil count increases, often with an increase in the percentage of immature cells (**a shift to the left**). This may represent a systemic bacterial infection, such as pneumonia (Table 37-2).
        (a) Certain viruses (e.g., chicken pox, herpes zoster), some **rickettsial diseases** (e.g., Rocky Mountain spotted fever), some **fungi,** and **stress** (e.g., physical exercise, acute hemorrhage or hemolysis, acute emotional stress) may also cause this response.
        (b) Other causes include **inflammatory diseases** (e.g., acute rheumatic fever, rheumatoid arthritis, acute gout), **hypersensitivity reactions to drugs, tissue necrosis** (e.g., from myocardial infarction, burns, certain cancers), **metabolic disorders** (e.g., uremia, diabetic ketoacidosis), **myelogenous leukemia,** and **use of certain drugs** (e.g., epinephrine, lithium).
      (3) Neutropenia, a decreased number of neutrophils, may occur with an **overwhelming infection of any type** (bone marrow is unable to keep up with the demand). It may also occur with **certain viral infections** (e.g., mumps, measles), with **idiosyncratic drug reactions,** and as a result of chemotherapy. Neutropenia is defined as an absolute neutrophil count (ANC) of less than 1000 cells/mm³. Some define absolute neutropenia as an ANC of less than 500 cells/mm³. The ANC is calculated by

Table 37-1. Normal Percentage Values for White Blood Cell (WBC) Differential

Cell Type	Normal Percentage Value
Polymorphonuclear leukocytes	50%–70%
Bands	3%–5%
Lymphocytes	20%–40%
Monocytes	0%–7%
Eosinophils	0%–5%
Basophils	0%–1%

Table 37-2. Examples of Changes in Total White Blood Cell (WBC) Count and WBC Differential in Response to Bacterial Infection

	WBC Count	
Cell Type	**Normal**	**With Bacterial Infection**
Total WBCs	8,000 (100%)	15,500 (100%)
Neutrophils		
Polymorphonuclear leukocytes	60%	82%
Bands	3%	6%
Lymphocytes	30%	10%
Monocytes	4%	1%
Eosinophils	2%	1%
Basophils	1%	0%

multiplying the percent of neutrophils by the total WBC count (e.g., WBC 4000/mm^3, neutrophils 60%; ANC = 4000 × 0.6 = 2400 cells/mm^3).

  b. Basophils stain deeply with blue basic dye. Their function in the circulation is not clearly understood; in the tissues, they are referred to as **mast cells.**

    (1) Basophilia, an increased number of basophils, may occur with chronic myelogenous leukemia (CML) as well as other conditions.

    (2) A decrease in basophils is generally not apparent because of the small numbers of these cells in the blood.

  c. Eosinophils stain deep red with acid dye and are classically associated with immune reactions. **Eosinophilia,** an increased number of eosinophils, may occur with such conditions as **acute allergic reactions** (e.g., **asthma, hay fever, drug allergy**) and **parasitic infestations** (e.g., trichinosis, amebiasis).

  d. Lymphocytes play a dominant role in immunological activity and appear to produce antibodies. They are classified as B lymphocytes or T lymphocytes; T lymphocytes are further divided into helper-inducer cells (T$_4$ cells) and suppressor cells (T$_8$ cells).

    (1) Lymphocytosis, an increased number of lymphocytes, usually accompanies a normal or decreased total WBC count and is most commonly caused by **viral infection.**

    (2) Lymphopenia, a decreased number of lymphocytes, may result from **severe debilitating illness, immunodeficiency,** or from **acquired immune deficiency syndrome (AIDS),** which has a propensity to attack T$_4$ cells.

    (3) Atypical lymphocytes (i.e., T lymphocytes in a state of immune activation) are classically associated with **infectious mononucleosis.**

  e. Monocytes are phagocytic cells. **Monocytosis,** an increased number of monocytes, may occur with **tuberculosis (TB), subacute bacterial endocarditis,** and during the recovery phase of some **acute infections.**

C. Platelets (thrombocytes). These are the smallest formed elements in the blood, and they are involved in **blood clotting** and vital to the formation of a hemostatic plug after vascular injury.

  1. Normal values for a platelet count are 150,000/mm^3–300,000/mm^3 (1.5–3.0 × 10^{11}/L).

  2. Thrombocytopenia, a decreased platelet count, can occur with a variety of conditions, such as idiopathic thrombocytopenic purpura or, occasionally, from such drugs as quinidine and sulfonamides.

    a. Thrombocytopenia is **moderate** when the platelet count is less than 100,000/mm^3.

    b. Thrombocytopenia is **severe** when the platelet count is less than 50,000/mm^3.

III. COMMON SERUM ENZYME TESTS. Small amounts of enzymes (catalysts) circulate in the blood at all times and are released into the blood in larger quantities when tissue damage occurs. Thus, serum enzyme levels can be used to **aid in the diagnosis of certain diseases.**

A. Creatine kinase (CK)

  1. CK, known formerly as creatine phosphokinase (CPK), is found primarily in heart muscle, skeletal muscle, and brain tissue.

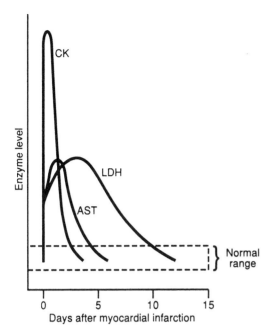

Figure 37-2. The graph shows the increase of serum creatine kinase (CK), lactate dehydrogenase (LDH), and aspartate aminotransferase (AST) levels after a myocardial infarction.

2. CK levels are used primarily to **aid in the diagnosis of acute myocardial** (Figure 37-2) **or skeletal muscle damage.** However, vigorous exercise, a fall, or deep intramuscular injections can cause significant increases in CK levels.

3. The **isoenzymes** of CK—**CK-MM,** found in skeletal muscle; **CK-BB,** found in brain tissue; and **CK-MB,** found in heart muscle—can be used to differentiate the source of damage.
   a. Normally, serum CK levels are virtually all the **CK-MM isoenzyme.**
   b. Increase in **CK-MB** levels provides a sensitive indicator of myocardial necrosis.

B. Lactate dehydrogenase (LDH)

1. LDH catalyzes the interconversion of lactate and pyruvate and represents a group of enzymes present in almost all metabolizing cells.

2. Five individual **isoenzymes** make up the total LDH serum level.
   a. **LDH$_1$** and **LDH$_2$** appear primarily in the heart.
   b. **LDH$_3$** appears primarily in the lungs.
   c. **LDH$_4$** and **LDH$_5$** appear primarily in the liver and skeletal muscles.

3. The distribution pattern of LDH isoenzymes may aid in diagnosing myocardial infarction, hepatic disease, and lung disease.

C. Alkaline phosphatase (ALP)

1. ALP is produced primarily in the **liver** and **bones.**

2. Serum ALP levels are **particularly sensitive to partial or mild biliary obstruction**—either extrahepatic (e.g., caused by a stone in the bile duct) or intrahepatic, both of which cause levels to increase.

3. **Increased osteoblastic activity,** as occurs in Paget's disease, hyperparathyroidism, osteomalacia, and others, also increases serum ALP levels.

D. Aspartate aminotransferase (AST)

1. AST, formerly known as **serum glutamic-oxaloacetic transaminase (SGOT),** is found in a number of organs, primarily in heart and liver tissues and, to a lesser extent, in skeletal muscle, kidney tissue, and pancreatic tissue.

2. Damage to the heart (e.g., from **myocardial infarction;** see Figure 37-2) results in increased AST levels about 8 hours after injury.

    a. Levels are **increased markedly** with **acute hepatitis;** they are **increased mildly** with **cirrhosis** and a **fatty liver.**

    b. Levels are also **increased** with **passive congestion of the liver** [as occurs in congestive heart failure (CHF)].

E. Alanine aminotransferase (ALT)

1. ALT, formerly known as **serum glutamic-pyruvic transaminase (SGPT),** is found in the liver, with lesser amounts in the heart, skeletal muscles, and kidney.

2. Although ALT values are **relatively specific for liver cell damage,** ALT is **less sensitive than AST,** and extensive or severe liver damage is necessary before abnormally increased levels are produced.

3. ALT also **increases less consistently and less markedly than AST** after an **acute myocardial infarction.**

F. Cardiac troponins (I, T, and C)

1. Troponins are a relatively new method to identify myocardial cell injury and thus assist in the diagnosis of acute myocardial infarction. These troponins may possess superior specificity in situations where false-positive elevations of CK-MB are likely.

2. Troponin T is found in cardiac and skeletal muscle, troponin I is found only in cardiac muscle, and troponin C is present in two isoforms found in skeletal and cardiac muscle. Troponin T has shown prognostic value in unstable angina and in detecting minor myocardial cell injury with greater sensitivity than CK-MB.

3. The normal value for troponin T is less than 0.1 ng/mL and I is less than 1.5 ng/mL.

IV. LIVER FUNCTION TESTS

A. Liver enzymes

1. Levels of certain enzymes (e.g., LDH, ALP, AST, ALT) **increase with liver dysfunction,** as discussed in III.

2. These **enzyme tests indicate only that the liver has been damaged.** They do not assess the liver's ability to function. Other tests provide indications of liver dysfunction.

B. Serum bilirubin

1. Bilirubin, a breakdown product of Hb, is the **predominant pigment in bile.** Effective bilirubin conjugation and excretion depend on **hepatobiliary function** and on the **rate of RBC turnover.**

2. Serum bilirubin levels are reported as **total bilirubin** (conjugated and unconjugated) and as **direct bilirubin** (conjugated only).

    a. Bilirubin is released by Hb breakdown and is bound to albumin as water-insoluble **indirect bilirubin** (unconjugated bilirubin), which is not filtered by the glomerulus.

    b. Unconjugated bilirubin travels to the liver, where it is separated from albumin, conjugated with diglucuronide, and then actively secreted into the bile as **conjugated bilirubin** (direct bilirubin), which is filtered by the glomerulus (Figure 37-3).

3. Normal values of total serum bilirubin are 0.1–1.0 mg/dl (2–18 mmol/L); of **direct bilirubin,** 0.0–0.2 mg/dl (0–4 mmol/L).

4. An increase in serum bilirubin results in **jaundice** from bilirubin deposition in the tissues. There are three major causes of increased serum bilirubin.

    a. Hemolysis increases total bilirubin; direct bilirubin (conjugated) is usually normal or slightly increased. Urine color is normal, and no bilirubin is found in the urine.

    b. Biliary obstruction, which may be intrahepatic (as with a chlorpromazine reaction) or extrahepatic (as with a biliary stone), increases total bilirubin and direct bilirubin; intrahepatic cholestasis (e.g., from chlorpromazine) may increase direct bilirubin as well. Urine color is dark, and bilirubin is present in the urine.

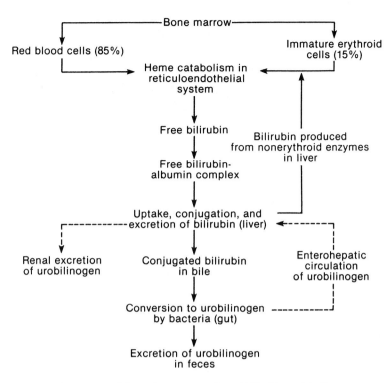

Figure 37-3. Schematic representation of bilirubin metabolism.

    c. Liver cell necrosis, as occurs in viral hepatitis, may cause an increase in both direct bilirubin (because inflammation causes some bile sinusoid blockage) and indirect bilirubin (because the liver's ability to conjugate is altered). Urine color is dark, and bilirubin is present in the urine.

C. Serum proteins

    1. Primary serum proteins measured are **albumin** and the **globulins** (i.e., alpha, beta, gamma).
        a. Albumin (4.0–6.0 g/dl) maintains serum oncotic pressure and serves as a transport agent. Because it is primarily manufactured by the liver, liver disease can decrease albumin levels.
        b. Globulins (23–35 g/L) function as transport agents and play a role in certain immunological mechanisms. A decrease in albumin levels usually results in a compensatory increase in globulin production.

    2. Normal values for total serum protein levels are 6.0–8.0 g/dl (60–80 g/L).

V. URINALYSIS. Standard urinalysis provides basic information regarding renal function, urinary tract disease, and the presence of certain systemic diseases. Components of a standard urinalysis include appearance, pH, specific gravity, protein level, glucose level, ketone level, and microscopic examination.

    A. Appearance. Normal urine is **clear** and ranges in color from **pale yellow to deep gold. Changes in color** can result from drugs, diet, or disease.

        1. A **red color** may indicate, among other things, the presence of blood or phenolphthalein (a laxative).

        2. A **brownish-yellow color** may indicate the presence of conjugated bilirubin.

        3. Other shades of red, orange, or brown may be caused by ingestion of various drugs (e.g., rifampin).

B. pH

1. **Normal pH** ranges from 4.5–9 but is typically **acidic** (around 6).

2. **Alkaline pH** may indicate such conditions as alkalosis, a *Proteus* infection, or acetazolamide use. It may also reflect changes caused by leaving the urine sample at room temperature.

C. Specific gravity

1. **Normal range** for specific gravity is 1.003–1.035; it is usually between 1.010 and 1.025.

2. Specific gravity is influenced by the number and nature of solute particles in the urine.
   a. **Increased specific gravity** may occur with such conditions as diabetes mellitus (DM; excess glucose in the urine) or nephrosis (excess protein in the urine).
   b. **Decreased specific gravity** may occur with diabetes insipidus, which decreases urine concentration.
   c. **Specific gravity, fixed at 1.010** (the same as plasma), occurs when the kidneys lose their power to concentrate or dilute.

D. Protein

1. **Normal values** for urine protein are 50–80 mg/24 hr, as the glomerular membrane prevents most protein molecules in the blood from entering the urine.

2. **Proteinuria** occurs with many conditions (e.g., renal disease, bladder infection, venous congestion, fever).
   a. The presence of a **specific protein** can help to identify a specific disease state (e.g., Bence Jones protein may indicate multiple myeloma).
   b. Most often, the protein in urine is **albumin.** Albuminuria may indicate abnormal glomerular permeability.

E. Glucose

1. The normal **renal threshold** for glucose is a blood glucose level of about 180 mg/dl; **glucose does not normally appear in urine** as detected by popular testing methods.

2. **Glycosuria** usually indicates diabetes mellitus. There are certain less common causes (e.g., a lowered renal threshold for glucose).

F. Ketones

1. Ketones **do not normally appear in urine.** They are excreted when the body has used available glucose stores and begins to metabolize fat stores.

2. The **three ketone bodies** are **betahydroxybutyric acid** (80%), **acetoacetic acid** (about 20%), and acetone (a small percentage). Some commercial tests (e.g., Ames products) measure only acetoacetic acid, but usually all three are excreted in parallel proportions.

3. **Ketonuria** usually indicates uncontrolled DM, but it may also occur with starvation and with zero- or low-carbohydrate diets.

G. Evaluation. Microscopic examination of centrifuged urine sediment normally reveals 0–1 RBC, 0–4 WBCs, and only an occasional cast per high-power field (HPF).

1. **Hematuria** (i.e., the presence of RBCs) may indicate such conditions as trauma, a tumor, or a systemic bleeding disorder. In women, a significant number of **squamous cells** suggests vaginal contamination (menstruation).

2. **Casts** (i.e., protein conglomerations outlining the shape of the renal tubules in which they were formed) may or may not be significant. Excessive numbers of certain types of casts indicate renal disease.

3. **Crystals,** which are pH dependent, may occur normally in acid or alkaline urine. **Uric acid crystals** may form in acid urine; **phosphate crystals** may form in alkaline urine.

4. **Bacteria** do not normally appear in urine. The finding of 50 or more bacteria per HPF may indicate a urinary tract infection (UTI); smaller values may indicate urethral contamination.

VI. COMMON RENAL FUNCTION TESTS

A. Introduction

1. Renal function may be assessed by measuring **blood urea nitrogen (BUN)** and **serum creatinine.** Renal function decreases with age, which must be taken into account when interpreting test values.
   a. These tests primarily evaluate glomerular function by assessing the **glomerular filtration rate (GFR).**
   b. In many **renal diseases,** urea and creatinine accumulate in the blood because they are not excreted properly.
   c. These tests also aid in determining **drug dosage** for drugs excreted through the kidneys.

2. **Azotemia** describes excessive retention of nitrogenous waste products (BUN and creatinine) in the blood. The clinical syndrome resulting from decreased renal function and azotemia is called **uremia.**
   a. **Renal azotemia** results from renal disease, such as glomerulonephritis and chronic pyelonephritis.
   b. **Prerenal azotemia** results from such conditions as severe dehydration, hemorrhagic shock, and excessive protein intake.
   c. **Postrenal azotemia** results from such conditions as ureteral or urethral stones or tumors and prostatic obstructions.

3. **Clearance**—a theoretical concept defined as the volume of plasma from which a measured amount of substance can be completely eliminated, or cleared, into the urine per unit time—can be used to estimate glomerular function.

B. BUN

1. **Urea,** an end product of protein metabolism, is produced in the liver. From there, it travels through the blood and is excreted by the kidneys. Urea is **filtered at the glomerulus,** where the tubules reabsorb approximately 40%. Thus, under normal conditions, **urea clearance** is about 60% of the true GFR.

2. **Normal values for BUN** range from 8 mg/dl to 18 mg/dl (3–6.5 mmol/L).
   a. **Decreased BUN levels** occur with **significant liver disease.**
   b. **Increased BUN levels** may indicate **renal disease.** However, factors other than glomerular function [e.g., protein intake, reduced renal blood flow, blood in the gastrointestinal (GI) tract] readily affect BUN levels, sometimes making interpretation of results difficult.

C. Serum creatinine

1. Creatinine, the metabolic breakdown product of muscle creatine phosphate, has a relatively constant level of daily production. Blood levels vary little in a given individual.

2. Creatinine is **excreted** by glomerular filtration and tubular secretion. **Creatinine clearance** parallels the GFR within a range of ±10% and is a **more sensitive indicator of renal damage than BUN levels** because renal impairment is almost the only cause of an increase in the serum creatinine level.

3. **Normal values for serum creatinine** range from 0.6–1.2 mg/dl (50–110 mmol/L).
   a. Values vary with the **amount of muscle mass**—a value of 1.2 mg/dl in a muscular athlete may represent normal renal function, whereas the same value in a small, sedentary person with little muscle mass may indicate significant renal impairment.
   b. Generally, the **serum creatinine value doubles with each 50% decrease in GFR.** For example, if a patient's normal serum creatinine is 1 mg/dl, 1 mg/dl represents 100% renal function, 2 mg/dl represents 50% function, and 4 mg/dl represents 25% function.

D. Creatinine clearance

1. Creatinine clearance, which represents the **rate at which creatinine is removed from the blood by the kidneys,** roughly approximates the GFR.
   a. The value is given in units of milliliters per minute, representing the volume of blood cleared of creatinine by the kidney per minute.
   b. **Normal values** for men range from 75 mL/min to 125 mL/min.

2. Calculation requires knowledge of **urinary creatinine excretion** (usually over 24 hours) and concurrent **serum creatinine levels. Creatinine clearance is calculated** as follows:

$$Cl_{CR} = \frac{C_U V}{C_{CR}}$$

Here, Cl_{CR} is the creatinine clearance in milliliters per minute, C_u is the concentration of creatinine in the urine, V is the urine volume (in milliliters per minute of urine formed over the collection period), and C_{CR} is the serum creatinine concentration.

3. Suppose the serum creatinine concentration is 1 mg/dl, and 1440 mL of urine were collected in 24 hours (1440 min) for a urine volume of 1 mL/min. The urine contains 100 mg/dl of creatinine. Creatinine clearance is calculated as:

$$\frac{100 \text{ mg/dl} \times 1 \text{ mL/min}}{1 \text{ mg/dl}} = 100 \text{ mL/min}$$

4. Incomplete bladder emptying and other problems may interfere with obtaining an accurate timed urine specimen. Thus, **estimations of creatinine clearance** may be necessary. These estimations require only a serum creatinine value. One estimation uses the method of **Cockroft and Gault,** which is based on body weight, age, and gender.

   a. This formula provides an **estimated value,** calculated for **males** as:

$$Cl_{CR} = \frac{(140 - \text{age in years}) \, (\text{body weight in kg})}{72(C_{CR} \text{ in mg/dl})}$$

   Again, Cl_{CR} is the creatinine clearance in milliliters per minute, and C_{CR} is the serum creatinine concentration.

   b. For **females,** use 0.85 of the value calculated for males.

   c. **Example:** A 20-year-old man weighing 72 kg has a $C_{CR} = 1.0$ mg/dl; thus,

$$C_{CR} = \frac{(140 - 20)(72)}{72(1)}$$

$$C_{CR} = 120 \text{ mL/min}$$

VII. ELECTROLYTES

A. Sodium (Na)

1. Na is the major cation of the **extracellular** fluid. Na along with chloride (Cl), potassium (K), and water is important in the regulation of osmotic pressure and water balance between intracellular and extracellular fluids. **Normal values** are 135–147 mEq/L or mmol/L.

2. The Na concentration is defined as the ratio of Na to water, not the absolute amounts of either. Laboratory tests for Na are used mainly to detect disturbances in water balance and body osmolality. The kidneys are major organs of Na and water balance.

3. An increase in Na concentration **(hypernatremia)** may indicate impaired Na excretion or dehydration. A decrease in Na concentration (hyponatremia) may reflect overhydration, abnormal Na loss, or decreased Na intake.

4. Patients with kidney, heart, or pulmonary disease may have difficulty with Na and water balance. In adults, changes in Na concentrations most often reflect changes in water balance, not salt imbalances. Therefore, Na concentration is often used as an indicator of fluid status, rather than salt imbalance.

5. Control of Na by the body is accomplished mainly through the hormones antidiuretic hormone (ADH) and aldosterone. ADH is released from the pituitary in response to signals from the hypothalamus. ADH's presence in the distal tubules and collecting ducts of the kidney causes them to become more permeable to the reabsorption of water, therefore concentrating urine. Aldosterone affects the distal tubular reabsorption of Na as opposed to water. Aldosterone is released from the adrenal cortex in response to low Na, high K, low blood volume, and angiotensin II. Aldosterone causes the spilling of K from the distal tubules into the urine in exchange for Na reabsorption.

6. **Hyponatremia** is usually related to total body depletion of Na (mineralocorticoid deficiencies, Na-wasting renal disease, replacement of fluid loss with nonsaline solutions, GI losses, renal losses, or loss of Na through the skin) or dilution of serum Na [cirrhosis, CHF, nephrosis, renal failure, excess water intake, or syndrome of inappropriate diuretic hormone (SIADH) release].

7. **Hypernatremia** usually results from a loss of free water, or hypotonic fluid or through excessive Na intake. Free water loss is most often associated with diabetes insipidus, but fluid loss can be via the GI tract, renal, skin, or respiratory systems. Excess Na intake can occur through the administration of hypertonic intravenous (IV) solutions, mineralocorticoid excess, excessive Na ingestion, or after administration of drugs high in Na content [e.g., ticarcillin, Na bicarbonate (HCO_3^-)].

B. Potassium

1. Potassium (K) is the most abundant **intracellular** cation (intracellular fluid K averages 141 mEq/L). Approximately 3500 mEq of K are contained in the body of a 70-kg adult. Only 10% of the body's K is extracellular. Normal values are 3.5–5.0 mEq/L or mmol/L.

2. The serum K concentration is not an adequate measure of the total body K because most of the body's K is intracellular. Fortunately, the clinical signs/symptoms of K deficiency [malaise, confusion, dizziness, electrocardiogram (ECG) changes, muscle weakness, and pain] correlate well with serum concentrations. The serum K concentration is buffered by the body and may be "normal" despite total body K loss. K depletion causes a shift of intracellular K to the extracellular fluid to maintain K concentrations. There is approximately a 100 mEq total body K deficit when the serum K concentration decreases by 0.3 mEq/L. This may result in misinterpretation of serum K concentrations as they relate to total body K.

3. The role/function of K is in the maintenance of proper electrical conduction in cardiac and skeletal muscles (muscle and nerve excitability), it exerts an influence on the body's water balance (intracellular volume) and plays a role in acid–base equilibrium.

4. K is regulated by:
   a. Kidneys (renal function)
   b. Aldosterone
   c. Arterial pH
   d. Insulin
   e. K intake
   f. Na delivery to distal tubule

5. **Hypokalemia** can occur. The kidneys are responsible for approximately 90% of the daily K loss. Other losses occur mainly through the GI system. Even in states of no K intake, the kidneys still excrete up to 20 mEq of K daily. Therefore, prolonged periods of K deprivation can result in hypokalemia. Hypokalemia can also result from K loss through vomiting or diarrhea, nasogastric suction, laxative abuse, and by diuretic use (mannitol, thiazides, or loop diuretics). Excessive mineralocorticoid activity and glucosuria can also result in hypokalemia. K can be shifted into cells with alkalemia and after administration of glucose and insulin.

6. **Hyperkalemia** most commonly results from decreased renal elimination, excessive intake, or from cellular breakdown (tissue damage, hemolysis, burns, infections). Metabolic acidosis may also result in a shift of K extracellularly as hydrogen ions move into cells and are exchanged for K and Na ions. As a general guideline, for every 0.1 unit pH change from 7.4, the K concentration will change by about 0.6 mEq/L. If a patient has a pH of 7.1 and a measured K of 4.5 mEq/L, the actual K concentration would be [(0.3 units less than 7.4) × 0.6 = 1.8; 4.5 − 1.8 = 2.7 mEq/L K concentration]. Correction of the acidosis in this situation will result in a dramatic decrease in K unless supplementation is instituted.

C. Chloride (Cl)

1. Cl is the major anion of the extracellular fluid and is important in the maintenance of acid–base balance. Alterations in the serum Cl concentration are rarely a primary indicator of major medical problems. Cl itself is not of primary diagnostic significance. It is usually measured to confirm the serum Na concentration. The relationship among Na, Cl, and bicarbonate (HCO_3^-) is described by the following: $Cl^- + HCO_3^- + R = Na^+$, where R is the anion gap. The **normal value** for Cl is 95–105 mEq/L or mmol/L.

2. **Hypochloremia** is a decreased Cl concentration, and it is often accompanied by metabolic alkalosis or acidosis caused by organic or other acids. Other causes include chronic renal failure, adrenal insufficiency, fasting, prolonged diarrhea, severe vomiting, and diuretic therapy.

3. **Hyperchloremia** is an increased Cl concentration that may be indicative of hyperchloremic metabolic acidosis. Hyperchloremia in the absence of metabolic acidosis is unusual because Cl retention is often accompanied by Na and water retention. Other causes include acute renal failure, dehydration, and excess Cl administration.

D. Bicarbonate/carbon dioxide content

1. The carbon dioxide (CO_2) content represents the sum of the bicarbonate (HCO_3^-) concentration and the concentration of CO_2 dissolved in the serum. The HCO_3^-/CO_2 system is the most important buffering system to maintain pH within physiological limits. Most disturbances of acid–base balance can be considered in terms of this system. Normal values are 22–28 mEq/L or mmol/L.

2. The relationship among this system is defined as follows: $HCO_3^- + H^+ \times H_2CO_3 \times H_2O + CO_2$ (bicarbonate ions bind hydrogen ions to form carbonic acid). Clinically, the serum HCO_3^- concentration is measured because acid–base balance can be inferred if the patient has normal pulmonary function.

3. **Hypobicarbonatemia** is usually caused by metabolic acidosis, renal failure, hyperventilation, severe diarrhea, drainage of intestinal fluid, and by drugs such as acetazolamide. Toxicity caused by salicylates, methanol, and ethylene glycol can also decrease the HCO_3^- level.

4. **Hyperbicarbonatemia** is usually caused by alkalosis, hypoventilation, pulmonary disease, persistent vomiting, excess HCO_3^- intake with poor renal function, and diuretics.

VIII. MINERALS

A. Calcium (Ca)

1. Ca plays an important role in nerve impulse transmission, muscle contraction, pancreatic insulin release, hydrogen ion release from the stomach, as a cofactor for some enzyme reactions and blood coagulation, and most importantly bone and tooth structural integrity. Normal values are: total Ca 8.8–10.3 mg/dl or 2.20–2.56 mmol/L.

2. The total Ca content of normal adults is 20–25 g/kg of fat-free tissue, and about 44% of this Ca is in the body skeleton. Approximately 1% of skeletal Ca is freely exchangeable with that of the extracellular fluid. The reservoir of Ca in bones maintains the concentration of Ca in the plasma constant. About 40% of the Ca in the extracellular fluid is bound to plasma proteins (especially albumin), 5%–15% is complexed with phosphate and citrate, and about 45%–55% is in the unbound, ionized form. Most laboratories measure the total Ca concentration; however, it is the free, ionized Ca that is important physiologically. Ionized Ca levels may be obtained from the laboratory. Clinically, the most important determinant of ionized Ca is the amount of serum protein (albumin) available for binding. The normal serum Ca range is for a serum albumin of 4 g/dl. A good approximation is that for every 1 g/dl decrease in albumin, 0.8 g/dl should be added to the Ca lab result. Doing this corrects the total plasma concentration to reflect the additional amount of free (active) Ca.

3. **Hypocalcemia** usually implies a deficiency in either the production or response to parathyroid hormone (PTH) or vitamin D. PTH abnormalities include hypoparathyroidism, pseudohypoparathyroidism, or hypomagnesemia. Vitamin D abnormalities can be caused by decreased nutritional intake, decreased absorption of vitamin D, a decrease in production, or an increase in metabolism. Administration of loop diuretics causing diuresis can also decrease serum Ca.

4. **Hypercalcemia** is an increased Ca concentration, and it is usually associated with malignancy or metastatic diseases. Other causes include hyperparathyroidism, Paget's disease, milk-alkali syndrome, granulomatous disorders, thiazide diuretics, excessive Ca intake, or vitamin D intoxication.

B. Phosphate (PO_4)

1. PO_4 is a major intracellular anion and is the source of phosphate for adenosine triphosphate (ATP) and phospholipid synthesis. Serum Ca and PO_4 are influenced by many of the same factors. It is useful to consider Ca and PO_4 together when interpreting lab results. Normal PO_4 values are 2.5–5.0 mg/dl or 0.80–1.60 mmol/L.

2. **Hyperphosphatemia** and **hypophosphatemia** can occur. The extracellular fluid concentration of phosphate is influenced by PTH, intestinal absorption, renal function, nutrition, and bone metabolism. Hyperphosphatemia is usually caused by renal insufficiency, although increased vitamin D or phosphate intake, hypoparathyroidism, and hyperthyroidism are also causes. Hypophosphatemia can occur in malnutrition, especially when anabolism is induced, after administration of aluminum-containing antacids or Ca acetate, in chronic alcoholics, and in septic patients. Hyperparathyroidism and insufficient vitamin D intake can also induce hypophosphatemia.

C. Magnesium (Mg)

1. Mg is the second most abundant intracellular and extracellular cation. It is an activator of numerous enzyme systems that control carbohydrate, fat and electrolyte metabolism, protein synthesis, nerve conduction, muscular contractility, as well as membrane transport and integrity. Normal values are 1.6–2.4 mEq/L or 0.80–1.20 mmol/L.

2. **Hypomagnesemia** and **hypermagnesemia** can occur. **Hypomagnesemia** is found more often than hypermagnesemia. Depletion of Mg usually results from excessive loss from the GI tract or the kidneys. Depletion can occur from either poor intestinal absorption or excessive GI fluid loss. Signs and symptoms include weakness, muscle fasciculations with tremor, tetany, and increased reflexes. Decreased intracardiac Mg may manifest as an increased QT interval with an increased risk of arrhythmia. **Hypermagnesemia** is most commonly caused by increased Mg intake in the setting of renal insufficiency. Other causes include excess Mg intake, hepatitis, and Addison's disease. Signs and symptoms of hypermagnesemia include bradycardia, flushing, sweating, nausea and vomiting, decreased Ca level, decreased deep-tendon reflexes, flaccid paralysis, increased pulse rate and QRS intervals, respiratory distress, and asystole.

STUDY QUESTIONS

Directions: Each of the numbered items or incomplete statements in this section is followed by answers or by completions of the statement. Select the **one** lettered answer or completion that is **best** in each case.

1. Hematological testing of a patient with acquired immune deficiency syndrome (AIDS) is most likely to show which of the following abnormalities?

(A) Basophilia
(B) Eosinophilia
(C) Lymphopenia
(D) Reticulocytosis
(E) Agranulocytosis

2. Hematological studies are most likely to show a low reticulocyte count in a patient who has which one of the following abnormalities?

(A) Aplastic anemia secondary to cancer chemotherapy
(B) Acute hemolytic anemia secondary to quinidine treatment
(C) Severe bleeding secondary to an automobile accident
(D) Iron-deficiency anemia 1 week after treatment with ferrous sulfate
(E) Megaloblastic anemia due to folate deficiency 1 week after treatment with folic acid

3. All of the following findings on a routine urinalysis would be considered normal EXCEPT

(A) pH: 6.5
(B) glucose: negative
(C) ketones: negative
(D) WBC: 3 per high-power field (HPF), no casts
(E) RBC: 5 per HPF

4. A 12-year-old boy is treated for otitis media with cefaclor (Ceclor). On the seventh day of therapy, he "spikes" a fever and develops an urticarial rash on his trunk. Which of the following laboratory tests could best confirm the physician's suspicion of a hypersensitivity (allergic) reaction?

(A) Complete blood count (CBC) and differential
(B) Serum hemoglobin (Hb) and reticulocyte count
(C) Liver function test profile
(D) Lactate dehydrogenase (LDH) isoenzyme profile
(E) Red blood cell (RBC) count and serum bilirubin

5. An increased hematocrit (Hct) is a likely finding in all of the following individuals EXCEPT

(A) a man who has just returned from a 3-week skiing trip in the Colorado Rockies
(B) a woman who has polycythemia vera
(C) a hospitalized patient who mistakenly received 5 L of intravenous (IV) dextrose 5% in water (D_5W) over the last 24 hours
(D) a man who has been rescued from the Arizona desert after spending 4 days without water
(E) a woman who has chronic obstructive pulmonary disease

6. A 29-year-old white man is seen in the emergency room. His white blood cell (WBC) count is 14,200 with 80% "polys." All of the following conditions could normally produce these laboratory findings EXCEPT

(A) a localized bacterial infection on the tip of the index finger
(B) acute bacterial pneumonia caused by *Streptococcus pneumoniae*
(C) a heart attack
(D) a gunshot wound to the abdomen with a loss of 2 pints of blood
(E) an attack of gout

7. A 52-year-old male construction worker who drinks "fairly heavily" when he gets off work is seen in the emergency room with, among other abnormal laboratory results, an increased creatine kinase (CK) level. All of the following circumstances could explain this increase EXCEPT

(A) he fell against the bumper of his car in a drunken stupor and bruised his right side
(B) he is showing evidence of some liver damage due to the heavy alcohol intake
(C) he has experienced a heart attack
(D) he received an intramuscular (IM) injection a few hours before the blood sample was drawn
(E) he pulled a muscle that day when lifting a heavy concrete slab

8. A 45-year-old man with jaundice has spillage of bilirubin into his urine. All of the following statements could apply to this patient EXCEPT

(A) his total bilirubin is increased
(B) his direct bilirubin is increased
(C) he may have viral hepatitis
(D) he may have hemolytic anemia
(E) he may have cholestatic hepatitis

Questions 9–11

A 70-year-old black man weighing 154 lb complains of chronic fatigue. Several laboratory tests were performed with the following results:

Blood urea nitrogen (BUN): 15 mg/dl
Aspartate aminotransferase (AST): within normal
    limits
White blood cell (WBC) count: 7500/mm³
Red blood cell (RBC) count: 4.0 million/mm³
Hematocrit (Hct): 29%
Hemoglobin (Hb): 9.0 g/dl

9. This patient's mean cell hemoglobin (Hb) concentration (MCHC) is

(A) 27.5
(B) 28.9
(C) 31.0
(D) 33.5
(E) 35.4

10. His mean cell volume (MCV) is

(A) 61.3
(B) 72.5
(C) 77.5
(D) 90.2
(E) 93.5

11. From the data provided above and from the calculations in questions 9 and 10, this patient is best described as

(A) normal except for a slightly increased blood urea nitrogen (BUN)
(B) having normochromic, microcytic anemia
(C) having sickle-cell anemia
(D) having hypochromic, normocytic anemia
(E) having folic acid deficiency

12. All of the following statements about sodium (Na) are true EXCEPT

(A) the normal range for Na is 135–147 mEq/L
(B) Na is the major cation of the extracellular fluid, and the laboratory test is used mainly to detect disturbances in water balance
(C) hyponatremia usually results from the total body depletion of Na or through a dilutional effect
(D) control of the Na concentration is mainly through regulation of arterial pH

13. A 53-year-old woman with diabetes mellitus is seen in the emergency room. Her blood glucose is 673 mg/dl and ketones are present in her blood. A diagnosis of diabetic ketoacidosis (DKA) is made. Other important laboratory values are: potassium (K) 4.8 mEq/L, 4+ glucose in urine, and an arterial pH of 7.1. All of the following statements apply to this patient EXCEPT

(A) her K value is normal; therefore, no K supplementation is likely to be necessary
(B) her K value should be corrected due to her acidosis; a corrected K would be 3.0 mEq/L
(C) K supplementation should be instituted because her total body K is depleted
(D) factors affecting K in this patient include glycosuria and arterial pH

14. A 50-year-old man presents with bicarbonate of 18 mEq/L. All of the following could be a cause of his low bicarbonate level EXCEPT

(A) metabolic acidosis
(B) salicylate toxicity
(C) diuretic therapy
(D) diarrhea

15. All of the following statements about calcium (Ca) and phosphorus (PO_4) are true EXCEPT

(A) an alcoholic with a serum albumin of 2 g/dl and a serum total Ca of 8.0 mg/dl has a corrected total Ca of 9.6 mg/dl
(B) Ca and PO_4 levels should be interpreted together because many of the same factors influence both minerals
(C) metastatic cancer often induces a decrease in serum Ca levels
(D) a patient with renal failure may present with hypocalcemia and hyperphosphatemia

16. All of the following are important functions of magnesium (Mg) EXCEPT

(A) nerve conduction
(B) phospholipid synthesis
(C) muscle contractility
(D) carbohydrate, fat, and electrolyte metabolism

Directions: Each item below contains three suggested answers, of which **one or more** is correct. Choose the answer

A	if **I only** is correct
B	if **III only** is correct
C	if **I and II** are correct
D	if **II and III** are correct
E	if **I, II, and III** are correct

17. Factors likely to cause an increase in the blood urea nitrogen (BUN) level include

I. intramuscular (IM) injection of diazepam (Valium)
II. severe liver disease
III. chronic kidney disease

18. A patient who undergoes serum enzyme testing is found to have an increased aspartate aminotransferase (AST) level. Possible underlying causes of this abnormality include

I. methyldopa-induced hepatitis
II. congestive heart failure (CHF)
III. pneumonia

19. Serum enzyme tests that may aid in the diagnosis of myocardial infarction include

I. alkaline phosphatase
II. creatine kinase (CK)
III. lactate dehydrogenase (LDH)

ANSWERS AND EXPLANATIONS

1. The answer is C *[II B 2 d (2)]*.
Valuable diagnostic information can be obtained through quantitative and qualitative testing of the cells of the blood. A finding of lymphopenia (i.e., decreased number of lymphocytes) suggests an attack on the immune system or some underlying immunodeficiency. Acquired immune deficiency syndrome (AIDS) attacks the T_4 population of lymphocytes and thus may result in lymphopenia.

2. The answer is A *[II A 5]*.
The reticulocyte count measures the amount of circulating immature red blood cells (RBCs), which provides information about bone marrow function. A low reticulocyte count is a likely finding in a patient with aplastic anemia—a disorder characterized by a deficiency of all cellular elements of the blood due to a lack of hematopoietic stem cells in bone marrow. A variety of drugs (e.g., those used in anticancer therapy) and other agents produce marrow aplasia. A high reticulocyte count would likely be found in a patient with hemolytic anemia or acute blood loss or in a patient who has been treated for an iron, vitamin B_{12}, or folate deficiency.

3. The answer is E *[V B, E–G]*.
Microscopic examination of the urine sediment normally shows fewer than 1 red blood cell (RBC) and from 0–4 white blood cells (WBCs) per high-power field (HPF). Other normal findings on urinalysis include an acid pH (i.e., around 6) and an absence of glucose and ketones.

4. The answer is A *[II B 2 c]*.
An allergic drug reaction will usually produce an increase in the eosinophil count (eosinophilia). This could be determined by ordering a white blood cell (WBC) differential.

5. The answer is C *[II A 2]*.
Overhydration with an excess infusion of dextrose 5% in water (D5W) produces a low hematocrit (Hct). The other situations described in the question result in increases of the Hct.

6. The answer is A *[II B 2 a]*.
The patient has leukocytosis with an increased neutrophil count (neutrophilia). A localized infection does not normally result in an increase in the total leukocyte count or neutrophil count. The other situations given in the question can produce a neutrophilic leukocytosis.

7. The answer is B *[III A]*.
Because creatine kinase (CK) is not present in the liver, alcoholic liver damage would not result in an increase in the level of this enzyme. CK is present primarily in cardiac and skeletal muscle. The other situations described in the question could all result in the release of increased amounts of CK into the bloodstream.

8. The answer is D *[IV B]*.
The patient with jaundice (deposition of bilirubin in the skin) usually has an increase in the total bilirubin serum level. Spillage of bilirubin into the urine requires an increased level of direct bilirubin, which is likely with viral hepatitis or cholestatic hepatitis. In hemolytic anemia, direct bilirubin is not usually increased, and therefore, there would be no spillage of bilirubin into the urine.

9–11. The answers are: 9-C *[II A 4 c]*, **10-B** *[II A 4 a]*, **11-B** *[II A 4; VI B 2]*.
The mean cell hemoglobin (Hb) concentration (MCHC) is calculated as follows:

$$MCHC = \frac{Hemoglobin\ (Hb) \times 100}{Hematocrit\ (Hct)} = \frac{9 \times 100}{29} = 31.0$$

The mean cell volume (MCV) is calculated as follows:

$$MCV = \frac{Hct\ (\%) \times 10}{RBC\ count\ (in\ millions)} = \frac{29 \times 10}{4} = 72.5$$

The patient described in the question is anemic because his Hb is 9 (normal: 14–18). The anemia is normochromic because the patient's MCHC of 31 is normal (normal range: 31–37), but the anemia is microcytic because the patient's MCV is 72.5 (normal: 80–100). The patient's blood urea nitrogen (BUN), 15 mg/dl, is within the normal range of 10–20 mg/dl.

12. The answer is D *[VII A 1, 5, 6, 7]*.
Sodium (Na), the major extracellular cation, is measured mainly to assist in the determination of fluid status/water balance. Regulation of Na is mainly through the kidneys via antidiuretic hormone (ADH) and aldosterone.

13. The answer is A *[VII B 2, 4, 6]*.
A "normal" potassium (K) level in the setting of metabolic acidosis, especially in a patient with diabetic ketoacidosis (DKA) should be treated appropriately. If the serum K level is corrected for the patient's acidosis, the corrected level is 3.0 mEq/L. This corresponds to a depletion in total body K stores. Once the acidosis and hyperglycemia begin to correct with appropriate treatment, K levels will decrease precipitously unless supplementation is begun. It is important to recognize that a laboratory value in the "normal" range may not actually be normal, especially when K is involved.

14. The answer is C *[VII D 3, 4]*.
Low bicarbonate (HCO_3^-) is usually found in patients with acidosis or renal failure and after hyperventilation or severe diarrhea. In general, disturbances in acid–base balance cause alteration in the serum HCO_3^- or carbon dioxide (CO_2) content. Diuretic therapy can cause an alkalosis and an increase in HCO_3^-.

15. The answer is C *[VIII A 2–4; B 2]*.
Malignancy or other metastatic diseases are most often associated with hypercalcemia, not hypocalcemia. Ionized calcium (Ca) is the free active form, and this level is increased in the setting of a low albumin. Therefore, the total Ca level must be adjusted to account for an increased ionized Ca in this setting. Both minerals are influenced by many of the same factors and thus are often interpreted together. Renal function is one such factor whereby a decrease in renal function (i.e., renal failure) can result in a low level of Ca and a high level of phosphorus (PO_4).

16. The answer is B *[VIII C 1]*.
Magnesium (Mg) is the second most abundant intracellular and extracellular cation. It is an activator of numerous enzyme systems that control carbohydrate, fat, and electrolyte metabolism, protein synthesis, nerve conduction, muscular contractility, as well as membrane transport and integrity. Phosphorus (PO_4), on the other hand, is important for adenosine triphosphate (ATP) and phospholipid synthesis.

17. The answer is B (III) *[VI B 2]*.
Chronic kidney disease can cause an increase in the blood urea nitrogen (BUN) level; a heavy protein diet and bleeding into the gastrointestinal (GI) tract are other factors that can produce this finding. Severe liver disease can prevent the formation of urea and, therefore, is likely to cause a decrease in the BUN level. Although an intramuscular (IM) injection of diazepam (Valium) may cause an increase in the serum creatine kinase (CK) or aspartate aminotransferase (AST) level, it would have no effect on the BUN.

18. The answer is C (I, II) *[III D]*.
A lung infection, such as pneumonia, normally would not cause an increase in the release of aspartate aminotransferase (AST), an enzyme primarily found in the liver and heart. In acute hepatitis, a marked increase of AST is a likely finding. AST levels also can be increased with passive congestion of the liver, as occurs in congestive heart failure (CHF).

19. The answer is D (II, III) *[III A–C]*.
Usually, the creatine kinase (CK), alanine aminotransferase (ALT), aspartate aminotransferase (AST), and lactate dehydrogenase (LDH) enzyme levels are increased after a myocardial infarction. Alkaline phosphatase is not present in cardiac tissue and, therefore, would not be useful in the diagnosis of a myocardial infarction.

38
Coronary Artery Disease

Alan H. Mutnick
Barbara Szymusiak-Mutnick

I. INTRODUCTION

A. Definition. Coronary artery disease (CAD) is a general term, which refers to a number of diseases other than atherosclerosis causing a narrowing of the major epicardial coronary arteries. **Ischemic heart disease (IHD)** is a form of heart disease with primary manifestations that result from myocardial ischemia due to atherosclerotic CAD. This term encompasses a spectrum of conditions, ranging from the asymptomatic preclinical phase to acute myocardial infarction and sudden cardiac death, and will be used throughout this chapter.

B. Incidence. IHD continues to be the leading single cause of death in the United States (231.1–297.9 deaths per 100,000) as compared to cancer, the second leading cause of death (159.1–228.1 deaths per 100,000).

1. IHD is responsible for 1 out of every 4.8 deaths in the United States, today.

2. Each year in the U.S., more than 1 million patients suffer an acute myocardial infarction (MI)

C. Economics. Based on models evaluating the costs associated with the treatment of Medicare patients with common IHD-related diagnosis, it has been estimated that the direct costs of hospitalization are more than $15 billion yearly, with an additional $4.5 billion yearly in diagnostic procedures.

D. Clinical guidelines. Due to the clinical, humanistic, and economic impact, which IDH has in the U.S., evidenced-based practice guidelines have evolved based on the differences in the diagnosis and management of IHD. The current chapter has relied very heavily on the use of these guidelines to assure the most up-to-date recommendations, based on the clinical literature. Guidelines developed, which are pertinent to daily pharmacy practice, include the following:

1. ACC/AHA 2002 Guideline Update for the Management of Patients with Chronic Stable Angina: a report of the American College of Cardiology/American Heart Association Task Force on Practice Guidelines (Committee to Update the 1999 Guidelines for the Management of Patients with Chronic Stable Angina). 2002. Available at http://www.acc.org/clinical/guidelines/stable/stable.pdf. Gibbons RJ, Abrams J, Chatterjee K, Daley J, Deedwania PC, Douglas JS, Ferguson TB Jr, Fihn SD, Fraker TD Jr, Gardin JM, O'Rourke RA, Pasternak RC, Williams SV.

2. ACC/AHA 2002 Guideline Update for the Management of Patients with Unstable Angina and Non-ST-Segment Elevation Myocardial Infarction: a report of the American College of Cardiology/American Heart Association Task Force on Practice Guidelines (Committee on the Management of Patients with Unstable Angina). 2002. Available at: http://www.acc.org/clinical/guidelines/unstable/unstable.pdg.

3. ACC/AHA/NHLBI Advisory on the Use and Safety of Statins: Pasternak RC, Smith SC Jr, Bairey-Merz CN, Grundy SM, Cleeman JI, Lenfant C. *J Am Coll Cardiol* 2002;40:567–572. Available at: American College of Cardiology: www.acc.org; American Heart Association: www.americanheart.org and the NHLBI: www.nhlbi.nih.gov/guidelines/ cholesterol.

4. AHA/ACC Guidelines for Preventing Heart Attack and Death in Patients with Atherosclerotic Cardiovascular Disease: 2001 Update: A statement for healthcare professionals from the American Heart Association and the American College of Cardiology. *Circulation.* 2001;104:1577–1579. Available at website: http://www.circulationaha.org.

5. Third Report of the National Cholesterol Education Program (NCEP): Detection, Evaluation, and Treatment of High Blood Cholesterol in Adults (Adult Treatment Panel III). Grundy

SM, Becker D, Clark LT, Cooper RS, Denke MA, Howard WJ, Hunninghake DB, Illingworth DR, Luepker RV, McBride P, McKenney JM, Pasternak RC, Stone NJ, Van Horn L. U.S. Department of Health and Human Services; NIH Publication No. 01-3670. May 2001. Available at website: http://www.nhlbi.nih.gov/guidelines/cholesterol/atp3xsum.pdf.

6. 1999 Update: ACC/AHA Guidelines for the Management of Patients with Acute Myocardial Infarction: Executive Summary and Recommendations: A Report of the American College of Cardiology/American Heart Association Task Force on Practice Guidelines (Committee on Management of Acute Myocardial Infarction). Ryan TJ, Antman EM, Brooks NH, Califf RM, Hillis LD, Hiratzka LF, Rapaport E, Riegel B, Russell RO, Smith EE, Weaver WD, Gibbons RJ, Alpert JS, Eagle KA, Gardner TJ, Garson A, Gregoratos G, Russell RD, Smith SC. Available at website: http://circ.ahajournals.org/cgi/content/full/100/9/1016.

E. Manifestations

1. **Angina pectoris,** an episodic, reversible oxygen insufficiency, is the most common form of IHD (see Section II).

2. **Acute ischemic (coronary) syndromes,** represents a term, which has evolved as a way to describe a group of clinical symptoms representing acute myocardial ischemia. The clinical symptoms include acute myocardial infarction, which might include ST-segment elevation (STEMI) or ST-segment depression (NSTEMI), it might include a Q-wave or non–Q-wave infarction, or it might be considered unstable angina (UA) [see Section III].

F. Etiology. The processes, singly or in combination, that produce IHD include decreased blood flow to the myocardium, increased oxygen demand, and decreased oxygenation of the blood. Generally speaking, significant IHD is defined angiographically as greater than or equal to a 70% diameter stenosis of at least one major coronary artery segment or 50% diameter stenosis of the left main coronary artery.

1. **Decreased blood flow.** (Coronary blood flow is illustrated in Figure 38-1.)
   a. **Atherosclerosis,** with or without coronary thrombosis, is the most common cause of IHD. In this condition, the coronary arteries are progressively narrowed by smooth-muscle cell proliferation and the accumulation of lipid deposits (plaque) along the inner lining (intima) of the arteries.

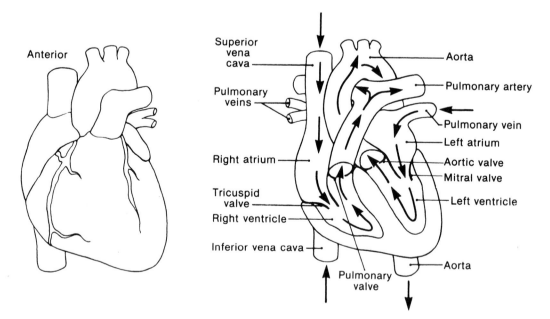

Figure 38-1. Oxygen and other nutrients are borne to the myocardium through the two major coronary arteries (the left and right) and their tributaries. The hemodynamic consequences of ischemic heart disease (IHD) depend on which of the coronary vessels are involved and what part of the myocardium that vessel supplies.

Table 38-1. Factors Affecting Cardiac Parameters That Control Myocardial Oxygen Demand

Factors	Heart Rate	Blood Pressure	Ejection Time	Ventricular Volume	Inotropic Effect
Exercise	Increase	Increase	Decrease	Increase or decrease	Increase
Cold	Increase	Increase	. . .	. . .	. . .
Smoking	Increase	Increase	Increase	. . .	Increase
Nitroglycerin	Increase	Decrease	Decrease	Decrease	Increase
β-Blockers	Decrease	Decrease	Increase	Increase	Decrease

    b. Coronary artery spasm, a sustained contraction of one or more coronary arteries, can occur spontaneously or be induced by irritation (e.g., by coronary catheter or intimal hemorrhage), exposure to the cold, and ergot-derivative drugs. One long-term study demonstrated that coronary spasm was most often associated with an atypical chest pain syndrome and cigarette smoking. These spasms can cause Prinzmetal's angina and even MI.

    c. Traumatic injury, whether blunt or penetrating, can interfere with myocardial blood supply (e.g., the impact of a steering wheel on the chest causing a myocardial contusion in which the capillaries hemorrhage).

    d. Embolic events, even in otherwise normal coronary vessels, can abruptly restrict the oxygen supply to the myocardium.

  2. Increased oxygen demand can occur with exertion (e.g., exercise, shoveling snow) and emotional stress, which increases sympathetic stimulation and, thus, heart rate. Some factors affecting cardiac workload, and therefore myocardial oxygen supply and demand, are listed in Table 38-1.

    a. Diastole. Under normal circumstances, almost all of the oxygen is removed (during diastole) from the arterial blood as it passes through the heart. Thus, little remains to be extracted if oxygen demand increases. To increase the coronary oxygen supply, blood flow has to increase. The normal response mechanism is for the blood vessels, particularly the coronary arteries, to dilate, thereby increasing blood flow.

    b. Systole. The two phases of systole—contraction and ejection—strongly influence oxygen demand.

      (1) The **contractile (inotropic) state of the heart** influences the amount of oxygen it requires to perform.

      (2) Increases in systolic wall tension, influenced by left ventricular volume and systolic pressure, increase oxygen demand.

      (3) Lengthening of ejection time (i.e., the duration of systolic wall tension per cardiac cycle) also increases oxygen demand.

      (4) Changes in heart rate influence oxygen consumption by changing the ejection time.

  3. Reduced blood oxygenation. The oxygen-carrying capacity of the blood may be reduced, as occurs in various anemias.

 G. Risk factors for IHD and goals for modification, where applicable, appear in Table 38-2.

 H. Therapeutic considerations. Because most IHD occurs secondary to atherosclerosis, which is a long-term, cumulative process, medical efforts focus on reducing risk factors through individual patient education and media campaigns. Once manifestations occur, treatment addresses their specific variables.

II. ANGINA PECTORIS

 A. Definition. The term **angina pectoris** is applied to varying forms of transient chest discomfort that are attributable to insufficient myocardial oxygen.

  1. Angina is a clinical syndrome characterized by discomfort in the chest, jaw, shoulder, back, and arms, which is usually aggravated by exertion or stress and relieved by nitroglycerin.

  2. Angina can occur in patients with valvular heart disease, uncontrolled hypertension, as well as in noncardiac organ systems such as the chest wall, esophagus, or lungs.

Table 38-2. Risk Factors for Ischemic Heart Disease and Guidelines for Their Modification, Where Applicable

---

Hyperlipidemia
  Excess serum cholesterol >200 mg/dl—Patients should be started on dietary therapy, and increased physical activity and weight management should be promoted.
  Low-density lipoprotein (LDL) cholesterol level >130 mg/dl—Use of an HMG-CoA reductase inhibitor for LDL cholesterol greater than 130 mg dl has been given a Class I* recommendation; lipid-lowering agents should be used if LDL cholesterol after diet is greater than 100 mg dL has been given a Class I* recommendation.
  High-density lipoprotein (HDL) cholesterol level <40 mg/dl—The use of a fibrate- or niacin-containing agent should be used if HDL is <40 mg/dl, occurring as an isolated finding or in combination with other lipid abnormalities, has been given a Class I* recommendation.
Hypertension—Control of hypertension to systolic/diastolic levels of less than 130 and 85 mm Hg, respectively, has been given a Class I* recommendation
Smoking—Smoking cessation has been given a Class I* recommendation
Diabetes mellitus—Tight control of hyperglycemia (HbA1c <7.0%) in diabetics has been given a Class I* recommendation
Obesity—Achievement and maintenance has been given a Class I* recommendation
Family history of ischemic heart disease (IHD)
Sedentary life style—Daily exercise has been given a Class I* recommendation
Chronic stress or type A personality (i.e., aggressive, ambitious, chronically impatient, competitive)
Age and gender (i.e., prevalence is higher among men than among premenopausal women and increases for both genders with age)
Oral contraceptive use
Gout

---

*Class I recommendation: "Conditions for which there is evidence and/or general agreement that a given procedure or treatment is useful and effective."

B. Common etiologies. Atherosclerotic lesions that produce a narrowing of the coronary arteries are the major cause of angina. However, tachycardia, anemia, hyperthyroidism, hypotension, and arterial hypoxemia can all cause an oxygen imbalance.

C. Types

  1. Stable (classic) angina
    a. In this most common form, exertion, emotional stress, or a heavy meal usually precipitates chest discomfort, which is usually relieved by rest, nitroglycerin, or both.
    b. Five components are usually considered: quality, location, and duration of pain; factors provoking pain and factors that relieve pain.
    c. Pain has been referred to as "squeezing," "griplike," "pressurelike," "suffocating," and "heavy," and is usually referred to as a discomfort rather than "pain."
    d. The anginal episode typically lasts for "minutes" and is usually substernal but has a tendency to radiate to the neck, jaw, epigastrium, or arms.
    e. Characteristically, the discomfort builds to a peak, radiating to the jaw, neck, shoulder, and arms, and then subsides without residual sensation. Angina is normally related to physical exertion, and the discomfort usually subsides quickly (i.e., in 3–5 minutes) with rest; if precipitated by emotional stress, the episode tends to last longer (i.e., about 10 minutes).
    f. Stable angina is characteristically due to a fixed obstruction in a coronary artery.

  2. Unstable angina—See also Section III
    a. In many patients who experience unstable angina, symptoms will be caused by significant coronary artery disease. Angina is considered unstable and requires further evaluation if patients experience:
      (1) Rest angina, which usually is prolonged >20 minutes occurring within a week of presentation
      (2) Severe new-onset angina refers to angina of at least Canadian Cardiovascular Society Classification (CCSC) to Class III severity, with onset within 2 months of initial presentation

(3) Increasing angina refers to previously diagnosed angina that is distinctly more frequent, longer in duration, or lower in threshold

(4) Decreased response to rest or nitroglycerin

b. Unstable angina predicts a higher short-term risk, represents a progressive clinical entity, may signal incipient MI, is referred to as an acute coronary syndrome, and should be reported promptly to a physician.

3. Angina decubitus (nocturnal angina)

a. This angina occurs in the recumbent position and is not specifically related to either rest or exertion.

b. Increased ventricular volume increases oxygen needs and produces angina decubitus, which may indicate cardiac decompensation.

c. Diuretics alone or in combination effectively reduce left ventricular volume and may aid the patient.

d. Nitrates such as nitroglycerin may relieve the paroxysmal nocturnal dyspnea associated with angina decubitus by reducing preload and improving left ventricular dysfunction.

4. Prinzmetal's angina (vasospastic or variant angina)

a. Coronary artery spasm that reduces blood flow precipitates this angina. The spasm may be superimposed on a coronary artery that already has a fixed obstruction due to thrombi or plaque formation.

b. It usually occurs at rest (i.e., pain may disrupt sleep) rather than with exertion or emotional stress.

c. Characteristically, an electrocardiogram (ECG) taken during an attack reveals a transient ST-segment elevation.

d. Calcium-channel blockers, rather than β-blockers, are most effective for this form of angina. Nitroglycerin may not provide relief, depending on the cause of vasospasm.

D. Physical examination is usually not revealing, especially between attacks. However, the patient's history, risk factors, and full description of attacks—precipitation pattern, intensity, duration, relieving factors—usually prove diagnostic.

E. Diagnostic test results

1. The **ECG** is normal in 50% or more of patients with stable angina pectoris, and a normal resting ECG does not exclude severe IHD. However, an ECG with evidence of left ventricular hypertrophy or ST-T–wave changes consistent with myocardial ischemia favor the diagnosis of angina pectoris. The presence of Q waves from a previous MI makes the diagnosis of IHD very likely. An ECG obtained during chest pain is abnormal in 50% of patients with angina who have a normal resting ECG. The ST segment can be either elevated or depressed.

2. Stress testing (exercise ECG) is a well-established procedure, which aids the diagnosis in patients who have normal resting ECGs. The most commonly used definition for a positive test is a ≥1-mm ST-segment depression or elevation for ≥60–80 milliseconds either during or after exercise. Exercise stress testing is preferable to other variations of the stress test (pharmacological) in patients who are able to exercise.

3. Pharmacological stress testing is useful in patients with suspected IHD who are unable to exercise.

a. Intravenous dipyridamole (coronary vasodilation), adenosine (coronary vasodilation) by inhibiting cellular uptake and degradation of adenosine increase coronary blood flow, and high-dose dobutamine (20–40 μg/kg/min) increase oxygen demand through increased heart rate, systolic blood pressure, and myocardial contractility causing an increase in myocardial blood flow are all able to induce detectable cardiac ischemia in conjunction with ECG testing.

b. Side effects occur for each of the agents and include: **dipyridamole** (angina—18–42%, arrhythmias—2%, headache—5–23%, dizziness—5–21%, nausea—8–12%, and flushing—3%), **adenosine** (chest pain—57%, headache—35%, flushing—25%, shortness of breath—15%, and first-degree atrioventricular [AV] heart block—18%), **dobutamine** (premature ventricular beats—15%, premature atrial beats—8%, supraventricular tachycardia and nonsustained ventricular tachycardia—3–4%, nausea—8%, anxiety—6%, headache—4%, and tremor—4%).

4. **Stress perfusion imaging** with ^{201}thallium or ^{99m}technetium can diagnose multivessel disease, localized ischemia, and may be able to determine myocardial viability. The added expense of the test makes it reserved for patients who have ECG abnormalities at rest. Coronary arteriography and cardiac catheterization are very specific and sensitive but are also invasive, expensive, and risky (the mortality rate is about 1%–2%); therefore, they must be used judiciously when trying to confirm suspected angina and to differentiate its etiology.

5. Various drugs can have an effect on the ECG and should be considered prior to, during, and after an exercise test is carried out. Examples include:
   a. Digoxin produces abnormal exercise-induced ST depression in 25%–40% of apparently healthy, normal subjects without ischemia.
   b. β-adrenergic blockers may delay the development of an abnormal ECG if patients receive them prior to or during a stress test. If possible, therapy should be slowly withheld from the patient at least four to five half-lives prior to the exercise testing. If it is not possible to withdraw therapy, the clinician needs to recognize that the test might be less reliable.
   c. Antihypertensives such as vasodilators can alter the stress test by altering the normal hemodynamic response of blood pressure. Additionally, short-term use of nitrates can attenuate angina and ST-segment changes associated with myocardial ischemia.

F. Treatment goals

1. To prevent MI and death, thereby increasing a patient's quality of life

2. To reduce symptoms of angina and occurrence of ischemia, which should improve a patient's quality of life

3. To remove or reduce **risk factors**

4. The management of angina pectoris includes therapies aimed at reversing cardiac risk factors.
   a. **Hyperlipidemia,** if present, should be treated. Reducing cholesterol and low-density lipoprotein (LDL) is associated with a reduced risk of cardiovascular disease and incidence of ischemic cardiac events, as demonstrated by several recent studies using 3-hydroxy-3-methylgutary–coenzyme A (HMG-CoA) reductase inhibitors. The National Cholesterol Education Program (NCEP) has published updated guidelines for treatment of high blood cholesterol (Adult Treatment Panel III [ATP-III]).
      (1) Total cholesterol is no longer the primary target of treatment; LDL cholesterol is now the primary target.
      (2) Current recommendations include the completion of a lipoprotein profile (total cholesterol, LDL cholesterol, high-density lipoprotein (HDL) cholesterol, and triglycerides) as the preferred initial test, rather than screening for total cholesterol and HDL alone.
      (3) If LDL is less than 100 mg/dl (goal of treatment), patients with IHD should be given instructions on diet and exercise and have levels monitored annually.
      (4) If LDL cholesterol is 101–129 mg/dl either at baseline or with LDL-lowering therapy, initiate or intensify lifestyle and/or drug therapies to lower LDL to less than 100 mg/dl. Additional emphasis should be placed on weight reduction and increased physical activity in persons with the **metabolic syndrome** (see below). Delay the use of intensifying LDL-lowering therapies and institute treatment of other lipid or non-lipid risk factors such as nicotinic acid or fibric acid if the patient has elevated triglyceride (>200 mg/dl) or low HDL levels (<40 mg/dl).
      (5) If triglycerides are 200–499 mg/dl; consider a fibrate or niacin after LDL-lowering therapy, but if ≥500 mg/dl, consider fibrate or niacin before LDL-lowering therapy.
      (6) The **metabolic syndrome** is closely linked to insulin resistance, where the normal actions of insulin are impaired. Excess body fat and physical inactivity promote the development of the syndrome; however, some individuals may be predisposed genetically. Patients with three or more of the following characteristics are referred to as having the metabolic syndrome and should be treated accordingly: abdominal obesity, triglycerides >150 mg/dl, HDL levels of <40 mg/dl for men and 50 mg/dl for women, blood pressure readings ≥130/85 mm Hg, and a fasting serum glucose level ≥110 mg/dl.
      (7) **Bile acid sequestrant resins**
         (a) **Mechanism of action.** These insoluble, nonabsorbable, anion-exchange resins bind bile acids within the intestines. Bile acids are synthesized from cholesterol.

(b) Indications. These agents have been shown to be safe and effective in lowering LDL-C especially in patients with modestly elevated levels, in primary prevention, in young adult men, and postmenopausal women. They are effective in combination with other agents.

(c) Precautions and monitoring effects

  (i) These resins are taken just before meals and present palatability problems in patients.

  (ii) Gastrointestinal (GI) intolerance, especially constipation, is frequent.

  (iii) Absorption of many other drugs can be affected. Other drugs should be taken 1 hour before or 4–6 hours after resins.

(8) Statins or HMG-CoA reductase inhibitors

  (a) Mechanism of action. These agents inhibit the enzyme, HMG-CoA, and reduce cholesterol production.

  (b) Indications. These agents are effective in lowering LDL levels, while increasing HDL levels and lowering triglyceride levels. They are primarily used to lower LDL cholesterol levels.

  (c) Precautions and monitoring effects

  (i) GI adverse effects are less frequently seen than with other classes of agents. Headache and dyspepsia frequently occur and should be evaluated, then followed up in 6–8 weeks, and then at each follow-up visit thereafter.

  (ii) These agents can elevate liver function tests (ALT, AST), which requires initial evaluation, then after approximately 12 weeks of therapy, then annually thereafter.

  (iii) Though the incidence of myopathy is believed to be low (0.08%) for lovastatin and simvastatin, elevations of creatine kinase (CK) greater than 10 times the upper limit of normal have been reported with pravastatin, with similar potential for the other members of the group. Consequently, routine monitoring is necessary in all patients, as follows: Evaluate muscle symptoms and check CK before starting therapy, evaluate in 6–12 weeks after starting therapy, and then at each follow-up visit. Patients presenting with muscle soreness, tenderness, or pain should have a CK measurement upon presentation, to minimize the develop of myopathies. Concurrent therapy with other agents, including cyclosporine, macrolide antibiotics, azole antifungals, niacin, fibrates, or nefazadone, may increase the risk.

(9) Fibric acid derivatives

  (a) Mechanism of action. These agents are presumed to inhibit cholesterol synthesis and lower LDL-C. They are effective at lowering triglycerides. In some patients, they modestly lower LDL-C and raise HDL-C.

  (b) Precautions and monitoring effects

  (i) GI effects are the most commonly experienced adverse effect.

  (ii) These agents can elevate liver function tests; routine monitoring should be carried out.

  (iii) Use with statins can lead to elevated CK, and monitoring is necessary to identify myopathies or rhabdomyolysis.

(10) Niacin

  (a) Mechanism of action. Numerous studies have demonstrated the role of niacin in the lowering of cholesterol and triglycerides through various mechanisms such as participation in tissue respiration oxidation-reduction reactions, which decreases hepatic LDL and very-low–density lipoprotein (VLDL) production; inhibition of adipose tissue lipolysis, decreased hepatic triglyceride esterification, and increases in lipoprotein lipase activity. Table 38-3 presents several agents and their effects on lipoproteins.

  (b) Indications. Niacin is valuable in treating patients with elevated total cholesterol and low LDL-C levels. It is used in combination therapy.

  (c) Precautions

  (i) Adverse GI effects are experienced with the use of niacin.

  (ii) Patients may experience flushing and itchy skin, which may be reduced with the administration of 325 mg aspirin about 30 minutes before the dose.

  (iii) Cases of severe liver toxicity have been reported. Liver function tests should be performed in patients receiving this drug.

Table 38-3. Selected Agents and Their Affects on Lipoproteins

Class/Agent	Lipid/Lipoprotein Effects	Daily Dose	Adverse Drug Effects
HMG-CoA reductase inhibitors (statins)	LDL—18–55% reduction HDL—5–15% increase TG—7–30% reduction	Lovastatin—20–80 mg Pravastatin—20–40 mg Simvastatin—20–80 mg Fluvastatin—20–80 mg Atorvastatin—10–80 mg	Myopathy, increased liver enzymes
Bile acid sequestrants	LDL—15–30% reduction HDL—3–5% increase TG—No change or increase	Cholestyramine—4–16 grams Colestipol—5–20 grams Colesevelam—2.6–3.8 grams	Gastrointestinal distress, constipation, decreased absorption of other drugs
Nicotinic acid	LDL—5–25% reduction HDL—15–35% increase TG—20–50% reduction	Immediate-release—1.5–3 grams Extended-release—1–2 grams Sustained-release—1–2 grams	Flushing, hyperglycemia, hyperuricemia (or gout), upper GI distress, hepatotoxicity
Fibric acids	LDL—5–20% reduction HDL—10–20% increase TG—20–50% reduction	Gemfibrozil—600 mg twice daily Fenofibrate—200 mg Clofibrate—1000 mg twice daily	Dyspepsia, gallstones, myopathy, unexplained non-CHD deaths in WHO study

Adapted from the Third Report of the National Cholesterol Education Program (NCEP): Detection, Evaluation, and Treatment of High Blood Cholesterol in Adults (Adult Treatment Panel III). Grundy SM, Becker D, Clark LT, Cooper RS, Denke MA, Howard WJ, Hunninghake DB, Illingworth DR, Luepker RV, McBride P, McKenney JM, Pasternak RC, Stone NJ, Van Horn L. U.S. Department of Health and Human Services; NIH Publication No. 01-3670. May 2001. Available at website: http://www.nhlbi.nih.gov/guidelines/cholesterol/atp3xsum.pdf.

(11) Ezetimibe (Zetia)

(a) **Mechanism of action.** First in a new class of lipid-lowering compounds approved by the FDA, which works by selectively inhibiting the intestinal absorption of cholesterol and related phytosterols, with a resultant decrease in intestinal cholesterol delivered to the liver, decreased hepatic cholesterol stores, and an increase in the clearance of cholesterol from the blood. Ezetimibe has demonstrated the ability to reduce total cholesterol, LDL, apolipoprotein B, and triglyceride levels while increasing HDL levels in patients with hypercholesterolemia.

(b) **Indications.** Ezetimibe as adjunctive therapy along with dietary measures, alone in patients with primary heterozygous familial and nonfamilial hypercholesterolemia, or in combination with the HMG-CoA reductase inhibitors (atorvastatin or simvastatin) in homozygous familial hypercholesterolemia.

(c) **Precautions.** As monotherapy, studies to date have not revealed significant side effects above those seen with placebo administration. However, when used in combination with HMG-CoA reductase inhibitors, reports have described an increased incidence (approximately 1.4%) in the elevation of liver transaminase levels (3 times the upper limit of normal) as compared to the incidence of 0.4% with HMG-CoA agents used alone.

(d) **Dose.** Normal dosing recommendations are a 10-mg dose given once daily.

b. **Hypertension.** Treatment of hypertension according to the Joint National Conference VI guidelines has received a Class I recommendation based on data from multiple randomized clinical trials with large numbers of patients (A—high) and should be controlled. Class I recommendations are based on evidence or general agreement that a given procedure or treatment is useful and effective **(see Chapter 39).**

c. **Smoking** should be stopped if at all possible and has received a Class I recommendation based on data derived from a limited number of randomized trials with small numbers of patients (B—intermediate).

(1) Transdermal use of nicotine-containing patches has become one strategy for aiding the cessation of smoking. Products such as Nicotrol, Habitrol, Nicoderm, and others are available in varying strengths to wean patients off the use of cigarettes over an 8–12-week period, using descending doses.

    (2) Nicotine gum (oral nicotine polacrilex chewing pieces) is available in 2-mg or 4-mg pieces. Nicorette is usually used for 3 months to aid in cessation of smoking.

    (3) Bupropion is a prescription antidepressant, which is also marketed under the brand name of Zyban as an aid to smoking cessation.

  d. Obesity should be reduced through diet and an appropriate exercise program in patients with hypertension, hyperlipidemia, or diabetes mellitus and has received a Class I recommendation based on expert consensus as the primary basis (C—low).

G. Therapeutic agents

  1. Recent evidence-based guidelines have provided recommendations for the treatment of patients with stable angina. Recommendations utilize 3 classes of guidelines [Class I (evidence or general agreement that a procedure or treatment is useful and effective), II (conflicting evidence or a divergence of opinion about the usefulness/efficacy of a procedure or treatment), and III (evidence and/or general agreement that the procedure/treatment is not useful/effective and in some cases may be harmful)], based on three levels of evidence (A [high], B [intermediate], C [low]).

    a. The following represent those therapies with Class IA recommendations: Aspirin in the absence of contraindications, β-adrenergic blockers in the absence of contraindications in patients with a previous heart attack (myocardial infarction), and angiotensin-converting enzyme (ACE) inhibitors in all patients with IHD who also have diabetes and/or left ventricular systolic dysfunction.

    b. The following represent those therapies with Class IB recommendations: β-adrenergic blockers in the absence of contraindications in patients without a previous heart attack (myocardial infarction), sublingual nitroglycerin or nitroglycerin spray for the immediate relief of angina, and calcium antagonists or long-acting nitrates as initial therapy for reduction of symptoms when β-adrenergic blockers are contraindicated.

    c. The following represent those therapies with Class IC recommendations: Calcium antagonists and long-acting nitrates as a substitute for β-adrenergic blockers if initial treatment with β-adrenergic blockers leads to unacceptable side effects.

    d. The following represent those therapies with Class IIa recommendations (conditions for which there is conflicting evidence or a divergence of opinion about the usefulness/efficacy of a procedure or treatment where the weight of evidence/opinion is in favor of usefulness/efficacy): Clopidogrel when aspirin is absolutely contraindicated, long-acting non–dihydropyridine calcium antagonists (diltiazem or verapamil) instead of β-adrenergic blockers as initial therapy, and ACE inhibitor in patients with IHD or other vascular disease.

    e. The following represent those therapies with Class IIb recommendations (conditions for which there is conflicting evidence or a divergence of opinion about the usefulness/efficacy of a procedure or treatment where usefulness/efficacy is less well-established by evidence/opinion): Low-intensity anticoagulation with warfarin in addition to aspirin.

    f. The following represent those therapies with Class III levels of evidence (conditions for which there is evidence and/or general agreement that the procedure/treatment is not useful/effective and in some cases may be harmful): Dipyridamole and chelation therapy.

  2. Nitrates (e.g., nitroglycerin)

    a. Mechanism of action

      (1) The primary value of nitrates is venous dilation, which reduces left ventricular volume (preload) and myocardial wall tension, decreasing oxygen requirements (demand).

      (2) Nitrates may also reduce arteriolar resistance, helping to reduce afterload, which decreases myocardial oxygen demand.

      (3) By reducing pressure in cardiac tissues, nitrates also facilitate collateral circulation, which increases blood distribution to ischemic areas.

      (4) Pharmacological effects have been shown to improve exercise tolerance, prolong the time to onset of angina, and the appearance of ST-segment depression during exercise testing.

    b. Indications

      (1) Acute attacks of angina pectoris can be managed with sublingual, transmucosal (spray or buccal tablets), or intravenous delivery.

      (2) Indications include the prevention of anticipated attacks, using tablets (oral or buccal) or transdermal paste or patches. Sublingual nitrates can be used before eating, sexual activity, or a known stressful event.

      (3) Nitrates are used in treatment of stable angina. They may not be effective as a single agent for treatment of Prinzmetal's angina, although some studies have shown nitrates to prevent or reverse vasospasm at varying doses. Intravenous nitroglycerin is used in the immediate treatment of unstable angina and is used for long-term therapeutic relief.

(4) Nitrates used in combination with β-adrenergic blockers have been shown to be more effective than nitrates or β-adrenergic blockers used alone.

c. Choice of preparation should be based on onset of action, duration of action, and patient compliance and preference because all nitrates have the same mechanism of action.

d. Precautions and monitoring effects

(1) To maximize the therapeutic effect, patients should thoroughly understand the use of their specific dosage forms (e.g., sublingual tablets, transdermal patches or pastes, tablets, capsules).

(2) Blood pressure and heart rate should be monitored because all nitrates can increase heart rate while lowering blood pressure.

(3) Preload reduction can be assessed through reduction of pulmonary symptoms such as shortness of breath, paroxysmal nocturnal dyspnea, or dyspnea.

(4) Nitrate-induced headaches are the most common side effect.

(a) Patients should be warned of the nature, suddenness, and potential strength of these headaches to minimize the anxiety that might otherwise occur.

(b) Compliance can be enhanced if the patient understands that the effect is transient and that the headaches usually disappear with continued therapy.

(c) Acetaminophen ingested 15–30 minutes before nitrate administration may prevent the headache.

e. Effective therapy should result in fewer anginal attacks without inducing significant adverse effects (e.g., postural hypotension, hypoxia). If maximal doses are reached and the patient still experiences attacks, additional agents should be administered.

f. Nitrate tolerance is a major problem with the long-term use of nitroglycerin and long-acting nitrates. Several agents such as ACE inhibitors (sulfhydryl-containing drugs), acetylcysteine, and diuretics have been shown to reverse nitrate tolerance by increasing the availability of sulfhydryl radicals. However, practical considerations suggest that less frequent administration (8–12 hours of nitrate-free intervals) is effective without introducing additional agents.

3. β-Adrenergic blockers

a. Mechanism of action. β-Blockers reduce oxygen demand, both at rest and during exertion, by decreasing the heart rate and myocardial contractility, which also decreases arterial blood pressure.

b. Indications

(1) These agents reduce the frequency and severity of exertional angina that is not controlled by nitrates.

(2) Nitrates have been combined with calcium antagonists, where slow-release dihydropyridines (e.g., felodipine, amlodipine) are preferred over diltiazem or verapamil. If patients need to receive a β-adrenergic blocker along with verapamil or diltiazem due to the added effects, they have to induce bradycardia, AV heart block, and fatigue.

c. Precautions and monitoring effects

(1) Doses should be increased until the anginal episodes have been reduced or until unacceptable side effects occur.

(2) β-Blockers should be avoided in Prinzmetal's angina (caused by coronary vasospasm) because they increase coronary resistance and may induce vasospasm.

(3) Asthma is a relative contraindication because all β-blockers increase airway resistance and have the potential to induce bronchospasm in susceptible patients.

(4) Patients with diabetes and others predisposed to hypoglycemia should be warned that β-blockers mask tachycardia, which is a key sign of developing hypoglycemia.

(5) Patients should be monitored for excessive negative inotropic effects. Findings such as fatigue, shortness of breath, edema, and paroxysmal nocturnal dyspnea may signal developing cardiac decompensation, which also increases the metabolic demands of the heart.

(6) Sudden cessation of β-blocker therapy may trigger a withdrawal syndrome that can exacerbate anginal attacks (especially in patients with IHD) or cause MI.

d. Choice of preparations. All β-blockers are likely to be equally effective for stable (exertional) angina. For further review of β-adrenergic blockers, see Chapter 40. For a list of agents and doses, see Table 38-4.

Table 38-4. Selected Agents and Their Affects on Lipoproteins

Class/Agent	Dose/Dosage Schedule	Comments
Nitrates		
Nitroglycerin sublingual tablets	0.3–0.6 mg up to 1.5 mg	Short-term effects: 1–7 minutes
Nitroglycerin spray	0.4 mg as needed	Similar to sublingual tablets
Nitroglycerin transdermal	0.2–0.8 mg/hr every 12 hours	Remove patch for 8–12 hours to reduce tolerance
Nitroglycerin intravenous infusion	5–200 µg/min	Short acting requiring continuous infusion and monitoring
Isosorbide dinitrate oral tablets	5–80 mg, 2–3 times daily	Longer acting up to 8 hours
Isosorbide dinitrate slow-release tablets	40 mg once or twice daily	Duration of activity up to 8 hours
Pentaerythritol tetranitrate sublingual tablets	10 mg as needed	Short acting as with nitroglycerin sublingual
Erythritol tetranitrate sublingual tablets	5–10 mg as needed	Short acting as with nitroglycerin sublingual
Erythritol tetranitrate oral tablets	10–30 mg three times daily	Longer duration of effect compared to sublingual tablets
β-Adrenergic Blockers		
Propranolol	20–80 mg twice daily	Possesses both β_1-and β_2-blocker effects
Metoprolol	50–200 mg twice daily	Possesses β_1-blocker effects
Atenolol	50–200 mg/day	Possesses β_1-blocker effects
Nadolol	40–80 mg/day	Possesses both β_1-and β_2-blocker effects
Timolol	10 mg twice daily	Possesses both β_1-and β_2-blocker effects
Acebutolol	200–600 mg twice daily	Possesses β_1-blocker effects
Betaxolol	10–20 mg/day	Possesses β_1-blocker effects
Bisoprolol	10 mg/day	Possesses β_1-blocker effects
Esmolol (intravenous)	50–300 µg/kg/min	Possesses β_1-blocker effects
Labetalol	200–600 mg twice daily	Possesses both α,- β_1-, and β_2-blocker effects
Pindolol	2.5–7.5 mg three times daily	Possesses both β_1- and β_2- blocker effects
Calcium-Channel Blockers		
Dihydropyridine derivatives		
Nifedipine	Immediate release; 30–90 mg daily	Short duration of action of 4–6 hours
Amlodipine	5–10 mg once daily	Long duration of action
Felodipine	5–10 mg once daily	Long duration of action
Isradipine	2.5–10 mg twice daily	Intermediate duration of action
Nicardipine	20–40 mg three times daily	Short duration of action
Nisoldipine	20–40 mg once daily	Short duration of action
Nitrendipine	20 mg once or twice daily	Intermediate duration of action
Miscellaneous		
Bepridil	200–400 mg once daily	Long duration of action
Diltiazem	Immediate release: 30–80 mg four times daily;	Short duration of action; important consideration necessary due to hypotension, bradycardia, and edema
	Slow release: 120–320 mg once daily	Long duration of action; important consideration necessary due to hypotension, bradycardia, and edema
Verapamil	Immediate release: 80–160 mg three times daily;	Short duration of action; important consideration necessary due to hypotension, bradycardia, edema, myocardial depression, and heart failure
	Slow release: 120–480 mg once daily	Long duration of action; important consideration necessary due to hypotension, bradycardia, edema, myocardial depression, and heart failure

4. Calcium-channel blockers
  a. Mechanism of action. Two actions are most pertinent in the treatment of angina.
    (1) These agents prevent and reverse coronary spasm by inhibiting calcium influx into vascular smooth muscle and myocardial muscle. This results in increased blood flow, which enhances myocardial oxygen supply.
    (2) Calcium-channel blockers decrease coronary vascular resistance and increase coronary blood flow, resulting in increased oxygen supply.
    (3) Calcium-channel blockers decrease systemic vascular resistance and arterial pressure; in addition, they decrease inotropic effects, resulting in decreased myocardial oxygen demand.
  b. Indications
    (1) Calcium-channel blockers are used in stable (exertional) angina that is not controlled by nitrates and β-blockers and in patients for whom β-blocker therapy is inadvisable. Combination therapy—with nitrates, β-blockers, or both—may be most effective.
    (2) These agents, alone or with a nitrate, are particularly valuable in the treatment of Prinzmetal's angina. They are considered the drug of choice in treatment of angina at rest.
  c. Individual agents
    (1) Diltiazem, verapamil, and bepridil
      (a) These drugs produce negative inotropic effects, and patients must be monitored closely for signs of developing cardiac decompensation (i.e., fatigue, shortness of breath, edema, paroxysmal nocturnal dyspnea). When coadministered with β-blockers or other agents that produce negative inotropic effects (e.g., disopyramide, quinidine, procainamide, flecainide), the negative effects are additive.
      (b) Patients should be monitored for signs of developing bradyarrhythmias and heart block because these agents have negative chronotropic effects.
      (c) Verapamil frequently causes constipation, which must be treated as needed to prevent straining at stool, which could cause an increased oxygen demand (Valsalva maneuver). Verapamil is not recommended in patients with sick sinus syndromes, atrioventricular (AV) nodal disease, or congestive heart failure (CHF).
    (2) Nifedipine
      (a) This calcium-channel blocker does not seem to have a strongly negative inotropic effect; therefore, it is preferred for combination therapy with agents that do. Nifedipine 10 mg (chewed or swallowed) has been used to treat Prinzmetal's angina or refractory spasm in patients who are not hypotensive. Controversy still exists as to the place that short-acting, rapid-release agents such as nifedipine have in patients with IHD.
      (b) Because nifedipine increases the heart rate somewhat, it can produce tachycardia, which would increase oxygen demand. Coadministration of a β-blocker should prevent reflex tachycardia.
      (c) Its potent peripheral dilatory effects can decrease coronary perfusion and produce excessive hypotension, which can aggravate myocardial ischemia.
      (d) Dizziness, light-headedness, and lower extremity edema are the most common adverse effects, but these tend to disappear with time or dose adjustment.
    (3) Amlodipine, felodipine, isradipine, nicardipine, nisoldipine, and **nitrendipine** are second-generation dihydropyridine derivative, calcium-channel blockers. They have been used effectively as once- or twice-a-day agents due to their long activity. Due to the potent negative inotropic effects of these agents, they are not recommended in patients with CHF (amlodipine has been shown to have less negative potential in CHF than other members of the class).

5. Antiplatelet agents
  a. Aspirin in doses of 75–325 mg daily should be routinely used in all patients with acute or chronic IHD with or without symptoms in the absence of any contraindications.
  b. Ticlopidine is a thienopyridine derivative that inhibits platelet aggregation induced by adenosine diphosphate. However, unlike aspirin, it has not been shown to decrease adverse cardiovascular events in patients with stable angina, and has been associated with thrombotic thrombocytopenic purpura on an infrequent basis.
  c. Clopidogrel is also a thienopyridine derivative related to ticlopidine, but it possesses antithrombotic effects that are greater than those of ticlopidine. Clopidogrel is a thera-

peutic option in those angina patients who can not take aspirin due to contraindications. Doses of 75 mg daily are recommended to prevent the development of acute coronary syndromes.

6. **Angiotensin Converting Enzyme Inhibitors** (ACE inhibitors)
   a. ACE inhibitors during the past 3–5 years have attracted continued attention as additional therapy in patients with IHD, as evidenced by the most recent guidelines, which provide a Class IIa recommendation for their use in patients with IHD or other vascular diseases.
   b. The Heart Outcomes Prevention Evaluation (HOPE) trial demonstrated that the ACE inhibitor ramipril (10 mg per day) reduced cardiovascular death, MI, and stroke in patients who were at high risk for or had vascular disease in the absence of heart failure.
   c. Current controversy on the use of ACE inhibitors centers around questions on therapeutic effects of each agent to determine if the beneficial effects seen in previous trials represent a class effect or if it is specific to those agents with proven benefit. Differences do exist among the currently available agents, and the need exists to determine the optimal dose necessary to induce the therapeutic effects appreciated from the HOPE, SAVE (captopril), and CONSENSUS I (enalapril) trials.
   d. Current guidelines do not suggest which agent to use, and it is anticipated that ongoing trials with additional agents will provide additional information regarding dosing regimens and potential differences that might exist among the class of drugs.

III. ACUTE CORONARY SYNDROME (ACS)

A. **Definition. ACS** is a relatively new term, which has been introduced into the medical literature to describe any pattern of clinical symptomatology that reflects the development of acute MI (See Figure 38-2a and 38-2b), and includes acute MI (AMI), which includes STEMI and NSTEMI, Q wave and non-Q wave) as well as unstable angina (UA).

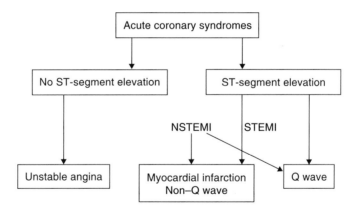

Figure 38-2a. The spectrum of clinical conditions representing the acute coronary syndromes. Patients presenting with acute myocardial ischemia present with either an elevated ST segment or no elevated ST segment on ECG. Evidenced-based practice guidelines demonstrate that the majority of patients presenting with ST-segment elevation (STEMI) eventually develop a Q-wave myocardial infarction as compared to the smaller group of ST-segment elevation patients who evolve into a non–Q-wave myocardial infarction (smaller arrow). The remaining patients categorized as ACS patients present with no ST-segment elevation on ECG and have either unstable angina or non–ST-segment elevated myocardial infarction (NSTEMI). Most NSTEMI patients evolve into a non–Q-wave myocardial infarction (larger arrow), with a smaller number of NSTEMI patients evolving into a Q-wave myocardial infarction. The spectrum of clinical conditions referred to as acute coronary syndromes includes unstable angina, non–Q-wave myocardial infarction (with either no ST-segment elevation or ST-segment elevation), and Q-wave myocardial infarction (with either ST-segment elevation or no ST-segment elevation). Adapted from ACC/AHA 2002 Guideline Update for the Management of Patients with Unstable Angina and Non-ST-Segment Elevation Myocardial Infarction: a report of the American College of Cardiology/American Heart Association Task Force on Practice Guidelines (Committee on the Management of Patients with Unstable Angina). 2002. Available at: http://www.acc.org/ clinical/ guidelines/unstable/unstable.pdg.

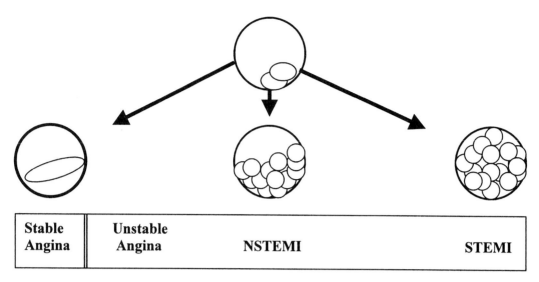

Figure 38-2b. Evolutionary progression of acute coronary syndromes. The graphic depicts the evolving changes taking place in IHD as advancing atherosclerosis (most common cause) and the resultant reduction in myocardial perfusion caused by coronary narrowing favor the development of the acute coronary syndrome due to either unstable angina, non–ST-segment elevation myocardial infarction (NSTEMI) or ST-segment elevated myocardial infarction (STEMI). Note the thrombi, which form in unstable angina and NSTEMI and STEMI are rich in both filrin and platelets. Adapted from University of Pittsburgh, School of Pharmacy Program, "Integrating New Fibrinolytic Findings into AMI Reperfusion and Combination Therapy: 2002 and Beyond." Vanscoy G, Rihn T, et al.

   B. Incidence. It has been estimated that nearly 8 million patients seen in emergency departments each year in the U.S. are seen for chest pain, and that up to 5 million of these patients are admitted to the hospital. More than 2 million of the patients admitted to the hospital are admitted with an ACS (400,000 with ST-segment–elevated MI, and 1.8 million with UA and NSTEMI).

   C. Classification of patients presenting with presumed ACS is critical to the appropriate determination of prognosis as well as clinical interventions. In ACS due to STEMI and NSTEMI, a portion of the cardiac muscle suffers a severe and prolonged restriction of oxygenated coronary blood. In the majority of patients, the cause is an occlusive or near-occlusive thrombus overlying or adjacent to a ruptured atherosclerotic plaque. This results in cellular ischemia, tissue injury, and tissue necrosis. One-and-a-half million people suffer an AMI each year. UA is believed to represent an impending AMI, and the goal of treatment is to prevent the development of the AMI.

      1. STEMI—A condition that requires immediate reperfusion therapy, if possible through either thrombolysis or percutaneous coronary intervention (PCI);

         a. The introduction of thrombolysis or PCI for the management of STEMI has demonstrated the ability to remove the offending thrombus from the affected coronary artery.

         b. Damage to the myocardial tissue is not routinely reversible as in the case of angina pectoris, due to potential death of myocardial tissue if reperfusion does not take place early enough.

      2. UA/NSTEMI—Similar conditions where evidence shows that no benefit in these patients is appreciated from reperfusion therapy. Specific guidelines have been developed for their diagnosis and management. Up to 25% of patients with NSTEMI and elevated cardiac enzymes go on to develop Q-wave MI, with the remaining patients having non–Q-wave MI. The development of UA carries a 10%–20% risk of progression to an MI in untreated patients where treatment has been shown to reduce the risk to 5%–7%.

   D. Diagnosis. The ECG is at the center of the decision pathway for the evaluation and management of patients with ACS, and is confirmed with serial cardiac markers in more than 90% of patents presenting with significant ST-segment elevation. Patients who present without ST-segment elevation are considered to have either UA or NSTEMI; the final diagnosis is made later, after the presence or absence of serial cardiac markers is determined. **Diagnostic test results.** The development of an ACS is a life-threatening emergency; diagnosis is presumed—and treatment is instituted—based on the patient's complaints and the results of an immediate 12-lead ECG. Laboratory tests and further diagnostic tests can rule out or provide confirmation of and help to identify the locale and extent of myocardial damage.

1. **Serial 12-lead ECG.** Abnormalities may be absent or inconclusive during the first few hours after presentation of the ACS and may not aid the diagnosis in about 15% of the cases. When present, characteristic findings show progressive changes.
    a. First, ST-segment elevation (injury current) appears in the leads, reflecting the injured area. Peaked upright or inverted T waves usually indicate acute myocardial injury; the early stages of a transmural Q-wave MI. Persistent ST depression may also indicate a non–Q-wave MI.
    b. Q waves developing (indicating necrosis) is generally diagnostic of an MI, but can be seen in other conditions.
    c. Unequivocal diagnosis can only be made in the presence of all three abnormalities. However, the manifestations depend on the area of injury. For example, in the non–Q-wave infarction, only ST-segment depression may appear.
    d. The most serious arrhythmic complication of an acute MI is ventricular fibrillation, which may occur without warning.
    e. Ventricular premature beats (VPBs) are the most commonly encountered arrhythmias and may require treatment.

2. **Cardiac enzymes**
    a. **Creatine kinase–heart** (CK-MB) is first elevated 3–12 hours after the onset of pain, peaks in 24 hours, and returns to baseline in 48–72 hours. Other causes can result in elevated CK-MB enzyme but do not demonstrate the typical pattern of rise and fall as seen in an MI. Until recently, CK-MB had been the principal serum cardiac marker used in the evaluation of ACS.
    b. **Cardiac troponin I** (cTnI) and **troponin T** (cTnT) are even more sensitive than MB-CK. They represent a powerful tool for risk stratification and have greater sensitivity and specificity than CK-MB. However, they do provide a low sensitivity in the early phases of MI (<6 hours after symptom onset) and require repeat measurements at 8–12 hours, if negative. Levels increase 3–12 hours after the onset of pain, peak at 24–48 hours, and return to baseline over 5–14 days.
    c. **Lactate dehydrogenase** (LDH) is followed for its characteristic patterns of rise and fall. The ratio of LDH_1/LDH_2 is helpful in diagnosing an MI. Cardiac troponin assays are replacing the use of LDH assays.

3. **Cardiac imaging.** As cardiac enzymes assays improve, the use of noninvasive cardiac imaging techniques are not indicated for initial diagnosis of an MI. Tests include ^{99m}Tc-pyrophosphate scintigraphy, myocardial perfusion imaging, radionucleotide ventriculography, two-dimensional echocardiography, and coronary angiography.

E. **Signs and symptoms**

1. Recent evidence-based clinical guidelines provide a Class I recommendation for patients with suspected ACS with chest discomfort at rest for longer than 20 minutes; hemodynamic instability or recent syncope or presyncope should be strongly considered for immediate referral to an emergency department or specialized chest pain unit. The foremost characteristic of ACS is persistent, severe chest pain or pressure, commonly described as crushing, squeezing, or heavy (likened to having an elephant sitting on the chest). The pain generally begins in the chest and, like angina, may radiate to the left arm, the abdomen, back, neck, jaw, or teeth. The onset of pain generally occurs at rest or with normal daily activities; it is not commonly associated with exertion.

2. Other common complaints include a sense of impending doom, sweating, nausea, vomiting, and difficulty breathing. In some patients, fainting and sudden death may be the initial presentation of ACS.

3. Observable findings include extreme anxiety, restless, agitated behavior, and ashen pallor.

4. Some patients, particularly those with diabetes or the elderly, may experience only mild or indigestion-like pain or a clinically silent MI, which may only manifest in worsening CHF, loss of consciousness, acute confusion, dyspnea, a sudden drop in blood pressure, or a lethal arrhythmia.

F. Overall treatment goals in ACS

1. To relieve chest pain and anxiety

2. To reduce cardiac workload and stabilize cardiac rhythm

3. To prevent/reduce myocardial damage by limiting the area affected and preserving pump function

4. To prevent or arrest complications, such as lethal arrhythmias, AMI, CHF, or sudden death

5. To reopen (or reperfuse) closed coronary vessels with thrombolytic drugs and/or PCI if indicated

G. Treatment of UA/NSTEMI

1. Anti-ischemic therapy
   a. Current evidence-based clinical guidelines provide Class I (conditions for which there is evidence and/or general agreement that a given procedure or treatment is useful and effective) recommendations for the following therapeutic interventions in patients with UA/NSTEMI:
   (1) Bed rest with continuous ECG monitoring for ischemia and arrhythmia detection in patients with ongoing rest pain
   (2) Nitroglycerin—sublingual, tablet, or spray followed by intravenous administration—for the immediate relief of ischemia and associated symptoms
   (3) Supplemental oxygen for patients with cyanosis or respiratory distress and continued need for supplemental oxygen in the presence of hypoxemia
   (4) Morphine sulfate intravenously when symptoms are not immediately relieved with nitroglycerin or when acute pulmonary congestion and/or severe agitation is present
   (5) A β-adrenergic blocker with the first dose administered intravenously if there is ongoing chest pain, followed by oral administration, in the absence of contraindications
   (6) In patients with continuing or frequently recurring ischemia when β-adrenergic blockers are contraindicated, a non–dihydropyridine calcium antagonist (i.e., diltiazem or verapamil) as initial therapy in the absence of severe left ventricular dysfunction or other contraindications.
   (7) An ACE inhibitor when hypertension persists despite treatment with nitroglycerin and a β-adrenergic blocker in patients with left ventricular dysfunction or CHF and in ACS patients with diabetes.
   b. Current evidence-based clinical practice guidelines provide a Class IIa (weight of evidence/opinion is in favor of usefulness/efficacy) recommendation for the following therapeutic interventions in patients with UA/NSTEMI:
   (1) Oral long-acting calcium antagonists for recurrent ischemia in the absence of contraindications and when β-adrenergic blockers and nitrates are used at their maximal doses
   (2) An ACE inhibitor for all post-ACS patients
   (3) Intra-aortic balloon pump counterpulsation for severe ischemia that is continuing or recurs frequently despite intensive medical therapy or for hemodynamic instability in patients before or after coronary angiography
   c. Current evidence-based clinical practice guidelines provide a Class IIb (usefulness/ efficacy is less well-established by evidence/opinion) recommendation for the following therapeutic interventions in patients with UA/NSTEMI:
   (1) Extended-release form of non–dihydropyridine calcium antagonists instead of a β-adrenergic blocker
   (2) Immediate-release dihydropyridine (nifedipine-like) calcium antagonist in the presence of a β-adrenergic blocker
   d. Current evidence-based clinical practice guidelines provide a Class III (conditions for which there is evidence and/or general agreement that the procedure/treatment is not

useful/effective and in some cases may be harmful) recommendation for the following therapeutic interventions in patients with UA/NSTEMI:

(1) Nitroglycerin or other nitrate within 24 hours of sildenafil (viagra) use

(2) Immediate-release dihydropyridine calcium antagonist in the absence of a β-adrenergic blocker

2. **Therapeutic agents.** See Table 38-4 for select agents and dosing regimens.

   a. **Nitrates (e.g., nitroglycerin).** See section II H.

   b. **Morphine**

   (1) **Mechanism of action.** Morphine causes venous pooling and reduces preload, cardiac workload, and oxygen consumption. Morphine should be administered intravenously, starting with 2 mg and titrating at 5–15-minute intervals until the pain is relieved or toxicity becomes evident.

   (2) **Indications.** Morphine is the drug of choice for myocardial pain and anxiety.

   (3) **Precautions and monitoring effects**

   (a) Because morphine increases peripheral vasodilation and decreases peripheral resistance, it can produce orthostatic hypotension and fainting.

   (b) Patients should be monitored for hypotension and signs of respiratory depression.

   (c) Morphine has a vagomimetic effect that can produce bradyarrhythmias. If ECG monitoring reveals excess bradycardia, it should be reversed by administering atropine (0.5–1 mg).

   (d) Nausea and vomiting may occur, especially with initial doses, and patients must be protected against aspiration of stomach contents.

   (e) Severe constipation is a potential problem with ongoing morphine administration. The patient may use a Valsalva maneuver while straining at the stool, which can produce a bradycardia or can overload the cardiac system and trigger cardiac arrest. Docusate (100 mg twice daily) is a useful prophylactic.

   c. **Oxygen** is required at 2–4 L/min via nasal cannula in any patient who has chest pain and who may be ischemic. Mild hypoxemia is common in acute MI patients. Increasing the oxygen content of the blood, thus improving oxygenation of the myocardium, is a top priority as continuing hypoxia rapidly increases myocardial damage.

   d. **Thrombolytic agents** have not demonstrated beneficial clinical outcomes in the absence of STEMI. Studies carried out to date have failed to show benefit with using thrombolytics in UA versus standard therapy to prevent MI. Additionally, thrombolytic agents actually increased the risk of MI in such patients. Therefore, based on current evidence-based guidelines, thrombolytic agents are not recommended in the management of ACS without ST-segment elevation.

3. **Antiplatelet and anticoagulation therapy** (See Table 38-5 select agents and dosing regimens)

   a. Current evidence-based clinical guidelines provide Class I (conditions for which there is evidence and/or general agreement that a given procedure or treatment is useful and effective) recommendations for the following therapeutic interventions in patients with UA/NSTEMI:

   (1) Antiplatelet therapy should be initiated promptly. Aspirin should be administered as soon as possible after presentation and continued indefinitely.

   (2) Clopidogrel should be administered to hospitalized patients who are unable to take aspirin because of hypersensitivity or major gastrointestinal intolerance.

   (3) In hospitalized patients in whom an early noninterventional approach is planned, clopidogrel should be added to aspirin as soon as possible on admission and administered for at least 1 month.

   (4) In patients for whom a PCI is planned, clopidogrel should be started and continued for at least 1 month and up to 9 months in patients who are not at high risk for bleeding.

   (5) In patients taking clopidogrel in whom elective coronary artery bypass grafting (CABG) is planned, the drug should be withheld for 5–7 days.

   (6) Anticoagulation with subcutaneous low-molecular–weight heparin (LMWH) or intravenous unfractionated heparin (UFH) should be added to antiplatelet therapy with aspirin and/or clopidogrel.

   (7) A platelet glycoprotein IIb/IIIa antagonist should be administered, in addition to aspirin and heparin, to patients in whom catheterization and PCI are planned. The agent may also be administered just prior to PCI.

Table 38-5. Antithrombotic Agents Used in the Treatment of IHD

Class/Agents	Dosing Regimen	Level of Evidence (Guidelines)
Oral Antiplatelets		
Aspirin	Initial dose of 162–325 mg followed by 75–160 mg/day	Class I
Clopidogrel	75 mg/day; a loading dose of 4–8 tablets (300–600 mg) can be used when rapid onset of action is required	Class I if patients are unable to tolerate aspirin
Ticlopidine	250 mg twice daily; a loading dose of 500 mg can be used when rapid onset of action is required; monitoring of platelet and white cell counts during treatment is required	Clopidogrel is preferred over ticlopidine due to its more rapid onset of action and better safety profile over ticlopidine.
Heparins		
Dalteparin (LMWH)	120 IU/kg subcutaneously every 12 hours (maximum of 10,000 IU twice daily)	Class I
Enoxaparin (LMWH)	1 mg/kg subcutaneously every 12 hours; the first dose may be preceded by a 30-mg IV bolus dose	Class I
Heparin (UFH)	Bolus dose of 60–70 U/kg (maximum of 5000 U) IV followed by infusion of 12–15 U/kg/hr (maximum 1000 U/hr) titrated to aPTT of 1.5–2.5 times control	Class I current guidelines suggest that the current evidence favors the use of enoxaparin over UHF as an anticoagulant unless CABG is planned within 24 hours.
Intravenous Antiplatelets		
Abciximab	0.25 mg/kg bolus followed by infusion of 0.125 mg/kg/min for 12–24 hr.	Class I recommendation for use in addition to aspirin and heparin in patients in whom catheterization and PCI are planned, and in patients just prior to PCI. Class III recommendation in patients in whom PCI is not planned.
Eptifibatide	180 µg/kg bolus followed by infusion of 2.0 µg/kg/min for 72–96 hr.	Class I recommendation for use in addition to aspirin and heparin in patients in whom catheterization and PCI are planned, and in patients just prior to PCI. Class IIa recommendation in addition to aspirin and LMWH or UFH in patients with continuing ischemia, an elevated troponin, or with other high-risk features in whom an invasive management strategy is not planned. Class IIb recommendation in addition to aspirin and LMWH or UFH in patients without continuing ischemia who have no other high-risk features and in whom PCI is not planned.
Tirofiban	0.4 µg/kg/min for 30 min followed by infusion of 0.1 µg/kg/min for 48–96 hr	Class I recommendation in addition to aspirin and heparin in patients in whom catheterization and PCI are planned, and in patients just prior to PCI. Class IIa recommendation in addition to aspirin and LMWH or UFH in patients with continuing ischemia, an elevated troponin, or with other high-risk features in whom an invasive management strategy is not planned. Class IIb recommendation in addition to aspirin and LMWH or UFH in patients without continuing ischemia who have no other high-risk features and in whom PCI is not planned.

b. Current evidence-based clinical guidelines provide Class IIa (weight of evidence/ opinion is in favor of usefulness/efficacy) recommendation for the following therapeutic interventions in patients with UA/NSTEMI:

(1) Eptifibatide or tirofiban should be administered, in addition to aspirin and LMWH or UFH, to patients with continuing ischemia, an elevated troponin, or other high-risk features in whom an invasive management strategy is not planned.

(2) Enoxaparin is preferable to UFH as an anticoagulant in patients with UA/NSTEMI, unless CABG is planned within 24 hours.

(3) A platelet glycoprotein IIb/IIIa antagonist should be administered to patients already receiving heparin, aspirin, and clopidogrel in whom catheterization and PCI are planned. The glycoprotein IIb/IIIa antagonist may also be administered just prior to PCI.

c. Current evidence-based clinical practice guidelines provide a Class IIb (usefulness/ efficacy is less well-established by evidence/opinion) recommendation for the following therapeutic interventions in patients with UA/NSTEMI: Eptifibatide or tirofiban, in addition to aspirin and LMWH or UFH, to patients without continuing ischemia who have no other high-risk features and in whom PCI is not planned.

d. Current evidence-based clinical practice guidelines provide a Class III (conditions for which there is evidence and/or general agreement that the procedure/treatment is not useful/effective and in some cases may be harmful) recommendation for the following therapeutic interventions in patients with UA/NSTEMI:

(1) IV thrombolytic therapy in patients without acute ST-segment elevation

(2) Abciximab administration in patients in whom PCI is not planned

H. STEMI

1. Approximately 90% of patients with acute MI and ST-segment elevation have complete thrombotic occlusion of the infarct-related artery. Atherosclerotic plaques are made up of lipid and fibrous proteins. When the lesion ruptures, the release of adenosine diphosphate alteplase (ADP), serotonins, and thromboxane A_2 is triggered, leading to platelet aggregation and the formation of the primary clot. Thromboplastin released from the injured vessel initiates the clotting cascade. The resulting fibrin traps red blood cells (RBCs), platelets, and plasma protein to form an intraluminal thrombus. Clot dissolution is caused by the conversion of plasminogen to plasmin mediated by plasminogen activators. All patients with STEMI should be considered for antithrombotic therapy, which includes thrombolytics, heparin, LMWH, glycoprotein IIb/IIIa antagonists, warfarin, aspirin, and direct thrombin inhibitors.

a. Mechanism of action. Administration of thrombolytic agents causes the thrombus clot to be lysed when administered early after symptom onset (<6–12 hours) and to restore blood flow.

b. Indications

(1) Thrombolytic agents were used in patients with STEMI with chest pain <6–12 hours. Successful early reperfusion has been shown to reduce infarct size, improve ventricular function, and improve mortality. However, benefits may be seen in patients using thrombolytic therapy as late as 12 hours after pain starts.

(2) Intravenous administration of streptokinase (SK), recombinant tissue-type plasminogen activator alteplase (t-PA), anisoylated plasminogen streptokinase activator complex (APSAC), reteplase (r-PA), and tenecteplase (TNK) may restore blood flow in an occluded artery if administered within 12 hours of an acute MI, although less than 6 hours is optimal. The goal of treatment of STEMI patients is to initiate thrombolytic therapy within 30–60 minutes of arrival in an emergency room.

(a) t-PA is relatively fibrin-specific and is able to lyse clots without depleting fibrinogen, and TNK has an even greater fibrin specificity. SK activates the fibrinolytic system and has a greater likelihood of causing systemic effects than t-PA. This effect may result in a greater degree of systemic bleeding as compared with t-PA, r-PA, and TNK.

(b) Though which agent—t-PA, SK, APSAC, r-PA, and TNK—is best is still controversial, most studies have shown that each agent, when used early, can reopen (reperfuse) occluded coronary arteries and reduce mortality from STEMI. However, considerations such as ease of use, onset of action, incidence of bleed, and cost play important factors in determining which agent to use for a given hospital and patient.

c. **Individual agents**
  (1) **Recombinant t-PA**
    (a) **Absolute contraindications** to t-PA include active internal bleeding; recent cerebrovascular accident (CVA); intracranial neoplasm; aneurysm; pregnancy; arteriovenous malformations; recent (within 2 months) intracranial surgery, spinal surgery, or trauma; and severe uncontrolled hypertension, bleeding diathesis, or hemorrhagic ophthalmic conditions.
    (b) A **"front-loaded" regimen**—the accelerated infusion, which consists of a total dose of 100 mg or less that is dosed over 1–1/2 hours—may be more beneficial. The initial dose of 15 mg is bolused, intravenously, 1–2 minutes, while an infusion is begun to:
      (i) Infuse t-PA at the rate of 0.75 mg/kg over 30 minutes (not to exceed 50 mg)
      (ii) Followed by t-PA infused at 0.5 mg/kg over 60 minutes (not to exceed 35 mg)
    (c) **An alternate dosing regimen is based on the patient's weight.**
      (i) **Dosage for patients over 65 kg.** A total of 100 mg of t-PA is generally administered to all patients who weigh over 65 kg over a 3-hour period. Though many regimens have been used, generally speaking, 6–10 mg of t-PA is given as an intravenous bolus dose over 1–2 minutes, followed by the remaining infusion rates over the next 3 hours: a 54–60-mg intravenous infusion over the first hour, a 20-mg intravenous infusion over the second hour, and a 20-mg intravenous infusion over the third hour.
      (ii) **Dosage for patients under 65 kg.** A dose of 1.25 mg/kg is given over a 3-hour period, with 10% of the total dose given initially as a bolus dose over 1–2 minutes.
  (2) **Streptokinase (SK)**
    (a) **Absolute contraindications** to SK include active internal bleeding, recent CVA, intracranial or intraspinal surgery, intracranial neoplasm, pregnancy, arteriovenous malformation, aneurysm, bleeding diathesis, and severe uncontrolled hypertension or hemorrhagic ophthalmic conditions.
    (b) **Precautions and monitoring effects**
      (i) Patients who have received SK within the previous 6 months have an added predisposition to allergic reactions as well as a refractory response to SK due to systemic antibody formation.
      (ii) Patients must be monitored for bleeding, arrhythmias, anaphylactoid reactions, and hypotension. Many patients develop arrhythmias, which do not require treatment, within 30–45 minutes of SK administration; these arrhythmias are called **reperfusion arrhythmias,** referring to a clot that has been removed and resulted in coronary reperfusion.
    (c) **Dosage.** An IV dose of 1.5 million IU is infused over 60 minutes. Other treatments are currently being used, including bolus doses followed by continuous infusions, as well as combination therapy with t-PA.
  (3) **Other agents**
    (a) APSAC at doses of 30 U is given by IV over 5 minutes.
    (b) Reteplase 10 U is given by IV bolus and repeated after 30 minutes.
    (c) Tenecteplase is the newest agent approved for use in acute treatment of MI at doses of 30–50 mg (based on the patient's weight) as a single IV bolus. Rapid rate of administration, fibrin specificity, fewer bleeding complications as compared to t-PA, and superiority over t-PA in late-treated patients make TNK a very likely candidate to replace t-PA as the agent of choice in STEMI.
d. **Postthrombolysis adjunctive therapy.** Antiplatelet and anticoagulant therapy following successful reperfusion is necessary to prevent reocclusion, ischemia, and reinfarction **(see Table 38-6).**
  (1) **Aspirin** administered (160–325 mg) during acute thrombolytic therapy has been shown to affect thrombolysis positively by preventing platelet aggregation and has reduced postinfarct mortality. Other agents include dipyridamole, ticlopidine, and clopidogrel.
  (2) **Heparin** has been administered along with the thrombolytics to prevent reocclusion once a coronary artery has been opened. It also appears to decrease mortality in patients with an MI even if they have not received thrombolytic therapy. In the United States, heparin has been given intravenously as a 4000-U bolus, followed by a con-

Table 38-6. Adjunctive Treatment Strategies and Their Associated Clinical Benefits in STEMI Patients

Class	Prevent Ischemia	Prevent Reocclusion	Preserve LV Function	Reduce Mortality
Antiplatelets	+	+		+
Anticoagulants	+	+		?
β-Blockers	+		+	+
ACE inhibitors			+	+
Statins				+

Adapted from University of Pittsburgh, School of Pharmacy Program, "Integrating New Fibrinolytic Findings into AMI Reperfusion and Combination Therapy: 2002 and Beyond." Vanscoy G, Rihn T, et al.

tinuous infusion of 1000 U/hour; the goal of therapy is to maintain the activated partial thromboplastin time (aPTT) 1.5–20 times control. Unless chosen for a specific clinical indication, heparin use with streptokinase is not recommended because of increased risk of hemorrhage. Patients who have not received thrombolytic therapy but are at risk for systemic or pulmonary embolism are candidates for continuous infusion of heparin. Other patients not receiving thrombolytic therapy may also benefit from low-dose SC heparin therapy until ambulatory. Low–molecular-weight heparins (e.g., enoxaparin, dalteparin) are currently being evaluated as alternatives to heparin.

(3) **Warfarin** is approved for the treatment of acute MI to reduce mortality and prevent recurrent MI and other thromboembolic complications such as stroke. The target INR is 2.5–3.5.

(4) **Antiplatelet agents** (e.g., abciximab, tirofiban, eptifibatide) act by inhibiting glycoprotein (GP) IIb/IIIa receptors. Fibrinogen acts with platelet GP IIb/IIIa receptors to mediate platelet aggregation. Combinations of these agents with thrombolytics have shown improved incidences and speed of reperfusion.

(5) **Heparin, enoxaparin, or dalteparin** along with aspirin should be used in hospitalized patients with unstable angina for at least 48 hours or until the unstable angina has resolved.

(6) **β-Adrenergic blockers**
  (a) If administered early in the acute phase, β-adrenergic blockers have been shown to reduce ischemia, reduce the potential zone of infarction, decrease oxygen demands, preserve left ventricular function, and decrease cardiac workload.
  (b) β-adrenergic blocker therapy has also been shown to significantly reduce post-MI mortality due to sudden death, risk of reinfarction, cardiac rupture, and ventricular arrhythmias.

(7) **ACE inhibitors**
  (a) Global left ventricular dysfunction has been determined to be an important marker of prognosis after MI. ACE inhibitors have clearly been shown to improve exercise capacity and reduce mortality in patients with moderate to severe congestive heart failure (CONSENSUS I, SOLVD trials).
  (b) ACE inhibitors (e.g., captopril, enalapril, ramipril) used after MI have aided in the prevention of progressive left ventricular dilation or "ventricular remodeling." These agents are beneficial in patients with MI presenting with left ventricular dysfunction.
  (c) The HOPE trial was conducted to evaluate the effects of ramipril in preventing the primary end point, a composite of CV death, MI, and stroke. The results demonstrated that ramipril resulted in an reduction of 22% over placebo in the primary end points (CV mortality, MI, stroke). Additionally, the benefits were observed in a broad range of patients without evidence of left ventricular dysfunction or heart failure who were at high risk for CV events.

(8) **"Statins."** Several large trials (4S, LIPID, CARE) have shown that when HMG-CoA reductase inhibitors are used aggressively to lower cholesterol levels, it resulted in a significant reduction in nonfatal MI or CHD (30%–40% reduction). Most recently, it has been recognized that inflammation is an important mechanism in ACS and that statins exert an important anti-inflammatory effect within coronary arteries (independent of their cholesterol-lowering effects).

    (9) Lidocaine should not be administered prophylactically, but should be used in patients who develop ventricular arrhythmias.

    (10) Calcium-channel blocking agents are not used in acute phases of MI and may be harmful to patients with impaired left ventricular function. They may decrease the incidence of reinfarction in patients with non–Q-wave infarcts.

    (11) Interventional therapy, coronary angiography, and PTCA may be of use in patients who have contraindications to thrombolytic therapy, for those in cardiogenic shock, for those in whom thrombolytic therapy has failed, or those with recurrent ischemia or hemodynamic instability.

        (a) Adjunct therapy includes antiplatelet drugs, anticoagulants, use of intracoronary stents, and intra-aortic balloon pumping.

        (b) Aspirin is given to reduce coronary reocclusion.

        (c) Heparin in large doses continues to be administered 48–72 hours after the procedure.

        (d) Intra-aortic balloon counter pulsation reduces recurrent ischemia and the incidence of reocclusion.

        (e) Clopidogrel is administered with the aspirin in patients with intracoronary stent placement.

        (f) Antiplatelet agents that bind to GP IIb/IIIa, such as abciximab, tirofiban, or eptifibatide, are used with heparin and aspirin.

I. Complications. MI potentiates many complications; the most common of these include:

  1. Lethal arrhythmias. Arrhythmias refractory to lidocaine may respond to procainamide, amiodarone, and other antiarrhythmics.

  2. Congestive heart failure (see Chapter 40 for a more detailed discussion).

    a. Left ventricular failure causes pulmonary congestion. Diuretics, especially furosemide, help reduce the congestion.

    b. Digitalis glycosides have a positive inotropic effect, which improves myocardial contractility, helping to compensate for myocardial damage.

  3. Cardiogenic shock

    a. In this life-threatening complication, cardiac output is decreased and pulmonary artery and pulmonary capillary wedge pressures are increased. This typically occurs when the area of infarction exceeds 40% of muscle mass and compensatory mechanisms only strain the already compromised myocardium.

    b. Vasopressors [e.g., norepinephrine, epinephrine, dopamine (high doses)] enhance blood pressure through α-receptor stimulation and may be indicated.

    c. Inotropic drugs [e.g., epinephrine, dopamine (middle doses), dobutamine, isoproterenol, digitalis] are rapidly acting agents used to increase myocardial contractility and improve cardiac output.

    d. Vasodilators (e.g., nitroprusside) reduce preload; they lower pulmonary capillary wedge pressure by dilating veins and reduce afterload by decreasing resistance to left ventricular ejection.

    e. Additional treatment may include invasive procedures such as intra-aortic balloon pumping.

STUDY QUESTIONS

Directions: Each of the numbered items or incomplete statements in this section is followed by answers or by completions of the statement. Select the **one** lettered answer or completion that is **best** in each case.

1. Exertion-induced angina, which is relieved by rest, nitroglycerin, or both, is referred to as

(A) Prinzmetal's angina
(B) unstable angina
(C) stable angina
(D) variant angina
(E) preinfarction angina

2. Myocardial oxygen demand is increased by all of the following factors EXCEPT

(A) exercise
(B) smoking
(C) cold temperatures
(D) isoproterenol
(E) metoprolol

3. Which of the following agents used in Prinzmetal's angina has spasmolytic actions, which increase coronary blood supply?

(A) Nitroglycerin
(B) Diltiazem
(C) Timolol
(D) Isosorbide mononitrate
(E) Propranolol

4. Patients with angina pectoris receiving propranolol plus diltiazem must be monitored for what adverse drug effect?

(A) Decreased cardiac output
(B) Decreased heart rate
(C) Increased heart rate
(D) Both A and B
(E) Both A and C

5. The development of ischemic pain occurs when the demand for oxygen exceeds the supply. Determinants of oxygen demand include all of the following choices EXCEPT

(A) contractile state of the heart
(B) myocardial ejection time
(C) left ventricular volume
(D) right atrial pressure
(E) systolic pressure

6. Myopathy is an adverse effect of all the following agents EXCEPT

(A) lovastatin
(B) simvastatin
(C) pravastatin
(D) gemfibrozil
(E) colestipol

7. Which of the following would not represent current therapeutic options in patients presenting with ACS who are classified as having NSTEMI?

(A) SL nitroglycerin
(B) β-adrenergic blockers
(C) Aspirin
(D) Morphine
(E) Tenecteplase

Directions: Each question below contains three suggested answers, of which **one or more** is correct. Choose the answer

A	if **I only** is correct
B	if **III only** is correct
C	if **I and II** are correct
D	if **II and III** are correct
E	if **I, II, and III** are correct

Questions 8–10

A 55-year-old man is approximately 6 hours after developing chest pain in the emergency room, in a local hospital with the signs and symptoms of an acute ST-segment elevated myocardial infarction (STEMI). This is the second such attack within the last 4 months, and the patient has not altered his life style to eliminate important risk factors. Previous therapy included a thrombolytic agent (name unknown), a blood thinner, and daily aspirin.

8. Which of the following thrombolytic agents would not be appropriate at this time?

I. Streptokinase (SK)
II. Tenecteplase
III. t-PA

9. Which of the following agents should be recommended during the acute MI to help prevent sudden death?

I. Atenolol
II. Metoprolol
III. Ramipril

10. Which of the following terms is considered a component of the ACS?

I. Unstable angina
II. NSTEMI
III. STEMI

Questions 11–15

For the following list of drugs provided, select the statement that best describes the drugs listed:

11. Tirofiban — A. Inhibition of intestinal absorption of cholesterol

12. Enoxaparin — B. Lowering of LDL, triglycerides, and increased HDL along with anti-inflammatory effects

13. Simvastatin — C. Glycoprotein IIb/IIIa antagonist that inhibits platelet aggregation

14. Clopidogrel — D. Recommended in ACS in those patients who can't tolerate aspirin

15. Ezetimibe — E. Recommended over UFH as an anticoagulant in patients with UA/NSTEMI

ANSWERS AND EXPLANATIONS

1. The answer is C *[II C 1 a–f].*
Classic, or stable, angina refers to the syndrome in which physical activity or emotional excess causes chest discomfort, which may spread to the arms, legs, neck, and so forth. This type of angina is relieved promptly (within 1–10 minutes) with rest, nitroglycerin, or both.

2. The answer is E *[I F 2; Table 38-1].*
Due to the β-adrenergic blocking effects of metoprolol (e.g., decreased heart rate, decreased blood pressure, decreased inotropic effect), there is a net decrease in myocardial oxygen demand. This is the direct opposite of the effects seen with the β-agonist isoproterenol. Exercise, cigarette smoking, and exposure to cold temperatures have all been shown to increase myocardial oxygen demand.

3. The answer is B *[II C 4 d].*
Calcium-channel blocking agents such as diltiazem have been shown to be capable of reversing spasm and, therefore, increasing coronary blood flow in Prinzmetal's angina. The calcium-channel blockers have proven benefit in the treatment of Prinzmetal's angina, a syndrome believed due more to a spastic event than to a fixed coronary occlusion.

4. The answer is D *[II G 4 c (I) (a) and II G 3 b (2)].*
Because propranolol (a β-adrenergic blocker) and diltiazem (a calcium-channel blocker) both reduce heart rate (a negative chronotropic effect) and reduce cardiac contractility (negative inotropic effect), patients receiving both drugs must be monitored for signs of decompensation (reduced cardiac output) and bradyarrhythmias.

5. The answer is D *[I F 2].*
As with most muscles in the body, the contractile force of the heart dictates the amount of oxygen that the heart needs to perform efficiently. Consequently, as contractility decreases, the oxygen needs of the heart increase. As contractility continues to decrease, the volume of fluid in the left ventricle increases due to poor muscle performance and increasing tension within the ventricle, resulting in additional oxygen requirements. As the amount of tension within the ventricle increases per cardiac cycle, there is again an added requirement for oxygen by the heart muscle.

6. The answer is E *[II F 4 a viii (c) (3).*
Myopathy is an adverse effect of all the HMG-CoA reductase inhibitors (lovastatin, simvastatin, pravastatin, atorvastatin, and fluvastatin), and the combination of the fibric acid derivatives (gemfibrozil, fenofibrate, and clofibrate) has been shown to increase the creatine kinase levels and predispose patients to myopathies and rhabdomyolysis.

7. The answer is E *[III G 2–3].*
Tenecteplase is the newest of the thrombolytics available for clinical use. The most recent guidelines for the treatment of unstable angina (UA) and non–ST-segment elevated myocardial infarction (NSTEMI) utilize expert opinion along with the clinical literature to provide evidence-based guidelines, and to date, thrombolytic agents have not demonstrated beneficial clinical outcomes in patients with UA or NSTEMI as compared to standard therapy. Additionally, thrombolytic agents actually increased the risk of MI in such patients. Therefore, based on current evidence-based guidelines, thrombolytic agents are not recommended in the management of ACS without ST-segment elevation.

8. The answer is A (I) *[III H C 2 b].*
Streptokinase (SK) is derived from exogenous substances, which initiate antibody formation after initial exposure. A patient receiving it within 6 months of previous exposure may have a refractory response to them due to excess antibody production. It has also been speculated that such patients may have an increased likelihood of developing an allergic reaction. Recombinant tissue-type plasminogen activator (t-PA) and tenecteplase represent recombinant DNA technology in which exogenous substances are not introduced into the body. The likelihood for antibody formation is nil, and these agents have been the preferred lytics based on evidence obtained from large clinical trials. Barring any contraindications, they would both be indicated for this patient. However, in a recent trial (ASSENT-2) comparing the two agents, tenecteplase was shown to have better clinical outcomes than t-PA in patients treated with a lytic more than 4 hours after symptom onset.

9. The answer is C (I and II) *[III H 1 d 6 (b)].*
Recent studies have made it relatively clear that when atenolol, metoprolol, and propranolol are given during the acute phases of a myocardial infarction (MI), there is a significant reduction in sudden death and overall mortality in the patients treated. Each of these β-adrenergic blockers is given intravenously, followed by oral therapy, in an attempt to eliminate sudden death as a consequence of MI. Because of the negative inotropic and chronotropic effects, it is still imperative to monitor the patient closely for signs of cardiac decompensation and bradyarrhythmias.

10. The answer is E (all) *[I E 2].*
During recent years, there has been an attempt to link the various clinical symptoms that represent IHD into key categories, based on the presentation and symptoms upon evaluation. ACS refers to those situations reflective of an acute ischemic event and includes unstable angina (UA) [potential impending MI] along with two forms of MIs, which are the non–ST-segment elevated MI (NSTEMI) and the ST–segment elevated MI (STEMI). Clinical guidelines have incorporated treatment modalities based on the three major presentations of the ACS in which UA/NSTEMI are combined with consistent therapy as compared to STEMI, which has different treatment guidelines. Stable angina is not considered one of the ACS but represents the starting point for the progression of atherosclerosis resulting in IHD.

11. The answer is C *[III H 1 d iv].*
Tirofiban is an antiplatelet that is referred to as a glycoprotein IIb/III, a receptor antagonist. This class of drugs works to prevent platelet aggregation by inhibiting the interaction between the primary binding site of platelets and has been shown to be effective in the prevention of thrombosis.

12. The answer is E *[III G 3 b (2), Table 38-5].*
Enoxaparin is an example of the class of drugs referred to as low–molecular-weight heparins, and as a group, a major advantage of them over the more traditional heparin is that they exhibit a more predictable anticoagulant response. Due to their lower molecular weight and decreased binding to plasma proteins, they have better bioavailability than heparin. Additionally, their decrease in plasma protein binding and binding to the endothelium results in half-lives that are 2–4 times longer than that of heparin. Current clinical practice guidelines recommend enoxaparin over heparin in patients with UA or NSTEMI unless CABG is planned within 24 hours.

13. The answer is B *[III H 1 d 8].*
Simvastatin is one of the 5 currently available HMG-CoA reductase inhibitors, which have been shown to significantly reduce LDL levels and nonfatal MI or CHD (30%–40% reduction). Recent studies have demonstrated that inflammation is an important mechanism involved in ACS and that statins exert an important anti-inflammatory effect within coronary arteries (independent of their cholesterol-lowering effects).

14. The answer is D *[III G 3 a (2)].*
Clopidogrel is a thienopyridine derivative related to ticlopidine that possesses antithrombotic effects that are greater than those of ticlopidine. Clopidogrel is a therapeutic option in those angina patients who can not take aspirin due to contraindications. Doses of 75 mg daily are recommended to prevent the development of acute coronary syndromes.

15. The answer is A *[II F 4 a 11].*
Ezetimibe is the first in a new class of lipid-lowering compounds approved by the FDA, which has a different mechanism of action that reduces cholesterol levels. By selectively blocking the intestinal absorption of cholesterol, it is able to stop one of the major pathways responsible for increasing available cholesterol within the body. Ezetimibe has demonstrated the ability to reduce total cholesterol, LDL, apolipoprotein B, and triglyceride levels while increasing HDL levels in patients with hypercholesterolemia.

39

Cardiac Arrhythmias

Alan H. Mutnick

I. INTRODUCTION. Sudden death from cardiac causes is believed to account for approximately 50% of all deaths from cardiovascular causes, with the majority of sudden deaths being caused by acute ventricular tachyarrhythmias. This would appear to create greater need for the knowledge necessary to appropriately utilize antiarrhymics for this high-risk patient population. However, recently conducted studies have cast doubt on the true place of antiarrhythmics in the treatment and prevention of cardiac arrhythmias. Studies such as the Cardiac Arrhythmia Suppression Trial (CAST) have demonstrated that certain classes of antiarrhythmics increased mortality in patients treated with antiarrhythmics as compared to placebo. Consequently, the use of trial and error to determine antiarrhythmic therapy has given way to an era of outcome-based antiarrhythmic drug decision making. By understanding the causes of arrhythmias and being aware of drug–drug and drug–target interactions, we are more likely to understand the key considerations in order to maximize therapeutic strategies while minimizing drug-induced toxicities.

A. Definition. Cardiac arrhythmias are deviations from the normal heartbeat pattern. They include **abnormalities of impulse formation,** such as heart rate, rhythm, or site of impulse origin, and **conduction disturbances,** which disrupt the normal sequence of atrial and ventricular activation.

B. Electrophysiology

1. **Conduction system**
   a. **Two electrical sequences** that cause the heart chambers to fill with blood and contract are initiated by the conduction system of the heart.
      (1) **Impulse formation,** the first sequence, takes place when an electrical impulse is generated automatically.
      (2) **Impulse transmission,** the second sequence, occurs once the impulse has been generated, signaling the heart to contract.
   b. **Four main structures** composed of tissue that can generate or conduct electrical impulses comprise the conduction system of the heart.
      (1) The **sinoatrial (SA) node,** in the wall of the right atrium, contains cells that spontaneously initiate an action potential. Serving as the main pacemaker of the heart, the SA node initiates 60–100 beats/min.
         (a) Impulses generated by the SA node trigger atrial contraction.
         (b) Impulses travel through internodal tracts—the anterior tract, middle tract (Wenckebach's bundle), posterior tract (Thorel's bundle), and anterior interatrial tract (Bachmann's bundle) [Figure 39-1].
      (2) At the **atrioventricular (AV) node,** situated in the lower interatrial septum, the impulses are delayed briefly to permit completion of atrial contraction before ventricular contraction begins.
      (3) At the **bundle of His**—muscle fibers arising from the AV junction—impulses travel along the left and right bundle branches, located on either side of the intraventricular septum.
      (4) The impulses reach the **Purkinje fibers,** a diffuse network extending from the bundle branches and ending in the ventricular endocardial surfaces. Ventricular contraction then occurs.
   c. **Latent pacemakers.** The AV junction, bundle of His, and Purkinje fibers are latent pacemakers; they contain cells capable of generating impulses. However, these regions have a slower firing rate than the SA node. Consequently, the SA node predominates except when it is depressed or injured, which is known as **overdrive suppression.**

2. **Myocardial action potential.** Before cardiac contraction can take place, cardiac cells must depolarize and repolarize.
   a. **Depolarization** and **repolarization** result from changes in the electrical potential across the cell membrane, caused by the exchange of sodium and potassium ions.

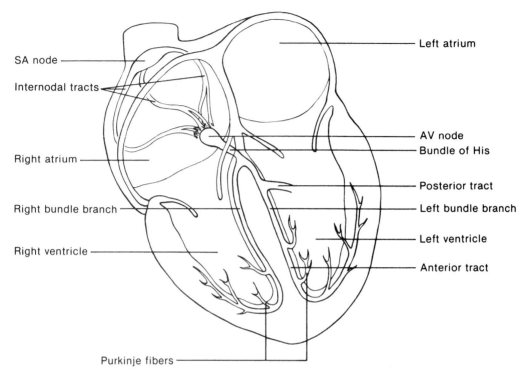

Figure 39-1. Electrical pathways of the heart. *SA* = sinoatrial; *AV* = atrioventricular.

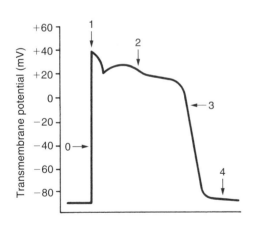

Figure 39-2. Myocardial action potential curve. This curve represents ventricular depolarization/repolarization. *0* = phase 0 (rapid depolarization); *1* = phase 1 (early rapid repolarization); *2* = phase 2 (plateau); *3* = phase 3 (final rapid repolarization); *4* = phase 4 (slow depolarization).

  b. Action potential, which reflects this electrical activity, has five phases (Figure 39-2).
  - **(1) Phase 0 (rapid depolarization)** takes place as sodium ions enter the cell through fast channels; the cell membrane's electrical charge changes from negative to positive.
  - **(2) Phase 1 (early rapid repolarization).** As fast sodium channels close and potassium ions leave the cell, the cell rapidly repolarizes (i.e., returns to resting potential).
  - **(3) Phase 2 (plateau).** Calcium ions enter the cell through slow channels while potassium ions exit. As the cell membrane's electrical activity temporarily stabilizes, the action potential reaches a plateau (represented by the notch at the beginning of this phase in Figure 39-2).
  - **(4) Phase 3 (final rapid repolarization).** Potassium ions are pumped out of the cell as the cell rapidly completes repolarization and resumes its initial negativity.
  - **(5) Phase 4 (slow depolarization).** The cell returns to its resting state with potassium ions inside the cell and sodium and calcium ions outside.

    c. During both depolarization and repolarization, a cell's ability to initiate an action potential varies.

        (1) The cell cannot respond to any stimulus during the **absolute refractory period** (beginning during phase 1 and ending at the start of phase 3).

        (2) A cell's ability to respond to stimuli increases as repolarization continues. During the **relative refractory period,** which occurs during phase 3, the cell can respond to a strong stimulus.

        (3) When the cell has been completely repolarized, it can again respond fully to stimuli.

    d. Cells in different cardiac regions depolarize at various speeds, depending on whether fast or slow channels predominate.

        (1) Sodium flows through fast channels; calcium flows through slow channels.

        (2) Where fast channels dominate (e.g., in cardiac muscle cells), depolarization occurs quickly. Where slow channels dominate (e.g., in the electrical cells of the SA node and AV junction), depolarization occurs slowly.

3. Electrocardiography. The electrical activity occurring during depolarization–repolarization can be transmitted through electrodes attached to the body and transformed by an **electrocardiograph (ECG) machine** into a series of waveforms (ECG waveform). Figure 39-3 shows a normal ECG waveform.

    a. The **P wave** reflects atrial depolarization.

    b. The **PR interval** represents the spread of the impulse from the atria through the Purkinje fibers.

    c. The **QRS complex** reflects ventricular depolarization.

    d. The **ST segment** represents phase 2 of the action potential—the absolute refractory period (part of ventricular repolarization).

    e. The **T wave** shows phase 3 of the action potential—ventricular repolarization.

C. Classification. Arrhythmias generally are classified by origin (i.e., supraventricular or ventricular).

1. Supraventricular arrhythmias stem from enhanced automaticity of the SA node (or another pacemaker region) or from reentry conduction.

2. Ventricular arrhythmias occur when an ectopic (abnormal) pacemaker triggers a ventricular contraction before the SA node fires (e.g., from a conduction disturbance or ventricular irritability).

3. Special note

    a. Torsades de Pointes has received increased attention during the last few years as a major proarrhythmic event, which has been reported with antiarrhythmic drug therapy. It is defined as a polymorphic ventricular tachycardia with a twisting QRS complex morphology, which sometimes occurs with drugs that prolong ventricular repolarization (QT interval widening). Though initial reports of Torsades de Pointes centered around antiarrhythmic drugs (quinidine), today more than 50 drugs, both antiarrhythmic agents as well as other classes of drugs such as antibiotics, have been shown to affect the duration of the QT interval and have been associated with this arrhythmia.

    b. Recently, a website referred to as "QTdrugs.org" was initiated and is currently maintained by Dr. Raymond Woosley. It is devoted to providing education and research on drug-induced arrhythmias, especially those due to prolongation of the QT interval on the electrocardiogram (ECG).

    c. Dr. Woosley and colleagues have established an International Registry for Drug-Induced Arrhythmias in which one can submit to the registry a suspected "drug-induced arrhythmia event" while also providing a list of drugs reported to prolong QT intervals or cause Torsades de Pointes (www.Torsades.org). Four separate drug lists were developed based on the relative risk of inducing Torsades de Pointes (dTp) or prolonged QT interval (See Table 39-1).

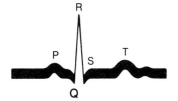

Figure 39-3. Normal ECG waveform.

Table 39-1. Drugs that Prolong the QT Interval and/or Induce Torsades De Pointes

List 1-Drugs that are generally accepted by authorities to have a risk of causing Torsades de Pointes

Drug (Generic)	Brand Names	Drug Class (Clinical Usage)	Comments
Amiodarone	Cordarone Pacerone	Antiarrhythmic/abnormal heart rhythm	F > M,TdP risk regarded as low
Arsenic trioxide	Trisenox	Anti-cancer/Leukemia	
Bepridil	Vascor	Anti-anginal/heart pain	F > M
Chlorpromazine	Thorazine	Antipsychotic/Antiemetic/ schizophrenia/nausea	
Cisapride	Propulsid	GI stimulant/heartburn	Restricted availability; F > M
Clarithromycin	Biaxin	Antibiotic/bacterial infection	
Disopyramide	Norpace	Anti-arrhythmic/abnormal heart rhythm	F > M
Dofetilide	Tikosyn	Antiarrhythmic/abnormal heart rhythm	
Domperidone	Motilium	Antinausea/nausea	
Droperidol	Inapsine	Sedative; Antinausea/anesthesia adjunct, nausea	
Erythromycin	E.E.S., Erythrocin	Antibiotic; GI stimulant/bacterial infection; increase GI motility	F > M
Halofantrine	Halfan	Antimalarial/malaria infection	F > M
Haloperidol	Haldol	Antipsychotic/schizophrenia, agitation	
Ibutilide	Corvert	Antiarrhythmic/abnormal heart rhythm	F > M
Levomethadyl	Orlaam	Opiate agonist/pain control, narcotic dependence	
Mesoridazine	Serentil	Antipsychotic/schizophrenia	
Methadone	Dolophine	Opiate agonist/pain control, narcotic dependence	F > M
Methadone	Methadose	Opiate agonist/pain control, narcotic dependence	F > M
Pentamidine	NebuPent, Pentam	Anti-infective/Pneumocystis pneumonia	F > M
Pimozide	Orap	Antipsychotic/Tourette's tics	F > M
Procainamide	Pronestyl, Procan	Antiarrhythmic/abnormal heart rhythm	
Quinidine	Quinaglute, Cardioquin	Antiarrhythmic/abnormal heart rhythm	F > M

List 2-Drugs that in some reports may be associated with Torsades de Pointes but at this time lack substantial evidence for causing Torsades de Pointes.

Drug (Generic)	Brand Names	Drug Class (Clinical Usage)
Amantadine	Symmetrel	Dopaminergic/Antiviral/Anti-infective/ Parkinson's Disease
Azithromycin	Zithromax	Antibiotic/bacterial infection
Chloral hydrate	Noctec	Sedative/sedation/insomnia
Dolasetron	Anzemet	Antinausea/nausea, vomiting
Felbamate	Felbatrol	Anticonvulsant/seizure
Flecainide	Tambocor	Antiarrhythmic/abnormal heart rhythm
Foscarnet	Foscavir	Antiviral/HIV infection
Fosphenytoin	Cerebyx	Anticonvulsant/seizure
Gaitfloxacin	Tequin	Antibiotic/bacterial infection
Granisetron	Kytril	Antinausea/nausea and vomiting
Indapamide	Lozol	Diuretic/stimulate urine & salt loss
Isradipine	Dynacirc	Antihypertensive/high blood pressure
Levofloxacin	Levaquin	Antibiotic/bacterial infection
Lithium	Eskalith, Lithobid	Antimania/bipolar disorder

Table 39-1. *Continued*

Drug (Generic)	Brand Names	Drug Class (Clinical Usage)
Moexipril/HCTZ	Uniretic	Antihypertensive/high blood pressure
Moxifloxacin	Avelox	Antibiotic/bacterial infection
Nicardipine	Cardene	Antihypertensive/high blood pressure
Octreotide	Sandostatin	Endocrine/acromegaly, carcinoid diarrhea
Ondansetron	Zofran	Antiemetic/nausea and vomiting
Quetiapine	Seroquel	Antipsychotic/schizophrenia
Risperidone	Risperdal	Antipsychotic/schizophrenia
Salmeterol	Serevent	Sympathomimetic/asthma, COPD
Tacrolimus	Prograf	Immunosuppressant/Immune suppression
Tamoxifen	Nolvadex	Anticancer/breast cancer
Telithromycin	Ketek	Antibiotic/bacterial infection
Tizanidine	Zanaflex	Muscle relaxant
Venlafaxine	Effexor	Antidepressant/depression
Voriconazole	VFend	Antifungal/antifungal
Ziprasidone	Geodon	Antipsychotic/schizophrenia

List 3- Drugs to be avoided for use in patients with diagnosed or suspected cogenital long QT syndrome. (Drugs on Lists 1 and 2 are also included here.)

Drug (Generic)	Brand Names	Drug Class (Clinical Usage)	Comments	List
Albuterol	Ventolin	Bronchodilator/Asthma		3
Albuterol	Proventil	Bronchodilator/Asthma		3
Amantadine	Symmetrel	Dopaminergic/Antiviral/Anti-infective/ Parkinson's Disease		2
Amiodarone	Cordarone, Pacerone	Antiarrhythmic/abnormal heart rhythm	F > M, TdP risk regarded as low	1
Arsenic trioxide	Trisenox	Anti-cancer/Leukemia		1
Azithromycin	Zithromax	Antibiotic/bacterial infection		2
Bepridil	Vascor	Antianginal/heart pain	F > M	1
Chloral hydrate	Noctec	Sedative/sedation/insomnia		2
Chlorpromazine	Thorazine	Antipsychotic/Antiemetic/ schizophrenia/ nausea	Restricted avail- ability; F > M	1
Cisapride	Propulsid	GI stimulant/heartburn		1
Clarithromycin	Biaxin	Antibiotic/bacterial infection		1
Cocaine	Cocaine	Local anesthetic		3
Disopyramide	Norpace	Antiarrhythmic/abnormal heart rhythm	F > M	1
Dobutamine	Dobutrex	Catecholamine/heart failure and shock		3
Dofetilide	Tikosyn	Antiarrhythmic/abnormal heart rhythm		1
Dolasetron	Anzemet	Antinausea/nausea, vomiting		2
Domperidone	Motilium	Antinausea/nausea		1
Dopamine	Intropine	Antiarrhythmic/abnormal heart rhythm		3
Droperidol	Inapsine	Sedative; Antinausea/anesthesia adjunct, nausea		1
Ephedrine	Rynatuss, Broncholate	Bronchodilator, decongestant/ allergies, sinusitis, asthma		3
Epinephrine	Primatene, Bronkaid	catecholamine, vasoconstrictor/ anaphylaxis, allergic reactions		3
Erythromycin	E.E.S., Erythrocin	Antibiotic; GI stimulant/bacterial infection; increase GI motility	F > M	1
Felbamate	Felbatrol	Anti-convulsant/seizure		2
Fenfluramine	Pondimin	Appetite suppressant/dieting, weight loss		3
Flecainide	Tambocor	Antiarrhythmic/abnormal heart rhythm		2

Table 39-1. *Continued*

List 3- Drugs to be avoided for use in patients with diagnosed or suspected cogenital long QT syndrome. (Drugs on Lists 1 and 2 are also included here.)

Drug (Generic)	Brand Names	Drug Class (Clinical Usage)	Comments	List
Foscarnet	Foscavir	Antiviral/HIV infection		2
Fosphenytoin	Cerebyx	Anticonvulsant/seizure		2
Gaitfloxacin	Tequin	Antibiotic/bacterial infection		2
Granisetron	Kytril	Antinausea/nausea and vomiting		2
Halofantrine	Halfan	Antimalarial/malaria infection		1
Haloperidol	Haldol	Antipsychotic/schizophrenia, agitation	F > M	1
Ibutilide	Corvert	Antiarrhythmic/abnormal heart rhythm	F > M	1
Indapamide	Lozol	Diuretic/stimulate urine & salt loss		2
Isoproterenol	Medihaler-Iso, Isupres	Catecholamine/allergic reaction		3
Isradipine	Dynacirc	Antihypertensive/high blood pressure		2
Levalbuterol	Xopenex	Bronchodilator/asthma		3
Levofloxacin	Levaquin	Antibiotic/bacterial infection		2
Levomethadyl	Orlaam	Opiate agonist/pain control, narcotic dependence		1
Lithium	Eskalith, Lithobid	Antimania/bipolar disorder		2
Mesoridazine	Serentil	Antipsychotic/schizophrenia		1
Metaproterenol	Metaprel, Alupent	Bronchodilator/asthma		3
Methadone	Dolophine, Methadose	Opiate agonist/pain control, narcotic dependence	F > M	1
Midodrine	ProAmatine	Vasoconstrictor/low blood pressure, fainting		3
Moexipril/HCTZ	Uniretic	Antihypertensive/high blood pressure		2
Moxifloxacin	Avelox	Antibiotic/bacterial infection		2
Nicardipine	Cardene	Antihypertensive/high blood pressure		2
Norepinephrine	Levophed	Vasconstrictor, Inotrope/shock, low blood pressure		3
Octreotide	Sandostatin	Endocrine/acromegaly, carcinoid diarrhea		2
Ondansetron	Zofran	Antiemetic/nausea and vomiting		2
Pentamidine	NebuPent, Pentam	Anti-infective/Pneumocystis pneumonia	F > M	1
Phentermine	Adipex, Fastin	Appetite suppressant/dieting, weight loss		3
Phenylephrine	Neosynephrine	Vasoconstrictor, decongestant/low blood pressure, allergies, sinusitis, asthma		3
Phenylpropanola mine	Acutrim, Dexatrim	Decongestant/allergies, sinusitis, asthma		3
Pimozide	Orap	Antipsychotic/Tourette's tics	F > M	1
Procainamide	Pronestyl	Antiarrhythmic/abnormal heart rhythm		1
Procainamide	Procan	Antiarrhythmic/abnormal heart rhythm		1
Pseudoephedrine	PediaCare	Decongestant/allergies, sinusitis, asthma		3
Pseudoephedrine	Sudafed	Decongestant/allergies, sinusitis, asthma		3
Quetiapine	Seroquel	Antipsychotic/schizophrenia	F > M	2
Quinidine	Quiniglute, Cardioquin	Antiarrhythmic/abnormal heart rhythm		1

Table 39-1. *Continued*

List 3- Drugs to be avoided for use in patients with diagnosed or suspected cogenital long QT syndrome. (Drugs on Lists 1 and 2 are also included here.)

Drug (Generic)	Brand Names	Drug Class (Clinical Usage)	Comments	List
Risperidone	Risperdal	Antipsychotic/schizophrenia		2
Ritodrine	Yutopar	Uterine relaxant/prevent premature labor		3
Salmeterol	Serevent	Sympathomimetic/asthma, COPD		2
Sibutramine	Meridia	Appetite suppressant/dieting, weight loss	F > M	3
Sotalol	Betapace	Antiarrhythmic/abnormal heart rhythm		1
Sparfloxacin	Zagam	Antibiotic/bacterial infection		1
Tacrolimus	Prograf	Immunosuppressant/Immune suppression		2
Tamoxifen	Nolvadex	Anti-cancer/breast cancer		2
Telithromycin	Ketek	Antibiotic/bacterial infection		2
Terbutaline	Brethine	Bronchodilator/asthma		3
Thioridazine	Mellaril	Antipsychotic/schizophrenia		1
Tizanidine	Zanaflex	Muscle relaxant		2
Venlafaxine	Effexor	Antidepressant/depression		2
Voriconazole	VFend	Antifungal/anti-fungal		2
Ziprasidone	Geodon	Antipsychotic/schizophrenia		2

List 4- Drugs that, in some reports, have been weakly associated with Torsades de Pointes but that, when used in usual dosages, are unlikely to be a risk for Torsades de Pointes.

Drug (Generic)	Brand Names	Drug Class (Clinical Usage)
Amitriptyline	Elavil	Tricyclic Antidepressant/depression
Amoxapine	Asendin	Tricyclic Antidepressant/depression
Ampicillin	Principen, Omnipen	Antibiotic/infection
Ciprofloxacin	Cipro	Antibiotic/bacterial infection
Clomipramine	Anafranil	Tricyclic Antidepressant/depression
Desipramine	Pertofrane	Tricyclic Antidepressant/depression
Doxepin	Sinequan	Tricyclic Antidepressant/depression
Fluconazole	Diflucan	Antifungal/fungal infection
Fluoxetine	Sarafem, Prozac	Anti-depressant/depression
Galantamine	Reminyl	Cholinesterase inhibitor/Dementia, Alzheimer's
Imipramine	Norfranil	Tricyclic Antidepressant/depression
Itraconazole	Sporanox	Antifungal/fungal infection
Ketoconazole	Nizoral	Antifungal/fungal infection
Mexiletine	Mexitil	Antiarrhythmic/Abnormal heart rhythm
Nortriptyline	Pamelor	Tricyclic Antidepressant/depression
Paroxetine	Paxil	Anti-depressant/depression
Protriptyline	Vivactil	Tricyclic Antidepressant/depression
Sertraline	Zoloft	Anti-depressant/depression
Trimethoprim-Sulfamethoxazole	Septra, Bactrim	Antibiotic/bacterial infection
Trimipramine	Surmontil	Tricyclic Antidepressant/depression

Reproduced with permission from Dr. Raymond Woosley, MD, PhD, Vice President for Health Sciences at the University of Arizona Health Sciences Center. At www.Torsades.org; viewed on October 21, 2002 and revised on June 6, 2003.

The University of Arizona Center for Education and Research on Therapeutics

Arizona Health Sciences Center; Most recently revised on 12/17/02.

Tucson, Arizona 85724-5018

Funded in part by Agency for Healthcare Research and Quality grant 1 U18 HS10385-01

Key:
- TdP: The FDA-approved labeling includes mention of cases or a risk of Torsades de Pointes (TdP).
- F > M (Females > Males): Substantial evidence indicates a greater risk (usually > two-fold) of TdP in women.

D. Etiology

1. **Precipitating causes.** Arrhythmias result from various conditions, including:
   a. Heart disease [e.g., infection, coronary artery disease (CAD), valvular heart disease, rheumatic heart disease, ischemic heart disease]
   b. Myocardial infarction (MI)
   c. Toxic doses of cardioactive drugs (e.g., digitalis preparations)
   d. Increased sympathetic tone
   e. Decreased parasympathetic tone
   f. Vagal stimulation (e.g., straining at stool)
   g. Increased oxygen demand (e.g., from stress, exercise, fever)
   h. Metabolic disturbances
   i. Cor pulmonale
   j. Systemic hypertension
   k. Hyperkalemia/hypokalemia
   l. Chronic obstructive pulmonary disease (COPD) [e.g., chronic bronchitis, emphysema]
   m. Thyroid disorders
   n. Drug therapy (both antiarrhythmic and nonantiarrhythmic drugs)

2. **Mechanisms of arrhythmias.** Abnormal impulse formation, abnormal impulse conduction, or a combination of both may give rise to arrhythmias.
   a. **Abnormal impulse formation** may stem from:
      (1) Depressed automaticity, as in escape beats and bradycardia
      (2) Increased automaticity, as in premature beats, tachycardia, and extrasystole
      (3) Depolarization and triggered activity, leading to sustained ectopic firing
   b. **Abnormal impulse conduction** results from:
      (1) A conduction block or delay
      (2) **Reentry** occurs when an impulse is rerouted through certain regions in which it has already traveled. Thus, the impulse depolarizes the same tissue more than once, producing an additional impulse (Figures 39-4 and 39-5). Reentry sites include the SA and AV nodes as well as various accessory pathways in the atria and ventricles (Figure 39-6). For reentry to occur, the following conditions must exist:
         (a) Markedly shortened refractoriness or a slow conduction area that allows an adequate delay so that depolarization recurs
         (b) Unidirectional conduction

E. Pathophysiology.
Arrhythmias may decrease cardiac output, reduce blood pressure, and disrupt perfusion of vital organs. Specific pathophysiological consequences depend on the arrhythmia present.

F. Clinical evaluation

1. **Physical findings.** Although some arrhythmias are silent, most produce signs and symptoms. Only an ECG can definitively identify an arrhythmia. However, physical findings may suggest which arrhythmia is present; they also yield information about the patient's clinical status and may help to identify associated complications. **Signs and symptoms** that typically accompany arrhythmias include:
   a. Chest pain
   b. Anxiety and confusion (from reduced brain perfusion)

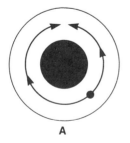 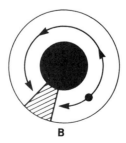 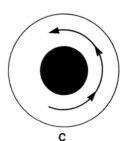

Figure 39-4. Reentry arrhythmias. *A* shows two waves of excitation going in opposite directions; *B* represents a unidirectional wave of excitation; *C* shows reexcitation of tissue in a slow conduction area.

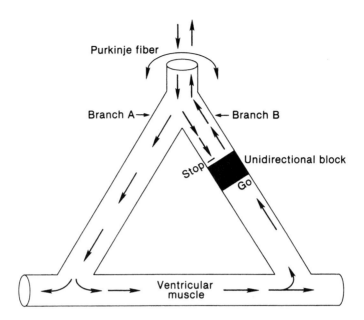

Figure 39-5. Ventricular reentry. This diagram shows a branched Purkinje fiber joining ventricular muscle. The *dark area* represents the site of a unidirectional block; in this depolarization region, the impulse heading toward the AV node continues upward, whereas the impulse traveling toward the muscle is blocked. Because retrograde conduction in *branch B* is slow, cells in *branch A* have time to recover and respond to the reentrant impulse.

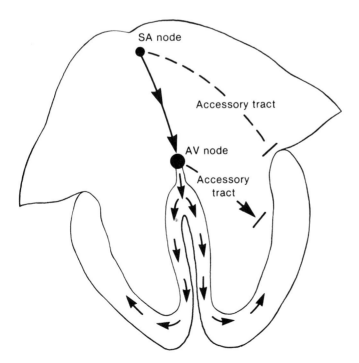

Figure 39-6. Reentry sites.

    c. Dyspnea
    d. Skin pallor or cyanosis
    e. Abnormal pulse rate, rhythm, or amplitude
    f. Reduced blood pressure
    g. Palpitations
    h. Syncope
    i. Weakness
    j. Convulsions
    k. Hypotension
    l. Decreased urinary output

  2. Diagnostic test results
    a. An **ECG** can identify a specific arrhythmia; usually, a 12-lead ECG is used.
    b. **Electrophysiological (EP) testing.** This intracardiac procedure determines the location of ectopic foci and bypass tracts and may help assess therapeutic response to antiarrhythmic drug therapy. It also can determine the need for a pacemaker or surgical intervention.
      (1) Intracardiac catheters and pacing wires are placed transvenously or transarterially.
      (2) The heart is divided into imaginary sections, and each section is stimulated until an arrhythmia is induced. The section in which the arrhythmia occurs is identified as the origin of the ectopic foci.
    c. **His bundle study,** a type of EP testing, can locate the origin of a heart block or reentry pattern.
    d. **Laboratory findings.** Some arrhythmias result from electrolyte abnormalities—most commonly, hyperkalemia and hypocalcemia.
      (1) A serum potassium level above 5 mEq/L reflects hyperkalemia; a serum calcium level below 4.5 mEq/L signifies hypocalcemia.
      (2) An ECG tracing may suggest an electrolyte abnormality. For example, prolonged QRS complexes, tented T waves, and lengthened PR intervals may signal hyperkalemia; prolonged QT intervals and flattened, or inverted, T waves suggest hypocalcemia.

 G. Treatment objectives
  1. Terminate or **suppress the arrhythmia** if it causes hemodynamic compromise or disturbing symptoms.
  2. Maintain adequate cardiac output and tissue perfusion.
  3. Correct or maintain fluid balance (some arrhythmias cause hypervolemia).

II. THERAPY. Antiarrhythmic agents directly or indirectly alter the duration of the myocardial action potential. Most antiarrhythmics fall into one of four classes, depending on their specific effects on the heart's electrical activity (Table 39-2).

 A. Class I antiarrhythmics
  1. Indications
    a. **Class IA drugs**
      (1) Quinidine is used to treat and prevent acute and chronic ventricular and supraventricular arrhythmias, especially paroxysmal supraventricular tachycardias (PSVTs), premature ventricular contractions (PVCs), premature atrial contractions (PACs), and ventricular tachycardia.
      (2) Procainamide is used for the same arrhythmias for which quinidine is given. It is used more frequently than quinidine because it can be administered intravenously and in sustained-release oral preparations. Quinidine poses added concern when used intravenously because of increased cardiovascular effects (i.e., hypotension, syncope, myocardial depression).
      (3) Disopyramide may be used as an alternative to quinidine or procainamide for treating ventricular arrhythmias (e.g., PVCs, moderate ventricular tachycardia).
    b. **Class IB drugs**
      (1) Lidocaine is used therapeutically for ventricular arrhythmias (especially PVCs and ventricular tachycardia) that result from acute MI and open-heart surgery. Controversy still exists as to the benefits of lidocaine when used prophylactically in patients with acute MI to prevent ventricular fibrillation. A recent analysis showed an increase in the number of deaths in patients receiving lidocaine during an acute MI as compared to placebo. Many feel that its current use prophylactically post-MI is no longer justified.

Table 39-2. Vaughan Williams' Classification of Antiarrhythmic Drugs Currently Available in the United States

Class	Action	Drugs
IA (fast-channel blockers)	Moderate depression of conduction, prolongation of repolarization, which results in an increase in the QRS interval and an increase in the QT interval	Disopyramide (Norpace, various), procainamide (Pronestyl, various), quinidine (Quinidex, Quinaglute, various)
IB	Modest depression of conduction, shortening of repolarization, which results in a decrease in the QT interval	Lidocaine (Xylocaine, various), mexiletine (Mexitil, various), phenytoin (Dilantin, various), tocainide (Tonocard)
IC	Strong depression of conduction, with mild or no effect on repolarization, which results in a very large increase in the QRS interval	Flecainide (Tambocor), moricizine (Ethomozin), propafenone (Rhythmol, various)
II (β-blockers)	β-adrenergic blockers slow sinus as well as AV nodal conduction, which results in a decrease in heart rate and a prolongation in the PR interval (atrial depolarization)	Propranolol* (Inderal, various), esmolol* (Brevibloc), acebutolol* (Sectral)
III	Prolongation of repolarization, which results in prolongation of the QT interval	Amiodarone (Cordarone, various), sotalol† (Betapace, various), ibutilide (Corvert), dofetilide (Tikosyn)
IV (slow-channel blockers)	Calcium-channel blockade in calcium-dependent channels, which results in reduced heart rate and an increase in the PR interval	Verapamil (Calan, Isoptin, various), diltiazem (Cardizem, Tiazac, various)
Other		Adenosine, atropine, digoxin, magnesium

*Only propranolol, esmolol, and acebutolol are currently approved for use as antiarrhythmics.
†Sotalol is a β-adrenergic blocker, which is available and has been classified as a type III antiarrhythmic.

(2) **Tocainide,** closely related to lidocaine, is used to treat and prevent ventricular arrhythmias, including frequent PVCs and ventricular tachycardia. It may be given after an acute MI.

(3) **Phenytoin** is most commonly used to treat digitalis-induced ventricular and supraventricular arrhythmias. It is also given to suppress ventricular arrhythmias associated with acute MI, open-heart surgery, or ventricular arrhythmias that are refractory to lidocaine or procainamide, but its efficacy is less significant for these indications than it is for digitalis-induced arrhythmias.

(4) **Mexiletine** is closely related to lidocaine, structurally with modifications, which reduce first-pass liver metabolism, making oral therapy possible. It is most commonly used to treat patients in whom a class I agent has failed and is moderately effective in suppressing ventricular ectopy, although comparable to quinidine.

c. **Class IC drugs**

(1) **Flecainide** suppresses PVCs and ventricular tachycardia; it may be used to treat some arrhythmias that are refractory to other agents. Flecainide is reserved for patients with refractory life-threatening ventricular arrhythmias who do not have CAD. It has also been shown to be effective in the treatment of supraventricular arrhythmias.

(2) **Propafenone** also suppresses PVCs and ventricular tachycardia and has been used successfully for treating sustained ventricular tachycardia when the arrhythmia is life-threatening. It has also been shown to be effective in the treatment of supraventricular arrhythmias.

(3) **Moricizine** is a difficult antiarrhythmic to classify based on the fact that it has properties of all three class I antiarrhythmic groups. Because it prolongs the QRS interval like other class IC agents, it has been classified as a class IC agent throughout this discussion. Moricizine is effective for suppressing PVCs and may offer some benefits over other agents because of a lower incidence of proarrhythmic effects.

2. Mechanism of action. As a class, all of the agents work by blocking the rapid inward sodium current and thereby slow down the rate of rise of the cardiac tissue's action potential. However, though this is a similar effect for all class I agents, differences in EP effects had led to a subclassification of the class I agents into three subsets (IA, IB, and IC), based on these EP effects.

    a. Class IA drugs moderately reduce the depolarization rate and prolong repolarization (refractory period).

    b. Class IB drugs shorten repolarization (refractory period); they also weakly affect the repolarization rate.

    c. Class IC drugs strongly depress depolarization but have a negligible effect on the duration of repolarization or refractoriness.

3. Administration and dosage

    a. Quinidine is administered orally, usually in three or four daily doses of 200–400 mg as a rapid-release sulfate salt (83% quinidine). However, sustained-release products in the form of a gluconate (62% quinidine) salt or a polygalacturonate (60% quinidine) salt in doses of 324–648 mg, which corresponds to 300–600 mg of the sulfate salt, may be given every 8 hours (polygalacturonate) or 12 hours (gluconate). (In special circumstances, it has been given intravenously or intramuscularly with caution.) To achieve an effective plasma concentration rapidly, a loading dose of 600–1000 mg may be administered in doses of 200 mg every 2 hours to a maximum of 1000 mg, or a 5–8 mg/kg intravenous infusion can be given at a rate of 0.3 mg/kg/min.

    b. Procainamide is available for oral, intravenous, or intramuscular use.

      (1) For **acute therapy,** intravenous administration is preferred.

        (a) Intermittent intravenous administration calls for the administration of an intravenous dose of 3–6 mg/kg infusion (up to 100 mg) over 2–4 minutes, repeated every 5–10 minutes until the arrhythmia is abolished, side effects occur, or 1 g has been given. The usual effective dose is 500–1000 mg.

        (b) Rapid intravenous administration calls for infusion of 1–1.5 g at a rate of 20–50 mg/min.

        (c) Once the arrhythmia is terminated, 1.5–5 mg/min is given as a continuous infusion.

      (2) For **long-term therapy,** oral administration is used. The usual daily dosage is 50 mg/kg in divided doses given every 6 hours as a sustained-release product or 3–6 g daily.

        (a) Capsules and tablets (Pronestyl, various) available as 250, 375, and 500 mg given in 4–6 divided doses

        (b) Sustained-release tablets (Pronestyl-SR) available as 250, 500, 750, and 1000 mg given in 6-hour doses

        (c) Sustained-release tablets (Procanbid) available as 500 and 1000 mg given in 12-hour doses

    c. Disopyramide is available in oral form.

      (1) Usually, 300–400 mg is given as a loading dose to attain an effective plasma level rapidly.

      (2) For maintenance therapy, doses of 400–800 mg/day are given in four doses every 6 hours (non–sustained-release capsule) or in two doses every 12 hours (sustained-release capsule).

    d. Lidocaine may be administered intravenously or intramuscularly.

      (1) An intravenous loading dose rapidly achieves a therapeutic plasma level.

        (a) Initially, 1–1.5 mg/kg (100 mg) is administered.

        (b) A second injection of half the initial dose may be required 5 minutes later, up to a maximum of 300 mg.

      (2) Continuous intravenous infusion of 2–4 mg/min produces an effective plasma level in 7–10 hours.

      (3) In an emergency, an intramuscular injection rapidly achieves an effective plasma level. The usual dosage is 300–400 mg injected into the deltoid muscle.

    e. Tocainide is administered orally and should be initiated in the hospital setting. Initially, 400 mg is given every 8 hours; then, 1200–1800 mg/day is given in two or three divided doses.

    f. Phenytoin is given orally or in intermittent intravenous doses.

      (1) For oral administration, a loading dose of 1 g is divided over the first 24 hours; for the next 2 days, 300–500 mg/day is administered. The maintenance dosage is 300–400 mg/day.

(2) For intermittent intravenous administration, 100 mg is given every 5 minutes at a rate not exceeding 25–50 mg/min, until the arrhythmia disappears, adverse effects develop, or 1 g has been given. The usual effective dosage is 700 mg.

g. Mexiletine is administered orally and should be initiated in the hospital setting.
   (1) A loading dose of 400 mg followed by maintenance dosage in 8 hours.
   (2) If this fails to control the arrhythmia, the dosage may be increased to 400 mg every 8 hours. (Alternatively, doses may be given every 12 hours.)
   (3) Normal maintenance doses are 200–300 mg every 8 hours.

h. Flecainide is administered orally and should be initiated in the hospital setting.
   (1) Initial dosage is 50 mg every 12 hours, and the dosage may be increased in twice-daily increments of 50 mg every 4 days to a maximum of 300 mg/day.
   (2) The usual maintenance dose is 100 mg every 12 hours.

i. Propafenone is administered orally and should be initiated in the hospital setting.
   (1) Initial dosage is 150 mg every 8 hours and can be increased every 3–4 days to the desired therapeutic effect or side effects.
   (2) The usual maintenance dose is 150–200 mg every 8 hours, up to a maximum of 1.2 grams/day.

j. Moricizine is administered orally and should be initiated in the hospital setting.
   (1) Initial dosage is 200 mg every 8 hours, increased every 3 days by 150 mg to the desired effect or side effects.
   (2) The usual maintenance dose is 200–300 mg divided into three equal doses throughout the day.

4. Precautions and monitoring effects

NOTE: Proarrhythmia (the ability to cause an arrhythmia) is the most important risk associated with the use of antiarrhythmic drug therapy. Bradyarrhythmias and ventricular tachyarrhythmias, such as Torsades de Pointes, can occur. These often take place during the initiation of antiarrhythmic drug treatment and should be considered when decision makers choose between outpatient and inpatient initiation of antiarrhythmic therapy.

a. Quinidine
   (1) This drug is contraindicated in patients with:
      (a) Complete AV block unless a ventricular pacemaker is in place
      (b) Marked prolongation of the QT interval or prolonged QT syndrome because ventricular tachyarrhythmia (torsades de pointes) may arise, resulting in quinidine syncope (i.e., syncope or sudden death)
   (2) An increase of 50% or more in the duration of the QRS complex necessitates dosage reduction.
   (3) Quinidine has a narrow therapeutic index. Therapeutic serum levels are in the range of 2–6 μg/mL depending on the specificity of the assay. Toxicity may cause acute cardiac effects, such as pronounced slowing of conduction in all heart regions; this, in turn, may lead to SA block or arrest, ventricular tachycardia, or asystole.
   (4) The ECG should be monitored during quinidine therapy to detect signs of cardiotoxicity. To counteract quinidine-induced ventricular tachyarrhythmias, catecholamines, glucagon, or sodium lactate may be given.
   (5) In patients receiving quinidine for atrial tachyarrhythmias, vagolytic effects may increase impulse conduction at the AV node, resulting in an accelerated ventricular response. To prevent this, agents that slow AV nodal conduction (e.g., verapamil, digoxin) may be administered.
   (6) The dosage should be reduced in elderly patients (over 60 years old) and in patients with hepatic dysfunction or congestive heart failure (CHF).
   (7) Embolism may occur upon restoration of normal sinus rhythm after prolonged atrial fibrillation. To prevent or minimize this complication, anticoagulants may be administered before quinidine therapy begins.
   (8) Quinidine may cause cinchonism at high serum concentrations, manifested by tinnitus, hearing loss, blurred vision, and gastrointestinal (GI) disturbances. In severe cases, nausea, vomiting, diarrhea, headache, confusion, delirium, photophobia, diplopia, and psychosis may occur.
   (9) GI reactions are the most common adverse reactions to quinidine. About 30% of patients experience diarrhea; nausea and vomiting may also occur. Arising almost immediately after the first dose, these symptoms sometimes warrant discontinuing the drug. However, aluminum hydroxide or use of the polygalacturonate salt may reverse this.

    (10) Hypersensitivity reactions include anaphylaxis, thrombocytopenia, respiratory distress, and vascular collapse.

b. Procainamide

    (1) This drug is contraindicated in patients with hypersensitivity to procaine and related drugs, myasthenia gravis, second- or third-degree AV block with no pacemaker, a history of procainamide-induced systemic lupus erythematosus (SLE), prolonged QT syndrome, or torsades de pointes.

    (2) An increase of 50% or more in the duration of the QRS complex necessitates dosage reduction.

    (3) Procainamide has a narrow therapeutic index. Therapeutic serum levels are reported in the range of 4–10 μg/mL. NAPA levels of 15–25 μg/mL are considered therapeutic. The active metabolite, N-acetylprocainamide possesses differing pharmacological cardiovascular effects, and serum levels need to be evaluated independently of procainamide. Toxicity may cause acute cardiac effects (e.g., pronounced slowing of conduction in all heart regions), which, in turn, may lead to SA block or arrest, ventricular tachycardia, or asystole.

    (4) High serum procainamide levels may induce ventricular arrhythmias (e.g., PVCs, ventricular tachycardia or fibrillation). The ECG should be monitored continuously to detect these problems. Catecholamines, glucagon, or sodium lactate may be administered to counteract these arrhythmias.

    (5) Hypotension may occur with rapid intravenous administration.

    (6) GI effects are less common than with quinidine therapy.

    (7) Hypersensitivity reactions are the most severe adverse effects of procainamide. These reactions include drug fever, agranulocytosis, and an SLE-like syndrome.

        (a) An SLE-like syndrome is manifested by fatigue, arthralgia, myalgia, and low-grade fever.

        (b) Antinuclear antibody titer is positive in 50%–80% of patients receiving procainamide. However, only 20%–30% of these patients develop symptoms of the SLE-like syndrome.

        (c) Drug discontinuation usually is necessary when symptomatic SLE-like syndrome occurs.

    (8) The dosage should be reduced and given over 6 hours to patients with renal or hepatic impairment, as the drug half-life is increased in these patients.

    (9) Lower doses may be needed in patients with CHF to adjust for the lower volume of distribution.

  (10) Embolism may occur upon restoration of normal sinus rhythm after prolonged atrial fibrillation. An anticoagulant is frequently administered before procainamide therapy begins to prevent this complication.

c. Disopyramide

    (1) This drug may cause marked hemodynamic compromise and ventricular dysfunction. It is contraindicated in patients with cardiogenic shock or second- or third-degree AV block with no pacemaker.

    (2) Disopyramide should be avoided or used with extreme caution in patients with CHF. It should also be used cautiously in patients with urinary tract disorders, myasthenia gravis, and renal or hepatic dysfunction.

    (3) In patients receiving this drug for atrial tachyarrhythmias, vagolytic effects may increase impulse conduction at the AV node, resulting in an accelerated ventricular response. To prevent this, agents that slow AV nodal conduction (e.g., verapamil, digoxin) may be given.

    (4) Anticholinergic effects of this drug include dry mouth, constipation, urinary hesitancy or retention, and blurred vision.

    (5) Therapeutic plasma levels range from 2–4 μg/mL.

d. Lidocaine

    (1) This drug may cause hemodynamic compromise in patients with severe cardiac dysfunction. Generally, however, it has few untoward cardiovascular effects.

    (2) Lidocaine should be used cautiously and in reduced dosage in patients with CHF or renal or hepatic impairment.

    (3) Central nervous system (CNS) reactions are the most pronounced adverse effects of lidocaine. These reactions may range from light-headedness and restlessness to confusion, tremors, stupor, and convulsions.

    (4) Tinnitus, blurred vision, and anaphylaxis have been reported.

    (5) Plasma lidocaine levels of 1.5–6.5 μg/mL are therapeutic.

(6) Lidocaine's metabolites—glycinexylidide and monoethylglycinexylidide—may have neurotoxic as well as antiarrhythmic effects.

e. Tocainide

(1) This drug is contraindicated in patients with hypersensitivity to lidocaine and related agents.

(2) Tocainide must be used cautiously in patients with CHF or reduced cardiac reserve.

(3) Neurological effects, including light-headedness, paresthesias, restlessness, confusion, and tremors, are encountered in 30%–50% of patients.

(4) Nausea, vomiting, epigastric pain, and diarrhea occur frequently.

(5) Other adverse effects of tocainide include hypotension, blurred vision, aplastic anemia, hepatitis, skin rash, and pulmonary fibrosis.

(6) Dosage reduction may be necessary in patients with renal or hepatic impairment.

(7) Plasma tocainide levels of 3–10 μg/mL are therapeutic.

f. Phenytoin

(1) This drug is contraindicated in patients with sinus bradycardia or heart block.

(2) Phenytoin must be used cautiously in patients with CHF, renal or hepatic impairment, myocardial insufficiency, respiratory depression, or hypotension.

(3) During acute therapy, this drug may cause CNS reactions (e.g., drowsiness, vertigo, nystagmus, ataxia, nausea). Cardiotoxicity also may occur, especially with fast intravenous infusion rates.

(4) Chronic phenytoin may lead to vestibular and cerebellar effects, behavioral changes, GI distress, gingival hyperplasia, megaloblastic anemia, and osteomalacia.

(5) Hypersensitivity reactions may be manifested by liver, skin, and hematological problems.

  (a) Toxic hepatitis may occur.

  (b) Skin reactions include exfoliative dermatitis, Stevens-Johnson syndrome, scarlatiniform or morbilliform rash, SLE, toxic epidermal necrolysis, eosinophilia, and erythema multiforme.

  (c) Hematological reactions include agranulocytosis, megaloblastic anemia, leukopenia, thrombocytopenia, and pancytopenia.

(6) Therapeutic plasma phenytoin levels range from 10–18 μg/mL.

g. Mexiletine

(1) This drug is contraindicated in patients with cardiogenic shock or second- or third-degree AV block with no pacemaker.

(2) Tremor is an early sign of mexiletine toxicity. Dizziness, ataxia, and nystagmus indicate an increasing plasma drug concentration.

(3) Hypotension, bradycardia, and widened QRS complexes may develop during mexiletine therapy.

(4) Adverse GI effects include nausea and vomiting.

(5) Therapeutic serum levels range from 0.50–2.0 μg/mL.

h. Flecainide

(1) This drug is contraindicated in patients with cardiogenic shock or second- or third-degree AV block with no pacemaker.

(2) The ECG should be monitored during flecainide therapy because this drug may exacerbate existing arrhythmias or precipitate new ones. Flecainide was shown in the CAST study to increase mortality in patients with asymptomatic ventricular arrhythmias and, therefore, should be reserved for patients with life-threatening ventricular arrhythmias that are refractory to other drugs.

(3) This drug has a significant negative inotropic effect and may bring on or worsen CHF and cardiomyopathy.

(4) Adverse CNS effects (e.g., dizziness, headache, tremor) and GI effects (e.g., nausea, abdominal pain) may occur.

(5) Blurred vision and dyspnea have been reported.

(6) Therapeutic serum levels recommended for flecainide are between 0.2 and 1.0 μg/mL.

i. Propafenone

(1) This drug, like other antiarrhythmic agents, may cause new or worsened arrhythmias. Such proarrhythmic properties range from an increased frequency of PVCs to the development of severe ventricular tachycardia, ventricular fibrillation, and torsades de pointes. This proarrhythmic effect has been under discussion for the class IC agents, and, thus, when used, these agents should be monitored closely. The findings from the CAST trial must be weighed against the benefits of using these agents for treating significant ventricular arrhythmias.

(2) Dizziness is a side effect that has been reported in as many as 10%–15% of patients taking the drug.

(3) Other associated side effects include vomiting; a metallic, bitter taste in the mouth; constipation; headache; and new or worsening CHF and asthma.

(4) Therapeutic serum levels recommended for propafenone are between 0.06 and 1.0 µg/mL.

j. Moricizine

(1) This drug has been reported to have proarrhythmic properties. However, it has been reported that the incidence of this effect may be less than with other antiarrhythmics. Patients predisposed to the development of such proarrhythmic effects include those with a history of coronary artery bypass surgery, pacemakers, CAD, CHF, and conduction abnormalities. As most patients receiving this agent have at least one of the previously mentioned risk factors, this agent must be used cautiously. The benefits of using this agent must be weighed against its associated risks.

(2) Dizziness is the most commonly reported adverse effect associated with the drug and has been reported in up to 15% of all patients.

(3) Other associated side effects include nausea, intraventricular conduction delays, headache, fatigue, palpitations, and shortness of breath.

(4) Further studies are necessary, as no specific concentrations have generally been defined.

5. Significant interactions

a. Quinidine

(1) Quinidine may increase serum levels of **digoxin** and increase the effects of **digitalis** on the heart, with a resultant increase in toxicity.

(2) Severe orthostatic hypotension may occur with concomitant administration of **vasodilators** (e.g., **nitroglycerin**).

(3) **Phenytoin, rifampin,** and **barbiturates** may antagonize quinidine activity and reduce its therapeutic efficacy.

(4) **Nifedipine** may reduce plasma quinidine levels.

(5) **Antacids, sodium bicarbonate,** and **sodium acetazolamide** may increase plasma quinidine levels, possibly resulting in toxicity.

(6) Quinidine may produce additive hypoprothrombinemic effects with **coumarin** anticoagulants.

b. Amiodarone and **cimetidine** may increase plasma procainamide levels, possibly leading to drug toxicity.

c. Phenytoin accelerates disopyramide metabolism, possibly reducing its therapeutic efficacy.

d. Lidocaine

(1) **Phenytoin** may increase the cardiodepressant effects of lidocaine.

(2) **β-Blockers** (class II antiarrhythmics) may reduce lidocaine metabolism, possibly leading to drug toxicity.

e. Phenytoin

(1) The risk of phenytoin toxicity increases with concomitant administration of **diazepam, antihistamines, isoniazid, chloramphenicol, dicumarol, cimetidine, salicylates, sulfisoxazole, phenylbutazone, amiodarone,** and **valproate.**

(2) **Carbamazepine** may enhance phenytoin metabolism and thus reduce plasma phenytoin levels and therapeutic efficacy. (Phenytoin has the same effect on carbamazepine.)

f. Mexiletine. Phenobarbital, rifampin, and **phenytoin** reduce plasma mexiletine levels and may decrease therapeutic efficacy.

B. Class II antiarrhythmics

1. Indications. These drugs—**β-adrenergic blockers**—are used mainly to treat systemic hypertension. Among the drugs in this class, propranolol, esmolol, and acebutolol are approved for antiarrhythmic use.

a. Propranolol may be given to:

(1) Control supraventricular arrhythmias (e.g., atrial fibrillation or flutter, PSVTs)

(2) Treat tachyarrhythmias caused by catecholamine stimulation (e.g., in hyperthyroidism, during anesthesia)

(3) Suppress severe ventricular arrhythmias in **prolonged QT syndrome**

(4) Treat digitalis-induced ventricular arrhythmias

(5) Terminate certain ventricular arrhythmias (e.g., PVCs in patients without structural heart disease)

    b. Esmolol is used to treat supraventricular tachycardias; it possesses a very short (9-minute) half-life and has been used to control the ventricular response to atrial fibrillation or flutter during or after surgery.

  2. Mechanism of action. Class II antiarrhythmics reduce sympathetic stimulation of the heart, decreasing impulse conduction through the AV node and lengthening the refractory period. Additionally, this class of antiarrhythmics slow the sinus rhythm without significantly changing the QT or QRS intervals, resulting in a reduced heart rate and a decrease in myocardial oxygen demand.

  3. Administration and dosage
    a. Propranolol may be given intravenously or orally when used as an antiarrhythmic.
      (1) Emergency therapy calls for slow intravenous administration of 1–3 mg diluted in 50 mL dextrose 5% in water or normal saline solution. This dose is infused slowly (no faster than 1 mg/min). A second dose of 1–3 mg may be given 2 minutes later.
      (2) For oral therapy, 10–80 mg/day is given in three or four doses. (However, 1000 mg or more may be required for resistant ventricular arrhythmias.)
    b. Esmolol is given intravenously. A loading dose of 500 µg/kg/min is infused over 1 minute, followed by a 4-minute maintenance infusion of 50 µg/kg/min. If a satisfactory response is not achieved within 5 minutes, the loading dose is repeated and followed by a maintenance infusion of 100 µg/kg/min.

  4. Precautions and monitoring effects
    a. Propranolol
      (1) This drug is contraindicated in patients with sinus bradycardia, second- or third-degree AV block, cardiogenic shock, severe CHF, or asthma.
      (2) The β-blocking effects of this drug may lead to marked hypotension, exacerbation of CHF and left ventricular failure, or cardiac arrest.
      (3) Blood pressure, heart rate, and the ECG should be monitored during intravenous infusion.
      (4) Embolism may occur upon restoration of normal sinus rhythm after sustained atrial fibrillation. An anticoagulant may be given before propranolol therapy begins to prevent this complication.
      (5) Propranolol may depress AV node conduction and ventricular pacemaker activity, resulting in AV block or asystole.
      (6) This drug may mask the signs and symptoms of hypoglycemia. It also may mask signs of shock.
      (7) Fatigue, lethargy, increased airway resistance, and skin rash have been reported.
      (8) Nausea, vomiting, and diarrhea may occur.
      (9) Sudden withdrawal of propranolol may lead to acute MI, arrhythmias, or angina in cardiac patients. Drug therapy is discontinued by tapering the dose over 4–7 days.
    b. Esmolol
      (1) This drug is contraindicated in patients with severe CHF or sinus bradycardia.
      (2) Hypotension occurs in approximately 30% of patients receiving esmolol. This effect can be reversed by reducing the dosage or stopping the infusion.
      (3) This drug is for short-term use only and should be replaced by a long-acting antiarrhythmic once the patient's heart stabilizes.
      (4) Dizziness, headache, fatigue, and agitation may occur.
      (5) Other adverse effects include nausea, vomiting, and bronchospasm.

  5. Significant interactions
    a. Propranolol
      (1) Severe vasoconstriction may occur with concomitant **epinephrine** administration.
      (2) **Digitalis** preparations can cause excessive bradycardia.
      (3) **Calcium-channel blockers** (e.g., **diltiazem, verapamil**) and other negative **inotropic** and **chronotropic drugs** (e.g., **disopyramide, quinidine**) add to the myocardial depressant effects of propranolol.
    b. Esmolol. Morphine may raise plasma esmolol levels.

C. Class III antiarrhythmics
  1. Indications
    a. Amiodarone is given to control malignant ventricular arrhythmias and has most recently within the new ACLS guidelines been recommended in the treatment of ventricular fibrillation and pulseless ventricular tachycardia, and may be used prophylactically

against both atrial and ventricular tachycardia and fibrillation. Unlike most other antiarrhythmics, with the exception of the β-adrenergic blockers, amiodarone has been shown to reduce arrhythmic deaths in patients after an MI.

   b. Bretylium is used solely to treat life-threatening ventricular arrhythmias, including ventricular tachycardia and ventricular fibrillation, that have not responded to other agents. It should be given only in intensive care facilities.

   c. Sotalol is used to treat supraventricular and ventricular tachyarrhythmias. Sotalol antagonizes both $β_1$- and $β_2$- adrenergic receptors, but also prolongs the Phase 3 action potential. It is this property that distinguishes it from other β-adrenergic blockers and is the reason why it is classified as a type III antiarrhythmic drug rather than a type II agent (β-adrenergic blocker).

   d. Ibutilide is used in the conversion of atrial fibrillation and flutter of recent onset (duration <30 days).

   e. Dofetilide is available in the U.S. under restricted access in the treatment of atrial fibrillation/flutter.

2. Mechanism of action. Class III antiarrhythmic drugs prolong the refractory period and action potential; they have no effect on myocardial contractility or conduction time.

3. Administration and dosage

   a. Amiodarone—Available for both oral and intravenous use and should only be initiated in the hospital setting. The Amiodarone in Out-of-Hospital Resuscitation of Refractory Sustained Ventricular Tachycardia (ARREST) study compared amiodarone with placebo in a blinded, randomized trial in patients with shock-refractory out-of-hospital ventricular fibrillation or pulseless ventricular tachycardia. This was the first large, randomized study to show a benefit of any antiarrhythmic drug over placebo in patients with out-of-hospital cardiac arrest. Amiodarone-treated patients had a significantly greater likelihood of surviving to hospital admission as compared to the placebo patients. Since publication of the ARREST trial, amiodarone has been incorporated into the most recent ACLS 2000 Guidelines and recommended by the expert panel members as the first-choice antiarrhythmic for shock-refractory ventricular fibrillation/ventricular tachycardia.

   (1) It is available for oral use where 800–1600 mg every 12 hours is given for 7–14 days, then 200–400 mg daily thereafter.

   (2) Oral treatment is used to suppress ventricular and supraventricular arrhythmias but can take days or weeks to take effect. Oral doses of 100–600 mg/day (usually 300–400 mg/day) for maintenance therapy in ventricular tachycardia and 100–200 mg/day for maintenance therapy for supraventricular tachycardias are given.

   (3) Intravenous formulation is available for treatment and prophylaxis of recurrent ventricular fibrillation or hemodynamically unstable ventricular tachycardia in refractory patients.

   (4) The intravenous form is rapidly distributed throughout the body. Recommended doses include a rapid loading infusion of 150 mg over 10 minutes, followed by a slow infusion of 1 mg/min for 6 hours (360 mg), and then a maintenance infusion of 0.5 mg/min for the remainder of the 24-hour period. Patients usually receive 2–4 days of infusions before conversion to oral form. However, a maintenance infusion can be continued for 2–3 weeks.

   b. Bretylium is used for short-term intravenous or intramuscular therapy.

   (1) For ventricular fibrillation, 5 mg/kg is given by rapid intravenous injection. As needed, the dosage may be increased to 10 mg/kg and repeated every 15–30 minutes up to a total of 30 mg/kg.

   (2) For other ventricular arrhythmias, 500 mg are diluted to 50 mL with dextrose 5% in water or normal saline solution and infused intravenously at 5–10 mg/kg over more than 8 minutes. The dose may be repeated in 1–2 hours, then given every 6–8 hours.

   (3) Bretylium has also been used successfully as a continuous infusion at a rate of 1–2 mg/min, after diluting 500 mg in 50 mL dextrose 5% in water or normal saline solution.

   (4) Intramuscular therapy calls for administration of 5–10 mg/kg undiluted. As needed, the dose may be repeated in 1–2 hours, then given every 6–8 hours.

   c. Sotalol is available commercially as an oral tablet, and therapy should be initiated within the hospital setting. Normal dosing of 80 mg twice daily initially and increasing doses at 2–3-day intervals to a maximum dose of 640 mg/day, given in two to three doses throughout the day.

d. Ibutilide is only available for injection in a 0.1 mg/mL 10-mL vial under the trade name of Corvert. Normal doses for the conversion of recent-onset atrial fibrillation to normal sinus rhythm is a dose of 1 mg (0.01 mg/kg for those <60 kg) over 10 minutes, with a repeat dose in 10 minutes if the arrhythmia does not end.

e. Dofetilide is only available for oral administration in 0.125-, 0.25-, and 0.5-mg capsules under the trade name of Tikosyn, and should only be initiated in a hospital setting with trained personnel and the equipment necessary to provide continuous cardiac monitoring during initiation of therapy.

   (1) A normal dose for the conversion of recent-onset atrial fibrillation to normal sinus rhythm is 0.5 mg twice daily for patients with creatinine clearance values greater than 60 mL/min with doses reduced 50% (0.25 mg) for those with creatinine clearance values of 40–60 mL/min, with doses reduced an additional 50% (0.125 mg) for those with creatinine clearance values of 20–40 mL/min.

   (2) Maintenance therapy is based on the ECG, with doses being reduced with Q-Tc prolongation exceeding 15% of the baseline value. Any patient developing a Q-Tc interval exceeding 500 msec should have therapy discontinued immediately.

   (3) Dofetilide should not be given to those with creatinine clearance values less than 20 mL/min.

4. Precautions and monitoring effects

   a. Amiodarone

   (1) Life-threatening pulmonary toxicity may occur during amiodarone therapy, especially in patients receiving more than 400 mg/day. Baseline as well as routine pulmonary function tests reveal relevant pulmonary changes.

   (2) Most patients develop corneal microdeposits 1–4 months after amiodarone therapy begins. However, this reaction rarely causes visual disturbance, but the patient should be monitored with routine ophthalmological examinations.

   (3) Blood pressure and heart rate and rhythm should be monitored for hypotension and bradyarrhythmias.

   (4) Patients should be monitored routinely for the possible development of hepatic dysfunction, thyroid disorders (e.g., hyperthyroidism, hypothyroidism), and photosensitivity.

   (5) CNS reactions include fatigue, malaise, peripheral neuropathy, and extrapyramidal effects.

   (6) Nausea and vomiting have been reported.

   (7) This drug has an extremely long half-life (up to 60 days). Therapeutic response may be delayed for weeks after oral therapy begins; adverse reactions may persist up to 4 months after therapy ends.

   b. Bretylium

   (1) This drug is contraindicated in digitalis-induced arrhythmias.

   (2) Severe hypotension, especially orthostatic hypotension, may develop when bretylium is administered intravenously for the treatment of acute arrhythmias.

   (3) Rapid intravenous injection may cause severe nausea and vomiting.

   (4) Patients with renal impairment may require dosage reduction.

   c. Sotalol

   (1) Side effects of this drug are directly related to β-blockade and prolongation of repolarization.

   (2) Transient hypotension, bradycardia, myocardial depression, and bronchospasm have all been associated with this drug.

   (3) This drug carries all the contraindications associated with other β-blockers along with those due to its electrophysiologic properties.

   d. Ibutilide

   (1) Infusion should be discontinued as soon as the atrial arrhythmia is terminated or if sustained or nonsustained ventricular arrhythmia or marked QT prolongation is documented.

   (2) Continuous ECG monitoring is required for at least 4 hours after discontinuing the infusion or until the QT interval returns to baseline.

   e. Dofetilide

   (1) Patients need to be monitored closely for the subsequent development of ventricular arrhythmias with increasing doses of dofetilide or with declining renal status. In clinical trials, ventricular tachycardias, including Torsades de Pointes, are the most frequently occurring arrhythmias due to dofetilide.

(2) Hypokalemia and those situations that might cause hypotension will predispose a patient to prolongation of the QT interval, which could put a dofetilide patient at risk for toxic arrhythmias.

5. **Significant interactions**
   a. **Amiodarone**
      (1) Amiodarone may increase the plasma levels of **quinidine, procainamide, diltiazem, digitalis,** and **flecainide.**
      (2) It may increase the pharmacological effect of **β-blockers, calcium-channel blockers,** and **warfarin.**
      (3) **SPECIAL NOTE:** Amiodarone has been reported to have numerous drug–drug interactions among all categories of drugs. To avoid the development of a significant drug–drug interaction a thorough patient medication profile should be carried out for each patient having amiodarone therapy initiated, as well as each time a patient currently receiving amiodarone is given an additional drug.
   b. **Bretylium. Antihypertensives** may potentiate bretylium-induced hypotension.
   c. **Sotalol**
      (1) Sotalol must be used cautiously in those patients receiving agents with cardiac-depressant properties.
      (2) Agents such as sotalol, which prolong the QT interval, may induce malignant arrhythmias when used in combination with other type IA antiarrhythmics, especially in the presence of low potassium levels.
   d. **Ibutilide** should be avoided with other agents that prolong repolarization or within 4 hours of administration.
   e. **Dofetilide** should be avoided in patients who have hypokalemia or preexisting QT prolongation.

D. **Class IV antiarrhythmics**

   1. **Indications**
      a. **Calcium-channel blockers** (e.g., verapamil, diltiazem) are used mainly to treat and prevent supraventricular arrhythmias.
         (1) They are first-line agents for the suppression of PSVTs stemming from AV nodal reentry.
         (2) They can rapidly control the ventricular response to atrial flutter and fibrillation.
      b. Other calcium-channel blockers available include nicardipine, nifedipine, bepridil, amLodipine, and felodipine, but these agents have primarily been used in the treatment of angina pectoris and hypertension. For information on these agents, see Chapters 38 and 40.

   2. **Mechanism of action.** Class IV antiarrhythmics are calcium-channel blockers. They inhibit AV node conduction by depressing the SA and AV nodes, where calcium channels predominate.

   3. **Administration and dosage**
      a. To control atrial arrhythmias, verapamil usually is administered intravenously. A dose of 5–10 mg is given over at least 2 minutes and may be repeated in 30 minutes, if necessary. A 5–10 mg/hr continuous intravenous infusion has also been used in treating arrhythmias.
      b. To prevent PSVTs, verapamil may be given orally in four daily doses of 80–120 mg each.
      c. To control atrial arrhythmias, diltiazem usually is administered intravenously. A dose of 20 mg (0.25 mg/kg) is given over 2 minutes. If an adequate response is not obtained, a second dose of 25 mg (0.35 mg/kg) is administered after 15 minutes. A 5–15 mg/hr intravenous continuous infusion has also been used in treating arrhythmias.

   4. **Precautions and monitoring effects**
      a. Verapamil and diltiazem are contraindicated in patients with AV block; left ventricular dysfunction; severe hypotension; concomitant, intravenous β-blockers; and atrial fibrillation with an accessory AV pathway.
      b. These drugs must be used cautiously in patients with CHF, sick sinus syndrome, MI, and hepatic or renal impairment.
      c. Because of the negative chronotropic effect, verapamil and diltiazem must be used cautiously in patients who have slow heart rates or who are receiving digitalis glycosides.

d. The ECG (especially the RR interval) should be monitored during therapy.

e. Patients over 60 years old should receive reduced dosages and slower injection rates.

f. Constipation and nausea have been reported with verapamil.

5. Significant interactions

a. Concomitant administration of **β-blockers** or **disopyramide** may precipitate heart failure.

b. Quinidine may increase the risk of calcium-channel blocker–induced hypotension.

c. Verapamil may increase serum **digoxin** concentrations, and diltiazem may do the same to a lesser extent.

d. Rifampin may enhance the metabolism of calcium-channel blockers, with a resultant decrease in pharmacological effect.

e. Verapamil and diltiazem may inhibit **theophylline** metabolism and may require reductions in theophylline dosage.

f. Diltiazem and verapamil inhibit the metabolism of **cyclosporine** and may require reductions in cyclosporine dosages.

E. Unclassified antiarrhythmics

1. Atropine

a. Indications. Atropine is therapeutic for symptomatic sinus bradycardia and junctional rhythm.

b. Mechanism of action. An anticholinergic, atropine blocks vagal effects on the SA node, promoting conduction through the AV node and increasing the heart rate.

c. Administration and dosage. For antiarrhythmic use, atropine is administered in a dose of 0.4–1 mg by intravenous push; the dose is given every 5 minutes to a maximum of 2 mg.

d. Precautions and monitoring effects

(1) Thirst and dry mouth are the most common adverse effects of atropine.

(2) CNS reactions (e.g., restlessness, headache, disorientation, dizziness) may occur with doses over 5 mg.

(3) Tachycardia and ophthalmic disturbances (e.g., mydriasis, blurred vision, photophobia) may occur with doses of 1 mg or more.

(4) Initial doses may induce a reflex bradycardia due to incomplete suppression of vagal impulses.

2. Adenosine

a. Indications. Adenosine is indicated for the conversion of acute supraventricular tachycardia to normal sinus rhythm.

b. Mechanism of action. Adenosine is a naturally occurring nucleoside, which is normally present in all cells of the body. It has been shown to:

(1) Slow conduction through the AV node

(2) Interrupt re-entry pathways through the AV node

(3) Restore normal sinus rhythm in patients with PSVTs

c. Administration and dosage. For antiarrhythmic effects, adenosine is given as a rapid bolus intravenous injection in a 6-mg dose over 1–2 seconds. If the first dose does not eliminate the arrhythmia within 1–2 minutes, the dose should be increased to 12 mg and again given as a rapid intravenous dose. An additional 12-mg dose may be repeated if necessary.

d. Precautions and monitoring effects

(1) The effects of adenosine are antagonized by methylxanthines, such as caffeine and theophylline. Theophylline has been successfully used for treating adenosine-induced side effects, such as hypotension, sweating, and palpitations. If side effects are encountered, aggressive therapy is not required because of the ultra-short half-life of the drug (10 seconds or less).

(2) The main side effect associated with adenosine use in up to 18% of patients is facial flushing, but this effect is normally very short-lived.

(3) Other side effects associated with adenosine use include shortness of breath, chest pressure, nausea, headache, and a metallic taste.

e. Additional use. Adenosine has been used as an adjunctive agent in patients undergoing various types of pharmacological stress testing (e.g., with thallium). In this situation, adenosine is given as a continuous infusion over a period of about 4–6 minutes and is able to provide a form of exercise tolerance test in patients not able to exert themselves due to age, fatigue, and various other physical handicaps.

STUDY QUESTIONS

Directions: Each of the numbered items or incomplete statements in this section is followed by answers or by completions of the statement. Select the **one** lettered answer or completion that is **best** in each case.

1. Strong anticholinergic effects limit the antiarrhythmic use of

(A) quinidine
(B) procainamide
(C) tocainide
(D) flecainide
(E) disopyramide

2. A pronounced slowing of phase 0 of the myocardial action potential results in a prolongation of either atrial depolarization causing a prolonged P wave on the electrocardiogram (ECG) or ventricular depolarization causing a prolonged QRS complex characterized by which class of antiarrhythmics?

(A) Type I
(B) Type II
(C) Type III
(D) Type IV
(E) Type V

3. Which of the following type III antiarrhythmics has been reported as causing the Torsades de Pointes type of ventricular tachycardia?

(A) Lidocaine
(B) Amiodarone
(C) Quinidine
(D) Flecainide
(E) Diltiazem

4. A patient receiving a class I antiarrhythmic agent on a chronic basis complains of fatigue, low-grade fever, and joint pain suggestive of systemic lupus erythematosus (SLE). The patient is most likely receiving

(A) lidocaine
(B) procainamide
(C) quinidine
(D) flecainide
(E) propranolol

5. Class IA antiarrhythmics do all of the following to the cardiac cell's action potential EXCEPT

(A) slow the rate of rise for phase 0 of depolarization
(B) delay the fast-channel conductance of sodium ions
(C) prolong phases 2 and 3 of repolarization
(D) inhibit the slow-channel conductance of calcium ions
(E) prolong the refractory period of the action potential

6. Which of the following drugs is a class IV antiarrhythmic that is primarily indicated for the treatment of supraventricular tachyarrhythmias?

(A) Ibutilide
(B) Mexiletine
(C) Verapamil
(D) Quinidine
(E) Propranolol

7. Which of the following agents was involved in the ARREST trial, and which resulted in the use of evidence-based practice to justify its addition as a first-line agent within the 2000 ACLS guidelines?

(A) Lidocaine
(B) Diltiazem
(C) Bretylium
(D) Amiodarone
(E) Dofetilide

8. Which of the following drugs is a class III antiarrhythmic agent that is effective in the acute management of atrial fibrillation or atrial flutter of recent onset?

(A) Bretylium
(B) Dofetilide
(C) Metoprolol
(D) Disopyramide
(E) Diltiazem

9. All of the following problems represent concerns when patients are started on amiodarone EXCEPT

(A) extremely long elimination half-life
(B) need for multiple daily doses
(C) development of hyper- or hypothyroidism
(D) development of pulmonary fibrosis
(E) interactions with other antiarrhythmic drugs

Directions: The group of items in this section consists of lettered options followed by a set of numbered items. For each item, select the **one** lettered option that is most closely associated with it. Each lettered option may be selected once, more than once, or not at all.

Questions 10–14
For each description of a phase of an action potential in Purkinje fibers, choose the corresponding letter in the accompanying diagram.

10. Slow-channel depolarization—calcium influx
11. Resting phase—diastole
12. Rapid repolarization
13. Fast-channel depolarization—sodium influx
14. Early repolarization

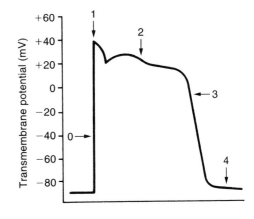

ANSWERS AND EXPLANATIONS

1. The answer is E *[II A 4 c (4)]*.
Disopyramide has anticholinergic actions about one-tenth the potency of atropine. Effects include dry mouth, constipation, urinary retention, and blurred vision. Therefore, it cannot be used in patients with glaucoma or with conditions causing urinary retention. Moreover, disopyramide has a negative inotropic effect and must, therefore, be used with great caution, if at all, in patients with preexisting ventricular failure.

2. The answer is A *[II A 2]*.
The class I antiarrhythmics (fast-channel blockers) slow impulse conduction by depressing the flow of sodium ions into cells during phase 0 of the action potential. Class II antiarrhythmics decrease impulse conduction through the AV node and lengthen the refractory period through their direct effects on the sympathetic nervous system. Class III antiarrhythmics prolong the refractory period and action potential and have no effect on conduction time throughout the AV and SA nodes. Class IV antiarrhythmics work directly on "slow-channel" ion conduction, which is more likely to take place during phase 2 (plateau), where calcium ions enter the cell through slow channels. Current classification of antiarrhythmics does not include a group of class V agents.

3. The answer is B *[I C 3 a, Table 39-1]*.
Torsades de Pointes is a form of ventricular tachyarrhythmia characterized by electrocardiographic changes, which include a markedly prolonged QT interval. This potentially fatal reaction has now been reported for both antiarrhythmics and nonantiarrhythmics. Antiarrhythmics, which have been reported to cause Torsades de Points, include amiodarone, disopyramide, dofetilide, flecainide, ibutilide, procainamide, quinidine, and sotalol. Additionally, drug classes such as antibiotics (e.g., erythromycin, levofloxacin, moxifloxacin, pentamidine, sparfloxacin), along with other agents such as dolasetron, felbamate, fluoxetine, fosphenytoin, indapamide, isradipine, paroxetine, sumatriptan, and tamoxifen, have been reported to be able to cause either a prolongation in the QT interval and/or induce torsades de pointes **(see Table 39-1)**. Of the agents listed, only amiodarone is a class III antiarrhythmic.

4. The answer is B *[II A 4 b (7)]*.
The patient's complaints are typical of a systemic lupus erythematosus (SLE)-like hypersensitivity reaction to procainamide. Symptoms of an SLE-like syndrome include fatigue, arthralgia, myalgia, a low-grade fever, and a positive antinuclear antibody titer. The patient's symptoms should subside if procainamide therapy is stopped and an alternative antiarrhythmic agent is given instead.

5. The answer is D *[II A 2]*.
Class IA antiarrhythmic agents delay phase 0 of depolarization. Fast-channel conduction of sodium and phases 2 and 3 of repolarization are also slowed. The net effect is to extend the refractory period of myocardial tissue. Class IA antiarrhythmic agents do not inhibit the slow-channel conductance of calcium ions; that is an action of class IV agents such as verapamil.

6. The answer is C *[II D 1 a]*.
Of the agents listed, verapamil is a calcium-channel blocker and represents the class IV antiarrhythmics. Verapamil has been used for its direct-acting effects on impulse conduction throughout the heart. Thus, verapamil is used to treat and prevent supraventricular arrhythmias. Ibutilide is a class III agent, quinidine is a class IA drug, mexiletine is a class IB agent, and propranolol, a β-adrenergic blocker, is class II. Mexiletine, quinidine, and propranolol are all also effective for supraventricular arrhythmias, while ibutilide is indicated for the treatment of atrial fibrillation/flutter of recent onset.

7. The answer is D *[II C 3 a]*.
In the ARREST trial, 44 percent of amiodarone-treated patients versus 34 percent of placebo-treated patients survived to hospital admission (P = 0.03) after shock-refractory cardiac arrest. The benefit was consistently observed in all major subgroups, regardless of the presenting cardiac-arrest rhythm. As a result of the trial, evidence of its findings were cited within the ACLS 2000 Guidelines, describing the lack of similar data for other antiarrhythmics, and the agreement by the expert panel that they would consider amiodarone as a first-line agent for such patients. Lidocaine and bretylium are the only other agents listed, which have been used in this patient population for ventricular tachyarrhythmias. However, the data have been lacking as to their efficacy compared to placebo.

8. The answer is B *[II C 1 e].*
Dofetilide, ibutilide, bretylium, amiodarone, and sotalol are class III antiarrhythmic agents. Class III agents, which prolong the refractory period and myocardial action potential, are used to treat ventricular arrhythmias. However, dofetilide and ibutilide are approved as type III agents indicated for the conversion from atrial fibrillation and flutter of recent onset to normal sinus rhythm.

9. The answer is B *[II C 3 a, 4 a, 5 a].*
Amiodarone, like bretylium, ibutilide, and sotalol, is a class III antiarrhythmic agent and acts by prolonging repolarization of cardiac cells. Amiodarone is given orally, often in once-a-day or twice-a-day maintenance dosage. Because of its very long elimination half-life, therapeutic response may be delayed for weeks. Therefore, an initial loading phase is often advisable. This requires hospitalization with close monitoring for desired effects, untoward reactions, and adjustments in dosage. Amiodarone may increase the plasma levels of quinidine, procainamide, diltiazem, and digitalis. During therapy with amiodarone, patients may develop hypo- or hyperthyroidism, pulmonary disorders, hepatic dysfunction, and various other unwanted effects. Because of amiodarone's extremely long half-life, adverse reactions may persist for months after therapy ends.

10–14. The answers are: 10-C, 11-E, 12-D, 13-A, 14-B *[I B 2 b].*
The action potential of cardiac Purkinje fibers reflects the depolarization and repolarization of the cardiac cells. This electrical activity involves the transport of sodium, calcium, and potassium ions across the cell membrane. The action potential has five phases. Phase 0 (rapid depolarization) is primarily dependent on the conduction of sodium ions into the cell through fast channels. Phase 0 is followed by phase 1 (early repolarization), which precedes phase 2, a slight notch that represents the inward flow of calcium ions into the cardiac cell via slow channels. Phase 3 (rapid repolarization) represents the inward flow of potassium ions. Phase 4 (slow repolarization), ending the action potential, represents electrical diastole.

40
Hypertension
Alan H. Mutnick

I. GENERAL CONSIDERATIONS

A. **Definition. Hypertension** is blood pressure elevated enough to perfuse tissues and organs. Elevated systemic blood pressure is usually defined as a systolic reading greater than or equal to 140 mm Hg and a diastolic reading greater than or equal to 90 mm Hg ($\geq$140/90). The most recent recommendations of the Seventh Report of the Joint National Committee on Detection, Evaluation, and Treatment of High Blood Pressure (JNC-7) has added a "Prehypertension" category, which includes individuals with systolic blood pressure readings of 120–139 or diastolic blood pressure readings of 80–89 mm Hg, and is now included in contemporary management strategies.

B. **Classification** of hypertension is shown in Table 40-1. This table reflects the latest recommendations of the JNC-7.

C. **Relationship between elevated blood pressure and cardiovascular disease** has been addressed in the JNC-7 report and formalizes the fact that the higher the blood pressure, the greater the chance of a myocardial infarction (MI), heart failure, stroke, or kidney disease. Table 40-2 reflects cardiovascular risk factors and/or lifestyle factors that affect the prognosis and treatment of hypertension, and the various types of target-organ damage associated with hypertension.

D. **Incidence. Hypertension is the most common cardiovascular disorder.** Approximately 43 million Americans have blood pressure measurements greater than 140/90. This number translates to almost 25% of the adult population. The incidence increases with age—that is, 60%–71% of people over age 60 have hypertension, according to data obtained from the Third National Health and Nutrition Examination Survey (NHANES III).

1. **Primary (or essential) hypertension,** in which no specific cause can be identified, constitutes more than 90% of all cases of systemic hypertension. The average age of onset is about 35 years.

2. **Secondary hypertension,** resulting from an identifiable cause, such as renal disease or adrenal hyperfunction, accounts for the remaining 2%–5% of cases of systemic hypertension. This type usually develops between the ages of 30 and 50.

E. **Physiology**

Blood pressure = (stroke volume $\times$ heart rate) $\times$ total peripheral vascular resistance (TPR)

Altering any of the factors on the right side of the blood pressure equation results in a change in blood pressure, as shown in Figure 40-1.

1. **Sympathetic nervous system. Baroreceptors** (pressure receptors) in the carotids and aortic arch respond to changes in blood pressure and influence arteriolar dilation and arteriolar constriction. When stimulated to constriction, the contractile force strengthens, increasing the heart rate and augmenting peripheral resistance, thus increasing cardiac output. If pressure remains elevated, the baroreceptors reset at the higher levels and so sustain the hypertension. Little evidence suggests that epinephrine and norepinephrine have a clear role in the etiology of hypertension. However, many of the drugs used to treat hypertension lower blood pressure by blocking the sympathetic nervous system.

2. **Renin–angiotensin–aldosterone system.** Decreased renal perfusion pressure in afferent arterioles stimulates the release of renin from juxtaglomerular apparatus of the kidney. The renin reacts with circulating angiotensinogen to produce angiotensin I (a weak vasoconstrictor). This, in turn, is hydrolyzed to form angiotensin II (a very potent natural vasoconstrictor). This

Table 40-1. Classification of Hypertension Based on the Seventh Report of the Joint National Committee on Detection, Evaluation, and Treatment of High Blood Pressure (JNC-7) for Adults ≥18 Years of Age

Blood Pressure Classification	Systolic Blood Pressure, mm Hg*		Diastolic Blood Pressure, mm Hg*	Lifestyle Modification	Management — Initial Drug Therapy	
					Without Compelling Indication	With Compelling Indications
Normal	<120	and	<80	Encourage		
Prehypertension	120–139	or	80–89	Yes	No antihypertensive drug indicated unless there is the presence of a compelling indication** requiring the use of drug therapy.	Drug(s) for the compelling indications
Stage 1 Hypertension	140–159	or	90–99	Yes	Thiazide-type diuretics for most; may consider ACE inhibitor, ARB, β-blocker, CCB, or combination	Drug(s) for the compelling indications
Other antihypertensive drugs (diuretics, ACE inhibitor, ARB, β-blocker, CCB) as needed
Stage 2 Hypertension	≥160	or	≥100	Yes	Two-drug combination for most (usually thiazide-type diuretic and ACE inhibitor or ARB or β-blocker, or CCB)	Drug(s) for the compelling indications
Other antihypertensive drugs (diuretics, ACE inhibitor, ARB, β-blocker, CCB) as needed

* Treatment is determined by the patient's highest blood pressure category.
** Select drug therapies (within parentheses) have been identified from clinical trials to possess positive clinical outcomes for specific clinical situations and represent "compelling indications" for their use. Such compelling indications include heart failure (diuretics, β-blockers, ACE inhibitors, ARB, aldosterone antagonist), postmyocardial infarction (β-blockers, ACE inhibitors, and aldosterone antagonist), high coronary disease risk (diuretic, β-blocker, ACE inhibitors, CCB), diabetes (diuretic, β-blockers, ACE inhibitors, ARB, CCB), chronic kidney disease (ACE inhibitors, ARB), and recurrent stroke prevention (diuretic, ACE inhibitors).
ACE—angiotensin-converting enzyme; ARB—angiotensin-receptor blocker; CCB—calcium-channel blocker.

Adopted from Special Communication; Clinician's Corner; *JAMA* 2003;289:2560–2572. The Seventh Report of the Joint National Committee on Detection, Evaluation, and Treatment of High Blood Pressure: The JNC-7 Report.

Table 40-2. Cardiovascular and/or Lifestyle Risk Factors for Consideration in the Management of Hypertension Based on the Seventh Report of the Joint National Committee on Detection, Evaluation, and Treatment of High Blood Pressure (JNC-7)

Major Risk Factors
  Hypertension
  Cigarette smoking
  Obesity (BMI ≥30, in which BMI refers to body mass index calculated as weight in kilograms divided by the square of height in meters)
  Physical inactivity
  Dyslipidemia (as a component of the metabolic syndrome)
  Diabetes mellitus (as a component of the metabolic syndrome)
  Microalbuminuria or estimated glomerular filtration rate (GFR) <60 mL/min
  Age (>55 years for men, >65 years for women)
  Family history of premature cardiovascular disease (men <55 years or women <65 years)

vasopressor stimulates aldosterone release from the adrenal gland (zona glomerulosa), which results in increased sodium reabsorption, fluid volume, and blood pressure.

3. **Mosaic theory** centers around the fact that multiple factors, rather than one factor alone, are responsible for sustaining hypertension. The interactions between the sympathetic nervous system, renin–angiotensin–aldosterone system, and potential defects in sodium transport within and outside the cell may all play a role in long-term hypertension. Additional factors contributing to the development include genetics, endothelial dysfunction, and neurovascular anomalies. Other vasoactive substances that are involved in the maintenance of normal blood pressure have also been identified; these include nitric oxide (vasodilating factor), endothelin (vasoconstrictor peptide), bradykinin [potent vasodilator inactivated by angiotensin-converting enzyme (ACE)], and atrial natriuretic peptide (naturally occurring diuretic).

4. **Fluid volume regulation. Increased fluid volume** increases venous system distention and venous return, affecting cardiac output and tissue perfusion. These changes **alter vascular resistance,** increasing the blood pressure.

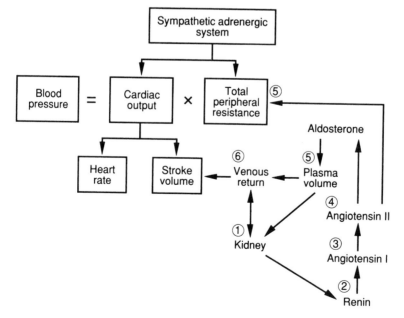

Figure 40-1. Blood pressure regulation. This figure depicts the various determinants of blood pressure as they relate to cardiac output and total peripheral resistance. Angiotensin II, a potent vasopressor, not only increases total peripheral resistance but also, by stimulating aldosterone release, leads to an increase in plasma volume, venous return, stroke volume, and ultimately an increase in cardiac output.

F. Complications. Untreated systemic hypertension, regardless of cause, results in inflammation and necrosis of the arterioles, narrowing of the blood vessels, and restriction of the blood flow to major body organs (Table 40-3). When blood flow is severely compromised, target-organ damage ensues.

1. **Cardiac effects**
   a. Left ventricular hypertrophy compensates for the increased cardiac workload. Signs and symptoms of heart failure occur, and the increased oxygen requirements of the enlarged heart may produce angina pectoris.
   b. Hypertension can be caused by accelerated atherosclerosis. Atheromatous lesions in the coronary arteries lead to decreased blood flow, resulting in angina pectoris. MI and sudden death may ensue.

2. **Renal effects**
   a. Decreased blood flow leads to an increase in renin–aldosterone secretion, which heightens the reabsorption of sodium and water and increases blood volume.
   b. Accelerated atherosclerosis decreases the oxygen supply, leading to renal parenchymal damage with decreased filtration capability and to azotemia. The atherosclerosis also decreases blood flow to the renal arterioles, leading to nephrosclerosis and, ultimately, renal failure (acute as well as chronic).

3. **Cerebral effects.** Decreased blood flow, decreased oxygen supply, and weakened blood vessel walls lead to transient ischemic attacks, cerebral thromboses, and the development of aneurysms with hemorrhage. There are alterations in mobility, weakness and paralysis, and memory deficits.

4. **Retinal effects.** Decreased blood flow with retinal vascular sclerosis and increased arteriolar pressure with the appearance of exudates and hemorrhage result in visual defects (e.g., blurred vision, spots, blindness).

Table 40-3. Target-Organ Damage Associated with Hypertension

Organ/Findings	Basis of Findings
Cardiovascular	
Blood pressure persistently ≥140 mm Hg systolic and/or ≥90 mm Hg diastolic	Constricted arterioles, causing abnormal resistance to blood flow
Angina pain	Insufficient blood flow to coronary vasculature
Left ventricular hypertrophy/dyspnea on exertion	Heart failure
Edema of extremities	Decrease in blood supply
Neurological	
Severe occipital headaches with nausea and vomiting, drowsiness, anxiety, and mental impairment	Vessel damage within the brain characteristic of dizziness, severe mental impairment, hypertension, resulting in transient ischemic attacks or strokes
Renal	
Polyuria, nocturia, and diminished ability to concentrate urine; protein and red blood cells in urine; elevated serum creatinine	Arteriolar nephrosclerosis (hardening of arterioles within the kidney)
Ocular	
Retinal hemorrhage and exudates	Damage to arterioles that supply the retina
Peripheral vascular	Absence of pulses in extremities with or without intermittent claudication; development of an aneurysm

Adopted from Special Communication; Clinician's Corner *JAMA* 2003;289:2560–2572. The Seventh Report of the Joint National Committee on Detection, Evaluation, and Treatment of High Blood Pressure: The JNC-7 Report.

II. SECONDARY HYPERTENSION

A. Clinical evaluation. Because most patients presenting with high blood pressure have primary rather than secondary hypertension, extensive screening is unwarranted. A thorough history and physical examination followed by an evaluation of common laboratory tests should rule out most causes of secondary hypertension. Patient age (primary hypertension normally seen between 30 and 55 years of age), sudden onset of worsening of hypertension, and blood pressure elevations not responding to treatment are findings consistent with secondary hypertension. If a secondary cause is not found, the patient is considered to have essential (primary) hypertension.

1. A patient's **history** and **other physical findings** suggest an underlying cause of hypertension. These include the following:
   a. Weight gain, moon face, truncal obesity, osteoporosis, purple striae, hirsutism, hypokalemia, diabetes, and increased plasma cortisol may signal Cushing's syndrome.
   b. Weight loss, episodic flushing, diaphoresis, increased urinary catecholamines, headaches, intermittent hypertension, tremors, and palpitations suggest pheochromocytoma.
   c. Steroid or estrogen intake, including oral contraceptives, nonsteroidal anti-inflammatory drugs (NSAIDs), nasal decongestants, tricyclic antidepressants, appetite suppressants, cyclosporine, erythropoietin, and monoamine oxidase (MAO) inhibitors, suggests drug-induced hypertension.
   d. Repeated urinary tract infections, elevated serum creatinine levels, nocturia, hematuria, and pain on urinating may signify renal involvement (e.g., chronic kidney disease).
   e. Abdominal bruits, recent onset, and accelerated hypertension indicate renal artery stenosis (e.g., renovascular disease).
   f. Muscle cramps, weakness, excess urination, and isolated hypokalemia may suggest primary aldosteronism.
   g. Sleep apnea, coarctation of the aorta, thyroid disease, and parathyroid disease have been included by the JNC-7 as additional secondary causes of hypertension.

2. **Laboratory findings**
   a. Blood urea nitrogen (BUN) and creatinine elevations suggest renal disease.
   b. Increased urinary excretion of catecholamine or its metabolites (e.g., vanillylmandelic acid, metanephrine) confirms pheochromocytoma.
   c. Serum potassium evaluation revealing hypokalemia suggests primary aldosteronism or Cushing's syndrome.

3. **Diagnostic tests**
   a. Renal arteriography or renal venography may show evidence of renal artery stenosis.
   b. Electrocardiography (ECG) may reveal left ventricular hypertrophy or ischemia.

B. Etiology

1. **Primary aldosteronism.** Hypersecretion of aldosterone by the adrenal cortex increases distal tubular sodium retention, expanding the blood volume, which increases total peripheral resistance.

2. **Pheochromocytoma.** A tumor of the adrenal medulla stimulates hypersecretion of epinephrine and norepinephrine, which results in increased total peripheral resistance.

3. **Renal artery stenosis.** Decreased renal tissue perfusion activates the renin–angiotensin–aldosterone system (see I E 2).

C. Treatment. Secondary hypertension requires treatment of the underlying cause (e.g., surgical intervention accompanied by supplementary control of hypertensive effects) [see III B].

III. ESSENTIAL (PRIMARY) HYPERTENSION

A. Clinical evaluation requires a thorough history and physical examination followed by a careful analysis of common laboratory test results.

1. **Objectives**
   a. To rule out uncommon secondary causes of hypertension
   b. To determine the presence and extent of target-organ damage
   c. To determine the presence of other cardiovascular risk factors in addition to high blood pressure

d. To reduce morbidity and mortality through multiple strategies that reduce blood pressure through life-style modifications with or without pharmacological treatment with minimal side effects.

2. **Predisposing factors**
   a. **Family history** of essential hypertension, stroke, and premature cardiac disease
   b. **Patient history** of intermittent elevations in blood pressure
   c. **Racial predisposition.** Hypertension is more common among African-Americans than Caucasians.
   d. **Obesity.** Weight reduction has been shown to reduce blood pressure in a large proportion of hypertensive patients who are more than 10% above ideal body weight.
   e. **Smoking,** resulting in vasoconstriction and activation of the sympathetic nervous system, is a major risk factor for cardiovascular disease.
   f. Stress
   g. High dietary intake of saturated fats or sodium
   h. Sedentary life-style
   i. Diabetes mellitus
   j. Hyperlipidemia
   k. Major risk factors according to the JNC-7 include smoking, diabetes mellitus, age >55 for men, age >65 for women, family history of cardiovascular disease, and dyslipidemia.
   l. Target-organ damage/clinical cardiovascular disease according to the JNC-7 includes heart disease (e.g., left ventricular hypertrophy, angina, prior MI, heart failure), stroke or transient ischemic attacks, nephropathy, peripheral artery disease, and retinopathy.

3. **Physical findings**
   a. Serial blood pressure readings greater than or equal to 140/90 should be obtained on at least two occasions before specific therapy is begun, unless the initial blood pressure levels are markedly elevated (i.e., >210 mm Hg systolic, >120 mm Hg diastolic, or both) or are associated with target-organ damage. A single elevated reading is an insufficient basis for a diagnosis.
   b. Essential hypertension usually does not become clinically evident—other than through serial blood pressure elevations—until vascular changes affect the heart, brain, kidneys, or ocular fundi.
   c. Examination of the ocular fundi is valuable; their condition can indicate the duration and severity of the hypertension.
      (1) **Early stages.** Hard, shiny deposits; tiny hemorrhages; and elevated arterial blood pressure occur.
      (2) **Late stages.** Cotton–wool patches, exudates, retinal edema, papilledema caused by ischemia and capillary insufficiency, hemorrhages, and microaneurysms become evident.

4. Untreated hypertension increases the likelihood of the development of numerous organ problems, which include left ventricular failure, MI, renal failure, cerebral hemorrhage or infarction, and severe changes in the retina of the eye.

B. **Treatment** (Tables 40-4 and 40-5; Figure 40-2)

1. **General principles.** Treatment primarily aims to lower blood pressure toward "normal" with minimal side effects and to prevent or reverse organ damage. Currently, there is no cure for primary hypertension. Treating systolic and diastolic blood pressures to targets that are less than 140/90 mm Hg is associated with a decrease in cardiovascular complications. For patients with hypertension who have diabetes or renal disease, the blood pressure goal recommended by the JNC-7 is 130/80 mm Hg.
   a. **Candidates for treatment**
      (1) All patients with a diastolic pressure of greater than 90 mm Hg, a systolic pressure of greater than 140 mm Hg, or a combination of both should receive antihypertensive drug therapy.
      (2) For those patients with a diastolic pressure of 80–89 mm Hg or a systolic pressure of 120–139 mm Hg (prehypertension), no drug treatment is indicated unless the patient has a compelling indication. However, life-style modifications such as weight reduction, dietary sodium reduction, increased physical activity, and moderation of alcohol consumption should be initiated.
   b. **Nonspecific measures.** Before initiating antihypertensive drug therapy, patients are encouraged to eliminate or minimize controllable risk factors (see III A 2).

Table 40-4. Common Antihypertensive Drugs

I. **Diuretics (Generic/Trade Name)**
   A. Thiazide diuretics
      • Bendroflumethiazide/Naturetin
      • Chlorothiazide/Diuril, various
      • Chlorthalidone/Hygroton, various
      • Hydrochlorothiazide/Hydrodiuril, various
      • Hydroflumethiazide/Saluron, various
      • Indapamide/Lozol, various
      • Methyclothiazide/Enduron, various
      • Metolazone/Zaroxolyn, Mykrox
      • Polythiazide/Renese
      • Trichlormethiazide/Naqua, various
   B. Loop diuretics
      • Bumetanide/Bumex, various
      • Ethacrynic acid/Edecrin
      • Furosemide/Lasix, various
      • Torsemide/Demadex, various
   C. Potassium-sparing diuretics
      • Amiloride/Midamor, various
      • Spironolactone/Aldactone, various
      • Triamterene/Dyrenium
II. **Vasodilators (direct acting)**
      • Diazoxide/Hyperstat, Proglycem
      • Hydralazine/Apresoline, various
      • Minoxidil/Loniten, various
      • Nitroprusside/Nitropress, various
III. **Angiotensin-converting enzyme (ACE) inhibitors**
      • Benazepril/Lotensin
      • Captopril/Capoten, various
      • Enalapril/Vasotec, various
      • Enalaprilat (IV)/Vasotec, various
      • Fosinopril/Monopril
      • Lisinopril/Prinivil, Zestril
      • Moexipril/Univasc
      • Perindopril/Aceon
      • Quinapril/Accupril
      • Ramipril/Altace
      • Trandolapril/Mavik
IV. **Angiotensin II receptor antagonists**
      • Candesartan cilexetil/Atacand
      • Eprosartan/Teveten
      • Irbesartan/Avapro
      • Losartan/Cozaar
      • Olmesartan/Benicar
      • Telmisartan/Micardis
      • Valsartan/Diovan
V. **Sympatholytics**
   A. β-Adrenergic blocking agents
      • Acebutolol/Sectral
      • Atenolol/Tenormin
      • Betaxolol/Kerlone
      • Bisoprolol/Zebeta
      • Carteolol/Cartrol
      • Carvedilol/Coreg
      • Labetalol/Normodyne, Trandate
      • Metoprolol/Lopressor, Toprol
      • Nadolol/Corgard
      • Penbutolol/Levatol
      • Pindolol/Visken
      • Propranolol/Inderal, various
      • Timolol/Blocadren
   B. Centrally acting α-agonists
      • Clonidine/Catapres, various
      • Guanabenz/Wytensin, various
      • Guanfacine/Tenex, various
      • Methyldopa/Aldomet, various
   C. Postganglionic adrenergic neuron blockers
      • Reserpine/various
   D. α-Adrenergic blocking agents
      • Doxazosin/Cardura, various
      • Prazosin/Minipress, various
      • Terazosin/Hytrin, various
   E. Calcium-channel blockers
      • Benzothiazepine derivatives
         Diltiazem/Cardizem, Dilacor, Tiazac, various
      • Diphenylalkylamine derivatives
         Verapamil/Isoptin, Calan, various
      • Dihydropyridines
         Amlodipine/Norvasc
         Felodipine/Plendil
         Isradipine/DynaCirc
         Nicardipine/Cardene
         Nifedipine/Procardia XL, Adalat CC
         Nisoldipine/Sular

   c. **Pharmacological treatment.** The recommendations of the JNC-7 suggest that recent clinical trials have demonstrated that most hypertensive patients will require two or more antihypertensive drugs.
      (1) Thiazide diuretics should be the initial choice of therapy, due to the fact that they have demonstrated a reduction in morbidity and mortality when used as initial monotherapy. They are the only drugs that have been shown to lower morbidity and mortality rates, have shown adequate long-term safety data, and have demonstrated patient tolerability.
      (2) Thiazide diuretics should be considered initial agents for treatment unless there are "compelling indications" for other medications.
      (3) Agents such as ACE inhibitors, angiotensin-receptor blockers, β-blockers, and calcium-channel blockers have all been recommended for patients who cannot receive a thiazide diuretic or in combination with a thiazide diuretic for adequate control of blood pressure. This may include the use of ACE inhibitors in hypertensive patients having systolic dysfunction after a myocardial infarction, a diabetic

Table 40-5. Common Combination Products for Hypertension

I. Diuretics
Hydrochlorothiazide—spironolactone (Aldactazide)
Hydrochlorothiazide—triamterene (Dyazide, Maxzide)
Hydrochlorothiazide—amiloride (Moduretic)

II. Diuretics—β-adrenergic blockers
Bendroflumethiazide—nadolol (Corzide)
Chlorthalidone—atenolol (Tenoretic)
Hydrochlorothiazide—propranolol (Inderide)
Hydrochlorothiazide—metoprolol (Lopressor HCT)
Hydrochlorothiazide—timolol (Timolide)
Hydrochlorothiazide—bisoprolol (Ziac)

III. Diuretics—angiotensin-converting enzyme (ACE) inhibitors
Hydrochlorothiazide—captopril (Capozide)
Hydrochlorothiazide—benazepril (Lotensin HCT)
Hydrochlorothiazide—lisinopril (Prinzide, Zestoretic)
Hydrochlorothiazide—enalapril (Vaseretic)
Hydrochlorothiazide—fosinopril (Monopril HCT)
Hydrochlorothiazide—moexipril (Uniretic)
Hydrochlorothiazide—quinapril (Accuretic)

IV. Diuretics—angiotensin II receptor antagonists
Hydrochlorothiazide—losartan (Hyzaar)
Hydrochlorothiazide—irbesartan (Avalide)
Hydrochlorothiazide—valsartan (Diovan HCT)
Hydrochlorothiazide—telmasartan (Micardis HCT)
Hydrochlorothiazide—candesartan (Atacand HCT)
Hydrochlorothiazide—eprosartan (Teveten HCT)

V. Angiotensin-converting enzyme (ACE) inhibitors—Calcium-channel blockers
Enalapril—felodipine (Lexxel)
Enalapril—diltiazem (Teczem)
Trandolapril—verapamil (Tarka)
Benazepril—amlodipine (Lotrel)

VI. Other
Chlorthalidone—clonidine (Combipres)
Chlorthalidone—reserpine (Regroton)
Chlorothiazide—reserpine (Diupres)
Chlorothiazide—methyldopa (Aldoclor)
Hydrochlorothiazide—methyldopa (Aldoril)
Hydrochlorothiazide—hydralazine (Apresazide)
Hydrochlorothiazide—guanethidine (Esimil)
Hydrochlorothiazide—reserpine (Hydropres)

nephropathy patient who might benefit from an ACE inhibitor in combination with a diuretic, or a patient with congestive heart failure (CHF).

  d. Monitoring guidelines. Specific monitoring guidelines for the various drug categories are covered in III B 2–7.

    (1) Blood pressure should be monitored routinely to determine the therapeutic response and to encourage patient compliance.

    (2) Clinicians must be alert to indications of adverse drug effects. Many patients do not link side effects to drug therapy or are embarrassed to discuss them, especially effects related to sexual function or effects that appear late in therapy.

  e. Patient compliance

    (1) Because hypertension is usually a symptomless disease, "how the patient feels" does not reflect the blood pressure level. In fact, the patient may actually report "feeling normal" with an elevated blood pressure and "abnormal" during a hypotensive episode because of the light-headedness associated with a sudden drop in blood pressure. Because essential hypertension requires a lifelong drug regimen, it is extremely difficult but necessary to impress on patients the need for compliance with their therapeutic regimen.

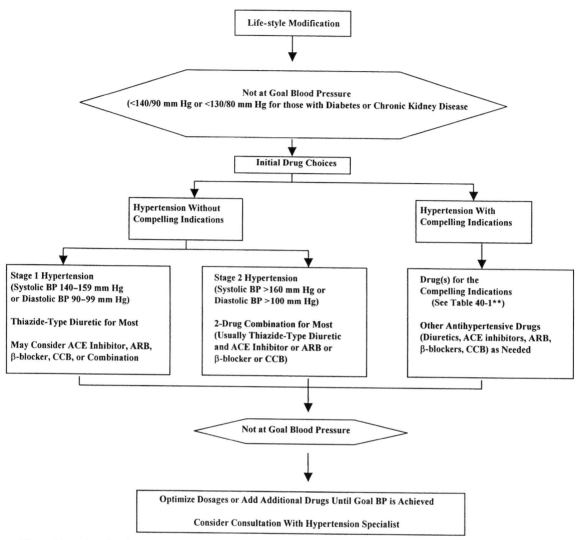

Figure 40-2. Algorithm for the treatment of hypertension. Based on the most recent recommendations from the Seventh Report of the Joint National Committee on Detection, Evaluation, and Treatment of High Blood Pressure (JNC-7).

   (2) Recognizing the seriousness of the consequences of noncompliance is key. Patients should be told that prolonged, untreated hypertension, known as the "silent killer," can affect the heart, brain, kidneys, and ocular fundi.

2. Diuretics
   a. Thiazide diuretics and their derivatives are currently recommended as initial therapy for hypertension. Recent recommendations include initiating therapy with a low dose (12.5 mg of hydrochlorothiazide or its equivalent), increasing the dose if necessary, and not exceeding a dose of 50 mg of hydrochlorothiazide or its equivalent.
      (1) Actions. Antihypertensive effects are produced by directly dilating the arterioles and reducing the total fluid volume. Thiazide diuretics increase the following:
         (a) Urinary excretion of sodium and water by inhibiting sodium and chloride reabsorption in the distal convoluted (renal) tubules
         (b) Urinary excretion of potassium and, to a lesser extent, bicarbonate
         (c) The effectiveness of other antihypertensive agents by preventing reexpansion of extracellular and plasma volumes
      (2) Significant interactions. NSAIDs, such as the now common over-the-counter forms of ibuprofen, interact to diminish the antihypertensive effects of the thiazide diuretics.

(3) Precautions and monitoring effects

(a) Potassium ion (K^+) depletion may require supplementation, increased dietary intake, or the use of a potassium-sparing diuretic.

(b) Uric acid retention may occur; this is potentially significant in patients who are predisposed to gout and related disorders.

(c) Blood glucose levels may increase, which may be significant in patients with diabetes.

(d) Calcium levels may increase because of the potential for retaining calcium ions.

(e) Patients with known allergies to sulfa-type drugs should be questioned to determine the significance of the allergy.

(f) Other common effects include fatigue, headache, palpitations, rash, vertigo, and transitory impotence.

(g) Hyperlipidemia, including **hypertriglyceridemia,** hypercholesterolemia, increased low-density lipoprotein (LDL) cholesterol, and decreased high-density lipoprotein (HDL) cholesterol, must be evaluated routinely to prevent an added risk for coronary artery disease.

(h) Fluid losses must be evaluated and monitored to prevent dehydration, postural hypotension, and even hypovolemic shock.

(i) Alterations in fluids and electrolytes (e.g., hypokalemia, hypomagnesemia, hypercalcemia) may predispose patients to cardiac irritability, with a resultant increase in cardiac arrhythmias. Electrocardiograms (ECGs) are performed routinely to prevent the development of life-threatening arrhythmias.

(4) Usual effective doses

(a) **Bendroflumethiazide**—2.5–15.0 mg daily

(b) **Benzthiazide**—50–150 mg daily

(c) **Chlorothiazide**—125–2000 mg daily

(d) **Chlorthalidone**—12.5–25 mg daily

(e) **Hydrochlorothiazide**—12.5–50 mg daily

(f) **Hydroflumethiazide**—25–100 mg daily

(g) **Indapamide**—1.25–2.5 mg daily

(h) **Methyclothiazide**—2.5–10.0 mg daily

(i) **Metolazone**—2.5–5.0 mg daily

(j) **Polythiazide**—2–4 mg daily

(k) **Quinethazone**—50–200 mg daily

(l) **Trichlormethiazide**—2–4 mg daily

b. Loop (high-ceiling) diuretics

(1) Indications. These agents are indicated when patients are unable to tolerate thiazides, experience a loss of thiazide effectiveness, or have impaired renal function (clearance <30 mL/min).

(2) Actions. Furosemide, ethacrynic acid, bumetanide, and **torsemide** act primarily in the ascending loop of Henle; hence, they are called "loop" diuretics. By acting within the loop of Henle, they decrease sodium reabsorption. Their action is more intense but of shorter duration (1–4 hours) than that of the thiazides; they may also be more expensive.

(3) Significant interactions. As with the thiazides, the antihypertensive effect of loop diuretics may be diminished by **NSAIDs.**

(4) Precautions and monitoring effects. Loop diuretics have the same effects as thiazides (see III B 2 a), in addition to the following:

(a) Loop diuretics have a complex influence on renal hemodynamics; thus, patients must be monitored closely for signs of hypovolemia. (*decrease blood volume*)

(b) Because these agents should be used cautiously in patients with episodic or chronic renal impairment, BUN and serum creatinine levels should be checked routinely.

(c) Transient deafness has been reported. If the patient is taking a potentially ototoxic drug (e.g., an aminoglycoside antibiotic), another class of diuretic (e.g., a thiazide diuretic) should be substituted.

(5) Usual effective doses

(a) **Bumetanide**—0.5–2.0 mg daily

(b) **Ethacrynic acid**—50–200 mg daily

(c) **Furosemide**—20–80 mg daily

(d) **Torsemide**—2.5–10 mg daily

c. Potassium-sparing diuretics

(1) Indications. The diuretics in this group—**spironolactone, amiloride, and triamterene**—are indicated for patients in whom potassium loss is significant and supplementation is not feasible. These agents are often used in combination with a thiazide diuretic because they potentiate the effects of the thiazide while minimizing potassium loss. **Spironolactone** is particularly useful in patients with hyperaldosteronism, as it has direct antagonistic effects on aldosterone (aldosterone-receptor blocker).

(2) Actions. Potassium-sparing diuretics achieve their diuretic effects differently and less potently than the thiazides and loop diuretics. Their most pertinent shared feature is that they promote potassium retention.

(3) Significant interactions. Coadministration with **ACE inhibitors** or **potassium supplements** significantly increases the risk of hyperkalemia.

(4) Precautions and monitoring effects

    (a) Potassium-sparing diuretics should be avoided in patients with acute renal failure and used with caution in patients with impaired renal function because they can retain potassium.

    (b) Triamterene should not be used in patients with a history of kidney stones or hepatic disease.

    (c) Hyperkalemia is a major risk, requiring routine monitoring of serum electrolytes. BUN and serum creatinine levels should be checked routinely to signal incipient excess potassium retention and impaired renal function.

(5) Usual effective doses

    (a) Amiloride—5–10 mg daily

    (b) Spironolactone—25–100 mg daily and 100–400 mg daily to treat hyperaldosteronism

    (c) Triamterene—50–100 mg daily

    (d) Eplerenone—50–100 mg daily

d. Combination products. Several products combine a thiazide and a potassium-sparing diuretic.

    (1) Aldactazide, 25 mg spironolactone/25 mg hydrochlorothiazide (one to two tablets daily)

    (2) Aldactazide–50, 50 mg spironolactone/50 mg hydrochlorothiazide (one tablet daily)

    (3) Moduretic, 5 mg amiloride/50 mg hydrochlorothiazide (one to two tablets daily)

    (4) Dyazide, 37.5 mg triamterene/25 mg hydrochlorothiazide (one to two capsules daily)

    (5) Maxzide, 75 mg triamterene/50 mg hydrochlorothiazide (one-half to one tablet daily)

    (6) Maxzide-25, 37.5 triamterene/25 mg hydrochlorothiazide

3. Sympatholytics

a. β-Adrenergic blockers

(1) Indications. β-Blockers are particularly effective in patients with rapid resting heart rates (i.e., atrial fibrillation, paroxysmal supraventricular tachycardia) or "compelling indications" such as heart failure, post-MI, high coronary disease risk, and diabetes.

(2) Actions. Proposed mechanisms of action include the following:

    (a) Stimulation of renin secretion is blocked.

    (b) Cardiac contractility is decreased, thus diminishing cardiac output.

    (c) Sympathetic output is decreased centrally.

    (d) Reduction in heart rate decreases cardiac output.

    (e) β-Blocker action may combine all of the above mechanisms.

(3) Epidemiology. Young (<45 years) whites with high cardiac output, high heart rate and normal vascular resistance respond best to β-blocker therapy.

(4) Precautions and monitoring effects

    (a) Patients must be monitored for signs and symptoms of **cardiac decompensation** (i.e., increasingly reduced cardiac output) because decreased contractility can trigger compensatory mechanisms, leading to CHF.

    (b) ECGs should be monitored routinely because all β-blockers can decrease electrical conduction within the heart.

    (c) Relative cardioselectivity is dose-dependent and is lost as dosages are increased. Therefore, **no β-blocker is totally safe in patients with bronchospastic disease** [e.g., asthma, chronic obstructive pulmonary disease (COPD)].

    (d) Suddenly stopping β-blocker therapy puts the patient at risk for a **withdrawal syndrome** that may produce:

        (i) Exacerbated anginal attacks, particularly in patients with coronary artery disease

(ii) MI

(iii) A life-threatening rebound of blood pressure to levels exceeding pretreatment readings

(e) β-Blocker therapy should be used with caution in patients with the following conditions:

  (i) **Diabetes.** β-Blockers can mask hypoglycemic symptoms, such as tachycardia.

  (ii) **Raynaud's phenomenon or peripheral vascular disease.** Vasoconstriction can occur.

  (iii) **Neurological disorders.** Several β-blockers enter the central nervous system (CNS), potentiating related side effects (e.g., fatigue, lethargy, poor memory, weakness, or mental depression).

(f) Hypertriglyceridemia, reduced HDL cholesterol, or increased LDL cholesterol have been reported as major consequences of β-blockers, which require routine lipid evaluations with chronic therapy.

(g) Impotence and decreased libido may result in reduced patient compliance.

(5) **Significant interactions.** β-Adrenergic blockers interact with numerous agents, requiring cautious selection, administration, and monitoring.

(6) **β-Blocker terms**

(a) **Relative cardioselective activity.** Relative to propranolol, β-blockers have a greater tendency to occupy the β_1-receptor in the heart, rather than the β_2-receptors in the lungs.

(b) **Intrinsic sympathomimetic activity.** These agents have the ability to release catecholamines and to maintain a satisfactory heart rate. Intrinsic sympathomimetic activity may also prevent bronchoconstriction and other direct β-blocking actions.

(7) **Specific agents**

(a) **Propranolol** was the first β-blocking agent shown to block both β_1- and β_2-receptors. The **average daily dose** is 40–480 mg. It is available both as a rapid-acting product and a long-acting product.

(b) **Metoprolol** was the first β-blocking agent with relative cardioselective blocking activity. The **average daily dose** is 50–300 mg.

(c) **Nadolol** was the first β-blocking agent that allowed once-daily dosing. It blocks both β_1- and β_2-receptors. The **average daily dose** is 40–320 mg.

(d) **Atenolol** was the first β-blocking agent to combine once-daily dosing with relative cardioselective blocking activity. The **average daily dose** is 25–100 mg.

(e) **Timolol** was the first β-blocking agent shown to be effective after an acute MI to prevent sudden death. It blocks both β_1- and β_2-receptors. The **average daily dose** is 20–60 mg.

(f) **Pindolol** was the first β-blocking agent shown to have high intrinsic sympathomimetic activity. The **average daily dose** is 10–60 mg.

(g) **Labetalol** was the first β-blocking agent shown to possess both α- and β-blocking activity. The **average daily dose** is 200–1200 mg. Labetalol is also effective for treating hypertensive crisis (Table 40-6).

(h) **Acebutolol** was the first β-blocking agent that combined efficacy with once-daily dosing, possessing intrinsic sympathomimetic activity and having relative cardioselective blocking activity. The **average daily dose** is 200–800 mg.

(i) **Esmolol** was the first β-blocking agent to have an ultrashort duration of action. This agent is not used routinely in treating hypertension owing to its duration of action and the need for intravenous administration. The **average daily dose** is 25–50 μg/kg/min up to 300 μg/kg/min intravenously.

(j) **Betaxolol** is a new β-blocker that possesses relative cardioselective blocking activity similar to metoprolol but has a half-life that allows for once-daily dosing. The **average daily dose** is 5–20 mg.

(k) **Carteolol** is a new β-blocking agent that has low lipid solubility so less drug penetrates the CNS, has moderate intrinsic sympathomimetic activity like pindolol, and allows for once-daily dosing. The **average daily dose** is 2.5–10.0 mg.

(l) **Penbutolol** is a new β-blocking agent that has weak intrinsic sympathomimetic activity like pindolol and allows for once-daily dosing. The **average daily dose** is 10–20 mg.

(m) **Bisoprolol** is a new β-blocking agent that is cardioselective and has no intrinsic sympathomimetic activity. It allows for once-daily dosing, and the **average daily dose** is 2.5–10 mg.

       (n) Carvedilol is a β-blocking agent that has β-blocking properties as well as α-blocking properties, with a resultant vasodilation. The drug is administered twice daily with a starting dose of 6.25 mg titrated at 7–14-day intervals to a dose of 25 mg twice daily. **Maximum daily doses** are 50 mg daily.

  b. Peripheral α$_1$-adrenergic blockers (e.g., prazosin, terazosin, doxazosin)

    (1) Indications. This group of drugs is available for hypertensive patients who have not responded to initial antihypertensive therapy.

    (2) Actions. The α$_1$-blockers (indirect vasodilators) block the peripheral postsynaptic α$_1$-adrenergic receptor, causing vasodilation of both arteries and veins. Also, the incidence of reflex tachycardia is lower with these agents than with the vasodilator hydralazine. These hemodynamic changes reverse the abnormalities in hypertension and preserve organ perfusion. Recent studies have also shown that these agents have no adverse effect on serum lipids and other cardiac risk factors.

    (3) Precautions and monitoring effects

      (a) First–dose phenomenon. A syncopal episode may occur within 30–90 minutes of the first dose; similarly associated are postural hypotension, nausea, dizziness, headache, palpitations, and sweating. To minimize these effects, the first dose should be limited to 1.0 mg of each agent and administered just before bedtime.

      (b) Additional adverse effects include diarrhea, weight gain, peripheral edema, dry mouth, urinary urgency, constipation, and priapism. Doxazosin in doses of 2–8 mg/day was one of the treatment arms in the recent Antihypertensive and Lipid-Lowering Treatment to Prevent Heart Attack Trial (ALLHAT), and the treatment was discontinued prematurely due to an apparent 25% increase in the incidence of combined cardiovascular disease outcomes than patients in the control group receiving the diuretic chlorthalidone. The added risk for CHF, stroke, and coronary heart disease were the major outcomes affected in the doxazosin arm.

    (4) The average daily doses are:

      (a) Prazosin, 2–30 mg in two doses

      (b) Terazosin, 1–20 mg in one dose

      (c) Doxazosin, 1–16 mg in one dose

  c. Centrally active α-agonists have been used in the past as alternatives to initial antihypertensives, but their use in mild to moderate hypertension has been reduced primarily due to other available agents. They act primarily within the CNS on α$_2$-receptors to decrease sympathetic outflow to the cardiovascular system.

    (1) Methyldopa

      (a) Actions. Methyldopa decreases total peripheral resistance through the above mechanism while having little effect on cardiac output or heart rate (except in older patients).

      (b) Precautions and monitoring effects

        (i) Common untoward effects include orthostatic hypotension, fluid accumulation (in the absence of a diuretic), and rebound hypertension upon abrupt withdrawal. Sedation is a common finding upon initiating therapy and when increasing doses; however, the sedative effect usually decreases with continued therapy.

        (ii) Fever and other flu-like symptoms occasionally occur and may represent hepatic dysfunction, which should be monitored by liver function tests.

        (iii) A positive Coombs' test develops in 25% of patients with chronic use (longer than 6 months). Less than 1% of these patients develop a hemolytic anemia. (Red blood cells, hemoglobin, and blood count indices should be checked.) The anemia is reversible by discontinuing the drug.

        (iv) Other effects include dry mouth, subtly decreased mental activity, sleep disturbances, depression, impotence, and lactation in either gender.

      (c) The **average daily dose** is 500 mg–3.0 g in two to four doses.

    (2) Clonidine

      (a) Indications. Clonidine is effective in patients with renal impairment, although they may require a reduced dose or a longer dosing interval.

      (b) Actions. Clonidine stimulates α$_2$-receptors centrally, decreasing vasomotor tone and heart rate.

      (c) Precautions and monitoring effects

Table 40-6. Rapid-Acting Parenteral Antihypertensive Agents for Hypertensive Crisis

Drug	Dose/Route	Onset of Action	Duration of Action	Comments
Vasodilators				
Sodium nitroprusside	0.3–10 mg/kg/min as IV infusion	0.5–1 minute	1–2 minutes	Immediate effect, very short duration; nausea, vomiting, muscle twitching, sweating, thiocyanate and cyanide intoxication
Nicardipine hydrochloride	5–15 mg/hr IV	<5–15 minutes	1–4 hours	Intermediate onset and duration; tachycardia may occur, headache, flushing, local phlebitis
Fenoldopam mesylate	0.1–0.3 μg/kg/min as IV infusion	<5 minutes	30 minutes	Intermediate onset and duration; action on dopamine D_1-receptors (dilation of renal/mesenteric vessels might be preferred over nitroprusside for long-term or with renal dysfunction; tachycardia, headache, nausea, flushing
Nitroglycerin	5–100 μg/min (0.3–6.0 mg/hr) as IV infusion	2–5 minutes	3–5 minutes	Useful in coronary artery disease; headache, vomiting, methemoglobinemia, tolerance with prolonged use
Enalaprilat	0.625–1.25 mg every 6 hours IV	15–30 minutes	4–6 hours	Useful in CHF, but avoid in renal impairment; precipitous fall in blood pressure in high-renin states
Hydralazine	10–20 mg IV; 10–50 mg IM;	10–20 minutes; 20–30 minutes	3–8 hours	Afterload reduction through arteriole dilation resulting in increased cardiac output; tachycardia, flushing headache, vomiting, aggravation of preexisting angina
Diazoxide	1–3 mg/kg over 30 seconds as an IV bolus, repeated every 5–15 minutes, or 10–30 mg/min infusion	2–4 minutes	3–12 hours	Useful in hypertensive encephalopathy, malignant hypertension, and eclampsia; flushing, nausea, tachycardia, and chest pain
Adrenergic Inhibitors				
Labetalol hydrochloride	20–80 mg IV bolus every 10 minutes, or 0.5–2.0 mg/min IV infusion	5–10 minutes	3–6 hours	Contraindicated in CHF, bronchospastic patients, or bradycardia; predictable hypotensive effect; vomiting, scalp tingling, burning in throat, heart block, orthostatic hypotension
Esmolol	250–500 μg/kg/min for 2 minutes, then 50–100 μg/kg/min for 4 minutes; may repeat if needed	1–2 minutes	10–20 minutes	β-adrenergic blocker with ultra-short duration of effect; primary use in perioperative situation due to short duration and quick onset; hypotension, nausea
Phentolamine	5–15 mg IV	1–2 minutes	3–10 minutes	α-Adrenergic blocker causing peripheral dilation; tachycardia, flushing, headache

IV = intravenous; IM = intramuscular; CHF = congestive heart failure.

(i) Intravenous administration causes an initial paradoxical increase in pressure (diastolic and systolic) that is followed by a prolonged drop. As with methyldopa, abrupt withdrawal can cause rebound hypertension.

(ii) Sedation and dry mouth are common but usually disappear with continued therapy.

(iii) Clonidine has a tendency to cause or worsen depression, and it heightens the depressant effects of alcohol and other sedating substances.

(d) The **average daily dose** is 0.2–1.2 mg in two to three doses.

(e) Patient compliance is a major issue for most hypertensive patients. The recently released once-weekly patch, which provides 0.1–0.3 mg per 24 hours, may improve compliance.

(3) Guanabenz and guanfacine

(a) Indications. These agents are recommended as adjunctive therapy with other antihypertensives for additive effects when initial therapy has failed.

(b) Actions. Guanabenz and guanfacine are centrally active α_2-agonists that have actions similar to clonidine.

(c) Precautions and monitoring effects. These agents should be used cautiously with other sedating medications and in patients with severe coronary insufficiency, recent MI, cerebrovascular accident (CVA), and hepatic or renal disease. Side effects include sedation, dry mouth, dizziness, and reduced heart rate.

(d) The **average daily doses** are 8–32 mg in two doses for guanabenz and 1–3 mg in one dose for guanfacine.

d. Postganglionic adrenergic neuron blockers. This class of antihypertensive drugs is best avoided unless it is necessary to treat severe refractory hypertension that is unresponsive to all other medications, because agents in this class are poorly tolerated by most patients.

(1) Reserpine

(a) General considerations. Because of the high incidence of adverse effects, other agents are usually chosen first. When used, reserpine is given in low doses and in conjunction with other antihypertensive agents. Reserpine in very low doses (0.05 mg) combined with a diuretic such as chlorothiazide (50–100 mg) may be an alternative to traditional doses of 0.05–0.25 mg/day.

(b) Actions. Reserpine acts centrally as well as peripherally by depleting catecholamine stores in the brain and in the peripheral adrenergic system.

(c) Precautions and monitoring effects

(i) A history of depression is a contraindication for reserpine. Even low doses, such as 0.25 mg/day, can trigger a range of psychic responses, from nightmares to suicide attempts. Drug-induced depression may linger for months after the last dose.

(ii) Peptic ulcer is also a contraindication for using reserpine. Even a single dose tends to increase gastric acid secretion.

(iii) Common adverse effects include drowsiness, dizziness, weakness, lethargy, memory impairment, sleep disturbances, and weight gain. Nasal congestion is also common but may decrease with continued therapy.

(d) The **average daily dose** of reserpine is 0.05–0.25 mg in one dose.

4. Vasodilators. These drugs are used as second-line agents in patients refractory to initial therapy with diuretics, β-blockers, or supplemental agents such as ACE inhibitors or calcium-channel blockers. Vasodilators directly relax peripheral vascular smooth muscle—arterial, venous, or both. The direct vasodilators should not be used alone owing to increases in plasma renin activity, cardiac output, and heart rate.

a. Hydralazine

(1) Actions. Hydralazine directly relaxes arterioles, decreasing systemic vascular resistance. It is also used intravenously or intramuscularly in managing hypertensive crisis.

(2) Precautions and monitoring effects

(a) Because hydralazine triggers compensatory reactions that counteract its antihypertensive effects, it is most useful when combined with a β-blocker, central α-agonist, or diuretic as a latter-step agent.

(b) Reflex tachycardia is common and should be considered before initiating therapy.

(c) Hydralazine may induce angina, especially in patients with coronary artery disease and those not receiving a β-blocker.

(d) Drug-induced systemic lupus erythematosus (SLE) may occur.

(i) Baseline and serial complete blood counts (CBCs) with antinuclear antibody titers should be followed routinely to detect SLE.

(ii) Slow acetylators of this drug have an increased incidence of SLE. Their risk may be reduced by administering doses of less than 200 mg/day.

(iii) Fatigue, malaise, low-grade fever, and joint aches may signal SLE.

(e) Other adverse effects may include headache, peripheral neuropathy, nausea, vomiting, fluid retention, and postural hypotension.

(3) The **average daily dose** is 50–300 mg in two doses.

b. **Minoxidil**

(1) **Actions.** A more potent vasodilator than hydralazine, minoxidil relaxes arteriolar smooth muscle directly, decreasing peripheral resistance. It also decreases renal vascular resistance while preserving renal blood flow. Effective in most patients, minoxidil is commonly used to treat patients with severe hypertension that has been refractory to conventional drug regimens.

(2) **Precautions and monitoring effects**

(a) Peripheral dilation results in a reflex activation of the sympathetic nervous system and an increase in heart rate, cardiac output, and renin secretion.

(b) Because this agent promotes sodium and water retention, particularly in the presence of renal impairment, patients should be monitored for fluid accumulation and signs of cardiac decompensation. Administering minoxidil along with a sympatholytic agent and a potent diuretic (e.g., furosemide) minimizes increased sympathetic stimulation and fluid retention.

(c) Hypertrichosis (i.e., excessive hair growth) is a common side effect, particularly if the drug is continued for more than 4 weeks.

(3) The **average daily dose** is 5–100 mg in one or two doses.

c. **Nitroprusside**

(1) **Actions.** A direct-acting peripheral dilator, this agent has potent effects on both the arterial and venous systems. It is usually used only in short-term emergency treatment of acute hypertensive crisis, when a rapid effect is required. Onset of action is almost instantaneous and is maximal in 1–2 minutes. Nitroprusside is administered intravenously with continuous blood pressure monitoring.

(2) **Precautions and monitoring effects.** To prevent acute hypotensive episodes, initial doses should be very low, followed by slow titration upward until the desired effect is achieved.

(a) Once the solution is prepared, it should be protected from light. Color changes are a signal that replacement is needed.

(b) Thiocyanate toxicity may develop with long-term treatment—particularly in patients with reduced renal activity—but can be treated with hemodialysis. Symptoms may include fatigue, anorexia, disorientation, nausea, psychotic behavior, or muscle spasms.

(c) Cyanide toxicity can occur (rarely) with long-term, high-dose administration. It may present as altered consciousness, convulsions, tachypnea, or even coma.

(3) The **average daily dose** is 0.5–10 μg/kg/min as a continuous intravenous infusion.

d. **Diazoxide**

(1) **Indications.** Diazoxide exerts a direct action on the arterioles but has little effect on venous capacity. It is used intravenously in the emergency treatment of acute hypertensive crisis.

(2) **Administration**

(a) Because the antihypertensive effect of diazoxide increases with the speed of infusion, recent recommendations suggest that a slow infusion spread over 15–30 minutes may achieve more predictable, controllable, hypotensive effects than rapid, high-dose administration.

(b) Alternatively, maximal reductions in mean arterial pressure may be obtained after 2 minutes through bolus injections of 50–150 mg for 5–10 seconds, repeated every 5–10 minutes, if needed. Additionally, the drug may be administered as a continuous infusion of 15–30 mg/min.

(3) **Precautions and monitoring effects**

(a) Diazoxide is closely related to the thiazides chemically; therefore, patients with thiazide sensitivity cross-react to diazoxide. In patients with impaired cerebral or cardiac function, the risks may outweigh the benefits of diazoxide administration.

(b) Diazoxide also produces transient hyperglycemia, requiring caution if administered to patients with diabetes.

(c) Hypotensive reactions may be severe.

(d) Unlike the thiazides, this agent promotes sodium and water retention, potentiating edema.

5. ACE inhibitors

a. General considerations. The ACE inhibitors (e.g., benazepril, captopril, enalapril, fosinopril, lisinopril, moexipril, perindopril, quinapril, ramipril, and trandolapril) are a rapidly growing group of drugs. Currently, 10 agents are available for use, but as the number of agents continues to grow, the differences among them must be considered. The recently completed Heart Outcomes Prevention Evaluation (HOPE) project demonstrated substantial clinical benefits in patients receiving ramipril, which could not be explained through its blood pressure–lowering effects alone.

b. Indications. Previous guidelines utilized the ACE inhibitors as first-line alternatives for treating hypertension in patients unable to tolerate thiazides or β-blockers. However, recent JNC-7 recommendations have identified specific patient populations that have "compelling indications" such as diabetes, post-myocardial infarction, high coronary disease risk, chronic kidney disease, and recurrent stroke prevention as where ACE inhibitors are indicated in the treatment of hypertensive or prehypertensive patients. This has been primarily because of studies documenting their clinical efficacy as well as minimal impact on patients' abilities to maintain normal function.

c. Actions

(1) These agents inhibit the conversion of angiotensin I (a weak vasoconstrictor) to angiotensin II (a potent vasoconstrictor), which decreases the availability of angiotensin II.

(2) ACE inhibitors indirectly inhibit fluid volume increases when interfering with angiotensin II by inhibiting angiotensin II–stimulated release of aldosterone, which promotes sodium and water retention. The net effect appears to be a decrease in fluid volume, along with peripheral vasodilation.

d. Significant interactions

(1) The antihypertensive effect of ACE inhibitors may be diminished by **NSAIDs** (e.g., over-the-counter forms of ibuprofen).

(2) Potassium-sparing diuretics increase serum potassium levels when used with ACE inhibitors, and potassium levels need to be very closely monitored in these patients.

e. Precautions and monitoring effects

(1) Neutropenia is rare but serious; there is an increased incidence in patients with renal insufficiency or autoimmune disease.

(2) Proteinuria occurs, particularly in patients with a history of renal disease. Urinary proteins should be monitored regularly.

(3) Serum potassium levels should be monitored regularly for hyperkalemia. The mechanism of action tends to increase potassium levels somewhat. Patients with renal impairment are at increased risk.

(4) Renal insufficiency can occur in patients with predisposing factors, such as renal stenosis, and when ACE inhibitors are administered with thiazide diuretics. Renal function should be monitored (e.g., through monitoring levels of serum creatinine and BUN).

(5) A dry cough may occur but disappears within a few days after the ACE inhibitor is discontinued. All ACE inhibitors have the potential to cause this side effect, but switching to an alternative agent may improve the symptoms.

(6) Other untoward effects include rashes, an altered sense of taste (dysgeusia), vertigo, headache, fatigue, first-dose hypotension, and minor gastrointestinal disturbances.

f. Specific agents

(1) Captopril. The original ACE inhibitor is given initially as a 6.25 mg dose three times daily and is increased to an **average daily dose** of 25–150 mg in two or three doses.

(2) Enalapril is a prodrug, which is rapidly converted to its active metabolite, enalaprilat. Initial doses are 5.0 mg daily, with an **average daily dose** of 5–40 mg. Additionally, the enalaprilat form of the drug has been used effectively for treating acute hypertensive crisis (see Table 40-6).

(3) Lisinopril is a long-acting analogue of enalapril, given initially as a 5–10 mg daily dose and adjusted to an **average daily dose** of 5–40 mg in one dose.

(4) Benazepril, fosinopril, moexipril, perindopril, quinapril, ramipril, and trandolapril have as their major benefit a longer duration of action, which in many patients may result in once-daily dosing and improved compliance. **Average daily doses** for these agents are:

(a) **Benazepril,** 10–40 mg in one to two doses

(b) **Fosinopril,** 10–40 mg in one dose

(c) **Moexipril,** 7.5–30 mg in one dose

(d) **Perindopril,** 4–8 mg in one to two doses

(e) **Quinapril,** 10–40 mg in one dose

(f) **Ramipril,** 2.5–20 mg in one dose

(g) **Trandolapril,** 1–4 mg in one dose

(5) Further study of these agents continues, and their use in other cardiovascular as well as noncardiovascular diseases continues to occur.

6. Calcium-channel blockers

a. Indications. The calcium-channel blockers are considered alternative drugs for the initial treatment of hypertension in select patient populations that are unable to take β-adrenergic–receptor blockers, such as patients with angina who also have bronchospastic disease or Raynaud's disease. Currently, eight agents (e.g., amlodipine, diltiazem, felodipine, isradipine, nicardipine, nifedipine, nisoldipine, verapamil) are available.

b. Actions

(1) Calcium-channel blockers inhibit the influx of calcium through slow channels in vascular smooth muscle and cause relaxation. Low-renin hypertensive, black, and elderly patients respond well to these agents.

(2) Although the calcium-channel blockers share a similar mechanism of action, each agent produces different degrees of systemic and coronary arterial vasodilation, sinoatrial (SA) and atrioventricular (AV) nodal depression, and a decrease in myocardial contractility.

c. Significant interactions. β-Adrenergic blockers, when used with calcium-channel blockers, may have an additive effect on inducing CHF and bradycardia. Electrical conduction to the AV node may be further depressed when patients are given agents such as verapamil and diltiazem along with β-blockers.

d. Precautions and monitoring effects

(1) Diltiazem and verapamil must be used with extreme caution or not at all in patients with conductive disturbances involving the SA or AV node, such as second- or third-degree AV block, sick sinus syndrome, and digitalis toxicity.

(2) Nifedipine use has been associated with flushing, headache, and peripheral edema; the patient may find these very troublesome, thus jeopardizing compliance. Using the sustained-release product once daily has been shown to effectively reduce these effects.

(3) Verapamil use has been associated with a significant degree of constipation, which must be treated to prevent stool straining and noncompliance.

e. Specific agents

(1) **Diltiazem.** The release of several extended-release products (Cardizem CD, Dilacor XR, Tiazac) has greatly increased this agent's role in the treatment of hypertension. Daily doses of 120–360 mg in two doses are effective for treating mild to moderate hypertension. Diltiazem already has proven efficacy as an antiarrhythmic and an antianginal agent.

(2) **Nifedipine.** The release of once-daily sustained-release preparations (Procardia XL, Adalat CC) has made this agent effective for long-term treatment of hypertension. A previously reported long list of side effects has been reduced with the sustained-release product at a daily dose of 30–120 mg as a single dose. Immediate-release nifedipine has been reported to cause ischemic events, and the current recommendation is to avoid its use if at all possible.

(3) **Verapamil.** This drug is similar to diltiazem in its actions (though with more potent effects on electrical conduction depression). Sustained-release products (Calan SR, Isoptin SR, Covera-HS, Verelan) at doses of 120–480 mg daily have been shown to be efficacious for long-term management of mild to moderate hypertension, while side effects such as dizziness, constipation, and hypotension are reduced.

(4) **Amlodipine, isradipine, felodipine, nicardipine,** and **nisoldipine** are second-generation calcium-channel blockers. These agents have been developed to produce more selective effects on specific target tissues than the first-generation agents diltiazem, nifedipine, and verapamil. These agents are chemically similar to nifedipine and are referred to as dihydropyridine derivatives. The daily dose ranges are:

   (a) Amlodipine, 2.5–10.0 mg in one dose
   (b) Isradipine, 5–20 mg in one dose
   (c) Felodipine, 2.5–20 mg in one dose
   (d) Nicardipine, 60–120 mg as an extended-release product
   (e) Nisoldipine, 10–40 mg in one dose

7. Angiotensin II type I receptor antagonists
   a. Indications. This class of drugs has been one of the fastest growing groups of drugs for the treatment of hypertension. Currently, seven agents are available and include candesartan cilexetil, eprosartan, irbesartan, losartan, olmesartan, telmisartan, and valsartan.
   b. Actions. This class of drugs works by blocking the binding of angiotensin II to the angiotensin II receptors. By blocking the receptor site, these agents inhibit the vasoconstrictor effects of angiotensin II as well as prevent the release of aldosterone due to angiotensin II from the adrenal glands. These two properties of angiotensin II have been shown to be important causes for developing hypertension. Clinically, angiotensin receptor blockers appear to be equally effective for the treatment of hypertension as ACE inhibitors.
   c. Precautions and monitoring effects
      (1) Similar to ACE inhibitors, increases in serum potassium levels can occur, especially in patients receiving potassium-sparing diuretics. When used alone, hyperkalemia has not been reported to be severe enough to require stopping its use. However, as in patients receiving ACE inhibitors, potassium levels need to be monitored closely in those with compromised renal function.
      (2) Cough associated with ACE inhibitors does not appear to occur with this group of drugs.
   d. Dosage guidelines for the available agents are as follows:
      (1) Candesartan cilexetil, 8–32 mg in one dose
      (2) Eprosartan, 400–800 mg in one to two doses
      (3) Irbesartan, 150–300 mg in one dose
      (4) Losartan, 25–100 mg in one to two doses
      (5) Olmesartan, 20–40 mg in one dose
      (6) Telmisartan, 20–80 mg in one dose
      (7) Valsartan, 80–320 mg in one dose
   e. Current status
      (1) Many authorities believe that in the treatment of hypertension, there do not appear to be significant differences between ACE inhibitors and angiotensin receptor blockers.
      (2) Familiarity and cost might very well provide the basis of the selection of one agent over another at this time.
      (3) There is little evidence that angiotensin II receptor blockers, like ACE inhibitors, prolong survival in patients with heart failure or after an MI.
      (4) Angiotensin receptor blockers should not be used in special hypertensive populations such as diabetics with nephropathy or CHF unless the patient cannot tolerate an ACE inhibitor.

IV. HYPERTENSIVE EMERGENCIES

A. Definition. A hypertensive emergency is a severe elevation of blood pressure (i.e., >200 mm Hg systolic or >140 mm Hg diastolic) that demands reduction—either immediate (within minutes) or prompt (within hours) in order to prevent or limit target-organ damage.

   1. Conditions requiring immediate reduction include hypertensive encephalopathy, acute left ventricular failure with pulmonary edema, dissecting aortic aneurysm, acute MI, and intracranial hemorrhage.

   2. Conditions requiring prompt reduction include malignant or accelerated hypertension.

B. Treatment

   1. The **reduction in blood pressure must be gradual** (e.g., a 15–mm Hg decrease in mean arterial pressure over the first hour) rather than precipitous to avoid compromising perfusion of critical organs, particularly cerebral perfusion.

   2. Specific agents used in hypertensive crisis are shown in Table 40-6; for further information on vasodilators, see III B 4.

STUDY QUESTIONS

Directions: Each of the numbered items or incomplete statements in this section is followed by answers or by completions of the statement. Select the **one** lettered answer or completion that is **best** in each case.

1. Which of the following agents represents a relatively new class of drugs used in treating hypertension?

(A) Trandolapril
(B) Carvedilol
(C) Irbesartan
(D) Moexipril
(E) Nitrendipine

2. Reflex tachycardia, headache, and postural hypotension are adverse effects that limit the use of which of the following antihypertensive agents?

(A) Prazosin
(B) Captopril
(C) Methyldopa
(D) Guanethidine
(E) Hydralazine

3. A 65-year-old man presents with stage I hypertension. The patient has diabetes mellitus and chronic kidney disease. Which of the following agents would be an appropriate selection for initial treatment in this patient based on the guidelines from the Seventh Report of the Joint National Committee on Detection, Evaluation, and Treatment of High Blood Pressure (JNC-7)?

(A) Chlorothiazide
(B) Propranolol
(C) Nitroprusside
(D) Lisinopril
(E) Clonidine

4. A hypertensive patient who has chronic obstructive pulmonary disease (COPD) and who is noncompliant would be best treated with which of the following β-blocking agents?

(A) Timolol
(B) Penbutolol
(C) Esmolol
(D) Acebutolol
(E) Propranolol

5. Long-standing hypertension leads to tissue damage in all of the following organs EXCEPT the

(A) heart
(B) lungs
(C) kidneys
(D) brain
(E) eyes

6. According to the Seventh Report of the Joint National Committee on Detection, Evaluation, and Treatment of High Blood Pressure (JNC-7), which of the following agents is suitable as initial therapy for treating stage I hypertension (assume no compelling indications for another type of drug)?

(A) Chlorothiazide
(B) Labetalol
(C) Atenolol
(D) Propranolol
(E) Bisoprolol

Directions: Each question below contains three suggested answers, of which **one or more** is correct. Choose the answer

A	if **I only** is correct
B	if **III only** is correct
C	if **I and II** are correct
D	if **II and III** are correct
E	if **I, II, and III** are correct

7. A patient treated with a thiazide diuretic should be monitored regularly for altered plasma levels of

  I. potassium
 II. glucose
III. uric acid

8. Before antihypertensive therapy begins, secondary causes of hypertension should be ruled out. Laboratory findings that suggest an underlying cause of hypertension include

  I. a decreased serum potassium level
 II. an increased urinary catecholamine level
III. an increased blood cortisol level

9. In an otherwise healthy adult with stage I hypertension, appropriate initial antihypertensive therapy would be

  I. chlorthalidone
 II. metoprolol
III. bisoprolol

Directions: Each group of items in this section consists of lettered options followed by a set of numbered items. For each item, select the **one** lettered option that is most closely associated with it. Each lettered option may be selected once, more than once, or not at all.

Questions 10–14

Match the adverse effects with the antihypertensive agent that is most likely to cause them.

(A) Ramipril
(B) Methyldopa
(C) Nitroprusside
(D) Prazosin
(E) Nadolol

10. Thiocyanate intoxication, hypotension, and convulsions

11. Bradycardia, bronchospasm, and cardiac decompensation

12. Cough, skin rash, and proteinuria

13. Postural hypotension, fever, and a positive Coombs' test

14. First-dose syncope, postural hypotension, and palpitations

Questions 15–19

Match each description of a β-blocker with the most appropriate β-adrenergic blocking agent.

(A) Esmolol
(B) Labetalol
(C) Bisoprolol
(D) Nadolol
(E) Pindolol

15. A β-blocker with intrinsic sympathomimetic activity

16. A β-blocker that also blocks α-adrenergic receptors

17. A β-blocker with an ultrashort duration of action

18. A β-blocker with a long duration of action and nonselective blocking activity

19. A β-blocker with relative cardioselective blocking activity

ANSWERS AND EXPLANATIONS

1. The answer is C *[III B 7 a].*
Irbesartan is one of the relatively new classes of drugs used in the treatment of hypertension referred to as an angiotensin II, type 1 receptor antagonist, which blocks the production of angiotensin II and consequently its effects as a powerful vasoconstrictor and stimulant for aldosterone release. Trandolapril and moexipril are angiotensin-converting enzyme inhibitors; carvedilol is a β-adrenergic blocking agent; and nitrendipine is a calcium-channel blocker.

2. The answer is E *[III B 4 a].*
Hydralazine is a vasodilator that works by directly relaxing arterioles, thereby reducing peripheral vascular resistance. Its effectiveness as an antihypertensive agent is compromised, however, by the compensatory reactions it triggers (e.g., reflex tachycardia) and by its other adverse effects (e.g., headache, postural hypotension, nausea, palpitations). Fortunately, the unwanted effects of hydralazine are minimized when it is used in combination with a diuretic agent and a β-blocker. Thus, hydralazine is most effective as a supplemental antihypertensive drug in combination with first-line therapy.

3. The answer is D *[III B 5 b].*
Lisinopril, an angiotensin-converting enzyme (ACE) inhibitor, acts by inhibiting the conversion of angiotensin I (a weak vasoconstrictor) to angiotensin II (a potent vasoconstrictor). Recent guidelines provided by the Seventh Report of the Joint National Committee on Detection, Evaluation, and Treatment of High Blood Pressure (JNC-7) call for the initial use of diuretics in the initial treatment of hypertension, unless the patient fits into a subtype group of patients that has "compelling indications," that have been shown to benefit from the use of ACE inhibitors. The patient has diabetes and chronic kidney disease and, therefore, an ACE inhibitor would be indicated in this case rather than a β-blocker (propranolol) or diuretic (chlorothiazide). Nitroprusside or clonidine are not indicated for the initial treatment of hypertension.

4. The answer is D *[III B 3 a (7) (h)].*
The β-adrenergic blocking agents are no longer considered initial treatment for hypertension unless there is a compelling indication shown to benefit from their use. A major feature of some of these agents is their relative selectivity for β_1-receptors (in the heart) rather than for β_2-receptors (in the lung), which provides advantages in the treatment of certain [e.g., chronic obstructive pulmonary disease (COPD)] patients. Of the β-blockers listed in the question, acebutolol is less likely than the rest to block β_2-receptors because of its relative cardioselective blocking activity. Acebutolol also has a long duration of action, which could be helpful in the noncompliant patient by requiring fewer doses per day. Penbutolol is a new β-blocker that has weak intrinsic sympathomimetic activity like pindolol but lacks relative cardioselectivity despite its long duration of action. Esmolol by nature of its continuous intravenous infusion would not lend itself to chronic ambulatory therapy. Timolol is a long-acting β-blocker but does not have the relative cardioselective properties that acebutolol possesses.

5. The answer is B *[I F; Table 40-3].*
Left untreated, hypertension can be lethal because of its progressively destructive effects on major organs, such as the heart, kidneys, and brain. The eyes also suffer damage; the lungs, however, do not. End-organ damage caused by hypertension includes left ventricular hypertrophy, congestive heart failure, angina pectoris, myocardial infarction, renal insufficiency caused by atherosclerotic lesions, nephrosclerosis, cerebral aneurysm and hemorrhage, retinal hemorrhage, and papilledema.

6. The answer is A *[III B 2 a].*
Thiazide diuretics are considered the first-line treatment choice for hypertension and should be used alone or in combination with other antihypertensives, if necessary. β-Blockers such as labetalol, atenolol, bisoprolol, nifedipine, and propranolol are no longer considered initial agents for treating hypertension. β-blockers have shown positive clinical outcomes in patients with heart failure, postmyocardial infarction, high coronary disease risk, and diabetes "compelling indications," and would be acceptable options for patients presenting with prehypertension or hypertension along with a compelling indication.

7. The answer is E (all) *[III B 2 a].*
Thiazide diuretics act directly on the kidneys by increasing the excretion of sodium and water and, to a lesser extent, the excretion of potassium. Patients who are treated with thiazides should be monitored

for hypokalemia, which may require potassium supplementation or addition of a potassium-sparing diuretic to the antihypertensive regimen. Thiazide diuretics have the opposite effect on uric acid and glucose excretion. Thus, patients receiving these drugs also should be monitored for increased plasma levels of uric acid (especially if they are predisposed to gout) and glucose (especially if they are predisposed to diabetes).

8. The answer is E (all) *[II A 1].*
Low serum potassium levels in a hypertensive patient suggest primary aldosteronism. Elevated urinary catecholamines suggest a pheochromocytoma; other signs and symptoms of this tumor include weight loss, episodic flushing, and sweating. Elevated serum cortisol levels suggest Cushing's syndrome; the patient is also likely to have a round (moon) face and truncal obesity. Secondary hypertension requires treatment of the underlying cause; supplementary antihypertensive drug therapy may also be needed.

9. The answer is A (I) *[III B 2 a, 3 a].*
Thiazide diuretics such as chlorthalidone are now considered, based on the JNC-7 report, to represent first-line therapy for hypertension barring any compelling indications such as heart failure, diabetes, chronic kidney disease, or post–myocardial infarction where other antihypertensive agents would be indicated. β-adrenergic blockers, such as metoprolol and bisoprolol, are no longer indicated as initial antihypertensive agents for treating hypertension.

10–14. The answers are: 10-C *[III B 4 c (2)],* **11-E** *[III B 3 a (4), (7) (a)],* **12-A** *[III B 5 e, f (4)],* **13-B** *[III B 3 c (1) (b)],* **14-D** *[III B 3 b (3), (4)].*
The goal of treatment in hypertension is to lower blood pressure toward "normal" with minimal side effects. All antihypertensive drugs can cause adverse effects. The primary purpose of the Seventh Report of the Joint National Committee on Detection, Evaluation, and Treatment of High Blood Pressure (JNC-7) guidelines is to acknowledge the long-term benefits of diuretics in the treatment of hypertension. However, at the same time, recognize that other agents may play a primary role in various clinical entities such as angiotensin-converting enzyme (ACE) inhibitors in diabetes, post–myocardial infarction, high coronary disease risk, and recurrent stroke prevention; calcium-channel blockers in patients with high coronary disease risk and diabetes, β-blockers in heart failure, post–myocardial infarction, high coronary disease risk, and diabetes.

15–19. The answers are: 15-E, 16-B, 17-A, 18-D, 19-C *[III B 3 a (7)].*
The β-adrenergic blocking agents are valuable for managing hypertension and are used as initial antihypertensives. The β-blockers are sympathetic antagonists. They act by blocking various receptors of the sympathetic nervous system. They differ in their selectivity for these sympathetic receptors. For example, β_1-blockers have relative cardioselective activity; that is, they block β_1-receptors (in the heart) rather than β_2-receptors (in bronchial smooth muscle) and, therefore, are highly useful antihypertensive agents. Intrinsic sympathomimetic activity also appears to reduce the problem of bronchoconstriction; moreover, drugs with this property can also maintain a satisfactory heart rate.

41
Heart Failure

Alan H. Mutnick

I. INTRODUCTION

A. Definition. Heart failure (HF) is a complex clinical syndrome that can result from any cardiac disorder that impairs the ability of the ventricle to deliver adequate quantities of blood to the metabolizing tissues during normal activity or at rest. The condition in the past has been referred to as "congestive heart failure" due to the **edematous state** commonly produced by the fluid backup resulting in shortness of breath, fatigue, limitation of exercise tolerance, and fluid retention. Fluid retention may lead to pulmonary and peripheral edema. Most recently, due to the fact that all patients do not necessarily present with fluid overload at the initial or follow-up evaluations, the term "heart failure" more adequately reflects the clinical syndrome.

B. Mortality rate. Approximately 300,000 patients die due to direct or indirect consequences of HF each year, and the number of deaths due to HF (primary or secondary causes) has increased steadily despite treatment advances. The risk of death is 5–10% annually in patients with mild symptoms and is as high as 30–40% in patients with advanced disease manifestations.

C. Incidence of HF. HF is a common medical condition that affects almost 5 million people in the United States, with about 500,000 new cases diagnosed each year. Approximately 1.5%–2.0% of the population has HF, and the incidence increases to 6%–10% in patients older than age 65. HF is the only major cardiovascular disorder that is increasing in incidence and prevalence. During the last 10 years, there has been a dramatic increase in the number of hospitalizations primarily due to HF (500,000 in 1991 to nearly 900,000 during 2001).

D. Cost of HF. Direct expenditures for the treatment of HF in the United States had been estimated at approximately $38 billion more than 10 years ago, which included physicians' and other health-care professionals' costs, hospital and nursing home services, medication costs, home health care, and other medical equipment. Currently in the United States, more than $500 million is spent annually on drugs used in the treatment of HF.

E. Etiology

1. Although the disease occurs most commonly among the elderly (80% of patients hospitalized with HF), it may appear at any age as a consequence of underlying cardiovascular disease.

2. There currently is no diagnostic test for HF, and the clinical diagnosis is normally based on patient history and physical examination.

3. HF should not be considered an independent diagnosis, as it is superimposed on an underlying cause.
   a. Coronary artery disease is the cause of HF in about two-thirds of patients with left ventricular systolic dysfunction.
   b. The remaining one-third of patients have a nonischemic cause of systolic dysfunction due to other causes of myocardial stress, which included trauma, disease, or other abnormal states (e.g., pulmonary embolism, infection, anemia, pregnancy, drug use or abuse, fluid overload, arrhythmia, valvular heart disease, cardiomyopathies, congenital heart disease).

4. The New York Heart Association (NYHA) had developed a classification system, still utilized today to quantify the functional limitations of HF patients (see below).
   a. Class I—Degree of effort necessary to elicit HF symptoms equals those that would limit normal individuals.
   b. Class II—Degree of effort necessary to elicit HF symptoms occurs with ordinary exertion.

c. Class III—Degree of effort necessary to elicit HF symptoms occurs with less-than-ordinary exertion.

d. Class IV—Degree of effort necessary to elicit HF symptoms occurs while at rest.

5. A criticism of the NYHA is its dependence on subjective assessments by the clinical practitioner, which changes frequently, and might not accurately reflect differing treatment options based on the degree of symptoms. Consequently, most recently, within the ACC/AHA Guidelines for the Evaluation and Management of Chronic Heart Failure, a new classification scheme was introduced that depicted HF as an evolving clinical entity and a progression characterized based on risk factors and structural changes, which may be asymptomatic and symptomatic, where specific treatments targeted at each stage can impact morbidity and mortality (Table 41-1).

F. Forms of HF. As mentioned above, HF is a complex syndrome and has been described in various ways. The following section provides several ways that have been used to describe the pathophysiology as well as the symptomatology involved in it. Though the terms low-output versus high-output and left-sided versus right-sided are not routinely used in the clinical setting, their use in this section is to help convey important educational aspects of HF, and are only presented for the purpose of simplifying the pathophysiology and symptomatology.

1. **Low-output versus high-output failure**

   a. If metabolic demands are within normal limits but the heart is unable to meet them, the failure is designated **low output** (the most common type).

   b. If metabolic demands increase (e.g., hyperthyroidism, anemia) and the heart is unable to meet them, the failure is designated **high output.** As compared to low-output failure, correction of the underlying cause of high-output failure is paramount as the initial treatment modality.

Table 41-1. Stages of HF Based on Evolution and Progression of Clinical Findings

Stage	Description	Examples
A	Patients at high risk of developing heart failure (HF) because of the presence of conditions that are strongly associated with the development of HF. Such patients have no identified structural or functional abnormalities of the pericardium, myocardium, or cardiac valves and have never shown signs or symptoms of HF.	Systemic hypertension; coronary artery disease; diabetes mellitus; history of cardiotoxic drug therapy or alcohol abuse; personal history of rheumatic fever; family history of cardiomyopathy
B	Patients who have developed structural heart disease that is strongly associated with the development of HF but who have never shown signs or symptoms of HF.	Left ventricular hypertrophy or fibrosis; left ventricular dilation or hypocontractility; asymptomatic valvular heart disease; previous myocardial infarction
C	Patients who have current or prior symptoms of HF associated with underlying structural heart disease.	Dyspnea or fatigue due to left ventricular systolic dysfunction; asymptomatic patients who are undergoing treatment for prior symptoms of HF
D	Patients with advanced structural heart disease and marked symptoms of HF at rest despite maximal medical therapy and who require specialized interventions.	Patients who are frequently hospitalized for HF and cannot be safely discharged from the hospital; patients in the hospital awaiting heart transplantation; patients at home receiving continuous intravenous support for symptom relief or being supported with a mechanical circulatory assist device; patients in a hospice setting for the management of HF

Adapted from Hunt SA, Baker DW, Chin MH, Cinquegrani MP, Feldman AM, Francis GS, Ganiats TG, Goldstein S, Gregoratos G, Jessup ML, Noble RJ, Packer M, Silver MA, Stevenson LW. ACC/AHA guidelines for the evaluation and management of chronic HF in the adult: executive summary: a report of the American College of Cardiology/American Heart Association Task Force on Practice Guidelines (Committee to Revise the 1995 Guidelines for the Evaluation and Management of Heart Failure). *J Am Coll Cardiol* 2001;38:2101–2113.

2. **Left-sided versus right-sided failure**
   a. **General symptomatology.** The signs and symptoms of HF usually result from the effects of blood backing up behind the failing ventricle (except in HF due to increased body demands).
   b. Left-sided and right-sided HF do not routinely exist as separate entities; however, the use of separate terms provides two distinct entities in order to best illustrate the systemic consequences as blood pools behind the respective "failing ventricle." In clinical practice, symptoms reflect systemic congestion rather than isolated left-sided or right-sided.
   c. This progression occurs because the cardiovascular system is a closed system (Figure 41-1); thus, over time, right-sided failure causes left-sided failure and vice versa.
   d. **Left-sided failure**
      (1) If blood cannot be adequately pumped from the left ventricle to the peripheral circulation and it accumulates within the left ventricle, the failure is designated **left-sided.**
      (2) Given this accumulation, the left ventricle is unable to accept blood from the left atrium and lung; therefore, the fluid portion of the blood backs up into the pulmonary alveoli, producing pulmonary edema.
   e. **Right-sided failure**
      (1) When blood cannot be pumped from the right ventricle into the lungs and accumulates within the right ventricle, the failure is designated **right-sided.**
      (2) When blood is not pumped from the right ventricle, the fluid portion of the blood backs up throughout the body (e.g., in the veins, liver, legs, bowels), producing systemic edema.

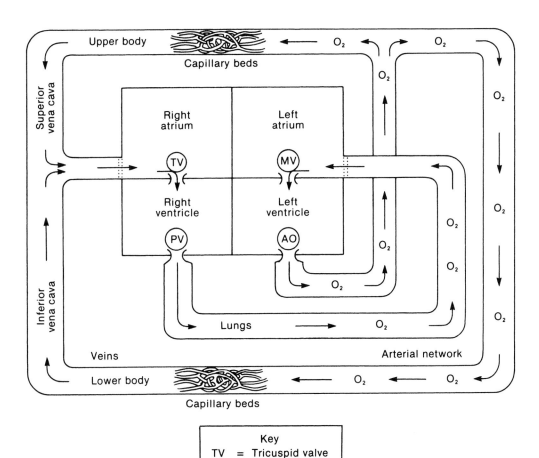

Figure 41-1. An overview of blood flow through the cardiovascular system.

Table 41-2. Substances That May Exacerbate Heart Failure

Promote Sodium Retention	Produce Osmotic Effect	Decrease Contractility
Androgens	Albumin	Antiarrhythmic agents (e.g., disopyramide, flecainide, quinidine)
Corticosteroids	Glucose	β-adrenergic blockers
Diazoxide	Mannitol	Select calcium channel blockers (e.g., diltiazem, nifedipine, verapamil)
Estrogens	Saline	Direct cardiotoxins (e.g., doxorubicin, ethanol, cocaine, amphetamines)
Licorice	Urea	Tricyclic antidepressants
Lithium carbonate		
NSAIDs		

G. **Treatment goals.** HF requires a two-pronged therapeutic approach, the overall goals of which are:

1. **To remove or mitigate the underlying causes or risk factors;** for example, by eliminating ingestion of certain drugs or other substances (Table 41-2) that can produce or exacerbate HF or by correcting an anemic syndrome, which can increase cardiac demands. Additionally, modifying risk factors, such as treatment of hypertension, diabetes, management of atherosclerotic disease, and control of conditions, such as smoking, alcohol, and illicit drug usage, that can cause cardiac injury.

2. **To relieve the symptoms and improve pump function by:**
   a. Reducing metabolic demands through rest, relaxation, and pharmaceutical controls
   b. Reducing fluid volume excess through dietary and pharmaceutical controls
   c. Administration of a combination of diuretics, ACE inhibitors, β-adrenergic blockers, and digitalis
   d. Promoting patient compliance and self-regulation through education
   e. Selecting appropriate patients for cardiac transplantation

3. During recent years, several sets of guidelines have been developed for the treatment of HF. Most recently, a panel of leading physicians and researchers in the field of HF provided recommendations within the following citation: Hunt SA, Baker DW, Chin MH, Cinquegrani MP, Feldman AM, Francis GS, Ganiats TG, Goldstein S, Gregoratos G, Jessup ML, Noble RJ, Packer M, Silver MA, Stevenson LW. ACC/AHA guidelines for the evaluation and management of chronic HF in the adult: executive summary: a report of the American College of Cardiology/American Heart Association Task Force on Practice Guidelines (Committee to Revise the 1995 Guidelines for the Evaluation and Management of Heart Failure). *J Am Coll Cardiol* 2001;38:2101–2113. The document is available on the websites of the American College of Cardiology (http://www.acc.org), the American Heart Association (http://www.americanheart.org), and the American College of Cardiology (http://www.acc.org/clinical/guidelines/failure/hf_index.htm). These guidelines represent the most up-to-date standards for the prevention, diagnosis, and treatment of HF (See Figure 41-3).

II. **PATHOPHYSIOLOGY.** HF and decreased cardiac output trigger a complex scheme of compensatory mechanisms designed to normalize cardiac output (cardiac output = stroke volume × heart rate). The principal manifestation of progression in cardiac dysfunction is a change in the geometry of the left ventricle resulting in ventricular dilation, as well as hypertrophy with a resultant increase in a more spherical shape referred to as "cardiac remodeling." This results in increases in ventricular wall tension, depression in mechanical performance, and retention of normal cardiac fluid, which worsen the remodeling process.

A. **Compensation.** A simplified figure reflecting these mechanisms is represented schematically in Figure 41-2.

1. **Sympathetic responses.** Inadequate cardiac output stimulates reflex (norepinephrine and epinephrine) activation of the sympathetic nervous system and an increase in circulating catecholamines. The heart rate increases, and blood flow is redistributed to ensure perfusion of the most vital organs (the brain and the heart).

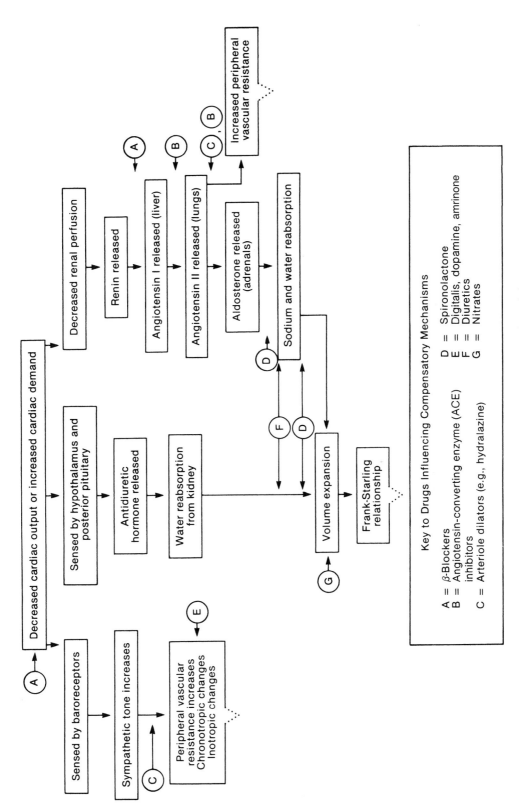

Figure 41-2. Compensatory mechanisms in congestive heart failure (CHF).

2. **Hormonal stimulation.** The redistribution of blood flow results in reduced renal perfusion, which decreases the glomerular filtration rate (GFR). Reduction in GFR results in:
   a. Sodium and water retention
   b. Activation of the renin–angiotensin–aldosterone system, which further enhances sodium retention and, thus, volume expansion

3. **Concentric cardiac hypertrophy** describes a mechanism that thickens cardiac walls, providing larger contractile cells and diminishing the capacity of the cavity in an attempt to precipitate expulsion at lower volumes (as described above, "ventricular remodeling").

4. **Frank-Starling mechanism.** The premise of this response is that increased fiber dilation heightens the contractile force, which then increases the energy released.
   a. Within physiological limits, the heart pumps all the blood it receives without allowing excessive accumulation within the veins or cardiac chambers.
   b. As blood volume increases, the various cardiac chambers dilate (stretch) and enlarge in an attempt to accommodate the excess fluid.
   c. As these stretched muscles contract, the contractile force increases in proportion to their distention. Then the extended fibers "snap back" (as a rubber band would), expelling the extra fluid into the arteries.
   d. Additional evidence suggests that the release of cytokines (e.g., tumor-necrosis factor) occurs in concert with elevated levels of circulating norepinephrine, angiotensin II, aldosterone, endothelin, and vasopressin, which may all play a role in adversely affecting the heart structure, resulting in depressed performance.

B. **Decompensation.** Over time, the compensatory mechanisms become exhausted and increasingly ineffective, entering a vicious spiral of decompensation in which the mechanisms surpass their limits and become self-defeating—as they work harder, they only exhaust the system's capacity to respond.

1. As the strain continues, total peripheral resistance and afterload increase, thereby decreasing the percentage of blood ejected per unit of time. Afterload is determined by the amount of contractile force needed to overcome intraventricular pressure and eject the blood.
   a. **Afterload** is the tension in ventricular muscles during contraction. In the left ventricle, this tension is determined by the amount of force needed to overcome pressure in the aorta. Afterload (also known as intraventricular systolic pressure) is sometimes used to describe the amount of force needed in the right ventricle to overcome pressure in the pulmonary artery.
   b. **Preload** is the force exerted on the ventricular muscle at the end of diastole that determines the degree of muscle fiber stretch. This concept is also known as ventricular end-diastolic pressure. Preload is a key factor in contractility because the more these muscles are stretched in diastole, the more powerfully they contract in systole.

2. As the fluid volume expands, so do the demands on an already exhausted pump, allowing increased volume to remain in the ventricle.

3. The resulting fluid backup (from the left ventricle into the lungs; from the right ventricle into peripheral circulation) produces the signs and symptoms of HF.

III. **CLINICAL EVALUATION.** Assessment of fluid status as well as left ventricular ejection fraction (usually less than 40% in patients with HF (see Figure 41-3).

A. **Fluid accumulation behind the left ventricle**

1. **Signs and symptoms**
   a. Dyspnea
      (1) As HF progresses, the amount of effort required to trigger **exertional dyspnea** lessens.
      (2) **Both paroxysmal nocturnal dyspnea** and **orthopnea** result from volume pooling in the recumbent position and can be relieved by propping up the patient with pillows or having the patient sit upright. (Orthopnea is often gauged by the number of pillows the patient needs to sleep comfortably.)
   b. Dry, wheezing cough

Stage A	Stage B	Stage C	Stage D
High risk of developing HF but no structural heart disease or symptoms of HF	Structural heart disease but without symptoms of HF	Structural heart disease with prior or current symptoms of HF	Refractory HF requiring specialized interventions
Therapy Treat hypertension Encourage smoking cessation Treat lipid disorders Encourage regular exercise Discourage alcohol intake, illicit drug use ACE inhibition in appropriate patients	**Therapy** All measures under stage A ACE inhibitors in appropriate patients β-Adrenergic blockers in appropriate patients	**Therapy** All measures under stage A Drugs for routine use: Diuretics ACE inhibitors β-Adrenergic blockers Digitalis Dietary salt restriction	**Therapy** All measures under stages A, B, and C Mechanical assist devices Heart transplantation Continuous (not intermittent) intravenous inotropic infusions for palliation Hospice care

Figure 41-3. Approach to heart failure. Adapted from Hunt SA, Baker DW, Chin MH, Cinquegrani MP, Feldman AM, Francis GS, Ganiats TG, Goldstein S, Gregoratos G, Jessup ML, Noble RJ, Packer M, Silver MA, Stevenson LW. ACC/AHA guidelines for the evaluation and management of chronic HF in the adult: executive summary: a report of the American College of Cardiology/American Heart Association Task Force on Practice Guidelines (Committee to Revise the 1995 Guidelines for the Evaluation and Management of Heart Failure). *J Am Coll Cardiol* 2001; 38:2101–2113.

    c. Exertional fatigue and weakness

    d. Nocturia. Edematous fluids that accumulate during the day migrate from dependent areas when the patient is in a recumbent position and renal perfusion increases.

2. Physical findings

    a. Rales (or crackles) indicate the movement of air through fluid-filled passages.

    b. Tachycardia is an early compensatory response detected through an increased pulse rate.

    c. S_3 ventricular gallop is a vibration produced by rapid filling of the left ventricle early in diastole.

    d. S_4 atrial gallop is a vibration produced by increased resistance to sudden, forceful ejection of atrial blood in late diastole; it does not vary with inspiration in left-sided failure and is more common in diastolic dysfunction.

3. Diagnostic test results

    a. Cardiomegaly (heart enlargement), left ventricular hypertrophy, and pulmonary congestion may be evidenced by chest radiograph, electrocardiogram (ECG), and reduction in left ventricular function via echocardiography and radionuclide ventriculography.

    b. Arm-to-tongue circulation time is prolonged.

    c. Transudative pleural effusion may be suggested by radiograph and confirmed by analysis of aspirated pleural fluid.

B. Fluid accumulation behind the right side of the heart

1. Signs and symptoms

    a. Complaints by the patient of tightness and swelling (e.g., "My ring is too tight," "My skin feels too tight") suggest edema.

    b. Nausea, vomiting, anorexia, bloating, or abdominal pain on exertion may reflect hepatic and visceral engorgement, resulting from venous pressure elevation.

2. Physical findings

    a. Jugular vein distention reflects increased venous pressure and is a cardinal sign of HF.

    b. S_3 ventricular gallop is described in III A 2 c.

    c. S_4 atrial gallop intensifies on inspiration in right-sided failure.

    d. Hepatomegaly (a tender, enlarged liver) is revealed when pushing on the edge of the liver results in a fluid reflux into the jugular veins, causing bulging (positive hepatojugular reflux).

    e. Bilateral leg edema is an early sign of right-sided HF; pitting ankle edema signals more advanced HF. However, edema is common to many disorders, and a pattern of associated findings, such as concurrent neck vein distention, is required for differential diagnosis.

    3. Laboratory findings. Elevated levels of hepatic enzymes [e.g., alanine aminotransferase (ALT)] reflect hepatic congestion.

IV. THERAPY

A. Bed rest

    1. Advantages
        a. Bed rest decreases metabolic needs, which reduces cardiac workload.
        b. Reduced workload, in turn, reduces pulse rate and dyspnea.
        c. Bed rest also helps decrease excess fluid volume by promoting diuresis.

    2. Disadvantages. Physical activity (except during acute decompensation) should be encouraged to avoid physical deconditioning and exercise intolerance. The risk of venous stasis increases with bed rest and can result in thromboembolism. Antiembolism stockings help minimize this risk, as do passive or active leg exercises, when the patient's condition permits.

    3. Progressive ambulation should follow adequate bed rest.

B. Dietary controls

    1. Consuming small but frequent meals (4–6 daily) that are low in calories and residue provide nourishment without unduly increasing metabolic demands.

    2. Moderate sodium restriction along with daily measurements of weight help maximize the lowest and safest doses of diuretics, a primary tool in reducing central volume in HF.
        a. Renal function should be evaluated to assess sodium conservation if severe sodium restriction is contemplated.
        b. Moderate sodium restriction (2–4 grams of dietary sodium/day) can be achieved with relative ease by limiting the addition of salt during cooking and at the table.
        c. The patient should be advised about medications and common products that contain sodium and cautioned about their use (e.g., antacids, sodium bicarbonate or baking soda, commercial diet food products, water softeners). Table 41-2 lists other substances that promote sodium retention.

C. Drug-related considerations. Therapeutic interventions might improve cardiac performance in the following ways:

    1. Drugs may increase the cardiac ejection fraction by directly stimulating cardiac contractility. The use of positive inotropic agents such as dopamine, dobutamine, and milrinone can produce immediate benefits; however, the long-term benefit has not been appreciated, and in some cases may actually increase morbidity and mortality.

    2. Drugs may increase the ejection fraction by decreasing the impedance to ejection through relaxation of peripheral blood vessels. The use of vasodilators such as hydralazine and other arteriol dilators may produce short-term benefit but do not necessarily produce clinical benefits in the long term.

    3. Drugs may improve the ejection fraction by affecting the cardiac remodeling process. Neurohormonal antagonists such as ACE inhibitors, β-adrenergic receptor blockers, and vasodilator-growth inhibitors such as nitrates may not produce immediate benefits, but long-term use might improve clinical status and decrease future cardiac events.

    4. ACE inhibitors, diuretics, β-adrenergic blockers, and usually digitalis form the basic core of treatment for HF.

D. Digitalis glycosides

    1. Digitalis, specifically digoxin, is now recommended in conjunction with diuretics, an ACE inhibitor, and a β-adrenergic blocker to improve the symptoms and clinical status of patients with HF due to left ventricular systolic dysfunction.

2. Digoxin had previously been recommended in patients with HF who had rapid atrial fibrillation to control the ventricular rate. Current guidelines suggest use of alternative agents for ventricular rate control rather than digoxin.

3. Digoxin can be used early to reduce symptoms in HF patients who have been started on ACE inhibitors or β-adrenergic blockers but have not yet responded to them.

4. Long-term trials of select patients with HF have demonstrated that treatment with digoxin had little effect on short-term mortality, but reduced the risk of death and hospitalization.

5. Therapeutic effects
   a. Positive inotropic effects were previously felt to provide most of the benefits through increased cardiac output, decreased cardiac filling pressure, decreased venous and capillary pressure, increased renal blood flow, and decreased heart size.
   b. Recent evidence suggests that digitalis acts by furthering the activation of neurohormonal systems rather than as a positive inotropic agent. This results in deactivation of renin–angiotensin–aldosterone compensation, which promotes diuresis, reduces fluid volume, decreases renal sodium reabsorption, and diminishes edema.
   c. Negative chronotropic effects accrue from the effect of digitalis on the sino-atrial (SA) node when given in doses that produce high total body stores (e.g., 15–18 μg/kg).

6. Choice of agent. All of the digitalis glycosides have similar properties; however, digoxin is the most commonly used preparation in the United States.
   a. Digoxin is available in tablet, injection, elixir, and capsule forms.
   b. Calculation of doses must factor in the differences in systemic availability among these forms. For example, digoxin solution in capsules is more bioavailable than digoxin tablets; therefore, 0.125-mg tablets are equivalent to 0.1-mg capsules. In the majority of patients, the dosage of digoxin should be the equivalent of 0.125–0.25 mg daily of the tablet formulation.

7. Dosage and administration. The range between therapeutic and toxic doses is extremely narrow. There is no "magic threshold" level for digoxin therapy, but serum concentrations of 0.8–2.0 ng/mL have been associated with therapeutic response and minimal toxicity.
   a. Rapid digitalization
      (1) In this method, the effects (and steady-state levels) are achieved within 24 hours, but the actual administration rate is usually slow and delivered in divided doses.
      (2) In the presence of an acute need for an immediate effect, intravenous digitalization with digoxin may be required—if the patient has not received any digitalis in the previous 2 weeks.
   b. Slow digitalization. When urgency is not the driving force, oral administration of maintenance doses should achieve steady-state levels in 7–8 days for the average patient (3–4 weeks in a patient with renal dysfunction).

8. Precautions and monitoring effects
   a. Potassium seems to antagonize digitalis preparations.
      (1) Decreased potassium levels favor digoxin binding to cardiac cells and increase its effect, thus increasing the likelihood of digitalis toxicity. This antagonism is particularly significant for the HF patient who is receiving a diuretic (many of which decrease potassium levels).
      (2) Conversely, increased potassium levels seem to decrease digoxin binding and decrease its effect. This is likely in patients taking potassium or a captopril-like agent (which increases potassium reabsorption).
   b. Calcium ions act synergistically with digoxin, and increased levels increase the force of myocardial contraction. At excessive levels, arrhythmias and systolic standstill can develop.
   c. Magnesium levels are inversely related to digoxin activity. As magnesium levels decrease, the predisposition to toxicity increases and, within reason, vice versa.
   d. Serum digoxin levels
      (1) In cardiac glycoside therapy, the patient's clinical state is the most practical barometer of a successful regimen. However, should questions arise as to compliance, absorption, or a drug–drug interaction, serum digoxin levels may be helpful.

   (2) After oral ingestion of digoxin, serum levels rise rapidly, then drop sharply as the drug enters the myocardium and other tissues. Therefore, a meaningful evaluation requires a determination of the relationship between serum digoxin levels and myocardial tissue levels.

   (3) The most meaningful results are obtained if serum samples are taken after steady state has been reached and 6–8 hours after an oral dose (3–4 hours after an intravenous dose).

   e. Renal function studies. Because the kidney is the primary metabolic route for **digoxin,** renal function studies such as serum creatinine levels aid the evaluation of elimination kinetics for digoxin.

9. Digitalis toxicity is a fairly common occurrence because of the narrow therapeutic range and can be fatal in a significant percentage of patients experiencing a toxic reaction.

   a. Risk of toxicity increases with coadministration of quinidine, verapamil, flecainide, propafenone, spironolactone, and amiodarone and is influenced by the electrolyte effects described previously.

   b. Signs of toxicity include:

   (1) Anorexia, a common and early sign

   (2) Fatigue, headache, and malaise

   (3) Nausea and vomiting

   (4) Mental confusion and disorientation

   (5) Alterations in visual perception (e.g., blurring, yellowing, a halo effect)

   (6) Cardiac effects, which include:

   (a) Premature ventricular contractions and ventricular tachycardia and fibrillation

   (b) SA and atrioventricular (AV) block

   (c) Atrial tachycardia with AV block

   c. Treatment of toxicity

   (1) Digitalis is discontinued immediately, as is any potassium-depleting diuretic.

   (2) If the patient is hypokalemic, potassium supplements are administered and serum levels are monitored to avoid hyperkalemia through overcompensation. However, potassium supplements are contraindicated in a patient with severe AV block.

   (3) Arrhythmias are treated with lidocaine (usually a 100-mg bolus, followed by infusion at 2–4 mg/min) or phenytoin (as a slow intravenous infusion of 25–50 mg/min, to a maximum of 1.0 g).

   (4) Cholestyramine, which binds to digitalis glycosides, may help prevent absorption and reabsorption of digitalis in the bile.

   (5) Patients with very high serum digoxin levels (such as those resulting from a suicidal overdose) may benefit from the use of purified digoxin-specific Fab fragment antibodies. One vial (40 mg) will bind 0.6 mg of digitalis. The dosage is calculated based on the estimated total body store of digitalis.

E. Diuretics

1. Diuretics should be prescribed for all patients with symptoms of HF who have evidence of or who have experienced fluid retention, since these drugs are the only ones that can correct fluid retention. Diuretics are generally best used in conjunction with an ACE inhibitor and/or a β-adrenergic blocker.

2. Diuretics have been shown to cause a reduction in jugular venous pressures, pulmonary congestion, peripheral edema, and body weight in short-term studies, and have been shown to improve cardiac function and exercise tolerance in intermediate-term studies.

3. The goal of diuretic therapy is to reduce and eventually eliminate signs and symptoms of fluid retention as assessed by JVD, peripheral edema, or both. Slow titration upward in doses may be necessary in order to minimize hypotension and should be continued until fluid retention is eliminated.

4. Body weight is an effective method of monitoring fluid losses and is best done on a daily basis by the patient.

5. Patients who experience diuretic resistance or tolerance to their effects might need intravenous administration, a combination of two agents with differing mechanisms (furosemide and metolazone) or the addition of agents such as dopamine or dobutamine, which increase renal blood flow. Additionally, evaluation of patient drug profiles may identify the addition of sodium-retaining agents such as NSAIDs.

6. All diuretics increase urine volume and sodium excretion, but differ in their pharmacolgical properties.

7. **Thiazide diuretics** are effective and commonly used, but they deplete potassium stores in the process. They are relatively weak, as they are able to increase the fractional excretion of sodium to only 5%–10% of the filtered load. However, they have been shown to lose their effectiveness in HF patients with moderately impaired renal function (creatinine clearance <30 mL/min).

8. The **loop** *diuretics* furosemide, ethacrynic acid, and bumetanide have become preferred diuretics that have the ability to increase sodium excretion to 20–25% of the filtered load and to maintain their efficacy until renal function is severely impaired (creatinine clearance <5 mL/min, plus the added advantage of reducing venous return independent of diuresis. Additionally, furosemide's action is more intense, and it is useful as a rapid-acting intravenous agent in reversing acute pulmonary edema, due to its direct dilating effects on pulmonary vasculature (see Table 41-3 for dosing).

9. **Potassium-sparing diuretics** may help avoid the exacerbating effects of hypokalemia, but they have a weaker diuretic effect than the other diuretics. As the number of HF patients receiving ACE inhibitor therapy continues to increase, fewer patients may require supplemental potassium therapy.

10. **Aldosterone antagonists.** Spironolactone was the first aldosterone antagonist available for clinical use in the United States. It has been shown to have direct blocking effects on the actions of aldosterone. Results from a large study, the Randomized Aldactone Evaluation Study (RALES), revealed that the addition of low doses (12.5–25 mg daily) to patients with class IV symptoms (NYHA) taking ACE inhibitors reduced the risk of death and hospitalization.
    a. Current guidelines recommend that spironolactone be considered in patients with severe HF (NYHA class IV) at rest despite the use of digoxin, diuretics, an ACE inhibitor, and a β-adrenergic blocker.

Table 41-3. Comparative Doses of Select Agents Used in the Treatment of Heart Failure (HF)

Drug	Initial Dose	Target Dose
Loop diuretics		
Bumetanide	0.5–1 mg once or twice daily	Titrate to achieve dry weight (up to 10 mg daily)
Furosemide	20–40 mg once or twice daily	Titrate to achieve dry weight (up to 400 mg daily)
Torsemide	10–20 mg once or twice daily	Titrate to achieve dry weight (up to 200 mg daily)
ACE inhibitors		
Benazepril	Currently not indicated in HF	
Captopril	6.25 mg three times daily	50 mg three times daily
Enalapril	2.5 mg twice daily	10–20 mg twice daily
Fosinopril	5–10 mg once daily	40 mg once daily
Lisinopril	2.5–5 mg once daily	20–40 mg once daily
Quinapril	10 mg twice daily	40 mg twice daily
Ramipril	1.25–2.5 mg once daily	10 mg once daily
β-Adrenergic receptor blockers		
Bisoprolol	1.25 mg once daily	10 mg once daily
Carvedilol	3.125 mg twice daily	25 mg twice daily; 50 mg twice daily for patients heavier than 85 kg
Metoprolol tartrate	6.25 mg twice daily	75 mg twice daily
Metoprolol succinate (extended release)	12.5–25 mg daily	200 mg once daily
Digitalis glycosides		
Digoxin	0.125–0.25 mg once daily	0.125–0.25 mg once daily

b. Due to the ability of spironolactone to increase potassium reabsorption by the kidney, candidates considered for spironolactone should have serum potassium levels evaluated and reduced to less than 5.0 mmol/L along with a serum creatinine level less than 2.5 mg/dl prior to initiation of therapy. Potassium supplements should be stopped as well, and routine potassium levels should be monitored to prevent the subsequent development of hyperkalemia.

c. At this time, the role of spironolactone in mild to moderate HF has not been evaluated and is not recommended in these individuals.

d. Σ-plerenone (Inspra) is a recently introduced aldosterone receptor antagonist indicated in the treatment of hypertension.

F. Vasodilators

1. These agents reduce pulmonary congestion and increase cardiac output by reducing preload and/or afterload. However, at the current time, there are no large-scale trials supporting the use of vasodilators (nitrates or hydralazine) alone in the treatment of HF.

2. Individual agents

a. Nitroprusside is administered intravenously in doses of 0.3–10 μg/kg/min to provide potent dilation of both arteries and veins.

b. Hydralazine. This arteriole dilator decreases afterload and increases cardiac output in patients with HF.

c. Prazosin. This α-adrenergic blocker acts as a balanced arteriovenous dilator.

d. Nitrates

(1) Venous dilation by nitrates increases venous pooling, which decreases preload.

(2) Their arterial effects seem to result in decreased afterload with continued therapy.

(3) Nitrates are available in many forms and doses. Because individual reactions vary widely, dosages have to be adjusted, but, in general, they are higher for HF than for angina. Table 41-4 provides examples of nitrate doses that have been used in HF.

e. Combination therapy. Hydralazine has been used with isosorbide dinitrate to reduce afterload (or with nitroglycerin to reduce preload) for treating chronic HF.

(1) The combination of these two agents should not be used as initial therapy over ACE inhibitors, but should be considered in those patients who are intolerant of ACE inhibitors.

(2) Suggested dosing regimens include hydralazine 25–40 mg four times daily and isosorbide dinitrate 20–40 mg three times daily.

(3) The combination has not been evaluated in patients already receiving ACE inhibitors, and alternative agents such as β-adrenergic blockers or angiotensin II receptor antagonists should be considered instead.

G. ACE inhibitors

1. Recent guidelines recommend the use of ACE inhibitors in all patients with HF due to left ventricular systolic dysfunction unless they have a contraindication to their use or have demonstrated intolerance to their use. Currently, they are considered the first-line agents in the treatment of HF and have been shown to have a beneficial effect on cardiac remodeling.

2. Relative contraindications include history of intolerance or adverse reactions, serum potassium >5.5 mEq/L, symptomatic hypotension, severe renal artery stenosis, and pregnancy.

Table 41-4. Examples of Nitrates That Have Been Used in Heart Failure

Form of Nitrate	Typical Dose	Dosing Interval
Intravenous nitroglycerin	5–200 μg/min	Continuous infusion
Nitroglycerin buccal tablets	1–3 mg	4–6 hours
Nitroglycerin capsules (sustained release)	6.5–19.5 mg	4–6 hours
Nitroglycerin ointment	1–3 inches	4–6 hours
Sublingual nitroglycerin	0.4 mg	1–2 hours
Oral isosorbide dinitrate	10–60 mg	4–6 hours
Sublingual isosorbide dinitrate	5–10 mg	4 hours

3. ACE inhibitors have been shown to reduce symptoms, improve clinical status, enhance the overall quality of life, and reduce death as well as the risk of death or hospitalization in mild, moderate, and severe HF patients with or without coronary artery disease.

4. Inhibit the enzyme responsible for the conversion of angiotensin I (a weak vasoconstrictor) to angiotensin II (a potent vasoconstrictor). This action significantly decreases total peripheral resistance, which aids in reducing afterload.

5. Inhibiting the production of angiotensin II interferes with stimulation of aldosterone release, thus indirectly reducing retention of sodium and water, which decreases venous return and preload.

6. In patients with a history of fluid retention or who present with fluid retention, an ACE inhibitor can be added to a diuretic. ACE inhibitors are also indicated for patients with left ventricular dysfunction without symptoms of HF.

7. ACE inhibitors are indicated for the long-term management of chronic HF and are generally recommended in combination with a β-adrenergic blocker, diuretic, and usually digoxin.

8. All ACE inhibitors that have been studied in the treatment of HF have shown benefit. The selection of agent and dose should be based on currently available large-scale studies where target doses of ACE inhibitors (captopril, enalapril, lisinopril, and ramipril) are different than those used to treat hypertension. See Table 41-3 for a comparative review of those ACE inhibitors currently used in the treatment of HF.

9. Common side effects to be monitored include hypotension (patients should be well hydrated prior to initiation of ACE inhibitors), dizziness, reduced renal function (increased serum creatinine of 0.5 mg/dl or more requires reassessment), cough, and potassium retention (if potassium levels are high without supplementation, discontinue the ACE inhibitor for several days and then try to restart at lower dose).

10. Recently, a new class of drugs, "angiotensin II receptor antagonists," has been approved for use in the treatment of mild to moderate hypertension. Candesartan cilexetil, eprosartan, irbesartan, losartan, olmesartan, telmisartan, and valsartan are the first such agents available, and currently studies are under way to assess their potential use for treating HF. Current guidelines suggest that ACE inhibitors should be preferred over the angiotensin II receptor antagonists, due to lack of available long-term trials demonstrating their benefit. However, they may be tried in those patients responding to ACE inhibitors who become intolerant to the ACE inhibitor cough.

H. β-Adrenergic blocking agents

1. Unlike ACE inhibitors, which strictly work by blocking the effects of the renin–angiotensin system, β-adrenergic blockers interfere with the sympathetic nervous system [i.e., norepinephrine-induced peripheral vasoconstriction, or norepinephrine-induced sodium excretion by the kidney, or norepinephrine-induced cardiac hypertrophy, or norepinephrine induced arrhythmia generation, or norepinephrine-induced hypokalemia, or norepinephrine-induced cell death (apoptosis) through increased stress due to norepinephrine stimulation].

2. β-adrenergic blockers, similar to ACE inhibitors, have been shown to decrease the risk of death or hospitalization as well as improve the clinical status of HF patients.

3. Current guidelines recommend the use of β-adrenergic blockers in all patients with stable HF due to left ventricular dysfunction unless they have a contraindication to their use or are unable to tolerate their effects due to hypotension, bradycardia, bronchospasm, and the like.

4. β-adrenergic blockers are generally used in conjunction with diuretics, ACE inhibitors, and usually digoxin. β-adrenergic blockers should not be taken without diuretics in patients with a current or recent history of fluid retention to avoid its development and to maintain sodium balance.

5. Side effects to β-adrenergic blockers may occur during the early days of therapy, but do not generally prevent their long-term use, and progression of the disease may be reduced, even if symptoms of the disease have not responded to β-adrenergic blocker therapy. Therapy should be initiated with low doses and titrated upward slowly as tolerated.

6. Patients should be monitored for signs of fluid retention by having patients weigh themselves daily and report any significant increases, which might warrant increases in diuretic doses. Additionally, fatigue, hypotension, bradycardia, and heart block are reported sides effects, which should be monitored to ensure appropriate attention and management.

7. Studies support the use of β-adrenergic blockers in patients with class I–IV HF, and not in the acute management of patients, as in an ICU, where other, shorter-term therapies such as digoxin may be more beneficial. Additionally, β-adrenergic blockers should be considered in patients who develop HF post–myocardial infarction if they are able to tolerate the negative inotropic effects.

8. Carvedilol is the first β-adrenergic blocker approved by the FDA for the management of chronic HF. However, doses for other select β-adrenergic blockers have been included in the current guidelines based on literature experiences (see Table 41-3).

   a. Initiation of carvedilol should not be undertaken until the patient is stable without fluid overload or hypotension, and on concomitant medications, which include diuretics, digoxin, and/or ACE inhibitors.

   b. Patients need to be monitored for bradycardia and the potential for heart block, in which case the dose will need to be decreased.

   c. Patient education is an important aspect for initiating carvedilol therapy, and patients need to be informed that they might not see positive effects for several months after obtaining the target dosage of carvedilol.

I. Calcium-channel blockers

1. Due to the lack of evidence supporting efficacy, calcium-channel blockers should not be used for the treatment of HF. Current guidelines list calcium-channel blockers as a class III recommendation, which states "that conditions [exist] for which there is evidence and/or general agreement that a procedure/therapy is not useful/effective and in some cases may be harmful."

2. Large-scale trials utilizing felodipine and amlodipine have not provided persuasive evidence that long-term treatment can improve the symptoms of HF or prolong survival. However, current guidelines suggest that amlodipine seems less likely to cause a worsening in nonischemic HF.

3. There are data that amlodipine does not adversely affect survival when given to patients with HF, but requires further study to evaluate potential benefits in a subset of patients referred to as "nonischemic cardiomyopathy."

J. Inotropic agents have been used in the emergency treatment of patients with HF and in patients refractory to, or unable to take, digitalis. However, current guidelines provide a class III recommendation, which states "that conditions [exist] for which there is evidence and/or general agreement that a procedure/therapy is not useful/effective and in some cases may be harmful." Current guidelines provide a class IIb recommendation for the use of continuous intravenous infusion of a positive inotropic agent for palliation of HF symptoms, which states, "conditions for which there is conflicting evidence and/or a divergence of opinion about the usefulness/efficacy of performing the procedure/therapy and that the usefulness/efficacy is less well established by evidence/opinion."

1. **Dopamine (intravenous)**

   a. **Low doses** of 2–5 μg/kg/min stimulate specific dopamine receptors within the kidney to increase renal blood flow, and thus increase urine output.

   b. **Moderate doses** of 5–10 μg/kg/min increase cardiac output in HF patients.

   c. **High doses**

      (1) As doses are raised above 10 μg/kg/min, alpha peripheral activity increases, resulting in increased total peripheral resistance and pulmonary pressures.

      (2) When the infusion exceeds 8–9 μg/kg/min, the patient should be monitored for tachycardia. If the infusion is slowed or interrupted, the adverse effect should disappear, as dopamine has a very short half-life in plasma.

2. **Dobutamine (intravenous)**

   a. Patients who are unresponsive to, or adversely affected by, dopamine may benefit from dobutamine in doses of 5–20 μg/kg/min.

b. Although dobutamine resembles dopamine chemically, its actions differ somewhat. For example, dobutamine does not directly affect renal receptors and, therefore, does not act as a renal vasodilator. It increases urinary output only through increased cardiac output.

c. Serious arrhythmias are a potential occurrence, although less likely to occur than with dopamine. Slowing or interrupting the infusion usually reverses this effect, as it does for dopamine.

d. Dobutamine and dopamine have been used together to treat cardiogenic shock, but similar use in HF has yet to be accepted.

3. **Inamrinone (intravenous)** is referred to as nonglycoside, nonsympathomimetic inotropic agents.

    a. A derivative of bipyridine, inamrinone has both a positive inotropic effect and a vasodilating effect.

    b. By inhibiting phosphodiesterase located specifically in the cardiac cells, it increases the amount of cyclic adenosine monophosphate (cAMP).

    c. Inamrinone has been used in patients with HF that have been refractory to treatment with other inotropic agents.

    d. Effective regimens have used loading intravenous infusions of 0.75 mg/kg over 3–4 minutes followed by maintenance infusions of 5–10 μg/kg/min.

    e. Precautions and monitoring effects

        (1) Inamrinone is unstable in dextrose solutions and should be added to saline solutions instead. Because of fluid balance concerns, this can be a potential problem in patients with HF.

        (2) Because of the peripheral dilating properties, patients should be monitored for hypotension.

        (3) Thrombocytopenia has occurred and is dose-dependent and asymptomatic.

        (4) Ventricular rates may increase in patients with atrial flutter or fibrillation.

4. **Milrinone (intravenous)** is similar to inamrinone. It possesses both inotropic and vasodilatory properties.

    a. This agent has been used as short-term management to treat patients with HF.

    b. Most milrinone patients in clinical trials have also been receiving digoxin and diuretics.

    c. Effective dosing regimens have used a loading dose of 50 μg/kg administered slowly over 10 minutes intravenously, followed by maintenance doses of 0.375 μg/kg/min by continuous infusion, based on the clinical status of the patient.

    d. Precautions and monitoring effects

        (1) Renal impairment significantly prolongs the elimination rate of milrinone, and infusions need to be reduced accordingly.

        (2) Monitoring is necessary for the potential arrhythmias occurring in HF, which may be increased by drugs such as milrinone and other inotropic agents.

        (3) Blood pressure and heart rate should be monitored when administering milrinone, due to its vasodilatory effects and its potential to induce arrhythmias.

        (4) Additional side effects include mild to moderate headache, tremor, and thrombocytopenia.

5. **Nesiritide (Natrecor)** is a recombinant form of human B-type natriuretic peptide, which is a naturally occurring hormone secreted by the ventricles. It is the first of this drug class to become available for human use in the United States.

    a. Nesiritide is approved for the intravenous treatment of patients with acutely decompensated HF associated with shortness of breath at rest or with minimal activity.

    b. Nesiritide binds to natriuretic peptide receptors in blood vessels, resulting in increased production of guanosine 3′5′-cyclic monophosphate (cGMP) in target tissues, which mediates vasodilation. In HF, nesiritide reduces pulmonary capillary wedge pressure and systemic vascular resistance.

    c. Initial treatment involves a bolus dose of 2 μg/kg followed by a continuous intravenous infusion of 0.01 μg/kg/min via continuous infustion to a maximum dose of 0.03 μg/kg/min.

    d. Monitoring for hypotension, elevated serum creatinine, headache, nausea, and dizziness is the key to successful use. Concomitant use of ACE inhibitors may increase the risk of symptomatic hypotension (systolic blood pressure <90 mm Hg and syncope).

K. Patient education

1. Patient should be made aware of the importance of taking their medications exactly as prescribed and should be advised to watch for signs of toxicity.

2. Patients should be educated on the need for life-style modifications, which will have a positive effect on reducing HF development as well as a reduction in HF symptoms and include dietary and life-style management, including daily weight monitoring, fluid management, sodium restriction, early intervention if symptoms appear, compliance with the treatment plan, modification of alcohol intake, and exercise and stress reduction.

3. The patient should understand the need for regular checkups and be able to recognize symptoms that require immediate physician notification, for example, an unusually irregular pulse rate, palpitations, shortness of breath, swollen ankles, visual disturbances, or weight gain exceeding 3–5 lb in 1 week.

4. The patient needs to be educated about drugs such as calcium-channel blockers; NSAIDs, which may cause a problem in HF by retaining fluid; and sodium. Additionally, the patient needs to be informed of the potential dangers of use of over-the-counter medications, which might also predispose him or her to HF symptoms and loss of symptom control. A thorough review of all medications (both prescription and over-the-counter) should be carried out as frequently as possible to ensure compliance with the treatment regimen.

STUDY QUESTIONS

Directions: Each of the numbered items or incomplete statements in this section is followed by answers or by completions of the statement. Select the **one** lettered answer or completion that is **best** in each case.

1. Which of the following groups of symptoms is most likely associated with the backing up of fluid behind a failing left ventricle?

(A) Nocturia, dry, wheezing cough, paroxysmal nocturnal dyspnea
(B) Paroxysmal nocturnal dyspnea, pedal edema, jugular venous distention, hepatojugular reflux
(C) Jugular venous distention, hepatojugular reflux, pedal edema, shortness of breath
(D) Hepatojugular reflux, jugular venous distention, pedal edema, abdominal distention
(E) Paroxysmal nocturnal dyspnea, jugular venous distention, abdominal distention, shortness of breath

2. Which of the following combinations of drugs, when used together, reduce both preload and afterload angiotensin-converting enzyme and might provide an alternative to (ACE) inhibitors in patient who are intolerant of them?

(A) Nitroglycerin and isosorbide dinitrate
(B) Hydralazine and isosorbide dinitrate
(C) Diltiazem and verapamil
(D) Prazosin and angiotensin II
(E) Hydralazine and methyldopa

3. When spironolactone is used in a patient with heart failure (HF), it works through what primary mechanism?

(A) Positive inotropic effect
(B) Positive chronotropic effect
(C) Aldosterone antagonism
(D) Negative inotropic effect
(E) Angiotensin II blockade

Questions 4–5

A 60-year-old hypertensive woman is currently being treated with nitroglycerin, carvedilol, furosemide, nifedipine, ramipril, aspirin, and digoxin. She is admitted with a diagnosis of HF.

4. Which agent is most likely to be discontinued in this patient?

(A) Nifedipine
(B) Carvedilol
(C) Aspirin
(D) Digoxin
(E) Furosemide

5. It is later found that the patient has developed HF as a result of a serious anemia due to aspirin-induced bleeding. What type of HF does the patient have?

(A) High-output
(B) Low-output
(C) Left-sided
(D) Right-sided
(E) Low-output, left-sided

6. Because of proven beneficial effects on "cardiac remodeling," these agents are now indicated as first-line therapy in HF patients. Which of the following is a representative of this group of drugs?

(A) Hydrochlorothiazide
(B) Lisinopril
(C) Losartan
(D) Carvedilol
(E) Furosemide

7. Which of the following statements is not correct, as it relates to the current status of HF in the United States?

(A) HF is the one cardiovascular disorder that is increasing in incidence and prevalence.
(B) Medication costs for treating HF in the United States approaches $38 billion.
(C) Patients with advanced disease have a 30%–40% risk of death annually.
(D) Current figures reveal approximately 5 million people in the United States who suffer from HF.
(E) Approximately 500,000 people each year are diagnosed with HF in the United States.

8. For treating the patient with HF, which of the following dosages of dopamine is selected for its positive inotropic effects?

(A) 2.0 µg/kg/min
(B) 5–10 µg/kg/min
(C) 10–20 µg/kg/min
(D) 40 µg/kg/min
(E) 40 mg/kg/min

9. The use of angiotensin-converting enzyme (ACE) inhibitors in HF centers around their ability to cause

(A) direct reduction in renin levels with a resultant decrease in angiotensin II and aldosterone levels
(B) indirect reduction in angiotensin II and aldosterone levels due to inhibition of ACE
(C) direct reduction in aldosterone secretion and angiotensin I production by inhibiting ACE
(D) increase in afterload due to an indirect decrease in angiotensin II as well as a decrease in preload due to an indirect reduction in aldosterone secretion
(E) inhibition of the angiotensin II receptor, which results in reduced angiotensin II levels and reduced secretion of aldosterone

Directions: Each item below contains three suggested answers, of which **one or more** is correct. Choose the answer

A	if **I only** is correct
B	if **III only** is correct
C	if **I and II** are correct
D	if **II and III** are correct
E	if **I, II, and III** are correct

10. Which of the following have been shown to be effective in the acute management of digitalis toxicity?

I. Cholestyramine resin
II. Fab fragment antibody
III. Potassium administration

11. Situations that predispose a digitalis-treated patient to toxicity include

I. hypercalcemia
II. hyperkalemia
III. hypermagnesemia

12. Guidelines necessary for monitoring the patient with HF include which of the following questions?

I. Does the patient have therapeutic blood levels of digoxin in the range of 0.8–2.0 ng/mL?
II. Is the patient taking a product that may decrease the effectiveness of therapy (e.g., antacids, baking soda)?
III. Does the patient have signs of digitalis toxicity or a digoxin–drug interaction?

13. Correct statements about dobutamine include which of the following?

I. Doses of 5–20 µg/kg/min have been associated with a positive inotropic effect in treating the patient with HF.
II. Patients receiving dobutamine should be monitored for increases in peripheral vascular resistance.
III. Dobutamine is considered a nonglycoside, nonsympathomimetic-positive inotropic agent.

ANSWERS AND EXPLANATIONS

1. The answer is A *[III A 1]*.
As mentioned within the text, due to the closed circulatory system, it is difficult to isolate signs and symptoms to strictly one side of the failing heart, as left-sided dysfunction will eventually result in right-sided dysfunction and vice versa. However, for the current question, of importance is that fact that fluid backing up behind a failing left ventricle would result in pulmonary signs and symptoms as compared to peripheral signs and symptoms when fluid backs up behind the failing right ventricle. The patient's symptoms and signs result from the pulmonary effects of fluid accumulation (e.g., rales, shortness of breath, paroxysmal nocturnal dyspnea, dry wheezing cough), versus those seen with fluid behind the failing right ventricle (peripheral accumulation of fluid within the liver, the legs, the abdomen, and the venous system in general).

2. The answer is B *[IV F 2 e]*.
The venous dilating properties of isosorbide dinitrate (preload) in conjunction with the arteriolar dilating effects of hydralazine (afterload) make this combination effective in reducing both preload and afterload. Recent guidelines suggest that the combination of the vasodilators hydralazine and isosorbide dinitrate should not be considered as initial therapy over ACE inhibitors, but should be considered in those patients unable to tolerate ACE inhibitors.

3. The answer is C *[IV E 10]*.
Spironolactone was the first aldosterone antagonist currently available for clinical use in the United States. In the recently completed RALES trial, spironolactone, given in 12.5–25 mg daily doses to HF patients with class IV symptoms taking ACE inhibitors, reduced the risk of death and hospitalization. It works in the distal convoluted tubule of the kidney and directly competes for binding to receptors at the sodium–potassium exchange site. Sodium is excreted while potassium is reabsorbed.

4. The answer is A *[IV I]*.
Because they have the potential to produce negative inotropic effects, calcium-channel blockers such as nifedipine must be used cautiously in patients who have HF. Agents such as amlodipine and felodipine have been studied in HF patients, but have not provided persuasive evidence of their benefits in HF. Of the currently available calcium-channel blockers, amlodipine has been shown to be less likely to cause a worsening in nonischemic HF. Carvedilol, despite being a β-adrenergic blocker, is suggested for use in treating HF in combination with diuretics (furosemide), ACE inhibitors (ramipril), and usually digoxin.

5. The answer is A *[I F 1 b]*.
In anemia, the lack of oxygen-carrying capacity by the red blood cells puts an added stress on the heart, which must work harder to provide better oxygenation to the metabolizing tissues. Initially, the heart may be able to compensate, either by increasing the heart rate or by increasing stroke volume through cardiac dilation and hypertrophy. However, if the anemia is allowed to continue, the heart is unable to meet the metabolic demands placed on it, resulting in the signs and symptoms of HF.

6. The answer is B *[IV G 1, H 1–2]*.
ACE inhibitors such as lisinopril have demonstrated, through inhibition of ACE, that a resultant decrease in angiotensin II is beneficial in decreasing morbidity and mortality in patients with HF. Evidence suggests that this has a beneficial effect to reduce "cardiac remodeling." Carvedilol is a β-adrenergic receptor blocker that functions similarly to ACE inhibitors by working on neurohormonal systems, but specifically is believed to work on the sympathetic system to decrease the damaging effects of norepinephrine on the heart.

7. The answer is B *[I B–D]*.
The actual costs involved in the treatment of HF, including medical care, home health care, medication costs, and hospitalization costs, reported in 1991 were approximately $38 billion. Medication costs alone are a bit less but are still reported to be more than $500 million annually.

8. The answer is B *[IV J 1]*.
Dopamine has shown great versatility in its effects. At doses of 2–5 μg/kg/min, it increases renal blood flow through its dopaminergic effects. At doses of 5–10 μg/kg/min, it increases cardiac output through

its β-adrenergic stimulating effect. At doses of 10–20 μg/kg/min, it increases peripheral vascular resistance through its α-adrenergic stimulating effects. There is no specific cutoff for any of these effects, so close titration is required to provide for individual response.

9. The answer is B *[IV G 3–4; Figure 41-2].*
By directly inhibiting the angiotensin-converting enzyme (ACE), production of angiotensin II is reduced, as is angiotensin II–mediated secretion of aldosterone from the adrenal gland. These effects are believed to have a beneficial effect on the prevention of "cardiac remodeling," which has been shown to have a detrimental effect on cardiac function.

10. The answer is E (all) *[IV D 9 c].*
Cholestyramine resin has been used in the acute situation to decrease the absorption of digoxin within the gastrointestinal tract. This results in lower digoxin levels if the resin is administered before all the digoxin has been absorbed. Potassium administration has been shown to be effective in protecting the myocardium from the toxic effects of digoxin while toxic levels return to normal. Fab fragment antibody, though expensive, has been shown to be effective in the management of very high serum digoxin levels, where 40 mg of drug are able to bind 0.6 mg of digitalis.

11. The answer is A (I) *[IV D 8 a–c].*
Calcium ions act synergistically with digitalis. Therefore, when hypercalcemia occurs, digitalis exerts an added pharmacological effect on the heart. This may present itself as toxic arrhythmias, cardiac standstill, and even death. Elevated potassium levels or elevated magnesium levels seem to aid in the prevention of digitalis-induced toxicity. There is building evidence that digitalis preparations need calcium ions to work, and consequently low calcium levels may negate the pharmacological potential of digoxin.

12. The answer is E (all) *[IV D 7–9].*
Digoxin has a narrow therapeutic range; serum levels of 0.8–2.0 ng/mL provide a therapeutic response with minimal toxicity. Monitoring serum digoxin levels is especially helpful during initial dosage titrations and when questions arise as to compliance, absorption, or a drug–drug interaction. Patients with HF must be informed of the need to take their medication appropriately and accurately so that blood levels for all drugs will be within the therapeutic range. Patients must also be told to inform their pharmacist of any additional drugs they are taking since these could aggravate the disease or interact with digoxin or with other drugs. Patients should also be monitored for those symptoms related to HF that effective therapy should prevent. Reporting symptoms such as swollen legs or shortness of breath enables the physician to add different drugs or increase the dosage of current medications.

13. The answer is A (I) *[IV J 2].*
Dobutamine in doses of 5–20 μg/kg/min is an inotropic agent that is useful in the treatment of HF. Dobutamine does not have the versatility that dopamine offers, lacking comparable effects on renal blood flow and peripheral vascular resistance. Rather, dobutamine has a peripheral dilating effect that offers a benefit to patients who have reduced cardiac output due to elevated peripheral resistance.

42
Thromboembolic Disease
James B. Groce III

I. DEFINITION. Venous thromboembolic disease (VTED) occurs when one or more of the elements of **Virchow's triad** are present, resulting in deep venous thrombosis (DVT) and/or pulmonary embolism (PE).

   A. Vascular injury

   B. Venous stasis

   C. Hypercoagulable state [i.e., decreased protein C, protein S, or antithrombin]

II. INCIDENCE. VTED is recognized in 260,000 patients annually. Less than 50% of patients who have VTED are symptomatic; therefore, the total annual incidence of VTED may exceed 500,000.

III. RISK FACTORS

   A. Patient-specific risk factors

   1. Older than 40 years of age

   2. Obesity

   3. Varicose veins

   4. Immobility (i.e., bed rest for more than 4 days)

   5. Pregnancy

   6. High-dose estrogen therapy

   7. Previous venous thromboembolism

   8. Deficiency of antithrombin, protein C, or protein S

   9. Activated protein C resistance

   10. Antiphospholipid antibody

   11. Lupus anticoagulant

   B. Risk factors associated with medical illness and surgical procedures

   1. Trauma or surgery, especially involving the pelvis, hip, and lower limbs

   2. Malignancy, especially pelvic, abdominal, and metastatic

   3. Major medical illness, especially:
      a. Heart failure or recent myocardial infarction (MI)
      b. Paralysis of the lower limbs
      c. Inflammatory bowel disease
      d. Sepsis
      e. Kidney disease
      f. Polycythemia
      g. Paraproteinemia
      h. Behçet's syndrome
      i. Homocysteinemia

IV. PREVENTION AND TREATMENT

   A. Nonpharmacological prevention. VTED can be prevented by reducing venous stasis with **external pneumatic compression** or **graduated compression stockings.**

B. Pharmacological prevention. VTED can be prevented by counteracting increased blood coagulability with **unfractionated heparin (UFH)** [see V A], **oral anticoagulant therapy** (see V B), **low–molecular-weight heparin (LMWH)** [see V C], or a **synthetic pentasaccharide** (see V D).

V. PHARMACOLOGICAL AGENTS

A. Unfractionated heparin

1. **Indications.** Patients with proven VTED should receive concomitant UFH for acute treatment and warfarin therapy acutely, followed by warfarin therapy for continued prevention of recurrence of VTED (Table 42-1), unless contraindications (e.g., pregnancy) are present.

2. **Mechanism of action.** The major mechanism by which heparin blocks coagulation is by catalyzing the inhibition of thrombin. UFH acts as an anticoagulant by catalyzing the **inactivation of thrombin (factor IIa), activated factor X (factor Xa),** and **activated factor IX (factor IXa) by antithrombin.**

3. **Pharmacokinetics.** The mechanisms of heparin clearance are complex.
   a. Heparin binds to a number of plasma proteins other than antithrombin that compete with antithrombin heparin binding.
   b. UFH is cleared by rapid-phase (cellular) elimination followed by a more gradual (renal) clearance, which can best be explained by a **combination of saturable and nonsaturable first-order kinetic models.**
   c. When administered in fixed doses, the anticoagulant response to UFH varies among patients and within the same patient (i.e., inter- and intrapatient variability). This variability is caused by differences in patients' plasma concentrations of heparin-neutralizing proteins and rates of heparin clearance.

4. **Administration and dosage**
   a. UFH's therapeutic effect is hastened by administration of a **loading dose,** which may be **empirically selected** (e.g., 5000-unit bolus given intravenously) or individualized by the patient's **dosing weight.**
      (1) The weight-based approach has resulted in the use of loading doses varying from 70–100 units/kg.
      (2) In some instances, the indication for which heparin therapy is being initiated is considered, with 70 units/kg being used for all thrombotic indications other than suspected or proved pulmonary embolism, for which up to 100 units/kg may be used.

Table 42-1. Guidelines for Anticoagulant Therapy with Unfractionated Heparin (UFH) and Warfarin in the Treatment of Venous Thromboembolic Disease (VTED)

Disease	Guideline
Suspected VTED	Obtain baseline aPTT, PT/INR, CBC
	Check for contraindications to heparin therapy
	Give 5000 units unfractionated heparin IV push; order imaging study
Proven VTED	If therapy indicated, rebolus with heparin, 80 units/kg IV, and start maintenance infusion at 18 units/kg/hr
	Check aPTT at 6 hr, and adjust to maintain a range corresponding to a therapeutic heparin level
	Check platelet count daily
	Start warfarin therapy on day 1; adjust subsequent daily dosing based on PT/INR
	Stop UFH after 4–5 days of overlap (UFH with warfarin), when INR is >2.0 for 2 consecutive days
	Anticoagulate with warfarin for 3–6 months (patient/disease-state specific)

Note that combined therapy (i.e., UFH and warfarin) should be continued for at least 4–5 days. *aPTT* = activated partial thromboplastin time; *CBC* = complete blood count; *INR* = international normalized ratio; *IV* = intravenous; *PT* = prothrombin time.

Used with permission from Hyers TM, et al. Antithrombotic therapy for venous thromboembolic disease. *Chest* 2001:119(Suppl):176s–193s.

    b. Variable approaches to continuous dosing have been employed.

        (1) Empiric dosing of 1000 units/hour may be used, but may result in subtherapeutic or supratherapeutic outcomes [i.e., activated partial thromboplastin time (aPTT) below or above the targeted range].

        (2) Another approach to continuous dosing includes commencing with a fixed dose (other than the empiric dose of 1,000 units/hour). One such approach may see an initial loading dose followed by 32,000 units/24 hours by continuous infusion.

        (3) Yet another approach validated in the medical and pharmaceutical literature uses a **weight-based dosing nomogram** for commencing UFH therapy that varies between 15 and 25 units/kg/hr.

            (a) Lower doses are used initially for most thrombotic indications other than pulmonary embolism.

            (b) Pulmonary embolism requires more aggressive therapy (i.e., up to 25 units/kg/hr) based on the consideration that the clearance of heparin may be increased, thus necessitating an increased dose.

        (4) Heparin dosing adjustment protocols have been developed to assist the initial weight-based dosing efforts. Such protocols should be developed for a specific aPTT reagent (Tables 42-2 and 42-3).

    5. Monitoring the effects of UFH. The anticoagulant effects of UFH are usually monitored by the **aPTT.** The aPTT should be monitored 6 hours after commencing heparin therapy. Subsequent dosing adjustments are based on the results of this and additional aPTTs.

        a. The aPTT ratio used to determine therapeutic effect is measured by dividing the observed aPTT by the mean of the normal laboratory control aPTT.

        b. For many aPTT reagents, a therapeutic effect is achieved with an **aPTT ratio of 1.5–2.5.**

        c. However, because aPTT reagents may vary in their sensitivity, it is **inappropriate to use the same aPTT ratio (i.e., 1.5–2.5) for all reagents.** The therapeutic range for each aPTT reagent should be calibrated to be equivalent to a **heparin level of 0.2–0.4 U/mL by whole blood (protamine titration) or to an antifactor Xa level (i.e., plasma heparin level) of approximately 0.3–0.7 U/mL.**

B. Oral anticoagulants—warfarin

    1. Indications

        a. Warfarin is proven effective in the:

        (1) Primary and secondary prevention of VTED

Table 42-2. Heparin Dosage Adjustment Protocol: Example 1

Patient's aPTT (sec)*	Repeat Bolus Dose (units)	Stop Infusion (min)	Change Rate of Infusion (mL/hr)† Units/24 hr	Timing of Next aPTT
<50	5000	0	+3 [2880]	6 hours
50–59	0	0	+3 [2880]	6 hours
60–85‡	0	0	0	Next morning
86–95	0	0	−2 [−1920]	Next morning
96–120	0	30	−2 [−1920]	6 hours
> 120	0	60	−4 [−3840]	6 hours

Starting dose of 5,000 units intravenous bolus followed by 32,000 units/24 hr as a continuous infusion. First aPTT performed 6 hours after the bolus injection, dosage adjustments made according to protocol and the aPTT repeated as indicated in the right-hand column.

aPTT = activated partial thromboplastin time.

*The normal range for aPTT with Dade Actin FS reagent is 27–35 seconds. This numerical range may vary based upon the sensitivity of the reagent.

†Concentration of heparin equal to 40 units/mL.

‡A therapeutic range of 60–85 seconds is equivalent to a heparin level of 0.2–0.4 units/mL by whole-blood protamine titration or 0.3–0.7 units/mL as a plasma antifactor Xa level. The therapeutic range varies with the responsiveness of the aPTT reagent to heparin.

Table 42-3. Heparin[†] Dosage Adjustment Protocol: Example 2*

Patient's aPTT (sec)[‡]	Dose Change (units/kg/hr)	Additional Action	Timing of Next aPTT (hr)
<35 (<1.2 × mean normal)	+4	Rebolus with 80 units/kg	6
35–45 (1.2–1.5 × mean normal)	+2	Rebolus with 40 units/kg	6
46–70[†] (1.5–2.3 × mean normal)	0	0	6[§]
71–90 (2.3–3.0 × mean normal)	−2	0	6
>90 (>3 × mean normal)	−3	Stop infusion for 1 hour	6

aPTT = activated partial thromboplastin time.

*Initial dosing: loading dose 80 units/kg; maintenance infusion: 18 units/kg/hr (aPTT in 6 hr).

†Heparin, 25,000 units in 250 mL of d5w. Infuse at rate indicated by body weight through an infusion apparatus calibrated for low flow rates.

‡The therapeutic range in seconds should correspond to a plasma heparin level of 0.2–0.4 IU/mL by protamine sulfate or 0.3–0.7 IU/mL by plasma-amiodolytic assay. When the aPTT is checked at 6 hours or longer, steady-state kinetics can be assumed.

§During the first 24 hours, repeat the aPTT every 6 hours. Thereafter, monitor the aPTT once every morning unless it is outside of the therapeutic range.

Used with permission from Hyers TM, et al. Antithrombotic therapy for venous thromboembolic disease. *Chest* 119(Suppl):176s–193s.

     (2) Prevention of systemic arterial embolism in patients with tissue and mechanical prosthetic heart valves or atrial fibrillation
     (3) Prevention of acute MI in patients with peripheral arterial disease
     (4) Prevention of stroke, recurrent infarction, and death in patients with acute MI
   b. Warfarin may also be used in patients with valvular heart disease to prevent systemic arterial embolism, although its effectiveness has never been demonstrated by a randomized clinical trial.

2. Mechanism of action
   a. Oral anticoagulants (e.g., warfarin) are vitamin K antagonists, producing their anticoagulant effect by **interfering with the cyclic interconversion of vitamin K and its 2,3-epoxide (vitamin K epoxide).**
   b. Inhibition of this process leads to the depletion of vitamin KH2 and **results in the production of hemostatically defective, vitamin K–dependent coagulant proteins or clotting factors (i.e., prothrombin or factors II, VII, IX, and X).**
   c. These vitamin K–dependent coagulant proteins or clotting factors (i.e., factors VII, IX, X, and II, respectively) decline over 6–96 hours.

3. Pharmacokinetics
   a. Warfarin is a **racemic mixture** of roughly equal amounts of two optically active isomers, the **R and S forms.**
   b. Warfarin is rapidly absorbed from the gastrointestinal tract and reaches maximal blood concentrations in healthy volunteers in 90 minutes.
   c. Dose response to warfarin is influenced by:
     (1) Pharmacokinetic factors (i.e., differences in absorption and metabolic clearance)
     (2) Pharmacodynamic factors (i.e., differences in the hemostatic response to given concentrations of warfarin)
     (3) Technical factors [e.g., inaccuracies in prothrombin time (PT) and international normalized ratio (INR) testing and reporting]
     (4) Patient-specific factors [e.g., diet (increased intake of green, leafy vegetables), poor patient compliance (missed doses, self-medication, alcohol consumption), poor communication between patient and physician (undisclosed use of drugs that may interact with warfarin)] (Table 42-4)

Table 42-4. Factors That May Potentiate or Inhibit Warfarin Effects

	Potentiate Anticoagulant Effect	Inhibit Anticoagulant Effect
Drugs	Phenylbutazone Metronidazole Sulfinpyrazone Trimethoprim-sulfamethoxazole Disulfiram Amiodarone Erythromycin Anabolic steroids Clofibrate Cimetidine Omeprazole Thyroxine Ketoconazole Isoniazid Fluconazole Piroxicam Tamoxifen Quinidine Vitamin E (large doses) Phenytoin	Cholestyramine Barbiturates Rifampin Griseofulvin Carbamazepine Penicillin
Other	Low vitamin K intake Reduced vitamin K absorption Liver disease Hypermetabolic states (e.g., thyrotoxicosis) Alcohol (acute use)	High vitamin K intake Alcohol (chronic use)

Table 42-5. Practical Oral Anticoagulation Dosing

Day	Rapid Anticoagulation	Anticoagulation*
1	5–10 mg	5 mg
2	5–10 mg	5 mg
3	2.5–7.5 mg (adjust based on INR results)	5 mg (adjust based on INR results)
	Adjust dosage based on INR results until the INR is stable and therapeutic	Adjust dosage based on INR results until the INR is stable and therapeutic

INR = international normalized ratio.
*Rapid anticoagulation is not required, or there is a risk of bleeding.

4. **Administration and dosage**
 a. **Warfarin,** a coumarin compound, is the most widely used oral anticoagulant in North America. Although it is primarily **administered orally,** an injectable preparation is available in the United States.
 b. Commence oral anticoagulant therapy with the **anticipated daily maintenance dose of warfarin,** which can be variable.
 c. **The initial dose of warfarin therapy can be flexible** (Table 42-5).
  (1) Patient-specific parameters that are used to determine the initial dose of warfarin include the patient's weight (e.g., obesity, concurrent use of interacting drugs known

to inhibit the anticoagulant effect of warfarin, and the desired rapid anticoagulant effect).

(2) Based on these patient-specific parameters, some clinicians may use a larger initial dose of warfarin (e.g., 7.5–10 mg), which should not be misconstrued as a loading dose.

d. The initial dose of warfarin should be **overlapped with UFH for 4–5 days** (see Table 42-1).

e. The **duration of warfarin therapy** is dependent on each patient's indication(s) for use (Table 42-6).

f. **Reversal of warfarin effects** may be necessary due to elevated INR or complications associated with oral anticoagulant therapy (Table 42-7).

5. Monitoring warfarin therapy. PT and INR monitoring are usually performed daily upon commencing oral anticoagulant therapy (e.g., warfarin), until such time that the INR has been found to be therapeutic.

a. Laboratory monitoring is performed by measuring the **PT** for calculation of the INR.

(1) The PT is **responsive to depression of three** of the four vitamin K–dependent procoagulant **clotting factors** (i.e., **prothrombin** or **factors II, VII, and X**).

(2) The common commercial PT reagents vary markedly in their responsiveness to coumarin-induced reduction in clotting factors; therefore, PT results reported using different reagents are not interchangeable between laboratories.

b. The problem of variability in responsiveness of PT reagents has been overcome by the introduction of a standardized test known as the **INR.**

(1) The INR is equal to the observed PT ratio [i.e., (patient PT/mean laboratory control PT)^{ISI}], where ISI (International Sensitivity Index) is a measure of the responsiveness of a given thromboplastin to reduction of the vitamin K–dependent coagulation factors. The **lower the ISI,** the **more responsive the reagent** and the closer the derived INR will be to the observed PT ratio.

(2) Guidelines of the American College of Chest Physicians (ACCP) Consensus Conference on Antithrombic Therapy recommend two levels of therapeutic intensity: a less intense range corresponding to an INR of 2.0–3.0, and a more intense range corresponding to an INR of 2.5–3.5. The range corresponds to the indication (Table 42-8).

(3) Once the desired therapeutic INR has been achieved for 2 consecutive days, (e.g., for concomitant heparin plus warfarin overlap therapy) follow-up INR monitoring can be performed according to the following protocol.

(a) Week 1: monitor INR two or three times

(b) Week 2: monitor INR two times

(c) Weeks 3–6: monitor INR once a week

(d) Weeks 7–14: monitor INR once every 2 weeks

(e) Week 15–end of therapy: monitor INR once every 4 weeks (if INR dose responsiveness remains stable; if dose adjustment is necessary, a more frequent monitoring schema is reemployed until stable dose responsiveness is achieved)

c. Upon commencing oral anticoagulant therapy, **prolongation of the PT/INR** does not occur until depletion of the vitamin K–dependent procoagulant clotting factors occurs. This delay is **variable over 2–4 days.** During this delay, if active venous thrombosis is present, either UFH or LMWH is concomitantly commenced to adequately anticoagulate the patient while awaiting the therapeutic effect of warfarin.

C. Low–molecular-weight heparin

1. Indications

a. LMWH indications vary by manufacturer.

b. Each of the LMWHs have been evaluated in a large number of randomized clinical trials and have been proven to be safe and efficacious for **the prevention and treatment of venous thromboembolism.**

c. To date, different LMWHs have been evaluated for their role in:

(1) Prevention of venous thrombosis

(2) Treatment of VTED

(3) Management of unstable angina pectoris/non–Q wave MI

2. Chemistry. LMWHs are fragments of standard commercial-grade heparin produced by either chemical or enzymatic depolymerization. LMWHs are approximately one-third the size of heparin. Like **heparin,** which has a **mean molecular weight of 15,000** daltons

Table 42-6. Duration of Warfarin Therapy*

Duration	Indications
3–6 months	First event with reversible[+] or time-limited risk factor (patient may have underlying factor V Leiden or prothrombin 20210
≥6 months	Idiopathic VTE, first event
12 months to lifetime	First event[‡] with: • Cancer (until resolved) • Anticardiolipin antibody • Antithrombin deficiency • Recurrent event, idiopathic or with thrombophilia

See Table 42-3 for factors that may influence warfarin effects.

*All recommendations are subject to modification by individual characteristics, including patient preference, age, comorbidity, and likelihood of recurrence.

†Reversible or time-limited risk factors: surgery, trauma, immobilization, estrogen use.

‡Proper duration of therapy is unclear in first event with homozygous factor V Leiden, homocystinemia, deficiency of protein C or S, or multiple thrombophilias; and in recurrent events with reversible risk factors.

Used with permission from Hyers TM, et al. Antithrombotic therapy for venous thromboembolic disease. *Chest* 2001:119(Suppl):176s–193s.

Table 42-7. Guidelines for Reversal of Warfarin Effects

Clinical Situation	Guidelines
INR > therapeutic range but <5.0, no clinically significant bleeding, rapid reversal not indicated for reasons of surgical intervention	
INR significantly above therapeutic range	Lower the dose or omit the next dose; resume warfarin therapy at a lower dose when the INR approaches desired range
INR minimally above therapeutic range	Dose reduction may not be necessary
INR >5.0 but <9.0, no clinically significant bleeding	
No additional risk factors for bleeding	Omit the next dose or two of warfarin; monitor INR more frequently; resume warfarin therapy at a lower dose when the INR is in therapeutic range
Increased risk of bleeding	Omit the next dose of warfarin; give vitamin K_1 (1.0–2.5 mg orally)
More rapid reversal needed before urgent surgery or dental extraction	Give vitamin K_1 (2–4 mg orally); give an additional dose of vitamin K_1 (1–2 mg orally) if the INR remains high at 24 hours
INR >9.0, no clinically significant bleeding	Give vitamin K_1 (3–5 mg orally); closely monitor INR; repeat dose of vitamin K_1 if INR not substantially reduced by 24–48 hours
INR >20.0, serious bleeding, major warfarin overdose requiring very rapid reversal of anticoagulant effect	Give vitamin K_1 (10 mg by slow IV infusion) with fresh frozen plasma transfusion or prothrombin complex concentrate, depending on urgency; vitamin K_1 injections may be needed every 12 hours
Life-threatening bleeding, serious warfarin overdose	Give prothrombin complex concentrate with vitamin K_1 (10 mg by slow IV infusion); repeat if necessary, depending on INR
Continuing warfarin therapy indicated after high doses of vitamin K_1	Give heparin until the effects of vitamin K_1 have been reversed and patient is responsive to warfarin

Adapted with permission from Ansell J, et al. Managing oral anticoagulant therapy. *Chest* 119(Suppl):22s–38s.

INR = international normalized ratio; IV = intravenous.

Table 42-8. Recommended Therapeutic Goal and Range for Oral Anticoagulant Therapy

	INR	
Indication	**Goal**	**Range**
Prophylaxis of venous thrombosis (high-risk surgery)	2.5	2.0–3.0
Treatment of venous thrombosis	2.5	2.0–3.0
Treatment of pulmonary embolism	2.5	2.0–3.0
Prevention of systemic embolism	2.5	2.0–3.0
Tissue heart valves	2.5	2.0–3.0
Anterior myocardial infarction (to prevent systemic embolism)	2.5	2.0–3.0
Anterior myocardial infarction (to prevent recurrent infarction)	3.0	2.5–3.5
Valvular heart disease	2.5	2.0–3.0
Atrial fibrillation	2.5	2.0–3.0
Mechanical prosthetic valves (high risk)	3.0	2.5–3.5
Bileaflet mechanical valve in the aortic position (with normal sinus rhythm)	2.5	2.0–3.0
Some patients with thrombosis and antiphospholipid syndrome	3.0	2.5–3.5

Adapted with permission from Hirsh J, et al. Oral anticoagulants: mechanism of action, clinical effectiveness, and optimal therapeutic range. *Chest* 119(Suppl):8s–21s.

Table 42-9. Pharmacokinetic and Pharmacodynamic Parameters of Different Low–Molecular-Weight Heparins (LMWHs)

LMWH	Brand Name	Average MW (daltons)	Bioavail-ability	Half-life	Xa:IIa Binding Affinity Ratio
Dalteparin	Fragmin	6000	87%	3–5 hours	2.7:1
Enoxaparin	Lovenox	4500	92%	4.5 hours	3.8:1
Tinzaparin	Inohep	6500	87%	3.9 hours	2.8:1

MW = molecular weight

(range 3,000–30,000 daltons), **LMWHs** are heterogeneous in size with a **mean molecular weight of 4,000–5,000** daltons (range 1,000–10,000 daltons).

3. **Mechanism of action**
   a. LMWHs achieve their **major anticoagulant effect by binding to antithrombin** through a unique pentasaccharide sequence that enhances the ability of antithrombin to inactivate factor IIa (thrombin) and factor Xa.
      (1) Heparin and **LMWHs catalyze the inactivation of factor IIa (thrombin) by binding to antithrombin through the unique pentasaccharide sequence and to thrombin to form a ternary complex.** A minimum chain length of 18 saccharides (including the pentasaccharide sequence) is required for ternary complex formation.
         (a) Virtually all heparin molecules contain at least 18 saccharide units.
         (b) Only 20%–50% of the different LMWHs contain fragments with 18 or more saccharide units.
         (c) Therefore, **compared with heparin, which has an antifactor Xa:antifactor IIa binding affinity ratio of approximately 1:1,** the various commercial **LMWHs have antifactor Xa:antifactor IIa binding affinity ratios varying from 2:1 up to 4:1,** depending on their molecular size distribution (Table 42-9).
      (2) In contrast, inactivation of factor Xa by antithrombin does not require binding of the heparin molecules to the clotting enzyme. Therefore, inactivation of factor Xa is

achieved by small–molecular-weight heparin fragments, provided that they contain the high-affinity pentasaccharide.

   b. The **antithrombotic and hemorrhagic effects** of heparin have been compared with LMWHs in a variety of **experimental animal models.**

      (1) When compared on a gravimetric basis, **LMWHs are said to cause decreased** potential for **hemorrhagic episodes.**

      (2) These differences in the relative antithrombotic:hemorrhagic ratios among these polysaccharides could be explained by the observation that **LMWHs have less inhibitory effects on platelet function** and vascular permeability.

  4. Pharmacokinetics. The plasma recoveries and pharmacokinetics of LMWHs differ from heparin because of differences in the binding properties of the two sulfated polysaccharides to plasma proteins and endothelial cells.

   a. LMWHs bind much less avidly to heparin-binding proteins than heparin, a property that contributes to the superior bioavailability of LMWHs at low doses and their more predictable anticoagulation effect.

   b. LMWHs do not bind to endothelial cells in culture, a property that could account for their longer plasma half-life and their dose-independent clearance. Principally, the renal route clears LMWHs; therefore, the biological half-life of LMWHs is increased in patients with renal failure.

  5. Administration and dosage

   Dosing of LMWHs is **disease-state** and **product specific,** with different doses administered based on the indication for use and the manufacturer of the specific LMWH. Table 42-10 shows the manufacturer's suggested, FDA approved dosing for specific indications. Figure 42-1 shows manufacturer's suggested, FDA-approved dosing for VTED.

Table 42-10. Manufacturer Recommendations for Dosing of Low–Molecular-Weight Heparin (LMWH) Based on Disease State

Approved Labeling and Dosing/SQ Administration	Dalteparin	Enoxaparin	Tinzaparin
Hip-replacement surgery Prophylaxis	5000 IU QD for 5–10 days	30 mg Q12h 120 IU/kg SQ or 40 mg QD for 7–10 days	n/a
Extended hip prophylaxis	n/a	40 mg QD for 3 weeks	n/a
Knee-replacement surgery	n/a	30 mg Q12h for 7–10 days	n/a
General surgery prophylaxis	2500 IU QD or 5000 IU QD (high risk) for 5–10 days	40 mg QD for 7–10 days	n/a
Prophylaxis in acute medically ill	n/a	40 mg QD for 6–14 days	n/a
Treatment of DVT with or without PE	n/a	1 mg/kg Q12h as a "bridge" to warfarin (O/P Tx permitted) until stable INR -or- 1.5 mg/kg Q24h as a "bridge" to warfarin (I/P only) until stable INR	175 IU/kg Q24h as a "bridge" to warfarin (O/P) Tx permitted until stable INR
Unstable angina and Non–ST segment elevated myocardial infarction	120 IU/kg Q12h for 5–8 days + aspirin indefinitely	1 mg/kg Q12h for 2–8 days + aspirin indefinitely	n/a

Adapted with permission from Rihn T, Vanscoy GJ. Low Molecular Weight Heparin: Formulary Drug Class Reviews. *Pharm & Therapeutics* 2001:26;486–492.

QD = daily; Q12h = every 12 hours; O/P = outpatient; Tx = treatment; INR = international normalized ratio; IU = International Units; n/a = not applicable.

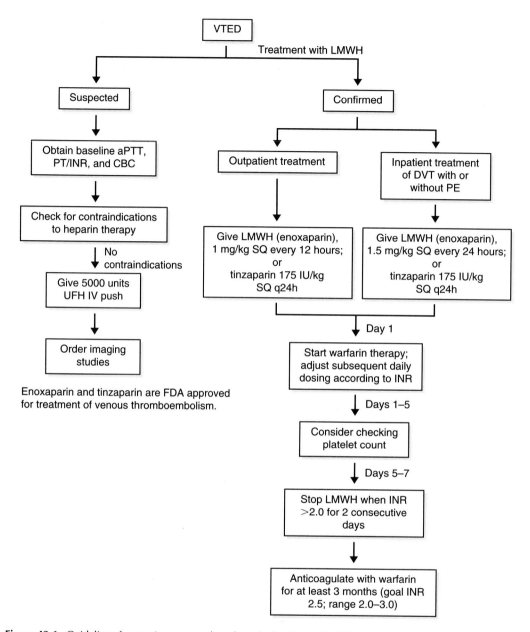

Figure 42-1. Guidelines for treating venous thromboembolic disease (VTED) with low–molecular-weight heparin (LMWH). Note that combined therapy (i.e., LMWH and warfarin) should be continued for at least 5–7 days. *aPTT* = activated partial thromboplastin time; *CBC* = complete blood count; *DVT* = deep venous thrombosis; *INR* = international normalized ratio; *IV* = intravenous; *PE* = pulmonary embolism; *PT* = prothrombin time; *SQ* = subcutaneous; *UFH* = unfractionated heparin. (Adapted with permission from Hyers TM, et al. Antithrombotic therapy for venous thromboembolic disease. *Chest* 2001;119(Suppl):176s–193s.)

D. Synthetic pentasaccharide

1. **Indications. Synthetic pentasaccharide** (fondaparinux—Arixtra, Organon Sanofi-Synthelabo LLC) is indicated for:

    (1) Thromboprophylaxis against DVT/PE after total hip-replacement surgery.

    (2) Thromboprophylaxis against DVT/PE after total knee-replacement surgery.

    (3) Thromboprophylaxis against DVT/PE after hip-fracture repair surgery.

2. **Chemistry.** Synthetic pentasaccharide is a selective **factor Xa inhibitor.** The molecular weight of the synthetic pentasaccharide product is 1728 daltons.

3. **Mechanism of action**
   a. The antithrombotic activity of fondaparinux is the result of antithrombin-mediated selective inhibition of factor Xa. Neutralization of factor Xa interrupts the blood coagulation cascade and thus inhibits thrombin formation and thrombus development.
   b. Fondaparinux does not inactivate thrombin (activated factor II) and has no known effect on platelet function.

4. **Pharmacokinetics**
   a. Following subcutaneous administration, the drug is completely bioavailable, with steady-state peak plasma levels achieved approximately 3 hours after administration of the dose.
   b. The elimination half-life is 17–21 hours, enabling once-daily dosing.
   c. Since the drug does not appear to be metabolized, at least a parenteral dose appears in the urine in active form and is renally eliminated.

5. **Adminstration and dosage**
   a. Fondaparinux must not be administered intramuscularly.
   b. The drug should not be used in patients with body weight less than 50 kg, as the incidence of major bleeding was found to double in this patient population during clinical trials.
   c. A usual dose of **2.5 mg subcutaneously once daily for 5–9 days** is recommended to prevent venous thromboembolism in patients undergoing total hip replacment, hip-fracture surgery, or knee-replacement surgery.
   d. The initial dose should be started 6–8 hours after surgery when hemostasis is established.

6. **Cautions**
   a. **Contraindications**
      (1) Prior sensitivity to fondaparinux
      (2) Active bleeding (risk of uncontrollable hemorrhage)
      (3) Severe renal impairment
      (4) Patients weighing less than 50 kg
      (5) Bacterial endocarditis
      (6) Thrombocytopenia associated with fondaparinux
   b. **Precautions**
      (1) Conditions or procedures that may enhance the risk of severe bleeding (e.g., trauma, hemophilia, gastrointestinal ulceration, concurrent use of antiplatelet agents, history of cerebrovascular hemorrhage, severe uncontrolled hypertension)
      (2) Renal impairment
      (3) Heparin-induced thrombocytopenia
      (4) Neuraxial anesthesia and indwelling epidural catheter use
      (5) Elderly patients
      (6) Pregnancy or breast-feeding (animal/human data unavailable)
      (7) Protamine is **ineffective** as an antidote

STUDY QUESTIONS

Directions: Each of the numbered items or incomplete statements in this section is followed by answers or by completions of the statement. Select the **one** lettered answer or completion that is **best** in each case.

1. A 67-year-old man weighing 100 kg (212 lb) and standing 60 inches tall presents to his physician after a transatlantic flight complaining of pain and swelling of his right lower extremity. The patient had total knee arthroplasty 2 weeks prior to his travel. His medical history reveals that he has an ejection fraction of 15%, he is in remission for non-Hodgkin's lymphoma, and he has had a previous myocardial infarction. His mother, father, and sister are all deceased from a stroke, pulmonary embolism, and childbirth, respectively. Given this patient's history, he is most likely suffering from which of the following?

(A) Ruptured Baker's cyst
(B) Deep venous thrombosis of the lower extremity
(C) Torn medial meniscus
(D) Septic arthritis

2. Prophylaxis against VTED may include

(A) Nonpharmacological prophylaxis
(B) Pharmacological prophylaxis
(C) Nonpharmacological and pharmacological prophylaxis
(D) Neither

3. Unfractionated heparin binds to antithrombin III and inactivates clotting factor(s)

(A) Xa
(B) IXa
(C) IIa
(D) All of the above
(E) None of the above

4. Initiation of unfractionated heparin therapy for the patient in question 1 would best be achieved with

(A) 5000-unit loading dose followed by 1000 units/hr
(B) 5000-unit loading dose followed by 1800 units/hr
(C) 8000-unit loading dose followed by 1800 units/hr
(D) 1000-unit loading dose followed by 1000 units/hr

Directions: Each item below contains three suggested answers, of which **one or more** is correct. Choose the answer

A   if **I only** is correct
B   if **III only** is correct
C   if **I and II** are correct
D   if **II and III** are correct
E   if **I, II, and III** are correct

Upon confirmation of diagnosis, the attending physician asks you, the pharmacist, to commence low–molecular-weight heparin (LMWH) therapy for the patient in question 1. Please answer the following questions regarding your pharmaceutical care for this patient.

5. When choosing an LMWH to treat the patient above, you would administer which of the following:

I. Enoxaparin 1 mg/kg/dose SQ q12h
II. Enoxaparin 1.5 mg/kg/dose SQ q24h
III. Tinzaparin 175 IU/kg/dose SQ q24h

6. Which of the following tests are used to monitor antithrombotic therapy?

I. International normalized ratio (INR)
II. Activated partial thromboplastin time (aPTT)
III. Heparin assay

7. A patient to be commenced on oral anticoagulant therapy for DVT would be treated with:

I. Oral anticoagulant therapy with warfarin for a goal international normalized ratio (INR) of 2–3
II. Oral anticoagulant therapy with warfarin for a goal INR of 2.5–3.5
III. Oral anticoagulant therapy with aspirin for a goal INR of 2–3

8. A patient on oral anticoagulant therapy is commenced on sulfamethoxazole-trimethoprim, double-strength twice daily. One may expect to see the INR

I. Increase
II. Decrease
III. Remain unchanged

9. If a patient has an INR greater than 20 and active bleeding that is clinically significant (i.e., hematuria), the pharmacist should

I. hold the drug therapy
II. administer vitamin K
III. administer fresh frozen plasma

10. When compared to unfractionated heparin, LMWHs have

I. preferential binding affinity to factor Xa relative to IIa (thrombin)
II. shorter half-lives
III. dose-dependent renal clearance

An 87-year-old woman weighing 49.0 kg (108 lb) and standing 66 inches tall has sustained a hip fracture requiring open reduction with internal fixation surgery. She has a documented serum creatine value recorded in the chart and in the laboratory results as 4.3 mg%. The orthopedic surgeon asks you (the pharmacist) what the appropriate fondaparinux dosing is for this patient to prevent venous thromboembolism after total hip-fracture repair surgery.

11. Which of the following are contraindications to the use of fondaparinux in this patient?

I. Patients weighing less than 50 kilograms
II. Patients with severe renal impairment
III. Patients who are elderly

ANSWERS AND EXPLANATIONS

1. The answer is B *[I A–C].*
The patient has the classical triad of risk factors predisposing to venous thromboembolic disease (VTED): injury (recent knee arthroplasty), venous stasis (transatlantic travel), and hypercoagulable state (family history of venous thromboembolic disease). The patient has other risk factors as well, including age >40 years, recent surgery, oncological disease (though in remission), heart failure, previous myocardial infarction with low ejection fraction, and obesity.

2. The answer is C *[IV A–B].*
Prophylaxis of VTED can involve a nonpharmacological approach, a pharmacological approach, or a combination of nonpharmacological and pharmacological approaches. The method of prophylaxis used is determined based on the patient's degree of risk. For example, a patient at high to extremely high risk for development of VTED requires nonpharmacological and pharmacological prophylaxis.

3. The answer is D *[V A 2].*
Unfractionated heparin acts as an anticoagulant by catalyzing the inactivation of thrombin (factor IIa), activated factor X (factor Xa), and activated factor IX (factor IXa) by antithrombin III.

4. The answer is C *[V A 4].*
Varying nomograms for dosing continuous-infusion unfractionated heparin exist in the medical and pharmaceutical literature. The loading dose is typically 70–100 units/kg. In this case [i.e., patient weighing 100 kg (212 lbs)], the loading dose is 80 units/kg. Maintenance doses of 15–25 units/kg/hr are typically used. In this case, the maintenance dose is 18 units/kg/hr.

5. The answer is E *[Table 42-10; Figure 42-1].*
Manufacturer's suggested, FDA-approved dosing for specific indication of VTED is reflective of appropriately conducted randomized perspective trials having been submitted and accepted by the FDA. Such trials have examined the role of low–molecular-weight heparin (LMWH) compared with unfractionated heparin. From these trials, evidence of efficacy and safety for these two LMWHs (enoxaparin and tinzaparin) at the treatment doses listed exists. Figure 42-1 shows manufacturer's suggested, FDA-approved dosing for VTED.

6. The answer is D *[V A 5].*
Unfractionated heparin may be appropriately monitored by either the activated partial thromboplastin time (aPTT) or heparin assay. Because different laboratories use aPTT reagents with varying sensitivities, the aPTT range and its corresponding ratio must be correlated to a heparin level of 0.2–0.4 units/mL [by whole-blood (protamine titration) assay]; or 0.3–0.7 units/mL by plasma-amidolytic assay. The safety and efficacy of low–molecular-weight heparin (LMWH) cannot be reliably evaluated by aPTT determinations. LMWH safety and efficacy can be evaluated by heparin assay. Because of the reliability of dose responsiveness seen with LMWH therapy, the need to perform heparin assays is controversial.

7. The answer is A *[V B 5; Table 42-6 and Table 42-8].*
Oral anticoagulant therapy is monitored by measuring the prothrombin time (PT). The PT is responsive to depression of three of the four vitamin K–dependent procoagulant clotting factors (prothrombin or factors II, VII, and X). These respective clotting factors take approximately 96 hours to be depleted, at which time the PT should be sufficient to arrive at an international normalized ratio (INR) of 2.0–3.0 for patients with deep venous thrombosis [i.e., by appropriately converting the PT ratio to the power of the International Sensitivity Index (ISI)]. Patients with mechanical prosthetic heart valves have INRs targeted in the 2.5–3.5 range. Aspirin therapy is not monitored by INR determinations.

8. The answer is A *[Table 42-4].*
Oral anticoagulant therapy with warfarin may be complicated by a myriad of drug–drug interactions owing to the highly protein-bound state of warfarin. Such drug interactions may potentiate (prolong) the prothrombin time/international normalized ratio (PT/INR), inhibit (shorten) the anticoagulant effect of warfarin, or have no effect on the actions of warfarin. Sulfamethoxazole-trimethoprim and other antibiotics have the potential to augment the anticoagulant effect of warfarin by eliminating bacterial flora and, thereby, producing vitamin-K deficiency.

9. The answer is E *[Table 42-7].*

Pharmacists may be called on to offer advice regarding reversal of warfarin therapy or may be empowered using Pharmacy and Therapeutics Committee or Medical Board approved protocols to reverse warfarin's effect. In all instances, the pharmacist must critically and clinically evaluate the situation and communicate with the physician regarding management issues. A need for immediate surgery or invasive procedures will always hasten the urgency of warfarin reversal. In the setting of active bleeding, its clinical significance must be demonstrated by consultation with the patient's physician. If the international normalized ratio is >20 and the patient has active bleeding that is clinically significant, the pharmacist must hold drug therapy, consider the most appropriate dose and route of vitamin K delivery, and administer fresh frozen plasma to replete the vitamin K–dependent clotting factors.

10. The answer is A *[V C 3 a (1) (c)].*

Compared with UFH, which has an antifactor Xa:antifactor IIa binding affinity ratio of approximately 1:1, the various commercial low–molecular-weight heparins (LMWHs) have antifactor Xa:antifactor IIa affinity ratios from 2:1 up to 4:1, depending on their molecular size distribution. This increased binding affinity for factor Xa relative to factor IIa (thrombin) is said to account for the improved ability of LMWHs to catalyze inactivation of thrombin, because the smaller fragments cannot bind to thrombin and therefore retain their ability to inactivate factor Xa. LMWHs have longer half-lives than UFH. LMWHs are cleared primarily via the kidneys, and their biological half-life is increased in patients with renal failure independent of dose.

11. The answer is C *[V D 5 b, 6 a (3), (4)].*

The synthetic pentasaccharide, fondaparinux is **contraindicated** in patients who have **severe renal impairment** and who **weigh less than 50 kg.** Calculation of the patient's estimated creatinine clearance (CrCl), by the method of Crockcoft-Gault reveals an estimated CrCl of approximately 8.5 cc/min which would be defined as severe renal impairment. Her stated weight is 49 kg. In this patient, her severe renal impairment and weight less than 50 kg constitute contraindications to the use of fondaparinux. It is recommended to use fondaparinux with *precaution* in this 87-year-old or in the elderly patient population.

43
Infectious Diseases

Paul F. Souney
Ron DeBellis
Anthony E. Zimmermann

I. PRINCIPLES OF ANTI-INFECTIVE THERAPY

A. Definition. Anti-infective agents treat infection by suppressing or destroying the causative microorganisms—bacteria, mycobacteria, fungi, protozoa, or viruses. Anti-infective agents derived from natural substances are called **antibiotics;** those produced from synthetic substances are called **antimicrobials.** These two terms now are used interchangeably.

B. Indications. Anti-infective agents should be used only when: Confirm the presence of infection by completing a careful history and physical, searching for signs and symptoms of infection as well as predisposing factors.

  1. A significant infection has been diagnosed or is strongly suspected.

  2. An established indication for prophylactic therapy exists.

C. Gram stain, microbiological culturing, and susceptibility tests should be performed before anti-infective therapy is initiated. Test materials must be obtained by a method that avoids contamination of the specimen by the patient's own flora.

  1. Gram stain. Performed on all specimens except blood cultures, the gram stain helps to identify the cause of infection immediately. By determining if the causative agent is gram-positive or gram-negative, the test allows a better choice of drug therapy, particularly when an anti-infective regimen must begin without delay.
    a. Gram-positive microorganisms stain **blue** or **purple.**
    b. Gram-negative microorganisms stain **red** or **rose-pink.**
    c. Fungi may also be identified by gram stain.

  2. Microbiological cultures. To identify the specific causative agent, specimens of body fluids or infected tissue are collected for analysis.

  3. Susceptibility tests. Different strains of the same pathogenic species may have widely varying susceptibility to a particular anti-infective agent. Susceptibility tests determine microbial susceptibility to a given drug and, thus, can be used to predict whether the drug will combat the infection effectively.
    a. Microdilution method. The drug is diluted serially in various media containing the test microorganism.
      (1) The lowest drug concentration that prevents microbial growth after 18–24 hours of incubation is called the **minimum inhibitory concentration (MIC).**
      (2) The lowest drug concentration that reduces bacterial density by 99.9% is called the **minimum bactericidal concentration (MBC).**
      (3) Breakpoint concentrations of antibiotics are used to characterize antibiotic activity: The interpretive categories are **susceptible, moderately susceptible (intermediate),** and **resistant.** These concentrations are determined by considering pharmacokinetics, serum and tissue concentrations following normal doses, and the **population distribution** of MICs of a group of bacteria for a given drug.
    b. Kirby-Bauer disk diffusion technique. This test is less expensive but less reliable than the microdilution method; however, it provides qualitative susceptibility information.
      (1) Filter paper disks impregnated with specific drug quantities are placed on the surface of agar plates streaked with a microorganism culture. After 18 hours, the size of a clear inhibition zone is determined; drug activity against the test strain is then correlated to zone size.
      (2) The Kirby-Bauer technique does not reliably predict therapeutic effectiveness against certain microorganisms (e.g., *Staphylococcus aureus, Shigella*).

D. Choice of agent. An anti-infective agent should be chosen on the basis of its pharmacological properties and spectrum of activity as well as on various host (patient) factors (Figure 43-1).

    1. Pharmacological properties include the drug's ability to reach the infection site and to attain a desired level in the target tissue.

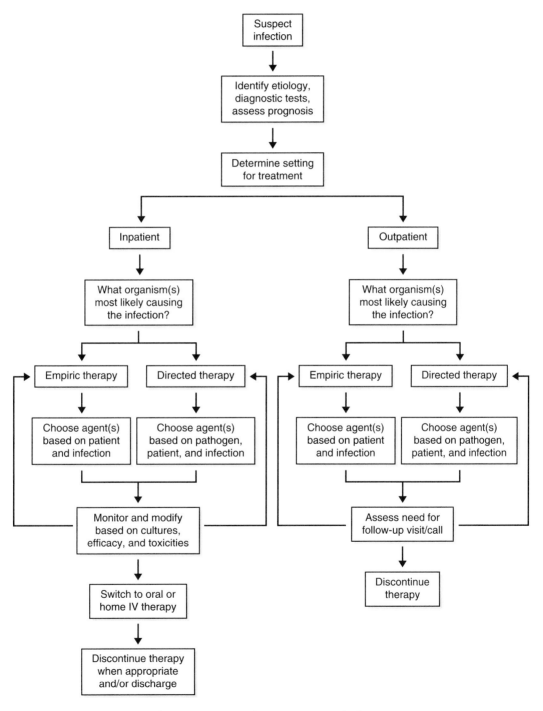

Figure 43-1. Approach to management of infection.

2. **Spectrum of activity.** To treat an infectious disease effectively, an anti-infective drug must be active against the causative pathogen. Susceptibility testing or clinical experience in treating a given syndrome may suggest the effectiveness of a particular drug.

3. **Patient factors.** Selection of an anti-infective drug regimen must take various patient factors into account to determine which type of drug should be administered, the correct drug dosage and administration route, and the potential for adverse drug effects.
   a. **Immunological status.** A patient with impaired immune mechanisms may require a drug that rapidly destroys pathogens (i.e., **bactericidal agent**) rather than one that merely suppresses a pathogen's growth or reproduction (i.e., **bacteriostatic agent**).
   b. **Presence of a foreign body.** The effectiveness of anti-infective therapy is reduced in patients who have prosthetic joints or valves, cardiac pacemakers, and various internal shunts.
   c. **Age.** A drug's pharmacokinetic properties may vary widely in patients of different ages. In very young and very old patients, drug metabolism and excretion commonly decrease. Elderly patients also have an increased risk of suffering ototoxicity when receiving certain antibiotics.
   d. **Underlying disease**
      (1) Preexisting **kidney** or **liver disease** increases the risk of nephrotoxicity or hepatotoxicity during the administration of some antibacterial drugs.
      (2) Patients with **central nervous system (CNS) disorders** may suffer neurotoxicity (motor seizures) during penicillin therapy.
      (3) Patients with **neuromuscular disorders** (e.g., myasthenia gravis) are at increased risk for developing neuromuscular blockade during aminoglycoside or polymyxin B therapy.
   e. **History of drug allergy or adverse drug reactions.** Patients who have had previous allergic or other untoward reactions to a particular antibiotic have a higher risk of experiencing the same reaction during subsequent administration of that drug. Except in life-threatening situations, patients who have had serious allergic reactions to penicillin, for example, should not receive the drug again.
   f. **Pregnancy and lactation.** Because drug therapy during pregnancy and lactation can cause unwanted effects, the mother's need for the antibiotic must be weighed against the drug's potential harm.
      (1) Pregnancy can increase the risk of adverse drug effects for both mother and fetus. Also, plasma drug concentrations tend to decrease in pregnant women, reducing a drug's therapeutic effectiveness.
      (2) Most drugs, including antibiotics, appear in the breast milk of nursing mothers and may cause adverse effects in infants. For example, sulfonamides may lead to toxic bilirubin accumulation in a newborn's brain.
   g. **Genetic traits**
      (1) Sulfonamides may cause hemolytic anemia in patients with glucose-6-phosphate dehydrogenase (G6PD) deficiency.
      (2) Patients who rapidly metabolize drugs (i.e., rapid acetylators) may develop hepatitis when receiving the antitubercular drug isoniazid.

E. **Empiric therapy.** In serious or life-threatening disease, anti-infective therapy must begin before the infecting organism has been identified. In this case, the choice of drug (or drugs) is based on clinical experience, suggesting that a particular agent is effective in a given setting.

   1. A **broad-spectrum antibiotic** usually is the most appropriate choice until the specific organism has been determined.

   2. In all cases, **culture specimens must be obtained** before therapy begins.

F. **Multiple antibiotic therapy.** A combination of drugs should be given only when clinical experience has shown such therapy to be more effective than single-agent therapy in a particular setting. A multiple-agent regimen can increase the risk of toxic drug effects and, in a few cases, may result in drug antagonism and subsequent therapeutic ineffectiveness. Indications for multiple-agent therapy include:

   1. **Need for increased antibiotic effectiveness.** The **synergistic** (intensified) effect of two or more agents may allow a dosage reduction or a faster or enhanced drug effect.

2. **Treatment of an infection caused by multiple pathogens** (e.g., intra-abdominal infection)

3. **Prevention of proliferation of drug-resistant organisms** (e.g., during treatment of tuberculosis)

G. **Duration of anti-infective therapy.** To achieve the therapeutic goal, anti-infective therapy must continue for a sufficient duration.

1. **Acute uncomplicated infection.** Treatment generally should continue until the patient has been afebrile and asymptomatic for at least 72 hours.

2. **Chronic infection** (e.g., endocarditis, osteomyelitis). Treatment may require a longer duration (4–6 weeks) with follow-up culture analyses to assess therapeutic effectiveness.

H. **Monitoring therapeutic effectiveness.** To assess the patient's response to anti-infective therapy, appropriate specimens should be cultured and the following parameters monitored.

1. **Fever curve.** An important assessment tool, the fever curve may be a reliable indication of response to therapy. Defervescence usually indicates favorable response.

2. **White blood cell (WBC) count.** In the initial stage of infection, the neutrophil count from a peripheral blood smear may rise above normal (neutrophilia) and immature neutrophil forms ("bands") may appear ("left shift"). In patients who are elderly, debilitated, or suffering overwhelming infection, the WBC count may be normal or subnormal.

3. **Radiographic findings.** Small effusions, abscesses, or cavities that appear on radiographs indicate the focus of infection.

4. **Pain** and **inflammation** (as evidenced by swelling, erythema, and tenderness) may occur when the infection is superficial or within a joint or bone, also indicating a possible focus of infection.

5. **Erythrocyte sedimentation rate (ESR or "sed rate").** Large elevations in ESR are associated with acute or chronic infection, particularly endocarditis, chronic osteomyelitis, and intra-abdominal infections. A normal ESR does not exclude infection; more often, ESR is elevated due to noninfectious causes such as collagen vascular disease.

6. **Serum complement concentrations,** particularly the C3 component, are often reduced in serious infections because of consumption during the host defense process.

I. **Lack of therapeutic effectiveness.** When an antibiotic drug regimen fails, other drugs should not be added indiscriminately or the regimen otherwise changed. Instead, the situation should be reassessed and diagnostic efforts intensified. Causes of therapeutic ineffectiveness include:

1. **Misdiagnosis.** The isolated organism may have been misidentified by the laboratory or may not be the causative agent for infection (e.g., the patient may have an unsuspected infection).

2. **Improper drug regimen.** The drug dosage, administration route, dosing frequency, or duration of therapy may be inadequate or inappropriate.

3. **Inappropriate choice of antibiotic agent.** As discussed in I D, patient factors and the pharmacological properties and spectrum of activity of a given drug must be considered when planning anti-infective drug therapy.

4. **Microbial resistance.** By acquiring resistance to a specific antibiotic, microorganisms can survive in the drug's presence. Many gonococcal strains, for instance, now resist penicillin. Drug resistance is particularly common in geographical areas where a specific drug has been used excessively (and perhaps improperly).

5. **Unrealistic expectations.** Antibiotics are ineffective in certain circumstances.
   a. Patients with conditions that require **surgical drainage** frequently cannot be cured by anti-infective drugs until the drain has been removed. For example, the presence of necrotic tissue or pus in patients with pneumonia, empyema, or renal calculi is a common cause of antibiotic failure.
   b. **Fever** should not be treated with anti-infective drugs unless infection has been identified as the cause. Although fever frequently signifies infection, it sometimes stems from noninfectious conditions (e.g., drug reactions, phlebitis, neoplasms, metabolic disorders,

arthritis). These conditions do not respond to antibiotics. One exception to this position is neutropenic cancer patients; such patients with no signs or symptoms of infection other than fever are widely treated with antimicrobial agents.

6. **Infection by two or more types of microorganisms.** If not detected initially, an additional cause of infection may lead to therapeutic failure.

J. Perioperative antibiotic prophylaxis

1. **Definition.** Perioperative antibiotic prophylaxis is a short course of antibiotic administered before there is clinical evidence of infection.

2. **General considerations**
   a. **Timing.** The antibiotic should be administered in order to ensure that appropriate antibiotic levels are available at the site of contamination before the incision. Initiation of prophylaxis is often at induction of anesthesia, just before the surgical incision. This ensures peak serum and tissue antibiotic levels.
   b. **Duration.** Prophylaxis should be maintained for the duration of surgery. Long surgical procedures (e.g., more than 3 hours) may require additional doses. There is little evidence to support continuation of prophylaxis beyond 24 hours.
   c. **Antibiotic spectrum** should be appropriate for the usual pathogens.
      (1) In general, **first-generation cephalosporins** (e.g., cefazolin) are the drugs of choice for most procedures and patients. These agents have an appropriate spectrum, a low frequency of side effects, a favorable half-life, and a low cost.
      (2) **Vancomycin** is a suitable alternative in penicillin-sensitive patients and in situations where methicillin-resistant *S. aureus* is a concern.
   d. **Route of administration.** Intravenous (IV) or intramuscular (IM) routes are preferred to guarantee good serum and tissue levels at the time of incision.

II. ANTIBACTERIAL AGENTS

A. **Definition and classification.** Used to treat infections caused by **bacteria,** antibacterial agents fall into several major categories: **aminoglycosides, carbapenems, cephalosporins, erythromycins, penicillins** (including various subgroups), **sulfonamides, tetracyclines, fluoroquinolones, urinary tract antiseptics,** and **miscellaneous antibacterials** (Table 43-1).

B. **Aminoglycosides.** These drugs, containing amino sugars, are used primarily in infections caused by gram-negative enterobacteria and in suspected sepsis. They have little activity against anaerobic and facultative organisms. The toxic potential of these drugs limits their use. Major aminoglycosides include **amikacin, kanamycin, gentamicin, neomycin, netilmicin, streptomycin,** and **tobramycin.**

1. **Mechanism of action.** Aminoglycosides are **bactericidal;** they inhibit bacterial protein synthesis by binding to and impeding the function of the 30S ribosomal subunit. (Some aminoglycosides also bind to the 50S ribosomal subunit.) Their mechanism of action is not fully known.

2. **Spectrum of activity**
   a. **Streptomycin** is active against both gram-positive and gram-negative bacteria. However, widespread resistance to this drug has restricted its use to the organisms that cause plague and tularemia, gram-positive streptococci (given in combination with penicillin), and *Mycobacterium tuberculosis* (given in combination with other antitubercular agents, as described in VI C 2).
   b. **Amikacin, kanamycin, gentamicin, tobramycin, neomycin,** and **netilmicin** are active against many gram-negative bacteria (e.g., *Proteus, Serratia,* and *Pseudomonas* organisms).
      (1) **Gentamicin** is active against some *Staphylococcus* strains; it is more active than tobramycin against *Serratia* organisms.
      (2) **Amikacin** is the broadest-spectrum aminoglycoside with activity against most aerobic gram-negative bacilli as well as many anaerobic gram-negative bacterial strains that resist gentamicin and tobramycin. It is also active against *M. tuberculosis* and *Mycobacterium avium-intracellulare (MAI).*
      (3) **Tobramycin,** as compared to gentamicin, may be more active against *Pseudomonas aeruginosa.*

Table 43-1. Some Important Parameters of Anti-Infective Drugs

Agent	Elimination Route	Half-Life	Administration Route	Common Dosage Range (Adults)
Aminoglycosides				
Amikacin	Renal	2–3 hours	IV, IM	15 mg/kg/day
Gentamicin	Renal	2 hours	IV, IM	3 mg/kg/day (standard dose); 6–7 mg/kg/day once daily
Kanamycin	Renal	2–4 hours	Oral, IV	15 mg/kg q 8–12 hours
Neomycin	Renal	2–3 hours	Oral, topical	50–100 mg/kg/day (oral); 10–15 mg/day (topical)
Netilmicin	Renal	2–7 hours	IV, IM	3–6 mg/kg/day
Streptomycin	Renal	2–3 hours	IM	15 mg/kg/day[†]
Tobramycin	Renal	2–5 hours	IV, IM	3–5 mg/kg/day (standard dose); 6–7 mg/kg/day, once daily
Carbapenems				
Imipenem	Renal	1 hour	IV	250 mg–1 g q 6 hours
Ertapenem	Renal	4 hours	IV, IM	1 g qd
Meropenem	Renal	1.5 hours	IV, IM	0.5–2 g q 8 hours
Cephalosporins				
First-generation				
Cefadroxil	Renal	1.5 hours	Oral	1–2 g/day
Cefazolin	Renal	1.4–2.2 hours	IV	250 mg–1 g q 8 hours
Cephalexin	Renal	0.9–1.3 hours	Oral	250–500 mg q 6 hours
Cephapirin	Renal (H)	0.6–0.8 hour	IV, IM	500 mg–2 g q 4–6 hours
Cephradine	Renal	1.3 hours	Oral, IV	250–500 mg q 6 hours
Second-generation				
Cefaclor	Renal (H)	0.8 hour	Oral	250–500 mg q 8 hours
Cefmetazole	Renal	72 minutes	IV	2 g q 6–12 hours
Cefonicid	Renal	4 hours	IV	1–2 g/day
Cefotetan	Renal	2.8–4.6 hours	IV, IM	1–2 g q 12 hours
Cefoxitin	Renal	0.8 hour	IV	1–2 g q 6–8 hours
Cefproxil	Renal	78 minutes	Oral	250–500 mg q 12–24 hours
Cefuroxime	Renal	1.5–2.2 hours	IV, IM	750 mg–1.5 g q 8 hours
Loracarbef	Renal	1 hour	Oral	200 mg q 12 hours or 400 mg/day
Third-generation				
Cefixime	Renal	3–4 hours	Oral	400 mg/day
Cefdinir	Renal	1.7–1.8 hours	Oral	300 mg q 12 hours
Cefoperazone	Hepatic	1.6–2.4 hours	IV	2–4 g q 12 hours
Cefotaxime	Renal (H)	1.5 hours	IV	1–2 g q 6–8 hours
Cefpodoxime	Renal	2.5 hours	Oral	100–400 mg q 12 hours
Ceftazidime	Renal	1.8 hours	IV, IM	1–2 g q 8–12 hours
Ceftibuten	Renal	2.5 hours	Oral	400 mg/day
Ceftizoxime	Renal	1.7 hours	IV	1–2 g q 8–12 hours
Ceftriaxone	Renal	8 hours	IV, IM	1–2 g/day
Fourth-generation				
Cefepime	Renal	2–2.3 hours	IV, IM	1–2 g q 12 hours
Erythromycins and other macrolides				
Azithromycin	Hepatic	68 hours	Oral	250 mg/day
Clarithromycin	Renal	3–7 hours	Oral	250–500 mg q 12 hours
Dirithromycin	Hepatic	8 hours	Oral	500 mg daily
Erythromycin base estolate, ethylsuc- cinate, and stearate	Hepatic	1.2–2.6 hours	Oral	250–500 mg q 6 hours

[†]Dosage applies to infections other than tuberculosis; for tuberculosis, dosage is 1g/day
[‡]Intravenous agent withdrawn from U.S. market

(Continued on next page)

Table 43-1. *Continued*

Agent	Elimination Route	Half-Life	Administration Route	Common Dosage Range (Adults)
Erythromycins and other macrolides (continued)				
Erythromycin glu- ceptate and lactobionate			IV	0.5–2 g q 6 hours
Troleandomycin	Hepatic (R)	1.05 hours	Oral	250–500 mg q 12 hours
Natural penicillins				
Penicillin G	Renal (H)	0.5 hour	Oral, IV, IM	200,000–500,000 units q 6–8 hours
Penicillin V	Renal	1 hour	Oral	500 mg–2 g/day
Penicillin G procaine	Renal	24–60 hours	IM	300,000–600,000 units/day
Penicillin G benzathine	Renal	24–60 hours	IM	300,000–600,000 units/day
Penicillinase-resistant penicillins				
Cloxacillin	Renal (H)	0.5 hour	Oral	250–500 mg q 6 hours
Dicloxacillin	Renal (H)	0.5–0.9 hour	Oral	500 mg–1 g/day
Methicillin	Renal (H)	0.5–1 hour	IV, IM	1–2 g q 4–6 hours
Nafcillin	Hepatic (R)	0.5 hour	Oral, IV, IM	0.25–2 g q 6 hours
Oxacillin	Renal (H)	0.5 hour	Oral, IV, IM	500 mg–2 g q 4–6 hours 500–875 mg q 12 hours
Aminopenicillins				
Amoxicillin	Renal (H)	0.9–2.3 hours	Oral	250–500 mg q 8 hours
Amoxicillin/ clavulanic acid	Renal	1 hour	Oral	250–500 mg q 8 hours
Ampicillin	Renal (H)	0.8–1.5 hours	Oral, IV, IM	250 mg–2 g q 4–6 hours
Ampicillin/ sulbactam	Renal	1–1.8 hours	IV, IM	1.5–3 g q 6 hours
Bacampicillin	Renal	1 hour	Oral	400–800 mg q 12 hours
Extended-spectrum penicillins				
Carbenicillin	Renal (H)	1.5 hours	IM, IV	1–5 g q 4–6 hours
Carbenicillin indanyl	Renal (H)	1.5 hours	Oral	382–764 mg qid
Mezlocillin	Renal (H)	0.6–1.2 hours	IV, IM	1–3 g q 4–6 hours
Piperacillin	Renal (H)	0.8–1.4 hours	IV, IM	1–1.5 mg/kg q 6–12 hours
Piperacillin/ tazobactam	Renal	0.7–1.2 hours	IV	3.375 g q 6 hours
Ticarcillin	Renal	0.9–1.5 hours	IV, IM	1–3 g q 4–6 hours
Ticarcillin/ clavulanic acid	Renal	1–1.5 hours	IV	3.1 g q 4–6 hours
Sulfonamides				
Sulfacytine	Renal	4–4.5 hours	Oral	250 mg q 6 hours
Sulfadiazine	Renal (H)	6 hours	Oral, IV	2–4 g/day
Sulfamethoxazole	Hepatic (R)	9–11 hours	Oral	1–3 g/day
Sulfisoxazole	Renal (H)	3–7 hours	Oral, IV	2–8 g/day
Sulfamethizole	Renal	—	Oral	0.5–1 g q 6–8 hours
Tetracyclines				
Demeclocycline	Renal	10–17 hours	Oral	300 mg–1 g/day
Doxycycline	Hepatic	14–25 hours	Oral, IV	100–200 mg q 12 hours
Methacycline	Renal	16 hours	Oral	150 mg q 6 hours to 300 mg q 12 hours
Minocycline	Hepatic	12–15 hours	Oral, IV	100–200 mg q 12 hours

Table 43-1. *Continued*

Agent	Elimination Route	Half-Life	Administration Route	Common Dosage Range (Adults)
Tetracyclines (continued)				
Oxytetracycline	Renal	6–12 hours	Oral, IM	250–500 mg q 6 hours 250–500 mg qid or 300 mg/ day in one or two divided doses
Tetracycline⁺	Renal	6–12 hours	Oral, IV, IM	1–2 g/day
Fluoroquinolones				
Alatrofloxacin*	Hepatic/ fecal	11 hours	IV	200–300 mg IV followed by 200 mg oral therapy
Ciprofloxacin	Renal (H)	5–6 hours	IV	200–600 mg q 12 hours
Enoxacin	Renal (H)	3–6 hours	Oral	200 mg/day–400 mg q 12 hours
Gatifloxacin	Renal	7 hours	Oral, IV	400 mg once daily
Grepafloxacin**	Hepatic	12 hours	Oral	400–600 mg once daily
Lomefloxacin	Renal	6.35–7.77 hours	Oral	400 mg/day
Levofloxacin	Renal	8 hours	IV, Oral	250–500 mg q 24 hours
Moxifloxacin	Hepatic	12 hours	Oral	400 mg once daily
Ofloxacin	Renal	5–7.5 hours	Oral	100 mg/day–400 mg
Sparfloxacin	Renal	20 hours	Oral	200 mg q 24 hours
Trovafloxacin	Hepatic/ fecal	11 hours	Oral	100–300 mg q 24 hours
Urinary tract antiseptics				
Cinoxacin	Renal	1–1.5 hours	Oral	250 mg q 6 hours or 500 mg q 12 hours
Fosfomycin	Renal/fecal	5.7 hours	Oral	One packet (3 g) in 90–120 ml water single dose
Methenamine hippurate and mandelate	Renal	1–3 hours	Oral	0.5–2 g qid
Nalidixic acid	Renal	8 hours	Oral	4 g/day
Nitrofurantoin	Renal	0.3–1 hour	Oral	5–7 mg/kg/day
Norfloxacin	Hepatic	3–4 hours	Oral	400 bid
Miscellaneous anti-infectives				
Atovaquone	Renal	—	Oral	750 mg tid × 21 days
Aztreonam	Renal	1.7 hours	Oral, IV	50–100 mg/kg/day
Clindamycin	Hepatic	2–4 hours	Oral, IM, IV	300–900 mg q 6–8 hours
Clofazimine	Hepatic	70 days	Oral	50–100 mg/day
Dapsone	Hepatic (R)	28 hours	Oral	50–100 mg/day
Lincomycin	Hepatic (R)	4.4–6.4 hours	IV, IM	600 mg–1 g q 8–12 hours
Linezolid	Renal	4–6 hours	Oral, IV	600 mg q 12 hours
Mupirocin	Renal	19–35 minutes	Topical	Apply q 8–12 hours
Quinupristin/ dalfopristin	Hepatic	1 hour/ 0.4–0.5 hour	IV	7.5 mg/kg q 8 hours
Spectinomycin	Renal	1.2–2.8 hours	IM	2–4 g (single dose)
Trimethoprim	Renal (H)	8–15 hours	Oral	100–200 mg/day
Vancomycin	Renal	6–8 hours	Oral, IV	500 mg q 6 hours
Antifungal agents				
Amphotericin B	Unknown	24 hours	IV	1–1.5 mg/kg/day
Caspofungin	Hepatic	9–11 hours	IV	70 mg on day 1, then 50 mg qd
Fluconazole	Renal	22–37 hours	IV, Oral	100–800 mg/day
Flucytosine	Renal	6 hours	Oral	50–150 mg/kg/day
Griseofulvin	Hepatic (R)	9–24 hours	Oral	300–375 mg/day

(Continued on next page)

Table 43-1. *Continued*

Agent	Elimination Route	Half-Life	Administration Route	Common Dosage Range (Adults)
Antifungal agents (continued)				
Intraconazole	Hepatic	24–42 hours	Oral	200–600 mg/day
Ketoconazole	Hepatic (Feces)	3.3 hours	Oral	200–400 mg/day bid
Miconazole	Hepatic	20–24 hours	Oral	200–400 mg/day
Nystatin	Feces	—	Oral	500,000–1,000,000 units tid
Terbinafine	Hepatic (R)	11–16 hours	Oral	250 mg/day
Voriconazole	Hepatic	6 hours	IV, PO	i.v. 6 mg/kg q 12 h × 2 doses, then 4 mg/kg q 12 h; p.o. 200 mg q 12 h for >40 kg, 100 mg q 12 h for <40 kg
Antiprotozol agents				
Atovaquone	Hepatic	67 hours	Oral	750 mg bid
Chloroquine	Renal (Feces)	72–120 hours	IM, Oral	Varied upon disease
Diloxanide	Renal	—	IM	500 mg tid
Eflornithine	Renal	3 hours	IV	100 mg/kg/dose q 6 hours
Emetine	Renal	4–7 days	SC, IM	1 mg/kg/day to 60 mg/day maximum
Fansidar	Renal	100–231 hours	Oral	1 tablet q week
Hydroxychloroquine	Renal	72–120 hours	Oral	310 mg q week
Iodoquinol	Fecal	—	Oral	650 mg tid for 20 days
Mefloquine	Hepatic	15–33 days	Oral	1250 mg single dose
Metronidazole	Hepatic (R)	6–14 hours	Oral, IV	250–500 mg q 6–8 hours
Paromomycin	Fecal	—	Oral	25–35 mg/kg/day
Pentamidine	Renal	6–9 hours	IM, IV, Inhalation	3–4 mg/kg q day IV, IM 300 mg q 4 weeks, inhalation
Primaquine	Hepatic	3.7–9.6 hours	Oral	15 mg (base)/day
Pyrimethamine	Renal	111 hours	Oral	25 mg q week
Quinacrine		5 days	Oral	100 mg/day
Quinine	Renal	12 hours	Oral	325 mg bid
Antitubercular agents				
Aminosalicylic acid	Renal	1 hour	Oral	150 mg/kg daily (maximum 12 g/day)
Capreomycin	Renal	4–6 hours	IM	15 mg/kg/day to 1 g/day maximum
Cycloserine	Renal	10 hours	Oral	15–20 mg/kg (maximum 1 g/day)
Ethambutol	Hepatic	3.3 hours	Oral	15–25 mg/kg/day
Ethionamide	Hepatic	3 hours	Oral	500 mg–1 g/day
Isoniazid	Hepatic	1–4 hours	Oral, IV	5–10 mg/kg daily (maximum dose = 300 mg)
Pyrazinamide	Hepatic	9–10 hours	Oral	15–30 mg/kg daily (maximum 2 g/day)
Antiviral agents				
Abacavir	Hepatic	1.5 hours	Oral	300 mg bid
Adefovir	Renal	7.5 hours	Oral	10 mg q day
Acyclovir	Renal	2.1–3.8 hours	Oral, IV, Topical	5–10 mg/kg q 8 hours (IV); 200–800 mg q 4 hours (oral)
Amprenavir	Hepatic	7–10 hours	Oral	1200 mg bid
Amantadine	Renal	12 hours	Oral	100–200 mg q day
Cidofovir	Renal	6.5 hours	IV	5 mg/kg week × 2 (induction); 5 mg/kg 2 weeks (maintenance)

Table 43-1. *Continued*

Agent	Elimination Route	Half-Life	Administration Route	Common Dosage Range (Adults)
Antiviral agents (continued)				
Delaviridine	Hepatic (R)	2–11 hours	Oral	400 mg tid
Didanosine	Hepatic (R)	1.5 hours	Oral	>60 kg 200 mg bid (tabs)
				>60 kg 250 mg bid (oral)
Enfuvirtide	NA	3.8 hours	SC	90 mg bid
Efavirenz	Hepatic	40–55 hours	Oral	600 mg q day
Famciclovir	Renal	2–2.3 hours	Oral	500 mg q 8 hours × 7 days
Foscarnet	Renal	2–8 hours	IV	40 mg/kg q 8 hours—HSV
				60 mg/kg q 8 hours—CMV
Ganciclovir	Renal	2.9 hours	IV	5 mg/kg q 12 hours
		4.8 hours	Oral	1000 mg tid (after induction)
Indinavir	Hepatic	1.8 hours	Oral	800 mg tid
Lamivudine	Renal	5–7 hours	Oral	150 mg bid or 300 mg daily
Lopinavir (+ ritonavir)	Hepatic	<1 hour	Oral	133 mg/33 mg per cap (3 caps bid) or 5 mL bid
Nelfinavir	Hepatic	3.5–5 hours	Oral	750 mg tid or 1250 mg bid
Nevirapine	Renal (H)	25–30 hours	Oral	200 mg q day × 14 days, then 200 mg bid
Oseltamivir	Renal	6–10 hours	Oral	75 mg bid for 5 days
Rimantadine	Renal	25 hours	Oral	100 mg bid
Ritonavir	Hepatic	3–5 hours	Oral	600 mg bid
Ribavirin	Renal	30–151 hours	Aerosol	6 g q 24 hours
Saquinavir	Hepatic	13 hours	Oral	1200 mg tid (Fortovase) 600 mg tid (Invirase)
Stavudine	Renal	1.5 hours	Oral	>60 kg 40 mg q 12 hours <60 kg 30 mg q 12 hours
Tenofovir	Renal	17 hours	Oral	300 mg daily
Valacyclovir	Renal	2.45–3.3 hours	Oral	1 g q 8 hours × 7 days
Valganciclovir	Renal	4.08 hours	Oral	900 mg bid induction, 900 mg daily maint.
Zalcitabine	Renal	1–3 hours	Oral	0.75 mg tid
Zanamavir	Renal	2.5–5.1 hours	Inhalation (Diskhaler)	2 inhalations (10 mg) bid × 5 days
Zidovudine	Renal (H)	1 hour	Oral	300 mg bid or 200 mg tid
Anthelmintics				
Albendazole	Hepatic	2.8–9 hours	Oral	100–800 mg daily
Diethylcarbamazine	Renal	30 hours	Oral	25 mg/day for 3 days, then 50 mg/day for 5 days, then 100 mg/day for 1 day, then 150 mg/day for 12 days
Mebendazole	Hepatic	2.8–9 hours	Oral	100–800 mg daily
Niclosamide	Fecal		Oral	2 grams/day
Oxamniquine	Renal	1–2.5 hours	Oral	12–15 mg/kg for 1 dose
Piperazine	Hepatic		Oral	65 mg/kg (maximum dose 2.5 g)
Praziquantel	Hepatic	0.8–1.5 hours	Oral	50 mg/kg in 3 divided doses on the same day
Pyrantel	Hepatic	—	Oral	11 mg/kg (maximum = 1 g) as a single dose
Thiabendazole	Hepatic	—	Oral	25 mg/kg for weight <70 kg, 1.5 g for weight >70 kg

*Alatrofloxacin is a prodrug rapidly converted in vivo to trovafloxacin.

**Removed from the U.S. market in 1999.

(4) Netilmicin may be active against gentamicin-resistant organisms; it appears to be less ototoxic than other aminoglycosides.

(5) Neomycin, in addition to its activity against such gram-negative organisms as *Escherichia coli* and *Klebsiella pneumoniae,* is active against several gram-positive organisms (e.g., *S. aureus, M. tuberculosis*). *P. aeruginosa* and most streptococci are now neomycin-resistant.

3. Therapeutic uses

a. Streptomycin is used to treat plague, tularemia, acute brucellosis (given in combination with tetracycline), bacterial endocarditis caused by *Streptococcus viridans* (given in combination with penicillin), and tuberculosis (given in combination with other antitubercular agents, as described in VI C 2).

b. Gentamicin, tobramycin, amikacin, and **netilmicin** are therapeutic for serious gram-negative bacillary infections (e.g., those caused by *Enterobacter, Serratia, Klebsiella, P. aeruginosa*), pneumonia (given in combination with a cephalosporin or penicillin), meningitis, complicated urinary tract infections, osteomyelitis, bacteremia, and peritonitis.

c. Neomycin is used for preoperative bowel sterilization; hepatic coma (as adjunctive therapy); and, in topical form, for skin and mucous membrane infections (e.g., burns).

4. Precautions and monitoring effects. Aminoglycosides can cause serious adverse effects. To prevent or minimize such problems, blood drug concentrations and blood urea nitrogen (BUN) and serum creatinine levels should be monitored during therapy.

a. Ototoxicity. Aminoglycosides can cause vestibular or auditory damage. Relative ototoxicity:

$$Streptomycin = kanamycin > amikacin = gentamicin = tobramycin > netilmicin$$

(1) Gentamicin and streptomycin cause primarily **vestibular** damage (manifested by tinnitus, vertigo, and ataxia). Such damage may be bilateral and irreversible.

(2) Amikacin, kanamycin, and neomycin cause mainly **auditory** damage (hearing loss).

(3) Tobramycin can result in both vestibular and auditory damage.

b. Nephrotoxicity. Because aminoglycosides accumulate in the proximal tubule, mild renal dysfunction develops in up to 25% of patients receiving these drugs for several days or more. Usually, this adverse effect is reversible.

(1) Neomycin is the most nephrotoxic aminoglycoside; streptomycin is the least nephrotoxic. Gentamicin and tobramycin are nephrotoxic to approximately the same degree.

(2) Risk factors for increased nephrotoxic effects include:

(a) Preexisting renal disease

(b) Previous or prolonged aminoglycoside therapy

(c) Concurrent administration of another nephrotoxic drug

(d) Impaired renal flow unrelated to renal disease (e.g., from hypotension, severe hepatic disease)

(3) Trough levels above 2 μg/mL for gentamicin and tobramycin and above 10 μg/mL for amikacin are associated with nephrotoxicity.

c. Neuromuscular blockade. This problem may arise in patients receiving high-dose aminoglycoside therapy.

(1) Risk factors for neuromuscular blockade include:

(a) Concurrent administration of a neuromuscular blocking agent or an anesthetic

(b) Preexisting hypocalcemia or myasthenia gravis

(c) Intraperitoneal or rapid IV drug administration

(2) Apnea and respiratory depression may be reversed with administration of calcium or an anticholinesterase.

d. Hypersensitivity and **local reactions** are rare adverse effects of aminoglycosides.

e. Therapeutic levels

(1) Gentamicin and tobramycin peak at 6–10 μg/mL for traditional dosing; when utilizing the once-daily administration (ODA) method, the gentamicin and tobramycin peak is 16–20 μg/mL or 8–10 times the MIC of targeted bacteria. Their trough level is 0.5–1.5 μg/mL for traditional or once-daily regimens.

(2) Amikacin peaks at 25–30 μg/mL. The trough level is 5–8 μg/mL.

5. **Significant interactions**
   a. **IV loop diuretics** can result in increased ototoxicity.
   b. **Other aminoglycosides, cephalothin, cisplatin, amphotericin B,** and **methoxyflurane** can cause increased nephrotoxicity when given concurrently with streptomycin.

C. **Carbapenems.** These agents are β-lactams that contain a fused β-lactam ring and a 5-membered ring system that differs from penicillins in being unsaturated and containing a carbon atom instead of a sulfur atom. The class has a broader spectrum of activity than do most β-lactams. Formerly known as thienamycin, **imipenem** was the first carbapenem compound introduced in the United States, followed by **meropenem** and most recently **ertapenem.** Because it is inhibited by renal dipeptidases, imipenem must be combined with **cilastatin** sodium, a dipeptidase inhibitor (cilastatin is not required with meropenem or ertapenem since these are not sensitive to renal dipeptidase).

1. **Mechanism of action.** Carbapenems are **bactericidal;** inhibit bacterial cell wall synthesis.

2. **Spectrum of activity.** These drugs have the broadest spectrum of all β-lactam antibiotics. The group is active against most gram-positive cocci (including many enterococci), gram-negative rods (including many *P. aeruginosa* strains), and anaerobes. This class has good activity against many bacterial strains that resist other antibiotics. These β-lactam antibiotics resist destruction by most β-lactamases.

3. **Therapeutic uses.** Carbapenems are most valued in the treatment of severe infections caused by drug-resistant organisms susceptible to these agents. These agents are effective against urinary tract and lower respiratory infections, intra-abdominal and gynecological infections, and skin, soft-tissue, bone, and joint infections.

4. **Precautions and monitoring effects**
   a. Carbapenems may cause nausea, vomiting, diarrhea, and pseudomembranous colitis.
   b. Seizures, dizziness, and hypotension may develop; seizures appear less frequently with meropenem or ertapenem (1.5% of patients receiving imipenem versus 0.5% of those receiving meropenem or ertapenem).
   c. Patients who are allergic to penicillin or cephalosporins may suffer cross-sensitivity reactions during carbapenem therapy.

D. **Cephalosporins.** These agents are known as **β-lactam antibiotics** because their chemical structure consists of a β-lactam ring adjoined to a thiazolidine ring. Cephalosporins generally are classified in four major groups based mainly on their spectrum of activity (Table 43-2).

1. **Mechanism of action.** Cephalosporins are **bactericidal;** they inhibit bacterial cell wall synthesis, reducing cell wall stability, thus causing membrane lysis.

2. **Spectrum of activity**
   a. **First-generation** cephalosporins are active against most gram-positive cocci (except enterococci) as well as enteric aerobic gram-negative bacilli (e.g., *E. coli, K. pneumoniae, Proteus mirabilis*).
   b. **Second-generation** cephalosporins are active against the organisms covered by first-generation cephalosporins and have extended gram-negative coverage, including β-lactamase–producing strains of *Haemophilus influenzae.*
   c. **Third-generation** cephalosporins have wider activity against most gram-negative bacteria, for example, *Enterobacter, Citrobacter, Serratia, Providencia, Neisseria,* and *Haemophilus* organisms, including β-lactamase–producing strains.
   d. **Fourth-generation** cephalosporins. Cefepime is the first member of this group to be marketed. Cefepime is highly resistant to β-lactamases and has a low propensity for selection of β-lactam–resistant mutant strains. It shows evidence of greater activity versus gram-positive cocci, *Enterobacteriacae,* and *Pseudomonas* than third-generation cephalosporins. Its clinical value continues to be defined.
   e. Each generation of cephalosporin has shifted toward increased gram-negative activity but has lost activity toward gram-positive organisms. Fourth-generation agents have improved activity toward gram-positive organisms over third-generation agents.

3. **Therapeutic uses**
   a. **First-generation** cephalosporins commonly are administered to treat serious *Klebsiella* infections and gram-positive and some gram-negative infections in patients with mild

Table 43-2. Classification of Cephalosporins

First-Generation	Second-Generation	Third-Generation	Fourth-Generation
Cefadroxil* (Duricef, Ultracef)	Cefaclor* (Ceclor)	Cefdinir (Omnicef)* Cefixeme (Suprax)*	Cefepime (Maxpime)
Cefazolin (Ancef, Kefzol)	Cefmetazole (Zefazone)	Cefoperazone (Cefobid)	
Cephalexin* (Keflex)	Cefonicid (Monocid)	Cefotaxime (Claforan)	
Cephapirin (Cefadyl)	Cefotetan (Cefotan)	Cefpodoxime proxetil* (Vantin)	
Cephradine* (Anspor, Velosef)	Cefoxitin (Mefoxin)	Ceftazidime (Fortax, Taxicef, Tazidime)	
	Cefuroxime (Zinacef)	Ceftibuten* (Cedax)	
	Cefuroxime axetil* (Ceftin)	Ceftizoxime (Cefizox)	
	Cefpodoxime* (Vantin)	Ceftriaxone (Rocephin)	
	Cefprozil* (Cefzil)	Cefditoren* (SpecTracef)	
	Loracarbef* (Lorabid)		

*Oral agents.

     penicillin allergy. These agents also are used widely in perioperative prophylaxis. For most other indications, they are not the preferred drugs.

  b. Second-generation cephalosporins are valuable in the treatment of urinary tract infections resulting from *E. coli* organisms and gonococcal disease caused by organisms that resist other agents.

    (1) Cefaclor is useful in otitis media and sinusitis in patients who are allergic to ampicillin and amoxicillin.

    (2) Cefoxitin is therapeutic for mixed aerobic–anaerobic infections, such as intra-abdominal infection. **Cefprozil, cefotetan, cefpodoxime,** and **loracarbef** are second-generation cephalosporins that can be administered twice daily but offer no important spectrum differences.

    (3) Cefuroxime commonly is administered for community-acquired pneumonia.

  c. Third-generation cephalosporins penetrate the cerebrospinal fluid (CSF) and, thus, are valuable in the treatment of meningitis caused by such organisms as meningococci, pneumococci, *H. influenzae,* and enteric gram-negative bacilli.

    (1) These agents also are used to treat sepsis of unknown origin in immunosuppressed patients and to treat fever in neutropenic immunosuppressed patients (given in combination with an aminoglycoside).

    (2) Third-generation cephalosporins are useful in infections caused by many organisms resistant to older cephalosporins.

    (3) These agents frequently are administered as empiric therapy for life-threatening infection in which resistant organisms are the most likely cause.

    (4) Initial therapy of mixed bacterial infections (e.g., sepsis) commonly involves third-generation cephalosporins.

  d. The **fourth-generation** agent, cefepime, is approved for treatment of urinary tract infections, uncomplicated skin and skin structure infections, pneumonia, and empiric use in febrile neutropenic patients. Cefepime has a spectrum of activity similar to third-generation agents, but is more resistant to some β-lactamases.

4. Precautions and monitoring effects

  a. Because all cephalosporins (except cefoperazone) are eliminated renally, doses must be adjusted for patients with renal impairment.

  b. Cross-sensitivity with penicillin has been reported in up to 10% of patients receiving cephalosporins. More recent information indicates that true cross-reactivity is rare.

    c. Cephalosporins can cause hypersensitivity reactions similar to those resulting from penicillin [see II E 1 e (1)]. Manifestations include fever, maculopapular rash, anaphylaxis, and hemolytic anemia.

    d. Other adverse effects include nausea, vomiting, diarrhea, superinfection, nephrotoxicity, and *Clostridium difficile*–induced colitis; with cefoperazone, cefmetazole, and cefotetan, (and formerly moxalactam and cefamandole), bleeding diatheses may occur. Bleeding can be reversed by vitamin K administration.

    e. Cephalosporins may cause false-positive glycosuria results on tests using the copper reduction method.

  5. Significant interactions

    a. Probenecid may impair the excretion of cephalosporins (except ceftazidime), causing increased cephalosporin levels and possible toxicity.

    b. Alcohol consumption may result in a disulfiram-type reaction in patients receiving cefmetazole, cefotetan, and cefoperazone.

    c. Aminoglycosides or loop diuretics may cause additive toxicity when administered with cephalothin.

    d. Plasma concentrations of cefaclor extended-release tablets, cefdinir, and cefpodoxime may be reduced by coadministration with **antacids.**

    e. H_2-antagonists may reduce plasma levels of cefpodoxime and cefuroxime.

    f. Iron supplements and **iron-fortified foods** reduce absorption of cefdinir by 80% and 30%, respectively.

E. Erythromycins. The chemical structure of these macrolide antibiotics is characterized by a lactone ring to which sugars are attached. Erythromycin base and the estolate, ethylsuccinate, and stearate salts are given orally; erythromycin lactobionate and gluceptate are given parenterally.

  1. Mechanism of action. Erythromycins may be **bactericidal** or **bacteriostatic;** they bind to the 50S ribosomal subunit, inhibiting bacterial protein synthesis.

  2. Spectrum of activity. Erythromycins are active against many gram-positive organisms, including streptococci (e.g., *Streptococcus pneumoniae*), and *Corynebacterium* and *Neisseria* species as well as some strains of *Mycoplasma, Legionella, Treponema,* and *Bordetella*. Some *S. aureus* strains that resist penicillin G are susceptible to erythromycins.

  3. Therapeutic uses

    a. Erythromycins are the preferred drugs for the treatment of *Mycoplasma pneumoniae* and *Campylobacter* infections, legionnaires' disease, chlamydial infections, diphtheria, and pertussis.

    b. In patients with penicillin allergy, erythromycins are important alternatives in the treatment of pneumococcal pneumonia, *S. aureus* infections, syphilis, and gonorrhea.

    c. Erythromycins may be given prophylactically before dental procedures to prevent bacterial endocarditis.

  4. Precautions and monitoring parameters

    a. Serious adverse effects from erythromycins are rare.

    b. Gastrointestinal (GI) distress (e.g., nausea, vomiting, diarrhea, epigastric discomfort) may occur with all erythromycin forms.

    c. Allergic reactions (rare) may present as skin eruptions, fever, and eosinophilia.

    d. Cholestatic hepatitis may arise in patients treated for 1 week or longer with erythromycin estolate; symptoms usually disappear within a few days after drug therapy ends. There have been infrequent reports of hepatotoxicity with other salts of erythromycin.

    e. IM injections of more than 100 mg produce severe pain persisting for hours.

    f. Transient hearing impairment may develop with high-dose erythromycin therapy.

  5. Significant interactions

    a. Erythromycin inhibits the hepatic metabolism of **theophylline,** resulting in toxic accumulation.

    b. Erythromycin interferes with the metabolism of **digoxin, corticosteroids, carbamazepine, cyclosporin,** and **lovastatin,** possibly potentiating the effect and toxicity of these drugs.

    c. Clarithromycin and erythromycin increase terfenadine and astemizole concentrations. Cardiac arrhythmia may result. Azithromycin and dirithromycin do not appear to interfere with terfenadine metabolism; however, if used concomitantly, patients should be closely monitored.

d. Clarithromycin may potentiate **oral anticoagulants** [monitor prothrombin time (PT)], increase **cyclosporine** levels with increased toxicity, and increase **digoxin** and **theophylline** levels.

e. Coadministration of clarithromycin and **cisapride** may increase risk of serious cardiac arrhythmias; coadministration is contraindicated.

f. Sudden deaths have been reported when clarithromycin was added to ongoing **pimozide** therapy; coadministration is contraindicated.

6. Alternatives to erythromycin

a. Clarithromycin, azithromycin, and **dirithromycin** are semisynthetic macrolide antibiotics. These expensive but well-tolerated alternatives to erythromycin are administered once daily.

(1) Clarithromycin

(a) Spectrum of activity. Clarithromycin is more active than erythromycin against staphylococci and streptococci. In addition to activity against other organisms covered by erythromycin, it is also active in vitro against MAI, *Toxoplasma gondii,* and *Cryptosporidium* species.

(b) Therapeutic uses. This agent is indicated for the prevention of *Mycobacterium avium* complex infection and is useful in otitis media, sinusitis, mycoplasmal pneumonia, and pharyngitis. Clarithromycin is also used with omeprazole or lansoprazole for *Helicobacter pylori* eradication.

(2) Azithromycin

(a) Spectrum of activity. Azithromycin is less active than erythromycin against gram-positive cocci but more active against *H. influenzae* and other gram-negative organisms. Azithromycin concentrates within cells, and tissue levels are higher than serum levels.

(b) Therapeutic uses. This agent is useful in nongonococcal urethritis caused by chlamydia, lower respiratory tract infections, *M. avium* complex infection and prophylaxis, pharyngitis, pelvic inflammatory disease, and legionnaires' disease. Azithromycin is also indicated for pediatric use.

(3) Dirithromycin is indicated for the treatment of acute exacerbations of chronic bronchitis, pharyngitis and tonsillitis caused by *Streptococcus pyogenes,* and uncomplicated skin and skin structure infections caused by *S. aureus.*

b. Troleandomycin is similar to erythromycin in most respects, but generally is less active against susceptible organisms.

F. Penicillins

1. Natural penicillins. As with cephalosporins and all other penicillins, natural penicillins are β-lactam antibiotics. Among the most important antibiotics, natural penicillins are the preferred drugs in the treatment of many infectious diseases.

a. Available agents

(1) Penicillin G sodium and potassium salts can be administered orally, intravenously, or intramuscularly.

(2) Penicillin V, a soluble drug form, is administered orally.

(3) Penicillin G procaine and **penicillin G benzathine** are repository drug forms. Administered intramuscularly, these insoluble salts allow slow drug absorption from the injection site and, thus, have a longer duration of action (12–24 hours).

b. Mechanism of action. Penicillins are **bactericidal;** they inhibit bacterial cell wall synthesis in a manner similar to that of the cephalosporins.

c. Spectrum of activity

(1) Natural penicillins are highly active against gram-positive cocci and against some gram-negative cocci.

(2) Penicillin G is 5–10 times more active than penicillin V against gram-negative organisms and some anaerobic organisms.

(3) Because natural penicillins are readily hydrolyzed by penicillinases (β-lactamases), they are ineffective against *S. aureus* and other organisms that resist penicillin.

d. Therapeutic uses

(1) Penicillin G is the preferred agent for all infections caused by *S. pneumoniae* organisms, including:

(a) Pneumonia

(b) Arthritis
(c) Meningitis
(d) Peritonitis
(e) Pericarditis
(f) Osteomyelitis
(g) Mastoiditis

(2) Penicillins G and V are highly effective against other streptococcal infections, such as pharyngitis, otitis media, sinusitis, and bacteremia.

(3) Penicillin G is the preferred agent in gonococcal infections, syphilis, anthrax, actinomycosis, gas gangrene, and *Listeria* infections.

(4) Administered when an oral penicillin is needed, penicillin V is most useful in skin, soft-tissue, and mild respiratory infections.

(5) Penicillin G procaine is effective against syphilis and uncomplicated gonorrhea.

(6) Used to treat syphilis infections outside the CNS, penicillin G benzathine also is effective against group Aβ-hemolytic streptococcal infections.

(7) Penicillins G and V may be used prophylactically to prevent streptococcal infection, rheumatic fever, and neonatal gonorrhea ophthalmia. Patients with valvular heart disease may receive these drugs preoperatively.

(8) There is emerging resistance to penicillin G by *S. pneumoniae* in some areas of the United States. The alternative therapy is vancomycin.

e. Precautions and monitoring effects
(1) **Hypersensitivity reactions.** These occur in up to 10% of patients receiving penicillin. Manifestations range from mild rash to anaphylaxis.
  (a) The rash may be urticarial, vesicular, bullous, scarlatiniform, or maculopapular. Rarely, thrombopenic purpura develops.
  (b) Anaphylaxis is a life-threatening reaction that most commonly occurs with parenteral administration. Signs and symptoms include severe hypotension, bronchoconstriction, nausea, vomiting, abdominal pain, and extreme weakness.
  (c) Other manifestations of hypersensitivity reactions include fever, eosinophilia, angioedema, and serum sickness.
  (d) Before penicillin therapy begins, the patient's history should be evaluated for reactions to penicillin. A positive history places the patient at heightened risk for a subsequent reaction. In most cases, such patients should receive a substitute antibiotic. (However, hypersensitivity reactions may occur even in patients with a negative history.)

(2) **Other adverse effects** of natural penicillins include GI distress (e.g., nausea, diarrhea), bone marrow suppression (e.g., impaired platelet aggregation, agranulocytosis), and superinfection. With high-dose therapy, seizures may occur, particularly in patients with renal impairment.

f. Significant interactions
(1) **Probenecid** increases blood levels of natural penicillins and may be given concurrently for this purpose.
(2) Antibiotic antagonism occurs when **erythromycins, tetracyclines,** or **chloramphenicol** is given within 1 hour of the administration of penicillin. The clinical significance of such antagonism is not clear.
(3) With penicillin G procaine and benzathine, precaution must be used in patients with a history of hypersensitivity reactions to penicillins because prolonged reactions may occur. Intravascular injection should be avoided. Procaine hypersensitivity is a contraindication to the use of procaine penicillin G.
(4) Parenteral products contain either potassium (1.7 mEq/million units) or sodium (2 mEq/million units).

2. **Penicillinase-resistant penicillins.** These penicillins are not hydrolyzed by staphylococcal penicillinases (β-lactamases). These agents include **methicillin, nafcillin,** and the **isoxazolyl penicillins—cloxacillin, dicloxacillin,** and **oxacillin.**
  a. Mechanism of action (see II E 1 b)
  b. Spectrum of activity. Because these penicillins resist penicillinases, they are active against staphylococci that produce these enzymes.
  c. Therapeutic uses
    (1) Penicillinase-resistant penicillins are used solely in staphylococcal infections resulting from organisms that resist natural penicillins.

(2) These agents are less potent than natural penicillins against organisms susceptible to natural penicillins and, thus, make poor substitutes in the treatment of infections caused by these organisms.

(3) Nafcillin is excreted by the liver and, thus, may be useful in treating staphylococcal infections in patients with renal impairment.

(4) Oxacillin, cloxacillin, and dicloxacillin are most valuable in long-term therapy of serious staphylococcal infections (e.g., endocarditis, osteomyelitis) and in the treatment of minor staphylococcal infections of the skin and soft tissues.

d. Precautions and monitoring effects

(1) As with all penicillins, the penicillinase-resistant group can cause hypersensitivity reactions [see II E 1 e (1)].

(2) Methicillin may cause nephrotoxicity and interstitial nephritis.

(3) Oxacillin may be hepatotoxic.

(4) Complete cross-resistance exists among the penicillinase-resistant penicillins.

e. Significant interactions. Probenecid increases blood levels of these penicillins and may be given concurrently for that purpose.

3. Aminopenicillins. This penicillin group includes the semisynthetic agents **ampicillin** and **amoxicillin** and their derivatives, **bacampicillin** and **cyclacillin.** Because of their wider antibacterial spectrum, these drugs are also known as **broad-spectrum penicillins.**

a. Mechanism of action (see II E 1 b)

b. Spectrum of activity. Aminopenicillins have a spectrum that is similar to but broader than that of the natural and penicillinase-resistant penicillins. Easily destroyed by staphylococcal penicillinases, aminopenicillins are ineffective against most staphylococcal organisms. Against most bacteria sensitive to penicillin G, aminopenicillins are slightly less effective than this agent.

c. Therapeutic uses. Aminopenicillins are used to treat gonococcal infections, upper respiratory infections, uncomplicated urinary tract infections, and otitis media caused by susceptible organisms.

(1) For infections resulting from penicillin-resistant organisms, **ampicillin** may be given in combination with sulbactam.

(2) Amoxicillin is less effective than ampicillin against shigellosis.

(3) Amoxicillin is more effective against *S. aureus, Klebsiella,* and *Bacteroides fragilis* infections when administered in combination with clavulanic acid (amoxicillin/potassium clavulanate) because clavulanic acid inactivates penicillinases.

d. Precautions and monitoring effects

(1) Hypersensitivity reactions may occur [see II E 1 e (1)].

(2) Diarrhea is most common with ampicillin.

(3) In addition to the urticarial hypersensitivity rash seen with all penicillins, ampicillin and amoxicillin frequently cause a generalized erythematous, maculopapular rash. (This occurs in 5%–10% of patients receiving ampicillin.)

e. Significant interactions (see II E 2 e)

4. Extended-spectrum penicillins. These agents have the widest antibacterial spectrum of all penicillins. Also called **antipseudomonal penicillins,** this group includes the **carboxypenicillins** (e.g., **carbenicillin, carbenicillin indanyl, ticarcillin**) and the **ureidopenicillins** (e.g., **mezlocillin, piperacillin**).

a. Mechanism of action (see II E 1 b)

b. Spectrum of activity. These drugs have a spectrum similar to that of the aminopenicillins but also are effective against *Klebsiella* and *Enterobacter* species, some *B. fragilis* organisms, and indole-positive *Proteus* and *Pseudomonas* organisms.

(1) Carbenicillin frequently is active against ampicillin-resistant *Proteus* strains and some other gram-negative organisms.

(2) Ticarcillin is two to four times as active as carbenicillin against *P. aeruginosa.* Combined with clavulanic acid, ticarcillin has enhanced activity against organisms that resist ticarcillin alone.

(3) Piperacillin is 10 times as active as carbenicillin against *Pseudomonas* organisms and is more active than carbenicillin against streptococcal organisms.

(4) Piperacillin and tazobactam. Tazobactam is a β-lactamase inhibitor that expands the spectrum of activity to include some organisms not sensitive to piperacillin alone (if resistance is due to β-lactamase production), including strains of staphylococci, *Haemophilus, Bacteroides,* and *Enterobacteriaceae.* Generally, tazobactam does not enhance activity versus *Pseudomonas.*

      (5) Mezlocillin and **piperacillin** are more active than carbenicillin against *Klebsiella* organisms.

  c. Therapeutic uses. Extended-spectrum penicillins are used mainly to treat serious infections caused by gram-negative organisms (e.g., sepsis; pneumonia; infections of the abdomen, bone, and soft tissues).

  d. Precautions and monitoring effects
    (1) Hypersensitivity reactions may occur [see II E 1 e (1)].
    (2) Carbenicillin and ticarcillin may cause hypokalemia.
    (3) The high sodium content of carbenicillin and ticarcillin may pose a danger to patients with heart failure (HF).
    (4) All inhibit platelet aggregation, which may result in bleeding.

  e. Significant interactions (see II E 2 e)

G. Sulfonamides. Derivatives of sulfanilamide, these agents were the first drugs to prevent and cure human bacterial infection successfully. Although their current usefulness is limited by the introduction of more effective antibiotics and the emergence of resistant bacterial strains, sulfonamides remain the drugs of choice for certain infections. The major sulfonamides are **sulfadiazine, sulfamethoxazole, sulfisoxazole, sulfacytine,** and **sulfamethizole.**

  1. Mechanism of action. Sulfonamides are **bacteriostatic;** they suppress bacterial growth by triggering a mechanism that blocks folic acid synthesis, thereby forcing bacteria to synthesize their own folic acid.

  2. Spectrum of activity. Sulfonamides are broad-spectrum agents with activity against many gram-positive organisms (e.g., *S. pyogenes, S. pneumoniae)* and certain gram-negative organisms (e.g., *H. influenzae, E. coli, P. mirabilis).* They also are effective against certain strains of *Chlamydia trachomatis, Nocardia, Actinomyces,* and *Bacillus anthracis.*

  3. Therapeutic uses
    a. Sulfonamides most often are used to treat urinary tract infections caused by *E. coli,* including acute and chronic cystitis, and chronic upper urinary tract infections.
    b. These agents have value in the treatment of nocardiosis, trachoma and inclusion conjunctivitis, and dermatitis herpetiformis.
    c. Sulfadiazine may be administered in combination with pyrimethamine to treat toxoplasmosis.
    d. Sulfamethoxazole may be given in combination with trimethoprim to treat such infections as *Pneumocystis carinii* pneumonia, *Shigella* enteritis, *Serratia* sepsis, urinary tract infections, respiratory infections, and gonococcal urethritis (see II J 7 c).
    e. Sulfisoxazole is sometimes used in combination with erythromycin ethylsuccinate to treat acute otitis media caused by *H. influenzae* organisms. For the initial treatment of uncomplicated urinary tract infections, sulfisoxazole may be given in combination with phenazopyridine for relief of symptoms of pain, burning, or urgency.
    f. Prophylactic sulfonamide therapy has been used successfully to prevent streptococcal infections and rheumatic fever recurrences.

  4. Precautions and monitoring effects
    a. Sulfonamides may cause blood dyscrasias (e.g., hemolytic anemia—particularly in patients with G6PD deficiency, aplastic anemia, thrombocytopenia, agranulocytosis, and eosinophilia).
    b. Hypersensitivity reactions to sulfonamides probably result from sensitization and most commonly involve the skin and mucous membranes. Manifestations include various types of skin rash, exfoliative dermatitis, and photosensitivity. Drug fever and serum sickness also may develop.
    c. Crystalluria and hematuria may occur, possibly leading to urinary tract obstruction. (Adequate fluid intake and urine alkalinization can prevent or minimize this risk.) Sulfonamides should be used cautiously in patients with renal impairment.
    d. Life-threatening hepatitis caused by drug toxicity or sensitization is a rare adverse effect. Signs and symptoms include headache, nausea, vomiting, and jaundice.
    e. Acquired immune deficiency syndrome (AIDS) patients have increased frequency of cutaneous hypersensitivity reactions to sulfamethoxazole.

  5. Significant interactions. Sulfonamides may potentiate the effects of **phenytoin, oral anticoagulants,** and **sulfonylureas.**

H. Tetracyclines. These broad-spectrum agents are effective against certain bacterial strains that resist other antibiotics. Nonetheless, they are the preferred drugs in only a few situations. The major tetracyclines include **demeclocycline, doxycycline, methacycline, minocycline,** and **chlortetracycline.**

1. **Mechanism of action.** Tetracyclines are **bacteriostatic;** they inhibit bacterial protein synthesis by binding to the 30S ribosomal subunit.

2. **Spectrum of activity.** Tetracyclines are active against gram-negative and gram-positive organisms, spirochetes, *Mycoplasma* and *Chlamydia* organisms, rickettsial species, and certain protozoa.
   a. ***Pseudomonas*** and *Proteus* organisms are now resistant to tetracyclines. Many coliform bacteria, pneumococci, staphylococci, streptococci, and *Shigella* strains are increasingly resistant.
   b. Cross-resistance within the tetracycline group is extensive.

3. **Therapeutic uses**
   a. Tetracyclines are the agents of choice in rickettsial (Rocky Mountain spotted fever), chlamydial, and mycoplasmal infections; amebiasis; and bacillary infections (e.g., cholera, brucellosis, tularemia, some *Salmonella* and *Shigella* infections).
   b. Tetracyclines are useful alternatives to penicillin in the treatment of anthrax, syphilis, gonorrhea, Lyme disease, nocardiosis, and *H. influenzae* respiratory infections.
   c. Oral or topical tetracycline may be administered as a treatment for acne.
   d. **Doxycycline** is highly effective in the prophylaxis of "traveler's diarrhea" (commonly caused by *E. coli*). Because the drug is excreted mainly in the feces, it is the safest tetracycline for the treatment of extrarenal infections in patients with renal impairment.
   e. **Demeclocycline** is used commonly as an adjunctive agent to treat the **syndrome of inappropriate antidiuretic hormone (SIADH)** secretion.

4. **Precautions and monitoring effects**
   a. GI distress (e.g., diarrhea, abdominal discomfort, nausea, anorexia) is a common adverse effect of tetracyclines. This problem can be minimized by administering the drug with food or temporarily decreasing the dosage.
   b. Skin rash, urticaria, and generalized exfoliative dermatitis signify a hypersensitivity reaction. Rarely, angioedema and anaphylaxis occur.
   c. Cross-sensitivity within the tetracycline group is common.
   d. Phototoxic reactions (severe skin lesions) can develop with exposure to sunlight. This reaction is most common with demeclocycline and doxycycline.
   e. Tetracyclines may cause hepatotoxicity, particularly in pregnant women. Manifestations include jaundice, acidosis, and fatty liver infiltration.
   f. Renally impaired patients may experience a significant increase in blood urea nitrogen (BUN) secondary to catabolic effects of tetracyclines.
   g. Tetracyclines may induce permanent tooth discoloration, tooth enamel defects, and retarded bone growth in infants and children.
   h. Use of outdated and degraded tetracyclines can lead to renal tubular dysfunction, possibly resulting in renal failure.
   i. Minocycline can cause vestibular toxicity (e.g., ataxia, dizziness, nausea, vomiting).
   j. IV tetracyclines are irritating and may cause phlebitis.

5. **Significant interactions**
   a. **Dairy products** and other foods, **iron preparations,** and **antacids** and **laxatives** containing aluminum, calcium, or magnesium can cause reduced tetracycline absorption. Absorption of doxycycline is not inhibited by these factors.
   b. **Methoxyflurane** may exacerbate the tetracyclines' nephrotoxic effects.
   c. **Barbiturates** and **phenytoin** decrease the antibiotic effectiveness of tetracyclines.
   d. Demeclocycline antagonizes the action of **antidiuretic hormone (ADH)** and may be given as a diuretic in patients with SIADH.

I. **Fluoroquinolones** are agents related to nalidixic acid [see II I 1 c, 2 c (1), 4 c (1)] and include **ciprofloxacin, enoxacin, lomefloxacin, norfloxacin, ofloxacin, sparfloxacin, gatifloxacin, moxifloxacin, grepafloxacin, levofloxacin,** and **trovafloxacin.** They are bactericidal for growing bacteria.

1. **Mechanism of action.** Fluoroquinolones inhibit DNAg

2. Spectrum of activity. Fluoroquinolones are highly active against enteric gram-negative bacilli, *Salmonella, Shigella, Campylobacter, Haemophilus,* and *Neisseria.*

    a. Ciprofloxacin has good activity against *P. aeruginosa,* but the fluoroquinolones as a group have variable activity against non–*P. aeruginosa.* Ciprofloxacin is active against many anaerobes; it has moderate activity against *M. tuberculosis.*

    b. Gram-positive organisms are less susceptible than gram-negative organisms but usually are sensitive, except for *Enterococcus faecalis* and methicillin-resistant staphylococci.

    c. Ofloxacin has the greatest activity against *Chlamydia.*

    d. Trovafloxacin has a broad spectrum including gram-positive and gram-negative anaerobes, *Chlamydia* species, and *M. pneumoniae.*

3. Therapeutic uses (Table 43-3)

    a. Norfloxacin is indicated for the oral treatment of urinary tract infections, uncomplicated gonococcal infections, and prostatitis.

    b. Ciprofloxacin, ofloxacin, levofloxacin, gatifloxacin, and trovafloxacin are available orally and intravenously. Ciprofloxacin is approved for use in urinary tract infections; lower respiratory infections; sinusitis; bone, joint, and skin structure infections; empiric use in febrile neutropenic patients; typhoid fever; urethral and cervical gonococcal infections; and infectious diarrhea. Ofloxacin is approved for use in lower respiratory infections, uncomplicated gonococcal and chlamydial cervicitis and urethritis, skin and skin structure infections, prostatitis, and urinary tract infections.

    c. Lomefloxacin, levofloxacin, gatifloxacin, trovafloxacin, and enoxacin are approved for the treatment of urinary tract infections. Lomefloxacin, sparfloxacin, gatifloxacin, moxifloxacin, grepafloxacin, levofloxacin, and trovafloxacin are also used in lower respiratory infections, and enoxacin and grepafloxacin are also used in uncomplicated gonococcal infections.

4. Precautions and monitoring effects

    a. Occasional adverse effects include nausea, dyspepsia, headache, dizziness, insomnia, cardiac QT prolongation, arthropathy, tendonitis, CNS effects, photosensitivity, and hypoglycemia.

    b. Infrequent adverse effects include rash, urticaria, leukopenia, and elevated liver enzymes.

Table 43-3. Quinolone Agents Classified by Generation

	Agent	Spectrum of Coverage	Site of Infection
First-generation	Cinoxacin (Cinoxacin, Cinobac) Enoxacin (Penetrex) Nalidixic acid (NegGram) Norfloxacin (Noroxin)	Gram negatives	Urinary tract
Second-generation	Lomefloxacin (Maxaquin)	Gram negatives Gram positives	Urinary tract
	Ciprofloxacin (Cipro) Ofloxacin (Floxin)	Gram negatives Gram positives	Systemic, urinary tract
Third-generation	Gatifloxacin (Tequin) Grepafloxacin (Raxar)* Levofloxacin (Levaquin) Moxifloxacin (Avelox) Sparfloxacin (Zagam)	Gram negatives Gram positives Atypicals	Systemic, urinary tract
Fourth-generation	Trovafloxacin (Trovan)	Gram negatives Gram positives Atypicals Anaerobes	Systemic, urinary tract

*Removed from the U.S. market in 1999.

    c. Crystalluria occurs with high doses at alkaline pH.

    d. Cartilage erosion has been observed in young animals; thus, fluoroquinolones should not be used in children or in women who are pregnant or nursing.

    e. Trovalloxacin has been associated with serious liver injury leading to liver transplantation and/or death. Liver injury has been reported with both short-term and long-term drug exposure. Trovafloxacin use longer than 2 weeks significantly increases risk. This agent should be reserved for serious life or limb-threatening infections.

5. Significant interactions

    a. Ciprofloxacin has been shown to increase **theophylline** levels. Variable effects on theophylline levels have been reported from other members of the group. In patients requiring fluoroquinolones, theophylline levels should be monitored.

    b. **Antacids** and **sucralfate** and divalent or trivalent cations such as iron may significantly decrease the absorption of fluoroquinolones.

    c. Fluoroquinolones may increase prothrombin times in patients receiving **warfarin.**

    d. Concurrent use with **nonsteroidal anti-inflammatory drugs** (NSAIDs) may increase the risk of CNS stimulation (seizures).

    e. Fluoroquinolones may produce prolonged QT interval when administered with **terfenadine, astemizole, cisapride,** and **antiarrhythmic agents.** Some fluoroquinolones (i.e., gatifloxacin, moxifloxacin) should be avoided in patients with known prolongation of the QTC interval, with uncorrected hopocalcemia, or who are receiving class IA or class III antiarrhythmic drugs.

    f. Some fluoroquinolones have been reported to enhance the effects of oral anticoagulants.

    g. Hyperglycemia and hypoglycemia have been reported in patients receiving quinolones and an antidiabetic agent. Blood glucose monitoring is recommended in such patients.

    h. Didanosine should be administered at least 4 hours after gatifloxacin.

J. Urinary tract antiseptics. Concentrating in the renal tubules and bladder, these agents exert local antibacterial effects; most do not achieve blood levels high enough to treat systemic infections. [However, some new quinolone derivatives, such as ciprofloxacin and ofloxacin, are valuable in the treatment of certain infections outside the urinary tract (see II H 3 b).]

1. Mechanism of action

    a. **Methenamine** is hydrolyzed to ammonia and formaldehyde in acidic urine; formaldehyde is antibacterial against gram-positive and gram-negative organisms. Mandelic and hippuric acids, with which methenamine is combined, provide supplementary antibacterial action.

    b. **Nitrofurantoin** is **bacteriostatic;** in high concentrations, it may be **bactericidal.** Presumably, it disrupts bacterial enzyme systems.

    c. **Quinolones. Nalidixic acid** and its analogues and derivatives—**oxolinic acid, norfloxacin, cinoxacin, ciprofloxacin,** and others—interfere with DNA gyrase and inhibit DNA synthesis during bacterial replication.

    d. **Fosfomycin tromethamine** is bactericidal in the urine at therapeutic doses. The bactericidal action is because of its inactivation of the enzyme enolpyruvyl transferase, thereby blocking the condensation of uridine diphosphate-N-acetylglucosamine with p-enolpyruvate, one of the first steps in bacterial cell wall synthesis.

2. Spectrum of activity

    a. **Methenamine** is active against both gram-positive and gram-negative organisms (e.g., *Enterobacter, Klebsiella, Proteus, P. aeruginosa, S. aureus*).

    b. **Nitrofurantoin** is active against many gram-positive and gram-negative organisms, including some strains of *E. coli, S. aureus, Proteus, Enterobacter,* and *Klebsiella.*

    c. **Quinolones** (see II H)

        (1) **Nalidixic acid** and **oxolinic acid** are active against most gram-negative organisms that cause urinary tract infections, including *P. mirabilis, E. coli, Klebsiella,* and *Enterobacter* organisms. These drugs are not effective against *Pseudomonas* organisms.

        (2) **Norfloxacin** is active against *E. coli, Enterobacter, Klebsiella, Proteus, P. aeruginosa, S. aureus, Citrobacter,* and some *Streptococcus* organisms.

        (3) **Cinoxacin** is active against *E. coli, Klebsiella, P. mirabilis, Proteus vulgaris, Proteus morganii, Serratia,* and *Citrobacter* organisms.

3. Therapeutic uses

    a. **Methenamine** and **nitrofurantoin** are used to prevent and treat urinary tract infections.

b. Quinolones are administered to treat urinary tract infections; some also are used in such diseases as osteomyelitis and respiratory tract infections.

c. Fosfomycin is indicated for treatment of uncomplicated urinary tract infection (acute cystitis) in women caused by susceptible strains of *E. coli* or *E. faecalis.*

4. Precautions and monitoring effects

a. Methenamine may cause nausea, vomiting, and diarrhea; in high doses, it may lead to urinary tract irritation (e.g., dysuria, frequency, hematuria, albuminuria). Skin rash also may develop.

b. Nitrofurantoin may cause various adverse effects.

(1) GI distress (e.g., nausea, vomiting, diarrhea) is relatively common.

(2) Hypersensitivity reactions to nitrofurantoin may involve the skin, lungs, blood, or liver; manifestations include fever, chills, hepatitis, jaundice, leukopenia, hemolytic anemia, granulocytopenia, and pneumonitis.

(3) Adverse CNS effects include headache, vertigo, and dizziness. Polyneuropathy may develop with high doses or in patients with renal impairment.

c. Quinolones

(1) **Nalidixic acid** and **oxolinic acid** may cause nausea, vomiting, abdominal pain, urticaria, pruritus, skin rash, fever, eosinophilia, and CNS effects, such as headache, dizziness, confusion, vertigo, drowsiness, and weakness.

(2) **Cinoxacin** may induce nausea, vomiting, diarrhea, headache, insomnia, skin rash, pruritus, and urticaria.

5. Significant interactions

a. The effects of methenamine are inhibited by **alkalinizing agents** and are antagonized by **acetazolamide.**

b. Nitrofurantoin absorption is decreased by **magnesium-containing antacids.** Nitrofurantoin blood levels are increased and urine levels decreased by **sulfinpyrazone** and **probenecid,** leading to increased toxicity and reduced therapeutic effectiveness.

c. Quinolones

(1) Cinoxacin urine levels are decreased by **probenecid,** reducing therapeutic effectiveness.

(2) Norfloxacin is rendered less effective by **antacids.**

K. Miscellaneous antibacterial agents

1. Aztreonam. This agent was the first commercially available monobactam (monocyclic β-lactam compound). It resembles the aminoglycosides in its efficacy against many gram-negative organisms but does not cause nephrotoxicity or ototoxicity. Other advantages of this drug include its ability to preserve the body's normal gram-positive and anaerobic flora, activity against many gentamicin-resistant organisms, and lack of cross-allergenicity with penicillin.

a. Mechanism of action. Aztreonam is **bactericidal;** it inhibits bacterial cell wall synthesis.

b. Spectrum of activity. This drug is active against many gram-negative organisms, including *Enterobacter* and *P. aeruginosa.*

c. Therapeutic uses. Aztreonam is therapeutic for urinary tract infections, septicemia, skin infections, lower respiratory tract infections, and intra-abdominal infections resulting from gram-negative organisms.

d. Precautions and monitoring effects

(1) Aztreonam sometimes causes nausea, vomiting, and diarrhea.

(2) Liver enzymes may increase transiently during aztreonam therapy.

(3) This drug may induce skin rash.

2. Chloramphenicol. A nitrobenzene derivative, this drug has broad activity against rickettsia as well as many gram-positive and gram-negative organisms. It also is effective against many ampicillin-resistant strains of *H. influenzae.*

a. Mechanism of action. Chloramphenicol is primarily **bacteriostatic,** although it may be bactericidal against a few bacterial strains.

b. Spectrum of activity. This agent is active against rickettsia and a wide range of bacteria, including *H. influenzae, Salmonella typhi, Neisseria meningitidis, Bordetella pertussis, Clostridium, B. fragilis, S. pyogenes,* and *S. pneumoniae.*

    c. Therapeutic uses. Because of its toxic side effects, chloramphenicol is used only to suppress infections that cannot be treated effectively with other antibiotics. Such infections typically include:

      (1) Typhoid fever

      (2) Meningococcal infections in cephalosporin-allergic patients

      (3) Serious *H. influenzae* infections, particularly in cephalosporin-allergic patients

      (4) Anaerobic infections (e.g., those originating in the pelvis or intestines)

      (5) Anaerobic or mixed infections of the CNS

      (6) Rickettsial infections in pregnant patients, tetracycline-allergic patients, and renally impaired patients

    d. Precautions and monitoring effects

      (1) Chloramphenicol can cause bone marrow suppression (dose-related) with resulting pancytopenia; rarely, the drug leads to aplastic anemia (non–dose-related).

      (2) Hypersensitivity reactions may include skin rash and, in extremely rare cases, angioedema or anaphylaxis.

      (3) Chloramphenicol therapy may lead to gray baby syndrome in neonates (especially premature infants). This dangerous reaction, which stems partly from inadequate liver detoxification of the drug, is manifested by vomiting, gray cyanosis, rapid and irregular respirations, vasomotor collapse, and, in some cases, death.

    e. Significant interactions

      (1) Chloramphenicol inhibits the metabolism of **phenytoin, tolbutamide, chlorpropamide,** and **dicumarol,** leading to prolonged action and intensified effect of these drugs.

      (2) Phenobarbital shortens chloramphenicol's half-life, thereby reducing its therapeutic effectiveness.

      (3) Penicillins can cause antibiotic antagonism.

      (4) Acetaminophen elevates chloramphenicol levels and may cause toxicity.

3. Clindamycin. This agent has essentially replaced lincomycin, the drug from which it is derived. It is used to treat skin, respiratory tract, and soft-tissue infections caused by staphylococci, pneumococci, and streptococci.

    a. Mechanism of action. Clindamycin is **bacteriostatic;** it binds to the 50S ribosomal subunit, thereby suppressing bacterial protein synthesis.

    b. Spectrum of activity. This agent is active against most gram-positive and many anaerobic organisms, including *B. fragilis.*

    c. Therapeutic uses. Because of its marked toxicity, clindamycin is used only against infections for which it has proven to be the most effective drug. Typically, such infections include abdominal and female genitourinary tract infections caused by *B. fragilis.*

    d. Precautions and monitoring effects

      (1) Clindamycin may cause rash, nausea, vomiting, diarrhea, and pseudomembranous colitis as evidenced by fever, abdominal pain, and bloody stools.

      (2) Blood dyscrasias (e.g., eosinophilia, thrombocytopenia, leukopenia) may occur.

    e. Significant interactions. Clindamycin may potentiate the effects of **neuromuscular blocking agents.**

4. Dapsone. A member of the sulfone class, this drug is the primary agent in the treatment of all forms of leprosy.

    a. Mechanism of action. Dapsone is **bacteriostatic** for *Mycobacterium leprae;* its mechanism of action probably resembles that of the sulfonamides.

    b. Spectrum of activity. This drug is active against *M. leprae;* however, drug resistance develops in up to 40% of patients. Dapsone also has some activity against *P. carinii* organisms and the malarial parasite *Plasmodium.*

    c. Therapeutic uses

      (1) Dapsone is the drug of choice for treating leprosy.

      (2) This agent may be used to treat dermatitis herpetiformis, a skin disorder.

      (3) Maloprim, a dapsone–pyrimethamine product, is valuable in the prophylaxis and treatment of malaria.

      (4) Dapsone, with or without trimethoprim, is used for prophylaxis of *P. carinii* pneumonia in patients with AIDS.

    d. Precautions and monitoring effects

      (1) Hemolytic anemia can occur with daily doses above 200 mg. Other adverse hematological effects include methemoglobinemia and leukopenia.

(2) Nausea, vomiting, and anorexia may develop.

(3) Adverse CNS effects include headache, dizziness, nervousness, lethargy, paresthesias, and psychosis.

(4) Dapsone occasionally results in a potentially lethal mononucleosis-like syndrome.

(5) Paradoxically, this drug sometimes exacerbates leprosy.

(6) Other adverse effects include skin rash, peripheral neuropathy, blurred vision, tinnitus, hepatitis, and cholestatic jaundice.

e. Significant interactions. Probenecid elevates blood levels of dapsone, possibly resulting in toxicity.

5. Linezolid is a synthetic oxazolidinone that has clinical utility in the treatment of infections caused by aerobic gram-positive bacteria.

a. Mechanism of action. Linezolid is bacteriostatic against *Enterococci* and *Staphylococci,* and bactericidal against *Streptococci.* Linezolid binds to the 23S ribosomal RNA of the 50S subunit and thus inhibits protein synthesis.

b. Spectrum of activity. The drug is active against vancomycin-resistant *Enterococcus faecium* and *S. aureus* (methicillin-susceptible and -resistant strains) as well as other aerobic gram-positive bacteria.

c. Therapeutic uses. Linezolid is indicated for treatment of infections caused by vancomycin-resistant *E. faecium,* nosocomial pneumonia caused by methicillin-susceptible and -resistant strains of *S. aureus,* community-acquired pneumonia caused by penicillin-susceptible strains of *S. pneumoniae,* and skin and skin structure infections due to these organisms.

d. Precautions and monitoring effects

(1) Safety data are limited. Adverse effects generally are minor (e.g., gastrointestinal complaints, headache, rash).

(2) Thrombocytopenia or a significant reduction in platelet count has been reported (2.4%) and is related to duration of therapy. Monitor platelets in patients with risk of bleeding, preexisting thrombocytopenia, platelet disorders (including those caused by concurrent medications) and in patients receiving linezolid lasting longer than 2 weeks.

e. Significant interactions. Patients receiving concomitant therapy with adrenergic or serotonergic agents or consuming more than 100 mg of tyramine a day may experience an enhancement of the drug's effect.

6. Spectinomycin. An aminocyclitol agent related to the aminoglycosides, this antibiotic is useful against penicillin-resistant strains of gonorrhea.

a. Mechanism of action. Spectinomycin is **bacteriostatic;** it selectively inhibits protein synthesis by binding to the 30S ribosomal subunit.

b. Spectrum of activity. This agent is active against various gram-negative organisms.

c. Therapeutic uses. Spectinomycin is used only to treat gonococcal infections in patients with penicillin allergy or when such infection stems from penicillinase-producing gonococci (PPNG).

d. Precautions and monitoring effects. Because spectinomycin is given only as a single-dose IM injection, it causes few adverse effects. Nausea, vomiting, urticaria, chills, dizziness, and insomnia occur rarely.

7. Trimethoprim. A substituted pyrimidine, trimethoprim is most commonly combined with sulfamethoxazole (a sulfonamide discussed in II F) in a preparation called co-trimoxazole. However, it may be used alone for certain urinary tract infections.

a. Mechanism of action. Trimethoprim inhibits dihydrofolate reductase, thus blocking bacterial synthesis of folic acid.

b. Spectrum of activity

(1) Trimethoprim is active against most gram-negative and gram-positive organisms. However, drug resistance may develop when this drug is used alone.

(2) Trimethoprim–sulfamethoxazole is active against a variety of organisms, including *S. pneumoniae, N. meningitidis,* and *Corynebacterium diphtheriae;* some strains of *S. aureus, Staphylococcus epidermidis, P. mirabilis, Enterobacter, Salmonella, Shigella, Serratia,* and *Klebsiella* species; and *E. coli.*

(3) The trimethoprim–sulfamethoxazole combination is synergistic; many organisms resistant to one component are susceptible to the combination.

c. Therapeutic uses

(1) Trimethoprim may be used alone or in combination with sulfamethoxazole to treat uncomplicated urinary tract infections caused by *E. coli, P. mirabilis,* and *Klebsiella* and *Enterobacter* organisms.

(2) Trimethoprim–sulfamethoxazole is therapeutic for acute gonococcal urethritis, acute exacerbation of chronic bronchitis, shigellosis, and *Salmonella* infections.

(3) Trimethoprim–sulfamethoxazole may be given as prophylactic or suppressive therapy in *P. carinii* pneumonia.

d. Precautions and monitoring effects

(1) Most adverse effects involve the skin (possibly from sensitization). These include rash, pruritus, and exfoliative dermatitis.

(2) Rarely, trimethoprim–sulfamethoxazole causes blood dyscrasias (e.g., acute hemolytic anemia, leukopenia, thrombocytopenia, methemoglobinemia, agranulocytosis, aplastic anemia).

(3) Adverse GI effects including nausea, vomiting, and epigastric distress glossitis may occur.

(4) Neonates may develop kernicterus.

(5) Patients with AIDS sometimes suffer fever, rash, malaise, and pancytopenia during trimethoprim therapy.

8. Vancomycin. This glycopeptide destroys most gram-positive organisms.

a. Mechanism of action. Vancomycin is **bactericidal;** it inhibits bacterial cell wall synthesis.

b. Spectrum of activity. This drug is active against most gram-positive organisms, including methicillin-resistant strains of *S. aureus*.

c. Therapeutic uses. Vancomycin usually is reserved for serious infections, especially those caused by methicillin-resistant staphylococci. It is particularly useful in patients who are allergic to penicillin or cephalosporins. Typical uses include endocarditis, osteomyelitis, and staphylococcal pneumonia.

(1) Oral vancomycin is valuable in the treatment of antibiotic-induced pseudomembranous colitis caused by *C. difficile* or *S. aureus* enterocolitis. Because vancomycin is not absorbed after oral administration, it is not useful for systemic infections. Because of resistance, the Centers for Disease Control and Prevention recommend vancomycin as the second choice to metronidazole for *C. difficile* infections.

(2) Because 1 g provides adequate blood levels for 7–10 days, IV vancomycin is particularly useful in the treatment of anephric patients with gram-positive bacterial infections.

d. Precautions and monitoring effects

(1) Ototoxicity may arise; nephrotoxicity is rare but can occur with high doses.

(2) Vancomycin may cause hypersensitivity reactions, manifested by such symptoms as anaphylaxis or skin rash.

(3) Therapeutic levels peak at 20–40 μg/mL. The trough is less than 15 μg/mL.

(4) "Red man's syndrome" may occur. This is facial flushing and hypotension due to too rapid infusion of the drug. Infusion should be over a minimum of 60 minutes for a 1 g dose.

(5) IV solutions are very irritating to the vein.

e. Vancomycin-resistant enterococci. A few strains of vancomycin-resistant enterococci are susceptible to teicoplanin (investigational by Hoechst Marion Roussel), linezolid (Zyvox), or quinupristin/dalfopristin (Synercid). These agents may be useful for multiple-drug–resistant *E. faecium*.

9. Clofazimine is phenazine dye with antimycobacterial and anti-inflammatory activity.

a. Mechanism of action. Clofazimine appears to bind preferentially to mycobacterial DNA, inhibiting replication and growth. It is **bactericidal** against *M. leprae,* and it appears to be **bacteriostatic** against *M. avium-intracellulare.*

b. Spectrum of activity. Clofazimine is active against various mycobacteria, including *M. leprae, M. tuberculosis,* and *M. avium-intracellulare.*

c. Therapeutic uses. Clofazimine is used to treat leprosy and a variety of atypical *Mycobacterium* infections.

d. Precautions and monitoring effects

(1) Pigmentation (pink to brownish) occurs in 75%–100% of patients within a few weeks. This skin discoloration has led to severe depression (and suicide).

(2) Urine, sweat, and other body fluids may be discolored.

(3) Other effects include ichthyosis and dryness of skin (8%–28%), rash and pruritus (1%–5%), and GI intolerance (e.g., abdominal/epigastric pain, diarrhea, nausea, vomiting) in 40%–50% of patients. Clofazimine should be taken with food.

10. Quinupristin/dalfopristin (Synercid) is an intravenous streptogramin antibiotic composed of two chemically distinct compounds.

  a. Mechanism of action. Quinupristin binds to the 50S subunit, and dalfopristin binds tightly to the 70S ribosomal particle.

  b. Spectrum of activity. Synercid has activity against *Staphylococci* species, including resistant strains. This combination has better activity against *E. faecium* than *Enterococcus faecalis* and is also active against some gram-negative organisms and anaerobes; activity has not been shown against *Enterobacteriaceae.*

  c. Therapeutic uses. It is used for treatment of vancomycin-resistant *E. faecium* (VREF) bacteremia and skin and skin structure infections caused by *S. aureus* and *S. pyogenes.*

  d. Precautions and monitoring effects

   (1) Reported side effects are generally mild and infusion related: pain, erythema, or itching at the infusion site; increases in pulse and diastolic pressure; headache; nausea or vomiting; and diarrhea. It may increase liver function tests slightly.

   (2) Drug interactions are a result of CYP3A4 inhibition. Potential drug interactions include **cyclosporin, nifedipine, midazolam, and terfenadine.**

   (3) Concomitant use of medications that may prolong QTc interval should be avoided.

   (4) Mild to life-threatening pseudomembranous colitis has been reported.

III. SYSTEMIC ANTIFUNGAL AGENTS

A. Definition. These agents treat systemic and local fungal (mycotic) infections—diseases that resist treatment with antibacterial drugs.

B. Amphotericin B. This polyene antifungal antibiotic is therapeutic for various fungal infections that frequently proved fatal before the drug became available. It is used increasingly in the empiric treatment of severely immunocompromised patients in certain clinical situations.

  1. Mechanism of action. Amphotericin B is both **fungistatic** in clinically obtained concentrations and may be fungicidal in the presence of very susceptible organisms. It binds to sterols in the fungal cell membrane, thereby increasing membrane permeability and permitting leakage of intracellular contents. Other mechanisms may be involved as well.

  2. Spectrum of activity. Amphotericin B is a broad-spectrum antifungal agent with activity against *Aspergillus, Blastomyces, Candida* species (*albicans, krusei tropicalis,* and *glabrata*), *Cryptococcus, Coccidioides, Histoplasma, Paracoccidioides, Phycomycetes* (*mucor*), and *Sporothrix.* It is also useful against some protozoa such as *Leishmania, Naegleria,* and *Acanthamoeba.*

  3. Therapeutic uses. Amphotericin B is the most effective antifungal agent in the treatment of systemic fungal infections, especially in immunocompromised patients.

   a. It is the treatment of choice for pulmonary *Aspergillus* infections; *Blastomyces* infections, which are life-threatening with AIDS or CNS involvement; deep-organ infections with *Candida; Coccidioides* infections with severe pulmonary involvement or with disseminated nonmeningeal immunocompetent or immunocompromised patients; all *Cryptococcus* infections; disseminated *Histoplasma* infections involving CNS or immunosuppressed patients; *Malassezia furfur* fungemia; pulmonary and extrapulmonary *Phycomycetes* (mucormycosis); *Penicillium marneffi;* and extracutaneous *Sporothrix.*

   b. This agent may be used to treat coccidioidal arthritis.

   c. Topical preparations are given to eradicate cutaneous and mucocutaneous candidiasis.

   d. It may be used as empiric therapy in febrile, neutropenic patients.

   e. It is used as secondary prophylaxis of fungal infections in patients with human immunodeficiency virus (HIV), guarding against recurrence of infection.

   f. It may be used prophylactically in neutropenic cancer patients, and bone marrow transplant or solid-organ transplant patients to reduce the incidence of *Aspergillus* and candida infections.

4. **Precautions and monitoring effects.** Because amphotericin B can cause many serious adverse effects, it should be administered in a hospital setting—at least during the initial therapeutic stage. The adverse effects are divided into infusion reactions and others.

    a. Infusion reactions occur while the drug is being administered and include fever, shaking chills, hypotension, anorexia, nausea, vomiting, headache, dyspnea, and tachypnea. Premedication with acetaminophen and diphenhydramine has been helpful in prophylaxing against infusion reactions. In addition, hydrocortisone 10–50 mg may be added to the infusion as prophylaxis against infusion-related reactions. Meperidine 25–50 mg IV is effective treatment of active shaking chills/rigors. Meperidine is also effective in prophylaxis of rigors.

    b. Nephrotoxicity frequently occurs. Dosage adjustment or drug discontinuation or changing to a liposomal amphotericin B product may be necessary as renal impairment progresses.

    c. Electrolyte abnormalities, including hypokalemia, hypomagnesemia, and hypocalcemia, are common. Monitor and replace electrolytes as needed.

    d. Normocytic, normochromic anemia will develop over long-term use (10 weeks). Monitor hematocrit periodically.

    e. Bronchospasm, wheezing, and anaphylaxis or anaphylactoid reactions have occurred. A test dose of 1 mg of amphotericin B is often administered prior to infusion of large quantities of the drug.

    f. Phlebitis or thrombophlebitis is reported with conventional amphotericin B. Heparin (500–1000 units) can be added to the infusion to aid in prevention.

    g. CNS effects include headache, peripheral neuropathy, malaise, depression, seizure, myasthenia, and hallucinations.

    h. Elevated liver transaminases, aspartate aminotransferase, alanine aminotransferase (AST), alkaline phosphatase (ALT), bilirubin, gamma glutamyl transferase (GGT), and lactate dehydrogenase (LDH) may occur.

    i. Amphotericin B parenteral use should only be mixed in dextrose 5% in water (D5W) and should be protected from light.

5. **Significant interactions.** Other nephrotoxic drugs (aminoglycosides, capreomycin, colistin, cisplatin, cyclosporine, methoxyflurane, pentamidine, polymyxin B, and vancomycin) may cause additive nephrotoxicity.

6. Amphotericin B lipid complex (Abelcet), amphoterecin B cholesterol sulfate complex (Amphotec), and liposomal amphotericin B (Ambisome) offer alternative formulations of amphotericin B for the treatment of severe fungal infections in patients who are intolerant of or whose disease is refractory to conventional treatment.

C. Caspofungin. This echinocandin systemic antifungal agent is used in patients with refractory aspergillosis and candida esophagitis.

1. **Mechanism of action.** Caspofungin works by causing fungal cell wall lysis. By being a noncompetitive inhibitor of beta (1,3) synthase, which is an essential component of fungal cell wall synthesis, it causes osmotic instability within the fungus and fungal cell wall lysis.

2. **Spectrum of activity.** Good in vitro activity has been demonstrated with caspofungin against *Aspergillus* spp., *Candida* spp. and *Histoplasma* spp. Caspofungin has also been shown to be effective against *Candida* spp. resistant to azoles and amphotericin B.

3. **Therapeutic uses.** Caspofungin may be used as an alternative to amphotericin B when treating patients with *Aspergillus*. It also plays a role in treating patients with resistant *Aspergillus* infections.

    a. Caspofungin is effective in treating patients with aspergillosis, particularly when using a prolonged course of therapy (approximately 1 month) with resistant strains of *Aspergillus*. Caspofungin may be used alone or in combination with itraconazole for this indication.

    b. More published data are necessary; however, good preliminary data exist for the use of caspofungin in treating *Candida* esophagitis. The duration of therapy is less with this disease (approximately 14 days).

4. **Precautions and monitoring effects.** Although this drug has adverse events associated with its use, the overall toxicity profile is significantly better than that of amphotericin B. The side effects may appear similar between the two drugs; however, these occur much more frequently with amphotericin B.

a. Infusion-vein complications (not defined by manufacturer) and thrombophlebitis has been seen upon infusion of caspofungin.

b. Hematological decreases in hemoglobin and hematocrit may occur; however, the incidence does not differ from that of having a fungal disease.

c. Headache may occur.

d. Slight decreases in serum potassium may occur, but nowhere near the magnitude of that caused by amphotericin B.

e. Anorexia, nausea, vomiting, and diarrhea have occurred.

f. Rare increases in serum creatinine; however, there have been no reported cases of nephrotoxicity.

g. Possible slight increases in serum aminotransferases

h. Allergic reactions occur in <5% of patients and anaphylaxis in <2% of patients.

i. Pregnancy category C embryotoxic reactions have occurred in animals.

5. Significant interactions

   a. When cyclosporine is combined with caspofungin, clinically significant rises in ALT were observed. Serum transaminases should be monitored, and this combination should be avoided in patients with preexisting liver disease.

   b. When used in combination, carbamazepine, nelfinavir, nevirapine, phenytoin, and rifampin increases the clearance of caspofungin. Higher doses of caspofungin (70 mg qd) should be considered when this combination is administered.

   c. Tacrolimus clearance will be increased when the combination is used; monitor tacrolimus serum levels closely.

D. Flucytosine. This fluorinated pyrimidine usually is given in combination with amphotericin B.

   1. Mechanism of action. Flucytosine penetrates fungal cells and is converted to fluorouracil, a metabolic antagonist. Incorporated into the RNA of the fungal cell, flucytosine causes defective protein synthesis. It is either **fungistatic** or **fungicidal,** depending on the concentration of the drug.

   2. Spectrum of activity. This drug is primarily active against *Cryptococcus* and *Candida.* It is most commonly used in conjunction with amphotericin B. Fungal resistance against flucytosine alone has been well documented. Flucytosine may also possess some activity against chromomycosis and some strains of *Aspergillus* (in vitro testing only).

   3. Therapeutic uses. Flucytosine is adjunctively used with amphotericin B for severe systemic infections (e.g., septicemia, endocarditis, pulmonary and urinary tract infections, meningitis). Use of flucytosine alone is not recommended.

   4. Precautions and monitoring effects
      a. Frequent adverse effects include GI intolerance with nausea, vomiting, and diarrhea.
      b. Occasional adverse reactions are more severe and include marrow suppression with leukopenia or thrombocytopenia (dose-related, especially with renal failure or concurrent amphotericin B use). Confusion, rash, hepatitis, enterocolitis, headache, and photosensitivity reactions can also occur.
      c. Rare reactions include hallucinations, blood dyscrasias with agranulocytosis and pancytopenia, fatal hepatitis, anaphylaxis, and anemia.
      d. Flucytosine may cause a markedly false elevation of serum creatinine if an Ektachem analyzer is used.

   5. Significant interactions. Beneficial drug interactions occur with flucytosine. Flucytosine has demonstrated synergy with **amphotericin B** and **fluconazole** against *Cryptococcus* and *Candida* species.

E. Griseofulvin. Produced from *Penicillium griseofulvum dierckx,* this drug is deposited in the skin, bound to keratin.

   1. Mechanism of action. This agent is **fungistatic;** it inhibits fungal cell activity by interfering with mitotic spindle structure. Its mechanism of action is similar to colchicine.

   2. Spectrum of activity. Griseofulvin is active against various strains of *Microsporum, Epidermophyton,* and *Trichophyton.*

848 *Chapter 43 III E*

3. **Therapeutic uses.** Griseofulvin is effective in tinea infections of the skin, hair, and nails (including athlete's foot, jock itch, and ringworm) caused by *Microsporum, Epidermophyton,* and *Trichophyton.*
   a. Generally, this agent is given only for infections that do not respond to topical antifungal agents.
   b. Griseofulvin is available only in oral form.
   c. It possesses vasodilatory activity and may be used in Raynaud's disease.
   d. It may also be used to treat gout.

4. **Precautions and monitoring effects**
   a. Griseofulvin rarely results in serious adverse effects. However, the following problems have been reported.
      (1) Common: headache, fatigue, confusion, impaired performance, syncope, and lethargy, which generally resolve with continued use
      (2) Occasional: leukopenia, neutropenia, and granulocytopenia
      (3) Rare: serum sickness, angioedema, urticaria, erythema, and hepatotoxicity
   b. The dosage is dependent on the particle size of the product: 250 mg of ultramicrosize is equivalent in therapeutic effects to 500 mg of microsize.

5. **Significant interactions**
   a. Griseofulvin may increase the metabolism of **warfarin,** leading to decreased prothrombin time.
   b. **Barbiturates** may reduce griseofulvin absorption.
   c. **Alcohol consumption** may cause tachycardia and flushing.
   d. **Oral contraceptives** may cause amenorrhea or increased breakthrough bleeding.

F. **Imidazoles.** The substituted imidazole derivatives **ketoconazole, miconazole, fluconazole,** and **itraconazole** are valuable in the treatment of a wide range of systemic fungal infections.

1. **Mechanism of action.** Imidazoles inhibit sterol synthesis in fungal cell membranes and increase cell wall permeability; this, in turn, makes the cell more vulnerable to osmotic pressure. These agents are **fungistatic.**

2. **Spectrum of activity.** These agents are active against many fungi, including yeasts, dermatophytes, actinomycetes, and some *Phycomycetes.*

3. **Therapeutic uses**
   a. **Ketoconazole,** an oral agent, successfully treats many fungal infections that previously yielded only to parenteral agents.
      (1) It is therapeutic for systemic and vaginal candidiasis, mucocandidiasis, candiduria, oral thrush, histoplasmosis, coccidioidomycosis, chromomycosis, dermatophytosis (tinea), and paracoccidioidomycosis.
      (2) Because ketoconazole is slow-acting and requires a long duration of therapy (up to 6 months for some chronic infections), it is less effective than other antifungal agents for the treatment of severe and acute systemic infections.
   b. **Miconazole,** primarily administered as a topical agent, also is available in parenteral form.
      (1) Topical miconazole is highly effective in vulvovaginal candidiasis, ringworm, and other skin infections.
      (2) Parenteral miconazole serves as a second-line agent in severe systemic fungal infections only when other antifungal drugs are ineffective or cannot be tolerated.
   c. **Fluconazole.** Available in oral and parenteral forms, fluconazole can be used against systemic and CNS infections involving *Cryptococcus* and *Candida. Candida* oropharyngeal infection and esophagitis may also be treated with fluconazole. *Aspergillus, Coccidioides,* and *Histoplasma* have demonstrated in vitro sensitivity.
   d. **Itraconazole** is available as an oral agent with activity against systemic and invasive pulmonary aspergillosis without the hematological toxicity of amphotericin B. Other deep mycotic infections susceptible to itraconazole include blastomycosis, coccidioidomycosis, cryptococcosis, and histoplasmosis.
   e. **Voriconazole.** Voriconazole is available as both an intravenous and oral agent for the treatment of fungal infections involving invasive aspergillosis, *Scedosporium apiospermum,* and *Fusarium* spp., including those species that are refractory to other therapy.

4. Precautions and monitoring effects

   a. **Ketoconazole** may cause nausea, vomiting, diarrhea, abdominal pain, and constipation. Rarely, it leads to headache, dizziness, gynecomastia, and fatal hepatotoxicity.

   b. **Parenteral miconazole therapy** frequently induces nausea, vomiting, diarrhea, phlebitis, pruritic rash, anaphylactoid reaction, CNS toxicity, and hyponatremia. Dose-related anemia and thrombocytosis may also occur.

   c. **Fluconazole** commonly causes GI disturbances (e.g., nausea, vomiting, epigastric pain, diarrhea). Reversible elevations in serum aminotransferase, exfoliative skin reactions, and headaches have been reported.

   d. **Itraconazole** may cause nausea, vomiting, hypertriglyceridemia, hypokalemia, rash, and elevations in liver enzymes.

   e. **Voriconazole.** Visual disturbances, fever, rash, vomiting, nausea, diarrhea, headache, sepsis, peripheral edema, abdominal pain, and respiratory disorders rarely occurred. Liver function test abnormalities have occurred.

5. Significant interactions

   a. Both **ketoconazole** and **miconazole** may enhance the anticoagulant effect of **warfarin.**

   b. **Ketoconazole** may antagonize the antibiotic effects of **amphotericin B.**

   c. **Fluconazole** has been shown to elevate serum levels of **phenytoin, cyclosporine, warfarin,** and **sulfonylureas.** Concurrent hepatic enzyme inducers, such as **rifampin,** have resulted in increased elimination of both fluconazole and itraconazole.

   d. Coadministration of **itraconazole** or **ketoconazole** with **astemizole** or **terfenadine** may result in increased astemizole or terfenadine levels, possibly leading to life-threatening dysrhythmias and death.

   e. Both **ketoconazole** and **itraconazole** need the presence of stomach acid for adequate absorption. Use with antacids, H_2-blockers, or proton pump inhibitors is contraindicated.

   f. Concomitant use of imidazole antifungal agents with **cisapride** may result in increased concentrations of cisapride, which has been associated with adverse cardiac events such as torsades de pointes leading to sudden death.

   g. **Voriconazole.** Cytochrome P4502C19 is the major enzyme involved in metabolism. Voriconazole inhibits cytochrome P4502C19, CYP2C9, and CYP3A4. Any medication that is metabolized via these routes may be affected, and monitoring of blood levels (if appropriate) or clinical signs and symptoms is necessary when taking concomitant medications.

G. Nystatin. A polyene antibiotic, nystatin has a chemical structure similar to that of amphotericin B.

1. Mechanism of action. Nystatin is **fungicidal** and **fungistatic;** binding to sterols in the fungal cell membrane, it increases membrane permeability and permits leakage of intracellular contents.

2. Spectrum of activity. Nystatin is active primarily against *Candida* species.

3. Therapeutic uses

   a. This drug is used primarily as a topical agent in vaginal and oral *Candida* infections.

   b. Oral nystatin is therapeutic for *Candida* infections of the GI tract, especially oral and esophageal infections; because the drug is not readily absorbed, it maintains good local activity.

4. Precautions and monitoring effects. Oral nystatin occasionally causes GI distress (e.g., nausea, vomiting, diarrhea). Rarely, hypersensitivity reactions occur.

H. Terbinafine is a synthetic allylamine with structure and activity related to naftifine.

1. Mechanism of action. Terbinafine inhibits squalene monooxygenase, leading to an interruption of fungal sterol biosynthesis. Terbinafine may be **fungicidal** or **fungistatic,** depending on drug concentration and species.

2. Spectrum of activity. Terbinafine has activity against dermatophytic fungi (*Trichophyton, Microsporum,* and *Epidermophyton*), filamentous fungi (*Aspergillus*), and dimorphic fungi (*Blastomyces*). It may also possess some activity against yeasts.

3. Therapeutic uses

a. Oral terbinafine is useful against infections of the toenail and fingernail (onychomycosis, tinea unguium). Time to cure is reduced over imidazole antifungals for these indications. It is useful in patients who may not tolerate the adverse effect profile of imidazole antifungals.

b. It is also used in tinea capitis and tinea corporis infections.

4. Precautions and monitoring effects. Adverse effects include taste or ocular disturbances, symptomatic hepatobiliary dysfunction, decrease in lymphocyte count and neutropenia, and serious skin reactions.

IV. TOPICAL ANTIFUNGAL AGENTS

A. Definition. These agents are for topical use for fungal infections.

B. Amphotericin B is available as a 3% cream or lotion or an oral suspension that is not absorbed through the GI tract.

1. Mechanism of action (see III B 1)

2. Spectrum of activity (see III B 2)

3. Therapeutic uses. Amphotericin B is used for oropharyngeal candidiasis, cutaneous and mucocutaneous candidal infections, or as a local irrigant for the bladder, and intrapleural or intraperitoneal areas.

4. Precautions and monitoring effects. Compared with systemic administration, the topical formulations have relatively low toxicity.

a. Dry skin and local irritation with erythema, pruritus, or burning, along with mild skin discoloration, has occurred with the lotion and cream.

b. Rash and GI effects (e.g., nausea, vomiting, steatorrhea, diarrhea) tend to occur with the suspension. In addition, there have been case reports of urticaria, angioedema, Stevens-Johnson syndrome, and toxic epidermal necrolysis.

C. Butenafine is a synthetic benzylamine related to the allylamine antifungal agents (naftifine, terbinafine).

1. Mechanism of action. Butenafine alters fungal membrane permeability and growth inhibition, interferes with sterol biosynthesis by allowing squalene to accumulate within the cell, and may be fungicidal in certain concentrations against susceptible organisms such as the dermatophytes.

2. Spectrum of activity. Butenafine is active against *Trichophyton rubrum, Trichophyton mentagrophytes, Microsporum canis, Sporothrix schenckii,* and yeasts including *Candida parapsilosis* and *Candida albicans.*

3. Therapeutic uses. The 1% cream is used in dermatophytoses, including tinea corporis, tinea cruris, and tinea pedis.

4. Precautions and monitoring effects. If clinical improvement of fungal infection does not improve after the treatment period, the diagnosis should be reevaluated.

D. Butoconazole is an azole antifungal cream available for vaginal use.

1. Mechanism of action. Butoconazole has fungistatic activity against susceptible organisms. The drug interferes with membrane permeability, secondary metabolic effects, and growth inhibition. Butoconazole contains antibacterial effects against some gram-positive organisms.

2. Spectrum of activity. Butoconazole is active against dermatophytes (*Trichophyton concentricum, T. mentagrophytes, T. rubrum, Trichophyton tonsurans, Epidermophyton floccosum, M. canis, Microsporum gypseum*), yeasts (*C. albicans, Candida glabrata*), and some gram-positive organisms (*S. aureus, E. faecalis,* and *S. pyogenes*).

3. Therapeutic uses. A 2% cream is used for vulvovaginal candidiasis and complicated, recurrent vulvovaginal candidiasis.

4. Precautions and monitoring effects
  a. Vulvovaginal burning and itching are the most common; however, their incidence is low. Headache, itching of fingers, urinary frequency and burning, and vulvovaginal discharge, irritation, soreness, stinging, odor, and swelling rarely occur.
  b. Butoconazole may damage birth-control devices such as condoms and diaphragms, leading to inadequate protection. Consider alternative methods of birth control.
  c. Tampon use should be avoided with the use of butoconazole.

E. Ciclopirox is a synthetic antifungal agent that is chemically unrelated to any other antifungal agent. The ethanolamine contained in ciclopirox appears to enhance epidermal penetration.

  1. Mechanism of action. Ciclopirox causes intracellular depletion of amino acids and ions necessary for normal cellular function.

  2. Spectrum of activity. Ciclopirox is active against dermatophytes, yeasts, some gram-positive and gram-negative bacteria, *Mycoplasma*, and *Trichomonas vaginalis*. Specifically, ciclopirox has activity against *T. mentagrophytes, T. rubrum, E. floccosum, M. canis, M. furfur,* and *C. albicans*.

  3. Therapeutic uses. Ciclopirox is used topically for the treatment of tinea pedis, tinea cruris, tinea corporis, tinea versicolor (from *Malassezia*), and cutaneous candidiasis (moniliasis) from *C. albicans*.

  4. Precautions and monitoring effects. Local irritation manifested by erythema, pruritus, burning, blistering, swelling, and oozing has occurred. If this occurs, ciclopirox should be discontinued.

F. Clioquinol is a topical antifungal in a 3% ointment that can be used alone or in combination with hydrocortisone.

  1. Mechanism of action. Unknown

  2. Spectrum of activity. It is active against dermatophytic fungi.

  3. Therapeutic uses. It is used topically against:
  a. Tinea pedis and tinea cruris (ringworm infections)
  b. Previously used to treat diaper rash; however, it is no longer recommended, and use in children less than 2 years of age is contraindicated

  4. Precautions and monitoring effects
  a. Local irritation, rash, and sensitivity reactions are common.
  b. Systemic absorption following topical application may occur.
  c. High doses of clioquinol over long periods of time have been associated with oculotoxic/neurotoxic effects, including optic neuritis, optic atrophy, and subacute myelo-optic neuropathy.

G. Clotrimazole is an azole antifungal agent that is an imidazole derivative. It is related to other azole antifungal agents such as **butoconazole, econazole, ketoconazole, miconazole, oxiconazole, sulconazole,** and **tioconazole.**

  1. Mechanism of action. Clotrimazole alters fungal cell membrane permeability by binding with phospholipids in the membrane.

  2. Spectrum of activity. It is active against yeasts, dermatophytes *(T. rubrum, T. mentagrophytes, E. floccosum, M. canis)*, and some gram-positive bacteria. At higher concentrations, clotrimazole inhibits *M. furfur, Aspergillus fumigatus, C. albicans,* and some strains of *S. aureus, S. pyogenes, Proteus vulgaris,* and *Salmonella*. At very high concentrations, clotrimazole has an effect on *Sporothrix, Cryptococcus, Cephalosporium, Fusarium,* and *T. vaginalis*.

  3. Therapeutic uses
  a. The lozenges, which are administered 5 times per day, are useful in treating oropharyngeal candidiasis. Lozenges are also used for primary prophylaxis of mucocutaneous candidiasis in HIV-infected infants or children with severe immunosuppression.
  b. The cream, lotion, or solution is used to treat dermatophytoses, superficial mycoses, and cutaneous candidiasis.
  c. Intravaginal dosage forms are useful in treating vulvovaginal candidiasis.

4. Precautions and monitoring effects

   a. Cutaneous reactions with topical administration may include blistering, erythema, edema, pruritus, burning, stinging, peeling, skin fissures, and general irritation.

   b. The vaginal tablets are associated with mild burning, skin rash, itching, vulval irritation, lower abdominal cramps, bloating, slight cramping, vaginal soreness during intercourse, and an increase in urinary frequency.

   c. Cross-sensitization occurs with imidazole; however, it is unpredictable.

   d. Abnormal liver function tests (elevated AST) have occurred in patients taking the lozenges.

H. Econazole is an azole antifungal agent that is an imidazole derivative.

   1. Mechanism of action. Econazole alters cell membranes and increases permeability (like many other azole agents).

   2. Spectrum of activity. Econazole is active against dermatophytes, yeasts, some gram-positive bacteria, and *T. vaginalis.*

   3. Therapeutic uses

   a. The 1% topical cream, lotion, or solution is useful in treating dermatophytoses and cutaneous candidiasis (tinea corporis and tinea cruris).

   b. Econazole is also used to treat pityriasis (tinea) versicolor (*M. furfur*).

   4. Precautions and monitoring effects. In general, there is a low incidence of toxicity. Topically, a patient may experience burning, stinging sensations, pruritus, and erythema (after 2–4 days).

I. Gentian violet is a dye that possesses the ability to kill fungi, yeasts, and some gram-positive bacteria.

   1. Mechanism of action. None known

   2. Spectrum of activity. Gentian violet is active against *Candida, Epidermophyton, Cryptococcus, Trichophyton,* and some *Staphylococcus* species.

   3. Therapeutic uses. It is used to treat cutaneous *C. albicans* infections (monilia or thrush).

   4. Precautions and monitoring effects

   a. Gentian violet may cause irritation or sensitivity reactions or possibly ulceration of the mucous membranes. If the solution is swallowed, esophagitis, laryngitis, or tracheitis may occur.

   b. Skin tattooing may occur if gentian violet is applied to granulation tissue.

   c. Gentian violet should not be used in areas of extensive ulceration.

   d. This drug is a dye and will stain clothing.

J. Ketoconazole is an imidazole-derived antifungal drug that is available topically as a cream and a shampoo.

   1. Mechanism of action (see III E 1)

   2. Spectrum of activity (see III E 2)

   3. Therapeutic uses

   a. The 2% topical cream is used in treating tinea corporis, tinea cruris, and tinea pedis caused by the dermatophytes (*E. floccosum, T. mentagrophytes,* and *T. rubrum*).

   b. It is used for cutaneous candidiasis.

   c. The 2% topical cream or 2% shampoo may be used in treating tinea versicolor (*M. furfur*). Selenium-based shampoos may also be useful in this area.

   d. The 2% topical cream is useful against sebhorreic dermatitis. The 2% shampoo is useful in reducing scaling due to dandruff.

   e. When combined with a steroid, ketoconazole is useful in treating the following: atopic dermatitis, diaper rash, eczema, folliculitis, impetigo, intertrigo, lichenoid dermatitis, and psoriasis.

   f. An ophthalmic suspension can be extemporaneously prepared to treat fungal keratitis.

   4. Precautions and monitoring effects

   a. Reactions from the 2% topical cream include local irritation, pruritus, and stinging. Contact dermatitis is possible and occurs with other imidazole derivatives.

b. The 2% shampoo may lead to increased hair loss, irritation, abnormal hair texture, scalp pustules, dry skin, pruritus, and oiliness or dryness of hair and scalp. It may in addition straighten otherwise curly hair.

K. Miconazole is an imidazole-derived antifungal drug that is available topically as a 2% aerosol, 2% aerosol powder, 2% cream, a kit, 2% powder and 2% tincture, 2% vaginal cream, and 100 mg and 200 mg vaginal suppositories.

  1. Mechanism of action (see III E 1)

  2. Spectrum of activity (see III E 2)

  3. Therapeutic uses. Miconazole is advantageous over other agents such as nystatin and tolnaftate in that its activity covers dermatophytes as well as *Candida*.
  a. Topical use is effective against tinea pedis, tinea cruris, and tinea corporis caused by dermatophytes (*T. mentagrophytes, T. rubrum,* and *E. floccosum*).
  b. It is also effective against tinea versicolor from *M. furfur.*
  c. Like other imidazole derivatives, it is useful in treating cutaneous fungal infections.
  d. The vaginal cream and vaginal suppositories are effective in treating vulvovaginal candidiasis.

  4. Precautions and monitoring parameters
  a. Topical creams have caused local irritation and burning.
  b. Vaginal preparations have led to vulvovaginal burning, itching, irritation, pelvic cramps, vaginal burning, headache, hives, and skin rash.
  c. If vulvovaginal candidiasis persists for longer than 3 days, seek further medical attention.
  d. Tampons should be avoided in patients using vaginal suppositories or cream; sanitary pads should be substituted.
  e. Vaginal suppositories are manufactured from a vegetable oil base that may interact with latex products. Avoid using diaphragms or condoms concurrently with suppositories. Seek an alternative form of birth control.

L. Naftifine is a synthetic allylamine similar to terbinafine. It is available as a 1% topical cream and a 1% topical gel.

  1. Mechanism of action. Naftifine is **fungistatic** and interferes with sterol biosynthesis by accumulating squalene in the fungal cell. Naftifine also possesses some local anti-inflammatory activity.

  2. Spectrum of activity
  a. Naftifine is active against *T. mentagrophytes, T. rubrum, T. tonsurans, Trichophyton verrucosum, Trichophyton violaceum, E. floccosum, Microsporum audouinii, M. canis,* and *M. gypseum.*
  b. *C. albicans, Candida krusei, Candida parapsilosis,* and *Candida tropicalis* are affected by naftifine; however, the concentrations of naftifine vary for *Candida* killing depending on the species.
  c. In vitro activity has been demonstrated against *Aspergillus flavus* and *Aspergillus fumigatus.* Others include *Sporothrix schenckii, Cryptococcus neoformans, Petriellidum boydii, Blastomyces dermatitidis,* and *Histoplasma capsulatum.*

  3. Therapeutic uses. Naftifine is active against dermatophytoses and cutaneous candidiasis.
  a. It is also used to treat tinea cruris, tinea pedis, tinea corporis, and tinea mannum (*T. mentagrophytes, T. rubrum, T. verrucosum, T. violaceum, E. floccosum,* or *M. canis*).
  b. It is also useful in treating tinea unguium (onychomycosis).

  4. Precautions and monitoring effects. Transient burning and stinging

M. Nystatin. A polyene antibiotic, nystatin has a chemical structure similar to that of amphotericin B. It is available as an oral suspension, tablet, lozenge, topical cream, ointment, topical powder, and vaginal tablet.

  1. Mechanism of action. Nystatin is **fungicidal** and **fungistatic;** binding to sterols in the fungal cell membrane, it increases membrane permeability and permits leakage of intracellular contents.

  2. Spectrum of activity. Nystatin is active primarily against *Candida* species.

3. Therapeutic uses. This drug is used primarily as a topical agent in vaginal and oral *Candida* infections.

4. Precautions and monitoring effects. Irritation has occurred in extremely rare instances.

N. Oxiconazole is an imidazole-derived antifungal drug that is available as a 1% topical cream or 1% topical lotion.

1. **Mechanism of action** (see III E 1)

2. **Spectrum of activity** (see III E 2)

3. **Therapeutic uses**
   a. The 1% cream or lotion is useful in treating tinea cruris, tinea corporis, tinea mannum, and tinea pedis from dermatophytes.
   b. Oxiconazole is also effective against tinea versicolor caused by *M. furfur.*

4. **Precautions and monitoring effects.** Adverse effects are rare and are confined to local irritation.

O. Sulconazole is an imidazole-derived antifungal drug that is available as a 1% topical cream and a 1% topical solution.

1. **Mechanism of action** (see III E 1). The antibacterial effects exerted by sulconazole are thought to be due to a direct physicochemical effect on the destruction of unsaturated fatty acids present in bacterial cell membranes.

2. **Spectrum of activity**
   a. Sulconazole has activity against dermatophytes, including *E. floccosum, M. audouinii, M. canis, M. gypseum, T. mentagrophytes, T. rubrum, T. tonsurans,* and *T. violaceum.* It also has activity against *M. furfur.*
   b. Sulconazole also has activity against selected gram-positive aerobes (*S. aureus, S. epidermidis, Staphylococcus saprophyticus, E. faecalis, Micrococcus luteus,* and *Bacillus subtilus*) and anaerobes (*Clostridium* and *Propionibacterium acnes, Clostridium perfringens, Clostridium tetani,* and *Clostridium botulinum*).

3. **Therapeutic uses**
   a. The 1% topical cream or 1% topical solution is useful in treating tinea corporis and tinea cruris.
   b. The 1% topical cream has been studied for use against tinea pedis; the solution has not been evaluated for this indication.
   c. The 1% cream is useful against tinea versicolor (*M. furfur*).
   d. There is not an approved indication for cutaneous candidiasis; however, sulconazole 1% is as effective as miconazole 2% or clotrimazole 1% in treating cutaneous candidiasis.
   e. Sulconazole is useful in treating infections caused by bacteria such as impetigo (*S. pyogenes*) and ecthyma (*S. aureus*).

4. **Precautions and monitoring effects.** Adverse reactions include local effects such as burning and irritation, skin edema, dryness, scaling, fissuring, cracking, generalized red papules, and severe eczema.

P. Terbinafine is a synthetic allylamine available as a 1% cream with structure and activity related to naftifine.

1. **Mechanism of action.** Terbinafine inhibits squalene monooxygenase, leading to an interruption of fungal sterol biosynthesis. Terbinafine may be **fungicidal** or **fungistatic,** depending on drug concentration and species.

2. **Spectrum of activity.** Terbinafine has activity against dermatophytic fungi (*Trichophyton, Microsporum,* and *Epidermophyton*), filamentous fungi (*Aspergillus*), and dimorphic fungi (*Blastomyces*). It may also possess some activity against yeasts.

3. **Therapeutic uses.** It is useful for tinea pedis, tinea corporis, and tinea cruris.

4. **Precautions and monitoring effects.** It can cause local irritation.

Q. Terconazole is an imidazole-derived antifungal drug that is available as a 0.4% and 0.8% vaginal cream and an 80-mg vaginal suppository.

1. **Mechanism of action.** It is **fungicidal** against *C. albicans.* Like other imidazole agents, terconazole alters cellular membranes, resulting in increased membrane permeability.

2. **Spectrum of activity.** It is active against dermatophytes, yeasts, and, at high concentrations, gram-positive and gram-negative bacteria.

3. **Therapeutic uses** are for complicated and uncomplicated vulvovaginal candidiasis.

4. **Precautions and monitoring effects.** Adverse reactions include burning, pruritus, irritation, headache, body pain, and pain of female genitalia.

R. Tioconazole is an imidazole-derived antifungal drug that is available as a 6.5% vaginal ointment.

1. **Mechanism of action.** Tioconazole is **fungicidal** against *C. albicans.* Like other imidazole agents, tioconazole alters cellular membranes, resulting in increased membrane permeability.

2. **Spectrum of activity**
   a. Activity against fungi includes most strains of *Candida* and the dermatophytes. There is also activity against *Aspergillus* and *C. neoformans.*
   b. Tioconazole is active against the following aerobic gram-positive bacteria: *Gardnerella vaginalis, Corynebacterium minutissimum, E. faecalis, S. aureus, S. epidermidis,* and some *Streptococci.* Gram-negative bacteria: it is active against *H. pylori, Haemophilus ducreyi, Moraxella catarrhalis, Neisseria gonorrhoeae,* and *N. meningitidis.*
   c. Other organisms that tioconazole has activity against are *T. vaginalis, Lymphogranuloma venereum,* and *Chlamydia trachomatis.*

3. **Therapeutic uses.** Tioconazole is used for simple and complicated vulvovaginal candidiasis. Other uses have been explored; however, topical creams for use in those scenarios are not available in the United States.

4. **Precautions and monitoring effects.** Local irritation has been manifested as vulvovaginal burning, vaginitis, and pruritus.

S. Tolnaftate is available topically as a 1% aerosol, 1% powder, 1% cream, and 1% solution.

1. **Mechanism of action.** It may distort hyphae and stunt mycelial growth in susceptible fungi.

2. **Spectrum of activity.** Tolnaftate may be either **fungistatic** or **fungicidal** to the following organisms: *M. gypseum, M. canis, M. audouinii, Microsporum japonicum, T. rubrum, T. mentagrophytes, Tricophyton schoenleinii, T. tonsurans, E. floccosum, Aspergillus niger, C. albicans, C. neoformans,* and *A. fumigatus.*

3. **Therapeutic uses.** Tolnaftate is used for dermatophytoses and tinea versicolor.

4. **Precautions and monitoring effects.** There may be slight local irritation.

V. ANTIPROTOZOAL AGENTS

A. Classification. These drugs fall into two main categories: **antimalarial agents,** used to treat malaria infection; and **amebicides** and **trichomonacides,** used to treat amebic and trichomonal infections.

B. Antimalarial agents. Still a leading cause of illness and death in tropical and subtropical countries, malaria results from infection by any of four species of the protozoal genus *Plasmodium.* Antimalarial agents are selectively active during different phases of the protozoan life cycle. Major antimalarial drugs include **chloroquine, hydroxychloroquine, primaquine, pyrimethamine, quinine, fansidar,** and **mefloquine.**

1. **Mechanism of action**
   a. **Chloroquine** and **hydroxychloroquine** bind to and alter the properties of microbial and mammalian DNA.

b. The mechanism of action of **primaquine, quinine, fansidar,** and **mefloquine** is unknown.

c. Pyrimethamine impedes folic acid reduction by inhibiting the enzyme dihydrofolate reductase.

2. Spectrum of activity

a. Chloroquine and **hydroxychloroquine** are suppressive blood **schizonticidal** agents and are active against the asexual erythrocyte forms of *Plasmodium vivax* and *Plasmodium falciparum* and gametocytes of *P. vivax, Plasmodium malariae,* and *Plasmodium ovale.*

b. Primaquine, a curative agent, is active against liver forms of *P. vivax* and *P. ovale* and the primary exoerythrocyte forms of *P. falciparum.*

c. Pyrimethamine is active against chloroquine-resistant strains of *P. falciparum* and some strains of *P. vivax.*

d. Quinine, a generalized protoplasmic poison, is toxic to a wide range of organisms. In malaria, this drug has both suppressive and curative action against chloroquine-resistant strains.

e. Fansidar is a blood **schizonticidal** agent that is active against the erythrocytic forms of susceptible plasmodia. It is also active against *T. gondii.*

f. Mefloquine is a blood **schizonticidal** agent that is active against *P. falciparum* (both chloroquine-susceptible and -resistant strains) and *P. vivax.*

3. Therapeutic uses

a. Chloroquine is the preferred agent used to suppress malaria symptoms and to terminate acute malaria attacks resulting from *P. falciparum* and *P. malariae* infections.

   (1) It is more potent and less toxic than quinine.

   (2) Except where drug-resistant *P. falciparum* strains are prevalent, chloroquine is the most useful antimalarial agent.

b. Hydroxychloroquine is used as an alternative to chloroquine in patients who cannot tolerate cloroquine or when chloroquine is unavailable.

c. Primaquine is used to cure relapses of *P. vivax* and *P. ovale* malaria and to prevent malaria in exposed persons returning from regions where malaria is endemic.

d. Pyrimethamine is effective in the prevention and treatment of chloroquine-resistant strains of *P. falciparum.* It is now used almost exclusively in combination with a sulfonamide or sulfone.

e. Quinine

   (1) Quinine sulfate, an oral form, is therapeutic for acute malaria caused by chloroquine-resistant strains.

   (2) Quinine dihydrochloride, a parenteral form, is used in severe cases of chloroquine-resistant malaria. (It is available only from the Centers for Disease Control and Preventional in Atlanta.)

   (3) Quinine is almost always given in combination with another antimalarial agent.

f. Fansidar

   (1) Fansidar is used for the suppression or prophylaxis of chloroquine-resistant *P. falciparum* malaria.

   (2) It has been used for the prophylaxis of *P. carinii* infections in AIDS patients unable to tolerate co-trimoxazole (trimethoprim–sulfamethoxazole).

g. Mefloquine is indicated for the treatment of acute malaria and the prevention of *P. falciparum* and *P. vivax* infections.

4. Precautions and monitoring effects

a. Chloroquine and hydroxychloroquine

   (1) Because these drugs concentrate in the liver, they should be used cautiously in patients with hepatic disease.

   (2) Chloroquine must be administered with extreme caution in patients with neurological, hematological, or severe GI disorders.

   (3) Visual disturbances, headache, skin rash, and GI distress have been reported.

b. Primaquine

   (1) This agent is contraindicated in patients with rheumatoid arthritis and lupus erythematosus and in those receiving other potentially hemolytic drugs or bone marrow suppressants.

   (2) Primaquine may cause agranulocytosis, granulocytopenia, and mild anemia. In patients with G6PD deficiency, it may cause hemolytic anemia.

   (3) Abdominal cramps, nausea, vomiting, and epigastric distress sometimes occur.

c. Pyrimethamine
  (1) In high doses, this drug may cause agranulocytosis, megaloblastic anemia, aplastic anemia, and thrombocytopenia.
  (2) Erythema multiforme (Stevens-Johnson syndrome), nausea, vomiting, and anorexia may develop during pyrimethamine therapy.
d. Quinine
  (1) Quinine is contraindicated in patients with G6PD deficiency, tinnitus, and optic neuritis.
  (2) Quinine overdose or hypersensitivity reactions may be fatal. Manifestations of quinine poisoning include visual and hearing disturbances; GI symptoms (e.g., nausea, vomiting); hot, flushed skin; headache; fever; syncope; confusion; shallow, then depressed, respirations; and cardiovascular collapse.
  (3) Quinine must be used cautiously in patients with atrial fibrillation.
  (4) Renal damage and anuria have been reported.
e. Fansidar
  (1) Severe, sometimes fatal, hypersensitivity reactions have occurred. In most cases, death resulted from severe cutaneous reactions, including erythema multiforme, Stevens-Johnson syndrome, and toxic epidermal necrolysis.
  (2) Adverse hematological and hepatic effects as seen with sulfonamides have been reported.
f. Mefloquine
  (1) Concomitant use of mefloquine with quinine, quinidine, or β-adrenergic blockade may produce electrocardiographic abnormalities or cardiac arrest.
  (2) Concomitant use of mefloquine and quinine or chloroquine may increase the risk of convulsions.

C. Amebicides and trichomonacides. These agents are crucial in the treatment of amebiasis, giardiasis, and trichomoniases—the most common protozoal infections in the United States. The major amebicides include **diloxanide, emetine, iodoquinol, metronidazole, paromomycin,** and **quinacrine.**

1. Mechanism of action
  a. Diloxanide, a dichloroacetamide derivative, is **amebicidal;** its mechanism of action is unknown. (It is available only from the Centers for Disease Control and Prevention in Atlanta.)
  b. Emetine, an alkaloid obtained from ipecac, is **amebicidal;** it kills amebae by inhibiting amebic protein synthesis.
  c. Metronidazole is a synthetic compound with direct **amebicidal** and **trichomonacidal** action; it works at both intestinal and extraintestinal sites. Its mechanism of action involves disruption of the helical structure of DNA.
  d. Quinacrine is an acridine derivative that inhibits DNA metabolism.
  e. Iodoquinol is a luminal or contact amebicide that is effective against the trophozoites of *Entamoeba histolytica* located in the lumen of the large intestines.
  f. Paromomycin is a poorly absorbed amebicidal aminoglycoside whose mechanism of action parallels other aminoglycosides (i.e., protein synthesis inhibitor). It is also effective against enteric bacteria *Salmonella* and *Shigella.*

2. Spectrum of activity and therapeutic uses
  a. Diloxanide
    (1) This drug is used to treat asymptomatic carriers of amebic and giardiac cysts.
    (2) Diloxanide is therapeutic for invasive and extraintestinal amebiasis (given in combination with a systemic or mixed amebicide).
    (3) Diloxanide is not effective as single-agent therapy for extraintestinal amebiasis.
  b. Emetine
    (1) This drug is widely used to treat severe invasive intestinal amebiasis, amebic abscess, and amebic hepatitis.
    (2) Because of its toxicity, emetine generally is used only when other drugs are contraindicated or have proven to be ineffective.
    (3) Usually, emetine is administered in combination with another amebicidal agent.
  c. Metronidazole
    (1) This agent is the preferred drug in amebic dysentery, giardiasis, and trichomoniasis.
    (2) Metronidazole also is active against all anaerobic cocci and gram-negative anaerobic bacilli.

(3) This agent is the treatment of choice by the Centers for Disease Control and Prevention for the treatment of *C. difficile* colitis infections due to the emerging use of broad-spectrum antibiotics. This therapy is cost-effective.

d. Quinacrine is useful in the treatment of giardiasis and tapeworms (see VIII H 2).

e. Iodoquinol is indicated for treatment of intestinal amebiasis. It is active against the protozoa *E. histolytica*.

f. Paromomycin is indicated for acute and chronic intestinal amebiasis; it is not useful for extraintestinal amebiasis because it is not absorbed. Paromomycin has been used for *Dientamoeba fragilis, Taenia saginata, Dipylidium caninum,* and *Hymenolepis nana.*

3. Precautions and monitoring effects

a. Diloxanide rarely causes serious adverse effects. Vomiting, flatulence, and pruritus have been reported.

b. Emetine

(1) This drug may induce potentially lethal systemic toxicity. Manifestations may be cardiovascular [e.g., electrocardiogram (ECG) abnormalities, tachycardia, hypotension, HF], GI (e.g., nausea, vomiting, diarrhea), or neurological (e.g., dizziness, headache, changes in central or peripheral nerve function).

(2) Emetine usually is contraindicated in patients with cardiac disease, renal impairment, muscle disease, and polyneuropathy; in children; and in patients who have taken the drug in the past 6–8 weeks.

(3) IV injection is contraindicated.

(4) Deep subcutaneous administration (preferred over the IM route) may cause muscle weakness at the injection site.

c. Metronidazole

(1) The most common adverse effects of this drug are nausea, epigastric distress, and diarrhea.

(2) Metronidazole is carcinogenic in mice and should not be used unnecessarily.

(3) Headache, vomiting, metallic taste, and stomatitis have been reported.

(4) Occasionally, neurological reactions (e.g., ataxia, peripheral neuropathy, seizures) develop.

(5) A disulfiram-type reaction may occur with concurrent ethanol use.

d. Quinacrine (see VIII H 4)

(1) This drug frequently causes dizziness, headache, nausea, and vomiting. Nervousness and seizures also have been reported.

(2) Quinacrine should not be taken in combination with primaquine because this may increase primaquine toxicity.

(3) Quinacrine should be administered with extreme caution in patients with psoriasis because it may cause marked exacerbation of this disease.

e. Iodoquinol may produce optic neuritis or atrophy or peripheral neuropathy with high-dose, long-term use. Protein-bound iodine levels may be increased during treatment and may interfere with the results of thyroid tests for 6 months after treatment. Iodoquinol should not be used in patients who are hypersensitive to 8-hydroxyquinolone (e.g., iodoquinol, iodochlorhydroxyquin) or iodine-containing agents or in patients with hepatic disorders.

f. Paromomycin may cause nausea, cramping, and diarrhea at high doses (more than 3 g/day). Inadvertent absorption through ulcerative bowel lesions may result in ototoxicity or renal damage.

D. Pentamidine isethionate is an aromatic diamide antiprotozoal agent. It can be administered intramuscularly, intravenously, or by inhalation.

1. Mechanism of action is not fully understood, but in vitro studies indicate interference with nuclear metabolism and inhibition of DNA, RNA, phospholipid, and protein synthesis.

2. Therapeutic uses

a. Pentamidine is indicated for the prevention and treatment of infections due to *P. carinii*.

b. Unlabeled uses include treatment of trypanosomiasis, visceral leishmaniasis, and babesiosis.

3. Precautions and monitoring effects

a. Nephrotoxicity, bronchospasm, and cough are the most common effects produced by intravenous or inhaled pentamidine.

b. Severe hypotension may occur after a parenteral dose of pentamidine. Cardiorespiratory arrest can occur after a single rapid infusion of the drug.

c. Pain, erythema, and tenderness may occur after an IM administration of the drug. This can be minimized by using the Z-track technique of drug administration. Phlebitis may occur following IV administration.

d. Hypoglycemia may occur with initial administration of drug via the IV, IM, or inhalational route. After the patient has been on the drug for a period of time, hyperglycemia will result. The effect of the drug may actually induce a reversible insulin-dependent diabetes mellitus.

e. Leukopenia and thrombocytopenia, which can be severe, occur occasionally.

f. Pentamidine may result in elevated liver function tests, AST, and ALT.

g. GI effects can also occur, including nausea, vomiting, abdominal discomfort, pain, diarrhea, and dysgeusia.

h. Neurological effects can occur with parenteral administration and may include dizziness, tremors, confusion, anxiety, insomnia, and seizures.

i. Hypocalcemia and fever have also been reported and may be severe at times.

E. Atovaquone is a hydroxynaphthoquinone initially synthesized as an antimalarial drug.

  1. Mechanism of action. Atovaquone blocks mitochondrial electron transport at complex III of the respiratory chain of protozoa, resulting in inhibition of pyrimidine synthesis.

  2. Spectrum of activity. It is active against *P. carinii, T. gondii, Cryptosporidium parvum, P. falciparum, Isosporidia,* and *Microsporidia.*

  3. Therapeutic uses. Atovaquone is used for second-line treatment of mild to moderate *P. carinii* pneumonia in patients intolerant of co-trimoxazole or other sulfonamides, or nonresponsive to co-trimoxazole.

  4. Precautions and monitoring effects
    a. Oral absorption significantly increases when administered with food (especially a high-fat meal).
    b. Rash, nausea, diarrhea, headache, fever, abdominal pain, dizziness, and elevated liver function tests commonly are reported.

  5. Significant interactions. Atovaquone is highly bound to plasma protein. It should be used with caution when administered with other highly protein-bound drugs with a narrow therapeutic range.

F. Eflornithine HCl is an IV antiprotozoal agent. Its activity has been attributed to the inhibition of the enzyme ornithine decarboxylase.

  1. Mechanism of action is a specific, enzyme-activated, irreversible inhibitor of ornithine decarboxylase.

  2. Spectrum of activity and therapeutic uses. Eflornithine is active in the treatment of the meningoencephalitic stage of *Trypanosoma brucei gambiense* (sleeping sickness).

  3. Precautions and monitoring effects
    a. Myelosuppression is the most frequent serious side effect.
    b. Seizures occur in about 8% of treated patients.
    c. Cases of hearing impairment have been reported.

VI. ANTITUBERCULAR AGENTS

A. Definition and classification. Drugs used to treat tuberculosis suppress or kill the slow-growing mycobacteria that cause this disease. Antitubercular agents fall into two main categories: **primary** and **retreatment** agents. Because the causative organisms tend to develop resistance to any single drug, combination drug therapy has become standard in the treatment of tuberculosis.

  1. The **incidence** of tuberculosis in the United States is increasing due to shifts in populations considered to be endemic for tuberculosis, the rise in HIV-positive patients, and drug resistance.

2. Agents chosen for **therapy** must eradicate mycobacterium. Agents available include isoniazid, streptomycin, quinolones, ethambutol, pyrazinamide, rifampin, and rifabutin. **Combination chemotherapy** is essential. Agents showing the lowest incidence of resistance (isoniazid, rifampin, streptomycin) are usually used in combination with pyrazinamide or ethambutol.

3. Choice of therapy is dependent on many patient and disease factors (e.g., duration of therapy needed, likelihood of drug resistance, and HIV status).

4. Most patients are started on isoniazid, rifampin, and pyrazinamide. A fourth drug (e.g., ethambutol, streptomycin) is added with suspected resistance (i.e., if patients were previously treated or if resistance is expected). Patients failing this therapy must be treated with five drugs (isoniazid, rifampin, pyrazinamide, ethambutol, and streptomycin). If one or more of these agents cannot be used, ethionamide, para-aminosalicylic acid, cycloserine, or capreomycin (older, more toxic, second-line agents) can be used.

5. **Treatment choices based on Centers for Disease Control and Prevention recommendations**
   a. The first choice is isoniazid, rifampin, and pyrazinamide for 8 weeks, then isoniazid and rifampin daily for 16 weeks or isoniazid and rifampin 2–3 times per week in areas where resistance is less than 4%. In cases of suspected isoniazid resistance or until resistance patterns are determined in areas of high resistance, add ethambutol or streptomycin for at least 6 months or cultures dictate otherwise. If resistance is present, continue ethambutol and streptomycin for 3 months after seroconversion.
   b. The second choice includes isoniazid, rifampin, pyrazinamide, and either streptomycin or ethambutol daily for 2 weeks, then two times a week for 6 weeks, followed by isoniazid and rifampin two times a week for 16 weeks. If smear or culture is positive after 3 months, consult a medical expert.
   c. The third choice is isoniazid, rifampin, pyrazinamide, plus either streptomycin or ethambutol three times a week for 6 months. If smear or culture is positive after 3 months, consult a medical expert.
   d. For HIV-positive patients, use any of the previous recommendations, but continue therapy for at least 9 months and at least 6 months beyond culture conversion.

B. **Primary agents.** These drugs, isoniazid, ethambutol, rifampin, pyrazinamide, and streptomycin, usually offer the greatest effectiveness with the least toxicity; they are successful in most tuberculosis patients. Frequently, two or three are administered together; in most cases, the combination of isoniazid, rifampin, and pyrazinamide is most effective.

1. **Ethambutol** is a synthetic water-based compound.
   a. **Mechanism of action.** This drug is **bacteriostatic.** Its precise mechanism of action is unknown; however, it has only demonstrated activity against susceptible bacteria actively undergoing cell division.
   b. **Spectrum of activity and therapeutic uses.** Ethambutol is active against many *M. tuberculosis* strains as well as many other mycobacterial species. However, drug resistance develops fairly rapidly when it is used alone. In most cases, ethambutol is given adjunctively in combination with isoniazid or rifampin for tuberculosis. It is also useful in combination with other agents such as clarithromycin or azithromycin and rifabutin in treating *Mycobacterium avium* complex (MAC).
   c. **Precautions and monitoring effects.** Rarely, ethambutol causes such adverse effects as reversible dose-related (= 15 mg/kg/day) optic neuritis, drug fever, abdominal pain, headache, dizziness, and confusion. Liver function tests should be periodically monitored. Visual testing and renal function (reduce dose with impairment) should also be monitored.

2. **Isoniazid** is a hydrazide of isonicotinic acid. The mainstay of antitubercular therapy, this drug should be included (if tolerated) in all therapeutic regimens.
   a. **Mechanism of action.** Isoniazid is **bacteriostatic** for resting bacilli and **bactericidal** for rapidly dividing organisms. Its mechanism of action is not fully known; the drug probably disrupts bacterial cell wall synthesis by inhibiting mycolic acid synthesis.
   b. **Spectrum of activity.** Isoniazid has activity only against organisms in the genus *Mycobacterium.* More specifically, it has demonstrated activity against *M. tuberculosis, M. bovis,* and select strains of *Mycobacterium kansasii.*
   c. **Therapeutic uses**
      (1) The most widely used antitubercular agent, isoniazid should be given in combination with another antitubercular drug (such as rifampin or ethambutol) to prevent drug resistance in tuberculosis.

    (2) For uncomplicated pulmonary tuberculosis and most cases of extrapulmonary tuberculosis, short-course regimens of isoniazid are recommended (minimum of 6 months). Isoniazid therapy may last 6 months to 2 years, depending on the severity of illness.

    (3) Prophylactic isoniazid may be administered alone for up to 1 year in adults or children who have a positive tuberculin test result but lack active lesions.

  d. Precautions and monitoring effects

    (1) The most common adverse effects of isoniazid are skin rash, fever, jaundice, and peripheral neuritis.

    (2) Hepatitis, an occasional reaction, can be severe and, in some cases, fatal. The risk of hepatitis increases with the patient's age and rises with alcohol abuse. Monitor liver function tests.

    (3) Blood dyscrasias (e.g., agranulocytosis, aplastic or hemolytic anemia, thrombocytopenia) may occur. Monitor complete blood count (CBC) routinely.

    (4) Adverse GI effects include nausea, vomiting, and epigastric distress.

    (5) CNS toxicity may result from pyridoxine deficiency. Signs and symptoms include insomnia, restlessness, hyperreflexia, and convulsions. Pyridoxine 15–50 mg/day should be administered to patients taking isoniazid to minimize the peripheral neuropathy associated with its use (especially in patients with diabetes, HIV, uremia, alcoholism, malnutrition, pregnancy, or seizure disorder).

  e. Significant interactions

    (1) With concurrent **phenytoin** therapy, blood levels of both phenytoin and isoniazid may increase, possibly causing toxicity.

    (2) **Aluminum-containing antacids** may reduce isoniazid absorption.

    (3) Concurrent **carbamazepine** therapy may increase the risk of hepatitis.

    (4) Use of isoniazid with other antitubercular agents, such as cycloserine or ethionamide, may cause additive nervous system effects.

    (5) There is the potential for the serotonin syndrome to exist when isoniazid is used in combination with selective serotonin-uptake inhibitors or in patients taking meperidine. Isoniazid has been shown to have some monoamine oxidase (MAO)-inhibiting activity.

3. Rifampin is a complex macrocyclic agent.

  a. Mechanism of action. This drug is **bactericidal;** it impairs bacterial RNA synthesis by binding to DNA-dependent RNA polymerase.

  b. Spectrum of activity. Rifampin has activity against most mycobacterial strains. In addition, rifampin has activity against many other organisms, including *N. meningitidis, S. aureus, H. influenzae, Legionella pneumophilia,* and *C. trachomatis.*

  c. Therapeutic uses

    (1) The combination of rifampin and isoniazid is the most effective therapy for tuberculosis. Rifampin should not be administered alone because this can lead to the emergence of highly drug-resistant organisms.

    (2) Prophylactic rifampin is effective when administered to carriers of *N. meningitidis* disease and chemoprophylaxis of patients with *H. influenzae* type b organisms.

    (3) Rifampin may be used in combination with dapsone for the treatment of leprosy.

  d. Precautions and monitoring effects

    (1) Serious hepatotoxicity may result from rifampin therapy. Liver function tests should be routinely conducted.

    (2) In rare cases, this drug induces an influenza-like syndrome.

    (3) Other adverse effects include skin rash, drowsiness, headache, fatigue, confusion, nausea, vomiting, and abdominal pain.

    (4) Rifampin colors urine, sweat, tears, saliva, and feces orange-red.

  e. Significant interactions

    (1) Rifampin induces hepatic microsomal cyP450 enzymes and, thus, may decrease the therapeutic effectiveness of **corticosteroids, warfarin, oral contraceptives, quinidine, digitoxin, protease inhibitors (PIs), nonnucleoside reverse transcriptase inhibitors, ketoconazole, verapamil, methadone, oral antidiabetic agents, cyclosporine, dapsone, chloramphenicol,** and **barbiturates.**

    (2) **Probenecid** may increase blood levels of rifampin.

    (3) **Aminosalicylic acid** may impair absorption of rifampin secondary to bentonite, an excipient used in preparation of aminosalicylic granules.

4. Streptomycin (see II B 3)

5. **Pyrazinamide** is a pyrazine analogue of nicotinamide.
   a. **Mechanism of action.** This drug is **bactericidal** and/or **bacteriostatic,** depending on the cell concentration achieved.
   b. **Spectrum of activity and therapeutic uses.** Pyrazinamide is a highly specific agent and has activity only against *M. tuberculosis.* Pyrazinamide is used as a primary agent with isoniazid and rifampin for at least 2 months, followed by isoniazid and rifampin.
   c. **Precautions and monitoring effects.** This agent may result in hepatotoxicity and, rarely, hepatic necrosis resulting in death. Anorexia, nausea, vomiting, malaise, and fever have been reported. Hyperuricemia may result in gouty exacerbations. Both liver function tests and uric acid levels should routinely be monitored.

C. Retreatment agents. These agents include aminosalicylic acid, capreomycin, cycloserine, ethionamide, and kanamycin. Retreatment agents are less effective, more toxic, and are used in combination with primary agents.

1. **Mechanism of action**
   a. **Aminosalicylic acid** is **bacteriostatic;** it probably inhibits the enzymes responsible for folic acid synthesis.
   b. **Cycloserine** can be **bacteriostatic** or **bactericidal,** depending on its concentration at the infection site; it impairs amino acid utilization, thereby inhibiting bacterial cell wall synthesis.
   c. The mechanism of action of capreomycin (**bacteriostatic**), ethionamide (**bactericidal**), and pyrazinamide (**bactericidal**) is unknown.

2. **Spectrum of activity and therapeutic uses.** Second-line antitubercular agents are active against various microorganisms, including *M. tuberculosis.* These agents generally are reserved for patients with extensive extrapulmonary or drug-resistant disease or for patients who need retreatment. These drugs are almost always administered in combination.

3. **Precautions and monitoring effects**
   a. Adverse effects of **aminosalicylic acid** include leukopenia, agranulocytopenia, thrombocytopenia, hemolytic anemia, mononucleosis-like syndrome, malaise, joint pain, fever, and skin rash.
   b. **Capreomycin** and **streptomycin** are ototoxic and nephrotoxic; they should not be administered together.
   c. **Cycloserine** may cause adverse CNS effects, including headache, suicidal and psychotic tendencies, hyperirritability, confusion, paranoia, and nervousness.
   d. **Ethionamide** may induce nausea, vomiting, orthostatic hypotension, metallic taste, epigastric distress, and peripheral neuropathy.

D. Alternative agents

1. **Rifater.** A combination of rifampin 120 mg, isoniazid 50 mg, and pyrazinamide 300 mg in one tablet is used in patients expected to have low compliance with tuberculosis drug therapy. One **disadvantage** is that many patients are required to take as many as 5–6 tablets daily, which may reduce compliance.

2. **Quinolones.** Ciprofloxacin and levofloxacin are used in tuberculosis therapy. Levofloxacin is preferred due to increased serum concentrations. Levofloxacin is usually used in combination with other tuberculosis agents for active treatment. For prophylaxis, levofloxacin is combined with pyrazinamide.

3. **Macrolides.** Clarithromycin and azithromycin have shown limited activity against *M. tuberculosis.*

4. **Rifabutin** is an antimycobacterial agent that is similar to rifampin, with activity against both tubercular and nontubercular mycobacterial, and offers no clear advantage over rifampin.
   a. **Mechanism of action.** In addition to its antimycobacterial activity against tubercular and nontubercular mycobacterial, rifabutin has been reported to inhibit reverse transcriptase and block the in vitro infectivity and replication of HIV.
   b. **Therapeutic uses.** Rifabutin is indicated for the prevention of disseminated MAI complex disease in patients with advanced HIV infections.
   c. **Precautions and monitoring effects.** The use of rifabutin has resulted in mild elevation of liver enzymes and thrombocytopenia.
   d. **Significant interactions**

(1) Rifabutin antagonizes and potentially negates the immune response mediated by the bacillus Calmette-Guérin (BCG) vaccine.

(2) Rifabutin may increase the clearance of drugs by inducing hepatic microsomal enzymes, but does so to a lesser extent than rifampin. The concentrations of the following drugs may be reduced while taking rifabutin: **cyclosporine, zidovudine, prednisone, digitoxin, quinidine, ketoconazole, protease inhibitors, propranolol, phenytoin, sulfonylureas, and warfarin.** Serum cyclosporine levels should be monitored in patients receiving both agents.

5. Amikacin (see II B)

VII. ANTIVIRAL AGENTS

A. Definition. These drugs treat viral infections by influencing viral replication. Because viruses lack independent metabolic activity and can replicate only within living host cells, antiviral agents tend to injure host as well as viral cells. Unlike antibacterial agents, few antiviral drugs have been introduced over the years; most are active against only one virus, either DNA or RNA viruses.

B. DNA viruses. Currently approved antiviral therapies against the *Herpesviridae* family of DNA viruses [herpes simplex virus (HSV)-1 and -2, varicella-zoster virus (VZV), cytomegalovirus (CMV)] are **virustatic** and arrest DNA synthesis by inhibiting viral DNA polymerase. With the exception of the broad-spectrum antiviral drug **foscarnet,** these agents are prodrugs and require viral and host cellular enzymes (e.g., thymidine, deoxyguanosine kinase) to phosphorylate them into the active triphosphate form before exerting their antiviral activity. Hence, a common mechanism of resistance is a deficiency or structural alteration in viral thymidine kinase (Table 43-4).

1. Acyclovir is a synthetic acyclic analogue of guanosine with activity against various herpes viruses.

   a. Mechanism of action. Acyclovir monophosphate is phosphorylated to the triphosphate, where it becomes incorporated into viral DNA and inhibits viral replication.

   b. Spectrum of activity. This agent is active against herpes viruses, particularly HSV-1, HSV-2, VZV, and chickenpox (varicella).

   c. Therapeutic uses

   (1) Acyclovir is used to treat initial and recurrent HSV-1 and -2 infections in immunocompromised patients and for acute treatment of herpes zoster (shingles) and chickenpox.

   (2) This agent is available in topical, oral, and IV forms. Topical acyclovir is applied directly on herpes lesions in primary herpes infection and in non–life-threatening mucocutaneous HSV infection in immunocompromised patients, but is less effective than oral therapy.

Table 43-4. Activity of Anti-DNA Viral Agents

Agent	HSV-1	HSV-2	VZV	CMV	Influenza A	Influenza B
Acyclovir*	+	+	+	- - -	- - -	- - -
Amantadine	- - -	- - -	- - -	- - -	+	- - -
Cidofovir	- - -	- - -	- - -	+	- - -	- - -
Famciclovir	+	+	+	- - -	- - -	- - -
Foscarnet	+	+	=	- - -	- - -	- - -
Ganciclovir*	- - -	- - -	- - -	+	- - -	- - -
Oseltamivir	- - -	- - -	- - -	- - -	+	+
Ribavirin	- - -	- - -	- - -	- - -	+	+
Rimantadine	- - -	- - -	- - -	- - -	+	- - -
Valacyclovir*	+	+	+	- - -	- - -	- - -
Valganciclovir*	- - -	- - -	- - -	+	- - -	- - -
Zanamivir	- - -	- - -	- - -	- - -	+	+

*Requires activation into triphosphate form.

(3) Acyclovir may be administered intravenously in the treatment of initial and recurrent mucocutaneous HSV infection, VZV infection in immunocompromised patients, and in the treatment of HSV encephalitis.

d. Precautions and monitoring effects
   (1) Oral acyclovir may induce nausea, vomiting, diarrhea, and headache.
   (2) IV administration may cause dose-dependent nephrotoxicity, neurological effects (e.g., lethargy, confusion, tremors, agitation, seizures, coma, obtundation), hypotension, rash, itching, and inflammation and phlebitis at the injection site.
   (3) Local discomfort and pruritus may result from topical administration.
   (4) Acyclovir is removed in hemodialysis. Doses should be adjusted in renal impairment and hemodialysis.

e. Significant interactions. Acyclovir may increase blood concentrations of theophylline, possibly causing toxicity.

2. **Amantadine** is a synthetic tricyclic amine with a unique chemical structure similar to rimantadine. It is effective against influenza A viral infection.
   a. Mechanism of action. Amantadine inhibits replication of the influenza A virus by interfering with viral attachment and uncoating.
   b. Spectrum of activity and therapeutic uses
      (1) Amantadine is effective in the prophylaxis and treatment of influenza A virus strains. However, an annual influenza virus vaccine is considered first line for prophylactic therapy.
      (2) Clinicians recommend that all nonimmunized high-risk patients receive this drug at the first sign of community influenza A activity.
      (3) Suppressive therapy should continue for 24–48 hours after influenza symptoms disappear or, if necessary, up to 90 days for repeated exposure to the virus.
      (4) This drug may be used to treat some patients with parkinsonism.
   c. Precautions and monitoring effects
      (1) The most pronounced adverse effects of amantadine are ataxia, nightmares, and insomnia. Other CNS effects include depression, confusion, dizziness, fatigue, anxiety, and headache. Patients with a history of epilepsy and psychiatric disorders should be monitored closely during therapy.
      (2) Anticholinergic reactions (e.g., dry mouth, blurred vision, tachycardia) have been reported.
      (3) Dosage adjustment is needed for patients with impaired renal function.

3. **Cidofovir** is a synthetic acyclic purine nucleotide.
   a. Mechanism of action. Cidofovir diphosphate suppresses CMV replication by selective inhibition of viral DNA synthesis.
   b. Spectrum of activity. In vitro activity has been demonstrated against CMV, VZV, Epstein-Barr virus (EBV), and HSV-1 and -2. Controlled clinical studies are limited to patients with AIDS and CMV retinitis.
   c. Therapeutic use includes the treatment, but not the cure of, CMV retinitis in patients with AIDS.
   d. Precautions and monitoring effects
      (1) Avoid using this drug in patients with serum creatinine greater than 1.5 mg/dl or creatinine clearance (CrCl) less than 55 mL/min.
      (2) Cidofovir is contraindicated in patients with a history of severe hypersensitivity to probenecid or other sulfa-containing medications.
      (3) The dose-limiting toxicity of cidofovir is nephrotoxicity; neutropenia, peripheral neuropathy, and diarrhea are common adverse effects.
      (4) Probenecid must be administered with each cidofovir dose. The patient must be hydrated with 1 L of saline before infusing. Cidofovir is available only in IV form.

4. **Famciclovir** is a prodrug of the antiviral agent penciclovir.
   a. Mechanism of action. Famciclovir is rapidly phosphorylated in virus-infected cells by viral thymidine kinase to penciclovir monophosphate. Penciclovir is a competitive inhibitor of viral DNA polymerase and prevents viral replication by inhibition of herpes virus DNA synthesis.
   b. Spectrum of activity and therapeutic uses
      (1) Famciclovir has activity against HSV-1, HSV-2, and VZV. The drug is indicated for management of acute herpes zoster (also known as shingles) and oral genital herpes.

(2) Therapy must be promptly initiated as soon as herpes zoster or genital herpes is diagnosed (within 48–72 hr), at a dose of 500 mg every 8 hours for 7 days. Treatment is for 5–7 days only.

  c. Precautions and monitoring effects

    (1) Common adverse events include fatigue, GI complaints such as nausea, diarrhea, vomiting, constipation, and anorexia. Headache is also commonly reported.

    (2) Dose adjustment is necessary in patients with renal dysfunction. Famciclovir is removed by hemodialysis.

5. Foscarnet (trisodium phosphonoformate hexahydrate, PFA) is a synthetic pyrophosphate analogue, which directly inhibits enzymes involved in viral DNA synthesis without incorporation into viral DNA. It is a broad-spectrum antiviral agent and is the drug of choice in cases of acyclovir or ganciclovir resistance.

  a. Mechanism of action

    (1) Viral DNA replication requires the addition of deoxynucleoside triphosphates at the end of the DNA strand by DNA polymerase and the subsequent cleavage of pyrophosphate from the newly attached nucleotide. Foscarnet competitively binds directly to DNA polymerase to form an inactive complex and prevents pyrophosphate cleavage. Viral DNA chain elongation is thus terminated.

    (2) Foscarnet is also active against HIV-1, an RNA retrovirus. It is a noncompetitive, reversible inhibitor of HIV reverse transcriptase, the enzyme responsible for converting viral RNA to viral DNA.

  b. Spectrum of activity and therapeutic uses. Foscarnet has in vitro activity against HSV-1 and -2, CMV, VZV, and EBV DNA polymerases, influenza polymerase, and HIV reverse transcriptase. Therapeutically, the drug may be used in HSV-1 and -2, VZV, CMV, and HIV-1 infections.

    (1) Either alone or in combination with gancyclovir, foscarnet is considered first-line treatment for CMV retinitis in immunocompromised patients. An initial induction therapy lasts 2–3 weeks. Maintenance therapy within 1 month after induction may be needed to prevent relapse.

    (2) Foscarnet is indicated for the treatment of acyclovir-resistant mucocutaneous HSV in immunocompromised patients. It is not, however, a cure for HSV infections.

    (3) Foscarnet is able to cross the blood–brain barrier.

  c. Precautions and monitoring effects

    (1) IV foscarnet is highly nephrotoxic, causing acute tubular necrosis. The incidence of acute renal failure can be markedly reduced if adequate hydration and daily monitoring of serum creatinine and BUN are maintained throughout therapy.

    (2) Other common adverse effects include electrolyte abnormalities (e.g., hypocalcemia, hypomagnesemia, hypophosphatemia, hypokalemia), anemia, fever, and seizures.

    (3) Foscarnet is not recommended for patients with CrCl less than 50 mL/min.

    (4) Foscarnet must be administered using an infusion pump over at least 1 hour. Do not administer the drug as an IV bolus.

  d. Significant interactions

    (1) Concomitant **cyclosporin** increases the risk of renal toxicity.

    (2) Foscarnet is exclusively eliminated by glomerular filtration and tubular secretion.

    (3) Concurrent nephrotoxic agents should be avoided whenever possible.

6. Ganciclovir is a synthetic purine nucleoside analogue that is approved for the treatment of CMV infections.

  a. Mechanism of action. After conversion to ganciclovir triphosphate, ganciclovir is incorporated into viral DNA, which inhibits viral DNA polymerase, thereby terminating viral replication.

  b. Spectrum of activity. Ganciclovir has in vitro activity against HSV-1 and -2, VZV, EBV, and CMV (due to its enhanced ability to penetrate host cells).

  c. Therapeutic uses. It is indicated for treatment of CMV infections, such as colitis, pneumonia, and retinitis. However, ganciclovir use in CMV infections of the CNS has not been successful, even though it is capable of CNS penetration.

    (1) Conversion into the triphosphate form is greater in infected host cells, even though drug penetration occurs in both uninfected and infected cells.

    (2) Inhibitory concentrations for the viral DNA polymerase are lower than those for the host cellular polymerase.

(3) It is available in oral and IV formulations. The oral formulation is only approved for prevention and maintenance treatment of CMV.

d. Precautions and monitoring effects

(1) Ganciclovir has **black box warnings** concerning increased potential for dose-limited neutropenia, anemia, and thrombocytopenia. It is also potentially teratogenic and carcinogenic.

(2) Adverse effects commonly include fever and photosensitivity reactions. Phlebitis and pain may occur at the site of infusion.

(3) Because ganciclovir is cleared by glomerular filtration and tubular secretion, renal function and adequate hydration should be monitored. Doses should be adjusted in cases of renal impairment and hemodialysis.

(4) Solutions of ganciclovir are extremely alkaline. Avoid direct contact with skin.

e. Significant interactions

(1) **Probenecid** may increase ganciclovir levels and possibly toxicity.

(2) **Zidovudine** in combination with ganciclovir may result in neutropenia; careful monitoring of granulocyte levels is required when they are taken concurrently with ganciclovir.

(3) **Imipenem–cilastatin** in combination with ganciclovir may induce generalized seizures.

7. Oseltamivir is pharmacologically similar to zanamivir but structurally different. Both of these agents are in a new class with a mechanism of action different from the other antiviral agents.

a. Mechanism of action. Oseltamivir is a prodrug that must be hydrolyzed to oseltamivir carboxylate in vivo to exert antiviral activity. It is a potent selective inhibitor of the influenza virus enzyme, neuraminidase. Inhibition of this enzyme prevents viral replication and spread to other host cells.

b. Spectrum of activity. This agent is active against both the influenza A and B viruses.

c. Therapeutic uses

(1) It is approved for the symptomatic treatment of influenza A and B infections in adults who present with symptoms within 48 hours.

(2) It is also approved for the prophylaxis of influenza infections in patients 13 years of age and older. Note: The influenza virus vaccine is still the gold standard for prophylaxis.

(3) No studies have compared the efficacy of neuraminidase inhibitors to amantadine or rimantidine.

(4) Oseltamivir has been shown to decrease the duration of symptoms by 1 day if taken within 48 hours of viral symptoms.

d. Precautions and monitoring effects

(1) The most common adverse effects are nausea and vomiting, followed by vertigo and insomnia.

(2) Dosage adjustments are required for patients with impaired renal function.

(3) Cross-resistance between oseltamivir and zanamivir has been reported.

8. Rimantadine is a synthetic antiviral agent and an α-methyl derivative of amantadine that blocks the early step in the replication of the influenza A virus.

a. Mechanism of action. Rimantadine inhibits the early viral replication cycle, possibly inhibiting the uncoating of the virus. It has the same mechanism of action and spectrum of activity as amantadine.

b. Spectrum of activity and therapeutic uses

(1) Rimantadine is safe and effective in the prophylaxis and treatment of infections caused by various strains of influenza A virus in adults and for prophylaxis in children >1 year old.

(2) The method of choice for prophylaxis against influenza is vaccination; however, in some cases vaccine is contraindicated or not available.

(3) Rimantadine therapy should be considered for people who develop flu-like symptoms during influenza A season. Therapy should be initiated within 48 hours of symptoms' onset.

c. Precautions and monitoring effects

(1) Use with caution. Rimantadine may increase the incidence of seizure.

(2) The most frequent adverse reactions include GI disturbance (e.g., nausea, vomiting, anorexia) and CNS toxicity (e.g., insomnia, dizziness, headache), which are less than those observed with amantadine.

(3) Dose reductions are recommended in patients with hepatic or renal dysfunction.

9. **Valacyclovir** is the L-valine ester (prodrug) of the antiviral agent acyclovir.
   a. **Mechanism of action.** Valacyclovir is rapidly converted to acyclovir. Acyclovir is selective for the thymidine kinase enzyme, beginning the conversion of acyclovir to acyclovir triphosphate, stopping the replication of herpes viral DNA.
   b. **Spectrum of activity and therapeutic uses**
      (1) Valacyclovir is active against HSV-1, HSV-2, and VZV.
      (2) This agent is used for the acute treatment of herpes zoster (shingles), herpes labialis (cold sore), and genital herpes in immunocompetent adults.
      (3) Advantages over acyclovir include oral dosing of only once to three times daily and attainment of higher plasma concentrations than oral acyclovir. A disadvantage is that there is no IV form available.
   c. **Precautions and monitoring effects**
      (1) Valacyclovir is not indicated in immunocompromised individuals (e.g., advanced HIV disease, bone marrow transplant) due to the occurrence of thrombotic thrombocytopenic purpura/hemolytic uremic syndrome.
      (2) Begin therapy within 72 hours of herpes zoster diagnosis (or rash onset).
      (3) Most commonly reported adverse reactions are mild and include nausea, headache, and vomiting. Dosage adjustment is needed in patients with renal dysfunction.

10. **Ribavirin** is a synthetic nucleoside analogue indicated in the treatment of respiratory syncytial virus (RSV).
   a. **Mechanism of action.** Ribavirin may inhibit RNA and DNA synthesis by depleting intracellular nucleotide reserves.
   b. **Spectrum of activity.** This agent is active in vitro against a broad spectrum of RNA and DNA viruses, including influenza A and B, RSV, and herpes simplex.
   c. **Therapeutic uses.** Administered in aerosol form, ribavirin is used to relieve symptoms and speed recovery in infants and young children with influenza A and B and in the treatment of infants and children with RSV.
   d. **Precautions and monitoring effects**
      (1) Ribavirin must be administered only with a specific small-particle aerosol generator (Viratek SPAG-2).
      (2) This agent is not recommended in patients using ventilators because it may precipitate on respirator valves and tubing, causing lethal malfunction. (However, use of a prefilter may permit ribavirin therapy in such patients.)
      (3) Serious adverse effects include cardiac arrest, deterioration of pulmonary function, bacterial pneumonia, and apnea.
      (4) Rash, conjunctivitis, and reticulocytosis have been reported.
      (5) Inhalation therapy is not indicated for use in adults.

11. **Valganciclovir** is the L-valine ester (prodrug) of the antiviral agent ganciclovir.
   a. **Mechanism of action.** Valganciclovir is converted in vivo to ganciclovir. After conversion to the active form, ganciclovir triphosphate, ganciclovir is incorporated into viral DNA, which inhibits viral DNA polymerase, thereby terminating viral replication.
   b. **Spectrum of activity and therapeutic uses**
      (1) For in vitro activity, see VII B 6 b.
      (2) Valganciclovir is indicated for the treatment of CMV retinitis in patients with AIDS.
      (3) Markedly increased bioavailability when given with food over oral ganciclovir may be an advantage, but the clinical significance is not currently known.
   c. **Precautions and monitoring effects**
      (1) Same **black box warnings** as for ganciclovir
      (2) Doses should be adjusted in cases of renal impairment. Do not use in hemodialysis patients; ganciclovir must be used.
      (3) Available only orally. Do not substitute doses of oral valganciclovir 1:1 for oral ganciclovir; they are not equivalent.
      (4) Is a potential carcinogen and teratogen. Common adverse effects are the same as for ganciclovir.
      (5) If the tablet is broken, avoid contact with skin due to teratogenic and carcinogenic potential.
   d. **Significant interactions.** Same as for ganciclovir; see VII B 6 e.

12. **Zanamivir** is the first of a new class of antiviral agents called neuraminidase inhibitors approved by the FDA for the treatment of influenza A and B infections.
   a. **Mechanism of action.** Zanamivir inhibits replication of the influenza A and B viruses by selective inhibition of the influenza virus neuraminidase enzyme.
   b. **Spectrum of activity.** This agent is active against both the influenza A and B viruses.
   c. **Therapeutic uses**
      (1) It is approved for the treatment of uncomplicated influenza A and B infection for patients who have been symptomatic for less than 48 hours.
      (2) Zanamivir is approved for oral inhalation use only, using the Diskhaler device provided by the manufacturer.
      (3) Use for prophylaxis of influenza A or B has not been approved to date.
      (4) Not approved for use in children under 12 years of age or during pregnancy.
      (5) Shown to decrease duration of symptoms by 1.3 days if taken within 48 hours of viral symptoms.
   d. **Precautions and monitoring effects**
      (1) For patients with a history of asthma or chronic obstructive pulmonary disease, a fast-acting inhaled bronchodilator such as albuterol should be on hand due to the increased potential for the development of acute bronchospasm with this inhaled product. Patients who experience worsening of their pulmonary disease should discontinue this agent and contact their physician immediately.
      (2) The most common adverse effects were mild and included diarrhea, nausea, and vomiting.
      (3) Do not puncture the Rotodisk blister until immediately before administering the dose to ensure full dosage. Manual dexterity required for this device.

C. **RNA viruses.** Currently, 4 classes of antiretroviral agents are approved. These drugs are active against HIV-1 and HIV-2 and include the nucleoside reverse transcriptase inhibitors (NRTIs) **abacavir, zidovudine, didanosine, zalcitabine, stavudine, and lamivudine;** the nucleotide reverse transcriptase inhibitor (NtRTI) **tenofovir DF;** the nonnucleoside reverse transcriptase inhibitors (NNRTIs) **delavirdine, efavirenz, and nevirapine;** the fusion inhibitor **enfuvirtide** as well as the PIs **amprenavir, lopinavir, nelfinavir, saquinavir, ritonavir,** and **indinavir.** These agents are virustatic and require lifelong therapy. They are currently approved for use as dual-, triple-, or quadruple-combination cocktails. Monotherapy with any single antiretroviral agent is no longer considered acceptable in the treatment of HIV infection (Table 43-5). Currently, before initiating therapy a minimum of 2 CD4$^+$ cell counts and 2 HIV RNA levels should be obtained to confirm the initial measurements. After initiating therapy, repeat these measurements in 2–8 weeks, followed by every 3–4 months thereafter. A minimum of 1.0-log decline in HIV RNA levels should be seen after the first 2–8 weeks of therapy for clinical response with a subsequent decrease to below detectable levels achieved by 24 weeks.

1. **Reverse transcriptase inhibitors** are either classified as nucleosides or nucleotides. These agents are competitive inhibitors of reverse transcriptase, which leads to chain termination when incorporated into the viral DNA chain. They are inactive until phosphorylated by human cellular kinases into the active triphosphate metabolite. Each agent in this class of antiretrovirals requires dosage adjustment in patients with renal dysfunction. **All agents in the nucleoside class have a black box warning concerning the potential for development of lactic acidosis and severe hepatomegaly with steatosis.**
   a. **Abacavir** is a synthetic carbocyclic nucleoside analogue indicated for the treatment of both adult and pediatric patients with HIV.
      (1) **Mechanism of action** (see VII C 1)
      (2) **Spectrum of activity and therapeutic uses.** Abacavir is approved for use in adults and children >3 months of age only in combination with other antiretroviral agents. It has good penetration into the cerebral spinal fluid, unlike other agents in this class.
      (3) **Precautions and monitoring effects.** Abacavir has a **black box warning** about a life-threatening hypersensitivity reaction that can lead to death. It occurs in approximately 5% of patients taking this drug, typically within the first 6 weeks of therapy. This reaction involves respiratory symptoms, fever, rash, and GI complaints. A high percentage of these reactions have occurred in females. Reexposure if these adverse effects occur is contraindicated.
      (4) **Significant interactions.** None reported currently

Table 43-5. Current National Guidelines for Anti-HIV Treatment

- **Treatment is based on the use of highly active antiretroviral therapy (HAART)**

When to begin treatment:
- Treat any symptomatic patient (severe symptoms or AIDS)
- Treat any asymptomatic or AIDS patients with CD4 <200 and any value of HIV RNA (RT–PCR).
- Offer treatment if asymptomatic patient with CD4 >200 but <350 and any value of HIV RNA.
  - Some recommend observing or treating asymptomatic patients with CD4 >350 and HIV RNA > 55,000.
- Observe and defer treatment of asymptomatic patients with CD4 >350 and HIV RNA <55,000 (RT–PCR).

Preferred regimen:
- Choose one from the protease inhibitor (PI)/NNRTI list plus one from the nucleoside reverse transcriptase inhibitor (NRTI) combinations list.

PI or NNRTI	*NRTI combinations*
Indinavir	Zidovudine + lamivudine
Nelfinavir	Zidovudine + didanosine
Ritonavir + indinavir	Stavudine + didanosine
Ritonavir + lopinavir	Stavudine + lamivudine
Ritonavir + saquinavir (soft or hard gel cap)	Didanosine + lamivudine
Efavirenz	

Recommended Alternative Regimens:

Use these in place of the PI or NNRTI above	**Use in place of one of the NRTI combinations above**
Abacavir	Zidovudine + zalcitabine
Amprenavir	
Delaviridine	
Nelfinavir + saquinavir (soft gel cap)	
Nevirapine	
Ritonavir	
Saquinavir (soft gel cap)	

The Following Agents or Combinations Should Not Be Offered:
All monotherapies
Ritonavir + amprenavir
Ritonavir + nelfinavir
Tenofovir
Saquinavir (hard gel cap)
Hydroxyurea in combination with other antiretroviral agents
Zalcitabine plus any of the following: didanosine, lamivudine, stavudine
Zidovudine + stavudine

Monitoring:
- Before initiating drug therapy, need to obtain CD4 and HIV RNA levels plus complete blood count, chemistry, lipid profile, and liver enzymes.
- If HIV RNA does not fall by a 1.0 log decrease at 2–8 weeks and undetectable levels (<50 copies/mL) at 4–6 months, consider a regimen change.

HIV = human immunodeficiency virus; RT–PCR = reverse transcriptase-coupled polymerase chain reaction

    b. Dideoxyinosine (didanosine; ddI), a synthetic purine analogue, inhibits HIV-1 replication and is unique in having a long intracellular half-life (8–24 hours versus 3 hours for zidovudine).
      (1) Mechanism of action (see VII C 1)
      (2) Spectrum of activity and therapeutic uses. Didanosine has demonstrated a dose-dependent activity against HIV-1, resulting in lower virus production (p24 antigens); increases in peripheral blood CD4$^+$ cell counts; and increases in appetite, weight, and energy without significant neutropenia.

(a) It is approved for the treatment of adult and children in combination with other antiretroviral agents. Clinical trials have shown improved efficacy when used in combination with a PI, NNRTI, or another NRTI.

(b) Didanosine crosses the blood–brain barrier.

(3) Precautions and monitoring effects

(a) Didanosine can cause reversible peripheral neuropathy and acute, potentially lethal pancreatitis **(black box warning).** Serum triglycerides should be monitored, and ddI should be withheld when potential pancreatitis-inducing agents (e.g., IV pentamidine, sulfonamides) are given. Transiently elevated serum amylase may not reflect pancreatitis.

(b) Other adverse effects include headaches, diarrhea, nausea, and hyperuricemia (because ddI is catalyzed to uric acid).

(c) Didanosine is available in a specially buffered oral formulation to prevent degradation at acidic pH. It must be taken on an empty stomach.

(d) Do not use in combination with zalcitabine due to additive potential for toxicity.

(4) Significant interactions. Pancreatitis-inducing drugs, such as **cimetidine, ranitidine, sulfonamides, pentamidine,** and **alcohol, or those known to cause peripheral neuropathy,** should not be used with ddI.

c. **Lamivudine (3TC)** is a synthetic nucleoside analogue structurally related to zalcitabine with activity against HIV infection.

(1) Mechanism of action (see VII C 1)

(2) Spectrum of activity and therapeutic uses. Lamivudine is indicated for use in adults and children >3 months of age in combination with other antiretroviral agents. It is also used for the treatment of chronic hepatitis B in patients with active liver inflammation and evidence of hepatitis B viral replication.

(3) Precautions and monitoring effects

(a) Reported adverse reactions are minor and include headache, fatigue, and GI reactions such as nausea, vomiting, and diarrhea. CNS toxicity includes neuropathy, dizziness, and insomnia. Lab test abnormalities such as neutropenia and elevations in liver enzymes have also been reported.

(b) As with other antiviral therapies used for the treatment of HIV infection, lamivudine is not a cure for HIV infection, and patients may continue to acquire illnesses associated with HIV infection.

(c) Lamivudine has not been shown to reduce the risk of transmission of HIV through sexual contact.

(d) Do not use in combination with zalcitabine due to antagonism of effects and overlapping toxicities.

(4) Significant interactions

(a) Coadministration with **zidovudine** results in increased levels of zidovudine.

(b) Coadministration with **Bactrim** results in increased lamivudine levels.

d. **Stavudine (d4T)** is a synthetic thymidine nucleoside analogue that is active against HIV infection.

(1) Mechanism of action (see VII C 1)

(2) Spectrum of activity and therapeutic uses. Stavudine is indicated for use in combination with other antiretroviral agents in adults and children.

(3) Precautions and monitoring effects

(a) The major toxicity with stavudine is a dose-related but reversible peripheral neuropathy occurring in up to 21% of patients.

(b) Other adverse effects include headache, rash, sleep disorders, and abdominal pain.

(c) Fatal episodes of pancreatitis have been reported.

(d) Do not use in combination with zidovudine or zalcitabine.

(4) Significant interactions. No drug interactions have been reported with this agent.

e. **Tenofovir disoproxil fumarate (DF)** is an acyclic nucleoside phosphonate diester analogue **(nucleotide)** with antiviral activity against HIV.

(1) Mechanism of action. Tenofovir DF (a prodrug) is rapidly hydrolyzed by plasma esterases to tenofovir, with subsequent conversion to the active tenofovir diphosphate. Note: NtRTIs are active as the diphosphate, unlike the NRTIs, which require conversion to the triphosphate.

(2) Spectrum of activity and therapeutic uses. Tenofovir is approved for use in combination with other antiretroviral agents for the treatment of HIV in adults. Tenofovir has shown activity against nucleoside-resistant strains of HIV. However, more studies are needed to identify its proper place in therapy.

(3) Precautions and monitoring effects

(a) Minor adverse effects have been reported. These include complaints of diarrhea, vomiting, and nausea.

(b) Do not use in patients with CrCl <60 mL/min.

(c) Tenofovir must be taken with meals since oral bioavailability is poor.

(4) Significant interactions. Tenofovir may increase didanosine serum concentrations.

f. Zalcitabine (ddC) is a synthetic pyrimidine nucleoside analogue that is active against HIV.

(1) Mechanism of action (see VII C 1)

(2) Spectrum of activity and therapeutic uses. Zalcitabine is indicated for combination therapy with zidovudine for the treatment of adult patients with advanced HIV infection (CD4$^+$ cell count <300/mm^3).

(3) Precautions and monitoring effects

(a) The major clinical toxicity of zalcitabine is peripheral neuropathy, which occurs in up to 35% of patients and may be potentially fatal.

(b) Documented cases of pancreatitis have occurred alone or in combination with zidovudine. Serum amylase must be monitored.

(c) Other adverse effects include esophageal ulcers, cardiomyopathy, anaphylactoid reactions, and impaired hepatic function.

(d) Do not use in combination with didanosine, lamivudine, or stavudine.

(4) Significant interactions

(a) Drugs that have the potential to cause peripheral neuropathy should be avoided. These include **chloramphenicol, cisplatin, dapsone, disulfiram, ethambutol, glutethimide, gold, hydralazine, isoniazid, lithium, metronidazole, nitrofurantoin, phenytoin, ribavirin,** and **vincristine.**

(b) Zalcitabine treatment should be interrupted when a drug with the potential to cause pancreatitis is needed (i.e., **pentamidine**).

(c) Do not take with magnesium-, calcium-, or aluminum-containing antacids.

(d) Cimetidine and probenecid may increase zalcitabine levels, causing increased zalcitabine toxicity.

g. Zidovudine is a synthetic thymidine analogue. Formerly called azidothymidine (AZT), this agent was the first available drug for the treatment of HIV infection in patients with AIDS and AIDS-related complex (ARC).

(1) Mechanism of action (see VII C 1)

(2) Spectrum of activity and therapeutic uses

(a) Zidovudine has been shown to slow HIV-1 production, alleviate symptoms, and prolong life in some patients with AIDS.

(b) It is indicated for the prevention of maternal–fetal HIV transmission.

(c) Zidovudine is indicated in the treatment of adults and children over 3 months of age and in combination with zalcitabine for the treatment of HIV.

(d) Zidovudine can cross the blood–brain barrier.

(3) Precautions and monitoring effects

(a) Zidovudine can cause severe bone marrow suppression, including anemia, granulocytopenia, and thrombocytopenia, in up to 41% of patients after the first 4–8 weeks of therapy.

(b) Erythropoietin can be used as an alternative adjunctive therapy in patients with zidovudine-induced anemia.

(c) Other adverse effects include headache, malaise, seizures, anxiety, dyschromia, fever, and rash.

(d) Prolonged use may lead to symptomatic myopathy.

(4) Significant interactions

(a) **Co-trimoxazole, atovaquone, valproic acid, methadone, and probenecid** may increase zidovudine levels, causing increased zidovudine toxicity.

(b) Other **cytotoxic drugs, such as ganciclovir, amphotericin B, and pentamidine,** can cause additive bone marrow suppression.

(c) Acetaminophen, ribavirin, rifabutin, and rifampin may decrease levels of zidovudine.

h. Zidovudine/lamivudine. This was the first combination product approved by the FDA in 1997 for the treatment of HIV. This "drug cocktail" manufactured under the name Combivir was designed to improve compliance in patients by decreasing the number of tablets typically ingested daily when administered as individual agents. Adverse effects and drug interactions are the same as described for each agent above. Administered as lamivudine 150 mg/zidovudine 300 mg per tablet twice daily.

i. Zidovudine/lamivudine/abacavir. This was the first triple nucleoside combination approved by the FDA used alone or in combination with other antiretroviral agents for the treatment of HIV. It is administered as abacavir 300 mg/lamivudine 150 mg/zidovudine 300 mg per tablet twice daily. Adverse effects and drug interactions are the same as described above for each individual agent.

2. Nonnucleoside reverse transcriptase inhibitors. The NNRTI class binds directly to and produces a noncompetitive inhibition of the HIV-1 reverse transcriptase, leading to chain termination. These agents are indicated for use in adults and pediatric patients in combination with either NRTIs or possibly PIs. Their place in HIV therapy is still yet to be determined. Efavirenz is considered first-line therapy, whereas the others are currently recommended as alternatives to protease inhibitors.

a. Delavirdine

   (1) Mechanism of action (see VII C 2)

   (2) Spectrum of activity and therapeutic uses. Delavirdine is approved for use in adults in the treatment of HIV-1 in combination with other antiretroviral agents.

   (3) Precautions, monitoring effects, and significant interactions

   (a) It inhibits its own metabolism by reducing CYP3A4 and CYP2C9 activity and levels of indinavir and saquinavir; increases levels of terfenadine, astemizole, and cisapride with potential for cardiac arrhythmias; increases levels of midazolam, alprazolam, and triazolam, leading to increased sedation; and increases levels of clarithromycin, nifedipine, quinidine, and warfarin.

   (b) Decreased levels are seen when it is administered with St. John's wort, carbamazepine, phenobarbital, phenytoin, or rifampin.

   (c) It is important to review all medications before starting this agent due to its potential for numerous drug interactions.

   (d) The most frequent adverse effects are minor and include rash, headache, and nausea.

b. Efavirenz

   (1) Mechanism of action (see VII C 2)

   (2) Spectrum of activity and therapeutic uses. Efavirenz is approved for use in combination with other antiretroviral agents for the treatment of HIV-1 infection in adults and pediatric patients (>3 years of age). Advantage over other NNRTIs is once-daily dosing.

   (3) Precautions and monitoring effects. Most common adverse effects are CNS (52%), including insomnia, dizziness, drowsiness, nightmares, and hallucinations, and skin rashes (25%), with highest incidence noted in the pediatric population.

   (a) Take at bedtime for the first 4 weeks to decrease the incidence of CNS side effects.

   (4) Significant interactions. Efavirenz induces CYP3A4 enzyme and should not be used concomitantly with astemizole, cisapride, midazolam, triazolam, or ergot derivatives.

c. Nevirapine was the first NNRTI approved for use by the FDA for the treatment of HIV-1 infection.

   (1) Mechanism of action (see VII C 2)

   (2) Spectrum of activity and therapeutic uses. Nevirapine is indicated in combination with NRTIs in adults and pediatric (>2 months old) HIV patients as an alternative agent in those who have deteriorated clinically.

   (3) Precautions and monitoring effects

   (a) Most frequent adverse effects include rash (including Stevens-Johnson syndrome) and hepatotoxicity **(black box warning).** Others include fever, nausea, and headache.

   (b) To decrease the frequency of rash, begin with a low dose and titrate up.

   (4) Significant interactions. Nevirapine may induce CPY3A enzymes, resulting in decreased concentrations of caspofungin, ketoconazole, itraconazole, oral contraceptives, and protease inhibitors.

3. Protease inhibitors. This class includes **amprenavir, indinavir, lopinavir, nelfinavir, ritonavir,** and **saquinavir.** These agents are either used together or in combination with other antiretroviral agents. Current recommendations include one or two protease inhibitors in combination with two NRTIs to block HIV replication at different stages in the intracellular life cycle.

a. **Mechanism of action.** These agents competitively inhibit the viral protease enzyme, preventing the enzyme from cleaving the gag pol polyprotein necessary for the production of the infectious virions.

b. **Spectrum of activity.** These agents are active against HIV-1 protease.

c. **Therapeutic uses.** All of these agents are approved in combination with other antiretroviral agents for the treatment of HIV infection when antiretroviral therapy is warranted. Saquinavir was the first protease inhibitor approved by the FDA.

   (1) Cross-resistance between indinavir and ritonavir can occur but are not often noted with nelfinavir, lopinavir, amprenavir, or saquinavir.

   (2) **Amprenavir** (ages 4 years and older), **lopinavir** (ages 6 months and older), **nelfinavir** (ages 2 years and older) and **ritonavir** (children) are the only PIs approved for use in the pediatric population.

   (3) Saquinavir, ritonavir, and indinavir are not approved for use in the pediatric population.

   (4) Amprenavir has the longest half-life of all the PIs.

d. **Precautions and monitoring effects**

   (1) The **most common adverse events** in clinical trials were diarrhea, nausea, and abdominal discomfort. These agents can produce hyperglycemia. Glucose monitoring should be performed regularly while patients are on these medications. Use caution in patients with hemophilia because of the potential for increased bleeding episodes.

   (2) **Saquinavir** hard gel caps should be administered with fatty foods to improve bioavailability because the oral bioavailability alone is only 4%. Fortovase, a soft gel cap formulation of saquinavir, has improved bioavailability and efficacy and is the currently recommended formulation. Adverse effects are the same.

   (3) **Ritonavir** can cause taste disturbances, anorexia, elevated triglycerides, hepatic transaminases, and peripheral paresthesias.

   (4) **Indinavir** causes mild elevation of indirect bilirubin in approximately 10% of patients, which usually resolves without intervention; kidney stones are reported in 2%–3% of patients. Patients should drink at least 48 ounces of water daily to prevent nephrolithiasis. Dosage reduction is needed in patients with severe hepatic insufficiency. Indinavir must be dispensed in the original container with a desiccant to protect the agent from moisture.

   (5) **Nelfinavir** has few adverse effects, with diarrhea the most commonly reported.

   (6) **Amprenavir** is a sulfonamide with cross-sensitivity with other drugs in the sulfa class. Adverse effects are similar to those with nelfinavir, mainly GI. Patients should *not* take supplemental vitamin E since a high content is contained in the amprenavir capsules and solution.

   (7) Amprenavir and ritonavir are the only two PIs that carry a **black box warning.** Ritonavir when coadministered with certain medications can result in life-threatening adverse effects. Amprenavir is contraindicated in certain patient populations due to the potential toxicity from high amounts of the excipient propylene glycol in the oral solution.

e. **Significant interactions.** Rifampin reduces saquinavir concentrations by 80%. Rifabutin, phenobarbital, phenytoin, dexamethasone, and carbamazepine also lower saquinavir plasma concentrations. Ketoconazole and clarithromycin have increased saquinavir levels by 130%–180%.

   (1) **All protease inhibitors** are competitive inhibitors of drugs metabolized by the CYP3A family. These agents are contraindicated with the following drugs: terfenadine, astemizole, cisapride (which may result in high concentrations, causing cardiac arrhythmias), and midazolam and triazolam (resulting in prolonged sedation).

   (2) Ritonavir and nelfinavir should be taken with food; indinavir and amprenavir should be taken 1 hour before or 2 hours after meals.

   (3) Ritonavir has the highest incidence for potential drug interactions and has a **black box warning.** Check product information for the most current interaction information; this drug has a high potential to interact with many drugs.

f. **Lopinavir/ritonavir.** This is the first PI combination approved by the FDA for use in combination with other antiretroviral agents for the treatment of HIV. It is formulated as a 4:1 ratio of lopinavir to ritonavir. Ritonavir markedly reduces the metabolism of lopinavir, resulting in increased plasma concentrations. This was important since lopinavir has the shortest half-life of the PIs. The product is dosed twice daily with food to increase bioavailability. Dosing in children should be based on the lopinavir component. Adverse effects are mainly GI and include diarrhea, nausea, abdominal pain, and asthenia. Adverse effects and drug interactions are the same as described above for ritonavir. Use caution; the solution contains 42% alcohol.

g. Fusion inhibitors. Enfuvirtide is the first of a new class of antiretrovirals. It inhibits the entry of HIV-1 into CD4+ cells by interfering with the fusion of viral and cellular membranes. Approved for ages 6 and older, with other antiretroviral agents for treatment of advanced HIV-1 despite ongoing therapy. Adverse effects include local injection site reactions (nodules), hypersensitivity reactions, and pneumonia. No drug interactions with the CYP450 enzyme system or cross-resistance with other antiretrovirals reported.

VIII. ANTHELMINTICS

A. Definition. These drugs are used to rid the body of worms **(helminths).** These agents may act locally to rid the GI tract of worms or work systemically to eradicate worms that are invading organs or tissues.

B. Mebendazole is a synthetic benzimidazole-derivative anthelmintic.

1. **Mechanism of action.** Mebendazole interferes with reproduction and survival of helminths by inhibiting the formation of microtubules and irreversibly blocking glucose uptake, thereby depleting glycogen stores in the helminth.

2. **Spectrum of activity.** Mebendazole is active against nematodes (roundworms), which are pathogenic to humans: *Ancylostoma duodenale* (hookworm), *Angiostrongylus cantonensis, Ascaris lumbricoides* (roundworm), *Capillaria philippinensis* (Phillipine threadworm), *Enterobius vermicularis* (pinworm), *Gnathostoma spinigerum, Necator americanus* (hookworm), *Strongyloides stercoralis* (threadworm), *Trichinella spiralis* (pork worm), and *Trichuris thrichiura* (whipworm). Mebendazole also has activity against some cestodes (tapeworms), including *Hymenolepis nana* (dwarf tapeworm), *Taenia saginata* (beef tapeworm), *Taenia solium* (pork tapeworm), and *Echinococcus granulosus* (hydatid cyst).

3. **Therapeutic uses.** Mebendazole is used for the treatment of single or mixed infections with the prior-mentioned helminths. Immobilization and subsequent death of helminths are slow, with complete GI clearance up to 3 days after therapy.

4. **Precautions and monitoring effects**
   a. In cases of massive infection, abdominal pain, nausea, and massive diarrhea associated with expulsion of organisms may result.
   b. Myelosuppression (neutropenia and thrombocytopenia) can occur with high doses (30–50 mg/kg/day).
   c. Migration of roundworms through the nose and mouth have also been reported.
   d. If the patient is not cured in 3 weeks, retreatment is necessary.

5. **Significant interactions.** Agents that may reduce the blood levels and subsequent efficacy of mebendazole include carbamazepine and hydantoins.

C. Albendazole is a synthetic benzimidazole-derivative anthelmintic.

1. **Mechanism of action** (see VIII B 1)

2. **Spectrum of activity.** Albendazole is active against *T. solium* (pork tapeworm) and *E. granulosus* (dog tapeworm).

3. **Therapeutic uses.** Albendazole is used to treat parenchymal neurocysticercosis in combination with corticosteroids, as well as cystic hydatid disease (prior to and after surgical removal of the disease).

4. **Precautions and monitoring effects**
   a. The drug should be administered with a fatty meal to achieve optimal absorption.
   b. Hepatotoxicity occurs in 16% of patients; liver function tests every 2 weeks are recommended while taking albendazole.
   c. Rarely, leukopenia, thrombocytopenia, granulocytopenia, pancytopenia, and agranulocytosis occur. CBC should be checked every 2 weeks while taking albendazole.

D. Diethylcarbamazine citrate

1. **Mechanism of action.** Diethylcarbamazine citrate is a synthetic organic compound highly specific for several common parasites.

2. **Spectrum of activity.** This agent is active against *Wuchereria bancrofti, Brugia malayi, Dipetalonema streptocerca, Mansonella perstans, Mansonella ozzardi, Dirofilaria immitis, Ascaris,* and *Loa loa.*

3. **Therapeutic uses.** Diethylcarbamazine citrate is used for the treatment of Bancroft's filariasis, tropical eosinophilia, and loiasis.

4. **Precautions and monitoring effects**
   a. Patients treated for *W. bancrofti* infection often present with headache and general malaise. Severe allergic phenomena in conjunction with a skin rash have been reported.
   b. Patients treated for onchocerciasis present with pruritus and facial edema (termed a Mazzotti reaction). Severe reaction may be noted after a single dose. For this reason, **ivermectin** is used to treat onchocerciasis.
   c. Children who are undernourished or are suffering from debilitating ascariasis infection may experience giddiness, malaise, nausea, and vomiting after treatment. Other drugs are available to treat *Ascaris* (mebendazole and albendazole).

E. Pyrantel is a pyrimidine-derivative anthelmintic.

1. **Mechanism of action.** Pyrantel is a depolarizing neuromuscular blocking agent that causes a spastic paralysis of the helminth.

2. **Spectrum of activity.** Pyrantel is active against *A. lumbricoides* (roundworm) and *E. vermicularis* (pinworm), *A. duodenale* (hookworm), *N. americanus* (hookworm), and *Trichostrongylus orientalis* (hairworm).

3. **Therapeutic uses.** Pyrantel is used for the treatment of roundworm, pinworm, and hookworm infections.

4. **Precautions and monitoring effects**
   a. Most commonly reported reactions include anorexia, nausea, vomiting, diarrhea, headache, and rash.
   b. A single dose may be mixed with food, milk, juice, or taken on an empty stomach.

5. **Significant interactions.** When **piperazine** is used with pyrantel, the agents are antagonistic.

F. Thiabendazole, a pyrazinoisoquinolone derivative, is a synthetic heterocyclic anthelmintic.

1. **Mechanism of action** is not known precisely. Thiabendazole is shown to inhibit the helminth-specific enzyme, fumarate reductase. Thiabendazole also demonstrates anti-inflammatory, antipyretic, and analgesic effects.

2. **Spectrum of activity.** It is active against most intestinal nematodes (roundworms): *Ancylostoma braziliense* (dog and cat hookworm), *Ancylostoma caninum* (dog hookworm), *A. duodenale* (hookworm), *A. lumbricoides* (roundworm), *C. philippinensis* (Philippine threadworm), *Dracunculus medinensis* (guinea worm), *E. vermicularis* (pinworm), *N. americanus* (hookworm), *T. trichiura* (whipworm), *T. spiralis;* and is active against the fungi *Trichophyton* and *Microsporum* species.

3. **Therapeutic uses.** Thiabendazole is used for the treatment of strongyloidiasis (threadworm), cutaneous larva migrans (creeping eruption), and toxocariasis visceral larva migrans. It is used for the treatment of uncinariasis (hookworm), *N. americanus, A. duodenale,* trichuriasis (whipworm), and ascariasis (large roundworm) when more specific therapy is unavailable or further treatment is required with a second agent.

4. **Precautions and monitoring effects**
   a. Adverse effects of thiabendazole are usually mild and transient, occurring 3–4 hours after the drug has been administered and lasting for 2–8 hours.
   b. Most common reactions include anorexia, nausea, vomiting, and dizziness.
   c. Giddiness, seizures, vertigo, paresthesias, and psychic disturbances may also occur, but less frequently.
   d. If hypersensitivity develops, the drug should be discontinued. Erythema multiforme (including Stevens-Johnson syndrome) has been reported.

5. Significant interactions. Serum **xanthine** levels (theophylline and caffeine) may increase.

G. Piperazine

1. **Mechanism of action.** Piperazine causes flaccid paralysis of the helminth by blocking the response of ascaris muscle to acetylcholine.

2. **Spectrum of activity.** It is active against *A. lumbricoides* (roundworm) and *E. vermicularis* (pinworm).

3. **Therapeutic uses.** Piperazine is used for the treatment of enterobiasis (pinworm) and ascariasis (roundworm).

4. **Precautions and monitoring effects**
   a. The most commonly reported reactions include GI and CNS effects. If these effects become significant, therapy should be discontinued.
   b. Piperazine should be taken on an empty stomach.
   c. Prolonged, repeated, and excessive therapy (particularly in children) should be avoided due to potential neurotoxicity.
   d. Allergic or severe hypersensitivity reactions can occur.
   e. Piperazine can also cause hemolytic anemia.

H. Quinacrine (see also V C)

1. **Mechanism of action.** Quinacrine eradicates intestinal cestodes.

2. **Spectrum of activity.** Quinacrine is active against *T. saginata* (beef tapeworm), *T. solium* (pork tapeworm), *H. nana* (dwarf tapeworm), *Diphyllobothrium latum* (fish tapeworm), and the protozoa *Giardia lamblia*.

3. **Therapeutic uses.** Quinacrine is used for the treatment of *giardiasis* and *cestodiasis.*

4. **Precautions and monitoring effects**
   a. This agent should be used with caution in patients with hepatic disease.
   b. It may cause a transitory psychosis and should, therefore, be used with caution in those individuals over 60 years of age or with a history of psychosis.

I. Niclosamide

1. **Mechanism of action.** Niclosamide inhibits the oxidative phosphorylation in the mitochondria of cestodes.

2. **Therapeutic uses.** Niclosamide is used against *T. saginata* (beef tapeworm), *D. latum* (fish tapeworm), and *H. nana* (dwarf tapeworm).

3. **Precautions and monitoring effects**
   a. This agent may cause nausea, vomiting, dizziness, and drowsiness.
   b. It is not active against cysticercosis because it affects the cestodes of the intestine only.

J. Oxamniquine

1. **Mechanism of action.** Oxamniquine eradicates male and female schistosomes. Although it is less effective against female schistosomes, the residual females cease to lay eggs and lose the parasitological activity.

2. **Therapeutic uses.** This agent is active against *Schistosoma mansoni* infection, including the acute and chronic phases with hepatosplenic involvement.

3. **Precautions and monitoring effects**
   a. Convulsions may occur within a few hours of the first dose in patients with a previous seizure history.
   b. Transitory dizziness, drowsiness, nausea, vomiting, and urticaria may occur.
   c. Oxamniquine should be taken with food to increase GI tolerance.

K. Praziquantel

1. **Mechanism of action.** Praziquantel increases cell membrane permeability in susceptible helminths, with loss of intracellular calcium and paralysis of their musculature. Vacuolization and disintegration of the schistosome tegument result, followed by attachment of phagocytes to the parasite and death.

2. **Spectrum of activity.** Praziquantel is active against trematodes (flukes), including all *Schistosoma* species and *Clonorchis sinensis, Opisthorchis viverrini,* and *Fasciola hepatica* (liver flukes*); Paragonimus westermani, Paragonimus uterobilateralis,* and *Paragonimus kellicotti* (lung flukes); *Metagonimus yokogawai, Nanophyetus salmincola, Fasciolopsis buski,* and *Heterophyes heterophyes* (intestinal flukes).

3. **Therapeutic uses.** Praziquantel is active in treating schistosomiasis, all types that are pathogenic to humans; clonorchiasis and opisthorchiasis (Chinese and southeast Asian liver flukes); many other types of infections involving intestinal, liver, and lung flukes; and cestodiasis (tapeworm) infections.

4. **Precautions and monitoring effects**
   a. Treatment of ocular cysticercosis is contraindicated because parasite destruction within the eyes may cause irreparable lesions.
   b. In general, adverse effects are generally mild and well tolerated. It is difficult to differentiate between effects caused by the praziquantal versus effects demonstrated by dying parasites.
   c. The most common side effects are transient and may include malaise, headache, dizziness, and abdominal discomfort.
   d. Hepatic transaminase elevations (AST and ALT) have also frequently occurred.
   e. Praziquantal may impair activities that require mental alertness.

STUDY QUESTIONS

Directions: Each of the numbered items or incomplete statements in this section is followed by answers or by completions of the statement. Select the **one** lettered answer or completion that is **best** in each case.

1. Isoniazid is a primary antitubercular agent that

(A) requires pyridoxine supplementation
(B) may discolor the tears, saliva, urine, or feces orange-red
(C) causes ocular complications that are reversible if the drug is discontinued
(D) may be ototoxic and nephrotoxic
(E) should never be used due to hepatotoxic potential

2. All of the following factors may increase the risk of nephrotoxicity from gentamicin therapy EXCEPT

(A) age over 70 years
(B) prolonged courses of gentamicin therapy
(C) concurrent amphotericin B therapy
(D) trough gentamicin levels below 2 mg/mL
(E) concurrent cisplatin therapy

3. In which of the following groups do all four drugs warrant careful monitoring for drug-related seizures in high-risk patients?

(A) Penicillin G, imipenem, amphotericin B, metronidazole
(B) Penicillin G, chloramphenicol, tetracycline, vancomycin
(C) Imipenem, tetracycline, vancomycin, sulfadiazine
(D) Cycloserine, metronidazole, vancomycin, sulfadiazine
(E) Metronidazole, imipenem, doxycycline, erythromycin

4. Spectinomycin is an aminoglycoside-like antibiotic indicated for the treatment of

(A) gram-negative bacillary septicemia
(B) tuberculosis
(C) penicillin-resistant gonococcal infections
(D) syphilis
(E) gram-negative meningitis due to susceptible organisms

5. A man has an *Escherichia coli* bacteremia with a low-grade fever (101.6°F). Appropriate management of his fever would be to

(A) give acetaminophen 650 mg orally every 4 hours
(B) give aspirin 650 mg orally every 4 hours
(C) give alternating doses of aspirin and acetaminophen every 4 hours
(D) withhold antipyretics, and use the fever curve to monitor his response to antibiotic therapy
(E) use tepid water baths to reduce the fever

6. A woman has an upper respiratory infection. Six years ago, she experienced an episode of bronchospasm following penicillin V therapy. The cultures now reveal a strain of *Streptococcus pneumoniae* that is sensitive to all of the following drugs. Which of these drugs would be the best choice for this patient?

(A) Amoxicillin/clavulanate
(B) Erythromycin
(C) Ampicillin
(D) Cefaclor
(E) Cyclacillin

7. All of the following drugs are suitable oral therapy for a lower urinary tract infection due to *Pseudomonas aeruginosa* EXCEPT

(A) norfloxacin
(B) trimethoprim–sulfamethoxazole
(C) ciprofloxacin
(D) carbenicillin
(E) methenamine mandelate

8. A woman's neglected hangnail has developed into a mild staphylococcal cellulitis. Which of the following regimens would be appropriate oral therapy?

(A) Dicloxacillin 125 mg q6h
(B) Vancomycin 250 mg q6h
(C) Methicillin 500 mg q6h
(D) Cefazolin 1 g q8h
(E) Penicillin V 500 mg q6h

9. Which of the following drugs has demonstrated in vitro activity against *Mycobacterium avium-intracellulare* (MAI)?

(A) Vancomycin
(B) Clarithromycin
(C) Erythromycin base
(D) Troleandomycin
(E) Erythromycin estolate

10. All of the following statements regarding pentamidine isethionate are true EXCEPT

(A) it is indicated for treatment or prophylaxis of infection due to *Pneumocystis carinii*
(B) it may be administered intramuscularly, intravenously, or by inhalation
(C) it has no clinically significant effect on serum glucose
(D) it is effective in the treatment of leishmaniasis

11. RE is a 23-year-old male with a history of influenza A infections. An outbreak of influenza A has just been reported in his community, and he is exhibiting initial symptoms of influenza A. Which agent would be the most useful to treat RE?

(A) Cidofovir
(B) Famciclovir
(C) Rimantidine
(D) Foscarnet
(E) Ribavirin

12. Dr. Jones requests your help in prescribing a protease inhibitor for his patient. He has heard that not all agents are the same and asks for your recommendation as to which agent would penetrate the blood–brain barrier. Which agent would you recommend?

(A) Saquinavir
(B) Ritonavir
(C) Indinavir
(D) Nelfinavir
(E) Amprenavir

Directions: Each item below contains three suggested answers, of which **one or more** is correct. Choose the answer

A	if **I only** is correct
B	if **III only** is correct
C	if **I and II** are correct
D	if **II and III** are correct
E	if **I, II, and III** are correct

13. Drugs usually active against penicillinase-producing *Staphylococcus aureus* include which of the following?

I. Timentin (ticarcillin–clavulanate)
II. Augmentin (amoxicillin–clavulanate)
III. Oxacillin

14. Antiviral agents that are active against cytomegalovirus (CMV) include which of the following?

I. Ganciclovir
II. Foscarnet
III. Acyclovir

Directions: The group of items in this section consists of lettered options followed by a set of numbered items. For each item, select the **one** lettered option that is most closely associated with it. Each lettered option may be selected once, more than once, or not at all.

Questions 15–17

Match the following statements about effects or dosages with the appropriate drug.

(A) Clofazimine
(B) Itraconazole
(C) Lomefloxacin
(D) Neomycin

15. It may be administered once per day for the treatment of urinary tract infections

16. It may cause pink-to-brownish skin pigmentation within a few weeks of initiation of therapy

17. Coadministration with astemizole or terfenadine may lead to life-threatening cardiac dysrhythmias

ANSWERS AND EXPLANATIONS

1. The answer is A *[V B 2 d (5)]*.
Isoniazid increases the excretion of pyridoxine, which can lead to peripheral neuritis, particularly in poorly nourished patients. Pyridoxine (a form of vitamin B_6) deficiency may cause convulsions as well as the neuritis, involving synovial tenderness and swelling. Treatment with the vitamin can reverse the neuritis and prevent or cure the seizures.

2. The answer is D *[II B 4 b]*.
Trough serum levels below 2 mg/mL are considered appropriate for gentamicin and are recommended to minimize the risk of toxicity from this aminoglycoside. Because aminoglycosides accumulate in the proximal tubule of the kidney, nephrotoxicity can occur.

3. The answer is A *[II E 1 e (2), J 5 d (2); III B 4 b; IV C 3 c]*.
Seizures have been attributed to the use of penicillin G, imipenem, amphotericin B, and metronidazole. Seizures are especially likely with high doses in patients with a history of seizures and in patients with impaired drug elimination.

4. The answer is C *[II J 6]*.
Although active against various gram-negative organisms, spectinomycin is approved only for the treatment of gonorrhea and is particularly recommended for treatment of uncomplicated forms of the disease.

5. The answer is D *[I H 1]*.
The fever curve is very useful for monitoring a patient's response to antimicrobial therapy. Antipyretics can be used to reduce high fever in patients at risk for complications (e.g., seizures) or, in some cases, to make the patient more comfortable.

6. The answer is B *[II D 3 b]*.
Amoxicillin, ampicillin, and cyclacillin are all penicillins and should be avoided in patients with histories of hypersensitivity to other penicillin compounds. Although the risk of cross-reactivity with cephalosporins (e.g., cefaclor) is now considered very low, most clinicians avoid the use of these agents in patients with histories of type I hypersensitivity reactions (e.g., anaphylaxis, bronchospasm, giant hives).

7. The answer is B *[II E 4, H 3 a, b, I 2 a, 3 a, J 7]*.
Norfloxacin, ciprofloxacin, carbenicillin, and methenamine mandelate achieve urine concentrations high enough to treat urinary tract infections due to *Pseudomonas aeruginosa*. Trimethoprim–sulfamethoxazole is not useful for treating infection due to this organism, although the combination is useful for treating certain other urinary tract infections.

8. The answer is A *[II C, E 1 c (3), 2 b, J 8]*.
Although vancomycin, methicillin, and cefazolin have excellent activity against staphylococci, they are not effective orally for systemic infections. Vancomycin is prescribed orally for infections limited to the gastrointestinal tract, but because it is poorly absorbed orally, it is not effective for systemic infections. Most hospital- and community-acquired staphylococci are currently resistant to penicillin V. Thus, of the drugs listed in the question, the most appropriate drug for oral therapy of staphylococcal cellulitis is dicloxacillin.

9. The answer is B *[II D 6 a, b]*.
Clarithromycin, an alternative to erythromycin, has demonstrated in vitro activity against *Mycobacterium avium-intracellulare* (MAI). Clarithromycin is also used against *Toxoplasma gondii* and *Cryptosporidium* species, and it is more active than erythromycin against staphylococci and streptococci. Vancomycin is used to treat staphylococci and streptococci, but has no demonstarted activity versus MAI. Troleandomycin is similar to erythromycin but is generally less active against these organisms.

10. The answer is C *[IV D]*.
Pentamidine isethionate is indicated for both treatment and prophylaxis of infection due to *Pneumocystis carinii*. It can be administered intramuscularly, intravenously, or by inhalation. Inhalation may produce bronchospasm. Blood glucose should be carefully monitored because pentamidine may produce either hyperglycemia or hypoglycemia.

11. The answer is C *[VI B 7].*
Cidofovir, famciclovir, and foscarnet have little or no in vivo activity against influenza A. Ribavirin has some activity but is a second-line agent for influenza A and is mainly indicated for treatment of RSV. Rimantidine is a derivative of amantidine with excellent activity against influenza A. It is indicated for the prophylaxis and treatment of influenza A viral infections.

12. The answer is D *[VI C 3 c].*
All are protease inhibitors, but only nelfinavir has been shown to cross the blood–brain barrier, a known reservoir for HIV viruses.

13. The answer is E (all) *[II E 2–4].*
Timentin and augmentin each include a β-lactamase inhibitor, combined with ticarcillin and amoxicillin, respectively. These combinations offer activity against *Staphylococcus aureus* similar to that of the penicillinase-resistant penicillins, such as oxacillin.

14. The answer is C (I and II) *[VI B, F, G].*
Only ganciclovir and foscarnet are active against cytomegalovirus (CMV) infections. These agents are virustatic and arrest DNA synthesis by inhibiting viral DNA polymerase. Although ganciclovir can penetrate the central nervous system (CNS), the use of ganciclovir in the treatment of CMV infections in the CNS has not been successful. Foscarnet is a broad-spectrum antiviral agent and is used in patients with ganciclovir resistance. Acyclovir is not clinically useful for the treatment of CMV infections because CMV is relatively resistant to acyclovir in vitro.

15–17. The answers are 15-C *[II H 3 c],* **16-A** *[II J 9],* **17-B** *[III E 5 d].*
Lomefloxacin may be administered daily for treating urinary tract infections. Enoxacin is another fluoroquinolone used to treat urinary tract infections. Compared to other fluoroquinolones, neither lomefloxacin nor enoxacin improves the spectrum of activity.

Because clofazimine contains phenazine dye, it can cause pink-to-brown skin pigmentation. This change in pigmentation occurs in 75%–100% of patients taking clofazimine, and it occurs within a few weeks of the initiation of therapy. The discoloration of skin has reportedly led to severe depression and even suicide in some patients. Clofazimine is used in the treatment of leprosy and several atypical *Mycobacterium* infections.

Administration of itraconazole or ketoconazole with astemizole or terfenadine may increase the level of astemizole or terfenadine, which can lead to life-threatening dysrhythmias and death. Itraconazole, which is an imidazole, is a fungistatic agent. Specifically, itraconazole can be taken orally to treat aspergillosis infections and other deep fungal infections, such as blastomycosis, coccidioidomycosis, cryptococcosis, and histoplasmosis.

44

Seizure Disorders

Azita Razzaghi

I. INTRODUCTION

A. Definitions

1. **Seizures** are characterized by an excessive, hypersynchronous discharge of cortical neuron activity, which can be measured by the electroencephalogram (EEG). In addition, there may be disturbances in consciousness, sensory motor systems, subjective well-being, and objective behavior; seizures are usually brief, with a beginning and an end, and may produce postseizure impairment.

2. **Epilepsy** is defined as a chronic seizure disorder, or group of disorders, characterized by seizures that usually recur unpredictably in the absence of a consistent provoking factor. The term epilepsy is derived from the Greek word meaning "to seize upon" or "taking hold of." It was first described by Hughlings Jackson in the 19th century as an intermittent derangement of the nervous system due to a sudden, excessive, disorderly discharge of cerebral neurons.

3. **Convulsions** are violent, involuntary contractions of the voluntary muscles. A patient may have epilepsy or a seizure disorder without convulsions.

B. Classification.
An alternative seizure classification is being developed that is purely symptom based. This consists of four categories: sensorial (auras), consciousness, autonomic, and motor. Also, the international league against epilepsy is establishing a 4-level descriptive seizure classification based on symptoms, apathophysiological seizure, an epileptic syndrome, and functional disability. At present, there are two systems of classification of seizure disorder: The first system is based on the seizure type and the characteristics of the seizures (Table 44-1), and the second system is based on the characteristics of the epilepsy, including age at onset, etiological factors, and frequency, as well as the characteristics of the seizures as in the first classification system (Table 44-2).

1. **Partial seizures** are the most common seizure type, occurring in approximately 80% of epileptic patients.
   a. **Clinical and EEG changes** indicate initial activation of a system of neurons limited to part of one cerebral hemisphere that may spread to other or all brain areas. Manifestations of the seizures depend on the site of the epileptogenic focus in the brain.
   b. Partial seizures are subclassified as **simple** (usually unilateral involvement) or **complex** (usually bilateral involvement). Impairment of consciousness is a feature of complex seizures. Consciousness is defined as the degree of awareness and responsiveness of the patient to externally applied stimuli.
      (1) **Simple partial seizures** generally do not cause loss of consciousness. **Signs and symptoms** of simple partial seizures may be primarily motor, sensory, somatosensory, autonomic, or behavioral. These signs and symptoms may help pinpoint the site of the abnormal brain discharge, for example, localized numbness or tingling reflects a dysfunction in the sensory cortex, located in the parietal lobe.
         (a) **Motor signs** include convulsive jerking, chewing motions, and lip smacking.
         (b) **Sensory and somatosensory manifestations** include paresthesias and auras.
         (c) **Autonomic signs** include sweating, flushing, and pupil dilation.
         (d) **Behavioral manifestations,** which are sometimes accompanied by impaired consciousness, include déjà vu experiences, structured hallucinations, and dysphasia.
      (2) **Complex partial seizures** are accompanied by impaired consciousness; however, in some cases, the impairment precedes or follows the seizure. These seizures have variable manifestations.
         (a) Purposeless behavior is common.
         (b) The affected person may have a glassy stare, may wander about aimlessly, and may speak unintelligibly.

Table 44-1. International Classification of Epileptic Seizures

I. Partial seizures (seizures beginning locally)
  A. Simple partial seizures (consciousness not impaired)
    1. With motor symptoms
    2. With somatosensory or special sensory symptoms
    3. With autonomic symptoms
    4. With behavioral symptoms
  B. Complex partial seizures (with impairment of consciousness)
    1. Beginning as simple partial seizures and progressing to impairment of consciousness
      a. Without automatisms
      b. With automatisms
    2. With impairment of consciousness at onset
      a. With no other features
      b. With features of simple partial seizures
      c. With automatisms
  C. Partial seizures (simple or complex), secondarily generalized
II. Generalized seizures (bilaterally symmetric, without localized onset)
  A. Absence seizures
    1. True absence seizures (petit mal)
    2. Atypical absence seizures
  B. Myoclonic seizures
  C. Clonic seizures
  D. Tonic seizures
  E. Tonic–clonic seizures (grand mal)
  F. Atonic seizures
III. Unclassified seizures

Reprinted from Commission on Classification and Terminology of the International League Against Epilepsy. Proposal for classification of epilepsies and epileptic syndromes. *Epilepsia* 1985;26(3):268–278.

    (c) Psychomotor (temporal lobe) epilepsy may lead to aggressive behavior (e.g., outbursts of rage or violence).
    (d) Postictal confusion usually persists for 1–2 minutes after the seizure ends.
    (e) Automatism (e.g., picking at clothes) is common and may follow visual, auditory, or olfactory hallucinations.
  2. Generalized seizures are diffuse, affecting both cerebral hemispheres.
    a. Clinical and EEG changes indicate initial involvement of both hemispheres.
      (1) Consciousness may be impaired, and this impairment may be the initial manifestation.
      (2) Motor manifestations are bilateral.
      (3) The ictal EEG patterns initially are bilateral and presumably reflect neuronal discharge, which is widespread in both hemispheres.
    b. There are three **types** of generalized seizures.
      (1) Idiopathic epilepsies have an age-related onset, typical clinical and EEG characteristics, and a presumed genetic etiology.
      (2) Symptomatic epilepsies are considered the consequence of a known or suspected underlying disorder of the central nervous system (CNS).
      (3) Cryptogenic epilepsy refers to a disorder whose cause is hidden or occult; it is presumed to be symptomatic, but the etiologic factors are unknown. It is age-related, but often does not have well-defined clinical and EEG characteristics.
    c. Signs and symptoms of generalized seizures may be minor or major.
      (1) Absence (petit mal) seizures present as alterations of consciousness (absences) lasting 10–30 seconds.
        (a) Staring (with occasional eye blinking) and loss or reduction in postural tone are typical. If the seizure takes place during conversation, the individual may break off in midsentence.
        (b) Enuresis and other autonomic components may occur during absence seizures.
        (c) Some patients experience 100 or more absences daily.

Table 44-2. Classification of Epilepsies and Epileptic Syndromes

I. **Localized-related (focal, local, partial) epilepsies** and **syndromes**
   A. **Idiopathic** (with age-related onset)
      1. Benign childhood epilepsy with centrotemporal spikes (rolandic epilepsy)
      2. Childhood epilepsy with occipital paroxysms
   B. **Symptomatic**
      1. Chronic progressive epilepsia partialis continua of childhood
      2. Syndromes characterized by specific modes of precipitation
      3. Temporal lobe epilepsies
      4. Frontal lobe epilepsies
      5. Parietal lobe epilepsies
      6. Occipital lobe epilepsies
   C. **Cryptogenic**
II. **Generalized epilepsies and syndromes**
   A. **Idiopathic** (with age-related onset)
      1. Benign neonatal familial convulsions
      2. Benign neonatal convulsions
      3. Benign myoclonic epilepsy in infancy
      4. Childhood absence epilepsy (pyknolepsy)
      5. Juvenile absence epilepsy
      6. Juvenile myoclonic epilepsy
      7. Epilepsy with generalized tonic–clonic seizures on awakening
      8. Other generalized idiopathic epilepsies not defined above
      9. Epilepsies with seizures precipitated by specific modes of activation
   B. **Cryptogenic or symptomatic** (in order of age)
      1. West syndrome (infantile spasms)
      2. Lennox-Gastaut syndrome
      3. Epilepsy with myoclonic–astatic seizures
      4. Epilepsy with myoclonic absences
   C. **Symptomatic**
      1. **Nonspecific etiology**
         a. Early myoclonic encephalopathy
         b. Early infantile epileptic encephalopathy with suppression burst
         c. Other symptomatic generalized epilepsies not defined above
      2. **Specific syndromes** and generalized seizures complicating other disease states
III. **Epilepsies and syndromes undetermined whether focal or generalized**
   A. **With both focal and generalized seizures**
      1. Neonatal seizures
      2. Severe myoclonic epilepsy in infancy
      3. Epilepsy with continuous spike waves during slow-wave sleep
      4. Acquired epileptic aphasia (Landau-Kleffner syndrome)*
      5. Other undetermined epilepsies not defined above
   B. **Without unequivocal generalized or focal features**
IV. **Special situations**
   A. Febrile convulsions
   B. Isolated seizures or isolated status epilepticus
   C. Seizures occurring only when there is an acute metabolic or toxic event due to such factors as alcohol, drugs, eclampsia, and nonketotic hyperglycemia

*Believed to be a localized-related epilepsy.

Reprinted from Bleck TP. Convulsive disorders: the use of anticonvulsant drugs. *Clin Neuropharmacol* 1990;13(3): 198–209.

        (d) Onset of this seizure type occurs from ages 3–16 years; in most patients, absence seizures disappear by age 40.

   (2) Myoclonic (bilateral massive epileptic myoclonus) seizures present as involuntary jerking of the facial, limb, or trunk muscles, possibly in a rhythmic manner.

   (3) Clonic seizures are characterized by sustained muscle contractions alternating with relaxation.

   (4) Tonic seizures involve sustained tonic muscle extension (stiffening).

(5) Generalized (grand mal) tonic–clonic seizures cause sudden loss of consciousness.

    (a) The individual becomes rigid and falls to the ground. Respirations are interrupted. The legs extend, and the back arches; contraction of the diaphragm may induce grunting. This tonic phase lasts for about 1 minute.

    (b) A clonic phase follows, marked by rapid bilateral muscle jerking, muscle flaccidity, and hyperventilation. Incontinence, tongue biting, tachycardia, and heavy salivation sometimes occur.

    (c) During the postictal phase, the individual may experience headache, confusion, disorientation, nausea, drowsiness, and muscle soreness. This phase may last for hours.

    (d) Some epileptics have serial grand mal seizures, regaining consciousness briefly between attacks. In some cases, grand mal seizures occur repeatedly with no recovery of consciousness between attacks (**status epilepticus**); this disorder is discussed in III A.

(6) Atonic seizures (drop attacks) are characterized by a sudden loss of postural tone so that the individual falls to the ground. They occur primarily in children.

C. Epidemiology

  1. Most common neurological disorder

  2. Epilepsy has a prevalence of approximately 1% (i.e., 500,000 cases per 50 million persons worldwide).

  3. In the United States, the prevalence of epilepsy is 6.42 cases per 1000 people.

  4. The onset of seizures is greatest during the first year of life; this probability decreases each decade after the first year until age 60. Approximately 1 of 50 children and 1 of 100 adults are affected.

  5. Approximately 70% of epileptics have only one seizure type; the remainder have two or more seizure types.

D. Etiology. Some seizures arise secondary to other conditions. However, in most cases, the cause of the seizure is unknown.

  1. Primary (idiopathic) seizures have no identifiable cause.

    a. This type of seizure affects about 75% of epileptics.

    b. The onset of primary seizures typically occurs before age 20.

    c. Birth trauma, hereditary factors, and unexplained metabolic disturbances have been proposed as possible causes.

  2. Secondary seizures (symptomatic or **acquired seizures)** occur secondary to an identifiable cause.

    a. Disorders that may lead to secondary seizures include:

      (1) Intracranial neoplasms

      (2) Infectious diseases, such as meningitis, influenza, toxoplasmosis, mumps, measles, and syphilis

      (3) High fever (in children)

      (4) Head trauma

      (5) Congenital diseases

      (6) Metabolic disorders, such as hypoglycemia and hypocalcemia

      (7) Alcohol or drug withdrawal

      (8) Lipid storage disorders

      (9) Developmental abnormalities

    b. Age at seizure onset is associated with specific etiologies (Table 44-3).

E. Pathophysiology. Seizures reflect a sudden, abnormal, excessive neuronal discharge in the cerebral cortex. Any abnormal neuronal discharge could precipitate a seizure (Figure 44-1).

  1. Normal firing of neurons, which usually originate from the gray matter of one or more cortical or subcortical areas, requires the following elements:

    a. Voltage-dependent ion channels are involved in action-potential propagation or burst generation.

    b. Neurotransmitters control neuronal firing, including excitatory neurotransmitters, acetylcholine, norepinephrine, histamine, corticotropin-releasing factors (CRFs), inhibitory

Table 44-3. Probable Causes of Recurrent Seizures by Age Group

Age at Seizure Onset	Probable Cause of Seizure
Birth–1 month	Birth injury or anoxia, congenital hereditary diseases, and metabolic disorders
1–6 months	As above, plus infantile spasms
6 months–2 years	Infantile spasms, febrile convulsions, birth injury or anoxia, meningitis, and head trauma
3–10 years	Birth injury or anoxia, meningitis, cerebral vessel thrombosis, and idiopathic epilepsy
10–18 years	Idiopathic epilepsy and head trauma
18–25 years	Idiopathic epilepsy, trauma, neoplasm, and withdrawal from alcohol or drugs
35–60 years	Trauma, neoplasm, vascular disease, and withdrawal from alcohol or drugs
Over 60 years	Vascular disease, neoplasm, degenerative disease, and trauma

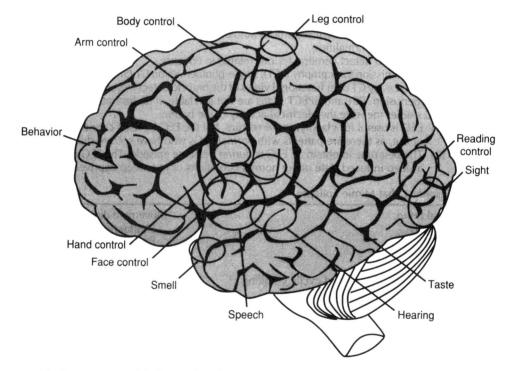

Figure 44-1. Gross anatomy of the brain. Clinical manifestation of seizures depends on the area of the cortex that is affected and its function, the degree of irritability, and the identity of the impulse.

neurotransmitters, γ-aminobutyric acid (GABA), and dopamine; therefore, for normal neuronal activity, there is a need for adequate ions (e.g., sodium, potassium, calcium); excitatory and inhibitory neurotransmitters; and glucose, oxygen, amino acids, and adequate systemic pH.

c. Epileptics may be **genetically** predisposed to a **lower seizure threshold.**

d. **A diencephalic nerve group** that normally suppresses excessive brain discharge may be deafferentated, hypersensitive, and vulnerable to activation by various stimuli in epileptics.

e. During seizures, there is an increased use of energy, oxygen, and, consequently, an increased production of carbon dioxide. Because of the limited capacity to increase the blood flow to the brain, the blood supply may be **oxygen deficient.** The ratio of supply to demand decreases when the seizure episode is prolonged, leading to increased ischemia and neuronal destruction. Thus, it is crucial to diagnose seizures and treat them as soon as possible.

2. **Abnormal electrical brain activity** occurring during a seizure usually produces **characteristic changes on the EEG.** Each part of the cortical area has its own function, and the clinical presentation of a seizure depends on the site, the degree of irritability of the area, and the intensity of the impulse.

3. Seizure activity may include three major **phases.**
    a. **A prodrome** may precede the seizure by hours or days.
        (1) Changes in behavior or mood typically occur during the prodrome.
        (2) This phase may include an aura—a subjective sensation, such as an unusual smell or flashing light.
    b. The **ictal phase** is the seizure itself. In some cases, its onset is heralded by a scream or cry.
    c. The **postictal phase** takes place immediately after the seizure.
        (1) Extensor plantar reflexes may appear.
        (2) The patient typically exhibits lethargy, confusion, and behavioral changes.

F. Clinical evaluation

1. **History** includes an evaluation of the seizure, including interviews of the patient's family and eyewitness accounts to establish:
    a. The frequency and duration of the episodes
    b. Precipitating factors
    c. The times at which episodes occur
    d. The presence or absence of an aura
    e. Ictal activity
    f. Postictal state

2. **Physical and neurological examinations** are the tools with which to identify an underlying etiology to rule out diseases that manifest as seizures (Table 44-4).

3. **Laboratory tests** may also identify an underlying etiology.
    a. Liver and kidney function tests, complete blood count (CBC), urinalysis, and serum drug levels (e.g., antidepressants and amphetamines may precipitate seizures) are necessary.
    b. Lumbar puncture may be required for evidence of cerebrospinal fluid (CSF) infection for the patient with a fever who has seizures.

4. **Neurological imaging studies,** including magnetic resonance imaging (MRI) or computed tomography (CT)–complement electrophysiological studies, can identify structural brain disorders (anatomical abnormalities).
    a. An MRI can detect cerebral lesions related to epilepsy and should be used in all cases, especially in patients with partial seizure, to exclude brain abnormalities.
    b. Positron-emission tomography (PET), single-photon-emission CT (SPECT), and stable xenon-enhanced x-ray CT offer functional views of the brain to detect hypometabolism or relative hypoperfusion. PET and SPECT scans are not available in all institutions.

Table 44-4. Disorders That Mimic Epilepsy

Gastroesophageal reflux	Movement disorders
Breath-holding spells	Shuddering attacks
Migraine	Paroxysmal choreoathetosis
Confusional	Nonepileptic myoclonus
Basilar	Tics and habit spasms
With recurrent abdominal pain and cyclic vomiting	Psychological disorders
Sleep disorders (especially parasomnias)	Panic disorder
Cardiovascular events	Hyperventilation attacks
Pallid infantile syncope	Pseudoseizures
Vasovagal attacks	Rage attacks
Vasomotor syncope	
Cardiac arrhythmias	

Reprinted from Scheurer ML, Pedley TA: The evaluation and treatment of seizures. *N Engl J Med* 1990;323:1469.

   c. EEG studies measure the electrical activity of the brain. These studies help to identify functional cerebral changes underlying structural abnormalities and are useful with MRI for patients considered for epilepsy surgery.

     (1) An EEG is useful for classifying the seizure or as an additional diagnostic tool, but the EEG by itself cannot rule seizures in or out, as there are patients with normal interictal EEGs who have seizure disorders.

     (2) The best time to obtain an EEG is *during* a seizure episode. EEG recordings done while the patient is asleep can often record the abnormal activity; therefore, EEGs performed during a sleep-induced state under normal conditions or in a sleep-deprived state can be more sensitive for making a diagnosis.

G. Treatment objectives

  1. To prevent or suppress seizures or reduce their frequency through drug therapy

  2. To control or eliminate the factors that cause or precipitate seizures

  3. To prevent serious consequences of seizures, such as anoxia, airway occlusion, or injury, by protecting the tongue and placing a pillow under the victim's head

  4. To encourage a normal lifestyle and prevent the patient from feeling like or being treated as an invalid

  5. Short- and long-term side effects

  6. Drug interactions

II. THERAPY

A. Principles of drug therapy

  1. Seizure control. Approximately 50% of epileptics achieve complete seizure control through drug therapy. In another 25%, drugs reduce the frequency of seizures. Epileptics generally require continuous drug therapy for at least 2 seizure-free years before the drug discontinuation can be considered.

  2. Initial treatment

    a. Before anticonvulsive drug treatment is instituted, treatable underlying causes of the seizure activity should be excluded.

    b. A single primary drug that is most appropriate for the seizure type must be selected. If there is more than one appropriate primary drug, then age, sex, and compliance of the patient must be considered.

    c. For patients with newly diagnosed epilepsy, administer low doses for a few days. Patients may respond to a dosage that is lower than that traditionally prescribed initially by their physicians, and this may have important implications in terms of limiting adverse effects. The incidence of adverse effects increases with increasing drug levels, even when the plasma concentrations are maintained within the so-called therapeutic or optimal range.

    d. Approximately one-fourth or one-third of the maintenance dose of a single medication is used to begin therapy; it is then increased over 3–4 weeks. The exceptions are phenytoin or phenobarbital, which can be started with the loading or maintenance dose. The dose should be titrated until seizure control or intolerable side effects occur.

    e. With the initiation of therapy, blood concentrations of medications should be measured:

     (1) To establish therapeutic ranges and dosage regimens based on symptomatic toxicity or seizure frequency

     (2) To assess the patient's compliance with therapy

     (3) To control the correlation among the dose, blood levels, and clinical therapeutic levels or toxicity

      (a) Phenytoin follows nonlinear kinetics, as drug levels increase dramatically (more than onefold) with only a small increase in the dose. However, prior to this twofold increase in drug level with a small increase in dose, there is a predictable linear increase with dose increases; for this reason, it is recommended to increase the dose in small increments to be able to predict when the drug follows the nonlinear kinetic. When this happens, that means the maximum rate of hepatic enzyme clearance is reached and the body can no longer clear the drug as it is introduced into the body.

(b) If physical examination reveals a new onset of nystagmus (except with phenytoin, in which nystagmus develops before clinical intoxication), ataxia, and unsteady, wide gait, the next dose increase should be minimal.

(c) There is no justification for increasing drug dosage when a patient's seizures are fully controlled, even if the plasma concentration is below the lower limit of the therapeutic range. If the patient continues to have seizures without any evidence of adverse effects at a plasma concentration near the toxic range, there are two approaches:

(i) Some increase the dosage according to clinical response up to the highest tolerated limit.

(ii) Some do not increase the dosage because of the likelihood of producing adverse effects.

(d) Carbamazepine has an autoinduction metabolism property, which means that if the dose is increased twofold, blood levels increase less than twofold because of increased metabolism.

(4) To determine the free drug level, which is helpful in patients who are in the therapeutic range but have side effects or no response. The plasma protein binding may be altered in these patients by some other disease state or medication. Because of this alteration, there is more free drug available in the system than the total level shows, especially with phenytoin, valproic acid, and carbamazepine.

3. **Paradoxical intoxication** occurs when a high concentration of a single drug causes an increased frequency of seizures without classical adverse events. This is common with hydantoins and carbamazepine. The proposed reason is that their effect on the cerebellum is blocked at high concentrations. Management usually requires no more than withholding enough doses of the drug to allow the concentration to drift down.

4. When seizures cannot be controlled, there are two options.
   a. The initial drug can be substituted with another agent. This is accomplished by gradually discontinuing the initial drug while simultaneously increasing the dosage of the second agent. Then the dosage of the second agent is titrated up to the maintenance level as the initial agent is gradually discontinued. There are three main advantages of gradual substitution:
   (1) It allows evaluation of the effects of individual drugs
   (2) It reduces the risk of toxicity
   (3) It reduces the risk of adverse drug interactions
   b. A second drug can be added. Combination therapy is reserved for patients with severe epilepsy in order to rapidly control the seizures. Rapid control can be important for psychosocial reasons as well as for the possibility of a more favorable prognosis.

5. **Long-term drug treatment.** Most physicians review the patient's condition when the patient has been seizure free for 2 years. This has important implications in children because early termination of treatment has better remission rates compared with adults. It is recommended to gradually decrease the dose, over at least 6 months. The age of onset of epilepsy, the presence of an underlying neurological condition, and any abnormal EEGs should be considered.

6. **Diseases and conditions that alter antiepileptic drug–protein bindings**
   a. Liver disease
   b. Hypoalbuminemia
   c. Burns
   d. Pregnancy
   e. High protein-binding drugs or antiepileptic agents. (Most important interactions are discussed under individual agents.)

7. **Medications.** There are medications that decrease levels of phenytoin, carbamazepine, phenobarbital, and primidone by enhancing their metabolism. These drugs also cause false decreases in thyroid function tests.
   a. Oral contraceptives
   b. Oral hypoglycemics

    c. Glucocorticoids
    d. Tricyclic antidepressants
    e. Azathioprine
    f. Cyclosporine
    g. Quinidine
    h. Theophylline
    i. Warfarin
    j. Doxycycline
    k. Levodopa

8. **Overview of drug therapy in seizure disorder**
   a. **Monotherapy.** Start the drug therapy as single agent.
   b. **Dosage Treatment**. Use a low dose for a few days. Patients with newly diagnosed epilepsy may respond to dosages that are lower than those prescribed initially by their physicians, and this may have important implications in terms of adverse effects. The incidence of adverse effects increases with increasing drug dosage, even when the plasma concentration is maintained within the so-called therapeutic or optimal range.
   c. **Drug monitoring**. There is no justification for increasing drug dosage when a patient is fully controlled, even if the plasma concentration is below the lower limit of the therapeutic range. If the patient continues to have seizures without any evidence of adverse effects at a plasma concentration near the toxic range, there are two approaches:
      (1) Some increase the dosage according to clinical response up to the highest tolerated limit.
      (2) Some do not increase the dosage because of the likelihood of producing adverse events.

9. **Adverse effects of anticonvulsive drugs**
   a. **Alternation in cognition and mentation**
      (1) **Sedation and depression** are the most common symptoms of overdose of anticonvulsive drugs, but they are difficult to assess. For example, barbiturates commonly cause depression, with primidone being the worst offender; diazepam and clorazepate are less likely to cause depression. Barbiturates, clonazepam, and trimethadione commonly cause cognitive impairment, ranging from sensation to confusion.
      (2) **Excitation** can be a paradoxical effect of barbiturates with younger children and the elderly. For example, felbamate can cause restlessness and hyperactivity.
   b. **Deterioration of motor performance and primary coordination** includes trembling hands, staggering when rounding corners, and mild limb ataxia. Drugs associated with these effects include hydantoins, methsuximide, carbamazepine, and primidone. These effects are less common with barbiturates and lamotrigine and are rarely seen with gabapentin.
   c. **Gastrointestinal symptoms** include nausea and vomiting. Two purposed mechanisms include:
      (1) A local effect on the stomach, as in the case of valproic acid; divalproex acid, however, has less incidence compared with valproic acid. These symptoms decrease in incidence if the drug is given with meals.
      (2) A brain stem effect, as in the cases of felbamate and carbamazepine. Nausea and vomiting caused by these drugs are associated with brain-stem involvement; therefore, drug levels play a role in these symptoms. Administration in smaller, more frequent doses decreases the incidence of these symptoms by lowering the transient peak concentration.
   d. **Appetite and body weight.** Few anticonvulsants affect appetite separate from nausea and vomiting, including anorexia or increased appetite.
      (1) **Drugs that cause anorexia** are felbamate, and to a lesser extent, carbamazepine, ethosuximide, and valproic acid.
      (2) **Drugs that cause increased appetite** are valproic acid, and to a lesser extent, carbamazepine.
   e. **Headache and dizziness**
      (1) **Diffuse headaches** may be caused by ethosuximide and, to a lesser extent, by methsuximide and felbamate.
      (2) **Dizziness** seen in association with anticonvulsants is caused by a combination of ataxia and loss of eye movement coordination, which is part of motor coordination symptoms.

B. Specific antiseizure agents. Table 44-5 lists the uses of antiepileptic medications based on seizure type. Table 44-6 lists classifications of anticonvulsive drugs.

  1. Carbamazepine
    a. Mechanisms of action. Carbamazepine is chemically related to tricyclic antidepressants. Its mechanism of action is unknown in the treatment of seizure disorders, but it is thought to act by reducing polysynaptic responses and blocking the posttetanic potentiation.
    b. Administration and dosage (Table 44-7)
      (1) Adults and children older than 12 years of age receive an initial oral dose of 200 mg twice daily. This may be increased gradually to 800–2000 mg daily (usually given in divided doses).
      (2) Children under age 12 usually receive 10–20 mg/kg daily in two or three divided doses.
    c. Precautions and monitoring effects
      (1) Carbamazepine should be used with caution in patients with bone marrow depression. A CBC should be obtained and platelets measured to determine baseline levels before therapy, and levels should be monitored during therapy. Aplastic anemia and agranulocytosis have been reported
      (2) Tricyclic antidepressants should be avoided if there is a history of hypersensitivity to tricyclics. Monoamine oxidase (MAO) inhibitors should be discontinued 2 weeks before carbamazepine therapy.

Table 44-5. Uses of Antiepileptic Medications Based on Seizure Type

	Choices of Drug Therapy			
Seizure Type	**Choice 1**	**Choice 2**	**Choice 3**	**Choice 4**
Simple partial	Carbamazepine (alone or combination)	Phenytoin	Primidone Lamotrigine	Gabapentin, levetiracetam Zonisamide
Complex partial	Carbamazepine Lamotrigine	Phenytoin	Phenobarbital Zonisamide	Valproic acid Primidone Topiramate Tiagabine
Primary generalized Tonic–clonic	Valproic acid Lamotrigine	Carbamazepine	Phenytoin Valproic acid	Phenobarbital Topiramate Tiagabine
Absence	Lamotrigine,* ethosuximide	Zonisamide, valproic acid		
Myoclonic	Valproic acid	Clonazepam	Zonisamide*	Felbamate* (alone or in combination)
Atonic	Valproic acid	Clonazepam		
Status epilepticus	Diazepam	Phenytoin	Phenobarbital	
Psychomotor	Phenytoin	Phenacemide		

*Also indicated for treatment of Lennox-Gastaut syndrome in children.

Table 44-6. Anticonvulsive Drug Classification

Barbiturates	Hydantoins	Succinimides	Oxazolidinediones	Benzodiazepine	Miscellaneous
Phenobarbital Primidone Mephobarbital	Phenytoin Mephenytoin Ethotoin Fosphenytoin	Ethosuximide Methsuximide Phensuximide Zonisamide	Paramethadione Trimethadione	Clonazepam Diazepam	Lamotrigine Felbamate Gabapentin Carbamazepine Valproic acid Phenacemide Topiramate Tiagabine Levetiracetam

Table 44-7. Dosages Characteristic of Antiepileptic Medications

Drug	Loading Dose	Usual Adult Dose (mg/day)	Half-life (hours)	Therapeutic Range of Total Plasma Concentration (μg/mL)	Major Mode of Elimination	Protein-Binding Level
Carbamazepine	No	800–2000	11*–22	4–12	Hepatic	40%–90%
Phenytoin	Yes	300–700	22–72 / 1–2 (free)	5–20	Hepatic	90%
Phenobarbital	Yes	90–300	100	15–40	Hepatic > Renal	50%
Primidone	No	750–3000	15*†	5–12	Hepatic	80%
Valproic acid	Yes	1000–3000	15–20	50–150	Hepatic	90%–95%
Ethosuximide	No	750–1000	30–60**	40–100	Hepatic > Renal	0%
Felbamate	No	2400	20–23	30–100	Hepatic > Renal	22%–25%
Gabapentin	Yes	900–1000	5–7	5–7	Renal	<3%
Lamotrigine	No	200–400	25 / 12.6[a] / 70[b]	2–6	Hepatic > Renal	55%
Topiramate	No	200–400	21	N/A	Renal > Liver	17%
Tiagabine	No	32–56	6–8	N/A	Liver	96%
Levetiracetam	Yes	500–3000	7	N/A	Renal	<10%
Zonisamide	No	100–600	63	N/A	Liver	50%

a = Receiving other enzyme-inducing drugs.
b = Valproic acid slows the metabolism.
* The half-life decreases autometabolism after chronic use.
† Metabolized in part to phenobarbital.
** Lower range in children and higher range in adults.

    (3) Carbamazepine should be used cautiously in patients with glaucoma because of its mild anticholinergic effects.

    (4) Carbamazepine is an enzyme inducer; therefore, the half-life decreases over 3–4 weeks ($t_{1/2}$18–54 hours; $t_{1/2}$10–25 hours); for maximal enzyme induction, levels should be rechecked to avoid breakthrough seizures.

    (4) Carbamazepine is metabolized in the liver to 10-11 epoxide, which also has anticonvulsant activity; carbamazepine may induce its own metabolism.

    (5) Adverse effects. The physician should be notified if any of the following adverse effects occur: jaundice, abdominal pain, pale stool, darkened urine, unusual bruising and bleeding, fever, sore throat, or an ulcer in the mouth. The most common side effects are dizziness, drowsiness, unsteadiness, nausea, and vomiting.

        (a) CNS effects. These include dizziness, ataxia, and diplopia. If diplopia and ataxia are common and occur after a dose, the schedule could be adjusted to include more frequent administration or a larger proportion of the dose at night. CNS side effects may decrease with chronic administration.

        (b) Gastrointestinal (GI) effects. These most commonly include nausea, vomiting, and anorexia.

        (c) Metabolic effects. Hyponatremia occurs after several weeks to months of therapy, and the incidence increases with age. The antidiuretic hormone (ADH) level may be low. Levels of 125–135 mEq/L without symptoms should be monitored. Fluid restriction should be instituted when levels decrease to less than 125 mEq/L with or without symptoms. Another agent should be used if fluid dose reduction does not help or the seizures recur.

        (d) Hematopoietic effects. Aplastic anemia is rare. Thrombocytopenia and anemia have a 5% incidence, and they respond to a cessation of drug therapy. Leukopenia is the most common hematopoietic side effect: 10% of cases are transient, and about 2% of patients have persistent leukopenia but do not seem to have increased infections even with white blood cell (WBC) counts of 3000/mL.

        (e) Dermatological effects. Pruritic and erythematous rashes, the Stevens-Johnson syndrome, and lupus erythematosus have been reported.

d. Significant interactions
   (1) Antiepileptic drugs, such as **phenytoin, primidone,** and **phenobarbital,** decrease the level of carbamazepine (increase metabolism). **Valproic acid** increases the level of carbamazepine (decreases metabolism).
   (2) Other medications such as **erythromycin, isoniazid, cimetidine, propoxyphene, diltiazem,** and **verapamil** increase the level of carbamazepine (decrease metabolism).

2. Phenytoin
   a. Mechanism of action
      (1) Phenytoin inhibits the spread of seizures at the motor cortex and blocks posttetanic potentiation by influencing synaptic transmission. There is an alternation of ion fluxes in depolarization, repolarization, and membrane stability phase and alternating calcium uptake in presynaptic terminals.
      (2) Phenytoin is effective for the treatment of generalized tonic–clonic (grand mal) seizures and for partial seizures, both simple and complex. It is not effective for absence seizures.
   b. Administration and dosage (see Table 44-7)
      (1) The usual daily dose for **adults** is 300–700 mg, with adjustments made as needed.
         (a) Regular daily doses above 500 mg are poorly tolerated.
         (b) A loading dose of 900 mg to 1.5 g may be given intravenously (IV). The infusion rate should not exceed 50 mg/min. (Alternatively, an oral loading dose may be given.)
      (2) The usual daily dose for children is 4–7 mg/kg divided every 12 hours. An IV loading dose of 15 mg/kg may be given.
      (3) Phenytoin sodium is available as capsules and parenteral solution. Phenytoin is available as tablets and oral suspension.
   c. Precautions and monitoring effects
      (1) IV phenytoin should not be used in patients with sinus bradycardia, sinoatrial block, second- and third-degree atrioventricular (AV) block, or Adams-Stokes syndrome.
      (2) Phenytoin should be used cautiously in patients with myocardial insufficiency and hypotension.
      (3) Elimination of phenytoin converts from first-order elimination (proportional to its concentration) to zero-order elimination (a fixed amount per unit time), usually at high therapeutic levels. The daily dose of phenytoin can be increased 100 mg daily until therapeutic blood levels are attained, after which increases of 30–50 mg will avoid two- to threefold increases in blood levels.
      (4) It is necessary to measure free drug levels or correct the total level when aluminum levels are abnormal or the patient has renal failure.
      (5) Adverse effects. The physician should be notified if any of the following adverse effects occur: swollen or tender gums, skin rash, nausea and vomiting, swollen glands, bleeding, jaundice, fever, or sore throat (i.e., signs of infection or bleeding).
         (a) CNS effects include ataxia (limiting side effect), dysarthria, and insomnia. Transient hyperkinesia may follow IV phenytoin infusion. Alcoholic beverages should be avoided while on this medication.
         (b) GI effects most commonly include nausea and vomiting. Phenytoin should be taken with food to enhance absorption and decrease GI upset.
         (c) Dermatological effects include maculopapular rashes sometimes with fever, Stevens-Johnson syndrome, and lupus erythematosus. Gingival hyperplasia may be reduced by frequent brushing and appropriate oral care.
         (d) Connective tissue disorders include a coarsening of the facial features.
         (e) Hematopoietic effects include thrombocytopenia, leukopenia, and granulocytopenia.
         (f) Miscellaneous effects include hyperglycemia and increased body hair.
   d. Significant interactions
      (1) Antiepileptic drugs, such as **carbamazepine, valproic acid, clonazepam,** and **phenobarbital,** decrease the level of phenytoin (increase metabolism). **Phenytoin** increases the conversion of primidone to phenobarbital (increases metabolism).
      (2) Other medications such as disulfiram, isoniazid, chloramphenicol, and propoxyphene increase the level of phenytoin (decrease metabolism). Drugs whose efficacy is impaired by phenytoin include **corticosteroids, digitoxin, doxycycline, estrogens, furosemide, oral contraceptives, quinidine, rifampin, theophylline, vitamin D,** and

enteral nutritional therapy. Coumarin and warfarin anticoagulants increase the serum phenytoin levels and prolong the serum half-life of phenytoin by inhibiting its metabolism.

3. Fosphenytoin
  a. Mechanism of action
    (1) Water-soluble prodrug of phenytoin. It is converted to phenytoin by the bloodstream phosphatases, with a half-life ($t_{1/2}$) of about 8 minutes in both adults and children.
    (2) It is indicated for patients who cannot take oral drugs, and in the acute treatment for status epilepticus.
    (3) Administered via IV or intramuscular (IM) injection
    (4) A dose conversion table should be used to convert the phenytoin dose to fosphenytoin.
    (5) Characteristics similar to phenytoin
    (6) Advantages
      (a) Fosphenytoin is an aqueous solution, unlike phenytoin, which is an alkaline solution; therefore, there is no need to add propylene glycol and ethanol to the solution.
      (b) Fosphenytoin causes less soft-tissue injury at the site of injection. When administered by IM injection, it is completely absorbed and has more predictable serum concentration than IM-injected phenytoin.

4. Valproic acid
  a. Mechanism of action
    (1) Increases levels of GABA
    (2) Potentiates a postsynaptic GABA response by inhibiting the enzymatic response for the catabolism of GABA
    (3) Affects the potassium channel, creating a direct membrane-stabilizing effect
  b. Administration and dosage (see Table 44-7)
    (1) For **adults,** valproic acid is administered orally in a usual dose of 1000–3000 mg daily in divided doses.
    (2) For **children,** valproic acid is administered orally in a dose of 15–60 mg/kg daily, divided into two or three doses.
    (3) Medication should be taken with food to reduce GI upset.
    (4) Tablets or capsules should be swallowed, not chewed, to avoid irritation of the mouth and throat.
  c. Precautions and monitoring effects. There are some reports of hepatotoxicity and increased liver function tests, which are mostly reversible. The severity and incidence of hepatotoxicity increase when the patient is younger than 2 years of age.
  d. Adverse effects. Contact the physician if abdominal pain, nausea, vomiting, or anoxia occurs; these could be symptoms of pancreatitis.
    (1) CNS effects include tremor, ataxia, diplopia, lethargy, drowsiness, behavioral changes, and depression.
    (2) GI effects include nausea and increased appetite. Enteric-coated divalproex sodium may reduce these side effects.
    (3) Dermatological effects include alopecia and petechiae.
    (4) Hematopoietic effects include thrombocytopenia, bruising, hematoma, and bleeding.
    (5) Hepatic effects include minor elevations of aspartate aminotransferase (AST), alanine aminotransferase (ALT), and lactate dehydrogenase (LDH).
    (6) Endocrine effects include decreased levels of prolactin, resulting in irregular menses, and secondary amenorrhea.
    (7) Pancreatic effects include acute pancreatitis.
    (8) Metabolic effects include hyperammonemia due to renal origin. Discontinuation may be considered if lethargy develops.
  e. Significant interactions
    (1) Antiepileptic drugs
      (a) Primidone decreases valproic acid clearance (increases metabolism).
      (b) Phenobarbital and **phenytoin** displace protein binding, resulting in an increased total phenytoin level and an increase or no change of free phenytoin.
      (c) Clonazepam increases CNS toxicity in patients on valproic acid.

(2) Other medications
  (a) Aspirin increases the level of valproic acid.
  (b) Warfarin inhibits the secondary phase of platelet aggregation.
  (c) Antacids increase the level of valproic acid.
(3) Laboratory tests
  (a) False-positive urine ketone tests may result in patients taking valproic acid; thus, diabetic patients must use caution when using urine tests.
  (b) Thyroid function tests may be altered by antiepileptic drugs.

5. **Phenobarbital**
  a. **Mechanism of action.** Phenobarbital increases the seizure threshold by decreasing postsynaptic excitation by stimulating postsynaptic GABA-A receptor inhibitor responses as a CNS depressant.
  b. **Administration and dosage** (see Table 44-7)
    (1) For **adults,** phenobarbital is administered orally at 90–300 mg daily (in three divided doses or as a single dose at bedtime).
    (2) Children typically receive 3–6 mg/kg daily in two divided doses. Adjustment is made as needed.
  c. **Precautions and monitoring effects**
    (1) Phenobarbital produces respiratory depression, especially with parenteral administration.
    (2) Phenobarbital should be used with caution in patients with hepatic disease who may need dose adjustments.
    (3) Phenobarbital has sedative effects in adults and produces hyperactivity in children.
    (4) Abrupt discontinuation of phenobarbital produces withdrawal convulsions. If the drug must be discontinued, another GABA-A agonist (e.g., benzodiazepine, paraldehyde) should be substituted.
    (5) Adverse effects. The physician should be notified if any of the following adverse effects occur: sore throat, mouth sores, easy bruising or bleeding, and any signs of infection.
      (a) CNS effects include agitation, confusion, lethargy, and drowsiness. Patients should avoid alcohol and other CNS depressants.
      (b) Respiratory effects include hypoventilation and apnea.
      (c) Cardiovascular effects include bradycardia and hypotension.
      (d) GI effects include nausea, diarrhea, and constipation. If GI upset is experienced, phenobarbital should be taken with food.
      (e) Hematological effects include megaloblastic anemia after chronic use (a rare side effect).
      (f) Miscellaneous effects include osteomalacia and Stevens-Johnson syndrome, both of which are rare.
  d. **Significant interactions**
    (1) Antiepileptic drugs, such as **valproic acid** and **phenytoin,** increase the level of phenobarbital (decrease metabolism).
    (2) Other drugs such as **acetazolamide, chloramphenicol, cimetidine,** and **furosemide** increase the level of phenobarbital (decrease metabolism). **Rifampin, pyridoxine,** and **ethanol** decrease the level of phenobarbital (increase metabolism).

6. **Primidone**
  a. **Mechanism of action.** Primidone is a metabolite of phenobarbital and phenylethylmalonamide (PEMA), which has some anticonvulsive effects. It has drug characteristics similar to phenobarbital, with some differences in dose and half-life.
  b. **Administration and dosage**
    (1) Primidone has a short half-life of 7 hours, which may require three-times daily dosing.
    (2) Primidone is tolerated better if started at 50 mg at night for 3 days until the target daily dose is reached.

7. **Ethosuximide**
  a. **Mechanism of action**
    (1) Ethosuximide may inhibit the sodium–potassium adenosine triphosphatase (Na^+–K^+ ATPase) system and the reduced form of nicotinamide-adenine dinucleotide phosphate (NADPH)–linked aldehyde reductase (which is necessary for the formation of γ-hydroxybutyrate, which is associated with the induction of absence seizures).

(2) Ethosuximide reduces or eliminates the EEG abnormality; however, absence seizures are the only seizures in which the normal EEG has clinical value (i.e., when the EEG abnormality is corrected, the seizures are also controlled).

(3) Ethosuximide is a relatively benign anticonvulsant with minimum protein binding.

b. Administration and dosage (see Table 44-7). Ethosuximide is usually given orally in an initial dose of 500 mg daily in adults and older children and 250 mg daily in children ages 3–6 years. The dose may be raised by 250 mg every week to a maximum of 1.5 g daily in adults.

c. Precautions and monitoring effects

(1) Blood dyscrasias have been reported, making periodic blood counts necessary.

(2) There have been reports of hepatic and renal toxicity; thus, periodic renal and liver function monitoring is necessary.

(3) Cases of systemic lupus erythematosus have been reported.

(4) **Adverse effects**

(a) **GI effects** include nausea and vomiting. Small doses may lessen these effects. Ethosuximide should be taken with food if GI upset occurs.

(b) **Hematopoietic effects** include eosinophilia, granulocytopenia, leukopenia, and lupus.

(c) **CNS effects** include drowsiness, blurred vision, fatigue, lethargy, hiccups, and headaches. Alcoholic beverages should be avoided with this medication.

(d) **Psychiatric–psychological** effects include confusion and emotional instability.

(e) **Dermatological effects include** pruritus, photosensitivity, urticaria, and Stevens-Johnson syndrome.

(f) **Genitourinary effects include** increased frequency of urination, vaginal bleeding, renal damage, and hematuria.

(g) **Miscellaneous effects include** periorbital edema and muscle weakness. Patients should also be advised of the risks of exposure to sunlight and ultraviolet light.

d. Significant interactions. Antiepileptic drugs, such as **carbamazepine,** decrease the level of ethosuximide (increases metabolism), and **valproic acid** increases the level of ethosuximide (decreases metabolism).

8. Clonazepam

a. Mechanism of action. Clonazepam is a potent GABA-A agonist, but its efficacy decreases over several months of treatment.

b. Administration and dosage

(1) For **adults,** clonazepam is an oral agent that may be given in an initial dose of 1.5 mg daily divided two or three times. The dose may be increased to a maximum of 20 mg daily.

(2) **Children** should receive 0.01–0.03 mg daily in two or three doses. The dosage may be increased to a maximum of 0.2 mg/kg daily.

c. Precautions and monitoring effects

(1) Patients with psychoses, acute narrow-angle glaucoma, and significant liver disease should use this medicine cautiously.

(2) **Adverse effects**

(a) **CNS effects** include drowsiness, ataxia, and behavior disturbances in children; these may be corrected by dose reduction.

(b) **Respiratory effects** include hypersalivation and bronchial hypersecretion.

(c) **Miscellaneous effects** include anemia, leukopenia, thrombocytopenia, respiratory depression, anorexia, and weight loss.

d. Significant interactions

(1) **Antiepileptic drugs,** such as **phenytoin,** increase the level of clonazepam (decrease metabolism).

(2) **Other drugs.** Clonazepam decreases the efficacy of **levodopa** and increases the serum level of **digoxin.**

9. Felbamate

a. Mechanism of action. A proposed mechanism of action is that the drug interacts with glycine modulatory site on *N*-methyl-D-aspartate (NMDA) receptors. Blockade of NMDA may contribute to neuroprotective effects of felbamate. Felbamate is used as monotherapy or adjunctive therapy or without secondary generalization in adults and generalized seizures associated with Lennox-Gastaut syndrome in children. The

United States Food and Drug Administration (FDA) recommended that use of felbamate be restricted to only those patients who are refractory to other medications and in whom the risk–benefit relationship warrants its use, because of severe hepatotoxicity.

b. Administration and dosage

(1) Adults and children older than 14 years of age

(2) Monotherapy, initially 1.2 g in three to four doses daily. The dosage may be increased in 600-mg increments every 2 weeks to 2.4 g daily based on clinical response and, thereafter, 3.6 g daily if necessary.

(3) Adjunctive therapy, 1.2 g in three to four doses daily, with reduction of the dosage of other antiepileptic drugs by 20%–33%. The dosage of felbamate may be increased in increments of 1.2 g at weekly intervals to a maximum of 3.6 g daily.

(4) Conversion to monotherapy initially 1.2 g daily in three to four doses, with reduction of the dosage of other antiepileptic drugs by 33% at week 3. The felbamate dosage may be increased to 3.6 g daily, and other antiepileptic drugs discontinued or dosage further reduced in stepwise fashion.

(5) Children 2–14 years of age with Lennox-Gastaut syndrome, as adjunctive therapy, initially 15 mg/kg daily in three to four doses. The dosage of other antiepileptic drugs is reduced by 20%. The amount of felbamate may be increased in increments of 15 mg/kg at weekly intervals to 45 mg/kg daily. Further reduction in the dosage of other antiepileptic drugs may be necessary.

c. Precaution and monitoring effects. There are two very serious toxic effects, aplastic anemia and liver failure, which lead to death for some patients.

(1) For aplastic anemia, the onset range from 5–30 weeks of initiation of therapy. Weekly or biweekly CBCs are recommended initially.

(2) For liver, toxicity time between initiation of treatment and diagnosis of these cases ranges from 14–257 days. It is recommended that liver function tests be performed before initiation of therapy to identify patients who have evidence of preexisting liver damage. Liver function tests should also be performed weekly or biweekly. The FDA recommends that this drug be used only in patients who are refractory to other medications and in whom the risk–benefit relationship warrants its use.

(3) Photoallergy or phototoxicity may occur; patients should take protective measures against exposure to ultraviolet light or sunlight.

(4) Instruct patients to store medication in its own tightly closed container at room temperature away from excessive heat, direct sunlight, and moisture.

(5) Adverse effects. Contact the physician if signs of infection, that is, bleeding or brusing, occur.

    (a) This drug has the potential to cause aplastic anemia (bone marrow).

    (b) The patient should be monitored for these toxicities by CBCs and liver function tests weekly or biweekly until discontinuation of any sign of these toxicities occurs.

    (c) CNS effects are insomnia, headache, anxiety, hyperactivity, and fatigue.

    (d) Cardiovascular effects are peripheral edema, vasodilation, hypotension, and hypertension.

    (e) Ocular effects are diplopia and blurred vision.

    (f) GI effects are anorexia, weight decrease, and nausea.

    (g) Hematological effects may include lymphadenopathy, leukopenia, and thrombocytopenia.

    (h) Metabolic/nutrition effects may include hypokalemia and hyponatremia.

d. Significant interactions

(1) Felbamate and phenytoin. Felbamate causes an increase in phenytoin plasma concentration. Phenytoin doubles felbamate clearance, resulting in 45% decrease in felbamate levels.

(2) Felbamate and carbamazepine. Felbamate causes a decrease in carbamazepine levels and an increase in carbamazepine metabolites. In addition, carbamazepine causes a 50% increase in felbamate clearance, resulting in a 40% decrease in steady-state trough levels.

(3) Felbamate and valproic acid. Felbamate causes an increase in valproic acid levels, but valproic acid does not affect felbamate levels.

(4) Adverse effects. Signs and symptoms associated with increased plasma level and toxicity are anorexia, nausea, vomiting, insomnia, and headache.

10. **Gabapentin**
    a. **Mechanism of action.** It is an analogue of GABA. It increases GABA turnover, but it does not bind to GABA or any other established neurotransmitter receptor. Its mechanism of action is currently unknown, although it binds to a specific receptor in the brain and inhibits voltage-dependent sodium currents. It has been shown to be effective as an add-on drug in patients with partial seizure with or without secondary generalization.
    b. **Administration and dosage**
        (1) Patients older than 12 years receive 900 mg to 1.8 g daily, administered as adjunctive therapy in three divided doses. Titrating to an effective dose normally can be achieved within 3 days by initiating therapy with 300 mg and then increasing the dose in 300-mg increments over the next 2 days to establish a dosage of 900 mg daily in three doses. If necessary, the dosage may be increased to 1.8 g daily. To minimize potential side effects, especially somnolence, dizziness, or fatigue, the first dose on day 1 may be administered at bedtime.
        (2) Patients 3–12 years of age should receive 10–15 mg/kg/day in 3 divided doses up to 25–50 mg/kg/day.
        (3) The drug is primarily excreted renally; therefore, the dosage should be adjusted for patients who have compromised renal function.
        (4) The drug does not bind to plasma protein. There are no significant pharmacokinetic interactions with other commonly used antiepileptic drugs.
        (5) If gabapentin is discontinued or an alternate anticonvulsant medication is added, it should be done gradually over a minimum of 1 week.
    c. **Precautions and monitoring effects**
        (1) The value of monitoring blood concentration has not been established and would not alter blood concentration of other antiepileptic drugs when used together.
        (2) It has a low level of toxic side effects, which include somnolence, dizziness, ataxia, and minimal interaction with other drugs.
        (3) Gabapentin is useful in patients who are taking other medications for epilepsy or other chronic diseases. It may be especially useful for elderly patients.
        (4) Gabapentin is well absorbed orally; it can be taken with or without food. However, patients who have GI problems might have problems with absorption.
        (5) **Adverse effects.** Common side effects are somnolence, dizziness, ataxia, fatigue, and nystagmus.
            (a) **CNS effects** are somnolence, dizziness, ataxia, and fatigue.
            (b) **GI effects** include dyspepsia, dryness of mouth, constipation, and increased appetite.
            (c) **Ocular effects** are diplopia, blurred vision, and nystagmus.
    d. **Significant interactions**
        (1) **Antacids and gabapentin.** Antacids reduce the bioavailability of gabapentin by 20%; gabapentin could be taken 2 hours after antacid use.
        (2) **Cimetidine and gabapentin.** Cimetidine decreases the renal excretion of gabapentin by 14% and consequently increases gabapentin plasma levels (however, this amount is not clinically significant).
        (3) **Oral contraceptives and gabapentin.** Oral contraceptives increase the level of norethindrone by 13%; this amount may not be clinically significant.

11. **Lamotrigine**
    a. **Mechanism of action.** Its antiepileptic effect is similar to that of phenytoin. Its effect may be due to inhibition of voltage-dependent sodium currents and reduction of sustained repetitive neuronal activity. It is indicated for the treatment of partial seizures and secondary generalized tonic–clonic seizures that are not controlled with other drugs. It is also used to treat Lennox-Gastaut syndrome. Lamotrigine is broad spectrum, as well tolerated as monotherapy, and probably the least teratogenic of the first-line agents. It may aggravate severe myoclonic epilepsy.
    b. **Administration and dosage**
        (1) Adults (older than 16 years), initially 50 mg/day in two divided doses [patients taking valproic acid (VPA) should be given 25 mg every other day], up to 100 mg/day (up to 25 mg daily with VPA treatment)
        (2) Patients 2–12 years 0.6 mg/kg/day in two divided dosed (0.15 mg/kg/day on VPA treatment), up to 1.2 mg/kg/day (up to 0.3 mg/kg/day with VPA treatment)
        (3) The smallest available chewable dispersible tablet is 5 mg. Then, after 2 weeks, increase by 0.3 mg/kg/day in one to two divided doses, up to 200 mg/day.

(4) Swallow chewable dispersible tablet whole, chewed, or in dispersing water or diluted fruit juice. If chewed, consume a small amount of water or dilute fruit juice to aid in swallowing. To disperse, add the chewable dispersible tablet to a small amount of liquid (1 teaspoon or enough to cover the medication). Approximately 1 minute later, when the tablet is completely dispersed, swirl the solution and consume the entire quantity immediately.

(5) For patients taking valproic acid, the initial dose is 50 mg daily for 2 weeks, followed by maintenance doses of 100–200 mg daily in two divided doses.

(6) Reduced clearance in the elderly necessitates dosage reduction.

(7) Patients with hepatic impairment may require dosage reduction because of reduction in metabolism.

c. Precautions and monitoring effects

(1) The value of monitoring plasma concentration has not been established.

(2) Caution should be used for patients taking this drug. It may adversely affect the patient's metabolism or complicate the elimination of the drug because of renal, hepatic, or cardiac impairment.

(3) Lamotrigine binds to melanin and can accumulate in melanin-rich tissue over time. Periodic ophthalmological monitoring is recommended.

(4) Photosensitization (photoallergy and phototoxicity) patients should take protective measures against exposure to ultraviolet light or sunlight.

(5) Serious rashes requiring hospitalization have been reported. The incidence of rashes, including Stevens-Johnson syndrome, is approximately 1% in patients less than 16 years old and 0.3% in adults. Rare cases of toxic epidermal necrolysis or rash-related death have occurred. Most rashes occur within 2–8 weeks of initial treatment.

(6) Adverse effects. The most common side effects are dizziness, diplopia, ataxia, blurred vision, nausea, and vomiting.

(a) CNS effects are headache, dizziness, and ataxia.

(b) GI effects are nausea, vomiting, diarrhea, and dyspepsia.

(c) Ocular effects are diplopia, blurred vision, and vision abnormality.

(d) Dermatological effects are pruritus, and a rash may form similar to that found when using phenytoin and carbamazepine. In many cases, the rash disappears during continued therapy, but 1%–2% of patients with the rash represent a more serious allergic reaction. Occasionally, patients have developed the Stevens-Johnson syndrome. Concomitant use with valproic acid may increase the likelihood of serious rash. The occurrences of life-threatening rash that were reported developed within 2–8 weeks following therapy; other cases of rash have been reported developing up to 6 months after therapy. The incidence of rash is higher in children than in adults.

(e) Monotherapy during pregnancy found no teratogenic effect.

d. Significant interactions

(1) Carbamazepine decreases lamotrigine concentration by 70% and increases carbamazepine levels.

(2) Phenobarbital or primidone decreases lamotrigine concentration by 40%.

(3) Valproic acid decreases the metabolism of lamotrigine and extends its half-life to 60 hours, which necessitates a dose reduction.

12. Topiramate

a. Mechanism of action. Topiramate is a derivative of fructose. It decreases rapid hippocampal neuronal firing, possibly because of sodium- or calcium-channel inhibition. It is also a weak carbonic anhydrase inhibitor and a sodium-channel blocking agent. Topiramate potentiates the activity of GABA. It has been shown to be effective adjunctive therapy for partial seizure treatment in adults, tonic–clonic seuizure, infantile spasms, and Lennox-Gastaut syndrome.

b. Administration and dosage

(1) 17 years and older, 25–50 mg/day, up to 400 mg/day in two divided doses. 2–16 years, 1–3 mg/kg/day, up to 5–9 mg/kg/day in two divided doses.

(2) Topiramate is 80% bioavailable, and food does not affect its bioavailability.

(3) Dose adjustment is necessary for patients with renal or hepatic impairments.

(4) Enzyme-inducing anticonvulsive drugs can decrease topiramate levels, but topiramate has a significant effect on metabolism of other anticonvulsive drugs.

(5) Initial treatment is 50 mg daily, followed by titration to an effective dosage. More than 400 mg daily has not been shown to improve response.

c. Precaution and monitoring effects
  (1) Increased incidence of kidney stones (renal calculus) in older patients who received this drug. Patients should be advised to increase intake of fluids while taking topiramate.
  (2) Paresthesia is a common side effect of anhydrase inhibitors.
  (3) Adverse effects
    (a) The physician should be notified if any of the following adverse effects occur:
      (i) Breast pain in females
      (ii) Nausea or tremor, which are dose-related side effects.
      (iii) Back pain, chest pain, dyspepsia, or leg pain
    (b) CNS effects include psychomotor slowing, difficulty with concentration and speech, somnolence, fatigue, asthenia, weight loss, cognitive disturbances and difficulties, tremors, dizziness, ataxia, and headache.
    (c) GI effects include upset, such as nausea, vomiting, and gastroenteritis.
    (d) Genitourinary effects include renal calculi.
    (e) CV effects include chest pain, palpitation, and vasodilation.
    (f) Ocular effects include abnormal vision, eye pain, and diplopia.
    (g) Hematological effects include anemia, epistaxis, leukopenia, and aplastic anemia.
d. Significant interactions
  (1) Phenytoin and carbamazepine will increase clearance.
  (2) Topiramate increases the clearance of other drugs that are cleared by cytochrome P_{450} (CYP450).

13. Tiagabine
  a. Mechanism of action. Tiagabine is designed to act on the inhibitory action of GABA by blocking its uptake, thereby prolonging its action after synaptic release. It is indicated as adjunctive therapy for partial seizures and secondary generalized tonic–clonic seizures.
  b. Administration and dosage
    (1) Starting dose of 4 mg daily for 2 weeks may be increased 4–8 mg weekly thereafter, to a maintenance dose of 32–56 mg daily.
    (2) Maximum recommended dosage for children is 32 mg daily; maximum recommended dosage for adults is 56 mg daily.
    (3) A high-fat meal decreases the rate of tiagabine absorption but does not affect the extension of absorption. Tiagabine should be taken with food.
  c. Precautions and monitoring effects
    (1) Generalized weakness: moderately severe to severe weakness has been reported. It resolves in all cases after reduction in dose or discontinuation of therapy.
    (2) Ophthalmic effects, as indicated by animal studies, include the possibility for residual binding to retina and melanin binding; this finding, however, has not been confirmed in human studies. Periodic ophthalmological monitoring is necessary.
    (3) Dermatological effects include the possibility of severe rash to Stevens-Johnson syndrome, as reported in clinical studies.
    (4) Adverse effects
      (a) CNS effects are confusion, dizziness, and fatigue.
      (b) GI effects are upset stomach, nausea, mouth ulceration, and anorexia.
  d. Significant interactions. Phenobarbital, phenytoin, and carbamazepine will increase tiagabine clearance.

14. Zonisamide
  a. Mechanism of action. It is not well known. It may block the sensitive sodium channels and T-type calcium channels. It is an effective agent for refractory partial seizure, generalized seizure indicated for adjunct therapy for partial seizure for adults, infantile spasm, mixed seizure types of Lennox-Gastaut syndrome, myoclonic, and generalized tonic–clonic seizure.
  b. Administration and dosage
    (1) Adults and children older than 16 years of age, 100 mg daily; within 2 weeks, increase to 200 mg/daily in 2-week bases, up to 600 mg daily.
    (2) Can be taken with or without food.
  c. Precautions and monitoring effects
    (1) May increase mean concentration of serum creatinine and BUN; renal function should be monitored periodically.
    (2) May increase serum alkaline phosphatase

(3) May produce drowsiness

(4) Side effects. The physician should be contacted if sudden pain or abdominal pain occurs or if blood in urine is detected; these symptoms could indicate a kidney stone. Increase fluid intake to decrease the risk of stone formation. Also, contact the physician if fever, sore throat, oral ulcer, or easy bruising is seen; these symptoms could be due to a hematological complication.

(5) Most commonly reported adverse events are somnolence, anorexia, dizziness, headache, nausea, and agitation.

(a) CNS: Ataxia, confusion, tremor, abnormal thinking

(b) Cardiovascular: palpitation, tachycardia, vascular insuffiency

(c) Dermatologic: Maculopapular rash, acne alopecia

(d) Other: bladder calculus and leukopenia

d. Significant interactions

(1) Zonisamide induces liver enzymes by increasing metabolism and through clearance of zonisamide and decreases half-life.

(2) Food will delay absorption but will not affect the bioavailability of the drug.

15. Levetiracetam

a. Mechanism of action. It is a pyrrolidone derivative and is chemically unrelated to other antiepileptic drugs. It displays inhibitory properties in the kindling model in rats. It is used as adjunctive therapy in the treatment of partial seizure in adult patients.

b. Administration and dosage. Starting dose of 1000 mg/day given in two divided doses may be increased every 2 weeks, to a maximum of 3000 mg/day.

c. Precautions and monitoring effects

(1) Hematological effects are minor, but there is a statistically significant decrease compared to placebo in total mean RBC count, mean hemoglobulin, and mean hematocrit.

(2) Decrease in WBC count and neurophil count

(3) It also causes drowsiness.

d. Side effects. Most commonly reported adverse events are somnolence, weakness (asthenia), infection, and dizziness.

(1) CNS: somnolence, dizziness, depression, nervousness

(2) Cardiovascular: palpitation, tachycardia, vascular insuffiency

(3) Respiratory: Pharyngitis, Rhinitis, increase cough

(4) Miscellaneous, weakness, headache and infection

e. Significant interactions. Levetiracetam does not influence the plasma concentration of existing antiepileptic drugs, and other antiepileptic drugs do not influence the pharmacokinetic effects of levetiracetam.

16. Less common drugs can be found in Table 44-8.

17. Vagus nerve stimulation (VNS)

a. It is used as adjunctive therapy for adults and children over 12 years of age whose partial seizures are refractory to antiepileptic medications.

b. A programmable signal generator that is implanted in the patient's left upper chest has a bipolar VNS lead that connects the generator to the left vagus nerve in the neck, a programming wand that uses radio-frequency signals to communicate noninvasively with the generator, and handheld magnets used by the patient or caregiver to manually turn the stimulator on or off.

c. The implantation procedure usually lasts 1 hour under general anesthesia. Once programmed, the generator will deliver intermittent stimulation at the desired setting until any additional programming is entered.

C. Surgery. If seizures do not respond to drug therapy, surgery may be performed to remove the epileptogenic brain region. The most commmon is cortical excision (lobectomy) Seventy to eighty percent of patients who have anterior temporal lobectomy have fewer seizures. Frontal lobectomy 30%–40% patients have fewer seizures.

1. Indications for surgery are intractable or disabling seizures recurring for 6–12 months. Should be considered for patients with medically refractory seizures.

2. In **stereotaxic surgery,** the surgeon uses three-dimensional coordinates to guide a needle through a hole drilled in the skull, then destroys abnormal pathways via small intracerebral incisions.

Table 44-8. Less Common Drugs Used in Practice

Drug	Labeled Indication	Half-Life (hours)	Total Plasma Concentration (mg/mL)	Therapeutic Range of Adult Dose (mg/day)	Usual Mode of Elimination	Major Protein-Binding Level
Mephobarbital	• Grand mal • Petit mal • Gets converted to phenobarbital • Indicated when phenobarbital must be d/c because of excessive drowsiness • Hyperexcitability • Mood disturbances	11–67	NA	400–600	Liver	40–60
Mephenytoin	• Tonic–clonic • Psychomotor • Status epilepticus • Used with phenytoin; together more sedative compared to phenytoin alone	95 (Active metabolite)	NA	200–600	Liver > > Renal	90
Ethotoin	• Tonic–clonic • Psychomotor • Used as second-line therapy; less toxic and less effective than phenytoin (alone or combined)	3–9a	15–50	2000–3000	Liver	NA
Phenacemide	• Severe mixed psychomotor • Toxic drug (hydantoin toxicity) • Second-line therapy	NA	NA	2000–3000	Liver	NA
Methsuximide	• Absence • Does not precipitate tonic–clonic (compared to other succinimides)	2–40b	NA	1200	Liver	NA
Phensuximide	• Absence • Less toxic and less effective compared to other succinimides	8b	NA	1000–3000	Urine, bile	NA
Paramethadione[c]	• Absence • Useful when other seizures exist with absence seizure • Note: Do not use with mephenytoin or phenacemide because of high toxicity	NA	NA	900–2400	Liver > Renal	NA
Trimethadione[c]	• Same as paramethadione	6–13 **days**	≥700	900–2400	Liver	0

a = At high doses, non-linear kinetic like phenytoin.

b = Active metabolite.

c = Possible fetal malformation if used during pregnancy.

3. **Other surgical approaches** include temporal lobe resection, removal of the temporal lobe tip, and cerebral hemispherectomy.

III. COMPLICATIONS

A. **Convulsive status epilepticus.** This disorder is characterized by rapid repetition of generalized tonic–clonic seizures with no recovery of consciousness between seizures. This life-threatening condition may persist for hours or even days; if it lasts longer than 1 hour, severe permanent brain damage may result.

1. **Causes** of status epilepticus include poor therapeutic compliance, intracranial infection or neoplasm, alcohol withdrawal, drug overdose, and metabolic imbalance.

2. **Management**
   a. A patent airway must be maintained.
   b. If the cause of the condition is unknown, dextrose 50% in water (25–30 mL) is given via IV in case hypoglycemia is the cause.
   c. If the seizures persist, **diazepam** (10 mg) is administered via IV at a rate not exceeding 2 mg/min until the seizures stop or 20 mg has been given.
   d. **Phenytoin or phosphenytoin** is then administered via IV no faster than 50 mg/min to a maximum dose of 11–18 mg/kg. Blood pressure is monitored to detect hypotension.
   e. If these measures do not stop the seizures, one of the following drugs is given.
      (1) **Diazepam** is given as an IV drip of 50–100 mg diluted in 500 mL dextrose 5% in water, infused at 40 mL/hr until the seizures stop.
      (2) **Phenobarbital** is given as an IV infusion of 8–20 mg/kg no faster than 100 mg/min.
   f. If seizures continue despite these measures, one of the following steps is then taken.
      (1) **Paraldehyde** is given via IV in a dosage of 0.10–0.15 mL/kg diluted to a 4% solution in normal saline solution.
      (2) **Lidocaine** is given in an IV loading dose of 50–100 mg, followed by an infusion of 1–2 mg/min.
      (3) **General anesthesia** is induced with ventilatory assistance and neuromuscular junction blockade.

B. **Nonconvulsive status epilepticus.** This condition presents as repeated absence seizures or complex partial seizures. The patient's mental state fluctuates; confusion, impaired responses, and automatisms are prominent. **Initial management** typically involves intravenous diazepam. Complex partial status epilepticus may also necessitate administration of such drugs as phenytoin or phenobarbital.

IV. SEIZURE DISORDER AND PREGNANCY

A. **Epidemiology.** About 0.5% of all pregnancies occur in women with epilepsy.

B. **Preconception counseling.** The risks for mother and fetus should be discussed, including the risks of fetal malformation associated with antiepileptic drugs and other genetic factors.

C. **Drug therapy**

1. If the patient is seizure free for at least 2 years, withdrawal of the drug should be considered. If antiepileptic drug therapy is necessary, a switch to monotherapy should be made if possible.

2. Five antiepileptic medications have been used or studied in pregnant patients: carbamazepine, phenobarbital, phenytoin, primidone, and valproic acid. Monotherapy of lamotrigine during pregnancy found no teratogenic effect. Congenital malformations associated with these drugs include craniofacial abnormalities, cardiac defects, and neuronal tube defects. Most of the studies did not consider paternal genetic factors, environmental factors, drug dosing, or combination therapy.

3. Antiepileptic drugs interfere with folate metabolism. Administration of folic acid, 4 mg daily, and multivitamins decreases the risk of malformation, especially of the neuronal tube.

4. Vitamin K, 10 mg per day for the last 1 or 2 months of gestation, will help to prevent neonatal hemorrhage, especially in cases of phenytoin or phenobarbital use.

5. Seizure disorder and oral contraceptives. Gabapentin, lamotrigine, levetiracetam, and tigabine do not affect the efficacy of oral contraceptives.

6. Seizure disorder and the elderly population. New generations of antiepileptic drugs such as levetiracetam and gabapentin may be more useful due to low levels of protein binding and safer side effects. Also, new generations have less potential for drug interactions than agents eliminated from the liver.

D. Monitoring

1. Free serum antiepileptic drug levels should be monitored monthly, immediately before the next dose, and the dose should be adjusted to the lowest dose providing adequate control.

2. Serum α-fetoprotein levels should be checked and ultrasonography should be performed at 16 weeks of gestation to evaluate for fetal neuronal tube defects. An alternative to these tests is amniocentesis, especially if the mother is taking valproate or carbamazepine.

3. Comprehensive ultrasonography should be performed at 18 and 22 weeks of gestation for patients taking antiepileptic drugs that cause cardiac anomalies

4. Intrapartum plans should include IV administration of a short-acting benzodiazepine. If there is concern about fetal or maternal respiratory depression, administering intravenous phenytoin or intramuscular phenobarbital should be considered. Clotting studies should be performed, and 1 mg vitamin K should be given to the infant. Nurses and physicians should be alerted for possible hemorrhage of the infant and apprised that the infant may experience antiepileptic drug withdrawal.

STUDY QUESTIONS

Directions: Each of the numbered items or incomplete statements in this section is followed by answers or by completions of the statement. Select the **one** lettered answer or completion that is **best** in each case.

1. Phenytoin is effective for the treatment of all of the following types of seizures EXCEPT

(A) generalized tonic–clonic
(B) simple partial
(C) complex partial
(D) absence
(E) grand mal

2. Which of the following anticonvulsants is contraindicated in patients with a history of hypersensitivity to tricyclic antidepressants?

(A) Phenytoin
(B) Ethosuximide
(C) Acetazolamide
(D) Carbamazepine
(E) Phenobarbital

3. Which of the following antiepileptic drugs is primary metabolized by the kidney?

(A) Phenytoin
(B) Gabapentin
(C) Topiramate
(D) Levetiracetam
(E) Answers B, C, and D

4. Which anticonvulsive drug treatment has a higher incidence of kidney stones?

(A) Phenytoin
(B) Carbamazepine
(C) Topiramate
(D) Tiagabine

5. What are the most common adverse effects of anticonvulsive drugs?

(A) Headache and dizziness
(B) Gastrointestinal symptoms
(C) Alternation of cognition and mentation
(D) Adverse effects on appetite and body weight
(E) All of the above

6. Which antiepileptic drug has the least effect on the efficacy of oral contraceptives?

(A) Phenytoin
(B) Tiagabine
(C) Gabapentin
(D) Lamotrigine
(E) Answers C and D

ANSWERS AND EXPLANATIONS

1. The answer is D *[I B 2 c (1), II B 2].*
Phenytoin (diphenylhydantoin) is the most commonly prescribed hydantoin for seizure disorders. It is one of the preferred drugs for generalized tonic–clonic (grand mal) seizures and for partial seizures, both simple and complex. However, phenytoin is not effective for absence (petit mal) seizures.

2. The answer is D *[II B 1 c (2)].*
Carbamazepine is structurally related to the tricyclic antidepressants (e.g., amitriptyline, desipramine, imipramine, nortriptyline, protriptyline) and should not be administered to patients with hypersensitivity to any of the tricyclic antidepressants.

3. The answer is B *[II B 5].*
Primidone's antiseizure activity may be partly attributable to phenobarbital. In patients receiving primidone, serum levels of both primidone and phenobarbital should be measured.

4. The answer is C *[II B 12]*
There is a higher incidence of kidney stones (renal calculus) with topiramate administration.

5. The answer is E *[II B 1-14, Table 44-8]*
Alternation in cognition and mentation, gastrointestinal symptoms, appetite and body weight, and headache and dizziness are all common adverse effects of anticonvulsive drugs.

6. The answer is C and D
Gabapetin and Lamotrigine do not increase the metabolism of oral contraceptives to be clinically significant; therefore, they could be used with oral contraceptives.

45
Parkinson's Disease

Azita Razzaghi

I. DISEASE STATE AND PATHOLOGY

A. Definition. Parkinson's disease is a slowly progressive degenerative neurological disease characterized by tremor, rigidity, bradykinesia (sluggish neuromuscular responsiveness), and postural instability. Parkinson's disease was first described by Dr. James Parkinson in 1817 as "shaking palsy."

B. Incidence

1. It has a prevalence of 1 to 2 per 1000 of the general population and 2 per 100 among people older than 65 years.

2. Onset generally occurs between age 50 and 65; it usually occurs in the 60s.

C. Pathogenesis. Parkinson's disease is a neurodegenerative disease associated with **depigmentation of the substantia nigra** and the **loss of dopaminergic input to the basal ganglia** (extrapyramidal system); it is characterized by distinctive **motor disability.** The basal ganglia are responsible for initiating, sequencing, and modulating motor activity.

1. In healthy individuals, dopamine is produced by neurons that project from the substantia nigra to the neostriatum (which include caudate and putamen) and globus pallidus. In these areas, dopamine acts as an inhibitory neurotransmitter.

2. Lewy bodies are widespread but occur especially in the basal ganglia, brain stem, spinal cord, and sympathetic ganglia.

3. In Parkinson's disease, the loss of dopamine-producing neurons in the substantia nigra results in an imbalance between dopamine, an inhibitory neurotransmitter, and the excitatory neurotransmitter acetylcholine. Alterations in the concentrations of other neurotransmitters, such as norepinephrine, serotonin, and γ-aminobutyric acid (GABA), are also involved in the pathophysiology of Parkinson's disease (Figure 45-1).

D. Etiology. Several forms of Parkinson's disease have been recognized.

1. **Primary (idiopathic) Parkinson's disease**
   a. This is also called classic Parkinson's disease or **paralysis agitans.**
   b. The cause is unknown, and while treatment may be palliative, the disease is incurable.
   c. Most patients suffer from this type of parkinsonism.
   d. **Hypotheses of neuronal loss** in idiopathic Parkinson's disease are:
      (1) **Absorption of highly potent neurotoxins,** such as carbon monoxide, manganese, solvents, and N-methyl-4-phenyl-1,2,3,6-tetrahydropyridine (MPTP), which is a product of improper synthesis of a synthetic heroin-like compound. Exposure to these agents, alone or in combination with the neuronal loss of age, may be the cause of Parkinson's disease.
      (2) **Exposure to the free radicals.** Normally, dopamine is catabolized by monoamine oxidase (MAO). Hydrogen peroxide and production of free radicals—both toxic to cells—are products of catabolism. Protective mechanisms, enzymes, and free radical scavengers, such as vitamins E and C, protect cells from damage. It is proposed that either a decrease in these protective mechanisms or an increase in the production of dopamine causes a destruction of the neurons by free radicals.

2. **Secondary parkinsonism—from a known cause**
   a. Only a small percentage of cases are secondary, and many of these are curable.
   b. Secondary parkinsonism may be caused by drugs, including dopamine antagonists, such as:
      (1) Phenothiazines (e.g., chlorpromazine, perphenazine)
      (2) Butyrophenones (e.g., haloperidol)
      (3) Reserpine

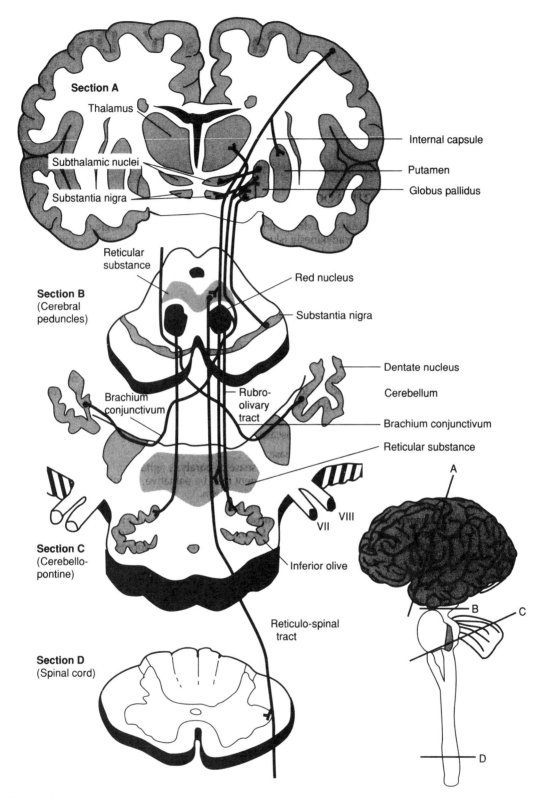

Figure 45-1. Extrapyramidal system involved in Parkinson's disease. (Reprinted from Netter F. Ciba Collection of Medical Illustrations. West Caldwell, NJ: Ciba Geigy Pharmaceuticals, 1983:69.)

    c. Poisoning by chemicals or toxins may be the cause; these include:
- **(1)** Carbon monoxide poisoning
- **(2)** Heavy metal poisoning, such as that by manganese or mercury
- **(3)** MPTP, a commercial compound used in organic synthesis and found (as a side product) in an illegal meperidine analogue

    d. Infectious causes include:
- **(1)** Encephalitis (viral)
- **(2)** Syphilis

    e. Other causes include:
- **(1)** Arteriosclerosis
- **(2)** Degenerative diseases of the central nervous system (CNS), such as progressive supranuclear palsy
- **(3)** Metabolic disorders, such as Wilson's disease

E. Signs and symptoms

    1. Tremor

      a. Tremor may be the initial complaint in some patients. It is most evident at rest **(resting tremor)** and with low-frequency movement. When the thumb and forefinger are involved, it is known as the **pill-rolling tremor.** Before pills were made by machine, pharmacists made tablets (pills) by hand, hence the name (Figure 45-2).

      b. Some patients experience **action tremor** (most evident during activity), which can exist with or before the resting tremor develops.

    2. Limb rigidity is present in almost all patients. It is detected clinically when the arm responds with a ratchet-like (i.e., cogwheeling) movement when the limb is moved passively. This is owing to a tremor that is superimposed on the rigidity.

    3. Akinesia or bradykinesia. Akinesia is characterized by difficulty in initiating movements, and bradykinesia is a slowness in performing common voluntary movements, including standing, walking, eating, writing, and talking. The lines of the patient's face are smooth, and the expression is fixed **(masked face)** with little evidence of spontaneous emotional responses (Figure 45-3).

    4. Gait and postural difficulties. Characteristically, patients walk with a stooped, flexed posture; a short, shuffling stride; and a diminished arm swing in rhythm with the legs. There may be a tendency to accelerate or festinate (Figure 45-4).

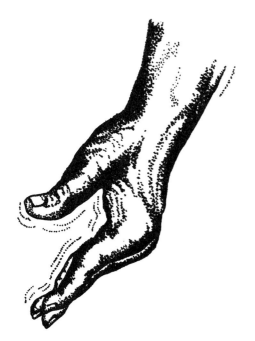

Figure 45-2. Resting (or static) tremors. (Adapted from Bates B. *A Guide to Physical Examination and History Taking.* 5th ed. Philadelphia: JB Lippincott, 1991:197.)

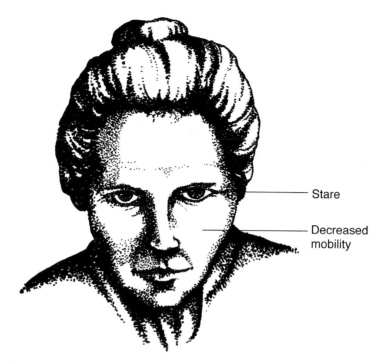

Figure 45-3. Masked face of Parkinson's disease. (Adapted from Bates B. *A Guide to Physical Examination and History Taking.* 5th ed. Philadelphia: JB Lippincott, 1991:197.)

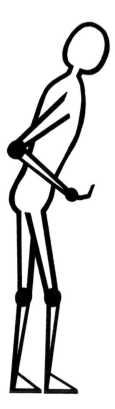

Figure 45-4. Characteristic walk of patients with Parkinson's disease. (Adapted from Bates B. *A Guide to Physical Examination and History Taking.* 5th ed. Philadelphia: JB Lippincott, 1991:553.)

Table 45-1. Stages of Parkinson's Disease

Stage 0:	No clinical signs evident
Stage I:	Unilateral involvement, including the major features of tremor, rigidity, or bradykinesia; minimal functional impairment
Stage II:	Bilateral involvement but no postural abnormalities
Stage III:	Mild to moderate bilateral disease, mild postural imbalance, but still ability to function independently
Stage IV:	Bilateral involvement with postural instability; patient requires substantial assistance
Stage V:	Severe disease; patient restricted to bed or wheelchair unless aided

Reprinted from Hoehn MM, Yahr MD. Parkinsonism: onset, progression, and mortality. *Neurology* 1967;17:427.

5. **Changes in mental status.** Mental status changes, including depression (50%), dementia (25%), and psychosis, are associated with the disease and may be precipitated or worsened by drugs.

6. **Unified Parkinson's disease rating scale (UPDRS)**
   a. **To evaluate the clinical efficacy** of antiparkinson drugs and **to monitor disease progression,** most investigators have used the UPDRS.
      (1) The disadvantages associated with the use of scales for rating the functional and motor disabilities of patients with Parkinson's disease include the potential of interrater variability and imprecision due to semiquantitative scoring.
      (2) The result of testing is highly dependent on the stage of the disease, whether the patient is being evaluated during an on- or off-period, and the relative distribution of the improvement across all the items evaluated.
   b. **Part I** of the UPDRS is an **evaluation of mentation, behavior, and mood.**
   c. **Part II** is a **self-reported evaluation of the activities of daily living (ADL)** and includes speech, swallowing, handwriting, ability to cut food, dressing, hygiene, falling, salivating, turning in bed, and walking.
   d. **Part III** is a **clinician-scored motor evaluation.**
      (1) Patients are evaluated for speech, rest-tremor facial expression and mobility, action or postural tremor of hands, rigidity, finger taps, hand movements, rapid alternative pronation–suppination movement of hands, leg agility, ease of arising from a chair, posture, postural stability, gait, and bradykinesia.
      (2) Each item is evaluated on a scale of 0–4.
         (a) **A rating of 0** on the motor performance evaluation scale indicates **normal performance.**
         (b) **A rating of 4** on the motor performance evaluation scale indicates **severely impaired performance.**
   e. **Part IV** is the **Hoehn and Yahr** staging of severity of Parkinson's disease (Table 45-1).
   f. **Part V** is the **Schwan and England ADL scale.**

F. **Diagnosis**

   1. Diagnosis depends on clinical findings.

   2. Tests (including imaging) are most often used to rule out an etiology of secondary Parkinson's disease.

   3. New technologies [e.g., positron emission tomography (PET) scan] are used to visualize dopamine uptake in the substantia nigra and basal ganglia. The PET scan measures the extent of neuronal loss in these areas, but it is not yet widely available.

   4. A specific form of single-photon–emission computed tomography (SPECT) can be helpful for diagnosis of Parkinsonian syndromes and non-parkinsonisms, particularly essential tremor.

G. **Treatment** (Figure 45-5)

   1. **Nondrug treatment**
      a. **Exercise** is an important adjunctive therapy and is most beneficial. Although exercise does not help with the symptoms of Parkinson's disease, regular focused exercise, stretching, and strengthening activities can have a positive effect on mobility and mood.

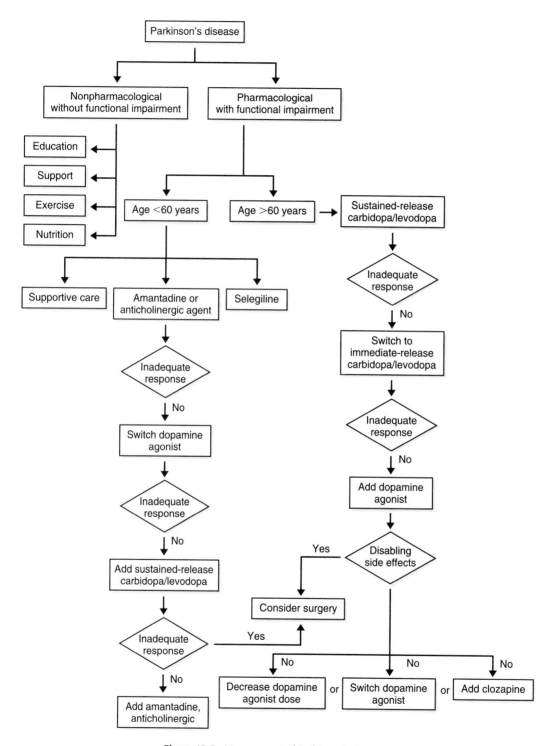

Figure 45-5. Management of Parkinson's disease.

b. Nutrition. Patients with Parkinson's disease are at increased risk of poor nutrition, weight loss, and reduced muscle mass. Examples of the beneficial effects of proper nutrition in this group of patients include:

(1) Sufficient fiber and fluid intake help prevent constipation associated with Parkinson's disease and the medications used to treat the disease.

(2) Calcium supplementation helps to maintain the existing bone structure.

(3) Excessive dietary protein in the late stages of the disease causes erratic responses to levodopa therapy.

(4) A large body of literature supports the pathophysiological role of antioxidants in the relief of oxidative stress in Parkinson's disease. High doses of antioxidants and α-tocopherol or vitamin E are recommended in this group of patients.

2. Drug therapy for symptomatic relief. Treatment is divided into two generalized categories: symptomatic therapies and preventive or protective measures. Neuroprotective strategies are used to slow the development and progression of the disorder.

H. Neuroprotective treatment:

1. MAO B such as selegiline and tocopherol (Vitamin-E) acts as a scavenger of free radicals.

2. Dopamine agonists serve as scavengers of free radicals and decrease dopamine turnover, which reduces oxidative stress. During early development of the disease, there are increases in oxidative stress. Four classes of drugs are available:

a. Anticholinergics (for resting tremor)

b. Precursor of dopamine (e.g., carbidopa/levodopa)

c. Direct-acting dopamine agonists (e.g., bromocriptine, pergolide)

d. Indirect-acting dopamine agonists

(1) Decrease reuptake (e.g., amantadine)

(2) Decrease metabolism (e.g., selegiline)

3. Drug therapy for treating associated symptoms

a. Tricyclic antidepressants are used to treat **depression.** They exhibit some dopaminergic and anticholinergic effects.

b. β–Blockers, especially **propranolol** with its high lipophilicity, **benzodiazepines,** and **primidone,** are medications used for **action tremor.** Usually, patients show a clinical response in low doses.

c. Antihistamines. Diphenhydramine hydrochloride has some mild anticholinergic effects and is used for symptomatic release of mild tremor; because of its adverse reaction in the CNS, it should be used with caution in the elderly.

4. General principles of drug therapy

a. If a patient does not respond to an agent in one class, another class should be tried. The two dopamine agonists, bromocriptine and pergolide, are two exceptions. Studies show that some patients respond to one agent when they fail to respond to another. This could be because of their different potencies or the limited information available on pergolide.

b. Therapy should be started with a low dose and titrated up. Response usually is seen within a few days after starting therapy.

c. If a second agent is added to the drug therapy, the dose of the first medication should be decreased to minimize side effects.

d. Drug therapy should never be discontinued suddenly because withdrawal may exacerbate the symptoms.

5. Definitions concerning drug therapy

a. Dyskinesias/dystonia are typically oral–facial movements, grimacing, or jerky and writhing movements of the trunk and extremities. They are always reversible with antiparkinsonian medications, and they decrease or diminish with dose reduction. Symptoms of Parkinson's disease may reappear by reducing the dose, and it is the clinical judgment of the physician or the preference of the patient whether to continue with the drug regimen or tolerate the side effects. There are three types of dyskinesias/dystonia: peak dose dyskinesia, biphasic dyskinesias, and off-period dystonia. All could benefit from sustained release preparations.

(1) Peak-dose dyskinesia

(a) Could be corrected with sustained-release preparations

    (b) Decrease L-dopa dose, or add COMT inhibitor.
    (c) Add amandatine.
    (d) Perform surgery.
   (2) Biphasic dyskinesias
    (a) Could be corrected with sustained-release preparations
    (b) Decrease L-dopa dose and increase dopaminergic dose. If symptoms are still present, a COMT inhibitor should be added.
    (c) Amandatine may be helpful.
   (3) Off-period dystonia
    (a) Decrease L-dopa dose.
    (b) Increase dopaminergic dose.
  b. On–off effect describes oscillations in response (at the receptor site) and sudden changes in mobility from no symptoms to full parkinsonian symptoms in a matter of minutes. No direct relationship between the on–off effect and drug levels has been found. Usually, a second drug is added to the therapy regimen to correct the effect. Reducing the dose of one drug and adding a second drug may also be useful.
  c. End-dose effect, known also as the **wearing-off effect,** occurs at a latter part of the dosing interval; it happens after a few years of L-dopa therapy. Reduce the single L-dopa dose and spread the total L-dopa dose over a larger number of single doses. Change to a dopamine agonist and use a sustained-release formulation of L-dopa.
  d. Drug holiday. Long-term levodopa use results in downregulation of dopamine receptors. A drug holiday allows striatal nigra dopamine receptors to be resensitized, although controversy exists regarding the consequences and the outcome of this "holiday."

 6. Physical rehabilitation restores patients' physical function and independence through physical and occupational therapy. These will help patients with managing big and small muscle groups by focusing on maintaining coordination, dexterity, flexibility, and range of motions.

 7. Psychological rehabilitation provides support for patients and their families. Keep in mind that patients with Parkinson's disease have a high incidence of depression and that, in later stages of the disease, they develop dementia (Table 45-2).

Table 45-2. Overview of Parkinson's Disease Management

Stage	Characteristics	Treatment Considerations	
		Physical	**Psychosocial**
Early	Fully functional May have unilateral tremor, rigidity	Preventive exercise program	Education Information
Early middle	Symptoms bilateral, bradykinesia, rigidity Mild speech impairment Axial rigidity, stooped posture, stiffness Gait impairment begins	Corrective exercise program	Counseling Support group Monitor for depression
Late middle	All symptoms worse but independent in ADLs[a] May need minor assistance Balance problems	Compensatory and corrective exercise Speech therapy Occupational therapy	Caregiver issues (medications, mobility) Monitor for dementia
Late	Severely disabled, impaired Dependent with ADLs	Compensatory exercise Dietary concerns Skin care Hygiene Pulmonary function	Dementia Depression

[a]ADLs = activities of daily living.

Reprinted from Custin TM. Overview of Parkinson's disease management. *Phys Ther* 1995;75:363–373.

8. **Secondary effects of Parkinson's disease include:**
   a. **Cardiovascular effects,** including orthostatic hypotension and arrhythmia
   b. **Gastrointestinal effects,** including constipation and hypersalivation
   c. **Genitourinary effects,** including increased urinary frequency and impotence
   d. **Central nervous system effects,** including hallucinations, depression, and psychosis

9. **Parkinson's disease late disabilities** can be divided into two groups.
   a. **Levodopa-related disabilities,** which include motor fluctuation, dyskinesia, neuropsychiatric toxicity, and reduced response
   b. **Non–levodopa-related disabilities,** which include cognitive impairment, instability resulting in more frequent falls, gait disturbance, incontinence, dysphagia, and speech disturbance
   c. Parkinson's disease late disabilities management therapies include:
      (1) Motor fluctuation. Altering the levodopa dosage and timing, alternative means of levodopa administration, delivery, and absorption; using direct-acting dopamine agonists or experimental agonists; altering metabolism of dopamine and levodopa parental agonists; using glutamate antagonists; and performing functional neurosurgery
      (2) Miscellaneous late disabilities and management therapies include:
         (a) Urinary urgency: oxybutynin
         (b) Urinary retention: apomorphine
         (c) Constipation: fiber, polyethylene glycols
         (d) Tenesmus: clonazepam, apomorphine
         (e) Hypersalivation: antihistamine, anticholinergic
         (f) Dysphagia: liquid levodopa
         (g) Sweating crises: β-blockers, anticholinergic agents
         (h) Daytime sleepiness: selegiline
         (i) Nightmares: amitriptyline, clonazepam
         (j) Panic attacks and depression: liquid levodopa, amitriptyline
         (k) Orthostatic hypotension: domperidone, desmopressin
         (l) Dysphonia: reduce levodopa dosage, speech therapy
         (m) Pain: amitriptyline, fluvoxamine

II. INDIVIDUAL DRUGS

A. **Anticholinergic agents** are used for mild symptoms, predominantly tremors.

1. **Mechanism of action.** This class of drugs blocks the excitatory neurotransmitter cholinergic influence in the basal ganglia. These drugs are more effective for tremor and rigidity than for bradykinesia and less effective for postural imbalance.

2. **Administration and dosage** (Table 45-3)

3. **Precautions and monitoring effects**
   a. Anticholinergics should be used with caution in patients with obstructed gastrointestinal (GI) or genitourinary (GU) tracts, narrow-angle glaucoma, or severe cardiac disease. Physicians should be notified if a rapid heartbeat or eye pain are experienced. (Frequent ophthalmological visits are recommended.)
   b. The sedative side effects of antihistamines may be beneficial in some patients.
   c. Alcohol and other CNS depressants should be used with caution.
   d. **Adverse effects** of anticholinergic therapy include the following:
      (1) Peripheral anticholinergic effects include dry mouth (hard candies may be helpful); decreased sweating, resulting in decreased tolerance to heat; urinary retention; constipation (stool softeners may be helpful); increased intraocular tension; and nausea. Because of patients' decreased tolerance to heat, these agents should be used with caution in hot weather. They should also be taken with food to minimize GI upset.
      (2) CNS effects include dizziness, delirium, disorientation, anxiety, agitation, hallucinations, and impaired memory. The incidence of CNS effects increases in elderly individuals.
      (3) Cardiovascular effects include hypotension and orthostatic hypotension.

4. **Significant interactions**
   a. Side effects may be potentiated by other drugs with anticholinergic activity such as **antihistamines, antidepressants,** and **phenothiazines.**

Table 45-3. Dosage Range and Characteristics of Drug Treatment

Drugs	Time to Peak Concentration (hours)	Half-Life (hours)	Daily Dosage Range (mg/day)
Anticholinergic agents			
Benztropine	Not available	Not available	1–6
Biperiden	1–1.5	18.4–24.3	2–8
Procyclidine	1.1–2	11.5–12.6	6–20
Trihexyphenidyl	1–1.3	5.6–10.2	2–15
Ethopropazine	Not available	Not available	50–400
Dopamine agents			
Carbidopa/levodopa	1	1–1.75	10/100–200/2000
Carbidopa/levodopa sustained-release	2	> standard treatment	10/400–25/1000 in 2–3 divided doses
Amantadine	4–8	9.7–14.5	100–400
Bromocriptine	1–3	3–8	2.5–40
Pergolide	2	27	0.1–5
Selegiline	0.5–2	2–20.5	5–108
Dopamine agents			
Non-ergot agents			
Pramipexole	1–2 3–4*	8–12†	1.5–4.5‡
Ropinirole	1–2 3–4*	6	3–24‡
COMT inhibitor	0.5–4	70	0.5–6
Tolcapone	2	2–3	300–600
Entacapone	1	2–3	200–1600

* = With food
† = Over 65 years of age.
‡ = In 3 divided doses.

    b. Anticholinergic agents increase **digoxin** levels.
    c. When anticholinergic agents are taken with **haloperidol,** the following occurs:
        (1) Schizophrenic symptoms may increase.
        (2) Haloperidol levels may decrease.
        (3) The severity of (not the risk of) tardive dyskinesia may increase.
    d. When **phenothiazines** are taken with anticholinergic drugs, the effects of the phenothiazines decrease and the anticholinergic symptoms increase.
    e. Patients on high doses of anticholinergics combined with **levodopa** should be watched for decreased levodopa activity because of a delayed gastric emptying time.

  B. Dopamine precursor. Levodopa/carbidopa is the most effective drug for managing Parkinson's disease; however, prolonged use decreases its therapeutic effects (there is a decline in efficacy after 3–5 years) and increases adverse drug reactions. Dopamine does not cross the blood–brain barrier; therefore, a precursor is used. Peripheral conversion of levodopa to dopamine causes adverse reactions like nausea, vomiting, cardiac arrhythmias, and postural hypotension. To decrease the peripheral conversion and peripheral adverse effects, a peripheral dopa decarboxylase inhibitor (carbidopa) is added to levodopa.

    1. Mechanism of action
      a. Levodopa is converted to dopamine by the enzyme dopa decarboxylase, which elevates CNS levels of dopamine.
      b. The sustained-release formulation is designed to release the drug over 4–6 hours, thereby inhibiting variation in plasma concentration and decreasing motor fluctuation "off" time, or to improve overall dose response in patients with advanced disease.

    2. Administration and dosage (see Table 45-3)
      a. It is necessary to give at least 100 mg daily of carbidopa to decrease the incidence of the peripheral conversion of levodopa and GI side effects (e.g., nausea) and increase the bioavailability of levodopa for the CNS.

b. If carbidopa is given in a separate dosage form, the dose of levodopa can be decreased by 75%.

c. If patients still complain of GI side effects after combination levodopa/carbidopa, plain carbidopa can be given.

d. Sustained-release preparations are approximately 30% less bioavailable as compared with levodopa/carbidopa. Because of this lower bioavailability, the daily dosage should be higher. If a patient is receiving a standard preparation and needs to be converted to the sustained-release dose, approximately 10% more levodopa should initially be added to the daily dosage and at least 3 days should pass between increased dosages; then gradually increase the levodopa dose up to 30% of standard preparation.

e. With the sustained-release preparation, the peak plasma concentration is lower and the trough plasma concentration is higher.

f. The sustained-release preparation could be divided in half at the scored point only. The tablet should not be chewed or crushed.

g. When carbidopa is given to patients being treated with levodopa, give the two drugs at the same time, starting with no more than 20%–25% of the previous daily dosage of levodopa and initiating therapy with carbidopa and levodopa.

h. Long-term treatment could lead to motor fluctuation and dyskinesias, especially at high doses.

3. **Precautions and monitoring effects**

   a. Levodopa must be used with caution in patients with narrow-angle glaucoma.

   b. Levodopa may activate a malignant melanoma in patients with suspicious undiagnosed skin lesions or a history of melanoma.

   c. The efficacy of levodopa declines with long-term therapy by desensitizing the receptors or because of the decreased number of receptors, resulting from the progression of the disease.

   d. **Adverse drug reactions**

      (1) GI effects include anorexia, nausea and vomiting, and abdominal distress. Levodopa should be taken with food to minimize stomach upset.

      (2) Cardiovascular effects include postural hypotension and tachycardia.

      (3) Musculoskeletal effects include dystonia or choreiform muscle movement.

      (4) CNS effects include confusion, memory changes, depression, hallucinations, and psychosis. Physicians should be notified if any of these symptoms occur.

      (5) Hematological effects include hemolytic anemia, leukopenia, and agranulocytosis (rare).

4. **Significant interactions**

   a. **Antacids** cause rapid and complete intestinal levodopa absorption (by decreasing gastric emptying time).

   b. **Hydantoin** decreases the effectiveness of levodopa.

   c. **Methionine** increases the clinical signs of Parkinson's disease.

   d. **Metoclopramide** increases the bioavailability of levodopa, which decreases the effects of metoclopramide on gastric emptying and on lower esophageal pressure. As a dopamine blocker, it may also precipitate parkinsonian symptoms.

   e. False-positive results are seen with the Coombs' test.

   f. The uric acid test increases with the calorimetric method but not with the uricase method.

   g. Hypertensive reactions may occur if levodopa is administered to patients receiving **MAO inhibitors** and **furazolidone.** MAO inhibitors must be discontinued 2 weeks before starting levodopa.

   h. Administering **papaverine** may decrease the effect of levodopa.

   i. **Tricyclic antidepressants** decrease the rate and extent of absorption of levodopa; hypertensive episodes have been reported when levodopa is combined with tricyclic antidepressants.

   j. **Food** decreases the rate and extent of absorption and transport to the CNS across the blood–brain barrier. A **protein-restricted diet** may also help to minimize the "fluctuations" (i.e., the decreased response to levodopa) at the end of each day or at various times of the day.

C. Direct-acting dopamine agonists are classified as ergot derivatives such as bromocriptine and pergolide and the non-ergolines such as pramipexole and ropinirole.

- Mimic dopamine agonist and reduce motor fluctuations
- Half life of drugs in this class varies and also varies among patients
- Are not metabolized by the oxidative pathway and do not produce free-radical metabolites
- May have a direct antioxidative effect
- Take longer than L-dopa to reach effective doses and require supplementary L-dopa for relief of symptoms after a varying period of time
- Common side effects are nausea and psychiatric side effects similar to L-dopa such as hallucinations and delusions; dyskinesias are less common.
- Other adverse effects are headache, nasal congestion, erythromelalgia, pleural and retroperitoneal fibrosis, pulmonary infiltrates, and vasospasm (except with new, non–ergot derivatives such as ropinirole).
- Annual chest radiographs have been recommended in patients on high-dose therapy with bromocriptine or pergolide to detect pleuropulmonary changes.
- New dopaminergic agonists (not ergot derivatives) cause postural hypotension, sleep disturbances, peripheral edema, constipation, nausea, dyskinesias, and confusion.

1. **Bromocriptine**
   a. **Mechanism of action.** Bromocriptine is responsible for directly stimulating postsynaptic dopamine receptors; it is most commonly used as an adjunct to levodopa therapy in patients:
      (1) With a deteriorating response to levodopa
      (2) With a limited clinical response to levodopa secondary to an inability to tolerate higher doses
      (3) Who are experiencing fluctuations in response to levodopa
   b. **Administration and dosage** (see Table 45-3)
      (1) Initially, patients are given one-half of a tablet twice daily, which is then increased to one tablet twice daily every 2–3 days.
      (2) Patients' responses are extremely variable. Many patients show a dopamine antagonist response at both low and high doses, with the desirable agonist response in the midrange.
      (3) Because postural hypotension may result from the first few doses of bromocriptine, the first dose should be administered with the patient lying down, and sudden changes in posture should be avoided.
   c. **Precautions and monitoring effects**
      (1) Bromocriptine may cause a first-dose phenomenon that can trigger sudden cardiovascular collapse. It should be used with caution in patients with a history of myocardial infarction or arrhythmias.
      (2) Early in therapy, dizziness, drowsiness, and fainting may occur, so patients should be cautious about driving or operating machinery. A physician should be notified if these symptoms appear.
      (3) **Cardiac dysrhythmias.** Patients on bromocriptine were found to have significantly more episodes of atrial premature contractions and sinus tachycardia.
      (4) **Other adverse effects**
         (a) **GI effects,** including anorexia, nausea, vomiting, and abdominal distress, may be decreased by taking bromocriptine with food.
         (b) **Cardiovascular effects** include postural hypotension (to which tolerance develops) and tachycardia. Blood pressure must be monitored, particularly for patients taking antihypertensive medication.
         (c) **Pulmonary effects,** including reversible infiltrations, pleural effusions, and pleural thickening, may develop after long-term treatment, so pulmonary function should be monitored in patients treated longer than 6 months.
         (d) **CNS effects,** including confusion, memory changes, depression, and hallucinations, as well as psychosis may be exacerbated by bromocriptine; thus, patients with psychiatric illnesses must be monitored.
   d. **Significant interactions**
      (1) A combination of **antihypertensive drugs** and bromocriptine could decrease blood pressure.
      (2) **Dopamine antagonists** increase the effect of bromocriptine.

2. Pergolide

  a. Mechanism of action. Pergolide is a semisynthetic ergosine derivative. In Parkinson's disease, it exerts its effect by directly stimulating postsynaptic dopamine receptors in the nigrostriatal system.

    (1) It is 1000 times more potent than bromocriptine on a milligram basis.

    (2) It inhibits the secretion of prolactin, increases the serum concentration of growth hormone, and decreases the serum concentration of luteinizing hormone.

    (3) It is most commonly used as adjunctive treatment to levodopa/carbidopa.

  b. Administration and dosage (see Table 45-3)

  c. Precautions and monitoring effects

    (1) Hypersensitivity reactions to pergolide and other ergot derivatives can occur.

    (2) Caution must be used with patients who are at high risk for ventricular arrhythmia, especially when doses higher than 3 mg/day are used.

    (3) Cardiac dysrhythmias. Adverse effects are similar to those experienced with bromocriptine [see II C 1 c (3)].

    (4) CNS effects include dyskinesia, hallucinations, somnolence, and insomnia.

    (5) GI effects include nausea, constipation, diarrhea, and dyspepsia.

    (6) Cardiovascular effects include premature atrial contractions and sinus tachycardia (alone or in combination with levodopa).

    (7) Miscellaneous effects include transient elevations of aspartate aminotransferase, alanine aminotransferase, and alkaline phosphatase, and pleural thickening.

  d. Significant interactions

    (1) Because pergolide is 90% protein bound, it must be used with caution with other highly **protein-bound drugs.**

    (2) Antipsychotic agents (e.g., phenothiazines, haloperidol, metoclopramide) combined with dopamine agonists decrease the dopamine action and decrease the therapeutic action of the antipsychotic agent.

D. Indirect-acting dopamine agonists

  1. Selegiline

    a. Mechanism of action

      (1) MAO catabolizes various catecholamines (e.g., dopamine, norepinephrine, epinephrine), serotonin, and various exogenous amines (e.g., tyramines) found in foods (e.g., aged cheese, beer, wine, smoked meat) and drugs. Lack of MAO in the intestinal tract causes absorption of these amines, creating a hypertensive crisis. MAO type A is predominantly found in the intestinal tract, and MAO type B in the brain. They differ in their substrate specificity and tissue distribution. This specificity decreases with selegiline as the dose increases. Most patients experience side effects at doses of selegiline higher than 30–40 mg/day.

      (2) Selegiline is a selective inhibitor of MAO type B, which prevents the breakdown of dopamine selectively in the brain at recommended doses.

      (3) Selegiline is most commonly used as an adjunct with levodopa/carbidopa when patients experience a "wearing-off" phenomenon; it decreases the amount of "off" time and decreases the dose needed of levodopa/carbidopa by 10%–30%.

      (4) Results of some studies show that selegiline delays the time before treatment with a more potent dopaminergic drug like levodopa is needed; the proposed mechanism of action is that an oxidation mechanism contributes to the emergence and progression of Parkinson's disease.

    b. Administration and dosage (see Table 45-3). Exceeding the recommended dose of 10 mg/day increases the risk of losing MAO selectivity. The precise selectivity dose is unknown but seems to be above 30–40 mg/day.

    c. Precautions and monitoring effects

      (1) Hypertensive crisis [see II D 1 a (1)]

      (2) Levodopa-associated side effects may be increased because the increased amounts of dopamine react with supersensitive postsynaptic receptors. Reducing the dose of levodopa/carbidopa by 10%–30% may decrease levodopa side effects.

      (3) Patients should be educated about foods and drugs containing tyramine and the signs and symptoms of hypertensive reactions.

      (4) CNS effects include dizziness, confusion, headache, hallucinations, vivid dreams, dyskinesias, behavioral and mood changes, and depression. Patients who experience insomnia should avoid taking the drug late in the day.

    (5) Cardiovascular effects include orthostatic hypotension, hypertension, arrhythmia, palpitations, sinus bradycardia, and syncope.

    (6) GI effects include nausea and abdominal pain and **lead to GI bleeding,** weight loss, poor appetite, and dysphagia.

    (7) GU effects include slow urination, transient nocturia, and prostatic hypertrophy.

    (8) Dermatological effects include increased sweating, diaphoresis, and photosensitivity.

    (9) Hepatic effects include mild and transient elevations in liver function tests.

  d. Significant interactions. MAO inhibitors are contraindicated with **meperidine** and other opioids. Because the mechanism of action is unknown, administration with opioids should be avoided.

  e. Death has occurred following initiation of selegiline shortly after discontinuation of fluoxetine. At least 5 weeks should elapse between discontinuation of fluoxetine and initiation of selegiline.

2. Amantadine

  a. Mechanism of action. Amantadine is an antiviral agent (used to prevent influenza).

    (1) Amantadine increases dopamine levels at postsynaptic receptor sites by decreasing presynaptic reuptake and enhancing dopamine synthesis and release.

    (2) It may also have some anticholinergic effects. It decreases tremor, rigidity, and bradykinesia.

    (3) It can be given in combination with levodopa as Parkinson's disease progresses.

    (4) Clinical effects of amantadine can be seen within the first few weeks of therapy, unlike the other antiparkinsonian medications (e.g., carbidopa/levodopa), which need weeks to months to show their full clinical effects.

  b. Administration and dosage (see Table 45-3)

    (1) Amantadine should be started at 100 mg/day. This may be increased to 200–300 mg/day as a maintenance dose.

    (2) Patients experiencing a decline in response may benefit from the following:

      (a) Discontinuing the drug for a few weeks, then restarting it

      (b) Using the drug episodically, only when the patient's condition most needs a therapeutic boost

    (3) Amantadine is also available in liquid form for patients with dysphagia.

  c. Precautions and monitoring effects

    (1) Amantadine should be used with caution in patients with renal disease, congestive heart failure (CHF), peripheral edema, history of seizures, and mental status changes. It may be necessary to modify dosages in patients with renal failure.

    (2) Tolerance usually develops within 6–12 months. If tolerance occurs, another drug from a different class can be added, or the dose may be increased.

    (3) Patients should be informed about the side-effect profile.

      (a) Peripheral anticholinergic effects include those mentioned in II A 3 d (1).

      (b) CNS effects include seizures as well as those mentioned in II A 3 d (2).

      (c) Cardiovascular effects. Patients may develop CHF. Periodic blood pressure monitoring and electrocardiograms (ECGs) are necessary in patients with myocardial infarction or arrhythmias.

      (d) Dermatological effects include **livedo reticularis,** a diffuse rose-color mottling of the skin, which is reversible upon discontinuation of the drug.

      (e) Hematological effects. Periodic complete blood counts (CBCs) should be done for patients with long-term therapy.

    (4) Renal function impairment. Dose adjustment is necessary in patients with renal function impairment.

  d. Significant interactions

    (1) Amantadine increases the anticholinergic effects of **anticholinergic drugs,** requiring a decrease in the dosage of the anticholinergic drug.

    (2) Hydrochlorothiazide plus **triamterene** decreases the urinary excretion of amantadine and increases its plasma concentration.

E. Non–ergot dopamine agonists

1. Pramipexole and ropinirole are indicated for both early and advanced stages of Parkinson's disease.

2. Both selectively bind to dopamine receptors and activate the D_2 receptor but have little or no affinity to the D_1 receptor. They have greater affinity for the D_3 receptor than for the D_2 receptor. The incidence of adverse events (such as pleuropulmonary fibrosis and retroperitoneal fibrosis, coronary vasoconstriction, erythromelalgia, and Raynaud's phenomenon), is low compared to nonselective dopamine agonists.

3. **Non–ergot dopamine agonists** have a low potential for the development of motor fluctuations and dyskinesia.
   a. **Pramipexole**
      (1) **Mechanism of action**
         (a) D_2 subfamily of dopamine receptors. Pramipexole fully stimulates the dopamine receptors to which it binds. Its action may be related to its capacity to function as an antioxidant and oxygen free-radical scavenger.
         (b) Pramipexole also has antidepressant activity in moderate depression, which may be related to its preferential binding to the dopamine D_1-receptor subtype.
         (c) Long-acting dopamine agonists appear to have a lower risk of inducing abnormal movements. Their use as initial treatment in early Parkinson's disease seems warranted, particularly for those with disease onset at a younger age.
      (2) **Administration and dosage**
         (a) Initial treatment: starting dose of 0.375 mg daily given in three divided doses
         (b) Do not increase more frequently than every 5–7 days.
         (c) Maintenance treatment: 1.5–4.5 mg daily in three divided doses with or without levodopa
         (d) When given in combination with levodopa, consider reduction of levodopa dose by an average of 27% from baseline
         (e) Titrate slowly to balance benefits and side effects, such as dyskinesia, hallucinations, somnolence, and dry mouth.
         (f) May be taken with food to reduce the occurrence of nausea. Food decreases the rate of absorption but not the extent of absorption.
         (g) Dosage adjustment is necessary in patients with renal function impairment.
         (h) Weak protein bound 15%
         (i) Not extensively metabolized. More than 90% of the dose is excreted unchanged in urine.
         (j) Dose needs to be decreased by 25% in the elderly
      (3) **Precautions and monitoring effects**
         (a) Dose reduction necessary in patients older than 65 years, and in patients with renal function impairment or failure
         (b) Symptomatic hypotension
            (i) Dopaminergic agents appear to impair the systemic regulation of blood pressure, which results in orthostatic hypotension.
            (ii) Monitoring and education of the patient is necessary, especially during dose-escalation periods.
         (c) Hallucinatory effects are increased in patients over 65 years of age with early or advanced stages of Parkinson's disease.
         (d) Other effects include nausea, insomnia, constipation, dizziness, somnolence, GI side effects, and visual hallucinations.
      (4) **Significant interactions**
         (a) Cimetidine reduces renal clearance of pramipexole.
         (b) No interaction with selegiline, probenecid, or domperidone.
         (c) When combined with levodopa, the dosage of levodopa must be decreased by 27%.
   b. **Ropinirole**
      (1) **Mechanism of action** is similar to pramipexole.
      (2) **Administration and dosage**
         (a) Initial treatment: 0.25 mg three times daily
         (b) Titrate weekly increments.
         (c) After week 4, if necessary, daily dosage may be increased by 1.5 mg/day on a weekly basis up to 9 mg/day, to a total of 24 mg/day.
         (d) Discontinue gradually over a 7-day period. Decrease the frequency of administration from three times to two times daily for 4 days, and then once daily for the remainder of the week.
         (e) When given in combination with levodopa, consider reduction of levodopa dose.
         (f) May be taken with food to reduce the occurrence of nausea. Food decreases the rate of absorption, but not the extent of absorption.
         (g) Metabolized by the liver (CYP1A2), and first-pass effect.

(h) Smoking induces the liver metabolism.
(i) 30%–40% protein bound
(3) Precautions and monitoring effects
  (a) Syncope. Bradycardia is observed in patients treated with ropinirole. Most cases occur within the first 4 weeks of therapy and are usually associated with a recent increase of dose.
  (b) Binds to melanin-containing tissues like the eyes and skin.
  (c) Symptomatic hypotension
    (i) Dopaminergic agents appear to impair the systemic regulation of blood pressure, which results in orthostatic hypotension.
    (ii) Monitoring and education of the patient is necessary, especially during dose-escalation periods.
  (d) Hallucinatory effects are increased in patients over 65 years of age with early or advanced stages of Parkinson's disease.
  (e) Other side effects include nausea, dizziness, somnolence, headache, fatigue, and abnormal vision.
(4) Significant interactions
  (a) Smoking induces the liver metabolism, but the affect of smoking on clearance of ropinirole has not been studied.
  (b) There is no interaction between levodopa, theophylline, digoxin, or domperidone.
  (c) Estrogens decrease the clearance of ropinirole by approximately 36%.
  (d) Ciprofloxacin increases ropinirole area under the curve by 84% and maximum plasma concentration by 60%.

4. Catechol-O-methyltransferase (COMT) inhibitors
  a. Tolcapone
    (1) Mechanism of action
      (a) Tolcapone is a selective and reversible inhibitor of COMT and is used as an adjunct to levodopa/carbidopa therapy.
      (b) Tolcopone inhibits COMT both peripheral and centrally.
      (c) COMT is the main enzyme responsible for peripheral and central metabolism of catecholamines, including levodopa. Addition of a COMT inhibitor results in the doubling of the elimination half-life of levodopa and in increased oral bioavailability of levodopa by 40%–50%.
      (d) Tolcapone is indicated as an adjunct therapy to carbidopa/levodopa therapy.
    (2) Administration and dosage
      (a) Starting dose of 100–200 mg, three times daily
      (b) Usual daily dose of 200 mg, three times daily
      (c) If patient fails to show expected benefit after 3 weeks of treatment, discontinue drug because of associated risk of liver failure. Rapid withdrawal or abrupt reduction dose could lead to hyperpyrexia and confusion symptoms such as high fever and severe rigidity similar to those in neuroleptic malignant syndrome.
    (3) Precautions and monitoring
      (a) Liver toxicity. High risk of fatal liver failure has been reported with tolcapone. Discontinue use if substantial benefit is not seen within 3 weeks of commencement of therapy.
      (b) Do not use in patients with liver disease or in patients who have two ALT or AST values greater than the upper limit of normal.
      (c) Advise patient regarding self-monitoring for liver disease (i.e., clay-colored stool, jaundice, fatigue, appetite loss, or lethargy).
      (d) Monitor AST and ALT every 2 weeks for the first year, then every 4 weeks for the next 6 months and every 8 weeks thereafter.
      (e) MAO and COMT are two major enzyme systems involved in the metabolism of catecholamines; combination of tolcapone with a non-selective MAO inhibitor will result in inhibition of the pathway responsible for normal catecholamine metabolism.
      (f) Tolcapone can be taken concomitantly with a selective MAO-B inhibitor, such as selegiline.
    (4) Other side effects
      (a) Orthostatic hypotension. Tolcapone enhances levodopa bioavailability, and therefore may increase the occurrence of orthostatic hypotension.

(b) Diarrhea usually manifests within 6–12 weeks after administration of tolcapone, but can develop as early as 2 weeks after administration. Diarrhea normally resolves after discontinuation of the drug.

(c) Hallucinations are sometimes accompanied by confusion, insomnia, and excessive dreaming. Hallucinatory effects usually occur after initiation of tolcapone and are usually resolved by decreasing the dose of levodopa.

(d) Tolcapone may potentiate the dopaminergic side effect of levodopa and may cause or exacerbate preexisting dyskinesia. Decreased doses of levodopa may or may not alleviate the symptoms.

(e) Severe cases of rhabdomyolysis have been reported, which present as fever, alternation of consciousness, and muscular rigidity.

(f) Others. Dyspepsia, abdominal cramping, mild paresthesia of the legs, and temporary discoloration of urine have also been noted but are not considered clinically important.

(g) Drug interactions. Although no drug interaction studies have been conducted, concurrent use of tolcapone and drugs that are metabolized by the COMT system (i.e., methyldopa, dobutamine, apomorphine) should be monitored. Tolcapone also has affinity for the CYP2C9 isoenzyme, similar to warfarin. Coagulation parameters should be monitored when tolcapone is administered with warfarin.

b. Entacapone

(1) Mechanism of action

(a) Entacapone is a selective and reversible inhibitor of COMT and permits additional levodopa to reach the brain. It does not have any anti-parkinson effect of its own.

(b) It acts only peripherally by inhibiting COMT.

(c) It improves the duration of "on" time and decreases the duration of "off" time.

(d) It is indicated as an adjunct to those on levodopa/carbidopa therapy who experience the signs and symptoms of end-of-dose "wearing-off."

(2) Administration and dosage

(a) 200 mg with each dose of L-dopa up to 8 times daily with a maximum dose of 1600 mg daily.

(b) Rapid withdrawal could lead to emergency signs and symptoms of Parkinson's disease such as hyperpyrexia and confusion (symptoms resembling neuroleptic malignant syndrome).

(3) Precautions and monitoring effects

(a) MAO. COMT and MAO are two major enzymes in the metabolism of catecholamines. Do not use together.

(b) Drugs metabolized by COMT. Drugs that are metabolized by this pathway, such as isoproterenol, epinephrine, norepinephrine, dopamine, and dobutamine, as well as methylodopa may interact and may result in increased heart rate, arrhythmias, and an excessive increase in blood pressure.

(c) Hepatic function impairment. The majority of the drug is metabolized by the liver; therefore, use caution in patients who have liver function abnormalities.

(d) Fibrotic complication. Cases of retroperitoneal fibrosis, pulmonary infiltrates, pleural effusion, and pleural thickening have been reported. These complications may resolve when the drug is discontinued, but complete resolution may not always occur.

(e) Biliary excretion: Entacapone is excreted by bile; therefore, use caution with drugs known to interfere with biliary excretion, such as probenecid, erythromycin, and ampicillin.

(4) Other side effects. Dyskinesia/hyperkenesia, nausea, urine discoloration (brownish-orange), diarrhea, and abdominal pain

(5) Drug interactions. May interact with drugs that are metabolized by the liver cytochrome P450.

III. SURGICAL TREATMENT. All surgeries require needle insertion into the brain, which in turn increases the risk of hemorrhage.

A. Globus pallidus internus (Gpi) pallidotomy

1. Definition. A pallidotomy entails the surgical resection of parts of the globus pallidus.

2. Advantage. Improves contralateral dyskinesia

3. Disadvantage. Increased risk of damage to other parts of the brain, including optic nerve and internal capsule, and risk of emotional, behavioral, and cognitive deficits

B. Deep-brain stimulation

1. Definition. High-frequency stimulation that induces functional inhibition of target regions of the brain by implanting an electrode into a target site and connecting the lead to a sub-cutaneously placed pacemaker.

2. Advantage. No destructive lesion is formed. Stimulation parameters can be readjusted at any time to improve efficacy or decrease adverse events.

3. Disadvantage. Side effects associated with equipment (such as lead breaks, infection, skin erosion, mechanical malfunction, and need for battery replacement). Other side effects include paresthesia limb dystonia, ataxia, intracerebral hemorrhage, seizure, and confusion.

C. Fetal nigral transplantation

1. Definition. Implantation of embryonic dopaminergic cells into the denervated striatum to replace degenerated neuronal cells.

2. Advantage. Implanted cells all survive, and innervation of the striatum is accomplished in an organotypic manner. Does not necessitate making a destructive lesion.

3. Disadvantage. Optimal transplant variables and target site not defined.

STUDY QUESTIONS

Directions: Each of the numbered items or incomplete statements in this section is followed by answers or by completions of the statement. Select the **one** lettered answer or completion that is **best** in each case.

1. Which of the following drugs is a COMT inhibitor and has reports of fatal liver toxicity with it?

(A) Tolcapone
(B) Entacapone
(C) Pergolide
(D) Selegiline

2. Levodopa is associated with which of the following problems?

(A) Gastrointestinal side effects
(B) Involuntary movements
(C) Decline in efficacy after 3–5 years
(D) All of the above

3. Amantadine has which of the following advantages over levodopa?

(A) More rapid relief over symptoms
(B) Higher success rate
(C) Better long-term effects

4. Which drug is a non-ergot dopamine agonist and has a side-effect profile different from the rest of the dopaminergic agents?

(A) Pergolide
(B) Levodopa/carbidopa
(C) Ropinirole
(D) Selegiline

5. Which of the following medications is indicated adjunct to carbidopa/levodopa therapy?

(A) Pramipexole
(B) Bromocriptine
(C) Amantadine
(D) Tolcapone

ANSWERS AND EXPLANATIONS

1. The answer is A *[II E 4 a, (3) (a)]*.
Severe cases of hepatocellular injury including fulminant liver failure, which causes death, have been reported. Patients should be monitored and instructed to look for signs of liver disease such as clay color stool, jaundice, fatigue, loss of appetite, and lethargy.

2. The answer is D *[II b 3 c, d]*.
Levodopa can cause gastrointestinal side effects such as nausea and vomiting, particularly when starting treatment. Bowel irregularity and gastrointestinal bleeding can also occur. With long-term levodopa therapy, involuntary choreiform movements can develop, and the efficacy of the drug declines. Other unwanted effects of levodopa include tachycardia and cardiac arrhythmias, postural hypotension, and psychiatric disturbances such as confusion or depression.

3. The answer is A *[II D 2a (4), c d]*.
Amantadine is most efficacious within the first few weeks, whereas benefits from levodopa may not be seen for weeks to months. Amantadine is more beneficial than the anticholinergics, but is less effective than levodopa. Unfortunately, the efficacy of amantadine declines after 6–12 months of therapy. The efficacy of levodopa declines after 3–5 years of therapy.

4. The answer is C *[II E 3 a, b]*.
Pramipexole and ropinirole, Dopamine receptor, non-ergot, are indicated for both early and advanced stages of Parkinson's disease. They selectively bind to dopamine receptors and activate the D_2 receptor, but have little or no affinity for the D_1 receptor. They have a greater affinity for the D_3 receptor than for the D_2 receptor. The incidence of adverse events (i.e., pleuropulmonary fibrosis and retroperitoneal fibrosis, coronary vasconstriction, erythromelalgia, and Raynaud's phenomenon) is low in comparison with nonselective dopamine agonists. Nonergot dopamine agonists have a low potential for the devlopement of motor fluctuations and dyskinesis.

5. The answer is D *[II E 4, a (1) (d)]*.
Tolcapone is an ihibitor of COMT enzyme used to metabolize catecholamines including levodopa; it is indicated as an adjunct therapy to carbidopa/levodopa therapy.

46
Schizophrenia

Faith L. Barnett
Penny S. Shelton

I. INTRODUCTION. Schizophrenia occurs in approximately 1% of the United States population and has a worldwide lifetime prevalence of 0.85%. It is a disease that produces multiple signs and symptoms involving thought, behavior, emotion, and perception. It is a disease that has significant socioeconomic impact, morbidity, and mortality. In the United States, there are more than 300,000 acute psychotic episodes secondary to schizophrenia each year. The cost of this disease is estimated to exceed $33 billion annually, with approximately one-half due to indirect costs such as loss of work hours. In recent decades, the care of patients with mental illness has increasingly been shifted to outpatient services. The deinstitutionalization of mental illness and inadequate care and shelter resources has contributed to the high prevalence of schizophrenia among the homeless population, an estimated 30%–50%.

II. PATHOPHYSIOLOGY. Although the actual cause of schizophrenia is unproved, theorized etiologies can be categorized broadly as genetic, neurophysiological, and psychosocial.

  A. Genetic studies have provided significant data supporting a genetic basis for schizophrenia. The risk factor in the general population is 0.5%–1% but increases to 5%–10% if one parent has a history of schizophrenia. It may be as high as 45% if both parents have the disorder. Monozygotic twin studies revealed a 40%–50% chance of developing schizophrenia in both twins if one developed the disease. However, genetics do not fully explain the etiology of schizophrenia; this is particularly evident in the less than 100% concordance rate among monozygotic twins.

  B. Neurophysiological theories center around various neurotransmitter deficits or hyperactivity. For many years, the **dopamine hypothesis** proposed an excess of dopamine to be the cause of schizophrenia. However, the dopamine hypothesis does not fully explain this disorder, because if we simply blocked dopamine activity, patients should get better, and this does not occur for all schizophrenics. Since this time, the hypofrontality theory has deduced that there is an excess of dopamine along the mesolimbic pathway; however, in the prefrontal, frontal, and temporal cortices, there is actually a decrease in dopamine activity. In addition, serotonin has also been found to play an etiological role in schizophrenia, particularly since the atypical antipsychotics, such as clozapine, block serotonin to a higher degree than dopamine. Furthermore, glutamate has been proposed as a cause of schizophrenia, particularly since glutamate is the dominant neurotransmitter in the cerebral cortex and one of its functions is to modulate dopamine activity.

  C. Psychosocial theories, though largely unproved, do exist. Among the proposed causes are stress, lack of interpersonal skills, conflicting and contradictory family communication, and socioeconomic influences. None of these theories are definitive, but may serve as triggers in individuals predisposed to the development of schizophrenia.

III. DIAGNOSIS AND CLINICAL PRESENTATION

  A. Schizophrenia is **diagnosed** using the *Diagnostic and Statistical Manual of Mental Disorders,* 4th ed. (DSM-IV-TR) criteria. Schizophrenia is basically a diagnosis by exclusion, meaning medical and drug-induced causes of psychosis must first be ruled out. The patient must have two or more of the characteristic symptoms: delusions, hallucinations, disorganized speech, disorganized or catatonic behavior, and negative symptoms. Continuous signs of active prodromal or residual psychosis must be present for 6 months, with at least 1 month of active symptoms. In addition, the symptoms must cause social or occupational dysfunction.

  B. The **types** of schizophrenia are defined in Table 46-1.

Table 46-1. Types of Schizophrenia

Type	Presentation
Catatonic	Marked psychomotor disturbances. The patient may demonstrate rigidity, immobility, or posturing and may also be withdrawn and silent. At the other extreme is characteristic excitement, such as pacing and shouting. Fluctuations between these two extremes may occur.
Disorganized	Marked incoherence with inappropriate responses or unresponsiveness. Delusions or hallucinations are disorganized and fragmented. The patient may giggle, grimace, and act in an incongruous or silly manner. Hypochondriacal behavior may be present.
Paranoid*	Most prominent characteristics are delusions of grandeur or persecution, during which the patient may be extremely anxious, aggressive, and/or argumentative.
Residual	The patient is not currently acutely psychotic, but has a history of at least one acute psychotic break and currently experiences residual symptoms such as vague associations, illogical thinking, withdrawal, or inappropriate affect. Living skills may be impaired.
Undifferentiated	May incorporate prominent delusions, hallucinations, incoherence, or grossly disorganized behavior. But overall, clinical presentation either does not meet the criteria for one of the specific types or meets the criteria for more than one type of schizophrenia.

*Denotes most common type.

    C. The **clinical features** are best categorized as **positive and negative** symptoms (Table 46-2). The most prominent symptoms are **hallucinations** and **delusions** (Table 46-3).

IV. TREATMENT OBJECTIVES. Because there is no known cure for schizophrenia, treatment is primarily aimed at relieving symptoms and restoring function. The **two major therapeutic approaches** are **psychotherapy** and **pharmacotherapy.** Together, these approaches attempt the following goals.

    A. Alleviate perception abnormalities such as delusions and hallucinations

    B. Help patients gain control of their thoughts and behavior

    C. Prevent self-inflicted harm

    D. Restore social and occupational function to the highest degree possible

    E. Prevent relapse and hospitalization

V. PHARMACOTHERAPY: ANTIPSYCHOTIC AGENTS

    A. Selection of an antipsychotic is based on the patient's history and the safety profiles of the available agents. In general, there are two types of antipsychotic agents: typical or traditional agents and the atypical agents. If a patient is experiencing his or her first psychotic episode and is newly diagnosed with schizophrenia, the American Psychiatric Association (APA) guidelines suggest initiating therapy with an atypical agent because of these agents' improved safety profile. However, if the patient has successfully been treated with a traditional agent in the past and tolerated it well, then using that agent again is appropriate. Generally, the positive symptoms respond better to antipsychotic therapy than the negative symptoms. Maximal improvement may take 6–8 weeks or longer. The duration of treatment is based on the number of psychotic episodes. With the first episode, treatment may be tapered to discontinuation after 6 months of therapy; however, continued therapy may improve long-term outcomes and quality of life.

Table 46-2. Positive and Negative Symptoms of Schizophrenia

Positive Symptoms	Negative Symptoms
Hallucinations	Affective flattening
Delusions	Alogia
Thought disorders	Apathy
Disorganized speech	Amotivation
Bizarre behavior	Anhedonia
Insomnia	Asocial behavior
Combativeness	Inattentiveness

Table 46-3. Delusions and Hallucinations

Psychotic Symptom	Delusion	Hallucination
Definition	Belief not based on fact or reality	Perception disturbance in sensory experiences of the environment
Types	Grandiose Religious Somatic Nihilistic Sexual Persecutory*	Auditory* Visual Olfactory Tactile

*Denotes most common.

B. Traditional antipsychotic agents

1. **Mechanism of action.** Although the exact mechanism is not fully understood, these agents are thought to exert their antipsychotic effect by blocking dopamine activity.

2. **High and low potency.** The traditional agents are typically classified by potency. High-potency agents tend to have more extrapyramidal symptoms (EPSs) associated with their use, whereas low-potency agents have more sedation, anticholinergic, and cardiovascular side effects.

3. **Efficacy** for these agents is similar when dosed using equipotent dosing. Potency, dosing, and dosing equivalents are in Table 46-4. When compared to the newer atypical agents, traditional agents are just as effective in treating positive symptoms. However, the atypical agents address the negative symptoms better than the traditional agents.

4. **Adverse effects.** When compared to the atypical agents, traditional antipsychotics are not well-tolerated.
   a. There are numerous adverse effects associated with these agents, and common **antipsychotic side effects** can be found in Tables 46-4 and 46-5.
   b. **Extrapyramidal side effects** may occur with any antipsychotic, except clozapine, but are more commonly associated with traditional high-potency agents.
      (1) **Acute dystonias** involve sudden muscle spasms. These reactions include torticollis (neck twisted to side), retrocollis (neck/head pulled back), trismus (clenched jaw), and oculogyric crisis (fixed upward gaze). These reactions can be very distressing to the patient and should be addressed immediately. The risk of acute dystonias is highest within the first 24–48 hours of therapy or following a dose increase. They are most likely to occur in young patients, in men, and in patients receiving high doses. Acute dystonias can be managed initially through intramuscular or intravenous administration of anticholinergic agents, such as diphenhydramine or benztropine. Further reactions may be prevented by reducing the dose, concomitant oral anticholinergic therapy, (benztropine, diphenhydramine, or trihexyphenldyl) or switching to an atypical agent.
      (2) **Akathisia** is associated with motor restlessness and inner tension and agitation. The patient has the sensation or need to move and typically manifests this as pacing or

Table 46-4. Properties of Traditional Antipsychotics

Antipsychotic Agent*	Equiv. Dose	Dose¹ (mg)	Sedation	EPS	Anticholinergic Side Effects	Orthostatic Hypotension
Phenothiazines						
Chlorpromazine	100	30–800	+++	++	++	+++
Trifluoperazine	5	2–40	+	+++	+	+
Thioridazine	100	150–800	+++	+	+++	+++
Mesoridazine	50	30–400	+++	+	+++	++
Perphenazine	10	12–64	++	++	+	+
Fluphenazine	2	0.5–40	+	+++	+	+
Thioxanthenes						
Thiothixene	4	8–30	+	+++	+	++
Butyrophenone						
Haloperidol	2	1–15	+	+++	+	+
Dihydroindolone						
Molindone	10	15–225	++	++	+	+
Dibenzoxazepine						
Loxapine	15	20–250	+	++	+	+

+++ = high, ++ = moderate, + = low.
*Most common traditional antipsychotic agents.
¹Adult daily dose range.

Table 46-5. Antipsychotic Side Effects

Anticholinergic side effects (blurred vision, constipation, dry mouth, urinary retention)
Sedation
Rash
Photosensitivity
Thermoregulation dysfunction
Lowered seizure threshold
Orthostatic hypotension
ECG changes
Hyperprolactinemia
Elevated liver transaminases
Blood dyscrasias
Weight gain
Sexual dysfunction
Extrapyramidal symptoms
Ocular opacities
Neuroleptic malignant syndrome

inability to keep legs and feet still. This side effect most commonly occurs within the first few weeks or months of therapy or following a dose increase. This extrapyramidal symptom may respond to lipophilic β-blockers, benzodiazepines, or anticholinergic agents. A dosage reduction or use of an atypical agent would also be beneficial.

(3) Pseudoparkinsonism clinically looks like idiopathic parkinsonism but is drug-induced by dopamine blockade agents, such as antipsychotics. Patients may present with shuffling gait, masked faces, cogwheel rigidity, and/or pill-rolling tremor. These movements typically occur within the first few weeks to months of therapy or following a dose increase. A dosage reduction should be attempted. Pseudoparkinsonism will typically improve with oral anticholinergic therapy. Changing the patient from the typical agent to an atypical agent may also be beneficial.

(4) Tardive dyskinesia (TD)

(a) Definition. As its name implies, TD is a latent extrapyramidal effect generally not occurring for months or years. This disorder is characterized by abnormal movements that can occur in any part of the body, including the face, tongue, shoulders, hips, extremities, fingers, and toes. The movements are of two general types: dystonic (fixed, held muscles) and choreoathetoid (writhing, rhythmic).

(b) Etiology. TD movements are thought to occur from prolonged dopamine blockade, which leads to upregulation of dopamine receptors and increased sensitivity to dopamine stimulation. Another theory involves the generation of free radicals from lipid peroxidation secondary to increased neurotransmitter turnover.

(c) Management of TD. Some cases of TD may become irreversible; therefore, the antipsychotic should be discontinued. However, upon initial tapering of the dose, the patient's movements may worsen. This is due to a lower dopamine blockade, which increases dopamine levels to interact with still up-regulated receptors. The opposite is true in that TD can be masked with an increase in the antipsychotic dose. The movements will improve or disappear, but the cause is still present and, in time, the movements will emerge again. There is no ideal treatment for TD other than removing the offending agent, although a number of agents have been attempted (Table 46-6). Anticholinergic agents should be used with caution, because these agents may be beneficial for dystonic TD movements but can worsen choreoathetoid movements.

(d) The best measure against TD is prevention. Patients treated with antipsychotics or other agents that have dopamine blockade should be monitored closely for the emergence of movement disorders. Measurement tools such as the Abnormal Involuntary Movement Scale (AIMS) or the Dyskinesia Identification System Condensed User Scale (DISCUS) are helpful and should be applied at baseline and every 3–6 months.

c. Neuroleptic malignant syndrome (NMS) is an uncommon but serious and potentially fatal complication of therapy. It is a syndrome of extrapyramidal effects, hyperthermia, altered consciousness, and autonomic changes (e.g., tachycardia, unstable blood pressure, diaphoresis, and incontinence). The onset is sudden, and recovery may take 5–10 days after discontinuation of the antipsychotic. Specific management includes discontinuing the antipsychotic, providing supportive measures, and drug therapy with dantrolene or bromocriptine.

d. QTc prolongation increases the risk for fatal ventricular arrhythmias, such as Torsades de Pointes. QTc prolongation may occur with any of the antipsychotics; however, an increased incidence associated with thioridazine and mesoridazine resulted in the issuance of a black box warning by the FDA.

Table 46-6. Pharmacotherapy for TD

Reserpine
Benzodiazepines
Baclofen
Valproic acid and derivatives
Vitamin E

C. Atypical antipsychotic agents

1. **General differences** between the traditional agents and atypical agents
   a. Traditional agents block dopamine$_2$ receptors, whereas atypical agents block serotonin receptors to a higher degree.
   b. Atypical agents have fewer extrapyramidal side effects than the traditional agents.
   c. As a class, the atypical agents treat negative symptoms better than traditional agents.
   d. Atypical agents do not produce sustained elevations of prolactin, whereas the traditional agents result in hyperprolactinemia.

2. To date, there are 5 atypical antipsychotics available on the U.S. market: **risperidone, olanzapine, quetiapine, clozapine, and ziprasidone.** Table 46-7 contains comparative information for these 5 agents.
   a. **Receptor affinity.** In general, all these agents have a higher affinity for 5-HT receptors as compared to dopamine receptors. But these agents differ in their affinity for other receptors; thus, they will have slightly different side effects. See receptor affinities and side effects in Table 46-8.
   b. **Clozapine** is the only antipsychotic proven, to date, to be effective in treatment of refractory patients. It is also the only atypical agent that is EPS/TD-free. However, clozapine is still reserved as last-line therapy because of its increased incidence of agranulocytosis and the need for frequent laboratory monitoring. Thus, patients must consent to the use of the drug and monitoring of complete blood count (CBC) weekly for the first 6 months of therapy and then every other week thereafter.
   c. **Ziprasidone injection** is the only parenteral atypical antipsychotic available. The recommended dose is 10 or 20 mg administered intramuscularly. The 10-mg dose may be repeated every 2 hours and the 20-mg dose may be repeated every 4 hours, up to a maximum total daily dose of 40 mg/day. Ziprasidone injection is an alternative to the parenteral traditional antipsychotics for the management of the acutely agitated patient with schizophrenia.

Table 46-7. Atypical Antipsychotics

	Clozapine	Risperidone	Olanzapine	Quetiapine	Ziprasidone
Starting Dose (mg/day)	12.5	2	2.5–5	25–50	40
Usual Adult Dose (mg/day)	300–900	4–16	10–20	250–750	120–160
Metabolic Pathway	1A2	2D6	1A2	3A4	3A4
Receptor Affinity	$\alpha_{1,2}$, $D_{1,2}$, 5-HT$_{2A,2c}$, M, H$_1$	D_2, 5-HT$_{2A,2c}$, $\alpha_{1,2}$, H$_1$	α_1, $D_{1,2,4}$, 5-HT$_{2A,2c}$, H$_1$	$\alpha_{1,2}$, $D_{1,2}$, 5-HT$_{2A}$, M, H$_1$	5-HT$_{2A,2C,1D}$, D_2, α_1, H$_1$
Sedation	+++	+	+++	++	+
EPS	0	+ to ++[1]	+	+	+
Anticholinergic Side Effects	+++	0	+++	0	0
Orthostatic Hypotension	++	+++	+	++	+
Weight Gain	++	+	++	+	0/+

+++ = high, ++ = moderate, + = low.
[1]EPS increases with doses >6 mg/day.

Table 46-8. Adverse Effects by Receptor Affinities

Receptor Antagonized	Adverse Effect
Histamine$_1$ (H$_1$)	Sedation
Serotonin$_{2c}$ (5-HT)	Weight gain
Dopamine$_2$ (D)	Extrapyramidal symptoms Hyperprolactinemia
Muscarinic (M)	Anticholinergic effects Cognitive/memory impairment Tachycardia
Alpha$_1$ (α)	Orthostatic hypotension Reflex tachycardia

    D. Rapid tranquilization is usually reserved for acutely psychotic patients with agitation and aggression. Injectable, traditional agents are typically used. For example: haloperidol 5–10 mg every hour may be given intramuscularly until acute symptoms are controlled, side effects occur, or patient falls asleep. Once control has been obtained, the patient can be converted to oral therapy and dosage adjusted in accordance to clinical response.

    E. Therapy in noncompliant patients. Patients who have a history of noncompliance with oral medication and frequent hospitalizations due to noncompliance may do better in the community setting with long-acting, depot antipsychotics. However, long-acting dosage forms only exist for two antipsychotics, and both are traditional agents (fluphenazine and haloperidol).

        1. Fluphenazine decanoate and **haloperidol** decanoate are both administered intramuscularly. Fluphenazine is given every 2–3 weeks, and haloperidol is given every 3–4 weeks.

        2. The dosage is based on the total daily oral dose of fluphenazine or haloperidol. Therefore, if a patient is taking any other oral antipsychotic, the dosage must first be converted to an equipotent fluphenazine or haloperidol dose using the chlorpromazine equivalents (see Table 46-4).

            a. Fluphenazine decanoate dosage is determined by the converting equation: 1.2–1.6 × (total daily dose of fluphenazine) = fluphenazine decanoate dose given every 2 weeks.

            b. Haloperidol decanoate dosage is determined by the converting equation: 10 × (total daily dose of oral haldol) = haloperidol decanoate dose given every 4 weeks. The first dose should not exceed 100 mg.

            c. These conversion equations are only rough estimates. It is important to monitor the patient carefully and to use the lowest effective dose.

    F. Switching treatment agents. A cross taper and titrate is used when changing from one antipsychotic to another. As you slowly titrate up with the newer agent, you are tapering down with the old agent. If the patient is being changed because of EPS in which an anticholinergic agent, like benztropine, was initiated, the patient can remain on the anticholinergic agent until the cross taper and titrate is complete. At that time, the patient should be reevaluated and the anticholinergic agent tapered to discontinuation. The only exception to this is in the case of clozapine being added as the new therapy. Clozapine has very high anticholinergic properties, and the anticholinergic agent should be discontinued when the cross taper and titration begins.

    G. Adjunctive therapy. The patient's symptoms should be carefully evaluated for response. If a partial or nonresponse occurs with an adequate trial of an antipsychotic, then another antipsychotic should be tried. Upon unsuccessful treatment with two or three antipsychotics, clozapine should be considered due to its proven efficacy in refractory patients. For those patients who cannot take clozapine or who do not respond to clozapine, augmentation therapy should be considered. The most common augmentative therapy is the addition of a mood stabilizer to the antipsychotic regimen, typically, valproic acid, carbamazepine, or lithium. Anxiolytics, particularly benzodiazepines, have also been used.

STUDY QUESTIONS

Directions: Each of the numbered items or incomplete statements in this section is followed by answers or by completions of the statement. Select the **one** lettered answer or completion that is **best** in each case.

1. Which of the following is NOT a positive symptom associated with schizophrenia?

(A) Hallucinations
(B) Anhedonia
(C) Delusions
(D) Disorganized thought

2. A 24-year-old white man presenting with his first psychotic episode is diagnosed with schizophrenia. The admitting physician requests your assistance in selecting an appropriate antipsychotic agent. According to the American Psychiatric Association guidelines, which of the following is the most appropriate for this patient?

(A) Chlorpromazine
(B) Thiothixene
(C) Clozapine
(D) Risperidone

3. A patient who has been treated with haloperidol for 3 weeks presents with muscle stiffness, tremor, and shuffling gait. This is most likely which type of extrapyramidal side effect?

(A) Akathisia
(B) Tardive dyskinesia
(C) Pseudoparkinsonism
(D) Acute dystonia

4. The atypical antipsychotics differ from the typical agents in various ways that define them as atypical. Which of the following is NOT a defining property of the atypical antipsychotics?

(A) Sustained hyperprolactinemia
(B) Improved efficacy in treating the negative symptoms
(C) Lower risk for extrapyramidal symptoms (EPSs)
(D) Greater serotonin receptor blockade than dopamine blockade

5. A 36-year-old woman diagnosed with schizophrenia about 15 years ago frequently presents to the hospital due to medication noncompliance. Which of the following is the most appropriate antipsychotic medication to improve patient compliance?

(A) Benztropine mesylate
(B) Chlorpromazine
(C) Haloperidol decanoate
(D) Trifluoperazine

6. A patient currently receiving fluphenazine for schizophrenia develops hyperthermia, tachycardia, diaphoresis, and muscle rigidity. Which of the following best describes this patient's presentation?

(A) Serotonin syndrome
(B) Neuroleptic malignant syndrome (NMS)
(C) Oculogyric crisis
(D) Serotonin withdrawal syndrome

7. Which of the following atypical antipsychotics would be the least sedating?

(A) Quetiapine
(B) Risperidone
(C) Olanzapine
(D) Clozapine

8. The typical antipsychotic agents are classified into high- and low-potency agents. Which of the following statements best defines high and low potency?

(A) High potency = more weight gain; low potency = weight loss
(B) High potency = fewer extrapyramidal symptoms (EPSs); low potency = more EPSs
(C) High potency = more EPSs; low potency = fewer EPSs
(D) High potency = high dose; low potency = low dose

9. Which of the following agents is NOT used to treat extrapyramidal symptoms (EPSs)?

(A) Donepezil (Aricept)
(B) Trihexyphenidyl (Artane)
(C) Diphenhydramine (Benadryl)
(D) Benztropine (Cogentin)

10. A 32-year-old patient with schizophrenia has been treated with haloperidol 10 mg twice a day for 10 weeks and benztropine 1 mg twice a day; however, persecutory delusions persist. The physician would like to change the patient to olanzapine. Which of the following statements is the preferred method for switching antipsychotic therapy?

(A) Discontinue both haloperidol and benztropine first, then start olanzapine.

(B) Discontinue benztropine first, then discontinue haloperidol by taper; finally, after haloperidol is discontinued, initiate the olanzapine.

(C) Decrease the haloperidol dose, and start the olanzapine dose in a cross taper and titration manner; continue the benztropine until the haloperidol has been discontinued.

(D) Start the olanzapine at full dose, and slowly decrease the haloperidol dose.

ANSWERS AND EXPLANATIONS

1. The answer is B *[III C; Table 46-2].*
With schizophrenia, it is common to have perception disorders as well as thought disorders. Anhedonia is one of the various negative symptoms that may be present.

2. The answer is D *[V A, C 2].*
The American Psychiatric Association (APA) now recommends an atypical antipsychotic for patients presenting with their first episode. From the choices provided, only clozapine and risperidone are atypical antipsychotics, and clozapine is reserved for treatment of refractory patients.

3. The answer is C *[V B 4 b (1)–(4)].*
All of the symptoms are extrapyramidal symptoms that can occur with antipsychotic therapy. Acute dystonia typically occurs within 24–48 hours of therapy. Akathisia is classified as motor restlessness. Tardive dyskinesia generally presents as various abnormal movements after months of therapy. This patient exhibits classic parkinsonian symptoms.

4. The answer is A *[V C 1].*
The atypicals have fewer extrapyramidal symptoms (EPSs), have greater affinity for serotonin receptors than dopaminergic, and treat negative symptoms better than the typical agents. However, the atypical agents do not cause sustained elevations in prolactin.

5. The correct answer is C *[V E].*
Haloperidol decanoate is a long-acting, injectable antipsychotic that is used to improve medication compliance and decrease rehospitalization. Fluphenazine and haloperidol are the only two antipsychotics available in the decanoate form.

6. The answer is B *[V B 4 c].*
Neuroleptic malignant syndrome (NMS) develops quickly and may persist for 5–10 days. The symptoms are classic features of NMS and require immediate medical attention.

7. The answer is B *[V C 2; Table 46-7].*
Risperidone causes less sedation than the other atypical antipsychotics because it has minimal histamine$_1$-receptor affinity as compared to the other atypicals.

8. The answer is C *[V B 2].*
High potency and low potency define the agent's propensity for causing extrapyramidal symptoms (EPSs). High-potency agents cause more EPSs but fewer anticholinergic side effects, sedation, and orthostatic hypotension, whereas low-potency agents cause fewer EPSs but more of the other side effects.

9. The answer is A *[V B 4 b].*
Anticholinergic agents such as trihexyphenidyl, diphenhydramine, and benztropine are used to treat extrapyramidal side effects. Donepezil is an acetylcholinesterase inhibitor that increases cholinergic function and has the potential to worsen EPSs.

10. The answer is C *[V F].*
The cross taper and titration method is the preferred method for changing antipsychotic therapy. This method should allow the new agent to be safely initiated without the reemergence of symptoms or exacerbation of side effects.

47
Mood Disorders

Faith L. Barnett
Penny S. Shelton

I. DEFINITIONS

A. Mood can be defined as one's sustained emotion and is typically described as euphoric, dysphoric, or euthymic (Figure 47-1).

B. Mood disorders can be defined as a sustained elevation or depression in mood that impairs the ability to function in society. These disorders cause significant morbidity and mortality, and increase the risk of suicide 10- to 20-fold. The predicted cost of mood disorders in the United States is $44 billion per year, with one-third of that amount attributable to diminished work performance. For the purpose of this chapter, two common mood disorders will be discussed: **major depression** and **bipolar disorder.**

II. MAJOR DEPRESSION

A. Incidence

1. Depression occurs **more often in women than in men** (2:1 ratio). It is predicted that 10%–25% of women and 5%–12% of men experience a depressive episode during their lifetime.

2. Although the initial episode of major depression generally occurs between the **ages of 25 and 44,** it can occur at any age. For example, 15% of the geriatric population residing in the community and up to 20% of the institutionalized geriatric population suffer from depression.

B. Etiology. Although the cause of depression has not been fully established, several theories have been proposed.

1. The **biogenic amine theory** was the first to be described and provides the basis for pharmacotherapy. These theories are based on the observation that patients taking **medications that deplete norepinephrine and serotonin** develop depression.

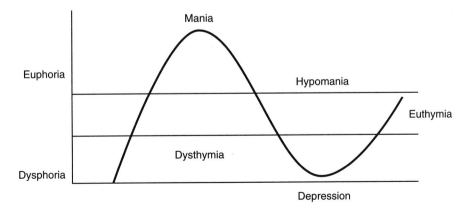

Figure 47-1. Euthymia is the range of normal fluctuation in mood. Euphoria describes the mood elevations above the normal range. Hypomania is another descriptive term that describes mood elevation; however, it is beneath the extreme mood elevation of mania. Dysphoria describes the mood depression below the normal range, and this can be further described as dysthymia or depression. Dysthymia is a less severe depression in mood, and depression is the lowest mood point.

2. However, in an attempt to explain the cyclic nature of depression, the **dysregulation theory** was formulated. This theory suggests that an **impaired balance of neurotransmitters,** not absolute decreases or increases in neurotransmitters, causes disruptions of mood.

3. An exact genetic link has not been discovered, but **familial history** of a mood disorder does increase the risk of being diagnosed with depression. Studies indicate that 8%–18% of depressed individuals have a first-degree relative with depression.

C. Diagnosis. Psychiatric diagnoses are made using the DSM-IV-TR criteria (*Diagnostic and Statistical Manual of Mental Disorders,* 4th edition text revision; published by the American Psychiatric Association, 2000). To be diagnosed with major depression, the patient must experience persistent symptoms (Table 47-1) for a period of at least 2 weeks.

D. Treatment. There are three types of treatment for depression: psychotherapy, pharmacotherapy, and electroconvulsive therapy. Pharmacotherapy (i.e., with **antidepressants**) is effective in 40%–70% of depressed patients.

1. Treatment phases. Pharmacotherapy has three phases: acute, continuation, and maintenance (Table 47-2). Failure to treat a patient with major depression through the continuation phase at the full therapeutic dose will very likely lead to relapse.

2. Drug selection. All antidepressants are equally effective in the treatment of depression; however, they have different mechanisms of action and side effects.
  a. If the patient has been successively treated in the past, reinstitute therapy with the previously used agent.
  b. If the patient has not received therapy in the past or was unsuccessfully treated with an antidepressant, select an antidepressant with a side-effect profile that complements the patient's disease process. For example, a depressed individual suffering from psychomotor agitation may benefit from a sedating antidepressant. However, if the clinical presentation includes psychomotor retardation, an activating antidepressant would be more appropriate.

3. Administration and dosage
  a. Initiating antidepressant therapy
    (1) Generally, therapy is initiated with half of the lowest dose in the target range to minimize side effects.
    (2) The dose is increased to the target range over a 1- to 2-week period.
    (3) Further dosage titration is based on clinical response.
      (a) The clinical response to antidepressants often lags behind drug initiation, with resolution of anxiety and insomnia in the first 1–2 weeks. The full effect may not be evident for 4–6 weeks. Alterations in postsynaptic receptor sensitivity have been proposed as the reason for this lag time between initiation of an antidepressant and clinical response.
      (b) Before determining an antidepressant as ineffective, the patient must have received the maximum tolerated dose for 4–6 weeks. When therapeutic failure occurs, it is generally recommended to try another antidepressant from another class.

Table 47-1. Clinical Features of Major Depression

One of the following must be present:
　　Depressed mood
　　Anhedonia (i.e., loss of interest or pleasure)
Plus four or more of the following:
　　Decreased or increased appetite
　　Unintentional weight loss or gain
　　Insomnia or hypersomnia
　　Psychomotor agitation or retardation (observable)
　　Fatigue or loss of energy
　　Feelings of worthlessness or excessive or inappropriate guilt
　　Diminished ability to think or concentrate or indecisiveness
　　Recurrent thoughts of death and/or suicidal ideation
　　Suicide attempt

Table 47-2. Treatment Phases for Depression

Treatment Phase	Duration	Goal
Acute	≈ 6 weeks	Resolve symptoms
Continuation	6–9 months	Prevent relapse
Maintenance	3–5 years or lifelong	Prevent recurrence in high-risk patients*

*Patients at high risk for recurrence include those who experienced their first episode when they were older than 50 years, patients older than 40 years who have experienced two or more episodes, and patients of all ages who have experienced three or more episodes.

    b. Changing antidepressant therapy. Caution is advised when changing antidepressant agents, because a potentially fatal interaction can occur as a result of "serotonin syndrome," when two serotonin-enhancing agents [e.g., monoamine oxidase inhibitors (MAOIs) and selective serotonin reuptake inhibitors (SSRIs)] are used concomitantly (Table 47-3).

    (1) A 2-week washout period is required:
        (a) Before starting or when discontinuing an MAOI
        (b) When switching from an MAOI to another antidepressant
    (2) A 5-week washout period is required when discontinuing fluoxetine due to the long half-life of its metabolite, norfluoxetine.

4. Therapeutic concentrations. Although therapeutic concentrations have been determined for most antidepressants, the correlation between levels and clinical response is unclear. Therapeutic levels do not guarantee the desired response or a lack of adverse effects; therefore, **patients should be evaluated by their clinical picture** (i.e., improvement in target symptoms and emergence of adverse effects).

5. Augmentation therapy. For patients unresponsive to two or more antidepressant trials, augmentation therapy is an option.
    a. Lithium, thyroid supplementation, and dual antidepressant therapy are options. However, combination antidepressant therapy is reserved as last-line therapy due to a lack of proved efficacy exceeding that of monotherapy.
    b. Low-dose (i.e., <100 mg) trazodone is commonly prescribed for insomnia, in combination with stimulating antidepressants.

Table 47-3. Clinical Manifestations of Serotonin Syndrome and Serotonin Withdrawal Syndrome

Classification of Dysfunction	Serotonin Syndrome	Serotonin Withdrawal Syndrome
Cognitive–behavioral dysfunction	Confusion Hypomania Agitation	None
Autonomic nervous system dysfunction	Diarrhea Shivering Fever Diaphoresis Changes in blood pressure Nausea and vomiting	Flu-like symptoms Dizziness Light headedness Chills Nausea and vomiting Sleep disturbances
Neuromuscular dysfunction	Myoclonus Hyperreflexia Tremor Seizure Death	Lethargy Myalgia Sensory disturbances (e.g., paresthesia)

6. **Therapeutic agents (i.e., antidepressants)**
   a. **Tricyclic amines (TCAs)** (Table 47-4)
      (1) **Indications.** TCAs should be reserved for:
         (a) A previous TCA responder
         (b) Medically healthy patients
         (c) Nonsuicidal patients
         (d) Patients refractory to newer agents
      (2) **Mechanism of action**
         (a) TCAs nonspecifically target the serotonin and norepinephrine receptors, blocking the reuptake of serotonin and norepinephrine.
         (b) In addition, TCAs bind to α-*adrenergic,* histaminergic, and cholinergic receptors, which accounts for many of the side effects seen with these agents.
      (3) **Administration and dosage**
         (a) The starting dose for most TCAs is 50 mg administered at bedtime.
         (b) Dose may be increased by 25–50 mg every 3–4 days. (See Table 47-4 for specific starting doses and target doses.)
      (4) **Precautions and monitoring effects**
         (a) Anticholinergic effects include blurred vision, urinary retention, constipation, and dry mouth.
         (b) α-Adrenergic blockade effects include orthostatic hypotension and dizziness.
         (c) Antihistamine effects include sedation.
         (d) TCAs also lower the seizure threshold and create cardiac conduction abnormalities that may manifest as T-wave flattening or prolongation of the QT, PR, or QRS intervals. Consequently, TCAs are potentially lethal if overdosed.
   b. **MAOIs** (see Table 47-4)
      (1) **Indications.** MAOIs are reserved for:
         (a) Patients suffering from atypical depression (i.e., hypersomnia, agitation, anxiety)
         (b) Patients who are refractory to other antidepressants

Table 47-4. Tricyclic Amines (TCAs), Monoamine Oxidose Inhibitors (MAOIs), and Miscellaneous Antidepressant Agents

Generic Name	Starting Dose (mg/day)	Target Dose* (mg/day)	Major Side Effects				
			Anticholinergic Effects	Sedation	Orthostatic Hypotension	Cardiac Effects	Weight Gain
TCAs							
Amitriptyline	50–75	100–300	++++	++++	++++	+++	++++
Doxepin	50–75	100–300	+++	++++	++	++	++++
Imipramine	50–75	100–300	+++	+++	++++	+++	++++
Trimipramine	50–75	100–300	++++	++++	+++	+++	++++
Protriptyline[†]	10–20	15–60	++	+	++	+++	+
Nortriptyline[†]	25–50	50–150	++	++	+	++	+
Desipramine[†]	50–75	100–300	+	++	++	++	+
MAOIs							
Phenelzine	10	15–90	++	++	++	+	+++
Isocarboxazid	20	20–40	++	++	++	+	++
Tranylcypromine	10	10–40	++	+	++	+	++
Miscellaneous Agents							
Amoxapine	50–100	100–400	++	++	++	++	++
Maprotiline	50–100	100–225	++	+++	+	++	++
Bupropion SR	150	300	–	–	–	+	–
Trazodone	50–100	150–600	–	++++	+++	+	++

++++ = very high; +++ = high; ++ = moderate; + = slight; – = none.

*The doses presented in this table are for normal adults. Dose adjustment is generally required for geriatric patients and patients with renal and hepatic impairment.
[†]These TCAs are secondary amines.

(2) Mechanism of action. These agents block the breakdown of biogenic amines by inhibiting the enzyme monoamine oxidase, thus increasing the concentrations of norepinephrine and 5-hydroxytryptamine (5-HT) in the brain.

(3) Administration and dosage. Therapy should be initiated cautiously and should follow various guidelines to ensure its safety, such as:

    (a) Providing an adequate washout period [see II D 3 b (1), (2)]

    (b) Initiating with low doses

    (c) Increasing doses gradually

    (d) Monitoring for potential drug–drug and drug–food interactions

(4) Precautions and monitoring effects

    (a) The side-effect profile for the MAOIs is quite comprehensive, including:

        (i) Orthostatic hypotension (minimized by slow-dosage titration)

        (ii) Weight gain

        (iii) Edema

        (iv) Sexual dysfunction

    (b) Isocarboxazid may cause hepatocellular damage; therefore, baseline and periodic liver function tests should be assessed. Discontinue therapy at the first signs of hepatic dysfunction or jaundice.

    (c) The nonselective inhibition of monoamine oxidase may result in accumulation of sympathomimetic amines. Therefore, ingestion of exogenous sources of sympathomimetic amines (e.g., decongestants, foods containing tyramine) while taking an MAOI places the patient at risk for hypertensive crisis. Patients should be educated about tyramine-containing foods (e.g., wine, aged cheese) and over-the-counter cold medications.

c. Bupropion (see Table 47-4)

  (1) Mechanism of action. Bupropion inhibits the reuptake of serotonin, norepinephrine, and dopamine, but its antidepressant mechanism is not fully understood.

  (2) Administration and dosage. Bupropion is available as an immediate-release product that is administered three times daily and as a sustained-release product that is administered twice daily.

  (3) Precautions and monitoring effects

    (a) Bupropion appears to have a stimulatory effect similar to the SSRIs [see II D 6 e], consequently causing agitation and insomnia. Therefore, it should not be given at bedtime.

    (b) This agent is also associated with an increased seizure risk, particularly in patients with eating disorders. Therefore, bupropion is contraindicated for use in patients with a history of anorexia, bulimia, or seizure disorder. Recommendations to minimize seizure risk include:

        (i) Keep dose increases to less than 100 mg/day

        (ii) Do not increase doses more frequently than every 3–4 days

        (iii) Single doses should not exceed 150 mg

        (iv) The maximum daily dose should be ≤450 mg

d. Trazodone (see Table 47-4)

  (1) Indications. Trazodone may be beneficial as a sleep aid for depressed patients with insomnia.

  (2) Mechanism of action. The mechanism of action has not been fully elucidated, but trazodone is thought to increase serotonin.

  (3) Administration and dosage. Antidepressant dosing is 150–400 mg/day administered two to three times daily.

  (4) Precautions and monitoring effects. Trazodone is associated with sedation, hypotension, nausea, and priapism. In fact, the side effects are often intolerable, limiting its use as an antidepressant.

e. SSRIs (Table 47-5)

  (1) Indications. SSRIs with an approved indication for depression are fluoxetine, sertraline, paroxetine, and citalopram.

  (2) Mechanism of action. SSRIs nonselectively increase serotonin by blocking the reuptake of this neurotransmitter.

  (3) Administration and dosage. Initial daily doses for the SSRIs are as follows: fluoxetine 10–20 mg, sertraline 25–50 mg, paroxetine 10–20 mg, citalopram 20 mg, and fluvoxamine 50 mg. (See Table 47-5 for dosage ranges). SSRIs should be administered in the morning due to their stimulatory effect, which may result in insomnia.

Table 47-5. Selective Serotonin Reuptake Inhibitors (SSRIs)

Generic Name	Dose Range and Frequency	Half-life	Cytochrome P450 Inhibition
Fluoxetine	20–80 mg/day once daily	2–3 days	2D6 and 2C9/10 (potent); 3A4 (mild)
Norfluoxetine*		7–9 days*	2D6 and 2C9/10 (potent); 3A4 (mild)
Sertraline	50–200 mg/day once daily	1 day	2D6 (mild)
Desmethylsertraline*		4 days*	2D6 (mild)
Paroxetine	20–60 mg/day once daily	21 hours	2D6 (potent)
Citalopram	20–40 mg/day once daily	1–2 days	2D6 (mild)
Fluvoxamine†	50–300 mg/day once daily‡	13–15 hours	3A4 (moderate); 2C9 and 1A2 (potent)

*Norfluoxetine is the active metabolite of fluoxetine with its corresponding half-life.

†Fluvoxamine is not approved by the United States Food and Drug Administration (FDA) for treatment of depression; however, it is approved for the treatment of obsessive-compulsive disorder (OCD).

‡The dose given is for the treatment of OCD, not depression.

    (4) Precautions and monitoring effects
        (a) The most common side effects include nausea, vomiting, sexual dysfunction, and insomnia. However, compared to TCAs and MAOIs, SSRIs are generally well tolerated.
        (b) Because SSRIs are metabolized via the "cytochrome P450" isoenzyme system, significant drug interactions may occur (see Table 47-5).
        (c) Abrupt discontinuation of an SSRI, with the exception of fluoxetine, can result in serotonin withdrawal syndrome (see Table 47-3). Therefore, these agents (except for fluoxetine) should be tapered to discontinuation.
  f. Venlafaxine (Table 47-6)
    (1) Mechanism of action. Venlafaxine increases 5-HT, norepinephrine, and, to some degree, dopamine by blocking the reuptake of these neurotransmitters.
    (2) Administration and dosage. Venlafaxine is available in two formulations, an immediate-release tablet, dosed two to three times daily, and an extended-release capsule, which may be given once daily.
        (a) When initiating therapy with the immediate-release product, start with 75 mg/day in two to three divided doses. You may increase by 75 mg/day every 4 days until within the usual adult dosage range of 150–375 mg/day. However, doses greater than 225 mg/day have not been proven to be more efficacious.
        (b) When switching from the immediate-release to the extended-release formulation, a direct conversion is performed to the extended-release formulation closest to the total daily dose of immediate-release venlafaxine.
    (3) Precautions and monitoring effects
        (a) Due to the serotonergic-enhancing abilities of venlafaxine, concomitant use with an MAOI is contraindicated.
        (b) The most common side effects include nausea, headache, somnolence, dry mouth, dizziness, and insomnia.
            (i) Nausea occurs frequently (25%–55% of patients) and is the most common cause of early discontinuation of therapy.
            (ii) Nausea is dose-related and tolerance may develop; however, initiating at lower doses and administering with food may alleviate this side effect.

Table 47-6. Newer Miscellaneous Antidepressants

Generic Name	Mechanism of Action	Dose Range and Frequency	Side Effects
Venlafaxine	5-HT and norepinephrine reuptake inhibitor	75–350 mg/day divided 2–3 times a day (once a day for the extended-release form)	Nausea, dry mouth, headache, sedation, dose-related hypertension (i.e., with doses >225 mg/day)
Nefazodone	Serotonin reuptake inhibitor; potent inhibitor (blocks 5-HT$_2$); potent inhibitor of cytochrome P4503A4 isoenzyme.	100–150 mg twice a day	Sedation, hypotension, priapism, nausea
Mirtazapine	Increases norepinephrine and 5-HT; blocks 5-HT$_2$ and 5-HT$_3$ receptors	15–45 mg/day once a day	Weight gain, sedation, dry mouth, dizziness, agranulocytosis (3/3000), sexual dysfunction (= placebo)

5-HT = 5-hydroxytryptamine.

      (c) Sustained hypertension (i.e., increases in supine diastolic blood pressure by 5.6 mm Hg) has been observed with venlafaxine at doses greater than 225 mg/day; hence, regular monitoring of blood pressure is recommended.

g. Nefazodone (see Table 47-6). Nefazodone is structurally similar to trazodone, yet has its own unique mechanism of action.

    (1) Mechanism of action. The antidepressant effects of nefazodone are due to increases in serotonin and 5-HT$_2$–receptor antagonism.

    (2) Administration and dosage

      (a) Nefazodone is initially dosed at 50 mg twice a day, with dosage titration over the first 1–2 weeks of therapy to 200–300 mg/day administered twice daily.

      (b) The maximum dose is 600 mg/day.

        (i) Doses above 300 mg/day have not been clearly associated with improved efficacy.

        (ii) However, side effects are noted to increase with higher doses.

    (3) Precautions and monitoring effects

      (a) The side-effect profile of nefazodone is better than that of trazodone and includes:

        (i) Orthostatic hypotension (caused by blocked α_1-adrenergic receptors)

        (ii) Sedation (less than trazodone)

        (iii) Sexual dysfunction equals that of placebo

        (iv) Dry mouth

        (v) Somnolence

        (vi) Nausea

        (vii) Dizziness

        (viii) Constipation

        (ix) Asthenia

      (b) Nefazodone exhibits the potential for drug–drug interactions.

        (i) Nefazodone is highly protein bound. Displacement interactions did not occur in vitro; however, interactions may occur in vivo, with other highly protein-bound medications such as phenytoin and warfarin.

        (ii) Nefazodone is a potent cytochrome P4503A4 isoenzyme (CYP3A4) inhibitor and will increase the concentration of medications that rely on CYP3A4 for metabolism.

      (c) Nefazadone has been associated with hepatic failure, therefore, monitoring liver function is imperative. Advise patients to notify their physician if they observe signs or symptoms (i.e., dark urine, jaundice) of hepatic dysfunction.

   h. Mirtazapine (see Table 47-6)
      (1) Mechanism of action
         (a) Mirtazapine inhibits presynaptic α_2-adrenergic receptors, which leads to increased central concentrations of norephinephrine and 5-HT.
         (b) Unlike the SSRIs, mirtazapine has a strong affinity for 5-HT$_1$ receptors while avoiding 5-HT$_2$ and 5-HT$_3$ receptors. This selectivity helps to diminish the incidence of common SSRI side effects (e.g., sexual dysfunction, agitation, insomnia).
         (c) However, mirtazapine does block histamine$_1$ (H$_1$) and 5-HT$_{2c}$ receptors, causing sedation and increased appetite, respectively.
      (2) Administration and dosage
         (a) Mirtazapine is dosed once daily, usually at bedtime.
         (b) The initial dose is 15 mg.
      (3) Precautions and monitoring effects
         (a) The more common side effects include:
            (i) Somnolence
            (ii) Dry mouth
            (iii) Weight gain
            (iv) Constipation
            (v) Dizziness
            (vi) Sedation/somnolence
         (b) Dose adjustments are necessary for the elderly and for the renally and hepatically impaired however, specific guidelines have not been established. Clinically monitor for increase in side effects with cautious dose escalation.

III. BIPOLAR DISORDER

A. Incidence

1. Bipolar disorder affects approximately 2% of the population in the United States.

2. Bipolar I disorder occurs equally among the genders, and bipolar II disorder affects females two times more frequently than males.

3. The age at onset is generally late teens to early twenties; however, patients may present with bipolar disorder at any age.

B. Etiology

1. Given that 80%–90% of patients with bipolar disorder have a positive family history, **genetics** is believed to play a role in its pathophysiology. However, a direct genetic link has not been discovered.

2. Like major depression, bipolar disorder is believed to be caused by an imbalance of neurotransmitters. However, in bipolar disorder, the **neurotransmitter levels fluctuate** and may be similar or reversed, depending on the patient's current clinical presentation.
   a. A manic episode is believed to result from elevations in norepinephrine.
   b. Depression has been associated with a decrease in norepinephrine.

3. A **dysregulation of γ-aminobutyric acid (GABA)** may play a role in bipolar disorder. A deficiency in GABA, an inhibitory neurotransmitter, may lead to mania due to unopposed excitatory neurotransmitters (e.g., dopamine, norepinephrine).

4. **Increased and decreased concentrations of calcium** in the cerebrospinal fluid (CSF) have been detected in depressed and manic individuals, respectively. Therefore, changes in the extracellular and intracellular calcium levels, which can effect the excitability of neurons, may be a factor in emotional variations and switches from depression to mania.

5. The latest research has focused on **G proteins** and their effects on mood stabilization. G proteins are involved in signal transduction and activation of second messenger systems for various neurotransmitters (e.g., norepinephrine, serotonin, dopamine).
   a. The current theory proposes that hyperactive G proteins cause mood instability; therefore, the normalization of G proteins will confer mood stability.
   b. G proteins and glutamate may also play a role in the long-term potentiation and cycling of mood disorders.

(1) Glutamate binding to G proteins linked to *N*-methyl-D-aspartate (NMDA) receptors may be involved in long-term potentiation. Lithium appears to inhibit this G protein–linked mechanism.

(2) Serotonin and norepinephrine are involved in bipolar illness, but the cycling and long-term potentiation may be mediated by glutamate and the medications that affect the glutamate system.

6. **Psychosocial and physical stressors** have been proposed as "triggers" for early episodes of bipolar disorder; however, later episodes may or may not be associated with similar stressors. A theory of increased sensitivity and kindling of the CNS has been suggested to explain the occurrence of later episodes and the cyclical nature of bipolar disorder.

C. Diagnosis

1. The diagnosis of bipolar disorder is made using the DSM-IV-TR criteria and reviewing the individual's history for episodes of mania, hypomania, or depression.

a. The diagnosis of **mania** requires the presence of an elevated, expansive, or irritable mood for at least 1 week (less time if it precipitates hospitalization). In addition, three or more of the symptoms described in Table 47-7 must be present and unrelated to substance abuse or a medical condition. Functional and social impairment must also be present.

b. The diagnostic criteria for **hypomania** include the same symptoms as mania; however, hypomania is less severe. Although changes in mood and affect are noticeable, the patient remains functional in society. Hypomania can continue to progress, or it can cycle into a manic episode.

c. The diagnostic criteria for **depression** are listed in Table 47-1.

d. A **mixed episode** is the coexistence of manic and depressive symptoms for at least 1 week. This is often referred to as **mood incongruent.**

2. Bipolar disorder is subdivided based on the combination of manic, depressive, hypomanic, and mixed episodes.

a. **Bipolar I disorder** is diagnosed if the patient has a history of at least one manic or mixed episode.

b. **Bipolar II disorder** is diagnosed if the patient has never experienced a manic episode, but has experienced one or more depressive episodes with at least one hypomanic episode.

c. **Cyclothymia** is diagnosed when the depressive and hypomanic symptoms persist for 2 years.

d. **Rapid cycling** is diagnosed when the patient has experienced at least four depressive, manic, hypomanic, or mixed (depressive and manic) episodes within a 12-month period.

D. Clinical course

1. In bipolar disorder, the length and severity of episodes vary. If untreated, manic episodes may last from days to months.

2. The time between episodes is unpredictable, but it is not unusual for episodes to occur at 1- to 2-year intervals.

3. The sequence of episodes is also unpredictable. Manic episodes do not necessarily follow depressive episodes.

Table 47-7. Symptoms of Mania

Grandiose ideations or expansive self-esteem
Decreased need for sleep
Pressured speech
Racing thoughts or flight of ideas
Distractability
Psychomotor agitation
Engaging in dangerous, high-risk activities

4. In general, the earlier the onset of disease, the worse the prognosis and the greater the likelihood of a progressive and chronic course of illness.

5. Concomitant substance abuse, mixed episodes, and rapid cycling all complicate the management of the disorder.

E. Treatment

1. Treatment phases. Acute, maintenance, and continuation phases are promoted in bipolar disorder as they are in the treatment of major depression (see Table 47-2). However, some promote the use of continuation or long-term prophylaxis after the first episode of bipolar disorder, particularly if it coincides with a positive family history.

2. Pharmacotherapy. Depending on the clinical presentation, antipsychotics, mood stabilizers, or antidepressants may have a role in treatment of patients with bipolar disorder. However, the primary therapeutic agents in the management of this disease are lithium and anticonvulsants, commonly known as mood stabilizers.

a. Atypical antipsychotics may be used adjunctively to the mood stabilizer during an acute manic espisode, particularly if psychotic symptoms are present. Olanzapine is the only atypical antipsychotic to be FDA approved for the treatment of acute mania; alternatively, risperidone, quetiapine, and ziprasidone may be used. Traditional antipsychotics, such as haloperidol, may be used if parenteral administration is necessary to manage acute agitation.

b. Antidepressants are to be used with caution in individuals with bipolar disorder. Lithium and lamotrigine are the first-line agents recommended for the treatment of bipolar depression. Some patients with severe depression or suicidal ideation may require augmentation with an antidepressant. In those cases, bupropion or paroxetine would be recommended first line due to less risk for conversion to mania; however, any of the other antidepressants may be chosen, with close monitoring to observe for signs of developing mania.

c. Benzodiazepines such as lorazepam are indicated for the short-term management of the acute agitation associated with mania.

3. Therapeutic agents

a. Lithium

(1) Indications. Lithium is first-line therapy for the treatment and prevention of bipolar disorder, except in the cases of mixed episodes or rapid cycling. In these cases, lithium may be helpful as augmentation therapy.

(2) Chemistry. Lithium is a monovalent cation, similar to sodium and potassium. Lithium carbonate and citrate are the two clinically relevant salt forms.

(a) Lithium carbonate is used more often in the treatment of bipolar disorder.

(b) Lithium citrate is available as a liquid and may be helpful in patients who are noncompliant with tablets or capsules.

(3) Pharmacokinetics

(a) The rate of absorption depends on the form administered.

(i) Lithium citrate (liquid) reaches a peak concentration in 15–45 minutes.

(ii) Immediate-release tablets and capsules peak in 1–3 hours.

(b) Bioavailability ranges from 0.8–1.0 for most products. Food can delay absorption but does not affect the extent of absorption. Some adverse effects (such as nausea, vomiting, and tremors) are related to the rapid rise in serum concentrations; therefore, administering lithium with food or giving lithium as an extended-release product may diminish such side effects.

(c) Lithium distributes into total body water and penetrates many body tissues, including the CNS, muscle, bone, kidney, saliva, and thyroid. Lithium follows a two-compartment model, and it takes at least 3 days for intracellular equilibration to occur. This helps to explain the lag time between initiation of therapy and clinical response.

(d) Lithium is not metabolized, and it is primarily eliminated through the kidneys. Lithium clearance is directly proportional to glomerular filtration rate, and its clearance is estimated to be approximately one-quarter of creatinine clearance.

(4) Mechanism of action. Although the mechanism of action for lithium remains unknown, there are several theories.

(a) Lithium is thought to help correct desynchronized biological rhythms in patients with bipolar disorder.

(b) Lithium may affect membrane stabilization.

(c) Lithium may augment homeostasis by enhancing the function of secondary messenger systems, particularly cyclic adenosine monophosphate (cAMP), cyclic guanosine monophosphate (cGMP), and phosphatidylinositol.

(d) Lithium is also noted to inhibit norepinephrine release and accelerate its metabolism.

(e) Lithium may also decrease receptor sensitivity and increase presynaptic reuptake of norepinephrine and 5-HT.

(5) Administration and dosage

(a) Lithium has a narrow therapeutic index. The **therapeutic range is approximately 0.5–1.5 mEq/L.**

   (i) In patients with **acute** mania, it is recommended to titrate the dose to the upper end of the therapeutic range (i.e., ≤0.8 mEq/L).

   (ii) In patients receiving lithium as **maintenance** therapy to prevent recurrence of mania or depression, it is recommended to target a concentration of (≤1.0 mEq/L).

(b) Adjust the dose to a concentration within the recommended **maintenance range** (0.6–1.0 mEq/L) once symptoms have remitted and the patient is stable.

(c) When **initiating therapy for acute episodes,** the recommended dose is 900 mg twice a day or 600 mg three times a day. Many patients may not be able to tolerate an initial daily dose of 1800 mg/day; therefore, in practice, many clinicians initiate therapy with **600 mg/day in divided doses.** Monitor serum levels every 3 days and titrate the dose to the appropriate therapeutic range to reduce the risk of side effects.

(d) Lithium may be **discontinued by taper** after 6 months of treatment, unless there is a history to support chronic therapy.

(6) Clinical response

(a) Patients presenting with mania generally show at least partial response to lithium within the first 2 weeks of therapy, assuming a therapeutic concentration has been reached.

(b) For patients presenting with depression, the time frame is considerably longer. It could be 4–6 weeks before a response is seen.

(7) Precautions and monitoring effects

(a) Contraindications to lithium include:

   (i) Acute renal failure and first trimester of pregnancy (absolute contraindications)

   (ii) Renal, cardiovascular, and thyroid disease (relative contraindications)

(b) Adverse effects (Table 47-8) can occur early in therapy or with chronic therapy, and individual patients may experience toxic effects despite a concentration ≤1.5 mEq/L.

Table 47-8. Adverse Events Associated with Lithium

Early Onset	Long-Term Use	Toxicity
Gastrointestinal upset	Weight gain	Severe drowsiness
Nausea	Altered taste	Coarse hand tremor
Polydipsia	Decreased libido	Muscle twitching
Polyuria	Hypothyroidism	Myoclonus
Nocturia	Rash	Choreoathetosis
Dry mouth	Acne	Cogwheel rigidity
Fine hand tremor	Psoriasis	Vomiting
Leukocytosis	Alopecia	Confusion
Muscle weakness	Nonspecific T-wave change	Ataxia
Difficulty concentrating	Premature ventricular contraction	Hyperreflexia
Sedation	(rare)	Nystagmus
	Nephrogenic diabetes insipidus	Seizure
	Nephrotoxicity (rare)	Coma
	Fine hand tremor	Death

Table 47-9. Factors That Change Lithium Concentrations

Decrease Lithium Concentrations	Increase Lithium Concentrations
Acetazolamide	Angiotensin-converting enzyme in hibitors
Methylxanthines (e.g., theophylline, caffeine)	Nonsteroidal anti-inflammatory drugs
Osmotic diuretics	Thiazides
Pregnancy (third trimester)	Dehydration
Sodium supplements	Renal dysfunction
Urine alkalinizers (e.g., sodium bicarbonate, potassium citrate)	Sodium loss
	Fluoxetine
	Postpartum

   (c) Toxicity is a potentially fatal medical emergency. Treatment of toxicity involves:
     (i) Holding or discontinuing lithium therapy
     (ii) Correcting water and electrolyte disturbances
     (iii) Attempting to empty the stomach by emesis or gastric lavage (acute toxicity) [Charcoal administration is ineffective.]
     (iv) Performing hemodialysis or peritoneal dialysis [only way to remove lithium in severe toxicity (i.e., ≥ 3 mEq/L)].
   (d) Significant interactions can occur that increase or decrease lithium concentrations (Table 47-9).
     (i) Concomitant use of lithium with antipsychotics or benzodiazepines may increase the risk for neurotoxicity, particularly with long-term combination therapy.
     (ii) Concomitant use of lithium with medications known to increase 5-HT may cause serotonin syndrome (see Table 47-3).
   (e) Monitor serum levels after dose increases and then every 6 months once the patient has stabilized, unless the patient's clinical status deteriorates.
     (i) Lithium concentrations should be drawn 12 hours after the initial dose. Drawing the sample in the morning before the first dose of the day is given is generally convenient.
     (ii) Renal and thyroid function should be assessed at baseline and every 2–3 months for the initial 6 months, and then every 6 months to yearly in patients maintained on lithium.
 b. Valproic acid (VPA)
   (1) Indications. VPA is an anticonvulsant that has demonstrated efficacy in mood disorders.
     (a) It can be used to treat acute mania, mixed mania, and rapid cycling.
     (b) It can be used as monotherapy in bipolar disorder or as adjunctive therapy with lithium or another mood stabilizer.
   (2) Mechanism of action. Although the mechanism of action is not fully understood, it is hypothesized to be related to GABA modulation and possibly second messenger systems.
   (3) Administration and dosage
     (a) There are **four formulations** available; the term VPA is used for all preparations.
       (i) The elixer is sodium valproate.
       (ii) The capsules are VPA.
       (iii) The enteric-coated preparation is a dimer (i.e., divalproex, divalproex ER)
       (iv) The injectable preparation is sodium valproate.
     (b) The **therapeutic range** for VPA was originally established for seizure disorders as 50–100 μg/mL. However, this range now serves as a guide in preventing toxicity and determining compliance with therapy in bipolar disorder. In general, VPA cannot be considered a therapeutic failure until a concentration of 80–120 μg/mL has been achieved for 4–6 weeks.
     (c) The dose of VPA for acute episodes can be loaded at 20 mg/kg/day to be administered in divided doses. The maintenance dose is based on clinical response and serum concentrations (to avoid toxicity). In the elderly or outpatient setting, therapy is initiated more cautiously, beginning at 250 mg administered three times a day and increased gradually based on response. Once stabilized, the

dose can be given once or twice daily to increase compliance. The extended-release formulations may be administered once daily with fewer side effects but may require a slightly higher dose due to less oral bioavailability.

(4) Precautions and monitoring effects

  (a) Common **dose-related side effects** include:

    (i) Nausea, vomiting, and stomach cramps (may be diminished by giving divalproex instead of sodium valproate and valproic acid)

    (ii) Lethargy

    (iii) Alopecia

    (iv) Thrombocytopenia

    (v) Elevation of liver function tests

  (b) Idiopathic side effects include:

    (i) Weight gain

    (ii) Hepatic failure

    (iii) Pancreatitis

    (iv) Agranulocytosis

  (c) Drug–drug interactions can occur with VPA.

    (i) Drugs known to increase VPA concentrations are cimetidine, chlorpromazine, erythromycin, felbamate, and salicylates.

    (ii) Drugs known to decrease VPA concentrations include rifampin, phenobarbital, lamotrigine, phenytoin, and carbamazepine (CBZ).

    (iii) VPA can increase warfarin and zidovudine concentrations.

    (iv) Concomitant use with CNS depressants may have additive effects.

  (d) Serum monitoring and laboratory assessment should be done according to the following schedule.

    (i) VPA concentration should be obtained every 7 days until the desired concentration is achieved and stable.

    (ii) Follow-up concentrations should be assessed every 2 weeks for the first 2 months, and then every 3–6 months, depending on the individual patient.

    (iii) Baseline complete blood count and liver function tests should be obtained and reassessed monthly for the first 2 months, and then every 6–12 months.

c. CBZ

  (1) Indications. CBZ is an anticonvulsant that has been found to work well as a mood stabilizer.

    (a) CBZ is typically reserved for use in bipolar patients with partial or no response to lithium. It may be considered first-line therapy in patients with a history of not responding to lithium or in patients with a history of mixed episodes or rapid cycling.

    (b) CBZ can be used as monotherapy or in combination with lithium or other mood stabilizers.

  (2) Mechanism of action. Although the mechanism of action is unknown, it may be related to the ability to modulate norepinephrine and G protein–linked second messenger systems, particularly cAMP.

  (3) Administration and dosage

    (a) The **therapeutic range** formerly established for CBZ as an anticonvulsant is now used to help avoid toxicity in bipolar patients.

      (i) The correlation between therapeutic concentration and clinical response is not as straightforward as it is with seizure disorders.

      (ii) Clinically, CBZ is only considered unsuccessful for mood stabilization when the patient has failed to respond and the serum concentration was well within the range of 6–12 μg/mL for 4–6 weeks.

    (b) For acute mania, initiate therapy with 200–400 mg/day and increase by 200 mg/day every 3–5 days to a usual dose of 600–1200 mg/day given in divided doses.

  (4) Precautions and monitoring effects

    (a) CNS-related side effects include:

      (i) Drowsiness

      (ii) Dizziness

      (iii) Ataxia

      (iv) Blurred vision

      (v) Diplopia

      (vi) Nystagmus

(vii) Confusion

(viii) Headache

(b) Dose-related side effects occur soon after initiating therapy or after a dose increase; therefore, it is possible to minimize these side effects by starting with low doses and titrating slowly. Dose-related side effects include:

    (i) Gastrointestinal effects (e.g., nausea, vomiting, diarrhea, constipation, anorexia, abdominal pain) [Decreasing the dose and giving with food may be helpful.]

    (ii) Hematological effects [blood dyscrasias (e.g., aplastic anemia, thrombocytopenia, neutropenia; rare), leukopenia (transient; fairly common)]

    (iii) Mild, transient elevations of liver function tests (monitor yearly)

(c) Non–dose-related side effects. Exfoliative dermatitis (e.g., Stevens-Johnson syndrome), agranulocytosis, and hepatic failure are rare but potentially fatal.

(d) CBZ induces enzymatic metabolism for many drugs, including itself. Autoinduction may begin as early as day 3 of therapy and continue for up to 30 days after the last dose of CBZ. For this reason, careful **monitoring of serum concentrations** and awareness of potential **drug interactions** is important.

    (i) Serum concentrations of CBZ should be obtained every 2 weeks for the first 2 months.

    (ii) Once a steady state is achieved, assessment may be reduced to every 2–3 months for 1 year.

    (iii) If the patient remains stable, the monitoring of CBZ may be reduced to every 6 months.

(e) Laboratory assessments (i.e., baseline complete blood count, liver function test, thyroid-stimulating hormone, electrolytes, and blood urea nitrogen/creatinine) should be obtained and periodically reassessed.

    (i) Additional laboratory monitoring includes baseline assessments of complete blood count, liver function tests, thyroid-stimulating hormone, electrolytes, and blood urea nitrogen/creatinine.

    (ii) Monitoring of these parameters may be repeated every 3–6 months and periodically as needed for changing clinical status.

d. Newer mood stabilizers (i.e., lamotrigine, gabapentin, and oxcarbazepine)

  (1) Indications. Mood elevations noticed during epilepsy studies with lamotrigine and gabapentin gave rise to the interest for their use in mood disorders.

  (2) Lamotrigine

    (a) Chemistry. The chemical structure of lamotrigine is similar to phenytoin and CBZ.

    (b) Mechanism of action. The mechanism of action is not fully understood, but lamotrigine appears to block sodium-mediated release of glutamate and aspartate at low concentrations. At higher concentrations, it blocks GABA and acetylcholine release.

    (c) Administration and dosage

      (i) Lamotrigine therapy (Table 47-10) should be initiated with a low dose and titrated slowly to decrease the risk of developing a rash. Because the risk is increased with the coadministration of VPA, in such cases, the dose titration must be increased even more cautiously.

      (ii) Subsequent dosage titration is based on desired mood response and the emergence of side effects.

      (iii) Doses greater than 50 mg/day should be administered in two divided doses.

Table 47-10. Dosing Lamotrigine

Lamotrigine added to regimens without valproic acid[1]	
Weeks 1 and 2	25 mg/day
Weeks 3 and 4	50 mg/day
Lamotrigine added to regimens containing valproic acid[1]	
Weeks 1 and 2	25 mg every other day
Weeks 3 and 4	25 mg every day

[1]Increase dose by 25–50 mg/day in 1- to 2-week increments.

(d) **Adverse effects.** Common side effects include dizziness, diplopia, blurred vision, nausea and vomiting, rash, photosensitivity, ataxia, and headache. The rash may be severe or potentially life-threatening; therefore, patients should be instructed to discontinue this medication at the first sign of a rash.

(3) Gabapentin

(a) **Chemistry.** Gabapentin is structurally similar to GABA but does not alter its function as an antagonist or agonist.

(b) **Mechanism of action.** The mechanism of action is currently unknown for its anticonvulsant and mood-stabilizing properties. However, its relatively clean profile makes gabapentin appealing as an adjunctive mood stabilizer.

(c) **Administration and dosage**

(i) Gabapentin is initiated with a 300-mg dose administered at bedtime to reduce side effects, with subsequent increases of 300 mg daily to 300 mg three times daily by the third day.

(ii) Although effective antiseizure maintenance doses are 900–1800 mg/day, dosing for mood stabilization is currently based on clinical response.

(iii) Because gabapentin has a short half-life, doses should not be separated by more than 12 hours.

(d) **Adverse effects.** Side effects such as somnolence, nystagmus, dizziness, ataxia, and fatigue have been associated with gabapentin. However, it is not metabolized; therefore, drug–drug interactions are virtually negligible.

(4) Oxcarbazepine is structurally and chemically similar to carbamazepine and is expected to have comparable efficacy in the management of bipolar disorder, with fewer side effects and better tolerability. Therefore, oxcarbazepine is considered to be an alternative to carbamazepine in the treatment of bipolar disorder. Generally, therapy is initiated with 150–300 mg twice daily, with subsequent dose increases based on response and tolerability, up to a maximum dose of 1200 mg/day.

4. Use of dual mood stabilizers

a. In patients who require more than one mood stabilizer, the combination of lithium and CBZ or VPA may be beneficial.

(1) Lithium may cause leukocytosis, and CBZ and VPA are known to cause leukopenia.

(2) Because CBZ and VPA are known to cause a variety of blood dyscrasias, the combination of these two agents is not recommended.

b. The more traditional mood stabilizers (i.e., lithium, VPA, and CBZ) may also be combined with one of the newer anticonvulsants (i.e., lamotrigine or gabapentin) for mood stabilization.

5. Mood stabilizers in pregnancy

a. Lithium, VPA, and CBZ can cause birth defects.

(1) Lithium, a category D drug, is particularly harmful during the first trimester, but may be used during the second and third trimesters.

(2) VPA and CBZ are category D drugs in pregnancy and should be used only when the benefit outweighs the risk. Folic acid supplementation may help minimize the fetal anomalies seen with VPA.

b. Lamotrigine, gabapentin, and oxcarbazepine are category C drugs, which indicates that anomalies have been seen in animal studies.

STUDY QUESTIONS

Directions: Each of the numbered items or incomplete statements in this section is followed by answers or by completions of the statement. Select the **one** lettered answer or completion that is **best** in each case.

1. Which of the following statements about depression is true?

(A) The incidence of depression is greater in men than in women.
(B) Approximately 5% of institutionalized elders develop depression.
(C) Depression has no genetic link.
(D) Depression is diagnosed using the DSM-IV-TR criteria.

2. A patient with major depression should receive antidepressant therapy for at least

(A) 2 weeks
(B) 6 weeks
(C) 2 months
(D) 6 months

3. Which of the following patients is most likely to require maintenance antidepressant therapy?

(A) A 22-year-old woman depressed about the loss of a parent
(B) A 33-year-old man presenting with his second episode of depression
(C) A 67-year-old man experiencing his first episode of depression
(D) A 34-year-old woman experiencing postpartum depression

4. A 36-year-old woman presents with a 2-month history of depressed mood, anhedonia, increased appetite, weight gain, hypersomnolence, and suicidal ideation. This is the patient's first episode of major depression. Which of the following antidepressants would be most appropriate in the treatment of this patient?

(A) Nortriptyline
(B) Sertraline
(C) Phenelzine
(D) Mirtazapine

5. Which of the following medications would most likely exacerbate a preexisting seizure disorder?

(A) Venlafaxine
(B) Trazodone
(C) Bupropion
(D) Paroxetine

6. A patient, who has received citalopram 40 mg/day for 2 weeks for the treatment of major depression, complains that the medication is not working and would like to be switched to another agent. What is the appropriate recommendation?

(A) Provide the patient with some information on MAOIs, and call the physician to recommend switching the patient to phenelzine
(B) Encourage the patient to continue with the current regimen, and inform the patient that it may take 4–6 weeks before the full response is evident
(C) Recommend adding lithium to augment the current regimen
(D) Recommend switching to mirtazapine due to a therapeutic failure with citalopram

7. A patient diagnosed with depression was unsuccessfully treated with fluoxetine. Fluoxetine was discontinued, and 14 days later, the patient started therapy with phenelzine. Three days after phenelzine was started, the patient presented with hyperreflexia, fever, elevated blood pressure, confusion, and diarrhea. What is the most likely cause of this clinical presentation?

(A) Serotonin syndrome
(B) Serotonin withdrawal syndrome
(C) Hypertensive crisis
(D) Neuroleptic malignant syndrome

8. A patient presents with pressured speech, inability to sleep for 72 hours, bizarre dress, inappropriate makeup, and grandiose delusions that interfere with social functioning. Which of the following is the most likely diagnosis?

(A) Depression
(B) Euthymia
(C) Hypomania
(D) Mania

9. Which of the following medications would be considered first-line monotherapy for the treatment of bipolar disorder?

(A) Gabapentin
(B) Lithium
(C) Risperidone
(D) Haloperidol

10. Which of the following is the appropriate therapeutic range for lithium in the treatment of acute mania?

(A) 0.6–1.0 mEq/L
(B) 0.6–1.5 mEq/L
(C) 0.6–0.8 mEq/L
(D) 0.8–1.2 mEq/L

11. Which of the following mood stabilizers would be most appropriate in a patient with liver disease?

(A) Lithium
(B) Valproic acid
(C) Carbamazepine
(D) None of the above

12. A 32-year-old, 70-kg man diagnosed with bipolar I disorder is being treated with valproic acid (VPA). Which of the following is a reasonable loading dose for VPA in this patient?

(A) 250 mg twice a day
(B) 500 mg twice a day
(C) 250 mg three times a day
(D) 500 mg three times a day

13. Which of the following factors may increase lithium concentration?

(A) Edema
(B) Osmotic diuretics
(C) Increased sodium intake
(D) Nonsteroidal anti-inflammatory drugs

ANSWERS AND EXPLANATIONS

1. The answer is D *[II C].*
The DSM-IV-TR criteria provide the diagnostic guidelines for psychiatric disorders. Depression occurs more often in women than in men, up to 20% of the institutionalized geriatric population experiences depression, and a higher incidence of depression occurs among patients with a positive family history supporting a genetic link.

2. The answer is D *[II D 1; Table 47-2].*
Patients should receive antidepressant therapy through the continuation phase, which is generally 6–9 months.

3. The answer is C *[Table 47-2].*
Patients at high risk for recurrent episodes of depression should receive maintenance therapy. Patients older than 50 years of age who are experiencing their first episode of depression are considered to be at high risk for recurrent episodes and should receive maintenance antidepressant therapy.

4. The answer is B *[II D 6 e].*
Sertraline, a selective serotonin reuptake inhibitor (SSRI), is a good first-line agent, particularly in patients who would benefit from the stimulatory side effects. Nortriptyline and mirtazapine would not be good alternatives due to this patient's hypersomnolence and weight gain. In addition, a tricyclic amine (TCA) [nortriptyline] is not recommended in patients at risk for suicide. Although some aspects of this patient's depression may be considered atypical, a monoamine oxidase inhibitor (MAOI) would not be selected as first-line therapy given that it is the patient's first episode of depression.

5. The answer is C *[II D 6 c (3) (b)].*
Although all antidepressants can lower the seizure threshold, bupropion is contraindicated in patients with seizure disorder. Bupropion is specifically discussed in the chapter as being contraindicated in patients with a seizure disorder. Paroxetine was associated with a 0.1% incidence of seizures during clinical trials. Seizure associated with venlafaxine occurs infrequently (1/100 to 1/1000 patients). The overdosage of trazodone may be associated with seizures, but at normal doses, trazodone is not thought to alter the seizure threshold.

6. The answer is B *[II D 3 a (3) (b)].*
An antidepressant must be given at the maximum tolerated dose for 4–6 weeks before it is considered a therapeutic failure; therefore, the best recommendation is to continue with the current regimen for at least 2 more weeks. MAOIs are reserved for refractory depressed patients and are not indicated in this patient scenario. Lithium is an appropriate augmentative agent but is not indicated until the patient has failed two or three different antidepressant trials.

7. The answer is A *[II D 3 b (2); Table 47-3].*
Serotonin syndrome may result when starting a monoamine oxidase inhibitor (MAOI) immediately after another agent that increases serotonin levels. Generally, a 2-week washout period is recommended; however, fluoxetine requires a 5-week washout period due to norfluoxetine (active metabolite).

8. The answer is D *[III C 1 a–c].*
The clinical presentation described is consistent with mania. Hypomania generally does not impair functioning. Euthymia implies normal mood, whereas depression typically involves more neurovegetative symptoms.

9. The answer is B *[III E 3 a (1)].*
Lithium is considered the first-line monotherapy for euphoric mania. Gabapentin has demonstrated utility as a mood stabilizer but is only considered an adjunctive therapy. Risperidone is an atypical antipsychotic that is used to treat psychosis associated with bipolar disorder; however, this should only be added to therapy when the patient exhibits psychotic symptoms. Haloperidol is a traditional antipsychotic that may be used parenterally to manage acute agitation but is not appropriate as first-line monotherapy.

10. The answer is D *[III E 3 a (5) (a) (i)].*
When using lithium in the treatment of acute mania, it is recommended to use the upper end of the therapeutic range (i.e., ≤0.8 mEq/L).

11. The answer is A *[III E 3 a (7) (a)].*
Lithium is not known to cause hepatic dysfunction, nor is it metabolized via the liver. However, both valproic acid and carbamazepine can impair liver function.

12. The answer is D *[III E 3 b (3) (c)].*
The appropriate loading dose for valproic acid (VPA) in acute mania is 20 mg/kg/day; therefore, in this patient, the appropriate loading dose is 1400 mg/day. This equation approximates the need for the patient, and it is appropriate to round up to available dosage forms.

13. The answer is D *[Table 47-9].*
Edema (increases in fluid volume), osmotic diuretics, and increased sodium intake all decrease lithium concentrations. Nonsteroidal anti-inflammatory drugs decrease renal blood flow and decrease lithium clearance, resulting in increased lithium concentrations.

48
Asthma and Chronic Obstructive Pulmonary Disease

Mona G. Tsoukleris
Brian G. Katona

I. ASTHMA

A. Definition. Asthma is a chronic inflammatory disorder of the airways. It involves complex interactions between many cells and inflammatory mediators that result in inflammation, obstruction (partially or completely reversible after treatment or resolves spontaneously), increased airway responsiveness (i.e., hyperresponsiveness), and episodic asthma symptoms (see I G 1).

B. Classification. Asthma severity classifications were revised by the National Institutes of Health (NIH) in the second expert panel report of the Heart, Lung, and Blood Institute to include **mild intermittent asthma** in addition to **mild, moderate, and severe persistent asthma** (Table 48-1). A patient's severity classification plays an important role in determining the most appropriate pharmacotherapeutic approach and is determined by:

1. Symptoms

2. Treatment requirements

3. Objective measurements of lung function, including diurnal variations

4. Frequency of nocturnal symptoms

C. Incidence. In 1999, approximately 16.9 million American adults reported having been told by a health-care professional that they had asthma.

1. It has been estimated that 7.8 million children age 18 years and younger have asthma.

2. Asthma improves in many children as they age, with 50% appearing to have "outgrown" asthma by their mid-teens. However, it is incorrect to consider that these individuals no longer have asthma, because many eventually have a return of symptoms.

3. In 1999, there were 10.8 million office and outpatient visits for asthma and 2.0 million asthma-related visits to emergency departments.

4. Although death from asthma remains uncommon, death rates were increasing in recent years, but appear to have reached a plateau. In 1999, there were 4,657 deaths attributed to asthma. The most common cause of death is believed to be inadequate assessment of the severity of airway obstruction by either practitioner or patient, leading to suboptimal therapy.

5. The cost to society of asthma is staggering. In 2000 alone, it is estimated that direct costs related to asthma exceeded $8.1 billion. These costs include $2.4 billion for medications and $3.5 billion for hospitalizations. Indirect costs of asthma are estimated at $4.6 billion.

D. Etiology. Precipitating factors of an acute asthma exacerbation may include:

1. Allergens (e.g., pollen, house dust mite, animal dander, mold, cockroach, food)
   a. Concurrent predisposition to allergy is highly prevalent in patients with asthma.
   b. For example, allergic rhinitis is reported in 45% of patients with asthma compared to 20% of the general population.

2. Occupational exposures (e.g., chemical irritants, flour, wood, textile dusts)

3. Viral respiratory tract infections

Table 48-1. Classification of Asthma Severity*

Classification	Characteristics†	Nighttime Occurrence of Symptoms	Lung Function
Severe persistent (step 4)	Continual symptoms; limited physical activity; frequent exacerbations	Frequent	FEV_1/PEF ($\leq$60%) predicted; PEF variability >30%
Moderate persistent (step 3)	Daily symptoms; daily use of inhaled short-acting β-agonist; exacerbations affect activity; exacerbations ≥ two times a week and may last days	> one night a week	FEV_1/PEF (>60%–80%) predicted; PEF variability >30%
Mild persistent (step 2)	Symptoms > two times a week but not every day; exacerbations may affect activity	> two nights a month	FEV_1/PEF ($\geq$80%) predicted; PEF variability 20%–30%
Mild intermittent (step 1)	Symptoms ≤ two times a week; asymptomatic between exacerbations; exacerbations brief (from a few hours to a few days); intensity of exacerbations may vary	≤ two times a month	FEV_1/PEF ≥80% predicted; PEF variability <20%; PEF normal between exacerbations

The characteristics noted in this table are general and may overlap because asthma is highly variable. (Adapted with permission from National Institutes of Health/National Heart, Lung, and Blood Institute. National Asthma Education and Prevention Program Expert Panel Report 2: Guidelines for the diagnosis and management of asthma. NIH Publication 97-4051, July 1997.

FEV_1 = forced expiratory volume in 1 second; PEF = peak expiratory flow.

*The presence of any one of the features of severity is sufficient to place a patient in that category. An individual should be assigned to the most severe grade in which any feature occurs.

†Patients at any level of severity can have mild, moderate, or severe exacerbations. For example, some patients with intermittent asthma experience severe, life-threatening exacerbations separated by long periods of normal lung function and no symptoms.

4. Exercise

5. Emotions (e.g., anxiety, stress, hard laughter or crying)

6. Exposure to irritants (e.g., strong odors, chemicals, fumes)

7. Environmental exposures (e.g., weather changes, cold air, sulfur dioxide, cigarette smoke)

8. Drugs
   a. Reactions to drugs may occur due to hypersensitivity or as an extension of the pharmacological effect.
   b. Problematic drugs include:
      (1) Aspirin and other nonsteroidal anti-inflammatory drugs
      (2) Antiadrenergic and cholinergic drugs (e.g., β-adrenergic blockers, bethanechol)
      (3) Medications (or foods) that contain tartrazine, sulfites, and other preservatives

E. **Pathology.** On postmortem examination of patients with asthma, the following characteristics have been identified:

1. Hypertrophy of smooth muscle

2. Airways containing plugs consisting of inflammatory cells and their debris, proteins, and mucus

3. Inflammatory cellular infiltrate with vasodilation, denuded airway epithelium, and microvascular leakage

4. Vasodilation of the vasculature

5. Denuded airway epithelium

6. Microvascular leakage

7. Collagen deposition in basement membranes

F. Pathophysiology (Figure 48-1)

   1. Major contributing processes

   a. Inflammatory cells (i.e., mast cells, eosinophils, activated T cells, macrophages, and epithelial cells) secrete mediators and influence the airways directly or via neural mechanisms.

   b. Airway obstruction is responsible for many of the clinical manifestations of asthma.

   (1) Severity of obstruction is variable and believed to be a result of bronchoconstriction, airway wall edema, mucus plug formation, airway remodeling, smooth muscle hypertrophy, and hyperplasia.

   (2) Airway obstruction reduces ventilation to some lung regions, which causes a ventilation/perfusion (V/Q) imbalance that leads to hypoxemia. This is reflected by a reduction in the partial pressure of arterial oxygen (PaO_2) observed in moderate to severe exacerbations.

   c. Hyperresponsiveness, an exaggerated response to certain stimuli, is an important feature of asthma and appears to correlate with clinical severity and medication requirements.

   (1) Increased levels of inflammatory mediators and infiltration by inflammatory cells are thought to be the primary mechanisms responsible for airway hyperresponsiveness.

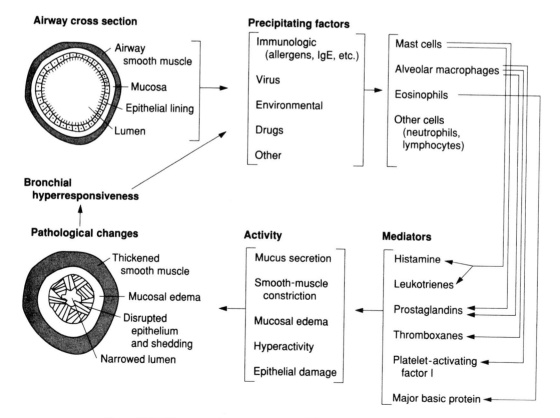

Figure 48-1. Diagrammatic representation of the pathophysiology of asthma.

(2) Additional mechanisms may include abnormal bronchial epithelial integrity, altered autonomic neural control (see I F 1 e), and a change in intrinsic bronchial smooth-muscle function.

d. Airway inflammation is crucial to development of asthma and contributes to airway hyperresponsiveness, airflow obstruction, respiratory symptoms, and disease chronicity. Inflammatory cells and their mediators are responsible for altered mucociliary function, epithelial disruption ranging from minor ciliary loss to severely denuded epithelium, increased airway permeability (to inhaled allergens, irritants, and inflammatory mediators), and reduced clearance of inflammatory mediators.

(1) Acute inflammation is associated with early recruitment of cells to the airway.

(2) Subacute inflammation is associated with recruited and resident cell activation, resulting in more persistent inflammation.

(3) Chronic inflammation is associated with persistent cell damage and ongoing repair, resulting in airway abnormalities that may become permanent.

e. Alteration in **autonomic neural control** also contributes to obstruction.

(1) Elevated parasympathetic tone and reflex bronchoconstriction may occur due to increased cholinergic sensitivity or a change in muscarinic receptor function.

(2) Increased smooth-muscle responsiveness may be due to smooth-muscle hypertrophy. Exposure of the nerve endings, caused by inflammation, may also contribute.

f. Airway remodeling can result from persistent inflammation when asthma is poorly controlled. The resulting damage can yield permanent airway abnormalities because of subbasement membrane collagen deposition and fibrosis. These events may occur even in the face of mild disease.

2. Sequencing of events in asthma. There are five main events that occur in asthma.

a. Triggering. After exposure to an allergic trigger, antigen binds to immunoglobulin E (IgE), which is attached to activated mast cells. Nonallergic factors (e.g., aspirin, viral infections) may also function as triggers.

(1) The **early asthmatic response** begins within 30 minutes of trigger exposure (usually only several minutes after exposure) and resolves within 2 hours. This response can be blocked by the administration of β-agonists or anti-inflammatory agents (i.e., cromolyn sodium or nedocromil).

(2) The **late asthmatic response** involves a second decline in lung function and may begin 4–8 hours after the initial trigger exposure. The late asthmatic response, characterized by persistent airflow obstruction, airway inflammation, and bronchial hyperresponsiveness, is found in approximately 50% of patients with asthma. The response may last several days, and bronchial hyperreactivity may persist for several weeks. This response can be blocked by the administration of corticosteroids or anti-inflammatory agents (i.e., cromolyn sodium or nedocromil).

b. Signaling. The activated mast cells and other signaling cells (e.g., lymphocytes, eosinophils, epithelial cells, macrophages) release chemical signals (e.g., cytokines, chemokines, eicosanoids, leukotrienes), which attract additional inflammatory cells to the airways.

c. Migration. An influx of inflammatory cells (e.g., eosinophils, lymphocytes, monocytes, granulocytes) begins.

(1) In addition to the migration of these cells to the airway, upregulation of adhesion molecules begins.

(2) These adhesion molecules affix themselves to cells in the circulation and attract these cells to the airways.

d. Cell activation is required before cells can release inflammatory mediators. Once present in the airways, eosinophils are activated. Leukotrienes appear to be important in this cell activation.

(1) These inflammatory mediators cause smooth-muscle constriction and set the stage for the late phase of the inflammatory process by initiating chemotaxis.

(2) Leukotrienes appear to be important in the development of bronchoconstriction, increased mucus production, increased vascular permeability, and hyperresponsiveness.

(3) Additional inflammatory mediators (e.g., eosinophil chemotactic factor, neutrophil chemotactic factor, basophil chemotactic factor, platelet-activating factor) participate in the late asthmatic response by recruiting additional inflammatory cells to the airways.

e. Tissue stimulation and damage occurs as a result of these inflammatory mediators released from activated cells. Neural alterations and damage to the airway epithelium itself also occurs. The epithelial damage is believed to contribute to airway hyperresponsiveness. Rather than resolving, airway inflammation may persist and result in a structural change to the lung known as airway remodeling.

G. Clinical evaluation

1. Physical findings

a. Acute exacerbations may have a sudden or gradual onset. Symptoms are frequently nocturnal or occur in the early morning hours.

(1) Common findings in an acute exacerbation include:
   (a) Shortness of breath
   (b) Wheezing (usually occurs at the end of exhalation, but may be heard throughout inspiration and exhalation in more severe asthma)
   (c) Chest tightness
   (d) Cough
   (e) Tachypnea and tachycardia
   (f) Pulsus paradoxus (severe exacerbations)

(2) Between acute asthma exacerbations, the patient may be asymptomatic.

b. Patients with **chronic, poorly controlled, severe asthma** may have evidence of chronic hyperinflation, including barrel chest and decreased diaphragmatic excursion.

c. Physical findings are dependent on the severity of the underlying disease and the severity of the exacerbation. Regardless of the underlying disease severity, patients can have mild, moderate, or severe exacerbations (Table 48-2).

2. Diagnostic test results

a. Pulmonary function tests determine the degree of airway obstruction and may be normal between exacerbations.

(1) Forced expiratory volume in 1 second (FEV$_1$) and forced vital capacity both decrease during an acute exacerbation.

(2) Residual volume (RV) and total lung capacity (TLC) may increase in asthma because of **air trapping** and subsequent **lung hyperinflation.**

(3) Peak expiratory flow rate (PEFR) correlates well with FEV$_1$. However, PEFR measurement is not used in making the diagnosis of asthma.

   (a) Uses of PEFR monitoring include assessment of therapy, trigger identification, and assessment of the need for referral to emergency care.

Table 48-2. Stages of Severity of an Acute Asthmatic Attack

Stage	Symptoms	FEV$_1$ or FVC	Arterial pH	PaO$_2$	PaCO$_2$
I: Mild	Mild dyspnea and wheezing	50%–80% of normal	Normal or ↑	Normal or ↓	Normal or ↓
II: Moderate	Respiratory distress at rest and marked wheezing	50% of normal	↑	↓	↓
III: Severe	Marked respiratory distress, loud wheezing, coughing, difficulty speaking, accessory chest muscle use, and chest hyperinflation	<50% of normal	Normal or ↓	↓	Normal or ↑
IV: Respiratory failure	Severe respiratory distress, confusion, lethargy, cyanosis, disappearance of breath sounds, and pulsus paradoxus >12 mm Hg	<25% of normal	↓↓	↓	↑↑

Arrows indicate changes: ↑ = increased; ↓ = decreased; ↑↑ = markedly increased; ↓↓ = markedly decreased.
FEV$_1$ = forced expiratory volume in 1 second; FVC = forced vital capacity; PaO$_2$ = partial pressure of arterial oxygen; PaCO$_2$ = partial pressure of arterial carbon dioxide.

      (b) PEFR monitoring is recommended for patients who have had severe exacerbations, who are poor perceivers of asthma symptoms, and who have moderate to severe disease.

      (c) PEFR is best measured in early morning, before medication administration. More frequent monitoring over a few weeks may also be indicated to identify specific patterns and to identify a patient's personal best PEFR measurement. In this case, measurements are taken before medications are taken in the morning (i.e., on awakening) and again at midday (i.e., after taking a short-acting β-agonist). **Diurnal variation** of greater than 20% in PEFR measured during the day suggests airway hyperresponsiveness and less-than-adequate asthma control.

    (4) Provocation testing with **histamine or methacholine challenge** may be performed to assess hyperresponsiveness and to rule out asthma in a patient who has had normal pulmonary function test results but in whom asthma is still suspected.

  b. Blood analysis typically shows a slightly increased white blood cell (WBC) count during an acute exacerbation; eosinophilia also may be present. Leukocytosis may be present because of WBC demargination that occurs when patients receive systemic corticosteroids.

  c. Sputum analysis may reveal:
    (1) Eosinophils
    (2) Curschmann's spirals (mucous casts of the small airways)
    (3) Charcot-Leyden crystals (products of eosinophil breakdown)
    (4) Creola bodies (clumps of epithelial cells)
    (5) Bacteria (if there is an infection)

  d. Pulse oximetry is a noninvasive means of assessing the degree of hypoxemia during an acute exacerbation. The oximeter measures oxygen saturation in arterial blood (SaO_2) and pulse.

  e. Arterial blood gas measurements may be required to help gauge the severity of the asthma exacerbation (see Table 48-2).
    (1) In the early stages of an asthma exacerbation, **hyperventilation** results in a decrease in the partial pressure of arterial carbon dioxide ($PaCO_2$). If the exacerbation progresses and the airways remain narrowed, respiratory muscles may fatigue.
    (2) Respiratory acidosis is a poor prognostic sign. It develops if hypoxemia worsens and the patient's respiratory rate is not maintained due to respiratory fatigue. This results in a rising $PaCO_2$ level.

  f. An **electrocardiogram (ECG)** may show sinus tachycardia. An ECG may be particularly useful in an older patient.

  g. A **chest radiograph** may be normal or could detect accompanying pneumothorax, atelectasis, or pneumonia. Evidence of hyperinflation may be present in acute asthma and in chronic, poorly controlled asthma. A chest radiograph may also be needed to exclude other causes of the patient's symptoms.

  h. Allergy skin tests and in vitro tests (e.g., **radioallergosorbent tests**) are helpful in identifying possible allergic triggers.

3. Signs of respiratory distress include:
  a. Use of accessory muscles
  b. Inability to speak in sentences or ambulate due to dyspnea
  c. Declining mental status
  d. PEFR less than 50% of predicted (or personal best)
  e. Cyanosis
  f. Suprasternal retractions
  g. Absence of respiratory sounds
  h. Increasing $PaCO_2$

4. Patients with **potentially fatal asthma** should be quickly identified and aggressively managed. These patients have the following characteristics:
  a. History of severe exacerbations, particularly exacerbations that develop suddenly
  b. Poor self-perception of asthma symptoms and severity
  c. History of intubation or intensive care unit (ICU) admission for asthma
  d. Two or more hospitalizations or three or more visits to the emergency department for asthma within 1 year
  e. Hospitalization or treatment in the emergency department for asthma within the last month

    f. Frequent β-agonist use (i.e., more than two canisters per month), current systemic steroid treatment, or recent systemic steroid withdrawal

    g. Concurrent conditions [e.g., cardiovascular or psychiatric disease, substance abuse, low socioeconomic status (particularly in urban areas)]

H. Therapy

1. Treatment objectives

    a. The goal of therapy is to provide symptomatic control with normalization of lifestyle and to return pulmonary function as close to normal as possible.

    b. The treatment goals listed in the NIH expert panel 2002 update report include:

      (1) Minimal or no chronic symptoms day or night

      (2) Peak expiratory flow rate >80% of personal best

      (3) No limitations of activities, no work/school missed

      (4) Minimal or no exacerbations

      (5) Minimal use of short-acting inhaled $beta_2$-agonist (<1 time daily, <1 canister/ month)

      (6) Minimal or no adverse effects from medications

2. Management of acute asthma exacerbations

    a. **Home-based** treatment of an acute asthma exacerbation (Figure 48-2)

    b. Treatment of an acute asthma exacerbation in the **hospital or emergency department** (Figure 48-3)

3. Management of persistent asthma

    a. A stepped approach based on severity of disease is used to manage persistent asthma (Table 48-3). Gaining control of asthma may be achieved with either a step-up or step-down approach (determined by severity of disease); however, the more aggressive step-down approach is advocated by the NIH expert panel.

      (1) **The step-down approach** starts with treatment one step above the patient's assessed asthma severity to give rapid disease control. For example, for step 2 asthma, start with the step 3 drug regimen, then review treatment every 1–6 months. Gradual stepwise reduction in treatment may be possible based on the patient's response to therapy.

      (2) **The step-up approach** begins with a treatment regimen at the same step as the patient's severity. The regimen is adjusted upward if the patient fails to respond to treatment. Consider the step-up approach if control is not maintained and after reviewing adherence to therapy, medication administration technique, and environmental control actions.

    b. At each step, patients should control their environment to avoid or control factors that make their asthma worse (e.g., allergens, irritants). This requires specific diagnosis and education.

    c. Inhaled β-agonists are used as needed for acute symptoms for all levels of severity.

      (1) Daily or increasing use of a short-acting inhaled $beta_2$-agonist suggests the need for additional long-term controller (i.e., anti-inflammatory) therapy.

      (2) Pretreatment with either an inhaled β-agonist, cromolyn sodium, or nedocromil may be used before exercise or allergen exposure.

    d. A rescue course of systemic corticosteroid may be needed at any time and at any step.

4. Prevention and treatment of exercise-induced bronchospasm (EIB)

    a. Steps to prevent EIB should be implemented in all patients with asthma.

    b. Patients should be advised that a warm-up period might be helpful in preventing EIB.

    c. If patients have EIB, it can usually be prevented with one of the following options.

      (1) Short-acting β-agonists (e.g., albuterol) should be administered 15 minutes before exercise.

      (2) Long-acting β-agonists (e.g., salmeterol) should be administered 30–60 minutes before exercise. When salmeterol is used chronically for EIB, some patients may lose protection toward the end of the 12-hour dosing interval. Because of its rapid onset, formoterol may be dosed 15 minutes before exercise.

      (3) Cromolyn sodium and nedocromil may be used to prevent EIB and exacerbations related to exposure to other asthma triggers. Cromolyn and nedocromil should be administered no more than 1 hour before exercise or exposure.

    d. Regardless of the prophylactic approach, all patients who experience EIB should have a short-acting β-agonist available for treatment of breakthrough symptoms.

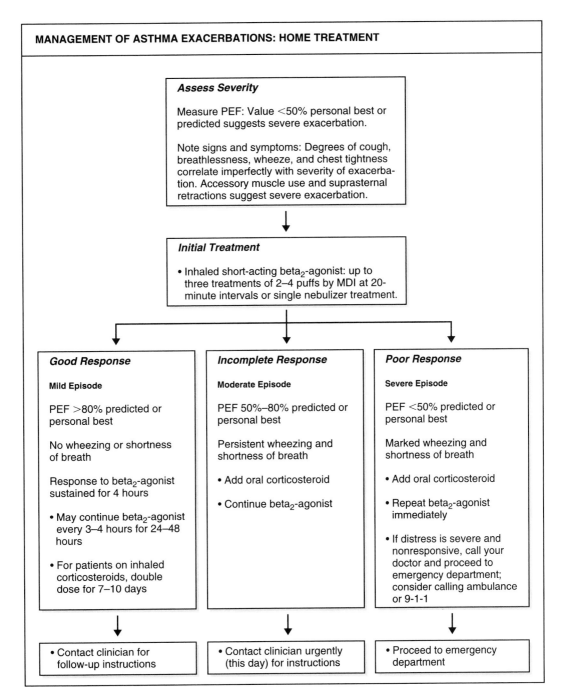

MANAGEMENT OF ASTHMA EXACERBATIONS: HOME TREATMENT

Assess Severity

Measure PEF: Value <50% personal best or predicted suggests severe exacerbation.

Note signs and symptoms: Degrees of cough, breathlessness, wheeze, and chest tightness correlate imperfectly with severity of exacerbation. Accessory muscle use and suprasternal retractions suggest severe exacerbation.

Initial Treatment

- Inhaled short-acting beta$_2$-agonist: up to three treatments of 2–4 puffs by MDI at 20-minute intervals or single nebulizer treatment.

Good Response

Mild Episode

PEF >80% predicted or personal best

No wheezing or shortness of breath

Response to beta$_2$-agonist sustained for 4 hours

- May continue beta$_2$-agonist every 3–4 hours for 24–48 hours

- For patients on inhaled corticosteroids, double dose for 7–10 days

- Contact clinician for follow-up instructions

Incomplete Response

Moderate Episode

PEF 50%–80% predicted or personal best

Persistent wheezing and shortness of breath

- Add oral corticosteroid

- Continue beta$_2$-agonist

- Contact clinician urgently (this day) for instructions

Poor Response

Severe Episode

PEF <50% predicted or personal best

Marked wheezing and shortness of breath

- Add oral corticosteroid

- Repeat beta$_2$-agonist immediately

- If distress is severe and nonresponsive, call your doctor and proceed to emergency department; consider calling ambulance or 9-1-1

- Proceed to emergency department

Figure 48-2. National Institutes of Health treatment algorithm for the home-based management of asthma exacerbations. (Adapted from NIH Highlights of the Expert Panel Report 2: Guidelines for the Diagnosis and Management of Asthma; NIH Publication No. 97-4051A, May 1997, Murphy S, et al., p. 41, Figure 3-8.

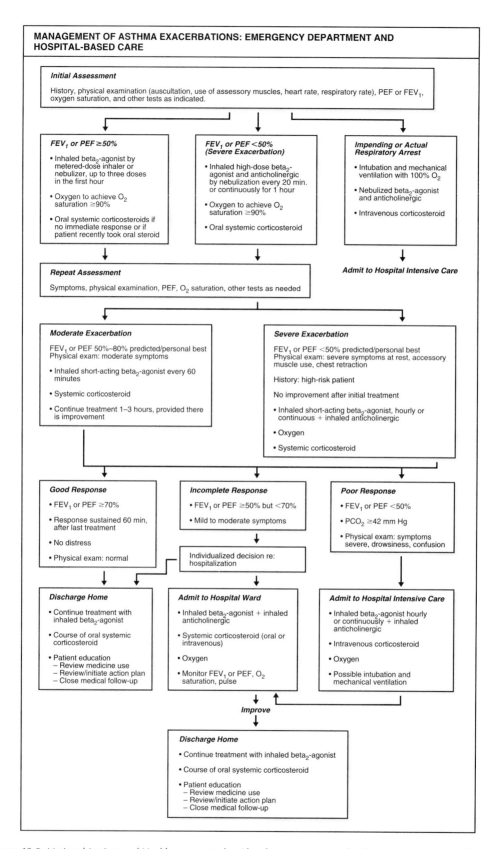

Figure 48-3. National Institutes of Health treatment algorithm for management of asthma exacerbations in the emergency department and hospital. (Adapted from NIH Highlights of the Expert Panel Report 2: Guidelines For the Diagnosis and Management of Asthma; NIH Publication No. 97-4051A, May 1997, Murphy S, et al., p. 46, Figure 3-11.

Table 48-3. Stepwise Approach for Managing Asthma in Adults and Children Older Than 5 Years of Age: Treatment Table from NHLBI EPR2 2002 Update. From NAEPP Expert Panel Report Guidelines for the Diagnosis and Management of Asthma—Update on Selected Topics 2002. NIH Publication No. 02-5075. June 2002.

Classify Severity: Clinical Features before Treatment or Adequate Control			Medications Required to Maintain Long-Term Control
	Symptoms/Day ———— Symptoms/Night	PEF or FEV₁ ———— PEF Variability	Daily Medications
Step 4 Severe Persistent	Continual ———— Frequent	≤60% ———— >30%	■ Preferred treatment: – High-dose inhaled corticosteroids AND – Long-acting inhaled beta₂-agonists AND, if needed, – Corticosteroid tablets or syrup long term (2 mg/kg/day, generally do not exceed 60 mg per day). (Make repeat attempts to reduce systemic corticosteroids and maintain control with high-dose inhaled corticosteroids.)
Step 3 Moderate Persistent	Daily ———— >1 night/week	>60%–<80% ———— >30%	■ Preferred treatment: – Low-to-medium dose inhaled corticosteroids and long-acting inhaled beta₂-agonists. ■ Alternative treatment (listed alphabetically): – Increase inhaled corticosteroids within medium-dose range OR – Low-to-medium dose inhaled corticosteroids and either leukotriene modifier or theophylline. If needed (particularly in patients with recurring severe exacerbations): ■ Preferred treatment: – Increase inhaled corticosteroids within medium-dose range, and add long-acting inhaled beta₂-agonists. ■ Alternative treatment (listed alphabetically): – Increase inhaled corticosteroids in medium-dose range, and add either leukotriene modifier or theophylline.
Step 2 Mild Persistent	>2/week but 1×/day ———— >2 nights/month	≥80% ———— 20%–30%	■ Preferred treatment: – Low-dose inhaled corticosteroids. ■ Alternative treatment (listed alphabetically): cromolyn, leukotriene modifier, nedocromil, OR sustained release theophylline to serum concentration of 5–15 mcg/mL.
Step 1 Mild Intermittent	≤2 days/week ———— ≤2 nights/month	≥80% ———— <20%	■ No daily medication needed. ■ Severe exacerbations may occur, separated by long periods of normal lung function and no symptoms. A course of systemic corticosteroids is recommended.
All Patients			■ Short-acting bronchodilator: 2–4 puffs short-acting inhaled beta₂-agonists as needed for symptoms. ■ Intensity of treatment will depend on severity of exacerbation; up to 3 treatments at 20-minute intervals or a single nebulizer treatment as needed. Course of systemic corticosteroids may be needed. ■ Use of short-acting inhaled beta₂-agonists on a daily basis, or increasing use, indicates the need to initiate or increase long-term control therapy.

Step down

Review treatment every 1 to 6 months; a gradual stepwise reduction in treatment may be possible.

Step up

If control is not maintained, consider step up. First, review patient medication technique, adherence, and environmental control.

■ Minimal or no chronic symptoms day or night
■ Minimal or no exacerbations
■ No limitations on activities; no school/work missed

■ PEF >80% of personal best.
■ Minimal use of inhaled short-acting beta₂-agonist (<1× per day, <1 canister/month)
■ Minimal or no adverse effects from medications

Note

■ The stepwise approach is meant to assist, not replace, the clinical decision making required to meet individual patient needs.
■ Classify severity: assign patient to most severe step in which any feature occurs (PEF is % of personal best; FEV₁ is % predicted.)
■ Gain control as quickly as possible (consider a short course of systemic corticosteroids); then step down to the least medication necessary to maintain control.
■ Provide education on self-management and controlling environmental factors that make asthma worse (e.g., allergens and irritants).
■ Refer to an asthma specialist if there are difficulties controlling asthma or if step 4 care is required. Referral may be considered if step 3 care is required.

5. **Concurrent diseases**
   a. **Allergic rhinitis, sinusitis,** and **gastroesophageal reflux disease** frequently coexist with asthma.
   b. Asthma control has been shown to improve if these conditions are adequately controlled.

I. **Therapeutic agents**

1. **β-Agonists** (e.g., albuterol, formoterol, levalbuterol, metaproterenol, pirbuterol, salmeterol)
   a. Short-acting β-agonists are best reserved for treatment of acute exacerbations and prophylaxis of EIB. Assessing the frequency of short-acting β-agonist use for rescue therapy can help determine the patient's level of asthma control. Those requiring regular use of short-acting β-agonists have uncontrolled disease and should receive more aggressive controller therapy.
   b. **Indications for long-acting β-agonists**
      (1) Maintenance treatment of moderate and severe persistent asthma in combination with inhaled corticosteroids, particularly for patients with frequent nocturnal symptoms
      (2) Prophylaxis of EIB
      (3) Patients with chronic obstructive pulmonary disease (COPD)
   c. **Therapeutic effects.** These sympathomimetic agents relieve bronchoconstriction during acute asthma exacerbations as well as during chronic therapy and prevent exacerbations from occurring during exercise.
   d. **Mechanism of action**
      (1) β-Agonists stimulate β_2-receptors, activating adenyl cyclase, which increases intracellular production of cyclic adenosine monophosphate (cAMP).
         (a) Increased intracellular cAMP, activation of cAMP—dependent protein kinases, and several other mechanisms result in bronchodilation, improved mucociliary clearance, and reduced inflammatory cell mediator release.
         (b) Stimulation of β_2-receptors in skeletal muscle accounts for tremor. Additional effects include gluconeogenesis, insulin secretion, and activation of Na^+, K^+-adenosine triphosphatase (ATPase).
      (2) β-Agonists differ in their affinity for the β_1- and β_2-receptors. Agents with greater β_1-receptor affinity are more likely to cause cardiac effects.
   e. **Administration and dosage**
      (1) Whenever possible, *agents* should be administered via inhalation to minimize systemic exposure and adverse reactions. Systemic administration should be reserved for patients who cannot use inhalation therapy.
      (2) When prescribed with other inhaled agents, β-agonists are usually administered first.
      (3) Regimens with long-acting agents should also include a concurrent inhaled corticosteroid, unless it is only being used to prevent EIB. All regimens containing long-acting agents should also include a short-acting agent for treatment of acute symptoms.
      (4) Dosage information is provided in Table 48-4.
   f. **Precautions and monitoring effects**
      (1) Common adverse effects of β-agonists include tremor, palpitation, tachycardia, nervousness, and headache.
      (2) Nonselective β-agonists (e.g., isoproterenol) may induce myocardial ischemia, myocardial necrosis, and arrhythmias because of excessive cardiac stimulation. Use of β_2-selective agents (e.g., albuterol, bitolterol, pirbuterol) is preferred.
      (3) **Tachyphylaxis** can occur with regular use of inhaled or oral β-agonists. Suggested mechanisms include:
         (a) A decrease in the number of active β-receptors due to movement of receptors from the cell surface into the cell (**downregulation**)
         (b) A decreased sensitivity in the β-receptors to stimuli, making them unable to activate adenyl cyclase
            (i) The clinical significance of this effect is unclear with normal doses of β-agonists.
            (ii) This effect may be reversed by adding corticosteroids to the regimen.
      (4) **Hypokalemia** may occur in some patients, particularly those receiving concurrent medications that cause hypokalemia (e.g., diuretics, amphotericin) and high doses, including inhaled agents.
      (5) **Paradoxical bronchoconstriction** found with β-agonists may be the result of a "cold-Freon effect" or the use of adjuvants.

Table 48-4. β-Adrenergic Agonists Used in the Treatment of Asthma or COPD

Agent	Severe Acute Pediatric	Severe Acute Adult	Chronic Pediatric	Chronic Adult	Site of Action	Duration of Action	Comments
Albuterol NEB: 0.5% (5 mg/mL)	ET: 0.15 mg/kg (minimum 2.5 mg) q 20 min × 3 doses, then 0.15–0.3 mg/kg up to 10 mg q 1–4 hr prn or 0.5 mg/kg/hr continuously QR: 0.05 mg/kg (minimum 1.25 mg; maximum 2.5 mg) in 2–3 cc saline q 4–6 hr	ET: 2.5–5.0 mg q 20 min × 3 doses, then 2.5–10.0 mg q 1–4 hr prn or 10–15 mg/hr continuously QR: 1.25–5.00 mg in 2–3 cc saline q 4–8 hr	Not currently recommended	Not currently recommended	β₁-receptors + β₂-receptors + + + +	3–8 hr inhalation 4–8 hr oral	May mix with cromolyn or ipratroprium NEB. May double dose for mild exacerbations.
MDI: 0.09 mg/puff	ET: 4–8 puffs q 20 min × 3 doses, then q 1–4 hr with spacer QR: 2 puffs tid-qid prn PT: 1–2 puffs 5 min before exercise	ET: 4–8 puffs q 20 min up to 4 hr, then q 1–4 hr prn QR: 2 puffs tid-qid prn PT: 2 puffs 5 min before exercise	Not currently recommended	Not currently recommended			
Rotahaler: 0.2 mg/capsule	QR: 1 capsule q 4–6 hr prn PT: 1 capsule before exercise	QR: 1–2 capsules q 4–6 hr prn PT: 1–2 capsules before exercise	Not currently recommended	Not currently recommended			
Oral: 4-mg sustained-release medication	Not currently recommended	Not currently recommended	0.3–0.6 mg/kg/day (maximum 8 mg/day)	4 mg q 12 hr			

(Continued on next page)

Table 48-4. Continued

Agent	Severe Acute — Pediatric	Severe Acute — Adult	Chronic — Pediatric	Chronic — Adult	Site of Action	Duration of Action	Comments
Bitolterol NEB: 0.2% (2 mg/mil)	ET: 0.15 mg/kg (minimum 2.5 mg) q 20 min × 3 doses, then 0.15–0.30 mg/kg up to 10 mg q 1–4 hr prn or 0.5 mg/kg/hr continuously	ET: 2.5–5.0 mg q 20 min × 3 doses, then 2.5–10.0 mg q 1–4 hr prn or 10–15 mg/hr continuously QR: 0.5–3.5 mg in 2–3 cc saline q 4–8 hr	Not currently recommended	Not currently recommended	β_1-receptors + β_2-receptors +++	6–8 hours	Dilute NEB with 2–3 cc normal saline. Do not mix NEB with other NEB solutions. Thought to be about half as potent as albuterol on a mg basis.
MDI: 0.37 mg/puff	ET: 4–8 puffs q 20 min × 3 doses, then q 1–4 hr with spacer QR: 2 puffs tid-qid prn PT: 1–2 puffs 5 min before exercise	ET: 4–8 puffs q 20 min min up to 4 hr, then q 1–4 hr prn QR: 2 puffs tid-qid prn PT: 2 puffs 5 min before exercise	Not currently recommended	Not currently recommended			
Epinephrine SC: 1:1000 (1mg/mL)	ET: 0.01 mg/kg/dose up to 0.3–0.5 mg q 20 min × 3 doses	ET: 0.3–0.5 mg/dose q 20 min × 3 doses	Not currently recommended	Not currently recommended	α-receptors +++ β_1-receptors +++ β_2-receptors +++	1–4 hr sc 1–3 hr inhalation	
Formoterol DPI: 12 mcg/caps for inhalation	Not currently recommended	Not currently recommended	≥5 years: 1 capsule q 12 h	1 capsule q 12 h	β_1-receptors + β_2-receptors ++++	10–12 hr	Approved for chronic treatment in children >5 years old and for prevention of EIB in children >12 years old. Use at least 15 minutes before exercise for EIB prophylaxis
Levalbuterol NEB: 0.63 mg, 1.25 mg	6–11 years: QR: 0.31 mg tid prn >11 years: 0.63–1.25 mg tid prn	QR: 0.63 mg tid (q 6–8 hr) up to 1.25 mg tid (q 6–8 hr)	Not currently recommended	Not currently recommended	β_1-receptors + β_2-receptors +++	6–8 hr	
Pirbuterol MDI: 0.2 mg/puff	ET: 4–8 puffs q 20 min × 3 doses, then q 1–4 hr with spacer QR: 2 puffs tid-qid prn PT: 1–2 puffs 5 min before exercise	ET: 4–8 puffs q 20 min up to 4 hr, then q 1–4 hr prn QR: 2 puffs tid-qid prn PT: 2 puffs 5 min before exercise	Not currently recommended	Not currently recommended	β_1-receptors + β_2-receptors +++	5 hr	Thought to be about half as potent as albuterol on a mg basis.

Salmeterol

MDI: 0.025 mg/puff	Not currently recommended	Not currently recommended	>4 years: 1–2 puffs q 12 hr	2 puffs q 12 hr	β_1-receptors + β_2-receptors ++++	10–12 hr	Not indicated for acute exacerbations. Take 30–60 min before exercise for EIB prophylaxis.
DPI: 0.05 mg/ inhalation	Not currently recommended	Not currently recommended	>4 years:1 inhalation q 12 hr	1 inhalation q 12 hr			

Terbutaline

MDI: 0.2 mg/puff	QR: 2 puffs tid–qid prn PT: 1–2 puffs 5 min before exercise	QR: 2 puffs tid–qid prn PT: 2 puffs 5 min before exercise	Not currently recommended	Not currently recommended	β_1-receptors + β_2-receptors ++++	3–6 hr inhalation 1.5–4 hr parenteral 4–8 hr oral	Parenteral solution not FDA-approved for nebulization
SC: 0.1% (1 mg/mL)	ET: 0.01 mg/kg q 20 min × 3 doses, then q 2–6 hr prn	ET: 0.25 mg q 20 min × 3 doses	Not currently recommended	Not currently recommended			

Adapted from NIH Expert Panel Report 2. Guidelines for the diagnosis and management of asthma. National Institutes of Health/National Heart, Lung, and Blood Institute. NIH Publication No. 97-4051. July 1997. Figure 3-5d p. 91. NIH ERR-2, Figure 3–5d.

DPI = dry-power inhaler; ET = emergency treatment; FDA = Food and Drug Administration; MDI = metered-dose inhaler; NEB = solution for nebulizer; PT = prophylactic treatment; QR = quick relief; SC = subcutaneous.

(6) Increased bronchial hyperreactivity to irritants such as methacholine and histamine has been observed with chronic β-agonist use. The S-isomer of albuterol has been implicated as a potential cause of this increased airway hyperresponsiveness. It is also possible that because of effective bronchoconstriction, patients continue to have untreated inflammation or continue to be exposed to asthma triggers.

(7) Unlike albuterol, which is a racemic mixture of albuterol's R- and S-isomers, levalbuterol HCl is comprised of the active R-enantiomer.

(8) Systemic adverse reactions when the recommended starting dose of levalbuterol is used appear to be similar to or *slightly less frequent* than the effects of albuterol. When the dose of levalbuterol is increased to 1.25 mg, however, the incidence of adverse reactions is similar to the corresponding dose of albuterol.

(9) It is important to be aware of **significant drug–drug interactions.**

(a) Concomitant use of systemic β-agonists with **monoamine oxidase inhibitors, tricyclic antidepressants, or methyldopa** may lead to severe hypertension. The risk with aerosolized agents may be smaller.

(b) β-Adrenergic blockers (e.g., propranolol) precipitate bronchospasm and increase the dose of β-agonist necessary to achieve bronchodilation. The risk of bronchospasm should be weighed against the potential benefits of β-blockers.

(c) β-Agonists should not be combined with other sympathomimetic agents because of additive cardiovascular effects. Vasoconstrictor and vasopressor effects of epinephrine are antagonized by **α-adrenergic blocking agents** (e.g., phentolamine).

(10) The effects of β-agonists should be closely monitored in the elderly and in patients with a history of hyperthyroidism, diabetes, seizures, arrhythmias, and coronary artery disease.

2. Corticosteroids

a. Therapeutic effects. Corticosteroids suppress the inflammatory response and decrease airway hyperresponsiveness.

b. Mechanism of action. Corticosteroids bind to glucocorticoid receptors on the cytoplasm of cells. The activated receptor **regulates transcription** of target genes.

(1) Corticosteroids reduce inflammation via:

(a) Inhibition of transcription and release of inflammatory genes

(b) Increased transcription of anti-inflammatory genes that produce proteins that participate in or suppress the inflammatory process

(2) Clinical effects include:

(a) Reduced production of inflammatory mediators

(b) Enhanced β-adrenergic receptor expression

(c) Decreased mucus production

(d) Prevention of endothelial and vascular leakage

c. Administration and dosage

(1) There is no significant difference in the clinical efficacy of the corticosteroid agents currently available. The **route of administration** is determined by the condition of the patient.

(a) Systemic corticosteroids are used for rapid response during an exacerbation. Improvement in pulmonary function may begin within 1–3 hours; however, the maximum effect is not achieved until approximately 6–9 hours after administration. Supplemental doses should be administered to patients who are already taking systemic corticosteroids when they experience an exacerbation, even if the exacerbation is mild. Systemic corticosteroids should have the following characteristics:

(i) Good glucocorticoid activity

(ii) Minimal mineralocorticoid activity

(iii) Short to intermediate duration of action

(b) Intravenous corticosteroids (e.g., methylprednisolone) are administered to patients who are unable to take oral medications. They are also used for patients believed to be in impending respiratory arrest and for initial treatment of exacerbations that require ICU admission. Large doses can be quickly administered; however, patients can usually be switched to oral therapy as soon as they show clinical improvement and can tolerate oral medication.

(c) Oral corticosteroids are acceptable as emergency treatment if the patient can tolerate the oral route and is not believed to be in imminent danger of respiratory arrest. **Prednisone and prednisolone are** the most frequently used oral corticosteroids.

  (i) Prednisone and prednisolone are frequently administered in short "bursts" over 3–10 days [see I I 2 c (2) (b)] to treat acute exacerbations in the outpatient setting and in the emergency department. This type of regimen may also be used to rapidly achieve asthma control.

  (ii) During "burst" therapy, these agents may be administered for 3–10 days in one or two daily doses and then discontinued. When used in this fashion, tapering is not usually necessary. However, if a patient's condition appears to worsen after the last dose has been administered, it is reasonable to re-institute the corticosteroid and then begin a tapering regimen.

(d) Because **inhaled corticosteroids** are least likely to produce adverse reactions, the inhaled route should be used whenever possible for chronic treatment. Inhaled corticosteroids should not be used to treat acute exacerbations.

  (i) The number of corticosteroids available for inhalation therapy is increasing. The two most recent additions include budesonide and fluticasone propionate.

  (ii) Dosages of inhaled corticosteroids are provided in Table 48-5. When asthma control is achieved, attempts should be made to use the lowest effective dose to maintain control (step-down therapy).

  (iii) Inhaled corticosteroids are considered first-line therapy for mild to severe persistent asthma in both adults and children.

(2) Treatment of asthma exacerbation in adults

(a) For treatment of a severe exacerbation, prednisone may be given at a dose of 2 mg/kg (maximum of 60 mg/day). For intravenous treatment, methylprednisolone is given at a dosage of 120–180 mg/day in three or four divided doses for 48 hours or until the patient can tolerate oral medications. The dosage is then reduced to 60–80 mg/day until PEFR reaches 70% predicted (or personal best).

(b) For outpatient "burst" therapy, the dosage of prednisone is 1–2 mg/kg/day (maximum of 60 mg/day) in one or two divided doses for 3–10 days.

Table 48-5. Estimated Comparative Daily Dosages for Inhaled Corticosteroids. From NAEPP Expert Panel Report Guidelines for the Diagnosis and Management of Asthma—Update on Selected Topics 2002. NIH Publication No. 02-5075. June 2002.

Drug	Low Daily Dose Adult	Low Daily Dose Child	Medium Daily Dose Adult	Medium Daily Dose Child	High Daily Dose Adult	High Daily Dose Child
Beclomethasone CFC 42 or 84 mcg/puff	168–504 mcg	84–336 mcg	504–840 mcg	336–672 mcg	>840 mcg	>672 mcg
Beclomethasone HFA 40 or 80 mcg/puff	80–240 mcg	80–160 mcg	240–480 mcg	160–320 mcg	>480 mcg	>320 mcg
Budesonide DPI 200 mcg/inhalation	200–600 mcg	200–400 mcg	600–1200 mcg	400–800 mcg	>1200 mcg	>800 mcg
Inhalation suspension for nebulization (child dose)		0.5 mg		1.0 mg		2.0 mg
Flunisolide 250 mcg/puff	500–1000 mcg	500–750 mcg	1000–2000 mcg	1000–1250 mcg	>2000 mcg	>1250 mcg
Fluticasone	88–264 mcg	88–176 mcg	264–660 mcg	176–440 mcg	>660 mcg	>440 mcg
MDI: 44, 110, or 220 mcg/puff						
DPI: 50, 100, or 250 mcg/inhalation	100–300 mcg	100–200 mcg	300–600 mcg	200–400 mcg	>7600 mcg	>400 mcg
Triamcinolone 100 mcg/puff	400–1000 mcg	400–800 mcg	1000–2000 mcg	800–1200 mcg	>2000 mcg	>1200 mcg

In all cases, the lowest dose to maintain control should be used. Some doses are outside package labeling.

DPI = dry-powder inhaler; MDI = metered-dose inhaler.

* MDI doses are actuator doses (i.e., amount leaving actuator).

(3) Treatment of asthma exacerbation in children

(a) For inpatient treatment of a severe exacerbation, prednisone, methylprednisolone, or prednisolone is given at a dosage of 1 mg/kg every 6 hours for 48 hours. The dosage is then reduced to 1–2 mg/kg/day (maximum of 60 mg/day) in two divided doses until PEFR is 70% predicted (or personal best).

(b) For outpatient "burst" therapy, the dosage of prednisone is 1–2 mg/kg/day (maximum of 60 mg/day) in one or two divided doses for 3–10 days.

d. Precautions and monitoring effects

(1) Systemic corticosteroids

(a) Careful monitoring is necessary in patients with diabetes, hypertension, congestive heart failure, peptic ulcer disease, immunosuppression, osteoporosis, chronic infections, cataracts, glaucoma, myasthenia gravis, and psychiatric diseases (e.g., depression, psychosis).

(b) If a prolonged course of systemic therapy is necessary to maintain asthma control, interference with the hypothalamic-pituitary-adrenal axis is minimized by a single morning dose (i.e., 6–8 A.M.) or alternate-day therapy. For alternate-day therapy, the dose is twice that of the single morning dose.

(c) Patients on regular systemic therapy should be closely monitored and should receive regular ophthalmological evaluations and osteoporosis screening and treatment (e.g., calcium, vitamin D) if indicated.

(2) Inhaled corticosteroids

(a) Local effects associated with inhaled corticosteroids include dry mouth, hoarseness, and fungal infection of the mouth and throat.

(b) The United States Food and Drug Administration (FDA) recently revised the warning labels on inhaled corticosteroid products to include dose-related slowing of growth velocity in children (approximately one-third inch per year). Shortly after the labeling was revised, two major publications demonstrated short-term growth suppression of approximately 1 cm in the first year of budesonide treatment, but without long-term effects on final adult height. Children should be treated with the lowest effective dose and should be reminded that poorly controlled asthma also slows growth.

(c) Large doses of inhaled corticosteroids may result in systemic effects such as reduced bone density, changes in adrenal function, skin changes, and cataract formation. Further study is needed to fully understand these effects and to determine their clinical significance. However, patients receiving high doses of inhaled corticosteroids should be closely monitored and should receive regular ophthalmological evaluations and osteoporosis screening and treatment (e.g., calcium, vitamin D) if indicated.

(d) Spacers should be prescribed for patients who receive moderate to high doses of inhaled corticosteroids via metered-dose inhalers (MDIs). Patients should also gargle, rinse their mouth and throat, and expectorate after administration. Both of these interventions minimize orpharyngeal drug deposition, local adverse reactions, and gastrointestinal absorption.

(3) Significant interactions

(a) Concurrent use of **hepatic microsomal enzyme inducers** (e.g., rifampin, barbiturates, hydantoins) causes enhanced corticosteroid metabolism, reducing therapeutic efficacy.

(b) Concurrent use of **estrogens, oral contraceptives, ketoconazole,** or **macrolide antibiotics** (e.g., erythromycin, clarithromycin) may decrease corticosteroid clearance.

(c) **Cyclosporine** may increase the plasma concentration of corticosteroids.

(d) Administration of **potassium-depleting diuretics** (e.g., thiazides, furosemide) or other potassium-depleting drugs (e.g., amphotericin) with corticosteroids causes enhanced hypokalemia. Serum potassium should be closely monitored, especially in patients on **digitalis glycosides.**

(e) Corticosteroids can decrease the serum concentrations of **isoniazid** and **salicylates** when the agents are used concurrently.

3. Leukotriene modifiers are the newest agents with anti-inflammatory properties to be approved for use in asthma. Leukotrienes are important participants in asthma pathophysiology. Cellular effects of leukotrienes include enhanced migration of eosinophils and neutrophils, increased adhesion of leukocytes, and increased monocyte and neutrophil aggregation. Leukotrienes also increase capillary permeability and cause smooth-muscle contraction.

a. **Leukotriene receptor antagonists** currently available in the United States include montelukast and zafirlukast.

   (1) **Therapeutic effects.** Leukotriene receptor antagonists have anti-inflammatory and bronchodilator activity. They may allow reduction in corticosteroid doses in some patients. Because they are less effective anti-inflammatory agents than inhaled corticosteroids, they are considered second-line agents. They may be useful in patients with concurrent allergic minitis.

   (2) **Mechanism of action.** The leukotriene receptor antagonists are selective cysteinyl leukotriene 1 (CysLT1) receptor antagonists; therefore, they prevent leukotrienes from interacting with their receptors.

   (3) **Administration and dosage**
      (a) The dosage of **zafirlukast** in children older than 12 years and adults is 20 mg twice daily. Food reduces bioavailability, so zafirlukast should be taken at least 1 hour before or 2 hours after meals. Children 5–11 years of age should receive 10 mg twice daily.
      (b) The dosage of **montelukast** in adolescents 15 years of age or older and adults is one 10-mg tablet once every evening. The dosage for children 6–14 years of age is one 5-mg chewable tablet once every evening. Children ages 2–5 should receive one 4-mg chewable tablet once every evening. Food does not appear to change bioavailability.

   (4) **Precautions and monitoring effects**
      (a) Adverse reactions to montelukast occur with a frequency similar to placebo and include headache, dizziness, and dyspepsia.
      (b) Adverse reactions associated with zafirlukast include headache, dizziness, nausea, and diarrhea.
      (c) **Churg-Strauss syndrome,** a form of eosinophilic vasculitis, has been associated with zafirlukast, montelukast, and pranlukast (available in Japan). It has usually, but not always, occurred in patients whose chronic steroid regimens were tapered and discontinued. At-risk patients should be monitored for vasculitic rash, eosinophilia, and increasing pulmonary, cardiac, and neuropathic symptoms.
      (d) **Significant drug–drug interactions** may occur.
         (i) **Aspirin** increases zafirlukast levels.
         (ii) **Erythromycin, theophylline,** and **terfenadine** decrease zafirlukast concentrations.
         (iii) Zafirlukast may increase the anticoagulant effect of **warfarin** and levels of dofetilide.
         (iv) Drug interactions appear to be less significant with montelukast. Patients who are receiving montelukast with **hepatic enzyme inducers** (e.g., rifampin, phenobarbital) should be monitored closely.
         (v) The chewable forms of montelukast (4- and 5-mg tablets) contain aspartame and should be avoided in patients with **phenylketonuria.**

b. The only **lipoxygenase inhibitor** approved by the FDA is **zileuton.** Zileuton may allow reduction in corticosteroid doses in some patients.

   (1) **Therapeutic effects.** Lipoxygenase inhibitors have anti-inflammatory and bronchodilator activity.

   (2) **Mechanism of action.** Lipoxygenase inhibitors prevent the formation of leukotrienes. Zileuton blocks 5-lipoxygenase, the enzyme responsible for leukotriene formation.

   (3) **Administration and dosage.** In adults and children 12 years of age and older, the dosage of zileuton is 600 mg four times daily. It may be taken without regard to meals.

   (4) **Precautions and monitoring effects**
      (a) Zileuton is contraindicated in patients with hepatic function impairment and should be monitored closely in patients who drink large quantities of alcohol.
      (b) Adverse effects include headache, abdominal pain, asthenia, nausea, dyspepsia, and myalgia. Drug therapy was discontinued in almost 10% of patients due to side effects, although this was similar to placebo.
      (c) **Significant drug–drug interactions** may occur.
         (i) Zileuton increases concentrations of **propranolol, terfenadine,** and **theophylline.**
         (ii) The anticoagulant effect of **warfarin** is increased by zileuton.

(d) Hepatic enzymes [e.g., alanine aminotransferase (ALT)] may become elevated during therapy, with most occurrences during the first several months of therapy. Symptomatic hepatitis has been reported. Therefore, the manufacturer recommends that serum ALT be checked before initiation of treatment, monthly for 3 months, and every 2–3 months for the rest of the first year. ALT should be checked periodically thereafter.

- **(i)** Patients should be monitored closely for signs or symptoms of liver dysfunction (e.g., right upper quadrant abdominal pain, flu-like symptoms, fatigue, nausea, lethargy, itching, jaundice).
- **(ii)** If ALT increases to more than five times the upper limit of normal, therapy should be discontinued and the patient should be monitored until enzymes normalize.

4. Cromolyn sodium and nedocromil sodium

  a. Therapeutic effects. Cromolyn sodium and nedocromil sodium are nonsteroidal drugs with anti-inflammatory properties. These medications are less effective in their anti-inflammatory properties than the inhaled corticosteroids; however, because of their excellent safety profile, they are frequently used in children.

  (1) When used prophylactically, cromolyn sodium and nedocromil sodium prevent the early and late response as well as asthma induced by exercise, cold air, and sulfur dioxide.

  (2) When used as maintenance therapy for asthma, these medications suppress nonspecific airway reactivity.

  b. Mechanism of action. Cromolyn sodium and nedocromil sodium are believed to act locally by stabilizing mast cells and thereby inhibiting mast cell degranulation. There is also evidence for inhibitory effects on inflammatory cells such as macrophages, eosinophils, neutrophils, monocytes, and platelets.

  c. Administration and dosage

  (1) Cromolyn sodium is available as an MDI (800 mg per inhalation), and a nebulizer solution (20 mg/2 mL). The required dosage is two puffs of the MDI or 20 mg of nebulizer solution. Because of the dosage needed to achieve asthma control, the nebulizer is preferred.

  (2) Nedocromil sodium is available as an MDI (1.75 mg per inhalation). The required dosage is two inhalations four times a day.

  (3) When used for prophylaxis of EIB, cromolyn sodium and nedocromil sodium should be administered 1 hour before exercise.

  (4) After administration, initial improvement is seen within 1–2 weeks; however, the maximum effect may take longer.

  d. Precautions and monitoring effects

  (1) Cromolyn sodium and nedocromil sodium are **not effective during an acute asthma exacerbation.** They should only be used for maintenance therapy of persistent asthma or for prevention of EIB.

  (2) Both drugs are well-tolerated, although paradoxical bronchospasm, wheezing, coughing, nasal congestion, and irritation or dryness of the throat may occur.

5. Theophylline compounds (methylxanthines)

  a. Indications

  (1) Theophylline compounds may be considered if β-agonists and corticosteroids fail to control an acute asthma exacerbation.

  (2) Theophylline is an alternative to long-acting β-agonists in the treatment of persistent asthma.

  (3) Theophylline is most beneficial as an adjuvant to inhaled corticosteroids in patients with nocturnal or early morning symptoms.

  b. Therapeutic effects

  (1) Theophylline compounds produce bronchodilation to a lesser extent than β-agonists.

  (2) Nonbronchodilator effects include reduced mucus secretion, enhanced mucociliary transport, improved diaphragmatic contractility, and possibly reduced fatigability.

  (3) There may also be some degree of anti-inflammatory activity, although the significance is unclear.

  c. Mechanism of action

  (1) The precise mechanism of action is still being debated. Although theophylline-induced phosphodiesterase inhibition results in increased levels of cAMP, this occurs in vitro only at concentrations greater than those achieved in vivo.

(2) Other suggested mechanisms include:
   (a) Alteration of intracellular calcium
   (b) Increased binding of cAMP to its binding protein
   (c) Adenosine antagonism
   (d) Increased circulating catecholamines
   (e) Inhibition of production of contractile prostaglandins (PGE_2 and $PGF_{2\alpha}$)
d. Administration and dosage
   (1) Oral therapy (e.g., sustained-release theophyllines) allows for a longer dosing interval and improves compliance. Compliance to oral theophylline also may be better than that of inhaled bronchodilators and corticosteroids.
      (a) Because theophylline does not distribute well into fatty tissue, dosages should be calculated using lean body weight.
      (b) The initial dose of theophylline for adults and children over age 1 is 10 mg/kg/day (maximum of 300 mg/day) given in divided doses. Usual dosage should be adjusted to achieve serum theophylline concentration of 5–15 μg/mL.
      (c) The dosage can be titrated slowly upward and the serum level monitored until a therapeutic level is obtained.
      (d) The usual maximal daily dose in adults is 800 mg/day.
      (e) The maximum recommended dosage in children under age 1 is 0.2 × (age in weeks) + 5 = mg/kg/day and in children 1 year of age and older is 16 mg/kg/day, given in divided doses.
      (f) In addition to theophylline, other methylxanthine compounds are available (e.g., oxtriphylline, dyphylline) but infrequently used. Dosing of these compounds is based on theophylline content (Table 48-6).
   (2) Intravenous therapy. Although frequently used in the past, IV administration is now uncommon. IV administration is generally used only in hospitalized patients in whom oral therapy is not possible (e.g., vomiting, NPO).
      (a) The usual **loading dose** for adults and children not previously receiving a methylxanthine is 5 mg/kg of theophylline administered over 20–30 minutes at a rate not exceeding 25 mg/min.
      (b) The usual **maintenance infusion** rate of theophylline in healthy nonsmoking adults on no interacting drugs is 0.4 mg/kg/hr. This rate should be adjusted for factors that affect theophylline metabolism and serum levels (see Table 48-7).
e. Precautions and monitoring effects
   (1) Theophyllines are contraindicated in patients with hypersensitivity to xanthine compounds and should be used cautiously in patients with a history of peptic ulcer or untreated seizure disorder.
   (2) Adverse effects include nausea, vomiting, diarrhea, anorexia, palpitations, dizziness, restlessness, nervousness, insomnia, seizures, reduced lower esophageal sphincter tone, and reduced control of gastroesophageal reflux disease. Patients who experience adverse gastrointestinal effects should be evaluated to rule out theophylline toxicity versus local gastrointestinal effect.
   (3) Theophylline clearance can be altered by several factors and drug interactions (Table 48-7). Close drug-level monitoring is required for patients with factors that alter theophylline clearance.

Table 48-6. Theophylline Content of Theophylline-Containing Products

Preparation	Theophylline Content	Equivalent Dose
Theophylline anhydrous (most oral solids)	100%	100 mg
Theophylline monohydrate (oral solutions)	91%	110 mg
Aminophylline anhydrous	86%	116 mg
Aminophylline hydrous	79%	127 mg
Oxtriphylline	64%	156 mg

Table 48-7. Factors That Alter Theophylline Clearance

Factors that increase theophylline clearance (decrease levels)
Age 1–9 years
Drugs
    Carbamazepine
    Phenobarbital
    Phenytoin
    Rifampin
Fever
Food (may delay or reduce absorption of some sustained-release products)
High-protein diet
Smoking (marijuana and tobacco)
Factors that decrease theophylline clearance (increase levels)
Age
    Elderly
    Premature neonates
    Term infants <6 months
Cor pulmonale
Congestive heart failure, decompensated
Drugs
    Alopurinol
    β-Blockers (nonselective)
    Calcium-channel blockers
    Cimetidine
    Clindamycin
    Fluoroquinolones (e.g., ciprofloxacin, grepafloxacin, norfloxacin, prulifloxacin)
    Influenza virus vaccine
    Macrolides (e.g., clarithromycin, erythromycin)
    Oral contraceptives
    Ticlopidine
    Zafirlukast
Fever/viral illness
Fatty foods (may increase rate of absorption of some products)
High-carbohydrate diet
Liver dysfunction (e.g., cirrhosis)

---

    (4) Careful monitoring is required in patients with hepatic disease, hypoxemia, hypertension, congestive heart failure, alcoholism, and in the elderly. Because of developmental changes in the neonate and child, dosing must be carefully established and monitored in these populations as well.

    (5) Therapeutic drug monitoring of serum levels, adverse reactions, and concomitant drug use is essential for long-term therapy due to theophylline's age- and condition-specific clearance.

        (a) Therapeutic effect is achieved and toxicity minimized by keeping drug concentrations at 5–15 mcg/mL.

        (b) Drug levels should be assessed at steady state, although pharmacokinetic analysis can be performed during a continuous infusion, before steady state, by using the proper pharmacokinetic equation. Steady-state drug levels can be measured at any time during an infusion.

        (c) During oral therapy, drug levels should be obtained at peak absorption, generally 1–2 hours after a dose for immediate-release products and 5–9 hours after a dose for most sustained-release formulations.

        (d) Dyphylline serum levels should be monitored during therapy because serum theophylline levels will not measure dyphylline. The minimal effective therapeutic concentration of dyphylline is 12 μg/mL.

    6. Anticholinergics. Bronchodilation occurs when these drugs block postganglionic muscarinic receptors in the airway. Response to anticholinergics is most pronounced in patients with fixed airway obstruction (e.g., COPD).

   a. Ipratropium bromide is a quaternary ammonium compound.
      (1) Indications
         (a) Ipratropium bromide is recommended for use in combination with β-agonists for the treatment of a severe, acute asthma exacerbation. However, benefits in the chronic management of asthma have not been established.
         (b) Ipratropium bromide may be particularly useful in older patients and patients with coexisting COPD.
         (c) Ipratropium bromide is an alternative bronchodilator in some patients who cannot tolerate β-agonists and in patients who present with bronchospasm induced by a β-blocker.
      (2) Administration and dosage
         (a) Closed-mouth MDI technique or the use of a spacer is recommended for patients receiving anticholinergic therapy via MDI.
         (b) The starting dose of the MDI is two inhalations four times a day. When administered via nebulizer, the dose is 500 μg (2.5 mL) four times a day.
      (3) Precautions and monitoring effects
         (a) If the anticholinergic spray contacts the eye, intraocular pressure may increase.
         (b) The onset of action (approximately 15 minutes) and peak effect (1–2 hours) are more delayed than for β-agonists.
   b. Aerosolized **atropine** is used rarely now that ipratropium bromide nebulization solution is available due to atropine's high incidence of adverse effects.
   c. Although not approved for use in asthma, **glycopyrrolate** is another quaternary ammonium compound that has been used in combination with β-agonists for the treatment of severe, acute asthma exacerbations.

7. **Antihistamines** are useful for patients with coexisting allergic rhinitis; however, their role in the treatment of asthma remains unclear. Antihistamines compete with histamine for histamine$_1$-receptor sites on effector cells and, thus, help prevent the histamine-mediated responses that influence asthma.

8. **Antibiotics** are not used for the treatment of asthma, per se. However, research is under way to determine the role of infection in asthma pathogenesis.

9. **Magnesium sulfate,** administered intravenously, may be useful in some patients because of its modest ability to cause bronchodilation. When administered intravenously, it also improves respiratory muscle strength in hypomagnesemic patients. Research has suggested that magnesium may reduce admission rate and improve FEV_1 in severe, acute asthma exacerbations and in stable, chronic asthma.

10. **Immunotherapy** improves asthma control in some patients and is ineffective in others. A recent meta-analysis demonstrated that immunotherapy may improve lung function, reduce symptoms, and decrease medication requirements in a significant number of patients.

11. Mucus may contribute to airway obstruction in asthma. However, because mucolytics may precipitate bronchospasm, they should not be used for the treatment of patients with asthma.

J. Drug delivery options

1. **MDIs**
   a. When administered with good technique and a spacer, the efficacy of MDIs is similar to that of nebulizers, despite the lower doses administered with an MDI and spacer. The only MDI that comes with a built-in spacer is the Azmacort (triamcinolone) inhaler.
   b. For small children to be able to use an MDI, a spacer with a facemask must be used.
   c. MDIs can be difficult to use. Steps for using an MDI properly are outlined in Table 48-8.
   d. MDIs can be administered to patients on mechanical ventilation with the use of a spacer designed for the mechanical ventilator circuit.
   e. Breath-actuated MDIs (e.g., Maxair Autohaler) require the patient to use a closed-mouth technique. When inhalation is begun, the medication is released automatically. This type of inhaler is useful for a patient who is having problems coordinating actuation and inhalation.

2. **Spacers and holding chambers** (e.g., Aerochamber, Aerosol Cloud Enhancer, AeroVent, Brethancer, Ellipse, E-Z Spacer, Inhal-Aid, InspirEase, OptiChamber, OptiHaler)
   a. Spacers and holding chambers reduce the amount of drug deposited in the upper airway and decrease oral absorption.

Table 48-8. Procedure for the Proper Use of Metered-Dose Inhalers (MDIs)

- Assemble MDI, if necessary.
- Remove cap, and inspect mouthpiece for foreign objects.
- Attach MDI to spacer (if applicable).
- Shake MDI (with spacer).
- Tilt head back slightly, and exhale normally.
- Position inhaler:
    Wrap lips around spacer mouthpiece.
    Position inhaler 1–2 inches from open mouth.
    Wrap lips around inhaler mouthpiece.
- Just as you begin to inhale, depress canister once to release medication.
- Continue inhaling slowly (over 3–5 seconds) until lungs are full.
- Hold breath for 10 seconds.
- Wait 1 minute before repeating steps to deliver additional puffs.

    b. The use of spacers and holding chambers minimizes local and systemic adverse reactions.

    c. Addition of a spacer in a patient with poor MDI technique improves pulmonary delivery of the agent.

    d. Spacers should be used in all patients who are receiving medium to high doses of inhaled corticosteroids.

    e. They are especially beneficial for patients with poor hand–lung coordination.

    f. Devices vary in construction and efficacy. The presence of a one-way mouthpiece valve, inhalation rate whistle, size, and durability are all factors that should be considered when selecting a particular spacer for a patient.

  3. Nebulizers

    a. Compared to MDI and spacer administration, nebulizers require less patient coordination during administration of multiple inhalations.

    b. Disadvantages of nebulizers include cost, preparation and administration time, size of the device, and drug delivery inconsistencies between devices.

    c. Despite the disadvantages, nebulization is recommended for delivery of high-dose β-agonists and anticholinergics in severe exacerbations and for delivery of cromolyn sodium to children.

  4. Dry-powder inhalers

    a. Dry-powder inhalers are coming to the market as a result of the international move to avoid the use of Freon propellants. They are also being used more frequently because many patients find them easier to use than an MDI.

    b. Dry-powder inhalers require the user to:

      (1) First load the dose into the delivery chamber

      (2) Inhale rapidly (versus slow inhalation required for MDI administration)

      (3) Use the closed-mouth technique

      (4) Avoid exhaling into the mouthpiece before inhalation.

    c. Spacers are not used with dry-powder inhalers.

    d. Patients should be advised to keep these devices away from moisture.

K. Nonpharmacological treatment

  1. Humidified oxygen is administered to all patients with severe, acute asthma to reverse hypoxemia. Although the fraction of inspired oxygen (FIO_2) administered is based on the patient's arterial blood gas status, 1–3 L/min is generally given via facemask or nasal cannula. The goal is to keep the SaO_2 greater than 90% (greater than 95% if the patient is pregnant or has heart disease).

  2. Heliox is a mixture of helium and oxygen that has a lower density than air. Because of its decreased airflow resistance, heliox may increase ventilation during acute asthma exacerbations. Because conflicting information has been published in studies using heliox, its role in asthma is unclear.

  3. Intravenous fluids and electrolytes may be required if the patient is volume depleted.

4. **Environmental control** and allergen avoidance are important in the management of a patient with asthma.
   a. Data are available that suggest that avoidance of known allergens can improve asthma control.
   b. Some measures include use of allergen-resistant mattress and pillow encasements, use of high-filtration vacuum cleaners, removal of carpets and draperies, and avoidance of furry pets.

5. **Vaccines** (e.g., influenza virus, polyvalent pneumococcals) are recommended to prevent infection, which may precipitate an exacerbation.

L. **Complications of asthma**

1. **Status asthmaticus** is a life-threatening condition that occurs when a severe asthma exacerbation fails to respond to usual treatment.
   a. **Findings** include altered consciousness, cyanosis (even with oxygen therapy), elevated $PaCO_2$, pulsus paradoxus (greater than 20 mm Hg), PEFR less than 100 L/min in adults, and FEV_1 less than 1 L.
   b. **Standard therapy** for status asthmaticus involves oxygen administration, intravenous rehydration, inhaled β-agonists and anticholinergics, and intravenous corticosteroids.
   c. **Aggressive therapy** is indicated for any patient with acute severe exacerbation and for patients who fail to respond to conventional therapy for acute exacerbation. If the patient has respiratory acidosis, intubation and mechanical ventilation may be indicated.

2. **Pneumothorax** is a condition characterized by accumulation of air in the pleural space, as sometimes occurs during an acute asthma exacerbation.
   a. **Symptoms** may include sudden pleuritic chest pain, dyspnea, hacking cough, and anxiety.
   b. **Physical findings** range from minor to severe and include tachypnea, hypotension, decreased fremitus, tympany on chest percussion, diaphoresis, and pallor.
   c. **Therapy** includes oxygen, aspiration of pleural air via a chest tube, and analgesics. However, a small pneumothorax may resolve spontaneously.

3. **Atelectasis,** or collapsed lung, inhibits gas exchange during respiration and may occur as a result of airway obstruction. In asthmatics, atelectasis usually involves the right middle lobe, but sometimes affects the entire lung.
   a. **Symptoms** include worsening dyspnea and anxiety.
   b. **Physical findings** include hyperventilation, diminished breath sounds, decreased chest excursion, mediastinal shift toward the affected side, and cyanosis.
   c. **Therapy** includes incentive spirometry, postural drainage, chest percussion, coughing and deep breathing exercises, and bronchodilators. Bronchoscopy may be necessary to remove secretions.

II. CHRONIC OBSTRUCTIVE PULMONARY DISEASE

A. **Definitions.** The National Heart, Lung, and Blood Institute/World Health Organization (NHLBI/WHO) Global Initiative for Chronic Obstructive Lung Disease (GOLD) definition of COPD is "a disease state characterized by airflow limitation that is not fully reversible. The airflow limitation is usually both progressive and associated with an abnormal inflammatory response of the lungs to noxious particles or gases." The American Thoracic Society definition is similar: a disease state characterized by the presence of airflow limitation due to chronic bronchitis or emphysema; the airflow obstruction is generally progressive, may be accompanied by airway hyperreactivity, and may be partially reversible. The two major forms of COPD—**chronic bronchitis** and **emphysema**—frequently coexist. COPD also coexists with asthma.

1. **Chronic bronchitis** is characterized by excessive mucus production by the tracheobronchial tree, which results in airway obstruction due to edema and bronchial inflammation. Bronchitis is considered chronic when the patient has a cough producing more than 30 mL of sputum in 24 hours for at least 3 months of the year for 2 consecutive years and other causes of chronic cough have been excluded.

2. **Emphysema** is marked by permanent alveolar enlargement distal to the terminal bronchioles and destructive changes of the alveolar walls. There is a lack of uniformity in airspace

enlargement, resulting in loss of alveolar surface area. The collapse of these small airways results in airflow limitation that is independent of exertion.

B. Incidence. Approximately 10.2 million Americans have COPD by the American Thoracic Society definition. Using more liberal European Respiratory Society criteria (airway obstruction only), this number increases to approximately 24 million. COPD is the fourth leading cause of death in the United States and the leading cause of hospitalization in the older population. It is most commonly diagnosed in older men; however, the incidence is increasing in women due to an increasing population of women smokers.

C. Etiology. Various factors have been implicated in the development of COPD, including:

1. **Cigarette smoking** is the primary etiologic factor for the development of COPD.
   a. One mechanism suggests that pulmonary hyperreactivity secondary to smoking results in persistent airway obstruction.
   b. There is also an increased risk of COPD in people who have α_1-antitrypsin (AAT) deficiency. One in three people with genetic AAT deficiency develop emphysema, usually as young adults.
      (1) AAT is a serine protease inhibitor, and it is also an acute-phase reactive protein. The major physiological function of AAT is inhibition of neutrophil elastase.
      (2) Smoking may contribute to disease development because smoking oxidizes methionine (Met) 358 and prevents AAT from binding with and inactivating elastase.
      (3) AAT deficiency should be suspected when emphysema develops early in the absence of a significant smoking history.

2. Exposure to irritants such as sulfur dioxide (as in polluted air), noxious gases, and organic or inorganic dusts

3. A history of respiratory infections or bronchial hyperreactivity

4. Social, economic, and hereditary factors

D. Pathophysiology

1. **Chronic bronchitis**
   a. **Respiratory tissue inflammation** results in vasodilation, congestion, mucosal edema, and goblet cell hypertrophy. These events trigger goblet cells to produce excessive amounts of mucus.
   b. **Changes in tissue** include increased smooth muscle, cartilage atrophy, infiltration of neutrophils and other cells, and impairment of cilia.
   c. Airways become blocked by thick, tenacious mucus secretions, which trigger a productive cough.
   d. Normally sterile airways become colonized with *Streptococcus pneumoniae, Hemophilus influenzae, Moraxella catarrhalis, Staphylococcus aureus,* and *Pseudomonas aeruginosa* species. Recurrent lung infections (viral and bacterial) reduce ciliary and phagocytic activity, increase mucus accumulation, weaken the body's defenses, and further destroy small bronchioles.
   e. As the **airways degenerate,** overall gas exchange is impaired, causing **exertional dyspnea.**
   f. Hypoxemia results from a V/Q imbalance and is reflected in an increasing arterial carbon dioxide tension (i.e., increasing $PaCO_2$).
   g. Sustained hypercapnia (increased $PaCO_2$) desensitizes the brain's respiratory control center and central chemoreceptors. As a result, compensatory action to correct hypoxemia and hypercapnia (i.e., a respiratory rate or depth increase) does not occur. Instead, hypoxemia serves as the stimulus for breathing.

2. **Emphysema**
   a. **Anatomical changes** are the result of loss of tissue elasticity.
      (1) **Inflammation** and **excessive mucus secretion** (as from long-standing chronic bronchitis) cause air trapping in the alveoli. This contributes to breakdown of the bronchioles, alveolar walls, and connective tissue.
      (2) As clusters of alveoli merge, the number of alveoli diminishes, leading to increased space available for air trapping.

(3) Destruction of alveolar walls causes collapse of small airways on exhalation and disruption of the pulmonary capillary beds.

(4) These changes result in V/Q abnormalities; blood is shunted away from destroyed areas to maintain a constant V/Q ratio, unlike the case in chronic bronchitis.

(5) Hypercapnia and respiratory acidosis are uncommon in emphysema because V/Q imbalance is compensated for by an increased respiratory rate.

  b. There are **specific lung regions** in which characteristic anatomical changes of emphysema occur.

(1) In **centrilobular** (centriacinar) emphysema associated with cigarette smoking, destruction is central, selectively involving respiratory bronchioles. Typically, bronchioles and alveolar ducts become dilated and merge.

(2) In **panlobular** (panacinar) emphysema, all lung segments are involved. The alveoli enlarge and atrophy, and the pulmonary vascular bed is destroyed. This form of emphysema is associated with AAT deficiency.

(3) In **paraseptal** emphysema, the lung periphery adjacent to fibrotic regions is the site of alveolar distention and alveolar wall destruction. This is associated with spontaneous pneumothorax.

E. Clinical evaluation

1. Physical findings

  a. **Predominant chronic bronchitis** typically has an insidious onset after age 45.

(1) A **chronic productive cough** is the hallmark of chronic bronchitis. It occurs first in winter, then progresses to year-round. It is usually worse in the morning.

(2) **Exertional dyspnea,** the most common presenting symptom, is progressive. However, the severity of this symptom does not reflect the severity of the disease.

(3) Other common findings include obesity, rhonchi and wheezes on auscultation, prolonged expiration, and a normal respiratory rate. As the disease progresses, right ventricular failure is common, which presents as jugular venous distention, peripheral edema, hepatomegaly, and cardiomegaly. Because patients tend to develop cyanosis, the term "blue bloater" is frequently used to describe patients with chronic bronchitis.

  b. **Predominant emphysema** has an insidious onset, and symptoms occur after age 55.

(1) The **cough** is chronic but less productive than in chronic bronchitis.

(2) **Exertional dyspnea** is progressive, constant, severe, more characteristic of emphysema than chronic bronchitis.

(3) Other common findings include weight loss, tachypnea, pursed-lip breathing, prolonged expiration, accessory chest muscle use, hyperresonance on percussion, diaphragmatic excursion, and diminished breath sounds. Because patients are able to maintain reasonably good oxygenation due to their tachypnea, the term "pink puffer" is sometimes used to describe patients with emphysema.

  c. Patients may have elements and physical findings from each of these diseases simultaneously.

2. Diagnostic test results

  a. **COPD** patients with characteristic symptoms of cough, dyspnea, sputum production, and/or exposure to known risk factors (e.g., smoking) should be evaluated for a COPD diagnosis. If the patient has FEV_1/FVC <70% and a postbronchodilator FEV_1 <80% predicted, he or she has airflow limitation that is not fully reversible.

  b. **Chronic bronchitis**

(1) Blood analysis usually reveals polycythemia due to erythropoiesis secondary to hypoxemia. With bacterial infection, the WBC count may be increased.

(2) Sputum inspection reveals thick purulent or mucopurulent sputum tinged yellow, white, green, or gray; an acute change in color is highly suggestive of infection. Microscopic analysis may detect neutrophils and microorganisms.

(3) Arterial blood gas studies may show a markedly decreased PaO_2 level (e.g., 45–60 mm Hg), reflecting hypoxemia and a $PaCO_2$ level that is normal or elevated (e.g., 50–60 mm Hg), reflecting hypercapnia.

(4) Pulmonary function tests may be normal in the early disease stages. Later, they show an increased RV, a decreased vital capacity, and a decreased FEV_1. Unlike emphysema, chronic bronchitis patients have normal diffusing capacity, normal static lung compliance, and normal TLC.

(5) Chest radiograph typically identifies lung hyperinflation and increased bronchovascular markings.
(6) An ECG may reveal right ventricular hypertrophy and changes consistent with cor pulmonale.

  c. Emphysema
    (1) Blood analysis may show a decreased AAT level. Although AAT deficiency is relatively uncommon, accounting for less than 5% overall of emphysema cases, AAT levels should be evaluated in patients who develop emphysema at a young age, particularly in the absence of a significant history of smoking.
    (2) Sputum inspection reveals scanty sputum that is clear or mucoid. Infections are less frequent than in chronic bronchitis.
    (3) Arterial blood gas studies typically indicate a reduced or normal PaO_2 level (e.g., 65–75 mm Hg) and, in late disease stages, an increased $PaCO_2$ level (e.g., 50–60 mm Hg).
    (4) Pulmonary function tests show normal or increased static lung compliance, reduced FEV_1 and diffusing capacity, and increased TLC and RV.
    (5) Chest radiograph usually reveals bullae, blebs, a flattened diaphragm, lung hyperinflation, vertical heart, enlarged anteroposterior chest diameter, decreased vascular markings in the lung periphery, and a large retrosternal air space.

F. Treatment objectives endorsed by GOLD include:

  1. Prevent disease progression (smoking cessation)
  2. Relieve symptoms and improve exercise tolerance (enable the patient to perform normal daily activities)
  3. Improve health status
  4. Prevent and treat exacerbations
  5. Prevent and treat complications
  6. Reduce mortality

G. Therapy

  1. Pharmacological treatment. Anticholinergics and β-agonists are the most commonly used agents. Methylxanthines are usually added when the response to other agents is inadequate. Corticosteroids are beneficial when an allergic component has been demonstrated. Fluticasone and budesonide have shown small benefits in FEV_1, but the majority of their benefit occurs in reducing the severity of exacerbations, not the number of exacerbations.
  a. Anticholinergics (e.g., ipratropium bromide, tiotropium bromide, atropine, glycopyrrolate)
    (1) Indications. Anticholinergics may be used as first-line bronchodilators or in conjunction with β-agonists in the treatment of COPD.
    (2) Mechanism of action. Ipratropium bromide, tiotropium bromide, and atropine produce bronchodilation by competitively inhibiting cholinergic responses. Ipratropium bromide and tiotropium bromide also reduce sputum volume without altering viscosity. Some studies have shown an increased response to these agents in COPD when they are combined with β-agonists.
    (3) Administration and dosage
      (a) Ipratropium bromide is three to five times more potent and has significantly fewer side effects than atropine, which is rarely used today since the development of nebulized ipratropium.
      (b) Initial MDI dosing of ipratropium bromide is two inhalations (40 μg) four times daily, but dosing can be increased to six inhalations four times daily without significant risk. These higher doses are often required to achieve therapeutic benefit. Administration should be via MDI with spacer or MDI alone using a closed-mouth technique.
      (c) Dosing of ipratropium bromide solution is 500 μg/2.5 mL (1 unit dose vial) or more via nebulizer four times daily.
      (d) Ipratropium should be administered regularly because of a slower onset and longer duration of action as compared with β-agonists.

(e) Tiotropium bromide capsules contain 22.5 μg tiotropium bromide monohydrate equivalent to 18 μg tiotropium. Tiotropium is an inhalation powder contained in a hard capsule. It should be administered once daily only via Handihaler device, which delivers 10 μg tiotropium.

(f) Glycopyrrolate can be nebulized in combination with β-agonists. The dose is 1–2 mg given every 8 hours.

b. β-Agonists (see I I 1; Table 48-4)

(1) Indications. Long-acting β-agonists may be used as first-line bronchodilators or in conjunction with anticholinergic agents in the maintenance treatment of COPD. Short-acting agents are used on an as-needed basis for episodic symptoms. Some patients may respond to the prolonged treatment with β-agonists even after demonstrating lack of acute reversibility (<12% or 200-cc increase in FEV_1) to short-acting agents.

(2) Mechanism of action. β-Agonists relieve dyspnea due to airway obstruction, although the response is not as significant as in asthmatic patients. These agents may also increase mucociliary clearance by stimulating ciliary activity.

(3) Administration and dosage

(a) β-Agonists are administered via inhalation (e.g., dry-powder inhaler, nebulizer, MDI with or without a spacer) unless the patient cannot use the drug properly; then an oral agent is used cautiously.

(b) β-Agonists of the same duration should not be used in combination because an adequate dose of a single agent provides peak bronchodilation. However, it is reasonable to administer a long-acting product (e.g., salmeterol, formoterol) on a regular basis with a short-acting agent reserved for as-needed, or rescue, therapy.

(c) Salmeterol and formoterol (long-acting β-agonists) are administered twice daily. They may also be used in combination with ipratropium bromide or tiotropium. Neither agent is used on an as-needed basis for rescue therapy, although formoterol does have a rapid onset of action.

c. Theophylline (see I I 5)

(1) Indications. Theophylline compounds typically are added to the drug regimen after an unsuccessful trial of ipratropium bromide and β-adrenergics.

(2) Mechanism of action. In COPD, theophylline compounds are used because they increase mucociliary clearance, stimulate the respiratory drive, enhance diaphragmatic contractility, improve the ventricular ejection fraction, and stimulate renal diuresis. Their bronchodilator properties are modest, at best.

(3) Administration and dosage. A trial of 1–2 months with the serum drug level maintained at 5–12 mcg/mL and maximized, if necessary, up to 20 mcg/mL is needed to assess therapeutic efficacy.

(a) Because of the nonbronchodilator effects of methylxanthines, they may be continued in the face of a clinical response, even in the absence of improved FEV_1.

(b) If no change occurs in the patient's clinical condition and/or FEV_1, theophylline therapy should be discontinued due to the potential for side effects.

(4) Precautions and monitoring effects. Serum drug levels should be closely monitored in patients with congestive heart failure and cor pulmonale due to reduced theophylline metabolism.

d. Corticosteroids (see I I 2; Table 48-5)

(1) Indications

(a) Systemic corticosteroids (preferably oral) are indicated in the treatment of acute COPD exacerbations.

(b) Inhaled corticosteroids play a less prominent role in COPD than in asthma.

(c) Candidates for prolonged use of inhaled corticosteroid therapy should:

(i) Be symptomatic and have a documented spirometric response (i.e., increase in FEV_1 of at least 15% and 200 mL after 6 weeks to 3 months of use)

(ii) Have an FEV_1 <50% predicted with a history of repeated exacerbations requiring systemic corticosteroids or antibiotics

(d) Long-term use of systemic steroids should be avoided.

(2) Administration and dosage

(a) For oral use in outpatient management of acute exacerbations, prednisolone is administered at a dosage of 40 mg/day for 10 days. The dose of oral (e.g., prednisolone) or intravenous corticosteroids (e.g., methylprednisolone) for hospital management of acute COPD exacerbations is not established. However, doses and duration of therapy should be limited (e.g., 30–40 mg/day of prednisolone for 10–14 days) to avoid significant adverse effects.

(b) The role of inhaled corticosteroids for chronic management of COPD is also limited [see II G 1 d (1) (c)]. In appropriate patients, corticosteroids may be administered via dry-powder inhaler or MDI with spacer. Response to oral corticosteroids is not predictive of response to inhaled corticosteroids.

e. Antibiotics

(1) **Indications**

(a) Antibiotics are used to treat exacerbations with suspected infection as evidenced by an increase in volume or change in color or viscosity of the sputum. Sputum cultures rarely offer additional information because COPD patients are often chronically seeded with the causative organism(s) [e.g., *S. pneumoniae, H. influenzae, M. catarrhalis, S. aureus,* and *P. aeroginosa*].

(b) Prevention of infection with chronic antibiotic therapy is controversial and should be considered only in patients with multiple exacerbations annually (i.e., more than two per year).

(2) **Antibiotic therapy**

(a) Ambulatory antibiotic treatment of exacerbations in patients with COPD is recommended when there is evidence of worsening dyspnea and cough with purulent sputum and increased sputum volume. Hospital or lab antibiograms should be reviewed when selecting an appropriate agent for *S. pneumoniae, M. catarrhalis,* and *H. influenzae.* Agents may include either a second-generation cephalosporin (e.g., cefuroxime, cefaclor), trimethoprim/sulfamethoxazole, a β-lactam with or without a β-lactamase inhibitor (e.g., amoxicillin, amoxicillin/clavulanate), or an oral fluoroquinolone (e.g., ciprofloxacin, levofloxacin, gatifloxacin).

(i) If infection with *M. pneumoniae* or *Legionella pneumophila* is a concern, a macrolide (e.g., erythromycin, clarithromycin, azithromycin) may be added.

(ii) If infection with *C. pneumoniae* is suspected, oral doxycycline is the drug of choice.

(b) Antibiotic treatment of pneumonia in hospitalized patients with COPD includes either a second- or third-generation cephalosporin (e.g., cefuroxime, ceftriaxone, cefotaxime) or a β-lactam with or without a β-lactamase inhibitor (e.g., ampicillin/sulbactam, piperacillin/tazobactam). If infection with *M. pneumoniae* or *L. pneumophila* is a concern, a macrolide (e.g., erythromycin, clarithromycin, azithromycin) may be added.

(c) *S. pneumoniae, H. influenzae,* and *M. catarrhalis* infections should be treated for approximately 7–10 days. Cases of *M. pneumoniae* may require longer therapy ranging from 10–14 days. Exceptions to this would be the use of azithromycin, whose uniquely long half-life allows 5 days of therapy.

f. Mucolytics (e.g., iodinated glycerol) may improve sputum clearance and disrupt mucus plugs, but their benefit is small, and they are not recommended.

g. Expectorants (e.g., guaifenesin) may be used, but the evidence of effectiveness is anecdotal. Potassium iodide should be avoided because of side effects associated with iodine therapy.

h. Antioxidants (e.g., *N*-acetylcysteine) may reduce exacerbation frequency. However, routine use cannot be recommended based on currently available data.

i. Vaccines

(1) **Influenza virus vaccine** is recommended because of its ability to reduce death and serious illness by almost 50%.

(2) **Polyvalent pneumococcal** vaccine is not currently recommended due to lack of evidence for efficacy.

2. Nonpharmacological treatment

a. Oxygen therapy (administered at low flow rate >15 hours/day) reverses hypoxemia, particularly during exercise and at night.

(1) Indications for home oxygen treatment include:

(a) PaO_2 <55 mm Hg or SaO_2 <88%

(b) PaO_2 of 55–60 mm Hg or SaO_2 <89% if evidence of cor pulmonale, pulmonary hypertension, or polycythemia (hematocrit >55%).

      (2) Patients hospitalized for COPD exacerbations should receive controlled oxygen to keep PaO_2 >60 mm Hg or SaO_2 >90%. ABGs should be performed 30 minutes after placing the patient on oxygen to identify and minimize CO_2 retention.

    b. Chest physiotherapy loosens secretions, helps reexpand the lungs, and increases the efficacy of respiratory muscle use. Techniques include postural drainage, chest percussion and vibration, coughing, and deep breathing. These efforts may help patients with lobar atelectasis or who produce large quantities (i.e., >25 mL/day) of sputum.

    c. Physical rehabilitation improves the patient's exercise tolerance and quality of life. A rehabilitation program usually includes physical conditioning and social, psychological, and nutritional interventions.

    d. Smoking cessation and avoidance of other irritants has been shown to slow the rate of decline in FEV_1 in COPD patients. Nicotine gum, patches, inhalers, buproprion, or clonidine may be useful in smoking cessation. Behavior intervention significantly enhances the effectiveness of pharmacological therapy in smoking cessation.

    e. Surgery. There is a growing body of evidence that lung volume reduction surgery may be beneficial to patients with severe COPD. Large clinical trials are under way to definitively answer this question.

H. Complications of COPD

    1. Pulmonary hypertension. With decreased pulmonary vascular bed space (due to lung congestion), pulmonary arterial pressure increases. In some cases, pressure increases enough to cause **cor pulmonale** (right ventricular hypertrophy) with consequent heart failure.

    2. Acute respiratory failure. In advanced stages of emphysema, the brain's respiratory center may become seriously compromised, leading to poor cerebral oxygenation and an increased $PaCO_2$ level. Hypoxia and respiratory acidosis may ensue. If the condition progresses, respiratory failure occurs.

    3. Infection. In chronic bronchitis, trapping of excessive mucus, air, and bacteria in the tracheobronchial tree sets the stage for infection. In addition, impairment of coughing and deep breathing, which normally cleanses the lungs, leads to destruction of respiratory cilia. Once an infection sets in, reinfection can easily occur.

    4. Polycythemia. An increase in red blood cells can lead to hypercoagulable states, embolism, and stroke.

STUDY QUESTIONS

Directions: Each of the numbered items or incomplete statements in this section is followed by answers or by completions of the statement. Select the **one** lettered answer or completion that is **best** in each case.

1. The symptoms of allergen-mediated asthma result from which of the following?

(A) Increased release of mediators from mast cells
(B) Increased adrenergic responsiveness of the airways
(C) Increased vascular permeability of bronchial tissue
(D) Decreased calcium influx into the mast cells
(E) Decreased prostaglandin production

2. Acute exacerbations of asthma can be triggered by all of the following EXCEPT

(A) bacterial or viral pneumonia
(B) hypersensitivity reaction to penicillin
(C) discontinuation of asthma medication
(D) hot, dry weather
(E) stressful emotional events

3. The National Institutes of Health (NIH) guidelines for the treatment of asthma recommend institution of routine inhaled corticosteroids when patients are classified as having greater than or equal to which type of asthma?

(A) Mild intermittent
(B) Mild persistent
(C) Moderate persistent
(D) Severe persistent

4. In the emergency department, the preferred first-line therapy for asthma exacerbation is

(A) theophylline
(B) a β-agonist
(C) a corticosteroid
(D) cromolyn sodium
(E) an antihistamine

5. The primary goals of asthma therapy include all of the following EXCEPT

(A) maintain normal activity levels
(B) maintain control of symptoms
(C) avoid adverse effects of asthma medications
(D) prevent acute exacerbations and chronic symptoms
(E) prevent destruction of lung tissue

6. Which of the following tests is used at home to assess therapy and determine if a patient with asthma should seek emergency care?

(A) Forced expiratory volume in one second (FEV_1)
(B) Forced vital capacity (FVC)
(C) Total lung capacity (TLC)
(D) Peak expiratory flow rate (PEFR)
(E) Residual volume (RV)

Directions: The question below contains three suggested answers, of which **one or more** is correct. Choose the answer

A	if **I only** is correct
B	if **III only** is correct
C	if **I and II** are correct
D	if **II and III** are correct
E	if **I, II, and III** are correct

7. The disease process of chronic bronchitis is characterized by

  I. the destruction of central and peripheral portions of the acinus
 II. an increased number of mucous glands and goblet cells
III. edema and inflammation of the bronchioles

Directions: The question in this section consists of lettered options followed by a set of numbered items. For each item, select the **one** lettered option that is most closely associated with it. Each lettered option may be selected once, more than once, or not at all.

Questions 8–10

(A) Cimetidine
(B) Albuterol
(C) Ipratropium bromide
(D) Epinephrine
(E) Atropine

Match the description with the appropriate agent.

8. Decreases theophylline clearance

9. Has anticholinergic activity with few side effects

10. Has high β_2-adrenergic selectivity

ANSWERS AND EXPLANATIONS

1. The answer is A *[I D 42 (A); Figure 48-1].*
In asthma, airborne antigen binds to the mast cell, activating the immunoglobulin E (IgE)-mediated process. Mediators (e.g., histamine, leukotrienes, prostaglandins) are then released, causing bronchoconstriction and tissue edema.

2. The answer is D *[I D; Figure 48-1].*
Exacerbations of asthma can be triggered by allergens, respiratory infections, occupational stimuli (e.g., fumes from gasoline or paint), emotions, and environmental factors. Studies have shown that cold air can cause release of mast cell mediators by an undetermined mechanism. Hot, dry air does not cause this release.

3. The answer is B *[Table 48-3].*
The National Institutes of Health (NIH) guidelines recommend routine use of inhaled corticosteroids in patients who have mild persistent asthma. Short-acting β-agonists should be used as needed for symptoms.

4. The answer is B *[Figure 48-3].*
In an emergency situation, the most rapidly acting agent is used first. Selection of the route of administration depends on the severity of the attack. An inhaled β-agonist administered in a nebulizer or administered as a subcutaneous agent is the most appropriate first-line therapy.

5. The answer is E *[I F, H 1; II D].*
Asthma is characterized by reversible airway obstruction in response to specific stimuli. Mast cells release mediators, which trigger bronchoconstriction. After an acute attack, in most cases symptoms are minimal, and pathological changes are not permanent. Unlike asthma, chronic obstructive pulmonary disease does cause progressive airway destruction, chronic bronchitis by excessive mucus production and other changes, and emphysema by destruction of the acinus.

6. The answer is D *[I G 2 a (3)].*
In monitoring of asthma therapy at home, peak expiratory flow rate (PEFR) is the best test for assessment of therapy, trigger identification, and the need for referral to emergency care. It is recommended for patients who have had severe exacerbations of asthma, who are poor perceivers of asthma symptoms, and those with moderate to severe disease.

7. The answer is D (II, III) *[II D 1, 2].*
Chronic bronchitis is characterized by an increase in the number of mucous and goblet cells due to bronchial irritation. This results in increased mucus production. Other changes include edema and inflammation of the bronchioles and changes in smooth muscle and cartilage. Emphysema is a permanent destruction of the central and peripheral portions of the acinus distal to the bronchioles. In this disease, adequate oxygen reaches the alveolar duct, due to increased rate of breathing, but perfusion is abnormal.

8–10. The answers are: 8-A *[Table 48-8],* **9-C** *[II G 1 a],* **10-B** *[Table 48-4].*
Cimetidine, a histamine$_2$-receptor antagonist, decreases theophylline clearance by inhibiting hepatic microsomal mixed-function oxidase metabolism, thus increasing serum theophylline concentrations. Theophylline clearance can be decreased by 40% during the first 24 hours of concurrent therapy. Anticholinergic agents such as atropine and ipratropium bromide produce bronchodilation by competitively inhibiting cholinergic receptors. The disadvantages of atropine include dry mouth, tachycardia, and urinary retention. Ipratropium bromide is three to five times more potent than atropine and does not have these side effects. Albuterol is one of the most β$_2$-selective adrenergic agents available. Other such agents include terbutaline, bitolterol, and pirbuterol. Agents with β$_2$-selectivity dilate bronchioles without causing side effects related to β$_1$-stimulation (e.g., increased heart rate).

49
Osteoarthritis and Rheumatoid Arthritis

Tina M. Harrison

I. INTRODUCTION

A. Definition and etiology

1. **Osteoarthritis (OA)** (formerly known as degenerative joint disease) is a common chronic condition of cartilage degeneration. Secondary changes can occur in the bone, leading to pain, decreased functioning, and even disability. OA affects nearly 21 million middle-aged and elderly Americans. It is the most common form of arthritis. Although not always symptomatic, most people over the age of 55 years have radiological evidence of the disease. Until age 55 years, OA affects men equally as women, but after age 55, women are more likely to have the disease.

2. **Rheumatoid arthritis (RA)** is a systemic disease that involves inflammation in the membrane lining of the joints and often affects internal organs. Most patients exhibit a chronic fluctuating course of disease that can result in progressive joint destruction, deformity, and disability. RA affects 1% of the U.S. population. It occurs two to three times more often in women, and the peak onset occurs between the fourth and sixth decades of life.

II. NORMAL JOINT ANATOMY AND PHYSIOLOGY

A. The **synovial joint** consists of two bone ends covered by articular cartilage. The role of articular cartilage includes:

1. Enabling frictionless movement of the joint

2. Distributing the load across the joint (shock absorber), to prevent damage

3. Promoting stability during use

B. **Cartilage** is avascular and aneural. It is metabolically active and undergoes continual internal remodeling. It is composed primarily of water but is also made from chondrocytes and extracellular matrix.

C. **Chondrocytes** control the synthesis and degradation of the matrix. They produce proteoglycans and collagen in the extracellular matrix to maintain the integrity of the matrix in healthy cartilage.

D. The **joint capsule** is a fibrous outer layer that encapsulates the joint. The joint capsule is lined by **synovium,** a membrane that produces a viscous fluid that lubricates the joint.

E. The **synovial fluid** is comprised, in part, of hyaluronic acid. Glucosamine is a component of hyaluronic acid. The role of hyaluronic acid is to maintain functional and structural characteristics of the extracellular matrix.

F. **Bursae** are small sacs that are lined with synovial membrane and filled with fluid to provide cushioning and lubrication for the movement of the joint.

OSTEOARTHRITIS

III. OSTEOARTHRITIS: PATHOPHYSIOLOGY

A. The disease is not a normal part of the aging process; however, there are many age-related changes that contribute to the development of OA.

1. The strength of tendons, ligaments, and muscles declines with advancing age and may contribute to the development of the disease.

2. The number of chondrocytes declines due to apoptosis (cell death), decreased proliferation, or both.

3. The synthesis of normal proteoglycans is reduced.

B. Chondrocytes lose the ability to promote healing and cartilage remodeling, resulting in cartilage matrix degradation. Proteoglycans are depleted.

C. Matrix metalloproteinases (MMPs) and proinflammatory cytokines promote cartilage degradation.

D. Interleukin-1 (IL-1) has several roles in the development of OA.

1. Responsible for the induction of chondrocytes and synovial cells to synthesize MMPs

2. Inhibits the synthesis of type II collagen and proteoglycans, preventing collagen from repairing itself

3. Enhances nitric oxide production and induces chondrocyte apoptosis

E. Pain occurs as a result of:

1. Osteophytes: spurs of cartilage and bone at the joint

2. Synovitis

3. Bursitis

4. Tendonitis

IV. RISK FACTORS for OA include advanced age, female gender, muscle weakness, obesity, joint trauma, heredity, congenital or developmental anatomical defects, and repetitive stress.

V. CLINICAL PRESENTATION. OA is characterized by a deep, localized ache in a joint. Pain and stiffness usually occurs with rest or immobility and lasts <30 minutes. Inflammation, if present, is mild. Patients will often complain of crepitus, a popping or cracking noise, heard in the joint upon moving.

VI. DIAGNOSIS

A. Physical examination. Joint tenderness, diminished range of motion, crepitus, abnormalities in joint shape

B. Laboratory tests. No specific lab tests are diagnostic for OA

C. Radiography. Narrowing of joint space (due to loss of cartilage) and the presence of osteophytes

D. The American College of Rheumatology (ACR) has developed **criteria for OA of the hip, knee, and hand:**

1. OA of the hip—characterized by hip pain and at least two of the following:
   a. Erythrocyte sedimentation rate (ESR) of less than 20 mm/hr
   b. Radiographic evidence of femoral or acetabular osteophytes
   c. Radiographic evidence of joint space narrowing

2. OA of the knee—knee pain and radiographic evidence of osteophytes and at least one of the following:
   a. Age >50 years
   b. Morning stiffness that lasts <30 minutes
   c. Articular crepitus on motion

   3. OA of the hand—hand pain, aching, or stiffness and three of the following:
     a. Hard-tissue enlargement of ≥2 of 10 selected joints*
     b. Hard-tissue enlargement of ≥2 distal interphalangeal joints
     c. Fewer than 3 swollen metacarpalphalenageal joints
     d. Deformity of at least 1 of 10 selected joints*

VII. TREATMENT

A. Goals

   1. Control pain and other symptoms

   2. Maintain or improve joint mobility

   3. Correct or minimize functional limitations and disability

B. Nonpharmacological treatments

   1. Weight loss (if overweight)—has been shown to decrease pain and symptoms of OA

   2. Aerobic exercise programs—bed rest and immobility are not necessary with OA

   3. Physical therapy for range-of-motion exercises and strengthening

   4. Assistive devices (e.g., canes, walkers, crutches) may help to decrease the load on a joint; however, patients should be instructed on their proper use for safety

   5. Joint protection—avoid prolonged standing, kneeling, and squatting

   6. Thermal therapy (hot or cold) (e.g., hot shower or tub, ice pack) may be of benefit for some patients with OA

C. Pharmacological treatment

   1. Acetaminophen is considered first-line therapy by the ACR for OA of the hip or knee. It has excellent analgesic and antipyretic activity, but no significant anti-inflammatory effects.
     a. Doses of ≤4 g/day is recommended to avoid toxicity. Concomitant use of other medications with acetaminophen should be evaluated closely to avoid an overdose.
     b. Hepatotoxicity can occur in patients taking >4 g of acetaminophen a day. Symptoms can include: nausea, vomiting, abdominal pain, malaise, and diaphoresis. In patients with chronic stable liver disease, doses of up to 4 g/day did not cause any evidence of hepatotoxicity.
     c. Because there is little, if any, inflammation in the OA joint, acetaminophen has been shown to be equally efficacious as ibuprofen and naproxen in patients with mild to moderate OA pain.

   2. Nonsteroidal anti-inflammatory drugs (NSAIDs) are indicated in OA treatment when the response to acetaminophen is inadequate. Examples are illustrated in Table 49-1.
     a. Mechanism of action. Nonselective inhibitors of cyclooxygenase-1 and -2, as well as thromboxane synthetase
     b. Analgesia is seen with a short treatment duration and at lower doses (e.g., ibuprofen ≤1200 mg/day)
     c. Anti-inflammatory response is seen with higher doses and usually requires several days of therapy to achieve anti-inflammatory affect
     d. Adverse effects
       (1) Gastrointestinal (GI) toxicity is caused by direct mucosal injury and inhibition of prostaglandins. Symptoms include dyspepsia, ulceration, and bleeding. People at risk of GI toxicity include the elderly, anyone with a history of peptic ulcer disease, chronic alcohol use, high-dose or multiple NSAID use, concomitant corticosteroid use, and NSAID treatment of <3 months.
       (2) Renal toxicity results from the inhibition of prostaglandins. While the risks are low (~5%), it does not appear to be dose dependent and is usually reversible. Effects can include hyperkalemia, hyponatremia, increased serum creatinine, sodium and

---

*Selected joints: 2nd and 3rd DIP, 2nd and 3rd PIP, 1st CMC of both hands.

Table 49-1. Selected Nonsteroidal Anti-Inflammatory Drugs

Generic (Brand)	Initial Daily Dose	Maximum Daily Dose
Nonacetylated Salicylates		
Salsalate (Disalcid)	500 mg three times a day	3000 mg
Magnesium salicylate (Doan's)	650 mg every 4 hours	4800 mg
NSAIDs		
Aspirin (various)	650 mg every 4 hours	6000 mg
Diclofenac (Voltaren)	75 mg twice a day	200 mg
Etodolac (Lodine)	300 mg twice a day	1200 mg
Ibuprofen (Motrin, Advil)	400 mg three times a day	3200 mg
Naproxen (Naprosyn, Aleve)	500 mg twice a day	1250 mg
Nabumeton (Relafen)	500 mg twice a day	2000 mg
Sulindac (Clinoril)	150 mg twice a day	400 mg
Tolmetin (Tolectin)	400 mg three times a day	1800 mg
COX-2 Inhibitors		
Celecoxib (Celebrex)	100 mg twice a day	400 mg
Rofecoxib (Vioxx)	25 mg daily	50 mg
Valdecoxib (Bextra)	10 mg daily	40 mg

water retention, as well as acute renal failure. People at risk for renal toxicity include the elderly, those with preexisting renal disease, hypertension, diabetes mellitus, congestive heart failure, cirrhosis, and volume depletion (e.g., hemorrhage, sepsis, diuretics, diarrhea).

(3) **Hematological** effects are due to decreased platelet aggregation.

(4) **Hepatic** toxicity, although not common, can include elevated liver enzymes and hepatotoxicity. Patients at risk include those with a history of hepatitis, alcoholism, and congestive heart failure.

(5) **CNS** effects can include sedation, confusion, and mental status changes and are primarily seen in the elderly.

(6) **Allergic reactions,** such as asthma, urticaria, and photosensitivity, may be seen. Cross-sensitivity has been seen in patients allergic to aspirin.

3. **Cyclooxygenase-2 specific inhibitors (COX-2 inhibitors)** are selective NSAIDs specific for the COX-2 enzyme and exhibit analgesic and anti-inflammatory properties.

   a. **Adverse effects**

      (1) **GI.** Due to the specificity of COX-2, these agents have fewer GI side effects (e.g., ulceration, bleeding) than their nonselective counterparts and may be an option in patients with a history of peptic ulcer disease.

      (2) **Hematological.** The COX-2 inhibitors have fewer effects on platelets like the nonselective NSAIDs.

      (3) **Renal, hepatic, CV, and CNS** effects are similar to those seen in traditional NSAIDs.

   b. These agents are very expensive and may not be covered by third-party insurance without special physician documentation.

4. **Other oral analgesics**

   a. **Tramadol (Ultram).** Considered a good choice when the patient's pain is unrelieved by NSAIDs, when the patient cannot take NSAIDs, or when the patient experiences breakthrough pain while taking NSAIDs.

      (1) **Mechanism of action.** Centrally acting analgesic that inhibits the reuptake of norepinephrine and serotonin, and mildly binds to the μ-receptor.

      (2) **Dose.** 50–100 mg every 4–6 hours, not to exceed 400 mg/day. In patients with impaired renal function (e.g., CrCl <30 mL/min), the dosage interval should be every 12 hours, with a maximum dose of 200 mg.

      (3) **Adverse effects.** Although it is not an opioid analgesic, its side effects are similar: nausea, constipation, rash, dizziness, somnolence, and orthostatic hypotension.

      (4) **Drug interactions.** Carbamazepine can decrease the effects of tramadol. Increased toxicity can occur with the concomitant use of quinidine, cimetidine, and SSRIs (e.g., paroxetine, sertraline, fluoxetine).

    b. Opiate analgesics (e.g., codeine, oxycodone) are usually reserved for patients who fail single- or multiple-analgesic therapy. They may also be useful for acute exacerbations of pain. Side effects can include constipation, sedation, nausea, respiratory depression, and confusion.

      (1) Propoxyphene. The use of propoxyphene is controversial, as it has demonstrated efficacy similar to acetaminophen. The clinician must also consider the acetaminophen content (650 mg) of propoxyphene/acetaminophen (e.g., Darvocet-N 100 mg) and the potential for overdose. Propoxyphene should be avoided in the elderly.

    c. Topical analgesics (e.g., capsaicin) are effective in relieving OA pain in some patients. Topical therapy can be used in conjunction with oral therapy or as monotherapy. Capsaicin is derived from hot chili peppers and with chronic use (>2 weeks) works by depleting stores of substance P. Patients should be counseled to wash hands thoroughly after application to avoid contact with other skin to avoid burning and stinging.

    d. Intra-articular injections

      (1) Corticosteroids may be useful in knee OA when fluid is present but are not routinely recommended in hip OA due to administration difficulties. Duration of action is up to 4 weeks. Due to adverse effects on the bone, injections should be limited to 3 or 4 per year.

      (2) Hyaluronic acid derivatives. Indicated for the treatment of knee OA when treatment failure to other therapies occurs. Intended to improve elasticity and viscosity of synovial fluid. **Sodium hyaluronate (Hyalgan)** [2 mL weekly for 5 weeks] and **hylan polymers (Synvisc)** [2 mL weekly for 3 weeks] are the two agents currently available. Most benefits are seen after the last dose; effects are superior to placebo and comparable to corticosteroid injections. These agents should be used with caution in patients with allergies to avian proteins, feathers, and egg products. Patients should be counseled to avoid strenuous or prolonged (>1 hr) weight-bearing activities within 48 hours following treatment.

    e. Adjunctive treatments

      (1) Glucosamine—acts as a substrate for and promotes the synthesis of the glycosaminoglycans; dose is 500 mg three times a day. **Side effects** may include GI discomfort, fatigue, skin rash, and hyperglycemia.

      (2) Chondroitin—helps protect against the breakdown of collagen and proteoglycans. Usually found in combination with glucosamine, but the added benefits are not clear; dose is 1200 mg/day. Side effects can include prolonged bleeding time and nausea.

      (3) S-adenosyl-methionine (SAMe)—the mechanism is unclear; however, it does play a role in maintaining cartilage. Dose is 600 mg/day × 2 weeks, then 400 mg/day.

    f. Surgical interventions (e.g., arthroscopy, joint replacement). Considered when pain is severe and not responding to medical treatment or when disability interferes with daily activities.

VIII. RHEUMATOID ARTHRITIS: ETIOLOGY AND PATHOGENESIS.

The cause of RA is unknown, but appears to be multifactorial. It is considered an autoimmune disease—where the body loses its ability to distinguish between synovial and foreign tissue. Other factors involved in RA are:

A. Environmental influences, such as bacterial and viral infections, are thought to have a role in the development of RA.

B. Genetic markers, such as HLA-DR4, a human leukocyte antigen, has been associated with triggering the inflammatory process in RA; however, it is not considered diagnostic, as up to 30% of people with this genetic marker never develop RA.

C. Tumor-necrosis factor–alpha (TNF-a), **interleukin-1** (IL-1), **IL-6,** and **growth factors** propagate the inflammatory process, and agents found to alter these cytokines show promise in reducing pain and deformity.

D. Inflamed synovium is a hallmark of the pathophysiology of RA. Synovium proliferates abnormally, growing into the joint space and into the bone—forming a pannus. The pannus migrates to the articular cartilage and into the subchondral bone. Through stimulation by the cytokines, the cells of the pannus produce proteolytic enzymes, which degrade cartilage. These same cytokines activate osteoclasts, which causes the demineralization of bone.

IX. CLINICAL MANIFESTATIONS

A. The onset of RA is insidious. In early disease, symptoms include malaise and anorexia, accompanied by symmetrically tender and swollen joints. Pain in the joints is common and aggravated by movement.

B. Most commonly, the joints first affected by RA include the metacarpophalangeal (MCP) and proximal interphalangeal (PIP) joints of the hands, metatarsophalangeal (MTP) joints of the feet, and wrists. Other areas affected by RA include the spine, shoulder, ankle, and hip.

X. CLINICAL COURSE. The severity of the disease is variable.

A. Within 4 months of diagnosis, irreversible joint damage is detectable on radiographic images. The rate at which joint damage occurs is greatest during the first year.

B. Prognosis is poorest with an early onset of the disease, significant functional disability during the first year, involvement of 20 or more joints, the presence of rheumatoid nodules, or extra-articular involvement.

C. Extra-articular manifestations can include rheumatoid nodules, anemia, peripheral neuropathy, kidney disease, CV, and pulmonary disease.

D. Osteoporosis may occur secondary to RA in patients receiving treatment with corticoste-roids.

XI. DIAGNOSIS AND CLINICAL EVALUATION

A. The ACR classifies RA by having at least four of the following seven criteria, and the first four criteria must have been present for at least 6 weeks:

1. Morning stiffness for $\geq$30 minutes—usually lasting for 1 hour before maximal improvement

2. Arthritis of three or more joint areas—at least three joint areas have simultaneous soft-tissue swelling

3. Arthritis of hand joints—swelling in at least one area in a wrist, MCP, or PIP joint

4. Symmetrical arthritis—simultaneous involvement of the same joint areas on both sides of the body

5. Rheumatoid nodules—observable subcutaneous nodules, over bony prominences or extensor surfaces

6. Serum rheumatoid factor—refer to laboratory assessment [X 1 B]

7. Radiological changes—refer to radiographic examination [X 1 C]

B. Laboratory assessment

1. **Rheumatoid factor (RF)** is found in more than 60% of patients with RA; however, as many as 5% of healthy individuals will also have elevated titers of RF. The most commonly found rheumatoid factors are IgM and IgG. IgA is also a good indicator since it correlates well with the ESR.

2. **Erythrocyte sedimentation rate (ESR) and C-reactive protein (CRP)** are markers of inflammation and are usually elevated in patients with RA. They can also help indicate the activity of the disease.

3. Since anemia is a common feature of RA, a **complete blood count (CBC)** should be regularly obtained. Anemia associated with RA tends to be hypochromic in 50%–100% of RA cases, and mild leukocytosis is evident in 25% of cases.

4. The **antinuclear antibody (ANA)** test is positive in 15% of patient with RA.

C. Radiographic examination. Baseline evaluations of the feet and hands are important to ascertain structural damage. As the disease progresses, evidence of periarticular osteopenia becomes apparent. The radiograph is a good indicator of the extent of bone erosion and cartilage loss. A magnetic resonance image (MRI) detects the proliferative pannus.

XII. TREATMENT OBJECTIVES. The goals in the management of RA are:

A. To prevent or control joint damage

B. To prevent loss of function

C. To decrease pain

D. To maintain the patient's quality of life

E. To avoid or minimize adverse effects of treatment

XIII. PROGNOSIS. Poor prognosis is suggested by a high RF titer, elevated ESR, >20 joints involved, onset of disease at an early age, and extra-articular involvement.

XIV. THERAPY

A. Nonpharmacological. Optimal therapy involves both drug- and nondrug therapy. Patients should be instructed on joint protection and range-of-motion exercises. Regularly scheduled rest periods are important to reduce physical stress on the joints. Physical therapy and occupational therapy may help patients maintain their activities of daily living. Arthritis support groups may help with psychological well-being.

B. Pharmacological. Drug therapy for RA involves the treatment of symptoms and disease modifying agents. Drugs with anti-inflammatory activity are the agents of choice for the symptomatic relief of RA.

    1. Salicylates, NSAIDs, and COX-2 inhibitors reduce joint pain and swelling, but they do not alter the course of the disease or prevent joint destruction (refer to Table 49-1).

    2. Corticosteroids. Low-dose systemic corticosteroids (e.g., prednisone, methylprednisolone) can work well either orally or parenterally. They have excellent anti-inflammatory activity and are immunosuppressants. The lowest effective dose should be utilized due to adverse effects. These agents do not alter the course of the disease; however, they are often used to "bridge" therapy as patients start on DMARDs (see below).

    3. Disease-modifying antirheumatic drugs (DMARDs)—Refer to Table 49-2.
      a. The objective of DMARD therapy is to reduce or prevent joint damage and preserve joint function.
      b. The ACR guidelines published in 2002 recommend that DMARD therapy be initiated, despite good control with NSAIDs, within 3 months.
      c. The onset for most of these agents is prolonged; therefore, anti-inflammatory drugs are usually given concurrently as a "bridge" until therapeutic effects occur.
      d. Factors such as cost, toxicity, compliance, and onset of action influence the selection of a DMARD.
      e. Inflammatory markers (e.g., ESR, CRP) are reduced significantly by DMARDs, but not by NSAIDs.
      f. Mechanism of action—not clearly defined; however, they act at different stages in the pathogenesis to control symptoms and modulate immune response.

    4. Newer DMARDs—Refer to Table 49-2. The newer agents have given significant advancement to the treatment of RA.
      a. Leflunomide (Arava) inhibits pyrimidine synthesis and is indicated as monotherapy for RA.
        (1) Hepatotoxicity is associated with the use of leflunomide. Contraindications include patients with impaired liver function and concomitant use with methotrexate. Liver

Table 49-2. DMARDs

Agent Brand (Generic)	Onset (months)	Dosing	Adverse Effects	Monitoring Parameters	Some Drug Interactions
MORE COMMONLY USED DMARDs					
Hydroxychloroquine (Plaquenil)	2–6	200–400 mg/day; max = 6.5 mg/kg/day	Nausea, HA, ocular toxicity, myopathy	Eye exam, CBC, LFTs	Cimetidine
Sulfasalazine (Azulfidine)	1–3	500 mg/day, may increase to a max of 3000 mg/day	Dizziness, nausea, diarrhea, HA, rash, abnormal LFTs	CBC, LFTs, SrCr	MTX, oral anticoagulants, digoxin, folic acid
Methotrexate (Rheumatrex)	1–2	5–20 mg/week	Nausea, diarrhea, mouth ulcers, rash, alopeica, abnormal LFTs, renal failure, leukopenia, myelosuppression	LFTs, SrCr, CBC, chest x-ray	Corticosteroids, cyclosporine, NSAIDs
LESS FREQUENTLY USED DMARDs					
Auranofin (Ridaura)	4–6	3–6 mg/day; may increase up to 9 mg/day	Itching, rash, stomatitis, conjunctivitis, proteinuria	SrCr avoid if CrCl <50 mL/min), u/a, CBC	Penicillamine, hydrochloroquine, immunosuppressants
Azathioprine (Imuran)	2–3	50–150 mg/day	Chills, fever, N/V, diarrhea, leukopenia, thrombocytopenia	CBC, LFTs	Allopurinol
Cyclosporine (Neoral)	2–4	3–10 mg/kg/day	HTN, HA, nausea, paresthesia, tremor, HA, leukopenia	BP, SrCr, LFTs, serum drug levels	CYP3A3/4 inhibitors, glucocorticoids, MTX, digoxin, allopurinol
Gold Salts (IM) (Aurolate)	3–6	25–50 mg IM q 2–4 weeks	Itching, rash, conjunctivitis, stomatitis, proteinuria	CBC w/diff, renal function, urinalysis	Penicillamine
D-Penicillamine (Cuprimine)	3–6	250–750 mg/day	Nausea, loss of taste, arthralgia, thrombocytopenia	u/a, CBC, LFTs	Gold, antimalarials, immunosuppressants, digoxin, iron, zinc, antacids
NEWER DMARDs					
Leflunomide (Arava)	1–4	100 mg/day PO x 3 days (load), then 20 mg/day	Diarrhea, respiratory tract infection, nausea, rash, HTN, alopecia	LFTs, SrCr, BP, eye exam	NSAIDs, MTX
Etanercept (Enbrel)	0.25–3	25 mg SQ twice a week	HA, injection site reaction, respiratory tract infection, infection, abdominal pain, weakness	s/s of infection	
Infliximab (Remicade)	0.25–4	3 mg/kg IV at weeks 0, 2, and 6, and then every 8 weeks	HA, fatigue, fever, nausea, abdominal pain, respiratory tract infection	s/s of infection	
Anakinra (Kineret)	0.25–1	100 mg/day SQ	HA, injection site reaction, infections	Neutrophil counts	

HA = headache; CBC = complete blood count; SrCr = serum creatinine, BP = blood pressure, N/V = nausea and vomiting; HTN = hypertenstion; LFTs = liver function tests; u/a = urinalysis; s/s = signs and symptoms; MTX = methotrexate.

function tests should be performed at baseline, and at least monthly intervals during the first 6 months of treatment, and then every 8 weeks thereafter.

  (2) **Significant weight loss** and **immunosuppression** may occur with therapy. Although rare, pancytopenia and Stevens-Johnson syndrome have been reported.

  (3) When adverse effects occur without using an elimination procedure (e.g., cholestyramine), it is important to remember that leflunomide can take up to 2 years to be eliminated from the body.

  (4) The average wholesale **cost of therapy** per year is $3200.

  b. Etanercept (Enbrel) binds to TNF-α and -β, inhibiting the inflammatory response mediated by immune cells. It is indicated as monotherapy or in conjunction with methotrexate.

  (1) **Immunosuppression** occurs with the use of etanercept. Other adverse effects can include pancytopenia, lupus-like symptoms, paresthesias, visual and gait disturbances, and confusion. Reactivation of latent tuberculosis has also been reported.

  (2) The average wholesale **cost of therapy** per year is $16,000.

  c. Infliximab (Remicade) binds to TNF-α and is only FDA approved in combination with methotrexate.

  (1) Like etanercept, **immunosuppression** is the most serious adverse effect. Tuberculosis has been associated with its use. Patients receiving concomitant therapy with other immunosuppressants should be closely monitored.

  (2) The average wholesale **cost of therapy** per year is $11,000.

  d. Anakinra (Kineret), the newest DMARD, is an interleukin-1 receptor antagonist. It is used as monotherapy or in conjunction with methotrexate.

  (1) **Immunosuppression** is the most serious adverse effect. Neutrophil counts should be monitored at baseline and monthly for 3 months, and quarterly for 1 year following initiation of therapy. The manufacturer cautions about the use of other immunosuppressants concurrently.

  (2) The average wholesale **cost of therapy** per year is $15,000.

C. Combination therapy—Concurrent use of several DMARD agents has been studied. Patients with new symptoms or whose current DMARD therapy has failed have benefited from combination DMARD therapy. It is unclear when combination therapy should be initiated; however, instead of using a "step up" approach to care, some evidence suggests using triple therapy (e.g., MTX, hydroxychloroquine, and sulfasalazine) and using a "step down" approach. Careful monitoring for adverse effects should be maintained.

D. Surgical treatment (e.g., carpal tunnel release, total joint arthroplasty, joint fusion) may be considered when pain is severe, range of motion is lost, or joint function is poor due to joint damage. Patients with good preoperative functional status generally have a faster rate of recovery.

STUDY QUESTIONS

Directions: Each of the numbered items or incomplete statements in this section is followed by answers or by completion of the statement. Select the **one** lettered answer or completion that is **best** in each case.

1. Which of the following statements best characterizes osteoarthritis?

 I. OA is a systemic disease that is characterized by profound, diffuse inflammation, resulting in joint destruction, deformity, and disability.
 II. OA is a common disorder characterized by cartilage degeneration that can cause joint pain, decreased functioning, and disability.
 III. OA, the most common form of arthritis, can result from age-related changes in the joint, loss of function of the chondrocytes, and proteoglycan depletion.

(A) I only
(B) III only
(C) I and II
(D) II and III
(E) I, II, and III

2. Which of the following factors is associated with a poor prognosis of RA?

(A) Absence of rheumatoid factor, minimal inflammation, limited joint involvement at the onset
(B) Age of disease onset ≥60 years, family history of the disease, high ESR
(C) Involvement of internal organs, poor response to aspirin, age of onset ≥60 years
(D) Good response to methotrexate, presence of rheumatoid factor, low ESR
(E) High RF titer, elevated ESR, age of onset ≤25 years

3. A 56-year-old woman has just been diagnosed with OA of the right knee. What nonpharmacological treatment would you recommend?

 I. Maintain her ideal body weight
 II. Aerobic exercise programs
 III. Limit activity to ≤30 minutes at one time, and rest the joint as often as possible

(A) I only
(B) III only
(C) I and II
(D) II and III
(E) I, II, and III

4. Risk factors for renal toxicity associated with NSAIDs and COX-2 inhibitors include all of the following EXCEPT:

(A) Orthostatic hypotension
(B) Cirrhosis
(C) Volume depletion
(D) Diabetes mellitus
(E) Age

5. All of the following statements are true about the use of hyaluronic acid derivatives EXCEPT:

(A) Injections must be given in weekly intervals, and optimal effects are seen after the last dose.
(B) These are viable options for patients with OA of the hip.
(C) Patients should avoid strenuous activities for 2 days following their treatment.
(D) Patient with an allergy to eggs or feathers should use caution when receiving these products.
(E) Considered second-line therapy when other treatments have failed.

6. Which of the following agents necessitates an ophthalmic examination to monitor for toxicity?

(A) Penicillamine
(B) Methotrexate
(C) Hydroxychloroquine
(D) Cyclosporine
(E) Auranofin

7. Which of the following DMARDs has the shorter onset of action?

(A) Penicillamine
(B) Hydroxychloroquine
(C) Etanercept
(D) Cyclosporine
(E) Auranofin

8. Osteoporosis is associated with the use of which of the following drugs used in RA?

(A) Leflunomide
(B) Prednisone
(C) Methotrexate
(D) Penicillamine
(E) Hydroxychloroquine

ANSWERS AND EXPLANATIONS

1. The answer is D *[III A and V]*.
Osteoarthritis is not considered a disease of inflammation. While there are times of minor inflammation (e.g., OA flare), it is localized to the affected joint.

2. The answer is E *[X 2]*.
Factors associated with a poor prognosis for RA include: more than 20 joints involved, extra-articular involvement, onset of the disease at an early age, high RF titers, and an elevated ESR.

3. The answer is D *[VII B]*.
Nonpharmacological treatment should include aerobic exercise, physical therapy, joint protection, thermal therapy, and weight loss, if someone is overweight.

4. The answer is A *[VII C 2 (b)]*.
Patients at higher risk of renal toxicity include the elderly; patients with HTN, DM, CHF, or cirrhosis; patients who are volume depleted; and patients who have preexisting renal disease.

5. The answer is B *[VII 4 d (ii)]*.
Hyaluronic acid derivatives are only indicated for OA of the knee.

6. The answer is C *[Table 49-2]*.
Ophthalmic exams are recommended when patients are receiving either hydroxychloroquine or leflunomide.

7. The answer is C *[Table 49-2]*.
All DMARDs have a fairly long onset of action; however, etanercept and infliximab are associated with the shortest onset of action.

8. The answer is B *[X 4]*.
Steroid (e.g., prednisone) use can lead to osteoporosis; therefore, patients taking prednisone should consider therapy with calcium.

50
Hyperuricemia and Gout

Larry N. Swanson

I. INTRODUCTION

A. Definitions

1. **Hyperuricemia** refers to a serum uric acid level that is elevated more than two standard deviations above the population mean. In most laboratories, the upper limit of normal is 7 mg/dl (uricase method). However, the level varies with the laboratory method used; the upper limit of normal is about 1 mg/dl lower for women than for men.

2. **Gout** is a disease that is characterized by recurrent acute attacks of urate crystal-induced arthritis. It may include **tophi**–deposits of monosodium urate–in and around the joints and cartilage and in the kidneys, as well as uric acid nephrolithiasis.

B. Incidence

1. Gout affects approximately 0.2%–1.5% of the population in the United States.

2. Most gout victims are men (approximately 95% of cases); most women with the disease are postmenopausal.

3. The mean age at disease onset is 47 years.

4. The risk of developing gout increases as the serum uric acid level rises. Virtually all gout patients have a serum uric acid level above 7 mg/dl.

5. Research shows that among patients with a serum uric acid level above 9 mg/dl, the cumulative incidence of gout reached 22% after 5 years.

6. Gout has a familial tendency; 10%–60% of cases occur in family members of patients with the disease.

7. Obesity, heavy alcohol consumption, and certain other life-style factors increase the chances of developing gout.

C. Uric acid production and excretion

1. Uric acid, an end product of **purine metabolism,** is produced from both dietary and endogenous sources. Its formation results from the conversion of adenine and guanine moieties of nucleoproteins and nucleotides (Figure 50-1).

2. **Xanthine oxidase** catalyzes the reaction that occurs as the final step in the degradation of purines to uric acid.

3. The body ultimately excretes uric acid via the kidneys (300–600 mg/day; two-thirds of total uric acid) and via the gastrointestinal (GI) tract (100–300 mg/day; one-third of the total uric acid).

4. Uric acid has no known biological function.

5. The body has a total uric acid content of 1.0–1.2 g; the daily turnover rate is approximately 600–800 mg.

6. At a pH of 4.0–5.0 (i.e., in urine), uric acid exists as a poorly soluble free acid; at physiological pH, it exists primarily as **monosodium urate salt.**

7. Uric acid filtration, reabsorption, and secretion sites are shown in Figure 50-2.

D. Etiology. Hyperuricemia and gout may be primary or secondary.

1. **Primary hyperuricemia** and **gout** apparently result from an innate **defect in purine metabolism** or **uric acid excretion.** The exact cause of the defect usually is unknown.
   a. Hyperuricemia may result from **uric acid overproduction, impaired renal clearance of uric acid,** or a **combination** of these.

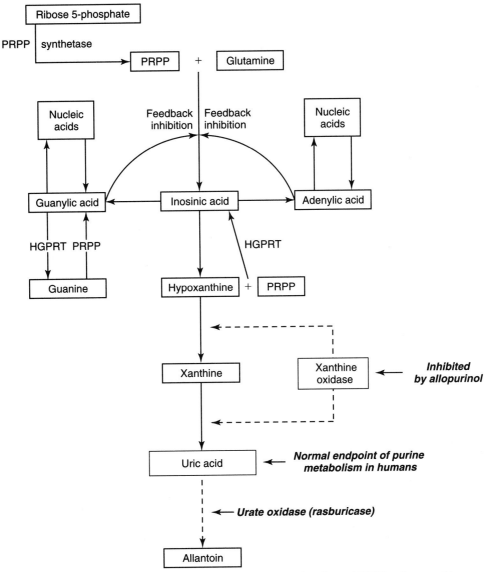

Figure 50-1. Uric acid formation. *PRPP* = phosphoribosyl-1-pyrophosphate; *HGPRT* = hypoxanthine–guanine phosphoribosyltransferase. (Adapted with permission from DiPiro J, Talbert R, Yee G, et al. *Pharmacotherapy—A Pathophysiologic Approach,* 5th ed. The McGraw-Hill Companies, 2002, p 1660.)

    b. Some patients with primary hyperuricemia and gout have a known enzymatic defect, such as hypoxanthine-guanine phosphoribosyltransferase (HGPRT) deficiency or phosphoribosyl-1-pyrophosphate (PRPP) synthetase excess (see Figure 50-1).

    c. Principally for therapeutic purposes, patients with primary hyperuricemia and gout can be classified as **overproducers** or **underexcretors** of uric acid.

        (1) Overproducers (about 10% of patients) synthesize abnormally large amounts of uric acid and excrete excessive amounts—more than 800–1000 mg daily on an unrestricted diet or more than 600 mg daily on a purine-restricted diet. These individuals generally have a markedly increased miscible urate pool (greater than 2.5 g).

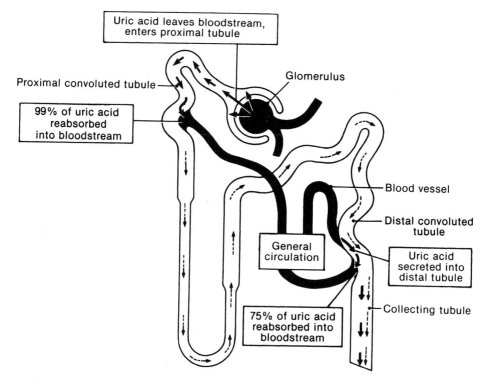

Figure 50-2. Uric acid filtration, reabsorption, and secretion sites. At the glomerulus, uric acid is filtered and enters the proximal tubule. Here, approximately 99% of uric acid is reabsorbed into the bloodstream. At the distal tubule, uric acid is secreted; subsequently, about 75% of the amount secreted is reabsorbed. Therefore, almost all urinary uric acid is excreted at the distal tubule.

       (2) Underexcretors (about 90% of patients) generally produce normal or nearly normal amounts of uric acid but excrete less than 600 mg daily on a purine-restricted diet. They generally have only a slightly increased miscible urate pool. Some underexcretors are also overproducers.

  2. Secondary hyperuricemia and **gout** develop during the course of another disease or as a result of drug therapy.

    a. Hematological causes of hyperuricemia and gout (associated with increased nucleic acid turnover and breakdown to uric acid)

      (1) Lymphoproliferative disorders

      (2) Myeloproliferative disorders

      (3) Certain hemolytic anemias and hemoglobinopathies

    b. Chronic renal failure. In this condition, reduced renal clearance of uric acid can lead to hyperuricemia.

    c. Drug-induced disease

      (1) Aspirin and **other salicylates** inhibit tubular secretion of uric acid when given in low doses (e.g., less than 2 g/day of aspirin). At high doses, these substances frequently cause uricosuria.

      (2) Cytotoxic drugs increase uric acid concentrations by enhancing nucleic acid turnover and excretion.

      (3) Diuretics (except spironolactone) may cause hyperuricemia; most likely, this occurs either via volume depletion, which, in turn, increases proximal tubular reabsorption, or via impaired tubular secretion of uric acid.

      (4) Ethambutol and **nicotinic acid** increase uric acid concentrations by competing with urate for tubular secretion sites, thereby decreasing uric acid excretion.

      (5) Cyclosporine decreases renal urate clearance, as do pyrazinamide and levodopa.

      (6) Ethanol alters uric acid metabolism both by **increasing uric acid production** through an increase in adenine nucleotide catabolism and by **suppressing renal uric acid excretion** as a result of lactate inhibition of renal tubular uric acid secretion.

    d. Miscellaneous disorders. Diabetic ketoacidosis, psoriasis, and chronic lead poisoning are examples of conditions that may cause hyperuricemia.

E. Pathophysiology

1. Gouty arthritis develops when **monosodium urate crystals** are deposited in the synovium of involved joints.

2. An **inflammatory response** to monosodium urate crystals leads to an attack of acute gouty arthritis; painful joint swelling is characterized by redness, warmth, and tenderness. A systemic reaction may accompany joint symptoms.

3. If gout progresses untreated, **tophi,** or **tophaceous deposits** (deposits of monosodium urate crystals) eventually lead to joint deformity and disability; kidney involvement may lead to renal impairment. However, these developments are uncommon in the general gout population and represent late complications of hyperuricemia.

4. **Renal complications** of hyperuricemia and gout can have serious consequences.
   a. Acute tubular obstruction. This complication may develop secondary to uric acid precipitation in the collecting tubules and ureters, with subsequent blockage and renal failure. It is most common in patients with gout secondary to myeloproliferative or lymphoproliferative disorders—particularly after chemotherapy when allopurinol is omitted. Another agent, urate oxidase (Rasburicase), may be used in the prophylaxis and treatment of hyperuricemia in pediatric patients with leukemia, lymphoma, and solid-tumor malignancies who are receiving anticancer therapy. This agent works by converting uric acid into allantoin, which is five times more soluble in urine than uric acid.
   b. Urolithiasis. Occurring in about 20% of gout patients, urolithiasis is characterized by formation of uric acid stones in the urinary tract. Low urine pH seems to be a contributing factor. The risk of urolithiasis rises as serum and urinary uric acid levels increase.
   c. Chronic urate nephropathy. In this complication, urate deposits arise in the renal interstitium. Most clinicians agree, however, that chronic hyperuricemia rarely, if ever, leads to clinically significant nephropathy. The presence of concomitant disease (e.g., diabetes mellitus, hypertension) may explain the finding of nephropathy in gout patients.

F. Clinical presentation. Clinical evaluation and the need for intervention depend on the clinical presentation.

1. **Asymptomatic hyperuricemia**

2. **Acute gouty arthritis**

3. **Intercritical gout**

4. **Chronic tophaceous gout**

II. ASYMPTOMATIC HYPERURICEMIA is characterized by an elevated serum uric acid level but has no signs or symptoms of deposition disease (arthritis, tophi, or urolithiasis).

A. Clinical presentation. No definitive evidence indicates that asymptomatic hyperuricemia is harmful. Serum urate levels of up to 13 mg/dl in men and 10 mg/L in women have not been shown to cause a deterioration in renal function. Clinicians cannot predict which asymptomatic patients will develop gout symptoms or hyperuricemia-related complications. However, the risk of symptom development and complications increases as the serum uric acid level rises.

B. Therapy. Asymptomatic hyperuricemia does not have any adverse effects before the development of gout. Therefore, **drug treatment is not required,** although it is prudent to determine the causes of the hyperuricemia and correct them, if possible. **Supportive interventions** may include maintenance of adequate urine output (to prevent uric acid stone formation), avoidance of high purine foods, and regular medical appointments to monitor the serum uric acid level and check for clinical evidence of deposition disease.

III. ACUTE GOUTY ARTHRITIS. This clinical presentation of gout is characterized by **painful arthritic attacks** of sudden onset.

A. Pathogenesis. Monosodium urate crystals form in articular tissues; this process sets off an inflammatory reaction. Trauma, exposure to cold, or another triggering event may be involved in the development of the acute attack.

B. Signs and symptoms

1. The **initial attack** is abrupt, usually occurring at night or in the early morning as synovial fluid is reabsorbed. This severe arthritic pain progressively worsens and generally involves only one or a few joints.
    a. The **affected joints** typically become hot, swollen, and extremely tender. Seventeenth-century British physician Thomas Sydenham described his personal experience with gout this way: "Now it is a violent stretching and tearing of the ligaments—now, it is a gnawing pain and now a pressure and tightening. So exquisite and lively . . . is the feeling of the part affected, that it cannot bear the weight of bedclothes nor the jar of a person walking in the room."
    b. The **most common site** of the initial attack is the first metatarsophalangeal joint; an attack there is known as **podagra.** Other sites that may be affected include the instep, ankle, heel, knee, wrist, elbow, and fingers.

2. The first few untreated attacks typically last 3–14 days. Later attacks may affect more joints and take several weeks to resolve.

3. During recovery, as edema subsides, local desquamation and pruritus may occur.

4. **Systemic symptoms** during an acute attack may include fever, chills, and malaise.

C. Diagnostic criteria

1. **Definitive diagnosis** of gouty arthritis can be made by demonstration of **monosodium urate crystals** in the synovial fluid of affected joints. These needle-shaped crystals are termed negatively birefringent when viewed through a polarized light microscope.

2. **Serum analysis** usually reveals an above-normal uric acid level; however, this finding is not specific for acute gout. Other **common serum findings** include leukocytosis and a moderately elevated erythrocyte sedimentation rate.

3. A **dramatic therapeutic response to colchicine** may be helpful in establishing the diagnosis, but this is not absolute because other causes of acute arthritis may respond as well.

4. When fluid cannot be aspirated from the affected joint, a **diagnosis of gout is supported by:**
    a. A prior history of **acute monarticular arthritis** (especially of the big toe) followed by a **symptom-free period**
    b. The presence of **hyperuricemia**
    c. Rapid **resolution of symptoms after colchicine** therapy

5. **Other conditions** that may **mimic** gout may include pseudogout (calcium pyrophosphate dihydrate crystal disease) or septic arthritis.

D. Treatment goals

1. To relieve pain and inflammation

2. To terminate the acute attack

3. To restore normal function to the affected joints

E. Therapy

1. **General therapeutic principles**
    a. The affected joint (or joints) should be immobilized.
    b. Anti-inflammatory drug therapy should begin immediately. For maximal therapeutic effectiveness, these drugs should be kept on hand so that the patient may begin therapy as soon as a subsequent attack begins.
    c. Urate-lowering drugs should not be given until the acute attack is controlled, as these drugs may prolong the attack by causing a change in uric acid equilibrium.

2. **Specific drugs.** Any of the following agents may be used:
    a. **Nonsteroidal anti-inflammatory drugs (NSAIDs)**
        (1) **Indications.** Most physicians consider these drugs the agents of choice, especially the newer NSAIDs. These drugs may be preferred when treatment is delayed significantly after symptom onset or when the patient cannot tolerate the adverse GI effects of colchicine.

(a) **Indomethacin** (Indocin) is usually given in a dose of 50 mg three times daily until pain is tolerable; then rapidly reduce the dose to complete cessation of the drug. Definite relief of pain usually occurs within 2–4 hours. Tenderness and heat usually subside in 24–36 hours, and swelling gradually disappears in 3–5 days. Do not use the sustained-release dosage form.

(b) **Other NSAIDs,** such as **naproxen** (Naprosyn) 750 mg followed by 250 mg every 8 hours until the attack subsides or **sulindac** (Clinoril) 200 mg twice a day to start and reducing dose with satisfactory response (7 days of therapy usually adequate), are specifically approved for this indication, but many other NSAIDs have been used successfully. There is no evidence that any particular NSAID is more effective than others in the treatment of an acute gouty attack.

(2) Precautions and monitoring effects

(a) **Adverse effects of indomethacin** usually are dose-related. These effects occur in 10%–60% of patients and may warrant drug discontinuation. They primarily include GI complaints of nausea and abdominal discomfort and central nervous system (CNS) effects of headaches and dizziness. Indomethacin should be taken with food or milk to minimize gastric mucosal irritation.

(b) **Precautions.** NSAIDs, in general, require cautious use in patients with a history of hypertension, CHF, peptic ulcer disease, or mild to moderate renal failure.

b. Colchicine. The traditional drug for relieving pain and inflammation and ending the acute attack, colchicine is most effective when initiated 12–36 hours after symptoms begin (the period of maximal leukocyte migration).

(1) Mechanism of action. Colchicine apparently **impairs leukocyte migration** to inflammed areas and disrupts urate deposition and the subsequent inflammatory response.

(2) Dosage and administration

(a) **Oral regimen**

(i) The effective dose of colchicine in patients with acute gout is close to that which causes GI symptoms. The drug usually is administered orally in a dose of 1 mg initially, followed by 0.5 mg every 2 hours until pain relief occurs or abdominal discomfort or diarrhea develops or a total dose of 8 mg has been administered. Except in patients who have renal or hepatic dysfunction or are elderly and frail, colchicine given in this way is safe, although it entails some discomfort for the patient.

(ii) Most patients have some pain relief by 18 hours and diarrhea by 24 hours; joint inflammation subsides gradually within 48 hours for 75%–80% of patients.

(iii) During **subsequent attacks,** patients may receive half of the total dose administered for the initial attack, then receive the remaining half as 0.5 mg every 1–2 hours.

(b) **Intravenous (IV) regimen.** This route is used rarely now but has advantages when NSAIDs are contraindicated or when patients cannot take oral medications.

(i) A single dose of 2 mg usually is given in 30 ml of normal saline solution and infused slowly over 5 minutes. Two additional doses of 1 mg each may be given at 6-hour intervals, but the total dose should never exceed 4 mg. The doses should be reduced by at least 50% in patients with hepatic or renal disease or in elderly patients. Because it causes tissue irritation, colchicine should **never be given intramuscularly or subcutaneously.**

(ii) IV administration may relieve acute gouty arthritis more rapidly than oral administration. However, severe toxicity may occur without warning because the early signs of toxicity (e.g., GI hypermobility) may not occur.

(3) Precautions and monitoring effects

(a) **GI distress** (e.g., nausea, abdominal cramps, diarrhea) occurs in up to 80% of patients receiving oral colchicine. This dosage form should be avoided in patients with peptic ulcer disease and other GI disorders.

(b) **Local extravasation** (causing local pain and necrosis) can occur with administration of IV colchicine. This risk can be reduced by use of a secure IV line.

(c) **Colchicine therapy** may cause bone marrow depression. This rare effect develops mainly in patients who receive excessive doses or who have underlying renal or hepatic disease. Excessively high acute doses (especially given intravenously) or long-term therapy may result in neurological, renal, hepatic, or other toxicity.

c. Corticosteroids

(1) Intra-articular injections of a corticosteroid are usually very effective in patients with acute monarticular gout, and their use is becoming more widespread as experience with the diagnostic aspiration of joints increases. Aspiration alone can sometimes greatly reduce the pain of gout. The appropriate dose of corticosteroids is related to the size of the joint: an intra-articular dose of **methylprednisolone acetate** (e.g., DepoMedrol) ranges from 5–10 mg (for a small joint) to 20–60 mg (for a large joint such as the knee), depending on the volume of the effusion.

(2) Systemic corticosteroid therapy is administered usually only when NSAIDs and colchicine have been ineffective or are contraindicated. There are reports of good responses, without a rebound effect, to **oral prednisone** (30–50 mg per day initially, with the dose tapered during a period of 7–10 days), **intramuscular corticotropin** (40 U) or **triamcinolone acetonide** (60 mg), or **IV methylprednisolone** (a daily dose of 50–150 mg administered during a 30-minute period, with the dose tapered over 5 days).

IV. INTERCRITICAL GOUT
is the symptom-free period after the first attack. This phase may be interrupted by the recurrence of acute attacks.

A. Onset of subsequent attacks varies.
In most patients, the second attack occurs within 1 year of the first, but in some it may be delayed for 5–10 years. A small percentage of patients never experience a second attack. If hyperuricemia is insufficiently treated, subsequent attacks may become progressively longer and more severe and may involve more than one joint.

B. Treatment goals

1. To reduce the frequency and severity of recurrent attacks

2. To minimize urate deposition in body tissues, thereby preventing progression to chronic tophaceous gout

C. Therapy.
Gout can be prevented by identifying and correcting the cause of hyperuricemia or by administering drugs that inhibit the synthesis of urate or increase its excretion.

1. Nondrug urate-reducing measures. Potentially reversible factors that contribute to increased urate production include a high-purine diet (e.g., all meats, including organ meats, seafood, beans, peas, asparagus), obesity, and regular alcohol consumption. The purine content of the diet does not usually contribute more than 1.0 mg/dl to the serum urate concentration, but moderation in dietary purine consumption should be considered. Weight reduction sometimes reduces the serum uric acid level slightly; however, "crash diets" should be avoided.

2. Prophylaxis after resolution of an acute gout attack may consist of **low-dose colchicine,** 0.5–1.0 mg daily. **Adverse effects** from colchicine at these doses are uncommon. **Low-dose NSAIDs** may also be used, but the incidence of side effects is typically higher than with low doses of colchicine.

3. Urate-reducing drug therapy. Gout may be prevented by reducing serum urate concentrations to values less than 6.0 mg/dl. A reduction to less than 5.0 mg/dl may be required for the resorption of tophi. The decision to begin drug therapy should be carefully considered, as urate-lowering drug treatment should be lifelong. Urate-reducing drugs include **uricosurics,** which increase renal uric acid excretion, and the xanthine oxidase inhibitor, **allopurinol,** which reduces uric acid production.

a. Indications for therapy with a drug that lowers serum urate concentrations should be considered when **all** of the following criteria are met:

(1) The cause of the hyperuricemia cannot be corrected or, if corrected, does not lower the serum urate concentration to less than 7.0 mg/dl.

(2) The patient has had two or three definite attacks of gout or has tophi.

(3) The patient is convinced of the need to take medication regularly and permanently.

b. Specific drugs

(1) Uricosurics include **probenecid** (Benemid) and **sulfinpyrazone** (Anturane). These drugs are preferred for underexcretors. Long-term uricosuric therapy reduces the incidence of gouty arthritis attacks, prevents formation of new tophi, and helps resolve existing tophi.

(a) Mechanism of action. Probenecid and sulfinpyrazone block uric acid reabsorption at the proximal convoluted tubule, thereby increasing the rate of uric acid excretion (see Figure 50-2).
(b) Indications. Uricosurics generally are used to reduce hyperuricemia in patients who excrete less than 600 mg of uric acid per day.
(c) Dosage and administration
　　(i) Probenecid is given initially in two daily oral doses of 250 mg for 1 week, then increased to 500 mg twice daily every 1–2 weeks until the serum uric acid level drops below 6 mg/dl. Most patients respond to a dose of 1.5 g/day or less.
　　(ii) Sulfinpyrazone is given initially in two daily oral doses of 50 mg, then increased by 100 mg weekly. Most patients respond to a dose of 200 mg/day or less.
(d) Precautions and monitoring effects
　　(i) Uricosuric therapy should not be initiated during an acute gout attack. During the first 6–12 months of therapy, these drugs may increase the frequency, severity, and duration of acute attacks (by changing the equilibrium of body urate). Therefore, some clinicians administer prophylactic colchicine concomitantly during the early months of uricosuric therapy.
　　(ii) The **risk** is **minimized** by concurrently administering prophylactic drugs (see IV C 2), delaying urate-lowering therapy until several weeks after the last attack of gout, and starting therapy with a low dose of the drug that is chosen. When used concurrently with urate-lowering drugs, colchicine may be discontinued after the serum urate level becomes normal and is stable for 2 or 3 months.
　　(iii) Patients should maintain a **high fluid intake** (at least 2 L/day) and a high urine output during uricosuric therapy to decrease renal urate precipitation. The **greatest potential risks** of therapy with uricosuric drugs are the formation of **uric acid crystals** in urine and the deposition of **uric acid** in the **renal tubules, pelvis,** or **ureter,** causing renal colic or the deterioration of renal function. These risks can be reduced by initiating therapy with a low dose and increasing the dose slowly and by maintaining a high urine volume (preferably of alkaline urine, which can be achieved with 1 g of sodium bicarbonate taken 3–4 daily; plus a high fluid intake of at least 2 L/day), particularly during the early weeks of therapy.
　　(iv) Uricosurics are **contraindicated** in patients with urinary tract stones.
　　(v) These drugs generally are ineffective in patients with creatinine clearances below 50–60 ml/min.
　　(vi) Aspirin and **other salicylates** antagonize the action of uricosurics.
　　(vii) Probenecid is well tolerated by most patients, but it occasionally causes **adverse effects** [e.g., GI distress (8%), hypersensitivity reactions (5%)].
　　(viii) Sulfinpyrazone causes GI distress in 10%–15% of patients. Hypersensitivity reactions occur rarely. Sulfinpyrazone reduces platelet adhesiveness and may cause blood dyscrasias; periodic blood counts should be done.
(2) The only **xanthine oxidase inhibitor** available is **allopurinol.**
　(a) Mechanism of action. Allopurinol and its long-acting metabolite, oxypurinol, block the final steps in uric acid synthesis by inhibiting xanthine oxidase, an enzyme that converts xanthine to uric acid. Thus, the drug reduces the serum uric acid level while increasing the renal excretion of the more soluble oxypurine precursors; this decreases the risk of uric acid stones and nephropathy.
　(b) Indications. Allopurinol is considered by many to be the drug of choice for lowering uric acid levels because of its effectiveness in both underexcretors and overproducers, but it is specifically the preferred urate-reducing agent for patients in the following categories:
　　(i) Patients who are clearly overproducers (overexcretors) of uric acid
　　(ii) Patients with recurrent tophaceous deposits or uric acid stones
　　(iii) Patients with renal impairment (but dose needs to be decreased)
　(c) Dosage and administration. Allopurinol is given initially in a daily dose of 100–300 mg (preferably as a single dose), then increased in weekly increments if needed. Typically, the uric acid level starts to fall after 1–2 days with maximal effect for a given dose in 7–10 days. A dose of 300 mg/day reduces serum urate

concentrations to normal values in 85% of patients with gout. A normal dose of 300 mg/day for a patient with normal renal function should be decreased to 200 mg/day for a patient with a CrCl of 60 ml/min and decreased to 100 mg/day for a patient with a CrCl of 30 ml/min.

   (d) **Precautions and monitoring effects.** Allopurinol is generally well-tolerated.

      (i) A **rash** develops in approximately 2% of patients treated with allopurinol and in approximately 20% of those receiving both allopurinol and ampicillin. The rash usually subsides after the allopurinol has been discontinued and may not recur if therapy is resumed with a lower dose.

      (ii) The most serious side effect of allopurinol, which occurs in less than 1 in 1000 cases, is **exfoliative dermatitis,** often with vasculitis, fever, liver dysfunction, eosinophilia, and acute interstitial nephritis. Up to 20% of patients with this type of reaction become very sick. It is more likely to occur in patients with renal disease or those receiving diuretic therapy. Prednisone seems to be effective in such patients, but the discontinuation of allopurinol and the use of supportive therapy may be sufficient in cases that are not severe.

      (iii) Allopurinol may induce more frequent acute gout attacks. This risk can be minimized by administration of low doses and concurrent colchicine therapy.

V. CHRONIC TOPHACEOUS GOUT.

This rare clinical presentation may develop if hyperuricemia and gout remain untreated for many years.

   A. **Pathogenesis.** Persistent hyperuricemia leads to the development of tophi in the synovia, olecranon bursae, and various periarticular locations. Eventually, articular cartilage may be destroyed, resulting in joint deformities, bone erosions, deposition of tophi within tissues, and renal disease.

   B. **Clinical evaluation**

      1. Patients may develop large subcutaneous tophi in the pinna of the external ear (the classic site) as well as in other locations.

      2. Typically, the urate pool is many times the normal size.

   C. **Therapy.** Allopurinol and probenecid may be given in combination to treat severe cases.

STUDY QUESTIONS

Directions: Each of the numbered items or incomplete statements in this section is followed by answers or by completions of the statement. Select the **one** lettered answer or completion that is **best** in each case.

1. All of the following statements concerning an acute gouty arthritis attack are correct EXCEPT

(A) the diagnosis of gout is assured by a good therapeutic response to colchicine because no other form of arthritis responds to this drug
(B) to be assured of the diagnosis, monosodium urate crystals must be identified in the synovial fluid of the affected joint
(C) attacks frequently occur in the middle of the night
(D) an untreated attack may last up to 2 weeks
(E) the first attack usually involves only one joint, most frequently the big toe (first metatarsophalangeal joint)

2. A 42-year-old obese man has been diagnosed with gout. He has had three acute attacks this year, and his uric acid level is presently 11.5 mg/dl (upper limit of normal is 7 mg/dl). He has no other diseases. Rational treatment of this patient during the interval period between gouty attacks might include any of the following EXCEPT

(A) acetaminophen or aspirin 650 mg as needed for joint pain
(B) probenecid
(C) colchicine
(D) allopurinol
(E) a decrease in caloric intake

3. A 45-year-old man is admitted to the hospital with the diagnosis of an acute attack of gout. His serum uric acid is 10.5 mg/dl (normal is 3–7 mg/dl). Which of the following would be the most effective initial treatment plan?

(A) Before treating this patient, immobilize the affected joint and obtain a 24-hour urinary uric acid level to determine which drug, either allopurinol or probenecid, would be the best agent to initiate therapy.
(B) Begin oral colchicine 1 mg initially, followed by 0.5 mg every 2 hours until relief is obtained, gastrointestinal distress occurs, or a maximum of 8 mg has been taken; also, begin probenecid 250 mg twice a day concurrently.
(C) Administer oral indomethacin 50 mg three times a day for 2 days; then gradually taper the dose over the next few days.
(D) Administer oral naproxen 750 mg, followed by 250 mg every 8 hours for 3 weeks.
(E) Give colchicine 0.5 mg intramuscularly followed by 1 mg intravenously piggyback every 12 hours for 2 weeks.

Directions: The question below contains three suggested answers, of which **one or more** is correct. Choose the answer

A   if **I only** is correct
B   if **III only** is correct
C   if **I and II** are correct
D   if **II and III** are correct
E   if **I, II, and III** are correct

4. Allopurinol is recommended rather than probenecid in the treatment of hyperuricemia in which of the following situations?

I. When the patient has several large tophi on the elbows and knees
II. When the patient has an estimated creatinine clearance of 15 ml/min
III. When the patient has leukemia and there is concern regarding renal precipitation of urate

ANSWERS AND EXPLANATIONS

1. The answer is A *[III B 1, 2, C 1, 3].*
Other forms of acute arthritis may respond to colchicine, so that the diagnosis of gout cannot be established unequivocally by a good response to this agent. A definitive diagnosis requires the presence of urate crystals in the affected joint, although the presence of other symptoms or laboratory findings may suggest a probable diagnosis of gout.

2. The answer is A *[I D 2 c (1); IV C].*
Aspirin in doses less than 2 g/day can inhibit uric acid secretion. Weight reduction, allopurinol, or probenecid to lower the serum uric acid levels, and prophylactic colchicine are all appropriate interventions in the interval phase to reduce the incidence of acute gouty attacks.

3. The answer is C *[III E 1 c, 2 a, 3 b (1) (d) (i); IV C].*
Of the selections, the most effective initial plan in treating an acute attack of gout is to administer indomethacin orally, giving 50 mg three times a day for 2–3 days, then gradually tapering the dosage over the next few days. Even though joint immobilization is an appropriate initial step, drugs for pain relief should be administered as soon as possible. Uric acid modification therapy (allopurinol or probenecid) should not be initiated until the acute attack is under control. Initiating therapy with probenecid at this point may prolong the resolution of an acute attack of gouty arthritis, which can usually be accomplished within 7 days of NSAID therapy. Colchicine should never be given intramuscularly because it causes tissue irritation.

4. The answer is E (all) *[IV C].*
In the treatment of hyperuricemia, allopurinol is indicated rather than probenecid when large tophi are present, when the creatinine clearance is less than 50–60 ml/min (probenecid would be ineffective, but allopurinol dosage would have to be decreased), when the patient is an overproducer of uric acid, and when there is a need to prevent the formation of large amounts of uric acid (e.g., when conditions such as leukemia are present).

51
Peptic Ulcer Disease and Related Acid-Associated Disorders

Paul F. Souney
Anthony E. Zimmermann

I. INTRODUCTION

A. Definition

1. **Peptic ulcer disease** (PUD) refers to a group of disorders characterized by circumscribed lesions of the mucosa of the upper gastrointestinal (GI) tract (particularly the stomach and duodenum). The lesions occur in regions exposed to gastric juices.

2. **Gastroesophageal reflux disease (GERD)** refers to the retrograde movement of gastric contents from the stomach into the esophagus. Reflux may occur without consequences and thus be considered a normal physiological process, or it may lead to profound symptomatic or histological conditions (e.g., GERD). When reflux leads to inflammation (with or without erosions or ulcerations) of the esophagus, it is called **reflux (erosive) esophagitis.** Most patients (50%–70%) report typical symptoms but lack evidence of esophageal mucosal injury **(nonerosive reflux disease, or NERD).**

3. **Dyspepsia** is defined as persistent or recurrent abdominal pain or abdominal discomfort centered in the upper abdomen.

B. Manifestations

1. **Duodenal ulcers** almost always develop in the duodenal bulb (the first few centimeters of the duodenum). A few, however, arise between the bulb and the ampulla.

2. **Gastric ulcers** form most commonly in the antrum or at the antral–fundal junction.

3. **Less common forms of peptic ulcer disease**
   a. **Stress ulcers** result from serious trauma or illness, major burns, coagulopathy not related to anticoagulant therapy, need for mechanical ventilation >48 hours, or ongoing sepsis. The **most common site** of stress ulcer formation is the proximal portion of the stomach.
   b. **Zollinger-Ellison syndrome** is a severe form of peptic ulcer disease in which intractable ulcers are accompanied by extreme gastric hyperacidity and at least one gastrinoma (a non–β-islet cell tumor of the pancreas or another site).
   c. **Stomal ulcers** (also called marginal ulcers) may arise at the anastomosis or immediately distal to it in the small intestine in patients who have undergone ulcer surgery and have experienced subsequent ulcer recurrence after a symptom-free period.
   d. **Drug-associated ulcers** occur in patients who chronically ingest substances that damage the gastric mucosa, such as nonsteroidal anti-inflammatory drugs (NSAIDs).

4. **Reflux esophagitis** is most often recognized by the presence of recurrent symptoms (e.g., heartburn) or altered epithelial morphology visualized radiologically, endoscopically, or histologically. Heartburn is substernal burning or regurgitation that may radiate to the neck. Other symptoms include belching, water brash, chest pain, asthma, chronic cough, hoarseness, and laryngitis. Endoscopic evaluation detected **Barrett's esophagus** in 6% of patients with frequent heartburn. Barrett's esophagus is a premalignant condition that may lead to adenocarcinoma of the esophagus or esophagogastric junction.

C. Epidemiology

1. **Incidence.** Peptic ulcer disease is the most common disorder of the upper GI tract.
   a. **Duodenal ulcers** affect approximately 4%–10% of the United States population; **gastric ulcers** occur in approximately 0.03%–0.05% of the population.

b. Nearly 80% of peptic ulcers are duodenal; the others are gastric ulcers.

c. Most duodenal ulcers appear in people between age 20 and 50; onset of gastric ulcers usually occurs between age 45 and 55.

d. The 1-year point prevalence of active gastric or duodenal ulcer in the United States in men and women is about 1.8%; the lifetime prevalence of peptic ulcer ranges from 11%–14% for men and 8%–11% for women.

e. Approximately 10%–20% of gastric ulcer patients also have a concurrent duodenal ulcer.

f. In the United States, 44% of the adult population experience **heartburn** at least once a month; 14% take some type of "indigestion" medication at least twice a week. Of patients with GERD symptoms who have undergone endoscopy, 50%–65% have apparent esophagitis.

g. The annual prevalence of dyspepsia in Western countries is approximately 25%; 2%–5% of primary care consultations are for dyspepsia.

2. Hospitalization

a. Hospitalization rates in the United States for peptic ulcers have been declining; these rates dropped from 25.2 per 10,000 in 1965 to 16.5 per 10,000 in 1981. This reflects a decrease in hospitalization for uncomplicated cases due to increased outpatient diagnosis and treatment. There has been little change in hospitalization rates since then.

b. There has been little or no decrease in duodenal ulcer perforations and only a slight decrease in hemorrhages.

3. Mortality

a. The mortality rate for gastric ulcers declined between 1962 and 1979 from 3.5 per 100,000 to 1.1 per 100,000.

b. For duodenal ulcer, the mortality rate declined from 3.1 per 100,000 to 0.9 per 100,000.

c. Although death from GERD is uncommon, morbidity is not, because of the prevalence of the well-recognized complications such as esophageal ulceration (5%), stricture formation (4%–20%), and the development of Barrett's columnar-lined esophagus (8%–20%).

D. Description

1. Ulcer size. The average duodenal ulcer typically has a diameter of less than 1 cm; most gastric ulcers are somewhat larger (1–2.5 cm in diameter).

2. Most ulcers are sharply demarcated and have a round, oval, or elliptical shape.

3. The mucosa surrounding the ulcer typically is inflamed and edematous.

4. Ulcers penetrate the **muscularis propria** and, in some cases, extend into the serosa or even into the pancreas.

5. Fibrous tissue, granulation tissue, and necrotic debris form the ulcer base. During ulcer healing, a scar forms as epithelium from the edges covers the ulcer surface.

6. Nearly all duodenal ulcers are benign; up to 10% of gastric ulcers are malignant.

E. Etiology. The two major observations regarding peptic ulcer disease are the causal relationship among NSAID intake, gastroduodenal mucosal injury, the pathogenesis of gastric ulcer and, to a lesser extent, duodenal ulcer, and the association of ***Helicobacter pylori*** infection in the pathogenesis of duodenal ulcer (and to a lesser extent, gastric ulcer).

1. ***H. pylori*** (formerly *Campylobacter pylori*) is a gram-negative microaerophilic, spiral bacterium with multiple flagella that lives and infects the gastric mucosa. This bacterium is able to survive in the acidic gastric environment by its ability to produce urease, which hydrolyzes urea into ammonia. Ammonia neutralizes gastric hydrochloric acid (HCl), creating a neutral cloud surrounding the organism.

a. In the United States, the **prevalence** of *H. pylori* increases with age from approximately 10% at 20 years of age to approximately 50% at 60 years of age; approximately 17% of *H. pylori*–positive individuals will develop a duodenal ulcer. Prevalence is higher in developing countries.

b. *H. pylori* is associated with several common GI disorders.

(1) Always present in the setting of active chronic gastritis

(2) Present in the vast majority of duodenal (more than 90%) and gastric (60%–90%) ulcers. Recent studies indicate a decline in the prevalence of *H. pylori* in duodenal ulcer patients.

(3) Sometimes present with non-ulcer dyspepsia (probably in 50% of cases); eradication of *H. pylori,* when present, leads to symptom improvement in only about one-half of treated patients.

(4) In gastric cancer, 85%–95% (Although the association is strong, no causal relationship has yet been proven in gastric cancer. The World Health Organization has classified *H. pylori* as a Group 1 carcinogen.)

c. *H. pylori* **eradication** can cure peptic ulcers and reduce ulcer recurrence; it can eliminate the need for maintenance therapy in many ulcer patients.

2. **Genetic factors**
   a. The lifetime prevalence of developing an ulcer in **first-degree relatives** of ulcer patients is about threefold greater than in the general population. This may be secondary to clustering of *H. pylori* within families.
   b. People with **blood type O** have an above-normal incidence of duodenal ulcers.

3. **Smoking.** Smokers have an increased risk of developing peptic ulcer disease. In addition, cigarette smoking delays ulcer healing and increases the risk and rapidity of relapse after the ulcer heals. Nicotine decreases biliary and pancreatic bicarbonate secretion. Smoking also accelerates the emptying of stomach acid into the duodenum.

4. **NSAIDs.** When ingested chronically, aspirin, indomethacin, and other NSAIDs promote gastric ulcer formation.
   a. These drugs may injure the gastric mucosa by allowing back-diffusion of hydrogen ions into the mucosa.
   b. NSAIDs also inhibit the synthesis of prostaglandins, which are substances with a cytoprotective effect on the mucosa.
   c. Selective COX-2 inhibitors, celecoxib or rofecoxib, are associated with fewer ulcers than nonselective NSAIDs, with rates comparable to placebo at 3 months. Questions regarding long-term safety of COX-2 inhibitors remain. With the recent documentation of increasing COX-2 expression with the progression of Barrett's esophagus (BE) to cancer, trials have been initiated using COX-2 selective inhibitors in BE patients to prevent development of cancer.

5. **Alcohol.** A known mucosal irritant, alcohol causes marked irritation of the gastric mucosa if ingested in large quantities at concentrations of 20% or greater. The only association between ethanol intake and ulcer disease exists in patients with portal cirrhosis.

6. **Coffee.** Both regular and decaffeinated coffee contains peptides that stimulate release of gastrin, a hormone that triggers the flow of gastric juice. However, a direct link between coffee and peptic ulcer disease has not been proven.

7. **Corticosteroids.** Controversy over whether systemic corticosteroid therapy is associated with increased risk for the development of peptic ulcer disease has, for the most part, been resolved. Evidence for this direct association has always been weak in previous retrospective reviews/trials and reflected the concurrent use of an NSAID. Current data support no link between steroids and peptic ulcer disease in the absence of concurrent NSAID use.

8. **Associated disorders.** Peptic ulcer disease is more common in patients with hyperparathyroidism, emphysema, rheumatoid arthritis, and alcoholic cirrhosis.

9. **Advanced age.** Degeneration of the pylorus permits bile reflux into the stomach, creating an environment that favors ulcer formation.

10. **Psychological factors.** Once assigned key roles in the pathogenesis of peptic ulcer disease, stress and personality type now are viewed as relatively minor influences.

F. Pathophysiology. Ulcers develop when an imbalance exists between factors that protect gastric mucosa and factors that promote mucosal corrosion. Approximately 90% of patients with duodenal ulcer and 70% of patients with gastric ulcer have *H. pylori* infection.

1. **Protective factors**
   a. Normally, the mucosa secretes a thick mucus that serves as a barrier between luminal acid and epithelial cells. This barrier slows the inward movement of hydrogen ions and allows their neutralization by bicarbonate ions in fluids secreted by the stomach and duodenum.

b. Alkaline and neutral pancreatic biliary juices also help buffer acid entering the duodenum from the stomach.

c. An **intact mucosal barrier** prevents back-diffusion of gastric acids into mucosal cells. It also has the capacity to stimulate local blood flow, which brings nutrients and other substances to the area and removes toxic substances (e.g., hydrogen ions). Mucosal integrity also promotes cell growth and repair after local trauma.

2. **Corrosive factors.** Peptic ulcer disease reflects the inability of the gastric mucosa to resist corrosion by irritants, such as pepsin, HCl, and other gastric secretions.
    a. Exposure to gastric acid and **pepsin** is necessary for ulcer development.
    b. Disrupted mucosal barrier integrity allows gastric acids to diffuse from the lumen back into mucosal cells, where they cause injury.

3. **Physiological defects associated with peptic ulcer disease.** Researchers have identified various physiological defects in patients with duodenal and gastric ulcers.
    a. Duodenal ulcer patients may have the following defects:
       (1) Increased capacity for gastric acid secretion
          (a) Some duodenal ulcer patients have up to twice the normal number of parietal cells (which produce HCl).
          (b) Nearly 70% of duodenal ulcer patients have elevated serum levels of **pepsinogen I** and a corresponding increase in pepsin-secreting capacity.
       (2) Increased parietal cell responsiveness to gastrin
       (3) Above-normal postprandial gastrin secretion
       (4) Defective inhibition of gastrin release at low pH, possibly leading to failure to suppress postprandial acid secretion
       (5) Above-normal rate of gastric emptying, resulting in delivery of a greater acid load to the duodenum
    b. Gastric ulcer patients typically exhibit the following characteristics:
       (1) Deficient gastric mucosal resistance, direct mucosal injury, or both
       (2) Elevated serum gastrin levels (in acid hyposecretors)
       (3) Decreased pyloric pressure at rest and in response to acid or fat in the duodenum
       (4) Delayed gastric emptying
       (5) Increased reflux of bile and other duodenal contents
       (6) Subnormal mucosal levels of prostaglandins (these levels normalize once the ulcer heals)

4. **GERD** requires both initiation and perpetuation of the reflux of gastric contents. Esophagitis develops when noxious substances in the refluxate (i.e., acid, pepsin) are in contact with the esophageal mucosa long enough to cause irritation and inflammation.
    a. In patients with GERD, 65% of reflux events occur via transient lower esophageal sphincter (LES) relaxation (TLESR). The main difference between normal individuals and those with GERD is the frequency of TLESR. GERD patients have more frequent and prolonged TLESR. TLESR represents a decrease in LES pressure that is not associated with swallowing or peristalsis.
    b. Other mechanisms of LES incompetence are increased abdominal pressure and spontaneous reflux during periods of very low LES pressure.
    c. Such motility problems are permissive; that is, they allow reflux of acid and other noxious substances.

5. Many diseases cause dyspeptic symptoms, including PUD, GERD, gastric cancer, and biliary tract disease. However, in many cases, no clear pathological reason for a patient's symptoms can be determined. Dyspepsia in the absence of an identifiable organic cause is frequently described as "functional" or "non-ulcer" dyspepsia.

G. Clinical presentation. Signs and symptoms of PUD vary with the patient's age and the location of the lesion. Only about 50% of patients experience classic ulcer symptoms. The remainder are asymptomatic or report vague or atypical symptoms.

1. **Pain.** Patients typically describe heartburn or a gnawing, burning, aching, or cramp-like pain. Some patients report abdominal soreness or hunger sensations. It is unclear whether peptic ulcer pain results from chemical stimulation or from spasm.
    a. Duodenal ulcer pain usually is restricted to a small, midepigastric area near the xiphoid. Pain may radiate below the costal margins into the back or the right shoulder. Pain from

a duodenal ulcer frequently awakens the patient between midnight and 2 A.M.; it is almost never present before breakfast.

b. Gastric ulcer pain is less localized. It may be referred to the left subcostal region. Gastric ulcer rarely produces nocturnal pain.

c. GERD patients most commonly present with heartburn, belching, regurgitation, or water brash; **atypical presentations** include chest pain, hoarseness/laryngitis, loss of dental enamel, asthma, chronic cough, or dyspepsia. Complications of GERD include esophageal ulceration, strictures, Barrett's esophagus, and adenocarcinoma of the esophagus or esophagogastric junction.

d. Dyspepsia applies broadly to a range of symptoms, including abdominal or retrosternal pain and discomfort, heartburn, nausea, vomiting, and other symptoms referable to the proximal GI tract.

e. Food usually relieves duodenal ulcer pain but may cause gastric ulcer pain. This finding may explain why duodenal ulcer patients tend to gain weight, whereas gastric ulcer patients may lose weight. Pain characteristically occurs 90 minutes to 3 hours after meals in duodenal ulcer patients, whereas pain in gastric ulcer patients is usually present 45–60 minutes after a meal. Food aggravates reflux disease.

2. Nausea and **vomiting** may occur with either ulcer type.

3. Disease course. Both duodenal and gastric ulcers tend to be chronic, with spontaneous remissions and exacerbations. Within a year of the initial symptoms, most patients experience a relapse.

a. In many cases, relapse is seasonal, occurring more often in the spring and autumn.

b. All patients with a confirmed duodenal or gastric ulcer should be tested for *H. pylori* infection. If the patient is *H. pylori*–positive, eradication therapy will reduce the recurrence rate significantly and preclude the need for maintenance medication.

c. GERD is also a chronic disease; most patients with reflux esophagitis who are healed with antisecretory drug therapy will experience a recurrence within 6 months of discontinuation of the healing regimen. Maintenance therapy reduces the recurrence of esophagitis.

H. Clinical evaluation

1. Physical findings. Patients with peptic ulcer disease may exhibit superficial and deep epigastric tenderness and voluntary muscle guarding. With duodenal ulcer, patients also may show unilateral spasm over the duodenal bulb. Gastric ulcer patients may have weight loss.

2. Diagnostic test results

a. Blood tests may show hypochromic anemia.

b. Stool tests may detect occult blood if the ulcer is chronic.

c. Gastric secretion tests may reveal hypersecretion of HCl in duodenal ulcer patients and normal or subnormal HCl secretion in gastric ulcer patients.

d. Upper GI series (barium x-ray) reveals the ulcer crater in up to 80% of cases. Duodenal bulb deformity suggests a duodenal ulcer.

e. Upper GI endoscopy, the most specific test, may be done if barium x-ray yields inconclusive results. This procedure confirms an ulcer in at least 95% of cases and may detect ulcers not demonstrable by radiography.

f. Biopsy might be necessary to determine whether a gastric ulcer is malignant.

g. *H. pylori* status is determined by noninvasive tests (not requiring endoscopy) or invasive methods (requiring endoscopy).

(1) Noninvasive. Serology, the test of choice when endoscopy is not indicated, is inexpensive. Several office tests are available. Breath tests can also be used to detect the organism and are uniquely suited as noninvasive means of confirming eradication of *H. pylori* after therapy. False-negative breath tests may occur in patients receiving proton pump inhibitors, antibiotics, or bismuth compounds.

(2) Invasive. These methods include histological visualization of *H. pylori* or measurement of urease activity, which require biopsy.

I. Treatment objectives

1. Relieve pain and other symptoms and promote healing

2. Prevent complications

3. Minimize recurrence (eradicate *H. pylori* in PUD)

4. Maintain adequate nutrition

5. Teach the patient about the disease to improve therapeutic compliance

6. Maintain the patient symptom free

II. THERAPY

A. **Drug therapy.** Peptic ulcer patients usually are treated with antacids, histamine$_2$ (H$_2$)-receptor antagonists, or proton pump inhibitors; other drugs are added as necessary. Drug regimens that suppress nocturnal acid secretion are found to result in the highest duodenal ulcer healing rates. Drug therapy typically provides prompt symptomatic relief and promotes ulcer healing within 4–6 weeks (Figure 51-1). GERD management requires more aggressive acid sup-

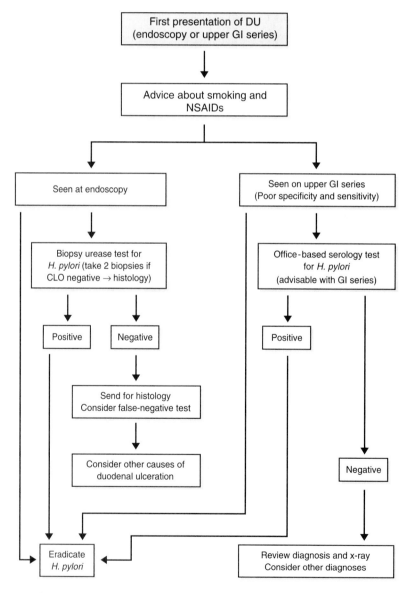

Figure 51-1. Treatment strategy for management of duodenal ulcer.

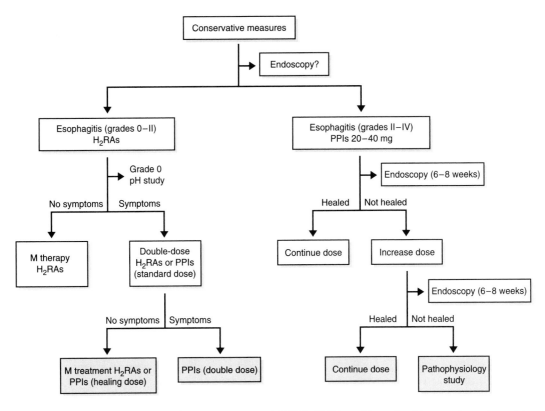

Figure 51-2. Treatment strategy for management of GERD. H_2RAs = histamine H_2-receptor antagonists; *PPI* = proton pump inhibitor; *M* = maintenance.

pression regimens; the pharmacodynamic end point is to maintain the pH in the esophagus at 4 or more (Figure 51-2).

1. **Antacids.** These compounds, which neutralize gastric acid, are used to treat ulcer pain and heal the ulcer. Studies show antacids and H_2-receptor antagonists to be equally effective. Antacids are available as **magnesium, aluminum, or calcium.** The most widely used antacids are mixtures of aluminum hydroxide and magnesium hydroxide (Table 51-1). Duodenal ulcers rarely occur in the absence of acid or when the hourly maximum acid output is less than 10 mEq. Peptic activity decreases as acidity decreases; experimental ulcer formation is inhibited by antacids; and acid-reducing operations cure ulcers.

   a. **Mechanism of action and therapeutic effects.** Antacids reduce the concentration and total load of acid in the gastric contents. By increasing gastric pH, antacids also inhibit pepsin activity. In addition, they strengthen the gastric mucosal barrier.

   b. **Choice of agent**

      (1) **Nonsystemic antacids** (e.g., magnesium or aluminum substances) are preferred to systemic antacids (e.g., sodium bicarbonate) for intensive ulcer therapy because they avoid the risk of alkalosis.

      (2) **Liquid antacid forms** have a greater buffering capacity than tablets. However, tablets are more convenient to carry. With either dosage form, the size and frequency of doses may limit patient compliance.

      (3) **Antacid mixtures** (e.g., aluminum hydroxide with magnesium hydroxide) provide more even, sustained action than single-agent antacids and permit a lower dosage of each compound. In addition, compounds in a mixture may interact so as to negate each other's untoward effects. For instance, the constipating effect of aluminum hydroxide may counter the diarrhea that magnesium hydroxide frequently produces.

Table 51-1. Comparison of Common Antacids

Brand Name	Acid-Neutralizing Capacity (mEq/mL or tab)	Therapeutic Amount (140 mEq) (mL or no. of tablets)	Sodium Content (mg/5 mL or tablet)
Concentrated Liquids			
Aluminum hydroxide, magnesium hydroxide			
Maalox TC	5.4	26	0.035
Aluminum hydroxide, magnesium hydroxide, simethicone			
Mylanta DS	5.0	28	0.050
Regular Liquids			
Aluminum hydroxide, magnesium hydroxide, simethicone			
Gelusil	2.4	58	0.090
Maalox Plus	2.6	54	0.040
Mylanta	2.5	56	0.030
Riopan Plus	3.0	47	0.013
Aluminum hydroxide			
Amphogel	2.0	70	0.100
Tablets			
Aluminum hydroxide, magnesium hydroxide, simethicone			
Gelusil II	21	6.7	0.00
Maalox Plus	11.4	12.2	0.00
Riopan Plus	13.5	10.4	0.00
Maalox Extra Strength	23.4	6.0	0.040
Calcium carbonate			
Tums	10.0	14	0.00
Tums E-X	15.0	9.3	0.11
Titralac	7.5	18.7	0.00
Calcium carbonate and magnesium hydroxide			
Rolaids	8.5	16.5	0.040
Mylanta Max Strength	24.0	5.8	0.026
Aluminum hydroxide			
Amphogel	16.0	8.75	0.080

(4) Calcium carbonate usually is avoided because it causes acid rebound, may delay pain relief and ulcer healing, and induces constipation. Another potential adverse effect of this compound is hypercalcemia; the risk is increased if calcium carbonate is taken with milk or another alkaline substance. The milk-alkali syndrome (i.e., hypercalcemia, alkalosis, azotemia, nephrocalcinosis) can also occur.

c. Administration and dosage

(1) Antacids differ greatly in acid-neutralizing capacity (ANC), defined as the number of milliequivalents (mEq) of a 1 N solution of HCl that can be brought to a pH of 3.5 in 15 minutes. With most duodenal ulcer patients, approximately 50 mEq/hr of available antacid is needed for ongoing neutralization of gastric contents. Therefore, the required dosage depends on the ANC of the specific antacid.

(2) In the fasting state, antacids have only a transient intragastric buffering effect (15–20 minutes). When ingested 1 hour after a meal, they have a much more prolonged effect, about 3–4 hours; therefore, they should optimally be taken 1 and 3 hours after meals and before sleep. Consequently, the typical antacid regimen calls for doses 1 and 3 hours after meals and at bedtime.

(3) Dosage

(a) Because the ANC of antacid products varies widely, no standard dosage can be given in terms of milliliters of suspension or number of tablets. However, patients with duodenal ulcers generally require individual dosages of 80–160 mEq of ANC (equivalent to 30–60 mL of Mylanta or Maalox). Thus, the total daily dosage may be as much as 420 mL of Mylanta or Maalox if the standard seven-times–daily dosing regimen is used. Because of the large doses required, increase in adverse effects, need for frequent administration, and poor patient compliance, their role in the management of PUD is limited.

(b) Antacid therapy usually continues for 6–8 weeks.

d. Precautions and monitoring effects

(1) Calcium carbonate– and magnesium-containing antacids should be used cautiously in patients with severe renal disease.

(2) Sodium bicarbonate is contraindicated in patients with hypertension, congestive heart failure (CHF), severe renal disease, and edema. It should not be used for ulcer therapy.

(3) All antacids should be used cautiously in elderly patients (particularly those with decreased GI motility) and renally impaired patients.

(4) Aluminum-containing antacids should be used cautiously in patients who suffer from dehydration or intestinal obstruction.

(5) The combination of calcium carbonate with an alkaline substance (e.g., sodium bicarbonate) and milk may cause the milk-alkali syndrome.

(6) Low-sodium antacids obviate the problem of fluid retention in hypertension and heart disease.

(7) Chronic administration of calcium carbonate–containing antacids should be avoided because of hypercalcemia and calcium ion stimulation of acid secretion.

(8) Aluminum or magnesium toxicity is unlikely in patients with normal renal function. The encephalopathy of tissue deposition of aluminum occurs only in dialysis patients receiving aluminum hydroxide for control of hyperphosphatemia. Chronic use of magnesium-containing antacids is not advisable in patients with renal insufficiency.

(9) Constipation can occur in patients using calcium carbonate– and aluminum-containing antacids.

(10) Diarrhea is a common adverse effect of magnesium-containing antacids. If diarrhea occurs, the patient may alternate the antacid mixture with aluminum hydroxide.

(11) Hypophosphatemia and osteomalacia can occur with long-term use of aluminum hydroxide, but these conditions can also occur with short-term use in severely malnourished patients, such as alcoholics.

e. Significant interactions. Because antacids alter gastric pH and affect absorption of ingested substances, they have a high potential for drug interactions. To ensure consistent absorption and therapeutic efficacy, orally administered drugs should be given 30–60 minutes before antacids.

(1) Antacids bind with **tetracycline and fluoroquinolones,** inhibiting the absorption and reducing therapeutic efficacy.

(2) Antacids may destroy the coating of **enteric-coated drugs,** leading to premature drug dissolution in the stomach.

(3) Antacids may interfere with the absorption of many drugs, including **cimetidine, ranitidine, digoxin, isoniazid, anticholinergics, iron products,** and **phenothiazines** [see II A 2 e (3)].

(4) Antacids may reduce the therapeutic effects of **sucralfate** (see II A 3 d).

2. H$_2$-receptor antagonists. These drugs may be preferred to other antiulcer agents because of their convenience and lack of effect on GI motility. Although reasonably effective in treating mild to moderate GERD symptoms, H$_2$-receptor antagonists are less reliable for healing erosive esophagitis. All current choices require multiple, divided doses for GERD management.

a. Mechanism of action and therapeutic effects. H$_2$-receptor antagonists (Table 51-2) competitively inhibit the action of histamine at parietal cell receptor sites, reducing the volume and hydrogen ion concentration of gastric acid secretions (Figure 51-3). These agonists accelerate the healing of most ulcers.

b. Choice of agent. Cimetidine, ranitidine, famotidine, or **nizatidine** may be administered to treat peptic ulcers or hypersecretory states (e.g., Zollinger-Ellison syndrome).

(1) **Cimetidine,** the first H$_2$-receptor antagonist approved for clinical use, reduces gastric acid secretion by approximately 50% (at a total daily dosage of 1000 mg).

(2) **Ranitidine,** a more potent drug, causes a 70% reduction in gastric acid secretion (at a total daily dosage of 300 mg).

(3) **Famotidine** is the most potent H$_2$-receptor antagonist. After a 40-mg dose, mean nocturnal gastric acid secretion is reduced by 94% for up to 10 hours.

Table 51-2. Histamine H_2-Receptor Antagonists

	Cimetidine (Tagamet)	Ranitidine (Zantac)	Famotidine (Pepcid)	Nizatidine (Axid)
Ring structure	Imidazole	Furan	Thiazole	Thiazole
Relative potency	1	4–10	4–10	20–50
Evening dose (mg)				
Active ulcer	800	300	40	300
Maintenance	400	150	20	150
Bioavailability (F)	60%–70%	50%–60%	40%–45%	90%–100%
Peak time (t_{max}) (hr)	1–3	1–3	1–3.5	0.5–3
Volume of distribution (L/kg)	1	1.4	1.1–1.4	0.8–1.6
Protein binding	20%	15%	15%–22%	32%–35%
Renal elimination	60%–75%	30% oral 70% intravenous	65%–70%	65%–75%
Half-life (hr)				
Normal	2	2–3	2.5–4	1.6
Anuric	4–5	4–10	20+	6–8.5
Clearance (L/h)	30–48	46	19–29	40–60

Reprinted from Hurwitz A. Clinical pharmacology of agents for the treatment of acid-related disorders. In: *Peptic Ulcer Disease and Other Acid-Related Disorders.* Zakim D, Dannenberg AJ, eds. New York, Academic Research Associates, 1991, p 343.

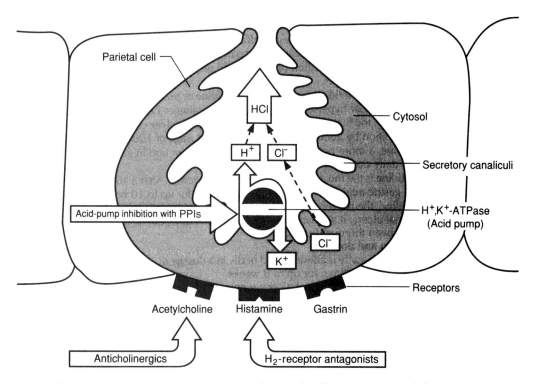

Figure 51-3. Schematic representation of parietal cell depicting sites of drug action.

(4) **Nizatidine,** the newest H$_2$-receptor antagonist, may be used to treat and prevent recurrence of duodenal ulcers.

c. **Administration and dosage**

(1) **Cimetidine** usually is administered orally in a dosage of 300 mg four times daily (with meals and at bedtime) for up to 8 weeks.

(a) Alternatively, duodenal ulcer patients may receive 400 mg twice daily or 800 mg at bedtime. An 800-mg bedtime dose is also effective in treating gastric ulcers.

(b) Hospitalized patients may receive parenteral doses of 300 mg intravenously every 6 hours.

(c) For duodenal ulcer prophylaxis, 400 mg may be given orally at bedtime. (However, in 20%–40% of patients, the ulcer recurs despite cimetidine prophylaxis.)

(2) **Ranitidine** usually is given orally in a dosage of 150 mg twice daily. Duodenal ulcer patients may receive 300 mg at bedtime, alternatively. Therapy continues for up to 8 weeks.

(a) Hospitalized patients may receive ranitidine by the intravenous (IV) or intramuscular route (50 mg every 6–8 hours).

(b) Prophylactic therapy may be administered to reduce the risk of ulcer recurrence. The approved prophylactic dosage is 150 mg at bedtime.

(c) Ranitidine 150 mg twice daily can be administered to maintain healing of erosive esophagitis; for this purpose, it is better than placebo but less effective than the proton pump inhibitors.

(d) Ranitidine bismuth citrate (RBC), combined with antibiotics such as clarithromycin, is indicated for eradication of *H. pylori* in patients with duodenal ulcer.

(3) **Famotidine,** administered to duodenal ulcer patients, is given in an oral dosage of 40 mg at bedtime for acute therapy for a maximum of 8 weeks. For prophylactic therapy, the dosage is 20 mg at bedtime.

(a) Hospitalized patients may receive an IV injection of 20 mg every 12 hours.

(b) As with cimetidine and ranitidine, the ulcer may recur after drug discontinuation.

(4) **Nizatidine,** for the treatment of duodenal ulcers, is given orally in a dosage of 300 mg once daily at bedtime or 150 mg twice daily for up to 8 weeks. For prophylactic therapy, the dosage is 150 mg at bedtime.

d. **Precautions and monitoring effects**

(1) Ranitidine must be used cautiously in patients with hepatic impairment. Hepatotoxicity is unusual and occurs most often during IV administration. Cimetidine has also been associated with hepatotoxicity.

(2) Cimetidine may cause such hematological disorders as thrombocytopenia, agranulocytosis, and aplastic anemia.

(3) All of these agents may cause headache and dizziness. Cimetidine additionally may lead to confusion, particularly if patients are over 60 years of age or if the dosage is not adjusted for patients with decreased kidney or liver function. All agents require dosage reductions in patients with impaired renal function.

(4) Cimetidine has a weak androgenic effect, possibly resulting in male gynecomastia and impotence.

(5) Cimetidine and ranitidine rarely can cause bradycardia, which is reversible on discontinuation of therapy.

(6) Evaluate *H. pylori* status in any patient with confirmed ulcer disease; eradication of *H. pylori* reduces the need for maintenance therapy in patients with duodenal or gastric ulcers. Patients with complicated ulcer disease should continue maintenance therapy until the eradication of *H. pylori.*

(7) Tolerance develops frequently to H$_2$RAs and may explain diminished responses to these agents over time.

e. **Significant interactions**

(1) Cimetidine binds the cytochrome P450 system of the liver and, thus, may interfere with the metabolism of such drugs as **phenytoin, theophylline, phenobarbital, lidocaine, warfarin, imipramine, diazepam,** and **propranolol.**

(2) Cimetidine decreases hepatic blood flow, possibly resulting in reduced clearance of **propranolol** and **lidocaine.**

(3) **Antacids** impair absorption of cimetidine and ranitidine and should be given 1 hour apart from these drugs.

(4) Cimetidine inhibits the excretion of procainamide by competing with the drug for the renal proximal tubular secretion site.

3. **Sucralfate.** This mucosal protectant is a nonabsorbable disaccharide containing sucrose and aluminum.
   a. **Mechanism of action and therapeutic effects.** Sucralfate adheres to the base of the ulcer crater, forming a protective barrier against gastric acids and bile salts.
      (1) Sucralfate's ulcer-healing efficacy compares favorably to that of the H_2-receptor antagonists.
      (2) Duodenal ulcers respond better than gastric ulcers to sucralfate therapy.
   b. **Administration and dosage**
      (1) An oral agent, sucralfate usually is given in a dosage of 1 g four times daily (1 hour before meals) and at bedtime. Unless radiography or endoscopy documents earlier ulcer healing, therapy continues for 4–8 weeks.
      (2) Continued sucralfate therapy after remission postpones ulcer relapse more effectively than does cimetidine therapy.
      (3) There is no evidence that combining sucralfate with H_2-receptor antagonists improves healing or reduces recurrence rates.
   c. **Precautions and monitoring effects.** Constipation is the most common adverse effect of sucralfate.
   d. **Significant interactions**
      (1) **Antacids** may reduce mucosal binding of sucralfate, decreasing its therapeutic efficacy and, thus, should be given 30–60 minutes apart from sucralfate if used in combination ulcer therapy.
      (2) Sucralfate may interfere with the absorption of orally administered **digoxin, tetracycline, phenytoin, iron, ciprofloxacin and other fluoroquinolones,** and **cimetidine** if doses are given simultaneously.

4. **GI anticholinergics** (e.g., belladonna leaf, atropine, propantheline) sometimes are used as adjunctive agents for relief of refractory duodenal ulcer pain. However, these agents have no proven value in ulcer healing.
   a. **Mechanism of action.** Anticholinergics decrease basal and stimulated gastric acid and pepsin secretion.
      (1) Given in combination with antacids, anticholinergics delay gastric emptying, thereby prolonging antacid retention. They are most effective when taken at night and in large doses.
      (2) Anticholinergics occasionally are used in patients who do not respond to H_2-receptor antagonists alone.
   b. **Administration and dosage**
      (1) Taken 30 minutes before food, anticholinergics inhibit meal-stimulated acid secretion by 30%–50% for a duration of 4–5 hours.
      (2) The optimal effective dose varies from patient to patient.
   c. **Precautions and monitoring effects**
      (1) All anticholinergics have side effects to varying degrees, such as dry mouth, blurred vision, tachycardia, urinary retention, and constipation.
      (2) These drugs are contraindicated in patients with gastric ulcers because they prolong gastric emptying. They also are contraindicated in patients with narrow-angle glaucoma and urinary retention.

5. **Prostaglandins** may prove valuable in ulcer therapy. These agents suppress gastric acid secretion and may guard the gastric mucosa against damage from NSAIDs. **Misoprostol** has been approved for use in the prevention of gastric ulcers caused by NSAIDs.
   a. **Mechanism of action.** Misoprostol has both antisecretory (inhibiting gastric acid secretion) and mucosal protective properties. NSAIDs inhibit prostaglandin synthesis, and a deficiency of prostaglandin within the gastric mucosa may lead to diminishing bicarbonate and mucus secretion, contributing to the mucosal damage caused by NSAIDs. Misoprostol increases bicarbonate and mucus production at doses of 200 mcg and above—doses that can also be antisecretory. Misoprostol also maintains mucosal blood flow.
   b. **Administration and dosage**
      (1) Misoprostol is indicated for the prevention of NSAID-induced gastric ulcers in patients at high risk for complications from gastric ulcers (e.g., patients over 60 years of age, patients with concomitant debilitating disease, patients with a history of ulcers).
      (2) Misoprostol has not been shown to prevent duodenal ulcers in patients taking NSAIDs.

(3) The recommended adult dosage is 200 mcg four times daily with food; it must be taken for the duration of NSAID therapy. If this dose cannot be tolerated, 100 mcg four times daily can be used.

(4) Adjustment of dosage in renally impaired patients is not routinely needed.

c. Precautions and monitoring effects

(1) Misoprostol is contraindicated in pregnant women because of its abortifacient property. Patients must be advised of the abortifacient property and warned not to give the drug to others.

(2) Misoprostol should not be used in women with childbearing potential unless the patient requires NSAID therapy and is at high risk of complications from gastric ulcers associated with use of the NSAIDs or is at high risk of developing gastric ulceration. In such a patient, misoprostol may be prescribed if the patient:

(a) Is capable of complying with effective contraceptive measures

(b) Has received both oral and written warnings of the hazards of misoprostol, the risk of possible contraception failure, and the danger to other women of childbearing potential should the drug be taken by mistake

(c) Had a negative serum pregnancy test within 2 weeks before beginning therapy

(d) Will begin misoprostol only on the second or third day of the next normal menstrual period

(3) The most frequent adverse effects are diarrhea (14%–40%) and abdominal pain (13%–20%). Diarrhea is dose-related, usually develops early in the course (more than 2 weeks), and is often self-limiting. Discontinuation of misoprostol is necessary in about 2% of patients. Administration with food minimizes the diarrhea.

d. Significant interactions. None has been reported.

6. Proton pump inhibitors (PPIs). Omeprazole was the first PPI available in the United States, followed by **lansoprazole, rabeprazole, pantoprazole, and esomeprazole** (Table 51-3). The intravenous form of pantoprazole has recently been approved by the United States Food and Drug Administration (FDA). Intravenous formulations of lansoprazole and esomeprazole are currently being developed.

a. Mechanism of action and therapeutic effects. The gastric proton pump H^+,K^+-ATPase has a sulfhydryl group near the potassium-binding site on the luminal side of the canalicular membrane. Omeprazole sulfenamide (the active form) forms a stable disulfide bond with this specific sulfhydryl, thereby inactivating the ATPase and shutting off acid secretion. All other PPIs exhibit a similar irreversible mechanism of action.

(1) Because of the potency and marked reduction in gastric acidity, the PPIs are more rapidly effective than other approved agents in treating peptic ulcer disease (i.e., PPIs tend to control symptoms and heal ulcers more rapidly than other antiulcer drugs). PPIs provide effective healing of duodenal ulcers; healing rates at 4 weeks are similar to those reported for H_2-receptor antagonist therapy at 8 weeks.

Table 51-3. Proton Pump Inhibitors

Pharmacokinetics of PPIs

Characteristic	Omeprazole (Prilosec)	Lansoprazole (Prevacid)	Rabeprazole (Aciphex)	Pantoprazole (Protonix)	Esomeprazole (Nexium)
Bioavailability (%)	30–40	80–85	52	77	64–89
Time to peak plasma concentration (hours)	0.5–3.5	1.7	2.0–5.0	1.1–3.1	1.56
Plasma elimination half-life (hours)	0.5–1	1.3–1.7	1.0–2.0	1.0–1.9	0.85–1.25
Protein binding (%)	95	97	96	98	97
Urinary excretion of oral dose (%)	77	14–23	30–35	71–80	80

(2) All PPIs are effective in healing erosive esophagitis, provide more rapid symptom relief and more consistent healing than H$_2$-receptor antagonists, and are also effective in maintenance of healing of erosive esophagitis.

(3) All PPIs except pantoprazole have been approved in various combinations of antibiotics for the eradication of *H. pylori* (Table 51-4).

(4) PPIs have resulted in significant improvement in patients with pathological hypersecretory conditions (e.g., Zollinger-Ellison syndrome) and GERD compared to H$_2$-receptor antagonists.

(5) Lansoprazole has been approved by the FDA for healing and prevention of NSAID-induced gastric ulcers.

(6) Omeprazole and lansoprazole have been approved by the FDA for use in infants and children for the short-term treatment of GERD and erosive esophagitis. Omeprazole is approved for use in children ages 2–16 years, and lansoprazole is approved for use in children 1–11 years old.

Table 51-4. Food and Drug Administration (FDA)-Approved Oral Regimens Used to Eradicate *Helicobacter pylori* and Reduce the Risk of Duodenal Ulcer Recurrence

Drug Combination	Dose and Frequency	Duration
Omeprazole	40 mg qd	Days 1–14
	20 mg qd	Days 15–28*
Clarithromycin	500 mg tid	Days 1–14
Omeprazole	20 mg bid	Days 1–10
	20 mg qd	Days 11–28*
Clarithromycin	500 mg bid	Days 1–10
Amoxicillin	1 g bid	Days 1–10
Ranitidine bismuth citrate	400 mg bid	Days 1–28
Clarithromycin	500 mg tid	Days 1–14
Lansoprazole**	30 mg tid	14 days
Amoxicillin**	1 g tid	14 days
Lansoprazole	30 mg bid	14 days
Amoxicillin	1 g tid	14 days
Clarithromycin	500 mg bid	14 days
Lansoprazole	30 mg bid	10 days
Amoxicillin	1 g bid	10 days
Clarithromycin	500 mg bid	10 days
Esomeprazole	40 mg qd	10 days
Amoxicillin	1 g bid	10 days
Clarithromycin	500 mg bid	10 days
Rabeprazole	20 mg bid	7 days
Amoxicillin	1 g bid	7 days
Clarithromycin	500 mg bid	7 days
Bismuth subsalicylate	525 mg qid	Days 1–14
Metronidazole	250 mg qid	Days 1–14
Tetracycline HCl	500 mg qid	Days 1–14
H$_2$RA of choice	Ulcer healing regimen	Days 1–28

*In patients with an ulcer present at the time of initiation of therapy, additional omeprazole treatment is recommended for ulcer healing and relief of symptoms.

** Approved for patients who are either allergic to or intolerant of clarithromycin or when resistance to clarithromycin is known or suspected.

H$_2$RA = histamine H$_2$-receptor antagonist.

b. Administration and dosage

(1) PPIs are more potent than H$_2$-blockers. In the usual dosage (omeprazole 20 mg daily), these agents inhibit more than 90% of 24-hour acid secretion in most patients, rarely producing achlorhydria. Esomeprazole 40 mg daily provided significantly higher intragastric pH values above 4 during 24-hour monitoring compared to lansoprazole 30 mg, rabeprazole 20 mg, omeprazole 20 mg, and pantoprazole 40 mg.

(2) Currently available PPIs should be taken in the morning before eating; food activates parietal cells, maximizing the effect of the PPI. Optimal binding to proton pumps occurs when the pumps are actively secreting.

(3) Recommended adult dosages

(a) Erosive esophagitis initially is healed with 20 mg omeprazole or equivalent doses of other PPIs for 8–12 weeks; only omeprazole has a demonstrated dose response in GERD patients (patients failing omeprazole 20 mg daily may benefit from higher doses; this has not been demonstrated with esomeprazole, lansoprazole, rabeprazole, or pantoprazole). Additionally, esomeprazole 40 mg qd has been shown to produce significantly higher healing rates than omeprazole 20 mg or lansoprazole 30 mg across all grades of erosive esophagitis.

(b) Esomeprazole 20 mg, lansoprazole 30 mg, omeprazole 20 mg, and pantoprazole 40 mg may be used to manage GERD symptoms in patients who have failed previous therapy with H$_2$-receptor antagonist therapy.

(c) The recommended dosage to maintain healing of erosive esophagitis is esomeprazole 20 mg, omeprazole 20 mg, lansoprazole 15 mg, pantoprazole 40 mg, or rabeprazole 20 mg daily for as long as medically necessary.

(d) Duodenal ulcer healing requires omeprazole 20 mg, lansoprazole 15 mg, or rabeprazole 20 mg once daily. Most patients heal within 4 weeks.

(4) Esomeprazole, lansoprazole, and omeprazole are delayed-release capsules and should be taken before eating, can be used concomitantly with antacids, and should not be chewed or crushed. Capsule contents can be sprinkled on foods (i.e., apple sauce) or mixed with acidic juices. Suspensions of omeprazole or lansoprazole in sodium bicarbonate have been used for administration to patients with nasogastric tubes.

(5) Rabeprazole and pantoprazole are available as enteric-coated tablets that should not be crushed or chewed.

(6) No dosing adjustments are necessary in patients with impaired renal or hepatic function or in the elderly.

(7) Intravenous pantoprazole is indicated for management of erosive esophagitis and treatment of Zollinger-Ellison syndrome. It is currently being widely used for the treatment of bleeding gastric ulcers, though not FDA approved.

c. Precautions and monitoring effects

(1) Headache, diarrhea, abdominal pain, nausea and vomiting, and flatulence have been reported in more than 1% of patients.

(2) Fever, fatigue, malaise, elevated liver enzymes, dizziness, vertigo, skin rash, and itching have been reported in less than 1% of patients.

d. Significant interactions

(1) Omeprazole interferes with the hepatic microsomal enzyme metabolism (cytochrome P450) of **diazepam, warfarin,** and **phenytoin, although clinically significant interactions are infrequent.**

(2) Lansoprazole may increase clearance of theophylline by approximately 10%.

(3) Because gastric pH plays a role in the bioavailability of **ketoconazole, ampicillin esters,** and **iron salts,** prolonged gastric acid inhibition with PPIs may decrease the absorption of these agents.

(4) Antacids may be used concomitantly with all PPIs.

(5) No clinically significant drug interactions have been reported to date with esomeprazole, rabeprazole, or pantoprazole.

(6) Food may reduce the bioavailability of esomeprazole and lansoprazole by 50%; food does not reduce the bioavailability of omeprazole or rabeprazole. Food may delay absorption of pantoprazole up to 2 hours.

7. Bismuth compounds. In the United States, bismuth subsalicylate (Pepto-Bismol) and RBC are the only available bismuth products. Colloidal bismuth subcitrate [CBS; tripotassium dicitratobismuthate (TDB)] is the preferred bismuth compound in other countries.

a. **Mechanism of action.** Bismuth prevents adhesion of *H. pylori* to gastric mucosa, decreases resistance when used with other anti–*H. pylori* agents, inhibits release of proteolytic enzymes, and suppresses *H. pylori* growth. Additionally, CBS blocks pepsin activity, binds mucus to retard hydrogen back-diffusion, and stimulates prostaglandin synthesis.

b. **Administration and dosage**
   (1) Bismuth subsalicylate or ranitidine bismuth citrate is highly effective when combined with PPIs and/or antibiotics. Eradication rates with these combinations are greater than 80% (see Table 51-4).
   (2) Preferred regimen with bismuth: bismuth subsalicylate 525 mg four times a day, metronidazole 250 mg four times a day, tetracycline 500 mg four times a day plus PPI (omeprazole 20 mg every day or lansoprazole 30 mg every day) for 2 weeks total. This regimen provides consistently high eradication rates (>90%) and may be useful for patients who have failed previous therapy. This regimen is not currently FDA approved.

c. Although not available in the United States, CBS provides intriguing features of ongoing interest.
   (1) CBS has been used since 1971 to treat gastric and duodenal ulcers. Efficacy rates are as follows:
      (a) **Duodenal ulcer:** 80% were healed at 4 weeks and 95% at 8 weeks.
      (b) **Gastric ulcer:** 68% were healed at 4 weeks and 81% at 8 weeks.
   (2) After healing by CBS, mucosal morphology is described as more normal in appearance than after H$_2$-blocker therapy; recurrence rates are also lower.
   (3) CBS precipitates at about pH 3.5, binding to ulcer craters. Animal studies have shown that this binding is unique to CBS among the bismuth compounds studied and does not occur with bismuth subsalicylate (Pepto-Bismol).

d. **Precautions and monitoring effects**
   (1) CNS toxicity with higher doses, including neurotoxicity
   (2) Dark stools and tongue, headache, diarrhea, rash, and abdominal pain
   (3) Tinnitus, hyperpyrexia, tachycardia, and confusion (salicylism) from high doses of bismuth subsalicylate

e. **Reversible proton pump inhibitors** are currently under development by a number of pharmaceutical companies (AstraZeneca and Altana). When compared with the currently available irreversible proton pump inhibitors, these agents are expected to offer more rapid symptom resolution, control pH more quickly, achieve higher pH levels, and sustain these more aggressive pH levels consistently over a 24-hour period.

8. **Prokinetic agents.** Cisapride is currently the only approved agent in this class; however, the manufacturer (Janssen Pharmaceutica) has **discontinued marketing** of cisapride in the United States due to highly arrhythmogenic potential. The manufacturer will supply cisapride through a limited-access program for those who meet specific eligibility criteria and for whom other therapies are not effective. Metoclopramide and erythromycin have well-studied prokinetic effects, and prucalopride is still under review by the FDA.
   a. **Mechanism of action.** Cisapride produces release of acetylcholine from the myenteric plexus and thereby may increase gastric emptying and LES pressure; cisapride does not affect TLESR. It does not increase or decrease gastric acid secretion.
   b. **Administration and dosage.** Cisapride is indicated for the relief of nocturnal symptoms of reflux; it is administered in doses of 10–20 mg four times a day.
   c. **Precautions and monitoring**
      (1) The **most common** side effects are diarrhea, abdominal pain, and headache. Other less common effects include bronchospasm, angioedema, and depression.
      (2) Cisapride is contraindicated in patients with a history of ischemic heart disease, respiratory failure, congestive heart failure, renal failure, severe dehydration, arrhythmias, or medications that prolong the QT interval. Serious cardiac arrhythmias, including ventricular tachycardia and Torsades de Pointes, have been reported.
   d. **Significant interactions**
      (1) **Ketoconazole** potently inhibits the metabolism of cisapride, resulting in an eightfold increase in the area under the curve (AUC) of cisapride. Coadministration of cisapride and ketoconazole can result in prolongation of the QT interval on the electrocardiogram (ECG). Coadministration of itraconazole, fluconazole, or miconazole IV is similarly contraindicated.

(2) The following oral or intravenous drugs are contraindicated with cisapride. These may lead to elevated cisapride blood levels and increased potential for arrhythmias.

    (a) Antibiotics: erythromycin, clarithromycin, troleandomycin, sparfloxacin

    (b) Antidepressants: nefazodone

    (c) Protease inhibitors: indinavir, ritonavir

    (d) Antiarrhythmics: quinidine, procainamide, sotalol

    (e) Antihistamines: astemizole

(3) The acceleration of gastric emptying by cisapride could affect the rate of absorption of other drugs. Patients receiving narrow therapeutic drugs or other drugs that require careful titration should be monitored closely.

(4) Coagulation times in patients receiving oral anticoagulants have increased in some cases.

(5) Cimetidine may increase peak plasma concentration and AUC of cisapride.

e. GABA$_B$ agonists (i.e., baclofen) have been shown to significantly reduce reflux episodes in healthy volunteers and GERD patients. Several compounds are under development that have greater peripheral specificity and are expected to provide fewer central nervous system–related adverse effects, while providing effective normalization of TRLESs.

f. Tegaserod, a selective 5-HT4–receptor agonist, is a promotility drug currently approved for irritable bowel syndrome. Early studies have demonstrated that tegaserod reduces esophageal acid exposure by enhancing esophageal acid clearance and gastric emptying and/or reducing TRLESs. More study is required.

9. Sedatives are useful adjuncts in promoting rest for highly anxious ulcer patients.

B. Other therapeutic measures

1. Modification of diet and social habits

a. Previously emphasized in ulcer therapy, strict dietary limitations now are considered largely unnecessary.

    (1) Bland or milk-based diets formerly were recommended; however, research indicates that these diets do not speed ulcer healing. In fact, most experts now advise ulcer patients to **avoid milk** because recent studies show that milk increases gastric acid secretion. Also, because milk leaves the stomach quickly, it lacks an extended buffering action.

    (2) Small, frequent meals, also previously recommended, can worsen ulcer pain by causing acid rebound 2–4 hours after eating.

b. Current dietary guidelines emphasize avoiding foods and beverages known to exacerbate gastric discomfort or promote acid secretion. This category typically includes coffee, caffeinated beverages, and alcohol.

c. Smoking. Patients who smoke should be encouraged to quit because smoking markedly slows ulcer healing, even during optimal ulcer therapy.

d. NSAIDs should be avoided by ulcer patients.

2. Surgery. An ulcer patient who develops complications may require surgery—sometimes on an emergency basis (see III). Incapacitating recurrent ulcers also may warrant surgery.

a. Types of surgical procedures for ulcer disease include antrectomy and truncal vagotomy (Billroth I procedure), partial gastrectomy and truncal vagotomy (Billroth II procedure), highly selective (proximal gastric) vagotomy, and total gastrectomy (the treatment of choice for Zollinger-Ellison syndrome that is unresponsive to medical management).

    (1) A **vagotomy** severs a branch of the vagus nerve, thereby decreasing HCl secretion.

    (2) An **antrectomy,** by removing the antrum, eliminates some acid-secreting mucosa as well as the major source of gastrin.

b. The general indications for antireflux surgery are failure of medical therapy to heal or prevent relapse of erosive esophagitis, inability of medical therapy to prevent recurrence of stricture, or a patient whose life-style is adversely affected by the need for medical therapy. **Fundoplication** successfully relieves symptoms and heals lesions in approximately 85% of patients. Recent studies have demonstrated that most patients require continued medical therapy after fundoplication.

3. Emerging endoscopic therapies. Several endoscopic techniques to treat GERD have recently been introduced.

a. Augmentation of LES pressure may be achieved by delivery of radio-frequency energy to the muscle of the gastroesophageal junction (Stretta procedure). The radio frequency is delivered by means of a flexible catheter comprising a bougie tip, a balloon-basket combination, and four-needle delivery sheaths.

b. Another endoscopic procedure to augment LES pressure uses an endoluminal-stitching technique. An endoscopic sewing machine mounted on a standard gastroscope is used to perform gastroplasty.

c. Early studies have demonstrated good feasibility in performing these procedures and an overall satisfactory safety profile. Further studies are necessary to assess long-term failure rate, early versus late complications, and success rate in the different GERD groups.

III. COMPLICATIONS of peptic ulcer disease cause approximately 7000 deaths in the United States annually.

A. Hemorrhage. This life-threatening condition develops from widespread gastric mucosal irritation or ulceration with acute bleeding.

1. Clinical features. The patient may vomit fresh blood or a coffee-grounds–like substance. Other signs include passage of bloody or tarry stools, diaphoresis, and syncope. With major blood loss, manifestations of **hypovolemic shock** may appear: The pulse rate may exceed 110, or systolic blood pressure may drop below 100.

2. Management
   a. Patient stabilization, bleeding cessation, and measures to prevent further bleeding are crucial.
      (1) Airway, breathing, and circulation must be ensured.
      (2) IV crystalloids and colloids (e.g., hetastarch) should be infused as needed.
      (3) The patient's electrolyte status must be monitored and any imbalances corrected promptly.
   b. Gastric lavage may be performed via a nasogastric or orogastric tube; iced saline solution is instilled until the aspirate returns free of blood.
   c. Vasoconstrictors, antacids, H_2-receptor antagonists, or proton pump inhibitors may be administered. **Vasopressin,** an agent that causes contraction of the GI smooth muscle, may be given to constrict vessels and control bleeding.
   d. Emergency surgery usually is indicated if the patient does not respond to medical management.

B. Perforation. Penetration of a peptic ulcer through the gastric or duodenal wall results in this acute emergency. Perforation most commonly occurs with ulcers located in the anterior duodenal wall.

1. Clinical features. Sudden acute upper abdominal pain, rigidity, guarding, rebound tenderness, and absent or diminished bowel sounds are typical manifestations. Several hours after onset, symptoms may abate somewhat; this apparent remission is dangerously misleading because peritonitis and shock may ensue.

2. Management. Emergency surgery is almost always necessary.

C. Obstruction. Inflammatory edema, spasm, and scarring may lead to obstruction of the duodenal or gastric outlet. The pylorus and proximal duodenum are the most common obstruction sites.

1. Clinical features. Typical patient complaints include postprandial vomiting or bloating, appetite and weight loss, and abdominal distention. Tympany and a succussion splash may be audible on physical examination. Gastric aspiration after an overnight fast typically yields more than 200 mL of food residue or clear fluid contents. (Gastric cancer must be ruled out as the cause of obstruction.)

2. Management
   a. Conservative measures (as in routine ulcer therapy) are indicated in most cases of obstruction.
   b. Patients with marked obstruction may require **continuous gastric suction** with careful monitoring of fluid and electrolyte status. A **saline load test** may be performed after 72 hours of continuous suction to test the degree of residual obstruction.

  c. If less than 200 mL of gastric contents are aspirated, liquid feedings can begin. **Aspiration** is performed at least daily for the next few days to monitor for retention and to guide dietary modifications as the patient progresses to a full regular diet.

  d. Surgery is indicated if medical management fails.

D. Postsurgical complications

 1. Dumping syndrome. Affecting about 10% of patients who have undergone partial gastrectomy, this disorder is characterized by rapid gastric emptying.

  a. Causes. The mechanism underlying dumping syndrome is poorly defined. However, intestinal exposure to hypertonic chyme may play a key role by triggering rapid shifts of fluid from the plasma to the intestinal lumen.

  b. Clinical features. The patient may experience weakness, dizziness, anxiety, tachycardia, flushing, sweating, abdominal cramps, nausea, vomiting, and diarrhea.

   (1) Manifestations may develop 15–30 minutes after a meal (early dumping syndrome) or 90–120 minutes after a meal (late dumping syndrome).

   (2) Reactive hypoglycemia may partly account for some cases of late dumping syndrome.

  c. Management. The patient usually is advised to eat six small meals of high protein and fat content and low carbohydrate content. Fluids should be ingested 1 hour before or after a meal but never with a meal. **Anticholinergics** may be given to slow food passage into the intestine.

 2. Other postsurgical complications include reflux gastritis, afferent blind loop syndrome, stomal ulceration, diarrhea, malabsorption, early satiety, and iron-deficiency anemia.

E. Refractory ulcers.
Ulcers that fail to heal on a prolonged course of drug treatment should not be confused with ulcers that recur after therapy is stopped. It is difficult to predict which patients will have a refractory ulcer.

 1. Differential diagnosis. Any compliant patient who continues to have dyspeptic symptoms after 8 weeks of therapy should have gastroscopy and biopsy to exclude rare causes of ulceration in the duodenum, such as Crohn's disease, tuberculosis, lymphoma, pulmonary or secondary carcinoma, and cytomegalovirus (CMV) infection in immunodeficient patients. Fasting plasma gastrin concentration should be measured to exclude Zollinger-Ellison syndrome.

 2. Treatment

  a. Available data indicate that only maximum acid inhibition, with a regimen such as omeprazole (20 mg twice a day) or lansoprazole (30 mg twice a day), offers advantages over continued therapy with standard antiulcer regimens.

  b. Eradication of *H. pylori* infection, when present, is likely to facilitate healing and alter the natural history of refractory ulcers.

  c. Every effort should be made to discover and reduce or eliminate NSAID use.

  d. Perform surgery.

F. Maintenance regimens

 1. Despite healing after withdrawal of therapy, 70% of ulcers recur in 1 year, and 90% in 2 years. Similarly, erosive esophagitis will recur in more than 80% of individuals within 1 year after discontinuation of antisecretory therapy.

 2. Candidates for long-term maintenance therapy include patients with serious concomitant diseases; four relapses per year; or a combination of risk factors, producing a more severe natural history of peptic disease (e.g., old age, male sex, a long history of aspirin or NSAID use, heavy alcohol intake, cigarette smoking, a history of peptic ulcer disease in an immediate relative, high maximal acid output, and a history of ulcer complications).

 3. Patients with confirmed ulcer disease should be evaluated for presence of *H. pylori*. Eradication of *H. pylori* minimizes the recurrence of ulcer disease. Patients with a history of complicated ulcer disease should have *H. pylori* eradication confirmed.

STUDY QUESTIONS

Directions: Each of the numbered items or incomplete statements in this section is followed by answers or by completions of the statement. Select the **one** lettered answer or completion that is **best** in each case.

1. Which of the following organisms has been implicated as a possible cause of chronic gastritis and peptic ulcer disease?

(A) *Campylobacter jejuni*
(B) *Escherichia coli*
(C) *Helicobacter pylori*
(D) *Calymmatobacterium granulomatis*
(E) *Giardia lamblia*

2. All of the following statements concerning antacid therapy used in the treatment of duodenal or gastric ulcers are correct EXCEPT

(A) antacids may be used to heal the ulcer but are ineffective in controlling ulcer pain
(B) antacids neutralize acid and decrease the activity of pepsin
(C) if used alone for ulcer therapy, antacids should be administered 1 hour and 3 hours after meals and at bedtime
(D) if diarrhea occurs, the patient may alternate the antacid product with aluminum hydroxide
(E) calcium carbonate should be avoided because it causes acid rebound and induces constipation

3. As part of a comprehensive management strategy to treat peptic ulcer disease, patients should be encouraged to do all of the following EXCEPT

(A) decrease caffeine ingestion
(B) eat only bland foods
(C) stop smoking
(D) avoid alcohol
(E) avoid the use of milk as a treatment modality

4. A gastric ulcer patient requires close follow-up to document complete ulcer healing because

(A) perforation into the intestine is common
(B) spontaneous healing of the ulcer may occur in 30%–50% of cases
(C) there is the risk of the ulcer being cancerous
(D) symptoms tend to be chronic and recur
(E) weight loss may be severe in gastric ulcer patients

5. Cisapride should not be used in combination with either fluconazole or indinavir because of increased potential for

(A) atrial fibrillation
(B) atrial flutter
(C) ventricular fibrillation
(D) torsades de pointes
(E) angina pectoris

6. All of the following provide acid suppression similar to omeprazole 20 mg every day EXCEPT

(A) lansoprazole 30 mg every day
(B) pantoprazole 40 mg every day
(C) rabeprazole 20 mg every day
(D) ranitidine 300 mg twice a day
(E) all provide equivalent acid suppression

Directions: Each item below contains three suggested answers, of which **one or more** is correct. Choose the answer

A	if **I only** is correct
B	if **III only** is correct
C	if **I and II** are correct
D	if **II and III** are correct
E	if **I, II, and III** are correct

7. Correct statements concerning cigarette smoking and ulcer disease include which of the following?

I. Smoking delays healing of gastric and duodenal ulcers
II. Nicotine decreases biliary and pancreatic bicarbonate secretion
III. Smoking accelerates the emptying of stomach acid into the duodenum

8. When administered at the same time, antacids can decrease the therapeutic efficacy of which of the following drugs?

I. Sucralfate
II. Ranitidine
III. Cimetidine

Directions: The group of items in this section consists of lettered options followed by a set of numbered items. For each item, select the **one** lettered option that is most closely associated with it. Each lettered option may be selected once, more than once, or not at all.

Questions 9–13

For each effect, select the agent that is most likely associated with it.

(A) Sodium bicarbonate
(B) Aluminum hydroxide
(C) Calcium carbonate
(D) Magnesium hydroxide
(E) Propantheline

9. May cause diarrhea

10. Cannot be used by patients with heart failure

11. Use with milk and an alkaline substance can cause milk-alkali syndrome

12. May cause dry mouth

13. Can be alternated with an antacid mixture to control diarrhea

ANSWERS AND EXPLANATIONS

1. The answer is C *[I E 1].*
Helicobacter pylori commonly is found in patients with peptic ulcer disease and always in association with chronic gastritis. Elimination of the organism has resulted in healing of the gastritis and the duodenal ulcer. More data, however, are needed before a definitive cause-and-effect relationship can be established.

2. The answer is A *[II A 1].*
Antacids have been shown to heal peptic ulcers, and their main use in modern therapy is to control ulcer pain. Antacids should be taken 1 hour and 3 hours after meals because the meal prolongs the acid-buffering effect of the antacid. If diarrhea becomes a problem with antacid use, an aluminum hydroxide product can be alternated with the antacid mixture; this takes advantage of the constipating property of aluminum. Because calcium carbonate causes acid rebound and constipation, its use should be avoided.

3. The answer is B *[II B 1 a (1)].*
Bland food diets are no longer recommended in the treatment of ulcer disease because research indicates that bland or milk-based diets do not accelerate ulcer healing. Studies show that patients can eat almost anything; however, they should avoid foods that aggravate their ulcer symptoms.

4. The answer is C *[I D 6].*
Five percent to 10 percent of gastric ulcers may be due to cancer. The ulcer may respond to therapy; however, failure of the ulcer to decrease satisfactorily in size and to heal with therapy may suggest cancer. Close follow-up is necessary to document complete ulcer healing.

5. The answer is D *[II A 8 d (2)].*
These combinations as well as many other potential interactions with cisapride may increase serum concentrations of cisapride, increasing the risk for torsades de pointes.

6. The answer is D *[II A 6 b (1)].*
Doses of omeprazole 20 mg, lansoprazole 30 mg, pantoprazole 40 mg, and rabeprazole 20 mg administered once daily provide similar levels of acid suppression. All provide significantly better acid inhibition than ranitidine, even at doses of 300 mg twice a day or more.

7. The answer is E (all) *[I E 3; II B 1 c].*
Clinical studies have shown that smoking increases susceptibility to ulcer disease, impairs spontaneous and drug-induced healing, and increases the risk and rapidity of recurrence of the ulcer. These findings may result in part from nicotine's ability to decrease biliary and pancreatic bicarbonate secretion, thus decreasing the body's ability to neutralize acid in the duodenum. Also, the accelerated emptying of stomach acid into the duodenum may predispose to duodenal ulcer and may decrease healing rates.

8. The answer is E (all) *[II A 1 e (3), 3 d].*
The mean peak blood concentration of cimetidine and the area under the 4-hour cimetidine blood concentration curve were both reduced significantly when cimetidine was administered at the same time as an antacid. The absorption of ranitidine is also reduced when it is taken concurrently with an aluminum magnesium hydroxide antacid mixture. To avoid this interaction, the antacid should be administered 1 hour before or 2 hours after the administration of cimetidine or ranitidine. Antacids may reduce mucosal binding of sucralfate, decreasing its therapeutic efficacy. Antacids should, therefore, be given 30–60 minutes before or after sucralfate.

9–13. The answers are: 9-D *[II A 1 b (3)],* **10-A** *[II A 1 d (2)],* **11-C** *[II A 1 d (5)],* **12-E** *[II A 4 c (1)],* **13-B** *[II A 1 b (3)].*
Magnesium-containing products tend to cause diarrhea, possibly because of magnesium's ability to stimulate the secretion of bile acids by the gallbladder. Because of its sodium content, sodium bicarbonate is contraindicated in patients with congestive heart failure (CHF), hypertension, severe renal disease, and edema. Sodium bicarbonate is no longer used in peptic ulcer therapy. In addition to causing acid rebound, calcium carbonate, if taken with milk and an alkaline substance for long periods, may cause milk-alkali syndrome. It also may cause adverse effects such as hypercalcemia, alkalosis, azotemia, and nephrocalcinosis. Propantheline, like other anticholinergic agents, may cause dry mouth, blurred vision, urinary retention, and constipation. These agents sometimes are used as adjuncts to relieve duodenal ulcer pain. They are contraindicated in gastric ulcer because they delay gastric emptying. Aluminum hydroxide is constipating and can be alternated with the patient's current antacid when that antacid product is causing diarrhea.

52
Diabetes Mellitus

Peggy C. Yarborough

I. INTRODUCTION

A. Definition. Diabetes mellitus (DM) is a chronic, progressive, systemic disease characterized by dysfunction in the following:

1. Metabolism of fats, carbohydrates, protein, and insulin

2. Function and structure of blood vessels and nerves

B. Classification. There are four clinical classes of diabetes: type 1, type 2, gestational (GDM), and other specific types (secondary DM). Although *not* a type of diabetes, prediabetes is included with the classification of glucose abnormalities.

1. **Type 1.** Also described as insulin-dependent diabetes mellitus (IDDM), juvenile-onset diabetes, or ketosis-prone diabetes
   a. Most common in children and in adults ≤30 years old, but may occur at any age.
   b. Predisposed to **ketoacidosis**—accumulation of ketone bodies in body tissues and fluids (see below).
   c. Dependent upon exogenous insulin-replacement therapy to prevent ketoacidosis and sustain life.
   d. The essential difference between type 1 and type 2 DM is that insulin production and secretion in type 1 is destroyed; in type 2 DM, insulin production and secretion may be altered or reduced but is not totally lacking.

2. **Type 2.** Also described as non–insulin-dependent diabetes mellitus (NIDDM) or adult-onset diabetes
   a. Approximately 90% of individuals with diabetes in the United States have type 2 diabetes, with a disproportionate representation among certain ethnic groups and the elderly.
   b. Usually diagnosed in adults >30 years old, but may occur at any age.
   c. The incidence of type 2 DM in adolescents is increasing, apparently related to an increasing incidence of obesity in this age group, decreasing exercise/physical activity, and genetic and other life-style factors.
   d. Endogenous insulin levels may appear normal, increased, or decreased, and the requirement for exogenous insulin is variable. In spite of apparently "normal" or "increased" insulin levels, β-cell dysfunction is manifest by a *relative insulin insufficiency* to maintain euglycemia, especially in the face of significant insulin resistance.
   e. Not prone to ketosis except during periods of severe physical stress such as infections, trauma, or surgery.
   f. Approximately 80% of patients are obese at the time of DM diagnosis.

3. **Gestational diabetes mellitus (GDM).** Defined as any degree of glucose intolerance that has its onset or is first detected during pregnancy.
   a. Occurs in approximately 2%–4% of pregnant women, generally during the second or third trimester.
   b. Six weeks after the pregnancy, a follow-up glucose tolerance test should be performed. Glucose regulation would then be reclassified as DM, IFG, IGT, or normoglycemia. In the majority of cases, glucose regulation returns to normal postpregnancy.
   c. Occurrence of GDM increases future risk for developing type 2 diabetes.

4. **Other specific types** (secondary diabetes). Broad term used to classify patients who have unusual causes of diabetes due to certain diseases of the pancreas, genetic defects, endocrinopathies, or drugs.

5. **Prediabetes.** Term used to refer to an intermediate metabolic stage between normal glucose homeostasis and diabetes. Prediabetes is a risk factor for future DM and cardiovascular disease (CVD).

C. Incidence. In the United States, an estimated 1%–5% of the population has DM, with a similar number of individuals remaining undiagnosed. Type 1 DM accounts for approximately 10% of cases and type 2 for about 90%.

D. Etiology. Various factors contribute to the development of DM.

1. **Type 1 DM.** Genetic predisposition, environmental factors, and autoimmunity have been proposed.
   a. **Genetics.** Certain genetic markers in the human leukocyte antigen (HLA) system have been strongly linked with type 1 DM, and the risk of developing diabetes is substantially increased in the offspring of individuals diagnosed with diabetes.
   b. **Environment.** Not all individuals at genetic risk for type 1 DM develop the disease. Some type of trigger, such as a virus (e.g., rubella) or toxic chemical, is needed for the expression of the genetic propensity for type 1 DM.
   c. **Autoimmunity.** An autoimmune component, perhaps stimulated by the environmental trigger, is involved in the development of type 1 diabetes. Anti-insulin or anti-β-cell antibodies are present in the blood of most individuals at the time of diagnosis of type 1 DM.

2. **Type 2 DM.** Genetic factors, a β-cell defect, and peripheral site defects have been implicated.
   a. **Genetics.** There is a greater than 90% concordance rate between monozygotic twins if one has type 2 diabetes. It has been estimated that offspring of individuals with type 2 diabetes have approximately a 15% chance of developing the disease.
   b. Diminished **β-cell function** is postulated to cause abnormalities in insulin secretion, resulting in a relative deficiency of insulin.
   c. A **peripheral site defect** is postulated to lead to **insulin resistance**—tissue insensitivity to the biological activity of insulin. This condition is thought to result primarily from postbinding abnormalities.

3. **Secondary diabetes** may arise from such conditions as endocrine disorders (e.g., Cushing's syndrome), pancreatic disease, and the use of drugs that antagonize insulin (e.g., thiazide diuretics, adrenocorticosteroids).

E. Pathophysiology

1. **Normal glucose regulation** involves both insulin and counterregulatory hormones.
   a. Insulin is responsible for a variety of effects throughout body tissues.
      (1) Stimulates glucose transport across cell membranes and promotes the storage of glucose as glycogen in muscle and liver cells
      (2) Enhances fat storage (lipogenesis) and prevents the mobilization of fat for energy (lipolysis and ketogenesis)
      (3) Inhibits production of glucose from liver or muscle glycogen (glycogenolysis)
      (4) Promotes incorporation of amino acids into proteins
      (5) Inhibits the formation of glucose from amino acids (gluconeogenesis)
      (6) Decreases the breakdown of fatty acids to ketone bodies
   b. Counterregulatory hormones: antagonize the glycemic effects of insulin.
      (1) Glucagon: produced in the α cells of the pancreas
      (2) Epinephrine
      (3) Norepinephrine
      (4) Growth hormone
      (5) Cortisol

2. **Abnormal glucose regulation** associated with diabetes. In untreated type 1 and type 2 DM, the disease follows a predictable progression from initial abnormalities of glucose metabolism to life-threatening diabetic ketoacidosis or hyperglycemic hyperosmolar nonketotic syndrome, as described below.
   a. **Diabetic ketoacidosis (DKA)** [type 1 DM]
      (1) Insulin deficiency results in hyperglycemia
         (a) Impaired glucose uptake in the peripheral tissues (primarily muscle)
         (b) Reduction in the conversion of glucose to glycogen (impaired **glycogenesis**), primarily in the liver
         (c) Impaired insulin-induced suppression of hepatic glucose production (**neoglucogenesis** and **glycogenolysis**)

(2) As blood glucose (BG) concentrations increase, the glucose reabsorptive capacity of the kidneys will be exceeded. This occurs at about 180 mg/dl, referred to as the **renal threshold for glucose.** Glucose is then excreted into the urine, resulting in an **osmotic diuresis** with subsequent **dehydration** and **electrolyte abnormalities.**

(3) Insufficient glucose uptake in the peripheral tissues (due to insulin deficiency) causes the cells to use protein and fat as energy sources rather than glucose.

(4) Breakdown of protein yields carbohydrate/glucose moieties, but with insufficient insulin, the additional glucose worsens hyperglycemia rather than serving as an energy source.

(5) Breakdown of triglycerides (the stored form of fat) yields **free fatty acids** and **glycerol** through the process of **lipolysis.** Without the administration of insulin, type 1 DM will progress to ketonemia and ketoacidosis, as described below:

(a) Increasing amounts of glycerol leads to enhanced hepatic glucose production, further worsening hyperglycemia.

(b) Free fatty acids are broken down in the liver into **ketone bodies,** which are excreted by the kidneys (**ketonuria**). Acetoacetate (a ketone body) is converted in the liver to acetone, which is excreted through the lungs. This is associated with a fruity odor and can sometimes be detected on the breath of the patient.

(c) As the utilization (breakdown) of adipose tissue continues, ketone production exceeds the capacity for excretion, leading to accumulation in the bloodstream (**ketonemia**).

(d) Increasing levels of free fatty acids contribute to the development and worsening of **acidosis.**

(e) Initially, there is compensation for acidosis by changes in breathing patterns (**Kussmaul breathing**) and by buffering systems of the blood (e.g., proteins, bicarbonate).

(f) As acidosis continues, breathing compensation and bicarbonate stores are insufficient or depleted. A state of ketosis with acidosis (**ketoacidosis**) then exists.

(g) If ketoacidosis is not promptly treated by insulin, coma and death will ensue in type 1 DM.

(h) The total lack of insulin in type 1 DM is a predisposing factor for DKA. Patients with type 1 DM are described as **ketosis-prone.**

b. Hyperglycemic hyperosmolar nonketotic (HHNK) syndrome [type 2 DM]

(1) Insulin deficiency, often with concomitant insulin resistance, results in hyperglycemia

(a) Impaired glucose uptake in the peripheral tissues (primarily muscle)

(b) Reduction in the conversion of glucose to glycogen (impaired **glycogenesis**), primarily in the liver

(c) Impaired insulin-induced suppression of hepatic glucose production (**neoglucogenesis** and **glycogenolysis**)

(2) Increasing blood glucose concentrations exceed the glucose reabsorptive capacity of the kidneys (occurs at about 180 mg/dl, referred to as the **renal threshold for glucose**). Glucose is then excreted into the urine, resulting in an **osmotic diuresis** with subsequent **dehydration** and **electrolyte abnormalities.**

(3) Insufficient glucose uptake in the peripheral tissues (due to insulin deficiency and/or insulin resistance) causes the cells to use protein as energy sources rather than glucose. Breakdown of protein yields carbohydrate/glucose moieties; however, with insufficient insulin, the additional glucose worsens hyperglycemia rather than serving as an energy source.

(4) In type 2 DM, the presence of even minimal blood levels of endogenous insulin usually prevents the breakdown of fats and subsequent ketonemia and ketoacidosis. Thus, patients with type 2 DM are described as **ketosis-resistant.**

(5) Although sufficient to suppress ketosis, endogenous insulin secretion in type 2 DM is insufficient for glycemic control. If insulin is not administered, profound dehydration with very high blood glucose levels may occur; this state is described as **hyperglycemic hyperosmolar nonketotic (HHNK) syndrome.** Coma and death may result.

F. Clinical evaluation

1. Physical findings

a. Symptom severity and onset help differentiate type 1 from type 2 DM.

(1) Type 1 DM typically presents with an abrupt onset and an acute presentation.

(2) Symptoms in individuals with type 2 DM generally develop gradually, with some patients being asymptomatic or having only mild symptoms upon diagnosis.
  b. Classic signs and symptoms of DM include polydipsia (excessive thirst), polyuria (excessive urination), and polyphagia (excessive hunger). Other common findings include dry skin, fatigue, weakness, frequent skin and vaginal infections, weight alterations, and visual disturbances.
  c. Individuals with type 1 DM may additionally present with unintentional weight loss, with or without signs and symptoms of ketoacidosis.
  d. Some of the progressive changes of long-standing DM may be evident at the time of diagnosis of type 2 DM: deterioration in function or structure of the retina, kidneys, peripheral nervous system, and integumentary system.

  2. Laboratory findings (reference)
    a. Diagnostic criteria: diabetes in nonpregnant adults
      (1) A random (casual) plasma glucose level ≥200 mg/dl with classic symptoms of DM, including polydipsia, polyuria, polyphagia, and weight loss.
      (2) A fasting plasma glucose (FPG) level of ≥126 mg/dl
      (3) A 2-hour plasma glucose ≥200 mg/dl during an oral glucose tolerance test (OGTT) using 75 g anhydrous glucose dissolved in water.
      (4) In the absence of unequivocal hyperglycemia with acute decompensation, the above criteria should be confirmed with repeat testing on a different day.
      (5) Note that these criteria do not distinguish between type 1 and type 2 DM; rather, they only identify the presence of clinical diabetes.
    b. Diagnostic criteria: gestational diabetes
      (1) Risk assessment for GDM should be undertaken at the first prenatal visit.
      (2) Glucose testing should be performed as soon as possible in women found to be at high risk for GDM (marked obesity, personal history of GDM, glycosuria, strong family history of DM). An FPG ≥126 mg/dl or casual PG ≥200 mg/dl, confirmed on a subsequent day, constitutes a diagnosis of DM.
      (3) High-risk women not found to have GDM at the initial screening and average-risk women should be tested between 24 and 28 weeks of gestation. Testing should follow one of two approaches:
        (a) One-step approach: perform a diagnostic OGTT
        (b) Two-step approach:
          (i) Initial screening of 50-gm oral glucose load (glucose challenge test, GCT). Perform OGTT on the subset of women exceeding the threshold value of 140 mg/dl (identifies ~80% of GDM) or 130 mg/dl (identifies 90% of GDM)
          (ii) Diagnostic OGTT: Following a 100-gm oral glucose load after an 8–14-hr fast, diagnosis of GDM may be made if two plasma glucose values equal or exceed the following:

Fasting	95 mg/dl
1 hr	180 mg/dl
2 hr	155 mg/dl
3 hr	140 mg/dl

Alternatively, a 75-gm glucose load may be used, but that test is not as well-validated for detection of GDM.
      (4) Low-risk women require no glucose testing, but this status is limited to individuals meeting *all* of the following criteria: less than 25 years of age, normal body weight before pregnancy, ethnic group with a low prevalence of GDM (e.g., *not* Hispanic, African-American, Asian, or Native American), no first-degree relative with DM, no history of poor obstetrical outcome.
    c. Diagnostic criteria: type 2 DM in children
      (1) Glucose testing should be performed in children at 10 years of age or at onset of puberty (if puberty occurs <10 years of age) who exhibit the following risk factors for DM:
        (a) Overweight, defined as: BMI >85th percentile for age and sex, weight for height >85th percentile, or weight >120% of ideal for height.
          –plus–
        (b) Any two of the following:
          (i) Family history of type 2 DM in first- or second-degree relative
          (ii) Race/ethnicity: Native American, African-American, Latino, Asian-American, or Pacific Islander

        (iii) Signs of insulin resistance or conditions associated with insulin resistance (e.g., acanthosis nigricans, hypertension, dyslipidemia, polycystic ovary syndrome)

    (2) Diagnostic criteria for DM are the same as listed for nonpregnant adults, above.

    (3) FPG is the preferred test for children because of its ease of testing and reproducibility.

    (4) Repeat every 2 years if testing is negative for DM.

  d. Diagnostic criteria: prediabetes in nonpregnant adults. Nonpregnant individuals not meeting the above criteria for diabetes but with abnormal test results, can be classified as having impaired fasting glucose (IFT) or impaired glucose tolerance (IGT). In 2002, IFG and IGT were offically termed **"prediabetes."** Use of this term better communicates to individuals the seriousness of this abnormality in the context of progression to DM.

    (1) IFT. Fasting plasma glucose level $\geq$110 mg/dl and <126 mg/dl

    (2) IGT. 2-hr OGTT plasma glucose $\geq$140 mg/dl and <200 mg/dl

II. DESIRED OUTCOMES OF DIABETES MANAGEMENT would include, but are not limited to, the following (adapt for individual patient):

A. Mortality outcomes Avoid diabetes-related premature death

  1. Life expectancy, American males: 74.1 years*

  2. Life expectancy, American females: 79.5 years*

B. Morbidity outcomes

  1. Retard progression of the disease.

  2. Prevent or in a timely manner treat acute complications.

  3. Prevent, detect early, or adequately treat vascular and neuropathic disease, and prevent or treat risk factors associated with those diseases (e.g., hypertension, tobacco use, triglycerides, cholesterol, obesity).

  4. Prevent or minimize drug-related problems.
    a. Side effects [adverse drug reactions (ADRs)]
    b. Toxicity
    c. Drug interactions (drug–drug, drug–disease, drug–food)

C. Behavioral outcomes

  1. Annual eye exams

  2. Routine self-monitoring of blood glucose (SMBG)

  3. Development of a consistent support system

  4. Adherence to medication regimen

  5. Routine and timely medical examinations and laboratory tests

  6. Avoidance of life-style or other behaviors [e.g., alcohol, caffeine, nicotine, certain over-the-counter (OTC) medications] that may increase the risk of diabetes-associated problems

D. Pharmacoeconomic outcomes

  1. Drug and treatment costs within patient resources

  2. Cost-effective and efficient use of health-care resources

E. Quality-of-life outcomes

  1. Match, or only minimally change, patient life-style and activities with disease treatment.

  2. Patient satisfaction with pharmaceutical care and health-care team

  3. Positive but realistic outlook for the future

III. DESIRED THERAPEUTIC END POINTS FOR DIABETES MANAGEMENT would include, but are not limited to, the following (adapt for the individual patient):

A. Nonpharmacological end points

1. Attain and/or maintain BMI <27.

2. Cessation of alcohol intake, or limit to no more than 1 oz in a day

3. Nicotine/tobacco cessation

4. Sodium restriction: no more than 2 gm/day

5. Routine, aerobic exercise no less than 3 times/week, 20–30 minutes per session

B. Pharmacological end points

1. Attain/maintain glycemic control.
   a. HbA1c <7% (based on 6% as upper limit of normal)
   b. SMBG standard deviation <40, based upon daily testing (at least once daily, alternating prebreakfast and presupper, with occasional 2 hr postprandial, largest meal)
   c. SMBG values: 50% within target of 70–140 mg/dl; NMT 30% above 200 mg/dl
   d. No more than 1–2 episodes of mild hypoglycemia per 1–2 weeks

2. Attain/maintain lipid profile within target range (reference).
   a. Low-density lipoprotein (LDL) <100 mg/dl
   b. Triglycerides (TG) <150 mg/dl
   c. High-density lipoprotein (HDL) >40 mg/dl male; >50 mg/dl female

3. Blood pressure (BP) <130/80 mm Hg, with minimal, or no, signs or symptoms of orthostatic hypotension

4. Minimal, or no, peripheral edema

5. Urinary albumin excretion <30 mcg albumin/mg creatinine in a spot collection (adjust end point based upon results of initial microalbumin test)

6. Retention of recognition of hypoglycemia symptoms

IV. THERAPY OF PREDIABETES. Modest weight loss and regular physical activity have been shown to reduce the rate of progression of prediabetes to type 2 DM (References B, C). Drug therapy (metformin [Reference C], acarbose [Reference D], and orlistat [Reference E]) have also been shown to reduce progression to DM in single trials, but not as effectively as intensive life-style interventions.

V. THERAPY OF DIABETES MELLITUS. Medical nutrition therapy, physical activity, pharmacotherapy, SMBG, and patient self-management education—especially concerning decision-making skills—are essential for successful management of the metabolic aspects of DM. Although some patients with "early" type 2 diabetes may not need pharmacotherapy for a while, the progressive nature of the disease ultimately results in the requirement of drug therapy.

A. Medical nutrition therapy (MNT). MNT incorporates the principles of good nutrition applied to the individual's diabetes control goals, eating preferences and habits, and concurrent medical conditions. An effective MNT plan will not be merely a "diet sheet" given to all people with diabetes. Some of the common approaches to diabetes MNT include the following:

1. **Carbohydrate (CHO) counting.** The individual is taught to identify and quantify the amounts of CHO foods consumed at each meal and throughout the day. Usually CHO intake is 45%–60% of total calories, based upon current diabetes control, TG levels, kidney function, and other medical concerns, as well as patient choice.
   a. When DM therapy includes a premeal short-acting insulin dose ("bolus"), patients may be taught to adjust the bolus dose to match the CHO intake.
   b. When bolus insulin is not employed, patients are taught to maintain consistent CHO intake at designated meals and across the day to match the antidiabetes effects of oral medications or intermediate-acting insulins.
   c. Sugar and simple CHOs would be "counted" as part of the CHO intake for the meal.

2. Limitations upon **fat intake** and **type of fat** consumed are important if weight loss is a goal or as part of therapy for hyperlipidemia. The primary dietary fat goal in diabetes is to reduce saturated fat and cholesterol intake. Saturated fat is the principal dietary determinant of plasma LDL cholesterol. Furthermore, persons with diabetes appear to be more sensitive to dietary cholesterol than the general public. Fat intake is generally targeted to the following levels: (Evidence-Based Nutrition Principles and Recommendations for the Treatment and Prevention of Diabetes and Related Complications. Diabetes Care, Vol. 26, Supp.1, Jan 2003)

   a. Less than 10% of total calories from saturated fats. In persons with persistent LDL cholesterol >100 mg/dl, consider lowering saturated fat intake to <7%.

   b. Dietary cholesterol intake <300 mg/day. For individuals with persistent LDL cholesterol >100 mg/dl, consider lowering dietary cholesterol to <200 mg/day.

   c. Minimize intake of trans-unsaturated fatty acids (hydrogenated vegetable oils). The effect of trans-unsaturated fatty acids is similar to saturated fats in raising plasma LDL cholesterol, and trans-fatty acids lower plasma HDL cholesterol.

   d. Polyunsaturated fat intake should be 10% of total caloric intake.

3. Limitations on **protein** and **type of protein** consumed are important in later phases of end-stage renal disease and may delay the need for dialysis. For individuals with glycemic control and normal renal function, protein should be eaten within the context of a healthy diet.

4. **Spaced intervals** between meals may be helpful for matching the hypoglycemic actions of insulin or insulin secretagogues or when postprandial glycemic normalization is delayed.

5. Consumption of dietary **fiber** (e.g., bran, beans, fruits, vegetables) is to be encouraged; however, there is no evidence that people with diabetes need a greater amount of fiber than other Americans. Very large amounts of fiber may benefit glycemic control, hyperinsulinemia, and plasma lipids, but the palatability and gastrointestinal side effects of such amounts of fiber may be unacceptable to most people.

6. **Dietary adjustment algorithms.** Alteration of dietary intake based upon factors that change the blood glucose level, such as stress, illness, or exercise. For example, consumption of additional carbohydrate and/or protein before vigorous exercise.

B. **Physical activity (exercise).** A carefully planned and consistent program of physical activity enhances glucose uptake to cells, thereby reducing the BG level. In addition, exercise may improve CHO metabolism and insulin sensitivity in patients with type 2 DM; may reduce levels of triglyceride-rich VLDL; may reduce blood pressure, especially in hyperinsulinemic subjects; may enhance weight loss and weight maintenance; and may prevent progression of pre-diabetes to DM.

1. Physical activity has potential problems for individuals with diabetes.

   a. Patients with severe (proliferative) retinopathy must consult an ophthalmologist before beginning any type of exercise program. Strenuous activity may precipitate vitreous hemorrhage or traction retinal detachment in these patients. These individuals should avoid anaerobic exercise and physical activity that involves straining, jarring, or Valsalva-like maneuvers.

   b. Patients with cardiovascular disease, those older than 35 years of age, or individuals with autonomic neuropathy, peripheral vascular disease, or microvascular disease should receive a cardiovascular evaluation and stress test before beginning an exercise program.

   c. Patients with significant peripheral neuropathy (with loss of protective sensation in the feet) should limit weight-bearing exercise. Repetitive exercise on insensitive feet can lead to ulceration and fractures. Treadmill exercises, jogging, prolonged walking, and step exercises are contraindicated; swimming, bicycling, rowing, chair exercises, arm exercises, and other non–weight-bearing exercise should be recommended.

   d. High-intensity or strenuous physical activity should probably be discouraged in individuals with overt nephropathy (>200 mg/min), unless blood pressure is carefully monitored during exercise.

2. **Aerobic activity** (e.g., swimming, walking, running) is the preferred type of exercise because of its desirable hypoglycemic effects (promotes utilization of glucose as fuel), as well as desirable effects upon cardiovascular health, hypertension, lipid profiles, circulation, and weight-loss efforts.

3. Anaerobic activity (e.g., weight lifting) should generally be avoided by people with diabetes unless it has been specifically approved by appropriate medical specialists such as a cardiologist (because it could have potential deleterious cardiovascular or blood pressure effects) or an ophthalmologist (because it could have potential deleterious effects upon underlying retinopathy).

4. The physical activity plan should be consistent with regard to frequency (daily, or at least 3–4 days per week), intensity, and duration.

5. General guidelines that may prove helpful in regulating the glycemic response to physical activity include:

    a. Assess metabolic control before physical activity. Avoid physical activity if glucose level is >250 mg/dl and ketosis is present; use caution if glucose level is >300 mg/dl with no ketosis. Ingest additional carbohydrate if glucose level is <100 mg/dl.

    b. Monitor blood glucose before and after physical activity (up to several hours post-exercise) to identify when/if changes in insulin or food intake are necessary and to learn individual glycemic responses to different physical activity conditions.

    c. Consume added carbohydrate as needed to avoid hypoglycemia; CHO-based food should be readily available during and after physical activity.

C. Pharmacotherapy: insulin and insulin analogues

  1. Indications. Insulin therapy is required for all patients with type 1 DM and for those with type 2 DM when oral antidiabetes therapy alone does not achieve the desired DM control. Insulin and insulin analogues may be used in combination with certain oral antidiabetes agents in type 1 or type 2 DM.

  2. Mechanism of action. Insulin lowers blood glucose and contributes to glucose homeostasis by a variety of physiological actions, including:

    a. ↑ glucose uptake and utilization by peripheral tissues

    b. ↑ glycogenesis (conversion of glucose to glycogen in liver and muscle)

    c. ↓ glycogenolysis (production of glucose from glycogen)

    d. ↓ gluconeogenesis (formation of glucose from noncarbohydrates, such as amino acids)

    e. ↓ lipolysis and ketogenesis (breakdown of fats to ketone bodies)

    f. ↑ formation of protein from amino acids

    g. ↑ formation of adipose tissue from triglycerides and fatty acids

  3. Descriptive terms

    a. Chemical sources of commercial insulin

      (1) Pork

      (2) Semisynthetic human. Produced by chemical alteration of pork insulin

      (3) Biosynthetic human. Produced by recombinant DNA techniques

      (4) Insulin analogue. Produced by chemical alteration of human insulin

      (5) Use of human insulin or insulin analogue is preferred for most individuals with diabetes because of reduced antigenicity.

    b. Concentration, products available in the United States

      (1) U-100. Refers to a concentration of 100 units/mL

      (2) U-500. Concentrated regular insulin 500 units/mL, for patients with insulin resistance. Due to its high concentration, bioactivity of U-500 regular insulin mimics an intermediate-acting insulin.

    c. Types of insulin. Refers to onset and duration of insulin preparation. See Table 52-1.

      (1) Rapid-acting insulin. Lispro insulin analogue and aspart insulin analogue

      (2) Short-acting insulin. Regular insulin

      (3) Intermediate-acting insulins. NPH (isophane insulin suspension) insulin and lente insulin

      (4) Long-acting insulin. Ultralente insulin (extended insulin zinc suspension) and glargine insulin analogue.

      (5) Premixed insulin products. Each give a rapid- or short-acting insulin as a pre-meal bolus plus an intermediate-acting insulin to control later hyperglycemia or the subsequent meal

        (a) 50/50 insulin. Mixture of 50% regular insulin with 50% NPH insulin

        (b) 70/30 insulin. Mixture of 30% regular insulin with 70% NPH insulin

        (c) 75/25 insulin analogue. Mixture of 25% lispro insulin analogue with 75% protamine lispro insulin analogue

Table 52-1. Time-Action of Insulin Types

	Onset (hr)	Peak (hr)	Duration (hr)	Variability in absorption and duration
Rapid acting				
Lispro	<0.25	0.5–1.5	3–4	Minimal
Aspart	<0.25	0.7–1	3–5	Minimal
Short-acting				
Regular	0.5–1	2–3	3–6+	Moderate
Intermediate-acting				
NPH	2–4	6–10	10–16	High
Lente	3–4	6–12	12–18	High
Long-acting				
Ultralente	6–10	10–16	18–20	High
Glargine	5	N/A	20–24	Minimal-moderate

From: Campbell RK, White JR. *Medications for the treatment of diabetes.* Alexandria, VA: American Diabetes Association, 2000.

    (d) 70/30 insulin analogue. Mixture of 30% aspart insulin analogue with 70% protamine aspart insulin analogue

  d. Extemporaneous mixtures. Two insulins mixed in one syringe, before administration. Extemporaneous mixtures allow the ratio to be tailor-made to match the patient's blood glucose reading, anticipated eating or physical activity, or other factors influencing the requirement for specific insulin action.

4. Administration and dosage

  a. Examples of initial doses of insulin, assuming a waking time in the morning, meals/snacks spaced consistently during the day and waking hours, and a late evening bedtime

    (1) Type 1 DM. Initial total daily dose (TDD) = 0.5 − 1.0 units/kg/day, given as three or four injections per day. Regimens employing only one or two injections per day do not achieve euglycemia in type 1 DM.

      (a) Three injections per day

        (i) Prebreakfast injection. Two-thirds of TDD. 25%–35% of the total breakfast dose is given as lispro, aspart, or regular insulin; 65%–75% of the total breakfast dose is given as NPH or lente insulin (1:2 ratio). May be mixed extemporaneously or may be a commercial premixed product.

        (ii) Presupper injection. 10%–20% of TDD, given as lispro, aspart, or regular insulin

        (iii) Bedtime (10 P.M.) injection. 10–25% of TDD, given as NPH or lente insulin

      (b) Four injections per day

        (i) Premeal injections (three injections). Total of 40%–50% of TDD. Total amount is divided between the three meals in a ratio proportional to the desired/usual ratio of CHO ingestion at those three meals. Given as lispro, aspart, or regular insulin before each meal.

        (ii) Bedtime injection. 50%–60% of TDD, given as NPH or glargine insulin. Caveat: If NPH insulin is used for the bedtime injection, the premeal insulin must be regular insulin.

      (c) Insulin pump therapy (use of external pump to provide continuous subcutaneous insulin infusion)

        (i) Premeal and pre-snack boluses. Dosage based on premeal BG level and anticipated CHO intake for the meal. Initial estimate would be similar to the initial estimate for the four-injection regimen described above. Given as lispro or aspart insulin.

        (ii) Basal insulin. Programmed to be delivered continuously. Initial estimate is 50%–60% of TDD, but may be subsequently altered to give differing basal infusions at certain times of the day. Initial rate is often 0.5–1.25 units/hr, given as lispro or aspart insulin.

(2) Type 2 DM. Initial TDD = 0.15 − 0.4 units/kg/day, but will vary greatly depending on degree of concomitant insulin resistance and degree of β-cell dysfunction.

(a) One injection per day. Bedtime insulin only, 0.25 units/kg/day, given as NPH or glargine insulin. Usually in combination with an oral antidiabetes medication, but may also be monotherapy.

(b) Two injections per day
(i) Prebreakfast injection. 2/3 of TDD, given as a premix insulin (70/30, 75/25, or 50/50–choice would depend on anticipated CHO intake at breakfast and lunch)
(ii) Presupper injection. 1/3 of TDD, given as a premix insulin (70/30, 75/25, or 50/50–choice would depend on anticipated CHO intake at supper)

(c) Three or four injections per day. Types, initial ratios, and regimens are similar to type 1, described above.

b. Initial doses and regimen adjusted accordingly, based upon ongoing SMBG, symptoms of hypoglycemia or hyperglycemia, and periodic glycosylated hemoglobin (AIC) results.

c. Alterations in insulin requirement
(1) Infection, exacerbations of other medical problems, weight gain, puberty, inactivity, hyperthyroidism, and Cushing's disease tend to increase insulin needs.
(2) Renal failure, adrenal insufficiency, nutrient malabsorption, hypopituitarism, weight loss, and increased exercise tend to reduce insulin needs.
(3) Drug–drug or drug–disease interactions may increase or decrease insulin requirements.

d. **Subcutaneous injection.** For routine administration of insulin
(1) Successful insulin therapy requires predictable and consistent insulin absorption and insulin action from day to day.
(a) In most patients, absorption of regular insulin is fastest from the abdomen, followed by the arm, buttocks, and thigh.
(b) Upon initiation of insulin therapy, patients should carefully monitor and record their own variations in absorption. If it is determined that the variation is sufficiently great, then a given injection (e.g, presupper dose) should always be given in the same anatomical region (e.g., arms). Random rotation of injection regions should be avoided in these individuals.
(c) Physical exercise increases blood flow to the exercising area, thus accelerating absorption of insulin injected at that site. To a lesser extent, hot showers, baths, and massage may have a similar effect. Patients should be advised to avoid giving an injection into a limb that will be subsequently exercised or heated. The abdomen may be preferable for the preexercise injection because that area is the least likely to have significant increases in absorption.
(2) Within an anatomical region, the injection site should be rotated to avoid lipohypertrophy and fibrosis.

e. **Continuous intravenous (insulin drip)** administration of regular insulin. Used for treatment of acute hyperglycemia, ketoacidosis, HHNK syndrome, or during surgical procedures or delivery.

f. **Continuous subcutaneous infusion (insulin pump therapy)**
(1) Short-acting or rapid-acting insulin is infused continuously during the day in a patient-specific pattern to deliver low doses of insulin (basal insulin) to offset the glycemic effects of daily patterns of counterregulatory hormones.
(2) Before each meal, the patient sets the pump to deliver a "bolus" dose of short-acting or rapid-acting insulin to control the glycemic effects of the meal. The bolus dose is determined by algorithms that consider the premeal glucose level, anticipated dietary intake, and activity.
(3) Offers the potential for tighter glycemic control.
(4) Indicated for selected diabetic individuals with widely fluctuating blood glucose levels, irregular or inconsistent work schedules, life-styles, or meals or who achieve less-than-desired control using frequent injection routines.
(5) Requires frequent SMBG, thorough training in the use of the infusion equipment, and an advanced understanding and application of exercise, dietary, and insulin adjustment protocols.

D. Pharmacotherapy. Insulin secretagogues (oral hypoglycemic agents)

1. Chemical classes
  a. Sulfonylureas
    (1) Ttolbutamide
    (2) Acetohexamide
    (3) Chlorpropamide
    (4) Glyburide
    (5) Glipizide
    (6) Glimepiride
  b. Meglitinides
    (1) Repaglinide
    (2) Nateglinide

2. Indications (labeled uses) and common clinical uses
  a. Type 2 DM
    (1) Monotherapy or in combination with other oral antidiabetes drugs or insulin
    (2) Use in type 2 DM predicated on
      (a) adequate control not attained by medical nutrition therapy and physical activity alone
      (b) —*or*— pharmacological intervention is required based on the presenting blood glucose levels and diabetes symptomatology
      (c) —*and*— there are sufficient numbers of functioning β cells.
  b. Type 1 DM. Not indicated. Pharmacological action depends on functioning β cells.

3. Mechanisms of action
  a. Predominant effect. Stimulate pancreatic secretion of insulin
  b. Improve "first phase" release of insulin/increase sensitivity of β cells to glucose stimulus
  c. Lessor effect. Increase hepatic sensitivity to insulin
  d. Lessor effect. Increase number and/or sensitivity of insulin receptors in muscle and adipose tissue
  e. Lessor effect. Reduce postreceptor defect ("transport defect") in muscle and adipose tissue

4. Choice of agent. The most clinically significant difference among sulfonylureas is duration of action (Table 52-2), which then impacts frequency of dosing and potential compliance issues. Other considerations include frequency and consistency of eating and exercise, additional patient-specific risk factors for severe hypoglycemia (e.g., hypoglycemia unawareness), patient-specific contraindications, and cost considerations.
  a. Glimepiride exhibits an insulin-sparing effect compared to other members of this class, reportedly by its relatively greater extrapancreatic effect.
  b. β-cell stimulation of insulin secretion is more glucose-dependent with repaglinide and nateglinide than with sulfonylurea agents. This action, along with its very short action, may present a reduced risk of late postprandial hypoglycemia for selected individuals.
  c. Chlorpropamide has the longest duration of action and poses a risk to patients with renal or hepatic impairment. It also causes more severe and frequent side effects (including hypoglycemia and hyponatremia) than other sulfonylureas.
  d. Glyburide has been associated with severe or prolonged hypoglycemia in the elderly.

5. Administration and dosage (see Table 52-2)

6. Significant precautions and adverse effects
  a. Insulin secretagogues are not recommended for children, pregnant and lactating women, or as monotherapy in patients without functioning pancreatic β-cells.
  b. Sulfonylurea agents are contraindicated in patients with allergy to sulfa agents.
  c. Insulin secretagogues should not be used for metabolic control during stressful conditions such as severe infection, injury, or surgery (all of which stimulate the release of counterregulatory hormones), which increase the risk of hyperglycemia. Insulin therapy should be instituted during these conditions.
  d. Certain agents should not be used in patients with severe renal or hepatic impairment.
  e. Sulfonylurea therapy has been associated with a possible increased risk of cardiovascular morbidity and mortality.

Table 52-2. Insulin Secretagogues: Monotherapy in Type 2 DM

Generic Name	Initial Daily Dose	Maximum Daily Dose	Duration of Action	Comments
Acetohexamide	250 mg single dose	1500 mg— Give in two doses when dose reaches 1000 mg	Intermediate 12–18 hr	Metabolized in liver to active metabolite (twice as potent as parent compound). Has diuretic activity. Has uricosuric activity.
Chlorpropamide	100 mg single dose	750 mg single dose (500 mg in older patients)	Very long 60 hr	70% metabolized in liver to less-active metabolites; 30% excreted intact by kidneys. Can potentiate ADH. One-third of patients have an Antabuse-like reaction with alcohol.
Tolazamide	100 mg single dose	1000 mg— Give in two doses when dose reaches 500 mg	Intermediate 12–24 hr	Metabolized in liver to less-active and inactive products. Has diuretic activity.
Tolbutamide	250–500 mg single dose	3000 mg in two or three doses	Short 6–12 hr	Metabolized in liver to inactive product.
Glipizide	5 mg single dose	40 mg—Give in two doses when dose reaches 15 mg	Intermediate 12–24 hr	Metabolized in liver to inactive products that are excreted in the urine and to a lesser extent, in the bile. Mild diuretic activity.
Glyburide	2.5 mg single dose	20 mg in one or two doses	Intermediate 16–24 hr	Metabolized in liver to weakly active and inactive products, excreted in urine and bile. Mild diuretic activity.
Glimepiride	1–2 mg single dose	8 mg	Short 8–12 hr	Metabolized in liver, renal eliminated, less stimulation of insulin secretion.
Repaglinide	0.5–2 mg tid ac	4 mg ac, or 12 mg/day	Very short 2–4 hr	Metabolized in liver to inactive metabolites. Action is dose-dependent and glucose-dependent.
Nateglinide	120 mg tid ac 60 mg tid ac for patients near target HbA1c	180 mg tid	Very short 4–6 hr	Metabolized in liver to less active metabolites, by CYP2C9 (70%) and CYP3A4 (30%). May elevate uric acid levels.

Facts and Comparisons (drug information monthly update service). St. Louis, MO: J. B. Lippincott Company, 2003.

f. Hypoglycemia and alcohol intolerance may occur during sulfonylurea therapy, most notably with chlorpropamide and tolbutamide. Alcohol intolerance is less common with the newer (second-generation) agents.

g. Adverse effects with insulin secretagogues include gastrointestinal (GI) disturbances (e.g., nausea, gastric discomfort, vomiting, constipation), tachycardia, headache, skin rash, and hematological problems (e.g., agranulocytosis, pancytopenia, hemolytic anemia).

h. Sulfonylureas pose a risk of cholestatic jaundice.

i. Primary failure. The agent fails to control hyperglycemia within the first 4 weeks after initiation. This most likely represents insufficient numbers of functioning β cells.

j. Secondary failure. The drug controls hyperglycemia initially but fails to maintain control. Approximately 5%–30% of initial responders experience secondary failure. In most instances, this represents progression of the DM, with a diminishing number of functioning β cells, rather than a "drug failure."

E. Pharmacotherapy. Insulin sensitizers

1. Chemical classes
   a. Biguanides: metformin
   b. Thiazolidinediones
      (1) Pioglitazone
      (2) Rosiglitazone
   c. Combination products
      (1) Metformin/glyburide
      (2) Metformin/glipizide
      (3) Metformin/rosiglitazone

2. **Indications (labeled uses) and common clinical uses**
   a. Insulin sensitizers are indicated in those individuals with a significant component of insulin resistance.
   b. Type 2 DM
      (1) Use in type 2 DM predicated on
         (a) adequate control not attained by medical nutrition therapy and physical activity alone
         (b) —*or*— pharmacological intervention is required based on the presenting blood glucose levels and diabetes symptomatology
         (c) —*and*— patient has adequate endogenous or exogenous insulin.
      (2) Monotherapy
      (3) Combination therapy, with other oral antidiabetes agents or insulin
   c. Type 1 DM. As adjunct to insulin; must not be used as monotherapy

3. Mechanisms of action
   a. These agents are pharmacologically "antihyperglycemic" agents rather than hypoglycemic agents.
   b. Increase hepatic sensitivity to insulin, thereby suppressing hepatic glucose production. Major action for metformin; secondary action for pioglitazone and rosiglitazone.
   c. Reduce postreceptor defect ("transport defect") in muscle and adipose tissue—this defect appears to be the major component of naturally occurring insulin resistance. Major action for pioglitazone and rosiglitazone; secondary action for metformin.
   d. Increase number and/or sensitivity of insulin receptors in muscle and adipose tissue, thereby addressing the cell-surface "binding defect"—this defect correlates most significantly with hyperinsulinemia. Major action for pioglitazone and rosiglitazone; secondary action for metformin.

4. **Administration and dosage.** (Table 52-3)

5. **Significant precautions and adverse effects**
   a. Metformin
      (1) Contraindicated in situations with potential for increased risk of lactic acidosis. Lactic acidosis is a rare but serious complication and is fatal in 50% of cases.
         (a) Renal dysfunction (SCr $\geq$1.4 mg/dl, female; SCr $\geq$1.5 mg/dl, male). Confirm adequate renal function in the elderly, even in the face of "low" SCr levels.
         (b) Hypoperfusion (hypoxic states)—for example:
            (i) During surgery
            (ii) Severe cardiovascular/pulmonary dysfunction
            (iii) Acute myocardial infarction or heart failure
         (c) Radiographic procedures using intravenous iodinated contrast agents (potential for transient renal dysfunction). Discontinue metformin during the procedure; reinitiate when renal function is reestablished and confirmed.
         (d) Chronic or binge ingestion of ethanol
         (e) Liver disease (hepatic function important for clearance of blood lactate)
      (2) Serum vitamin B_{12} levels may decline, usually without clinical manifestations
      (3) Follow labeled recommendations for monitoring liver function, renal function, and vitamin B_{12} status
      (4) Most notable subjective side effect: GI disturbances—loose stools or diarrhea, usually subsiding after 7–10 days
   b. Thiazolidinediones
      (1) Contraindicated in hepatic disease
         (a) Idiosyncratic hepatic failure, a rare but serious event, has occurred during therapy with troglitazone, a thiazolidinedione removed from the U.S. market in

Table 52-3. Insulin Sensitizers

Generic Name	Initial Dose	Maximum Dose	Half-Life (Plasma)	Comments
Metformin	500 mg bid	1000 mg bid is optimal therapeutic dose 850 mg tid is labeled maximum dose	Approx 6 hr	Usually taken with meals to lessen GI effects. Excreted unchanged in urine. Warnings against use in situations with potential for lactic acidosis.
Pioglitazone	15 or 30 mg qd	45 mg	3–7 hr (parent); 16–24 hr (metabolites)	May be taken without regard to meals. Food slightly delays the time to peak concentration, but does not reduce the extent of absorption. Protein binding >99%, mostly to albumin. Metabolized in liver (CYP2C8 and 3A4); excreted primarily through feces. Animal studies suggest some active metabolites.
Rosiglitazone	4 mg qd	8 mg qd	103–158 hr	May be taken without regard to meals. Protein binding >99%, mostly to albumin. Metabolized by CYP2C8 (major) and 2C9 (minor); metabolites excreted via urine and feces. Metabolites are active, but less active than the parent.

1999. Because of their strutural similarity to troglitazone, pioglitazone and rosiglitazone should be used cautiously in patients with hepatic disease. Clinical data have not shown evidence of drug-induced hepatoxicity from pioglitazone or rosiglitazone.

    (b) Follow labeled guidelines for routine monitoring of liver function (baseline, every 2 months during the first year, periodically thereafter).

  (2) Warning for use in patients with severe heart failure (NYHA Class III or IV cardiac status), due to possible increase in plasma volume (found in human studies) and heart enlargement (found in animal studies).

  (3) Premenopausal anovulatory women may resume ovulation during therapy, placing the patient at risk of pregnancy.

  (4) Most notable subjective side effects: edema, weight gain, headache, fatigue

 c. Safety in children or during pregnancy has not been established.

 d. Metformin is excreted into breast milk. Animal studies suggest that pioglitazone and rosiglitazone are secreted in breast milk, but it is not known if these drugs or metabolites are excreted in human milk.

F. Pharmacotherapy: α-glucosidase inhibitors

  1. Agents in this class

    a. Acarbose

    b. Miglitol

  2. Indications

    a. Used in individuals with significant postprandial hyperglycemia. These drugs have minimal effect on preprandial or fasting blood glucose levels.

    b. Type 2 DM

      (1) Monotherapy or in combination with insulin or other oral antidiabetes agents, notably insulin secretagogues

Table 52-4. α-Glucosidase Inhibitors

Generic Name	Initial Dose	Maximum Dose	Half-Life	Comments
Acarbose	25 mg with 1–3 meals/day	150 mg/day for pts <60 kg weight 300 mg/day for pts ≥60 kg weight	Intestinal action approx 2 hr	Take with first bite of meal. Negligible absorption of unchanged drug. Metabolized in GI tract; 35% of metabolites are absorbed and excreted in urine.
Miglitol	25 mg with 1–3 meals/day	300 mg/day	Intestinal action approx 2 hr	Take with first bite of meal. Not metabolized. Degree of absorption is dose-dependent. Excreted by kidneys (absorbed) and feces (unabsorbed).

        (2) Use in type 2 DM predicated on
            (a) adequate control (especially postprandial) not attained by medical nutrition therapy and physical activity alone
            (b) —*or*— pharmacological intervention is required based on the presenting postprandial blood glucose levels and diabetes symptomatology
            (c) —*and*— patient has adequate endogenous or exogenous insulin.
      c. Type 1 DM:
          (1) As an adjunct to insulin therapy; may be useful in individuals with delayed absorption of subcutaneous insulin
          (2) Not to be used as monotherapy

    3. Mechanism of action
      a. Inhibits the intestinal enzyme α-glucosidase (a class of enzymes). Intestinal absorption of complex carbohydrates such as starch, dextrins, and disaccharides (e.g., sucrose, maltose) requires the action of intestinal α-glucosidase.
      b. Inhibition of α-glucosidase retards the degradation and thus the absorption of carbohydrates, resulting in a slower and smaller rise in blood glucose following the meal.

    4. Administration and dosage (Table 52-4)

    5. Significant precautions and adverse effects
      a. Not indicated during pregnancy, in breast-feeding women, or in children.
      b. Contraindicated in inflammatory bowel disease, colonic ulceration, or obstructive bowel disorders; chronic intestinal disorders of digestion or absorption; or any medical condition that might deteriorate with increased intestinal gas formation.
      c. Contraindicated in cirrhosis of the liver.
      d. Follow labeled recommendations for routine liver function monitoring.
      e. Oral sugar sources other than glucose or lactose are unsuitable for rapid correction of hypoglycemia, because these drugs blunt the digestion of complex sugars to glucose.
      f. Most notable subjective side effects. Gastrointestinal effects, occurring primarily at initiation of therapy or when dosage is increased: diarrhea, abdominal pain, and flatulence (about 30%, 10%–20%, and 42%–77%, respectively). Usually self-limiting, transient, and can be minimized by starting with a low dose and slow upward titration of dosage.

VI. PATIENT EDUCATION AND SELF-CARE. Patient education about the disease and patient participation in medical care are the most important aspects of DM management. *Without patient involvement and participation, even the "ideal" pharmacotherapy, dietary, or other interventions will fail.* **Patient education** improves understanding of the disease, promotes optimal patient choices regarding diet, medication, and exercise, and facilitates decision-making skills. National, state, and local diabetes professional groups have published guidelines to ensure thorough and effective teaching content and methods. Examples of patient education topics include, but are not limited to, the following:

    A. Prevention, recognition, and treatment of acute hypoglycemic and hyperglycemic episodes.

B. Reduction of modifiable risk factors for the development of chronic complications

    1. Achievement of A1c <7% (based on upper limit of normal = 6%)

    2. Smoking cessation

    3. Normalization of blood pressure

    4. Normalization of blood lipid profile

    5. Reduction of weight to at least a BMI of 27, if applicable

    6. Routine assessment/screening for, and early treatment of, chronic complications

C. Pattern control. Adjustment algorithms for diet, exercise, and/or medications based on trends in BG control.

D. Implementation of **specific self-care measures**

    1. Foot care. Neuropathy, peripheral vascular disease, trauma, and infection increase the risk for lower-extremity complications and amputation, causing hospitalizations, disability, morbidity, and mortality.

        a. Inspect feet and interdigital areas daily, looking for changes in color or skin integrity.

        b. Inspect shoes daily before putting them on, to detect loose objects or rough shoe materials that may injure or irritate the skin.

        c. Clean feet daily, and dry thoroughly. Use forearm, elbow, or a thermometer to check water temperature if the patient has neuropathy-induced sensation loss.

        d. Moisturize dry skin with hand lotion or vaseline. Avoid area between the toes.

        e. Cut toenails straight across, or follow the natural curve of the toe.

        f. Avoid self-treatment of corns, calluses, or ingrown toenails.

        g. Wear well-fitting shoes and soft cotton socks. Avoid going barefoot.

        h. Seek prompt medical attention for any problems identified (e.g., cuts, blisters, calluses, unhealing wounds, or signs of infections such as redness, swelling, drainage, pus, or fever).

    2. Skin care. Dry skin occurs frequently in individuals with DM due to dehydration (secondary to hyperglycemia-induced diuresis) and/or anhidrosis (secondary to autonomic neuropathic condition, resulting in little or no perspiration). Elevated blood glucose levels and impaired circulation also increase the risk for the development of skin infections.

        a. Inspect skin daily for abrasions, pain, or swelling. Consult the health-care provider promptly if problems are noted.

        b. Keep skin clean using a mild soap and warm (not hot) water.

        c. Use moisturizing lotion (alcohol-free and not oiled-based) on dry skin areas.

        d. Use sunscreen products throughout the year. As a physical stress, severe sunburn may raise BG.

        e. Avoid situations with potential for local trauma, especially to legs and feet. If injury occurs, the lesion should be covered with sterile gauze and first-aid measures applied.

    3. Dental care. Periodontal disease is often accelerated in people with long-standing or poorly controlled diabetes.

        a. A yearly dental exam is recommended.

        b. Effective brushing and flossing is essential.

    4. Eye care. Diabetes is a leading cause of vision impairment in the United States and the leading cause of blindness for individuals between the ages of 20 and 74 years of age. A yearly dilated eye exam is recommended, with more frequent follow-up guided by the severity of disease.

VII. ASSESSMENT OF GLYCEMIC CONTROL

A. Self-monitoring of blood glucose (SMBG)

    1. Indicated for all individuals with diabetes. The frequency and time of testing will vary according to type of diabetes, type of antidiabetes medication, and goals of therapy.

    2. Involves the patient in the treatment process

3. Allows the patient and the health-care provider to assess the individual's response to various factors (e.g., life-style modifications, nutritional alterations, medication adjustments, stress, illness, infection, trauma, changes in physical activity).

4. Gives immediate feedback and data for the patient to use in the application of diet, exercise, or insulin adjustment algorithms (decision-making skills).

5. A variety of testing products and product features are available. The use of meters with test memory functions and the capacity to download (via computer) SMBG results provides efficient access and analysis of SMBG trends.

B. Urine glucose testing. No longer recommended since it only provides retrospective information and does not reflect current blood glucose. Reserved only for those individuals unable or unwilling to perform SMBG.

C. Urine ketone monitoring. An essential component of diabetes management, particularly during the following conditions:

1. During illness in all patients with diabetes, since even those with type 2 DM can become ketotic during periods of severe stress, infection, or trauma

2. Patients with type 1 DM when blood glucose is consistently >240 mg/dl

3. Pregnant women with diabetes (including gestational diabetes)

4. Individuals actively trying to lose weight by calorie restriction

D. Long-term monitoring of glycemic control:

1. **Hemoglobin A1C test (glycohemoglobin; glycosylated hemoglobin test)**
   a. Reflects average blood glucose level over the preceding 2–3 months.
   b. Based on an upper limit of normal being 6% for the A1C, a hemoglobin A1C level of 7.0% or lower indicates good overall glycemic control, whereas a level >7.0% reveals the need for additional intervention.
   c. Underlying hemoglobinopathies may cause anomalous values.
   d. In general, the frequency of A1C testing is at least 1–2 times per year in patients with stable glycemic control and at least quarterly in patients whose therapy has recently changed or who are in poor control.

2. **Glycosylated fructosamine test**
   a. Measures glycemic control over the preceding 2–3 weeks
   b. Useful for short-term follow-up of recently implemented interventions, when timely assessment of the intervention is important (e.g., changes in diabetes therapy during pregnancy).

VIII. ACUTE CHANGES IN GLYCEMIC CONTROL

A. Hyperglycemia

1. *Mild to moderate ↑ BG,* rapid onset (within hours), no metabolic abnormalities:
   a. **Acute ↑ BG,** due to unplanned event such as illness, emotional distress, or excessive caloric intake
   b. **↑ BG following prolonged or severe hypoglycemia**—Somogyi effect or rebound hyperglycemia
   c. **↑ BG occurring as a pattern in the early morning,** caused by counterregulatory hormones (i.e., dawn phenomenon).

2. *Moderate to severe ↑ BG* (>250 mg/dl), short duration (one to several days), with acidosis and ketosis: **ketoacidosis (DKA)** (see I B E 2a)
   a. Often the presenting disorder in children with previously undiagnosed type 1 DM.
   b. **Precipitating factors** include stress, infection, exercise, excessive alcohol consumption, improper insulin therapy, and dietary noncompliance.
   c. **Physical findings** include Kussmaul's respirations, acetone breath odor, dehydration, dry skin, poor skin turgor, reduced level of consciousness (ranging from confusion to coma), and abdominal pain.

      d. Laboratory findings include hyperglycemia, ketosis, low arterial pH and carbon dioxide partial pressure (PCO_2) values, and abnormal serum electrolyte values.

      e. Therapy involves fluid, intravenous insulin by continuous infusion, and electrolyte replacement. Without treatment, death ensues.

  3. *Severe* ↑ *BG* (>500 mg/dl) intermediate duration (days to weeks), with profound dehydration, ↓ CNS function and ↑ serum osmolality, without ketosis or acidosis: **HHNK** coma (see I B E 2b).

    a. Occurs primarily in type 2 DM

    b. Has a higher mortality rate than DKA

    c. Precipitating factors include illnesses and conditions that increase insulin requirements and predispose the patient to dehydration.

      (1) Examples include severe burns, GI bleeding, central nervous system (CNS) injury, and acute myocardial infarction.

      (2) Use of glucogenic drugs (e.g., steroids, glucagon, thiazide diuretics, cimetidine, propranolol)

      (3) Medical procedures or hypertonic high-glucose products such as intravenous hyperalimentation, peritoneal dialysis, and enteral nutrition

    d. Physical findings include polyuria, polydipsia, dehydration, hypotension, rapid respirations, abdominal discomfort, nausea, vomiting, tachycardia, palpitations, and profound signs of neurological deficits such as confusion, coma, generalized or focal seizures, myoclonic jerking, and hemiparesis.

    e. Laboratory findings include hyperglycemia (often substantially above 500 mg/dl), absence of ketosis, and serum osmolarity of ≥280 mOsm.

    f. Therapy involves fluid, insulin, and electrolyte replacement.

B. Hypoglycemia

  1. Mild hypoglycemia. Primarily adrenergic symptoms (tachycardia, palpitations, shakiness) or cholinergic (sweating) symptoms, or effects of mild CNS glucopenia (inability to concentrate, dizziness, hunger, blurred vision), but symptoms are not severe enough to interfere with self-medication for the hypoglycemia.

  2. Moderate hypoglycemia. The CNS is more markedly deprived of glucose, eliciting symptoms of confusion, inappropriate behavior, and impairment of motor function. The patient is minimally capable of self-treatment, and assistance is usually needed. The patient is NOT unconscious.

  3. Severe hypoglycemia. Coma, seizure, and/or impairment of motor function to the extent that self-treatment is not possible.

  4. Pseudohypoglycemia. Patient perceives hypoglycemic symptoms (usually adrenergic), but BG may be normal, or slightly above normal, and may be rapidly falling.

  5. Hypoglycemia unawareness. Patient perceives no or minimal symptoms. Family or coworkers may notice neurological impairment or sweating. BG may be low to seriously low.

  6. Precipitating factors

    a. Relative or absolute excess of insulin or oral hypoglycemic agent

    b. Delayed or insufficient food intake

    c. More exercise than usual

    d. Alcohol ingestion

    e. Drug interaction resulting in potentiation of hypoglycemic medication or a direct hypoglycemic effect

    f. Subtle causes, such as

      (1) *Hormonal changes* (e.g., drop in progesterone level as part of menstrual cycle)

      (2) Patient switches to a new bottle of insulin and, unknown to the patient or physician, the previous bottle had lost some of its potency

      (3) *Gastroparesis* (delayed emptying of the stomach following a meal), an autonomic neuropathy complication of diabetes

      (4) *Change in insulin injection sites*—especially if injection was given at a subcutaneous site associated with muscles used for exercise (blood flow, and thus insulin absorption, is increased due to the exercising muscle)

g. Treatment
> **(1) Conscious patient.** 10–15 gm fast-acting (simple) oral carbohydrate, such as 4 oz fruit juice, milk, or regular soda; 2–4 glucose tablets or hard candy. Honey or a glucose gel product may be placed into the patient's mouth, if the person is too confused or unresponsive for self-treatment. Treatment may be repeated in 10–15 minutes if BG does not return to normal.
>
> **(2) Unconscious patient**
> > **(a)** Intravenous glucose, using 10% or 50% dextrose solution
> > **(b)** Glucagon injection: 0.5–1 mg given subcutaneously, intramuscularly, or intravenously

IX. LONG-TERM COMPLICATIONS

A. Macrovascular complications (coronary artery, cerebrovascular and peripheral vascular disease)

1. Atherosclerosis (coronary, cerebrovascular, and peripheral vessels) occurs at an earlier age than nondiabetic individuals. Women with diabetes lose their gender protection from atherosclerosis.

2. Peripheral vascular disease may lead to pain (intermittent claudication), chronic "cold feet," or insufficient circulation to enable healing of distal lesions (ultimately leading to gangrene and amputation).

3. Hypertension (HTN)
> **a.** Coexistence of HTN and DM strikingly increases the risk of **cardiovascular disease,** doubles the risk of cardiovascular death, and increases incidence of **stroke** and **transient ischemic events** in DM individuals.
> **b.** Severity or lability of hypertension is determined by factors such as age, race, sex, greater body mass, duration of DM, and persistence of proteinuria.
> **c.** Associated with acceleration of retinopathy, nephropathy, and atherosclerosis
> **d.** Hyperinsulinemia and/or insulin resistance may be a significant factor in the development of DM hypertension.

4. Mortality from **coronary artery disease** (CAD) is two- to fourfold greater in both men and women with diabetes than those without DM, and mortality from cerebrovascular disease is three to five times greater.

5. May present as atypical presentation of CAD, including **silent myocardial infarction** and lack of chest pain (due to autonomic neuropathy). Symptoms may be limited to nausea, shortness of breath, sweating, and vomiting.

6. Modifiable risk factors include hyperglycemia, hypertension, dyslipidemia, tobacco use, obesity, nutrition, increased insulin levels, physical inactivity, and increased homocysteine levels.

7. Prevention and treatment strategies to slow the development and/or progression of disease.
> **a.** Aggressive management of hypertension, hyperlipidemia, and hyperglycemia
> **b.** Smoking cessation
> **c.** Increased physical activity
> **d.** Daily aspirin therapy for those individuals with no contraindications
> **e.** Drug therapy appropriate for the complication, including ACE-inhibitor therapy as a component of HTN therapy and a cardioselective β-blocker agent for cardiac disease.

B. Eye diseases

1. Diabetic **retinopathy**
> **a.** A consequence of microvascular changes
> **b.** Most prevalent eye complication and is often detectable within 5 years following the diagnosis of DM. Present in more than 90% of patients with type 1 and 55%–80% of patients with type 2 DM, after 15 years of diabetes.
> **c.** Leading cause of new blindness in the United States

   d. Categories of retinopathy
   (1) Nonproliferative (background) retinopathy. Vascular abnormalities include retinal microaneurysms (early, mild stage), blot hemorrhages, and retinal edema with or without "hard" exudates. May progress to macula edema.
   (2) Preproliferative retinopathy. With increasing abnormality of the tiny vessels, retinal ischemia occurs, giving rise to the appearance of white patches of oxygen-starved retina, known as soft or "cotton wool" spots.
   (3) Proliferative retinopathy
   (a) In response to the lack of oxygen, new but weak vessels begin to grow (neovascularization).
   (b) The new vessels grow (proliferate) out from the retinal surface, into the vitreous cavity. These vessels are fragile and may bleed into the vitreous. Hemorrhages into the vitreous can obscure vision, but they are usually reabsorbed in 1–3 months.
   (c) Traction retinal detachment. Scar tissue, and more new blood vessels, continue to grow onto the vitreous. The vitreous pulls (traction) on the retina and detaches it.
   e. Generally does not result in visual alterations until advanced stages are reached
   f. Treatment. Loss of vision can be reduced by 50% with laser photocoagulation if ocular changes are identified and treated in a timely manner.

2. Other ocular complications include cataracts, primary open-angled glaucoma, and ischemic optic neuropathy.

3. Modifiable risk factors include hyperglycemia, hypertension, dyslipidemia, and nicotine use.

4. Prevention strategies
   a. Aggressive management of hypertension, hyperlipidemia, and blood glucose
   b. Smoking cessation
   c. Routine ophthalmologic screening and follow-up, including an annual dilated eye exam

C. Diabetic nephropathy

1. DM is the most common single cause of end-stage renal disease (ESRD) in the United States and Europe.

2. Renal failure occurs in approximately 30–40% of individuals with type 1 DM within 30 years after diagnosis and approximately 20–30% of patients with type 2 DM.

3. Findings/progression
   a. First evidenced by the presence of elevated microalbuminuria (>30 mg albumin/24 hr)
   b. "Clinical" or dipstick positive albuminuria (>300 mg/24 hr)
   c. Proteinuria often associated with hypertension, which accelerates the rate of nephropathic changes
   d. Progressive decrease in glomerular filtration rate with rising serum creatinine until ESRD occurs.

4. Modifiable risk factors include hyperglycemia, hypertension, tobacco use, and excessive dietary protein intake.

5. Prevention and treatment strategies to slow the development and/or progression of disease.
   a. Aggressive management of HTN and blood glucose
   b. Initiation of ACE inhibitor therapy
   c. Smoking cessation
   d. Some data suggest restriction of daily dietary protein intake to 0.6–0.8 g/kg of IBW; however, low-protein meal plans should be used with caution to avoid malnutrition and associated muscle weakness.
   e. Early identification and aggressive treatment of urinary tract infections
   f. Yearly assessment of kidney function, including urinalysis for detection of microalbuminuria
   g. For ESRD, fluid and electrolyte restriction, as well as intermittent or chronic dialysis treatments, as indicated by severity of pathology, laboratory findings, and patient symptomatology

    h. For ESRD, patient and caregiver counseling to prepare them for the psychosocial, financial, physical, medical, and quality-of-life changes that accompany dialysis and possible kidney transplantation

D. Diabetic neuropathies

  1. Peripheral neuropathy

    a. The sensorimotor nervous system is most often affected, but sympathetic or parasympathetic abnormalities may be present also.

    b. Sensory deficits and symptoms originate in the distal portions of the lower extremities and gradually progress to the upper extremities, creating a "stocking-glove" distribution of pain and diminished sensation.

    c. Signs and symptoms depend on the class and stage of nerve fiber loss.

      (1) Small-fiber involvement impairs perception of pain and temperature and may lead to numbness/tingling or loss of sensation.

      (2) Large-fiber involvement produces impaired balance and diminished proprioception.

      (3) Motor nerve damage results in muscle weakness/atrophy.

      (4) The majority of patients experience damage to more than one type of nerve.

  2. Autonomic neuropathy involves multiple systems throughout the body.

    a. Genitourinary impairment may lead to neurogenic bladder and sexual dysfunction in both males (impotence, retrograde ejaculation) and females (diminished vaginal lubrication and orgasm frequency).

    b. Gastrointestinal impairment may lead to gastroparesis, nocturnal diarrhea, fecal incontinence, or chronic constipation.

    c. Cardiovascular impairment may lead to orthostatic hypotension or cardiac denervation syndrome.

  3. Modifiable risk factors include hyperglycemia, alcohol use, tobacco use, and hypertension.

  4. Prevention strategies

    a. Aggressive management of blood pressure and blood glucose.

    b. Smoking and alcohol cessation.

    c. Proper foot care to prevent development of lower-extremity complications in the presence of peripheral neuropathy and diminished circulation.

E. Foot, skin, and mucous membrane complications stem from vascular changes and peripheral neuropathy that cause alterations in the nerves that control blood flow and skin hydration.

  1. Individuals with DM are at increased risk for the development of skin infections caused by staphylococci, β-hemolytic steptococci, and fungus.

  2. Common infections include:

    a. Cutaneous infections such as furunculosis and carbuncles.

    b. Candida infections of the genitalia, upper thighs, and under the breasts.

    c. Cellulitis and/or lower-extremity vascular ulcers.

  3. Atrophic lesions (round painless lesions) and diabetic dermopathy (reddish-brown papular spots) are common, especially on the lower extremities.

  4. An ulcerating necrotic lesion called **necrobiosis lipoidica diabeticorum** may develop on the anterior leg surface or the dorsum of the ankle.

  5. Approximately 50% of patients with DM of 15 years, duration have peripheral neuropathy that may result in a loss of protective sensation and inability to detect even minor trauma. This places the patient at significant risk for the development of ulcers.

  6. Injury, infection, neuropathy, vascular disease, or ischemia may lead to gangrene, which is 20 times more common in people with DM.

  7. Prevention strategies

    a. Good glycemic control

    b. Proper foot care (see section VI D1) and early detection/intervention of identified problems.

    c. Proper skin care (see section VI D2)

d. Sensory exam of feet utilizing a 5.07 (10 gm) monofilament to identify patients with loss of protective sensation

e. Patient education concerning protective footwear (e.g., deep-soled shoes, individually molded shoes, orthotics) and avoidance of foot injury, especially when a loss of protective sensation is noted.

F. Importance of glycemic control as preventive of chronic complications

1. The Diabetes Control and Complications Trial (DCCT, 1993) demonstrated that intensive treatment of type 1 diabetic patients delays the onset and progression of diabetic retinopathy, nephropathy, and neuropathy.

2. The United Kingdom Prospective Diabetes Study (UKPDS, 1998) similarly demonstrated that the complications of type 2 DM may be reduced by strict glycemic control, regardless of the therapeutic agent chosen to attain that control.

X. SIGNIFICANT DRUG INTERACTIONS AFFECTING GLYCEMIC CONTROL

A. Potential hyperglycemia, as a dose-dependent, direct glucogenic effect. Corticosteroids, nicotinic acid, phenytoin, pentamidine (long-term effect), protease inhibitors, sympathomimetics, isoniazid, furosemide, thiazide diuretics

B. Potential hypoglycemia, as a direct hypoglycemic effect; monoamine oxidase (MAO) inhibitors, fluoxetine, salicylates (large doses), fenfluramine, alcohol, pentamidine (initial effect)

C. Prolonged hypoglycemia and masking of hypoglycemic symptoms. β-blockers

D. Altered protein binding of, or other drug interaction with, sulfonylurea agents. Alcohol, salicylates, nonsteroidal anti-inflammatory drugs (NSAIDs), methyldopa, chloramphenicol, MAO inhibitors, clofibrate, probenecid

XI. SPECIAL ISSUES IN DIABETES. These situations cause unique problems in the management of diabetes, but are beyond the length allocated for this chapter. Readers are encouraged to learn about these, as they will need to be dealt with as part of the reader's practice of pharmacy.

A. Pregnancy in DM (not GDM)

B. Pediatrics

C. Adolescence

D. Geriatrics

E. Surgery

F. DM management during hemodialysis or peritoneal dialysis

G. Kidney transplantation

H. Self-care issues (e.g., SMBG, injections) in the visually impaired or blind DM patient

I. DM patients in institutionalized facilities

J. Pancreas and islet cell transplantation

XII. REFERENCES

A. American Diabetes Association. Standards of medical care for patients with diabetes mellitus. *Diabetes Care* 2003;26:S33–S50.

B. Tuomelehto J, et al. Prevention of type 2 diabetes mellitus by changes in lifestyle among subjects with impaired glucose tolerance. *NEJM* 2000;344:1343–1350.

C. Diabetes Prevention Program Research Group. Reduction in the incidence of type 2 diabetes with lifestyle intervention or metformin. *NEJM* 2002;346:393–403.

D. Chiasson JL, et al. Acarbose for prevention of type 2 diabetes mellitus: the STOP-NIDDM randomized trial. *Lancet* 2002;359:2072–2077.

E. American Diabetes Association. Evidence-based nutrition principles and recommendations for the treatment and prevention of diabetes and related complications. *Diabetes Care* 2003;26: S51–S61.

STUDY QUESTIONS

Directions: Each of the numbered items or incomplete statements in this section is followed by answers or by completions of the statement. Select the **one** lettered answer or completion that is **best** in each case.

1. Current criteria used in the diagnosis of diabetes mellitus (DM) include all of the following symptoms EXCEPT

(A) fasting hyperglycemia
(B) polyuria
(C) polydipsia
(D) tinnitus
(E) weight loss

2. The most useful glucose test used in monitoring diabetes mellitus (DM) therapy is

(A) urine monitoring
(B) blood monitoring
(C) renal function monitoring
(D) cardiovascular monitoring
(E) vascular monitoring

3. Which of the following statements concerning insulin replacement therapy is most likely true?

(A) Most commercial insulin products vary little with respect to time, course, and duration of hypoglycemic activity.
(B) Regular insulin cannot be mixed with NPH (isophane insulin suspension).
(C) Regular insulin cannot be given intravenously.
(D) Regulating carbohydrate consumption is a necessity for all diabetic patients.
(E) Insulin therapy does not have to be monitored closely.

4. A mass of adipose tissue that develops at the injection site is usually due to the patient's neglect in rotating the insulin injection site. This is known as

(A) lipoatrophy
(B) hypertrophic degenerative adiposity
(C) lipohypertrophy
(D) atrophic skin lesion
(E) dermatitis

5. Sulfonylureas are a primary mode of therapy in the treatment of

(A) insulin-dependent (type 1) diabetes mellitus (IDDM) patients
(B) diabetic patients experiencing severe hepatic or renal dysfunction
(C) diabetic pregnant women
(D) patients with diabetic ketoacidosis
(E) non–insulin-dependent (type 2) DM (NIDDM) patients

6. Patients taking chlorpropamide should avoid products containing

(A) acetaminophen
(B) ethanol
(C) vitamin A
(D) penicillins
(E) milk products

7. The standard recommended dose of glyburide is

(A) 0.5–2 mg/day
(B) 1.25–20 mg/day
(C) 50–100 mg/day
(D) 200 mg/day
(E) 200–1000 mg/day

Questions 8–12

A 20-year-old previously healthy man presents to the emergency room with a 2-week history of polyuria, polydipsia, and a 20-lb unintentional weight loss. He complains of weakness, fatigue, nausea, and abdominal pain. Physical examination reveals dry, parched mucous membranes. Blood pressure is 110/70 mm Hg and pulse is 90 beats per minute (bpm) supine; blood pressure is 90/60 mm Hg, and pulse is 120 bpm upright. Temperature is 100°F (axillary); respiratory rate is 24 breaths per minute. General examination of the heart and lungs is unremarkable. No retinopathy is present. The abdomen is soft with mild tenderness but no rebound. Laboratory values are as follows:

Blood glucose: 420 mg/dl
Sodium (Na): 130 mEq/L(A)
Potassium (K): 3.7 mEq/L
Chloride (Cl): 97 mEq/L
Bicarbonate ($HCO_3{}^2$): 10 mEq/L
Arterial blood gas: 7.20 (pH)
Urinalysis: +3 glucose and moderate ketones
Chest radiograph: Unremarkable
Abdominal radiography (KUB): Unremarkable

8. What is the most likely diagnosis in this patient?

(A) Type 2 diabetes mellitus (DM) with hyperosmolar state
(B) Type 1 DM with diabetic ketoacidosis
(C) Type 2 DM without hyperosmolar state
(D) Type 1 DM without diabetic ketoacidosis

9. Initial appropriate therapy includes

(A) intravenous fluids and a sulfonylurea agent
(B) intravenous fluids alone
(C) intravenous fluids, 10 units of subcutaneous regular insulin, and discharge to home
(D) intravenous fluids, intravenous regular insulin by continuous drip at 6 units/hr, and hospital admission

10. After the acute illness has resolved, what further therapy would be appropriate?

(A) None, observe only
(B) Start a second-generation sulfonylurea
(C) Daily administration of a regimen of NPH (isophane insulin suspension) and regular insulin plus dietary modification
(D) Dietary modification alone

11. Appropriate follow-up of the patient once discharged to home includes all of the following EXCEPT

(A) periodic monitoring of hemoglobin A1C levels
(B) periodic opthalmologic examinations
(C) home glucose monitoring with a glucose meter
(D) weight-loss diet and an attempt to wean from insulin

12. The patient is at risk for developing all of the following complications EXCEPT

(A) hypoglycemia
(B) coronary artery disease
(C) retinopathy
(D) nonketotic hyperglycemia hyperosmolar state

ANSWERS AND EXPLANATIONS

1. The answer is D *[F 1 b, F 2 a 2]*.
Frequent urination (polyuria), thirst (polydipsia), and weight loss are all common signs of diabetes. When these symptoms are present, it is necessary to have a fasting or random (casual) blood glucose level drawn to determine a diabetic state. A fasting blood glucose level of 126 mg/dl or greater on more than one occasion is diagnostic of a diabetic state.

2. The answer is B *[II C 2, II D 1, 2]*.
Blood glucose monitoring is the most useful form of monitoring glucose levels. Urine monitoring provides only gross estimates of the current status and cannot rule out hypoglycemia. Renal function and cardiovascular functions provide evidence of long-standing disease and are not useful for monitoring daily progress.

3. The answer is D *[V A 1, V C 3 C, B 1 c (3) (a)]*.
Many commercial insulin preparations vary with respect to duration of activity and time for peak plasma level. Regular insulin can be mixed with NPH (isophane insulin suspension) and can be given intravenously. All insulin therapies should be monitored closely and on a daily basis. Careful regulation of carbohydrate intake is very important for all diabetic patients—carbohydrate consumption plays a major role in the balance of glucose metabolism and antagonizes the effects of insulin therapy.

4. The answer is C *[V C 4 d (2)]*.
Lipohypertrophy consists of masses of adipose tissue that develop at the injection site, usually in patients who do not rotate the injection sites properly. The masses gradually disappear if injection in these sites is avoided.

5. The answer is E *[V D 2 b, V D 2 a (2)]*.
Sulfonylureas should not be used as primary therapy in insulin-dependent (type 1) diabetes mellitus (IDDM) patients, in those who have severe hepatic or renal dysfunction, or in those patients who are pregnant. Diabetic ketoacidosis (DKA) should never be treated with sulfonylureas; this condition must be treated with insulin, fluids, and electrolyte replacement. However, sulfonylureas help to reduce blood glucose levels in type 2 DM that does not respond to diet alone.

6. The answer is B *[V D 6 f]*.
Acute ingestion of ethanol (alcohol) by patients who are taking any antidiabetic agent carries the risk of severe hypoglycemia particularly due to the potential hypoglycemic effects of ethanol (especially if consumed in the fasting state). In addition, the interaction of chlorpropamide and ethanol (disulfiram-like reaction) is notable with this agent.

7. The answer is B *[V D 5; Table 52-2]*.
The standard recommended dose of glyburide is 1.25–20 mg/day. Doses greater than 20 mg are not recommended by the manufacturer. Patients may be started on a low dose (e.g., 1.25 mg/day) and titrated up to an effective oral dose, as clinically indicated.

8–12. The answers are: 8-B *[I F 1]*, **9-D** *[V C 4 e]*, **10-C** *[V C 1, 1 B 1]*, **11-D** *[II C 1, VII D 1 1 B 1]*, **12-D** *[III A 2]*.
Type 1 diabetes mellitus (DM) with diabetic ketoacidosis (DKA) is the most likely diagnosis in the patient described in the question. The patient presented with high blood sugar, weight loss, acidosis, and positive urine ketones (high level). This is a typical presentation of DKA.

Type 1 DM always requires insulin therapy; it can never be left untreated or treated with diet or liquids alone and can never be treated with sulfonylurea agents. DKA requires hospitalization and should be treated with an insulin drip until the acidosis clears. Patients with DKA are dehydrated and must be given intravenous fluids.

All diabetic patients should be followed with periodic hemoglobin A1c measurements and ophthalmologic examination annually. Home glucose monitoring is the optimal way to follow a patient's level of control. Weight loss and an attempt to wean from insulin are appropriate only for type 2 DM. Those patients with type 1 diabetes cannot be weaned from insulin therapy.

Hypoglycemia is a possible complication of insulin therapy. All diabetic patients are at risk for coronary artery disease and retinopathy. Nonketotic hyperglycemic hyperosmolar coma is typically a complication of type 2 DM.

Thyroid Disease

John E. Janosik

I. PHYSIOLOGY

A. Thyroid hormone regulation

1. The thyroid gland synthesizes, stores, and secretes hormones that are important to growth, development, and the metabolic rate. These hormones are **thyroxine (T$_4$)** and **triiodothyronine (T$_3$).**

2. The thyroid gland also secretes **calcitonin,** which reduces blood calcium ion concentration.

3. Thyroid hormone secretion and transport are controlled by **thyroid-stimulating hormone (thyrotropin; TSH).** TSH is released by the anterior pituitary gland, which is triggered by **thyrotropin-releasing hormone (TRH),** secreted from the hypothalamus.
   a. The process produces increased levels of thyroid hormone (circulating free T$_4$ and free T$_3$), which, in turn, signals the pituitary to stop releasing TSH **(negative feedback).**
   b. Conversely, low blood levels of free hormone trigger pituitary release of TSH, which stimulates the thyroid gland to secrete T$_4$ and T$_3$ until free hormone levels return to normal. At this point, the pituitary gland ceases to release TSH, which completes the feedback loop (Figure 53-1).
   c. This homeostatic mechanism attempts to maintain the level of circulating thyroid hormone within a very narrow range.

B. Biosynthesis (Figure 53-2)

1. Essential to synthesis of thyroid hormones is dietary iodine, reduced to **inorganic iodide,** which the thyroid actively extracts from the plasma through iodide trapping **(iodide pump).** Some of this iodide is stored within the colloid; some diffuses into the lumen of thyroid follicles.

2. Iodide is oxidized by peroxidase and bound to tyrosyl residues within the thyroglobulin molecule in a process called **organification.**

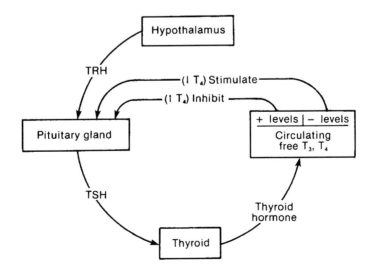

Figure 53-1. Thyroid hormone regulation loop. This carefully balanced hormone regulation system uses both positive (stimulating) and negative (inhibiting) feedback to maintain homeostasis. Disruption of any of these elements can produce serious consequences, such as myxedema crisis (under availability of thyroid hormone) or thyroid storm (overabundance of thyroid hormone). *TRH* = thyroid-releasing hormone; *TSH* = thyroid-stimulating hormone; *T$_4$* = thyroxine; *T$_3$* = triiodothyronine.

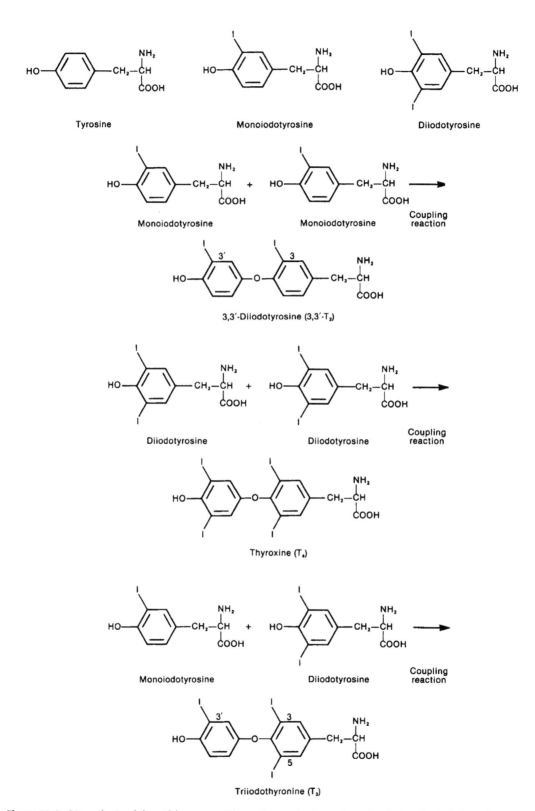

Figure 53-2. Biosynthesis of thyroid hormones. The major products are thyroxine (T₄) and triiodothyronine (T₃). These are formed in the follicle cells of the thyroid gland by iodination of tyrosine residues. Monoiodo- and diiodotyrosine residues are formed first. These then react to form T₃ and T₄.

    a. The synthesis begins with iodide binding to tyrosine, forming **monoiodotyrosine (MIT).**

    b. MIT then binds another iodide to form **diiodotyrosine (DIT).**

    c. Then, slowly, a coupling reaction binds MIT and DIT, producing T_3 and T_4.

C. Hormone transport

    1. After TSH stimulation of the thyroid gland, T_3 and T_4 are cleaved from thyroglobulin and released into the circulation.

    2. When in the circulation, thyroid hormone is transported bound to several plasma proteins, a process that:

        a. Helps to protect the hormone from premature metabolism and excretion

        b. Prolongs its half-life in the circulation

        c. Allows the thyroid hormone to reach its site of action

    3. Most thyroid hormone is transported by **thyroxine-binding globulin (TBG). Prealbumin** and **albumin** also serve as carriers.

D. Hormone metabolism

    1. Peripheral conversion of T_4 to T_3 occurs in the pituitary gland, liver, and kidneys and accounts for about 80% of T_3 generation.

    2. Deiodination accounts for most hormone degradation. The major steps in this process are shown in Figure 53-3.

    3. Deiodinated hormones are excreted in feces and urine.

    4. Minor nondeiodination pathways of metabolism include conjugation with sulfate and glucuronide, deamination, and decarboxylation.

E. Hormone function. Although the effects of thyroid hormones are known, the basic mechanisms producing these effects elude precise definition; however, they seem to activate the messenger

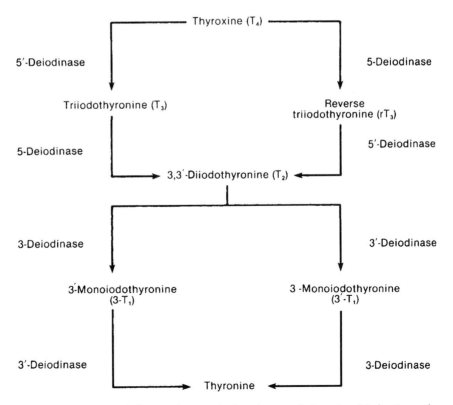

Figure 53-3. Thyroxine metabolism: major steps in the primary and alternative deiodination pathways.

RNA (mRNA) transcription process and can promote protein synthesis or (in excessive amounts) protein catabolism. **Thyroid hormones** affect the following:

1. Growth and development

2. Calorigenics by increasing the rate of basal metabolism

3. Cardiovascular system by increasing the metabolic rate, which increases blood flow, cardiac output, and heart rate (may be related in part to an increased tissue sensitivity to catecholamines)

4. The central nervous system (CNS) by increasing or diminishing cerebration

5. Musculature by causing a fine tremor

6. Sleep by inducing fatigued wakefulness with hyperthyroidism or somnolence with hypothyroidism

7. Lipid metabolism by stimulating lipid mobilization and degradation

F. Thyroid function studies (Table 53-1)

1. **Serum total thyroxine (TT$_4$)**
   a. This test provides the most direct reflection of thyroid function by indicating hormone availability to tissues. Total (free and bound) T$_4$ is determined by radioimmunoassay, which is sensitive and rapid.
   b. Changes in thyroid globulin concentration, particularly TBG, which increases during pregnancy, alter the total concentration of T$_4$ and may produce a misleading high or low test result.
   c. However, these changes in TBG do not affect the concentration of free T$_4$. Therefore, to clarify thyroid function, either protein-binding (T$_3$ uptake test) or free T$_4$ must be measured.
   d. An elevated TT$_4$ level indicates hyperthyroidism; a decreased TT$_4$ level, hypothyroidism. However, the TT$_4$ level in a euthyroid patient can be altered by other factors, such as pregnancy or febrile illnesses (which elevate the TT$_4$), nephrotic syndrome or cirrhosis (which lower it), and various drugs (Table 53-2).

2. **Serum total triiodothyronine (TT$_3$)**
   a. This sensitive and highly specific test measures total (free and bound) T$_3$.
   b. Serum T$_3$ and T$_4$ usually rise and fall together; however, hyperthyroidism commonly causes a disproportionate rise in T$_3$, and the TT$_3$ can rise before the TT$_4$ level. Therefore, TT$_3$ is useful for early detection or to rule out hyperthyroidism. Many of the symptoms associated with hyperthyroidism are due to elevated TT$_3$.
   c. This test may not be diagnostically significant for hypothyroidism, in which TT$_3$ levels may fall but stay within the normal range. The TT$_3$ may be low in only 50% of patients with hypothyroidism.
   d. If there is an abnormality in binding proteins, this test can yield the same misleading results as the TT$_4$ readings. Other factors affecting test results include pregnancy (which increases TT$_3$ levels), malnutrition or hepatic or renal disease (which lower TT$_3$ levels), or various drugs (see Table 53-2).

3. **Resin triiodothyronine uptake (RT$_3$U)**
   a. This test clarifies whether abnormal T$_4$ levels are due to a thyroid disorder or to abnormalities in the binding proteins because it evaluates the binding capacity of TBG.

Table 53-1. Test Results in Thyroid Disorders

Thyroid Function Test	Hypothyroidism	Hyperthyroidism
Serum resin triiodothyronine uptake (RT$_3$U)	↓ (<35%)	↑ (>45%)
Serum total thyroxine (TT$_4$)	↓ (<5 µg/dl)	↑ (>12 µg/dl)
Serum total triiodothyronine (TT$_3$)	↓ (<80 ng/dl)	↑ (>180 ng/dl)
Free thyroxine index (FTI)	↓ (<5.5)	↑ (<10.5)
Serum thyrotropin (TSH)	↑ (>6 µU/mL)	↓ (<0.5 µU/mL)
Sensitive thyrotropin (TSH) assay	↑ (>5 µU/mL)	↓ (<0.2 µU/mL)*

↑ = increased levels; ↓ = decreased levels.
*Some tests detect 0.001–0.002 mIU/L.

b. If an abnormal amount (high or low) of thyroid hormone is present in the blood, the RT_3U results **change in the same direction** as the altered level—elevated in hyperthyroidism, decreased in hypothyroidism.

c. However, if abnormalities in binding proteins underlie the abnormal levels of TT_4, TT_3, or both, the RT_3U results **change in the opposite direction**—decreasing as TBG increases, increasing as TBG decreases.

d. Various drugs can cause spurious changes in the RT_3U (see Table 53-2).

4. Serum thyrotropin (TSH) and sensitive TSH assays

a. Serum TSH assay

(1) This test is the **most sensitive** test for detecting the hypothyroid state because the hypothalamic–pituitary axis compensates very quickly for even slight decreases in circulating free hormone by releasing more TSH. The TSH levels may be elevated even before low circulating levels of TT_4 are detectable by diagnostic testing.

(2) Serum TSH is not a reliable test for hyperthyroidism (in which TSH is suppressed) because low levels and low–normal levels of TSH may be indistinguishable with this technology.

(3) Effects of drugs on the serum TSH are shown in Tables 53-2 and 53-3.

b. Sensitive TSH assay

(1) The sensitive TSH assay uses monoclonal antibodies referred to as immunoradiometric or immunometric (IMA) methodology (instead of the older radioimmunoassay techniques) and demonstrates greater sensitivity in the detection of thyroid disease than older tests.

(2) This assay is usually **more expensive** and **more commonly used** to monitor patients receiving replacement therapy to control overtreatment. [Overtreatment may contribute to excessive bone demineralization, electrocardiogram (ECG) changes, or elevation of liver function tests.]

(3) The sensitivity of the assay has improved since its first introduction in the late 1980s. Nomenclature established by the American Thyroid Association (ATA) has classified the improvement in sensitivity based on the lower limit of detection. The new classification follows a generational format, as shown in Table 53-4.

(4) The IMA technique is very sensitive. The fourth-generation IMA can detect TSH levels in the range of 0.001–0.002 mIU/L.

(5) The IMA or sensitive assays should not be used to assess thyroid function in hospitalized patients because some studies have reported abnormally high or low TSH levels in otherwise euthyroid patients.

(6) TSH levels may also be influenced by psychiatric illness. Current findings in human immunodefiency virus (HIV)-infected patients are uncertain. However, autoimmune thyroid disease appears to be more prevalent in HIV-infected patients.

5. Free thyroxine index (FTI)

a. This is not a separate test but rather an estimation of the free T_4 level through a mathematical interpretation of the relationship between RT_3U and serum T_4 levels.

$$FTI = \frac{TT_4 \times RT_3U}{\text{mean serum } RT_3U}$$

b. FTI values are elevated in hyperthyroidism, when TBG is low and decreased in hypothyroidism, or when TBG is elevated.

c. Effects of drugs on FTI are shown in Table 53-2.

G. Strategies and cost considerations for testing

1. The **most frequently** used and **least expensive** tests for screening are the TT_4 and the RT_3U, which are used to calculate the FTI. A serum TSH assay may also be used but at an additional cost (Figure 53-4).

2. Thyroid disease screening for the otherwise generally healthy population has been shown to **not be cost-effective** based on the rate of detection and cost associated with massive screening. However, with increased use and improvements in technology, costs have been falling (Figure 53-5).

3. The most appropriate **target population** for screening includes elderly patients hospitalized for exacerbations of chronic diseases or who are coincidentally diagnosed with a chronic

Table 53-2. Effects of Drugs on Thyroid Function Tests

Drug	Serum T4	Resin T3 Uptake	Free Thyroxine Index (FTI)	Serum T3	Serum TSH	Comment
p-Aminosalicylic acid (PAS)	→	(nd)	→	(nd)	↑ *	Antithyroid effect, rarely, with long-term use
Aminoglutethimide (Cytadren)	→	(nd)	(nd)	(nd)	↑	Inhibits peripheral conversion of T4 to T3
Amiodarone[1]	←	(nd)	(nd)	→	(nd)	Decreased serum TBG
Anabolic steroids and androgens	→	↑	0	→ *	(nd)	
Antithyroid drugs: Propylthiouracil (PTU) or methimazole (Tapazole)	→	→	→	→	0 or ↑	TSH may increase if patient becomes hypothyroid
Asparaginase (Elspar)	→	↑	(nd)	↓ *	↑ *	Decreased serum TBG
Barbiturates	↓[a]	(nd)	↓	(nd)	(nd)	Stimulates T4 metabolism
Calcium carbonate[2]	→	(nd)	(nd)	0	↑	Subclinical signs of hypothyroidism; separate time of ingestion of calcium and levothyroxine
Contraceptives, oral	←	→	0	←	0	TBG usually increased
Corticosteroids	0 or ↓	0 or ↑	0 or ↓	→	→	Usual doses decrease TBG; high doses may increase TBG
Danazol (Danocrine)	→	↑	0[b]	→	0 or ↓	Decreased serum TBG
Estrogens	←	↓	0	←	0	Increased serum TBG
Ethionamide (Trecator-sc)	←	(nd)	↓ *	(nd)	↑ *	Antithyroid effect
Fluorouracil (Adrucil)	←[c]	↓	↑ *	←	0	Patients clinically euthyroid; TBG increased
Heparin, intravenous	0[d]	0 or ↑ / 0[d]	0[d]	0	(nd)	FTI is increased with some measures
Hypoglycemics (sulfonylureas)	0	0[d]	0	(nd)	(nd)	
Iodides, inorganic	0	0	0	(nd)	(nd)	
Iodides, organic	0	0	0	(nd)	(nd)	
Levodopa and levodopa-carbidopa (Sinemet)	0	0	0	0	↓[e]	
Levothyroxine (Levothroid)	↑ (s)[f,g]	↑ or 0 or ↓ [f,g]	0 or ↑ [f,g]	↑ or 0[f,g]	↑ or 0[f]	
Liothyronine (Cytomel)	0[f] or ↓ (s)	0 or ↓[f]	↓[f]	↑ or ↓[f,g]	0[f]	
Liotrix (Thyrolar)	0[f] or ↓ (s)	0[f]	0[f]	0[f,g]	0[f]	
Lithium carbonate (Eskalith)	0 or →	0 or →	0 or →	0 or ↓	0 or ↑	
Methadone (Dolophine)	↑ (s)	↓	0 / 0*	←	0	Increased serum TBG
Mitotane (Lysodren)	→	0	0*	(nd)	(nd)	
Nitroprusside (Nipride)	→	(nd)	(nd)	(nd)	(nd)	Clinical hypothyroidism

Drug						Comments
Oxyphenbutazone (*Oxalid*) and phenylbutazone (*Butazolidin*)	0 or ↓	↑	↓		(nd)	↑ *	May compete with T4 for TBG binding, rarely, overt hypothyroidism and goiter may occur
Perphenazine (*Trilafon*)		0 or ↑ (s)	↑↓		↑	0*	Stimulates T4 metabolism and
Phenytoin (*Dilantin*)		0 or ↓ (s)	0 or ↓ (s)		↑↓	0	may compete with T4 for TBG binding
Propranolol (*Inderal*)	0 or ↑[h] ↓↓	0[i] ↓↑	(nd) ↓↓		↓[j] ↓↓	0 ↑	
Resorcinol (excessive topical use)						0*	Compete with T4 for TBG binding
Salicylates (large doses)	↑ (s)	*	↓↓		↓	0*	

↑ = increased; ↓ = decreased; 0 = no effect; (s) = slight effect; (nd) = no data. (Adapted from *The Medical Letter* 1981; 23:31.)

SC = subcutaneous; T3 = triiodothyronine; T4 = thyroxine; TBG = thyroxine-binding globulin; TSH = thyroid-stimulating hormone.

*Effect deduced rather than based on reported clinical evidence.

aPatients requiring thyroid replacement therapy have decreased serum thyroxine when barbiturates are given.

bFree thyroxine index may increase slightly but usually remains in the normal range.

cT4 assay by competitive protein binding is spuriously increased, but T4-RIA is probably not affected. Free thyroxine measured by dialysis may be increased.

dMay occasionally decrease serum T4 and increase resin T3 uptake.

eSlight decrease in euthyroid patients; but in long-standing hypothyroid patients, levodopa considerably decreases the elevated TSH.

fIn a patient on adequate doses for thyroid replacement.

gIncreased T4, FTI, and T3 tend to return to normal after several months of therapy with levothyroxine. After liothyronine, T3 may be elevated 2 hours after a dose and depressed 24 hours after a dose.

hIncreased T4 levels are reported in one study, but not in others.

iWith short-term propranolol in hyperthyroid patients.

jIn euthyroid patients, the decreased serum T3 returns to normal with continued propranolol therapy.

1Taken from Rae P, Farrar J, Beckett G, Toft A. Assessment of thyroid status in elderly people. *BMJ* 1993;307:177–180.

2Taken from Singh N, Singh P, Hershman JM. Effect of calcium carbonate on the adsorption of levothyroxine. *JAMA* 2000;283:2822–2825.

Table 53-3. Medications Influencing TSH Levels

Agent	Mechanisms	Potential Clinical Thyroid Effect(s)	Effect on TSH	Effect on Other Thyroid Function Tests	Comments
Dopamine and dopamine agonists	Central suppression of TSH release	Minimal or none	Suppression	Normal or decreased hormone levels	Prolonged use of dopamine in high doses may potentiate the low thyroxine state of critical illness
Dopamine antagonists	Release of central TSH inhibition	Minimal or none	Elevation	Usually normal	Effects not well-characterized
Somatostatin and analogues	Central suppression of TSH release	Minimal or none	Suppression	Usually normal	Effects not well-characterized
Calcium carbonate	Adsorption of levothyroxine to calcium in acid environment	Subclinical hypothy-roidism	Elevation	Decrease free T_4 and total T_4	
Corticosteroids	Central suppression of TSH release Reduction of thyroid iodine uptake Inhibition of T_4 to T_3 conversion Reduction of thyroid-binding globulin levels	Minimal or none	Suppression	Usually within normal range, although total T_4, free T_4, T_3 reduced and reverse T_3 increased from baseline	Compensatory mechanisms lead to normalization of TSH levels with chronic exposure
Lithium salts	Inhibition of iodo-thyronine biosyn-thesis Reduction of thyroid iodine concentration Suppression of thyroid hormone release Induction of thyroid autoimmunity	Clinical or sub-clinical hypothy-roidism	Elevation	Normal or decreased thyroid hormone levels	Some sources recommend thyroid function testing at 6-month intervals while on therapy

Drug	Mechanism	Clinical effect	TSH	Thyroid hormone levels	Comments
Iodine	Inhibition of iodine uptake and organification Impairment of thyroid hormone Inhibition of T_4 to T_3 conversion Induction of thyroid autoimmunity	Clinical or sub-clinical hypothyroidism Hyperthyroidism	Elevation Suppression	Decreased thyroid hormone levels Elevated thyroid hormone levels	Clinical hypothyroidism most common in those with underlying organification defects such as those seen in autoimmune thyroiditis or previous radioiodine therapy; iodine-induced hyperthyroidism is generally confined to those with iodine deficiency or auto-immune thyroid disease
Radiographic contrast media	Iodine effects (as above) Direct inhibition of T_4 to T_3 conversion	Minimal or none	Elevation	Normal or decreased thyroid hormone levels Elevation of reverse T_3 levels	Alterations are maximal 3–4 days after administration and may persist for up to 2 weeks
Amiodarone	Iodine effects (as above) Direct inhibition of T_4 to T_3 conversion Direct toxic effects on thyroid Induction of thyroid autoimmunity	Clinical or sub-clinical hypothyroidism Hyperthyroidism	Usual pattern is mild elevation for first 8–12 weeks of therapy followed by normalization: marked elevation seen with hypo-thyroidism; sup-pression with hyper-thyroidism	Increased total T_4 levels Increased free T_4 levels Increased reverse T_3 levels Decreased total and free T_3	Biochemical changes in thyroid function noted in a majority of patients on therapy, requiring frequent monitoring
Interferon	Unclear; likely due to immunomodul-ating properties and stimulation of autoimmunity	Hypothyroidism (silent thyroiditis, Graves' disease) Hyperthyroidism (with or without autoantibodies)	Elevation Suppression	Decreased thyroid hormone levels Increased thyroid hormone levels	No apparent direct influence on TSH secretion: pre-treatment detectable anti-microsomal antibodies may represent a risk factor for interferon-induced thyroid disease

T_3 = triiodothyronine; T_4 = thyroxine; TSH = thyroid-stimulating hormone.

Table 53-4. Sensitive TSH Assay Nomenclature

Generation	Lower Level of Detection
First	1–2 mIU/L
Second	0.1–0.2 mIU/L
Third	0.01–0.02 mIU/L
Fourth	0.001–0.002 mIU/L

TSH = thyroid-stimulating hormone.

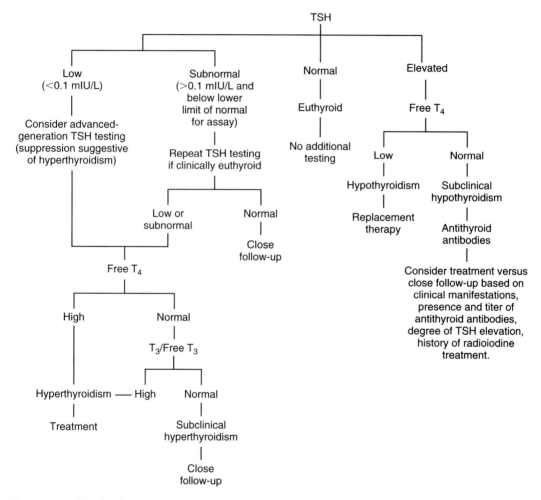

Figure 53-4. Algorithm for utilizing a sensitive thyroid-stimulating hormone (TSH) assay as a single test of thyroid function. The algorithm assumes a clinically intact hypothalamic–pituitary axis, absence of medications known to influence TSH or other thyroid indices, and generally good physical and psychiatric health. The TSH assay should meet the American Thyroid Association criteria for a sensitive assay and/or have a known functional sensitivity limit at the second generation (0.1 mIU/L) level or greater. "Close follow-up" is defined as clinical observation for signs and symptoms of hyperthyroidism or hypothyroidism and repeated TSH determinations at intervals of 6 to 12 months. T_3 = triiodothyronine; T_4 = thyroxine.

    disease [e.g., congestive heart failure (CHF), rheumatoid arthritis], mental status changes, or psychosocial problems.

    4. The ATA recommends a free thyroxine (FT_4) and a sensitive TSH assay as the primary laboratory tests to diagnose thyroid disease. The sensitive TSH assay is useful in detecting patients at risk of receiving an excess amount of thyroxine as replacement therapy.

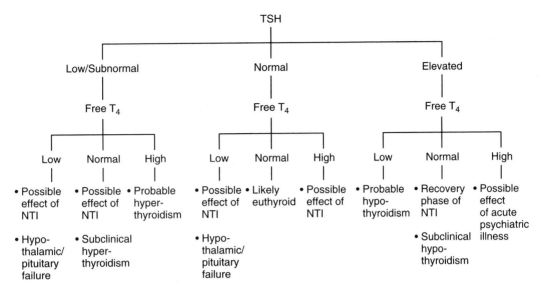

Figure 53-5. Algorithm for the use of sensitive thyroid-stimulating hormone (TSH) testing in patients with nonthyroidal illness (NTI). The TSH assay should meet the American Thyroid Association criteria for a sensitive assay and/or have a known functional sensitivity limit at the second-generation (0.1 mIU/L) level or greater. Medications known to alter TSH levels (i.e., corticosteroids, dopamine) must be considered in interpretation.

II. **HYPOTHYROIDISM.** The inability of the thyroid gland to supply sufficient thyroid hormone results in varying degrees of hypothyroidism from mild, clinically insignificant forms to the life-threatening extreme, myxedema coma.

   A. **Classification**

   1. **Primary hypothyroidism** is due to:
      a. Gland destruction or dysfunction caused by disease or medical therapies (e.g., radiation, surgical procedures)
      b. Failure of the gland to develop or congenital incompetence (i.e., **cretinism**)

   2. **Secondary hypothyroidism** is due to a pituitary disorder that inhibits TSH secretion. The thyroid gland is normal but lacks appropriate stimulation by TSH.

   3. **Tertiary hypothyroidism** refers to a condition in which the pituitary–thyroid axis is intact, but the hypothalamus lacks the ability to secrete TRH to stimulate the pituitary.

   B. **Causes**

   1. **Hashimoto's thyroiditis,** which is a chronic lymphocytic thyroiditis that is considered to be an autoimmune disorder

   2. **Treatment of hyperthyroidism,** such as radioactive iodine therapy, subtotal thyroidectomy, or administration of antithyroid agents

   3. **Surgical excision**

   4. **Goiter** (enlargement of the thyroid gland)
      a. **Endemic goiter** results from inadequate intake of dietary iodine. This is common in regions with iodine-depleted soil and in areas of endemic malnutrition.
      b. **Sporadic goiter** can follow ingestion of certain drugs or foods containing **progoitrin** (L-5-vinyl-2-thio-oxazolidone), which is inactive and converted by hydrolysis to goitrin. Goitrins inhibit oxidation of iodine to iodide and prevent iodide from binding to thyroglobulin, thereby decreasing thyroid hormone production. Progoitrin has been isolated in cabbage, kale, peanuts, brussels sprouts, mustard, rutabaga, kohlrabi, spinach, cauliflower, and horseradish. **Goitrogenic drugs** include propylthiouracil (PTU), iodides, phenylbutazone, cobalt, and lithium.

   c. **Less common causes** include acute (usually traumatic) and subacute thyroiditis, nodules, nodular goiter, and thyroid cancer.

C. Signs and symptoms

   1. Early clinical features tend to be somewhat vague: lethargy, fatigue, forgetfulness, sensitivity to cold, unexplained weight gain, and constipation.

   2. Progressively, the characteristic features of myxedema emerge: dry, flaky, inelastic skin; coarse hair; slowed speech and thought; hoarseness; puffy face, hands, and feet; eyelid droop; hearing loss; menorrhagia; decreased libido; and slow return of deep tendon reflexes (especially in the Achilles tendon). If untreated, myxedema coma will develop.

D. Laboratory findings (see Table 53-1)

E. Treatment goal is replacement therapy using oral agents (Table 53-5).

F. Therapeutic agents

   1. **Desiccated thyroid preparations**
      a. At one time the agent of choice, desiccated thyroid has fallen out of favor since standardized synthetic levothyroxine preparations have become available.
      b. Desiccated thyroid preparations are not considered bioequivalent; they have evidenced varying amounts of active substances. Although they met established *United States Pharmacopeia (USP)* criteria for iodine content, variation in activity was noted. The content assay, while specific for iodine, was unable to specify the ratio of T_3 to T_4, and this ratio varies with the animal source. Porcine gland preparations have a higher T_3 to T_4 ratio than those from ovine or bovine sources.

   2. **Fixed ratio (liotrix) preparations.** In an effort to standardize the T_3 to T_4 ratio, substances that mimic glandular content were developed. However, the T_3 component proved unnecessary (because T_4 is metabolized to T_3) and even disadvantageous because of T_3-induced **adverse effects** (e.g., tremor, headache, palpitations, diarrhea).

   3. **Levothyroxine**
      a. Predictable results and lack of T_3-induced side effects have made levothyroxine the agent of choice.
      b. The **two major brands** of levothyroxine preparations (Levothroid, Synthroid) have been compared for bioequivalence and were shown to be equivalent in patients with hypothyroidism.
      c. Recent studies in patients with hypothyroidism have compared brand and generic formulations of levothyroxine, which include Synthroid, Levoxyl, and generic formulations manufactured by Pharmaceutical Basics and sold by Geneva Generic and Rugby. Bioequivalence has been demonstrated with these formulations. However, when switching formulations, it is recommended to monitor the patient closely because there may be some individual patient variability between formulations (Figure 53-6).
      d. The **average adult maintenance** dose is 75–150 μg/day. The dose range has been shown to be 1.5–1.7 μg/kg/day or an average of 1.6 μg/kg/day for otherwise healthy adults.
      e. **Elderly** or **chronically ill patients** require an average dose of 50–100 μg/day, which is 25–50 μg/day less than otherwise healthy adults of the same height and weight.
      f. Thyroxine levels return to normal within a few weeks. Clinical improvement begins in 2 weeks with full resolution of signs and symptoms of hypothyroidism by 3–6 months of therapy.
      g. TSH levels begin to decrease after starting thyroid replacement. TSH remains elevated for some time after T_4 levels return to normal. Generally, TSH levels return to normal after a minimum of 6–8 weeks, but may continue to fall over 6–12 months (see Figure 53-6).

G. Precautions and monitoring effects

   1. Adult patients with a history of cardiac disease and elderly patients should begin therapy with lower doses (e.g., 25 μg/day of levothyroxine). After 2–4 weeks, the dose should be increased gradually to an individually adjusted maintenance dose (usually less than 100 μg daily).

Table 53-5. Thyroid Replacement Preparations

Preparation	Trade Names	Advantage	Disadvantage	Comments	Source
Dessicated thyroid	Thyroid USP Thyroid Strong Armour Thyroid Thyrar S-P-T	Low cost	Some preparations have unpredictable results Inconsistent T_3:T_4 ratio T_3 increases adverse effects	Contains T_3 Some brands are standardized by iodine content*	Porcine, bovine, or ovine thyroid glands
Liothyronine	Cytomel	Predictable results Useful for myxedema crisis	Lacks T_4	Usually reserved for myxedema crisis	Synthetic
Liotrix	Thyrolar	Standardized formulation	T_3 increases adverse effects Expensive	Fixed T_3:T_4 ratio of 1:4 Metabolism of T_4 to T_3 renders T_3 component unnecessary	Synthetic
Levothyroxine	Levothroid Synthroid† Levoxyl†	Predictable results, intravenous preparation available	Expensive	Agent of choice Does not contain T_3 All preparations may be interchangeable	Synthetic

*Iodine content, as well as T_3:T_4 ratio, varies with species.

†Generic formulations manufactured by Pharmaceuticals Basics for Geneva Generics and Rugby have been shown to be bioequivalent to Synthroid and Levoxyl. (Dong BJ, et al. *JAMA* 1997;277:1205–1213.)

T_3 = triiodotyronine; T_4 = thyroxine.

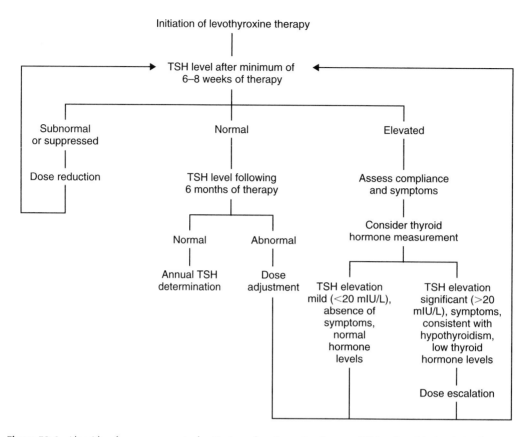

Figure 53-6. Algorithm for management of patients on levothyroxine therapy. *TSH* = thyroid-stimulating hormone.

2. Patients should be observed on initiation of therapy for possible **cardiac complications,** such as angina, palpitations, or arrhythmias.

3. Serum thyroid levels should be monitored, particularly T_4, sensitive TSH and RT_3U levels, as well as the FTI. Serum thyroxine tests remain elevated during the first few months of treatment even with the presence of clinical symptoms. Serum thyroxine tests do not predict the clinical state. Testing is unnecessary unless noncompliance is suspected.

4. It is recommended to monitor the sensitive TSH test 2–6 months after the last dose change. However, this test continues to change for up to 1 year. Testing early may result in overtreatment. Refer to the treatment algorithm for the management of patients on levothyroxine therapy (see Figure 53-6).

5. Levothyroxine administration, particularly long-term therapy, can induce thyrotoxicosis; T_4 levels can rise even though the dosage remains unchanged. Monitor for clinical signs of thyroid disease.

6. **Accelerated bone loss** has been associated with overtreatment. Patients receiving replacement therapy with low TSH values may have lower bone mineral density since excess hormone accelerates the rate of remodeling (rate of resorption > rate of formation) and may contribute to an increased incidence of nontraumatic fracture.

7. **Drug interactions. Cholestyramine,** a bile acid sequestrant, can contribute to a decrease in **thyroxine** bioavailability when administered concomitantly. Cholestyramine should be administered at least 6 hours after oral thyroxine to reduce the potential for this clinically significant drug interaction. Calcium carbonate can reduce thyroxine bioavailability by adsorption in an acid environment. These should be administered separately to avoid interaction.

H. Myxedema coma is a life-threatening complication with a high mortality rate.

   1. It is **most common** in elderly patients with preexisting, although usually undiagnosed, hypothyroidism.

   2. Precipitating factors include alcohol, sedative, or narcotic use; overuse of antithyroid agents; abrupt discontinuation of thyroid hormone therapy; infection; exposure to cold temperatures; and iatrogenic insult due to radiation therapy or thyroid surgery.

   3. The patient usually declines from profound lethargy to coma, hypothermia, and a significant decrease in respiratory rate, potentially leading to respiratory failure as the crisis progresses. Hypometabolism produces a fluid and electrolyte imbalance that leads to fluid retention and hyponatremia. **Cardiac effects** include decreased heart rate and contractility, decreasing cardiac output.

   4. Treatment consists of rapid restoration of T_3 and T_4 levels to normal.
   a. A loading dose of levothyroxine 400–500 μg is given as an intravenous (IV) bolus. Liothyronine, 25 μg, is then given orally every 6 hours.
   b. Treatment is continued until improvement is noted. Then, liothyronine is discontinued, and levothyroxine is changed to the oral preparation. A maintenance dose is then determined (see II G).

III. HYPERTHYROIDISM is the overabundance of thyroid hormone. **Thyrotoxicosis** is the general term applied to overactivity of the thyroid gland.

   A. Graves' disease (diffuse toxic goiter)

   1. The **most common form** of hyperthyroidism, Graves' disease occurs primarily, but not exclusively, in **young women.**

   2. The basis of this disease is an **autoimmune disorder** in which antibodies bind to and activate TSH receptors, resulting in the overproduction of thyroid hormone.
   a. These antibodies are termed **long-acting thyroid stimulators (LATS)** because their duration of action extends beyond that of TSH. As TSH is only mimicked, not overabundant, neither testing for TSH nor attempts to influence it are productive.
   b. Antibody titers often are elevated in patients with Graves' disease.

   3. Signs and symptoms characteristic of Graves' disease include:
   a. Diffusely enlarged nontender goiter
   b. Nervousness, irritability, anxiety, and insomnia
   c. Heat intolerance and profuse sweating
   d. Weight loss despite increased appetite
   e. Tremor and muscle weakness
   f. Palpitations and tachycardia
   g. Exophthalmos, stare, and lid lag (slow upper lid closing)
   h. Diarrhea
   i. Thrill or bruit over the thyroid
   j. Periorbital edema

   B. Plummer's disease (toxic nodular goiter)

   1. This **form of thyrotoxicosis** is less common than Graves' disease. Its underlying cause remains unknown, but its incidence is highest in patients over 50 years of age, and it arises usually from a long-standing nontoxic goiter.

   2. The thyrotoxicosis is a result of one or more adenomatous nodules autonomously secreting excessive thyroid hormone, which suppresses the rest of the gland. Scanning confirms the diagnosis if it indicates that activity and iodine uptake are confined to the nodular mass, unless TSH is introduced.

   3. Signs and symptoms are essentially the same as for Graves' disease except that one or more nodular masses are found, rather than diffuse glandular enlargement, and ophthalmopathy is usually absent. **Cardiac abnormalities** (e.g., CHF, tachyarrhythmias) are commonly seen with Plummer's disease.

C. Less common forms of hyperthyroidism

1. **Jodbasedow phenomenon** is an overproduction of thyroid hormone following a sudden, large increase in iodine ingestion—through either a sudden reversal of an iodine-deficient diet or the introduction of iodide or iodine in contrast agents or drugs (e.g., the anti-arrhythmic agent amiodarone).

2. **Factitious hyperthyroidism** occurs with abusive ingestion of thyroid replacement agents, usually in a misguided effort to lose weight. Diagnosis is aided by the absence of glandular swelling and of exophthalmos and the lack of autoimmune activity found in Graves' disease.

D. Laboratory findings (see Table 53-1)

E. Treatment goal. Symptomatic relief is provided until definitive treatment can be effected.

F. Therapeutic agents

1. **β-Adrenergic blocking agents—propranolol**
   a. Propranolol reduces some of the peripheral manifestations (e.g., tachycardia, sweating, severe tremor, nervousness) of hyperthyroidism.
   b. In addition to providing symptomatic relief, propranolol inhibits the peripheral conversion of T_4 to T_3.

2. **Antithyroid agents—propylthiouracil (PTU) and methimazole**
   a. **Action.** These agents may help attain remission through direct interference with thyroid hormone synthesis. Both agents inhibit iodide oxidation and iodothiouracil coupling. In addition, PTU (but not methimazole) diminishes peripheral deiodination of T_4 to T_3.
   b. **Therapeutic uses** of these drugs include:
      (1) **Definitive treatment** in which remission is achieved
      (2) **Adjunctive therapy** with radioactive iodine until the radiation takes effect
      (3) **Preoperative preparation** to establish and maintain a euthyroid state until definitive surgery can be performed
   c. **Dosages**
      (1) **Propylthiouracil**
         (a) For **adults,** the initial dose is 300–450 μg/day in three divided doses (i.e., 100–150 μg every 8 hours). Adult patients with severe disease may require as much as 600–1200 μg/day initially.
         (b) The initial dose is continued for about 2 months; then a maintenance dose of 100–150 μg/day is given, as a single dose or divided into two doses.
         (c) Maintenance therapy is continued for approximately 1 year, then gradually discontinued over 1–2 months while the patient is monitored for signs of recurrent hyperthyroidism. The patient may remain in remission for several years. A recurrent episode of hyperthyroidism is most likely to occur within 3–6 months of drug discontinuation.
         (d) If hyperthyroidism recurs after drug therapy is stopped, the agent should be restarted and alternative therapy should be considered (e.g., thyroid gland ablation or removal).
      (2) **Methimazole**
         (a) The initial dose range is 5–60 μg/day in three divided doses, depending on disease severity. After 2 months of therapy, a maintenance dose of 5–30 μg/day is initiated.
         (b) Maintenance therapy is continued for approximately 1 year at which time the drug is gradually discontinued, usually over 1–2 months.
   d. **Precautions and monitoring effects**
      (1) Serum thyroid levels and the FTI should be monitored for a return to normal.
      (2) Goiter size should decrease with reduced hormone output.
      (3) The incidence of **adverse effects** is less than 1% with PTU and less than 3% with methimazole. The adverse effects are similar for the two agents.
         (a) The most bothersome are **dermatologic reactions** (e.g., rash, urticaria, pruritus, hair loss, skin pigmentation). Others include headache, drowsiness, paresthesia, nausea, vomiting, vertigo, neuritis, loss of taste, arthralgia, and myalgia.
         (b) **Severe adverse effects**—agranulocytosis, granulocytopenia, thrombocytopenia, drug fever, hepatitis, and hypoprothrombinemia—occur less frequently. Patients

receiving methimazole who are over 40 years old and are receiving doses above 40 μg/day are at increased risk of developing agranulocytosis. Patients receiving PTU who are over 40 years old are at increased risk of developing agranulocytosis, but no dose association has been established.

3. **Radioactive iodine (RAI)**
   a. **Action.** The thyroid gland picks up the radioactive element iodine-131 (^{131}I) as it would regular iodine. The radioactivity subsequently destroys some of the cells that would otherwise concentrate iodine and produce T_4, thus decreasing thyroid hormone production.
   b. **Advantages**
      (1) **High cure rate**—almost 100% for patients with Graves' disease and only slightly less for patients with Plummer's disease
      (2) **Avoids surgical risks**—such as adverse reaction to anesthetics, hypoparathyroidism, nerve palsy, bleeding, and hoarseness
      (3) **Less expensive**—avoids cost of hospitalization
   c. **Disadvantages**
      (1) Risk of delayed hypothyroidism
      (2) Slight, though undocumented, risk of genetic damage
      (3) Multiple doses, which may be required, may delay therapeutic efficacy for a long period (many months or a year).
   d. **Dosage.** A dose of 80–100 mCi of ^{131}I per estimated gram of thyroid gland is recommended. Some protocols use lower dosages, but these may be less effective, requiring retreatment. When the dose is higher, there is a potential risk that hypothyroidism will develop.
   e. **Precautions and monitoring effects**
      (1) Radioiodine therapy generally is reserved for patients past the childbearing years because effects on future offspring are not known.
      (2) Response to ^{131}I is hard to gauge, and patients must be monitored early for recurrence of hyperthyroidism, and later for hypothyroidism, which may develop even 20 years or more after therapy.

4. **Subtotal thyroidectomy.** Partial removal of the thyroid gland may be indicated if drug therapy fails or radioactive iodine is undesirable. This is a difficult procedure, but the success rate is high and the cure rapid. Risks include those mentioned in III F 3 b (2), precipitating thyroid storm, and permanent postoperative hypothyroidism. The risk of inducing thyroid storm can be minimized by obtaining a euthyroid state through use of antithyroid agents (see III F 2) or propranolol (see III F 1).

G. **Complications**

1. **Hypothyroidism** may occur iatrogenically or, it has been proposed, as a natural sequel to Graves' disease.

2. **Thyroid storm (thyrotoxic crisis)** is a sudden exacerbation of hyperthyroidism caused by rapid release (leakage) of thyroid hormone. It is invariably fatal if not treated rapidly. In this crisis, unchecked hypermetabolism leads ultimately to dehydration, shock, and death.
   a. **Precipitating factors** include thyroid trauma or surgery, RAI therapy, infection, and sudden discontinuation of antithyroid therapy.
   b. **Characteristics.** It is characterized by a TT_4 level of 25–30 μg/dl, rapidly rising fever, tachycardia disproportionate to the fever, and unexplained, pronounced restlessness and tremor.
   c. **Treatment**
      (1) **PTU,** in doses of 150–250 μg orally every 6 hours, is the preferred agent because PTU blocks peripheral deiodination of T_4 to T_3, whereas methimazole does not. However, if necessary, **methimazole,** 15 mg orally every 6 hours, can be used instead.
      (2) **Propranolol,** in doses of 20–200 mg orally every 6 hours or 1–3 mg intravenously every 4–6 hours, should be administered unless contraindicated (e.g., if the patient has CHF).
      (3) **Potassium iodide,** in doses of 50–100 mg every 12 hours, is given (after PTU) to minimize intrathyroidal iodine uptake.
      (4) **Other supportive therapy** includes rehydration, cooling, antibiotics, rest, and sedation.

STUDY QUESTIONS

Directions: Each of the numbered items or incomplete statements in this section is followed by answers or by completions of the statement. Select the **one** lettered answer or completion that is **best** in each case.

1. What is the correct formula to use for calculating the free thyroxine index (FTI)?

(A) T_4 x RT_3U/mean serum RT_3U
(B) T_3 x T_3/mean serum RT_3U
(C) T_3 x RT_3U/mean serum RT_3U
(D) T_4 x RT_3U x mean serum RT_3U
(E) T_3 x RT_3U x mean serum RT_3U

2. What is the necessary precursor besides dietary iodine required for thyroxine biosynthesis?

(A) Triiodothyronine (T_3)
(B) Threonine
(C) Tyrosine
(D) Thyrotropin (thyroid-stimulating hormone)
(E) Thyroxine-binding globulin (TBG)

3. All of the following conditions are causes of hyperthyroidism EXCEPT

(A) Graves' disease
(B) Hashimoto's thyroiditis
(C) toxic multinodular goiter
(D) triiodothyronine toxicosis
(E) Plummer's disease

4. Which of the following preparations is used to attain remission of thyrotoxicosis?

(A) Propranolol
(B) Liotrix
(C) Levothyroxine
(D) Propylthiouracil
(E) Desiccated thyroid

5. The thyroid gland normally secretes which of the following substances into the serum?

(A) Thyrotropin-releasing hormone (TRH)
(B) Thyrotropin (thyroid-stimulating hormone)
(C) Diiodothyronine (DIT)
(D) Thyroglobulin
(E) Thyroxine (T_4)

6. All of the following conditions are causes of hypothyroidism EXCEPT

(A) endemic goiter
(B) surgical excision
(C) Hashimoto's thyroiditis
(D) goitrin-induced iodine deficiency
(E) Graves' disease

7. Common tests to monitor patients receiving replacement therapy for hypothyroidism include all of the following EXCEPT

(A) thyrotropin (TSH) stimulation test
(B) sensitive TSH assay
(C) free thyroxine index (FTI)
(D) resin triiodothyronine uptake (RT_3U)
(E) total thyroxine (TT_4)

8. Which of the following pairs of preparations has been studied for bioequivalence?

(A) Levoxyl—Thyrolar
(B) Thyroglobulin—Proloid
(C) Levothroid—Synthroid
(D) Cytomel—Synthroid
(E) Desiccated thyroid—Armour thyroid

9. The inhibition of pituitary thyrotropin secretion is controlled by which of the following?

(A) Free thyroxine (T_4)
(B) Thyroid-releasing hormone (TRH)
(C) Free thyroxine index (FTI)
(D) Reverse triiodothyronine (rT_3)
(E) Total thyroxine (TT_4)

10. Which of the following agents has been shown to interact with oral thyroxine (T_4) replacement therapy?

(A) Propylthiouracil
(B) Cholestyramine
(C) Thyrotropin
(D) Levothyroxine
(E) Lovastatin

11. What laboratory tests are currently recommended by the American Thyroid Association to diagnose thyroid disease?

(A) Resin triiodothyronine uptake (RT_3U) and total thyroxine (TT_4)
(B) Thyrotropin (TSH) and free thyroxine index (FTI)
(C) Total thyroxine (TT_4) and sensitive TSH assay
(D) Free T_4 and sensitive TSH assay
(E) Free T_4 and RT_3U

12. What patient population should be screened for thyroid disease?

(A) Hospitalized patients
(B) Elderly patients with chronic disease
(C) Elderly hospitalized patients
(D) College students
(E) Women over 20 years old

13. What is the average replacement dose of levothyroxine for an otherwise healthy adult?

(A) 25–50 μg/day
(B) 50–100 μg/day
(C) 75–150 μg/day
(D) 100–200 μg/day
(E) 200–400 μg/day

14. What factors affect the optimal replacement dose of levothyroxine?

(A) Age, height, and weight
(B) Duration of hypothyroidism
(C) Pretreatment thyroid-stimulating hormone (TSH) level
(D) Presence of chronic illness
(E) All of the above

15. Which of the values represents the lower level of detection for the fourth-generation sensitive TSH assay as established by the American Thyroid Association?

(A) 0.5–5 mIU/L
(B) 1–2 mIU/L
(C) 0.01–0.02 mIU/L
(D) 0.001–0.002 mIU/L
(E) 0.0001–0.0002 mIU/L

16. In which of the following clinical presentations should the sensitive TSH assay be used?

(A) Population screening for thyroid disease
(B) Screening hospitalized patients
(C) Patients receiving thyroid replacement after 6–8 weeks of therapy
(D) Patients who are human immunodeficiency virus (HIV) positive
(E) Screening patients with psychiatric illness

17. Which of the following agents has been shown to interact with oral thyroxine (T_4) replacement therapy?

(A) Propranolol
(B) Levothyroxine
(C) Calcium carbonate
(D) Thyrotropin
(E) Lovastatin

ANSWERS AND EXPLANATIONS

1. The answer is A *[I F 5].*
The free thyroxine index (FTI) is a mathematical interpretation of the relationship between the resin tri-iodothyronine uptake (RT_3U) and serum thyroxine (T_4) levels, compared to the mean population value for RT_3U. The FTI is calculated using reported values for total thyroxine (TT_4) and RT_3U. The normal FTI value in euthyroid patients is 5.5–12.

2. The answer is C *[I B].*
Biosynthesis of thyroid hormones begins with iodide binding to tyrosine, which forms monoiodotyrosine (MIT). MIT binds another iodide atom to form diiodotyrosine (DIT). When MIT and DIT are formed, a coupling reaction occurs, which produces triiodothyronine (T_3), thyroxine (T_4), reverse triiodothyronine (rT_3), and other by-products.

3. The answer is B *[II B 1; III A, B]*
Hashimoto's thyroiditis (chronic lymphocytic thyroiditis) is a cause of hypothyroidism. The incidence of Hashimoto's thyroiditis is 1%–2%, and it increases with age. It is more common in women than in men and more common in whites than in blacks. There may be a familial tendency. Patients with Hashimoto's thyroiditis have elevated titers of antibodies to thyroglobulin: A titer of greater than 1:32 is seen in more than 85% of patients. Two variants of Hashimoto's thyroiditis have been described: gland fibrosis and idiopathic thyroid atrophy, which is most likely an extension of Hashimoto's thyroiditis.

4. The answer is D *[III F 1, 2].*
In hyperthyroid patients, remission of thyrotoxicosis is achieved with propylthiouracil (PTU) by two mechanisms: (1) interference of iodination of the tyrosyl residues, ultimately reducing production of thyroxine (T_4) and (2) inhibition of peripheral conversion of T_4 to triiodothyronine (T_3). Propranolol is commonly used as an adjunct to PTU for symptomatic management of hyperthyroidism.

5. The answer is E *[I A 1].*
The major compounds secreted by the thyroid gland, after its stimulation by thyrotropin, are triiodothyronine (T_3) and thyroxine (T_4). When released from the thyroid, T_3 and T_4 are transported by plasma proteins, namely thyroxine-binding globulin (TBG), thyroxine-binding prealbumin, and albumin.

6. The answer is E *[II B; III A 1].*
Graves' disease (diffuse toxic goiter) is the most common form of hyperthyroidism. It occurs most often in women in the third and fourth decades of life. There is a genetic and familial predisposition. The etiology is linked to an autoimmune reaction between immunoglobulin G (IgG) and the thyroid.

7. The answer is A *[II G 3].*
The thyrotropin (TSH) stimulation test measures thyroid tissue response to exogenous TSH. It is not commonly used to monitor thyroid replacement therapy. It may be useful in the initial diagnosis of hypothyroidism.

8. The answer is C *[II F 3 b-c].*
Many brands of levothyroxine are currently available. Both generic and trade name preparations have been studied, with an emphasis on Levothroid and Synthroid. The importance of bioequivalence becomes apparent when patients have received different brands of levothyroxine and have exhibited changes in therapeutic response to equivalent replacement doses.

9. The answer is A *[I A 3 a].*
An increase in the blood level of thyroid hormone [circulating free thyroxine (T_4) and free triiodothyronine (T_3)] signals the pituitary to stop releasing thyroid-stimulating hormone (thyrotropin; TSH). The free fraction of T_4 is available to bind at the pituitary receptors.

10. The answer is B *[II G 7].*
Euthyroid patients receiving oral replacement therapy have become hypothyroid after concomitant administration of bile acid sequestrant therapy. It appears that bioavailability is reduced as a result of administering these agents at close dosing intervals. It is recommended that at least 6 hours pass before administration of a bile acid sequestrant. It would be preferable to select another nonbile acid sequestrant when clinically possible.

11. The answer is D *[I G 4]*.

The free thyroxine (free T_4) and the sensitive thyrotropin (TSH) assay should be used only for the diagnosis of patients most likely to have thyroid disease based on clinical presentation and relative risk (e.g., age, sex, family history), not for population screening. The sensitive TSH assay is also useful to monitor replacement therapy and to minimize overtreatment and the corresponding risk of accelerated bone loss.

12. The answer is B *[I G 3]*.

Cost versus benefit is critical to the decision of choosing to screen entire populations. Because the frequency of detection has been proven to be higher in elderly patients (2%–5%) with chronic disease, the relative minor costs associated to obtain resin triiodothyronine uptake (RT_3U) and serum total thyroxine (TT_4) to calculate a free thyroxine index (FTI) are worth the cost. A serum thyrotropin (TSH) assay can be reserved for patients with an abnormal FTI. Another consideration is to use the sensitive TSH assay for diagnosis in place of the serum TSH assay at a higher cost but without the necessity of retesting. If patients admitted to the hospital for an acute illness were screened, but the results are misleading, they may be prescribed inappropriate therapy because acute illness may be associated with the temporary effects causing abnormal test results.

13. The answer is C *[II F 3 d]*.

The average adult maintenance dose is 75–150 µg/day, which has been shown to be 1.5–1.7 µg/kg/day. The dose is usually adjusted in increments of 25–50 µg/day every 4 weeks. The total daily dose used to be 100–200 µg/day, which resulted in overtreatment after the introduction of the sensitive TSH assay. Elderly or chronically ill patients require an average dose of 50–100 µg/day, which is 25–50 µg/day less than otherwise healthy adults of the same height and weight.

14. The answer is E *[II F 3 e]*.

Elderly or chronically ill patients require an average dose of 50–100 µg/day, which is 25–50 µg/day less than otherwise healthy adults of the same height and weight. Because the average dose for replacement therapy is between 1.5 and 1.7 µg/kg/day, weight affects the total daily dose.

15. The answer is D *[I F 4 b (4)]*.

The American Thyroid Association has established standard nomenclature that indicates each technological improvement and the ability to detect lower levels of TSH using monoclonal antibodies. As the sensitivity of the assay improves, the lower level of detection is reported as a range in mIU/L. The most sensitive test is currently the fourth-generation immunometric assay, with a reported lower level of detection of 0.001–0.002 mIU/L.

16. The answer is C *[I F 4 b, (5), (6); II 64 Figure 53-6]*.

The sensitive TSH assay is not indicated for use in hospitalized patients who are not suspected to have thyroid disease. Studies have indicated that abnormally high or low TSH levels are detected in euthyroid hospitalized patients. Psychiatric illness may also influence TSH levels.

17. The answer is C *[II G 7]*.

Patients receiving oral replacement therapy who take calcium carbonate concomitantly have been shown to experience decreased free T_4 and total T_4 levels that resulted in an elevated TSH. The mechanism appears to be adsorption of levothyroxine to calcium carbonate at acid pH levels, which may reduce bioavailability. It is recommended to separate the time of ingestion of each product to reduce the chance of this interaction.

I. ACUTE RENAL FAILURE

A. Definition. Acute renal failure (ARF) is the sudden, potentially reversible interruption of kidney function, resulting in retention of nitrogenous waste products in body fluids.

B. Classification and etiology. ARF is classified according to its cause.

1. **Prerenal ARF** stems from impaired renal perfusion, which may result from:
   a. Reduced arterial blood volume [e.g., dehydration, hemorrhage, vomiting, diarrhea, other gastrointestinal (GI) fluid loss]
   b. Urinary losses from excessive diuresis
   c. Decreased cardiac output [e.g., from congestive heart failure (CHF) or pericardial tamponade]
   d. Renal vascular obstruction (e.g., stenosis)
   e. Severe hypotension

2. **Intrarenal ARF (intrinsic or parenchymal ARF)** reflects structural kidney damage resulting from any of the following conditions.
   a. **Acute tubular necrosis (ATN),** the leading cause of ARF, may be associated with:
      (1) Exposure to nephrotoxic aminoglycosides, anesthetics, pesticides, organic metals, and radiopaque contrast materials
      (2) Ischemic injury (e.g., surgery, circulatory collapse, severe hypotension)
      (3) Pigment (e.g., hemolysis, myoglobinuria)
   b. Acute glomerulonephritis
   c. Tubular obstruction, as from hemolytic reactions or uric acid crystals
   d. Acute inflammation (e.g., acute tubulointerstitial nephritis, papillary necrosis)
   e. Renal vasculitis
   f. Malignant hypertension
   g. Radiation nephritis

3. **Postrenal ARF** results from obstruction of urine flow anywhere along the urinary tract. Causes of postrenal ARF include:
   a. Ureteral obstruction, as from calculi, uric acid crystals, or thrombi
   b. Bladder obstruction, as from calculi, thrombi, tumors, or infection
   c. Urethral obstruction, as from strictures, tumors, or prostatic hypertrophy
   d. Extrinsic obstruction, as from hematoma, inflammatory bowel disease, or accidental surgical ligation

C. Pathophysiology. ARF progresses in three phases.

1. **Initiating phase**
   a. The initiating phase is defined as the time between the renal insult and the point at which extrarenal factors no longer reverse the damage caused by the obstruction or other cause of ARF. This phase may not be well-defined clinically and may escape notice or diagnosis.
   b. **Urine output** may drop markedly to 400 mL/day or less **(oliguria).** In some patients, urine output falls below 100 mL/day **(anuria).** Oliguria may last only hours or as long as 4–6 weeks. However, it has been shown that 40%–50% of ARF patients are not oliguric or anuric.
   c. **Nitrogenous waste products** accumulate in the blood.
      (1) **Azotemia** reflects urea accumulation due to impaired glomerular filtration and concentrating capacity.
      (2) Serum creatinine concentration, sulfate, phosphate, and organic acid levels climb rapidly.

d. The **serum sodium concentration** falls below normal from intracellular fluid shifting and dilution.

e. Hyperkalemia occurs due to the accumulation of organic acids (metabolic acidosis). If potassium intake is not restricted or body potassium is not removed, hyperkalemia results. Without treatment, hyperkalemia may lead to neuromuscular depression and paralysis, impaired cardiac conduction, arrhythmias, respiratory muscle paralysis, cardiac arrest, and ultimately death.

2. Maintenance phase

a. This phase begins when urine output rises above 500 mL/day—typically after several days of oliguria. A rise in urine output or a "diuretic response" may not be seen in non-oliguric patients. Increased urinary output does not signal recovery of renal function.

b. Urine output rises in increments of several milliliters to 300–500 mL/day. Urine output may double from day to day in the initial recovery period.

c. Azotemia and associated laboratory findings may persist until urine output reaches 1000–2000 mL/day.

d. The maintenance phase carries a risk of fluid and electrolyte abnormalities, GI bleeding, infection, and respiratory failure.

3. Recovery phase. During the recovery phase, renal function gradually returns to normal. Most recovered renal function appears in the first 2 weeks; however, recovery of renal function may continue for a year. Residual impairment may persist indefinitely.

D. Clinical evaluation

1. Physical findings. Initially, ARF causes azotemia and, in 50%–60% of cases, oliguria. Later, electrolyte abnormalities and other severe systemic effects occur.

a. Urine output typically is **low,** from 20–500 mL/day. Complete anuria is rare.

b. Signs and **symptoms of hyperkalemia,** resulting from metabolic acidosis and reduced potassium excretion by impaired kidneys, include:

(1) Neuromuscular depression (e.g., paresthesias, muscle weakness, paralysis)

(2) Diarrhea and abdominal distention

(3) Slow or irregular pulse

(4) Electrocardiographic changes with potential cardiac arrest

c. Uremia, caused by excessive nitrogenous waste retention, leads to nausea, vomiting, diarrhea, edema, confusion, fatigue, neuromuscular irritability, and coma.

d. Metabolic acidosis, a common complication of ARF, is evidenced by:

(1) Deterioration of mental status, obtundation, coma, and lethargy

(2) Depressed cardiac contractility and decreased vascular resistance, leading to hypotension, pulmonary edema, and ventricular fibrillation

(3) Nausea and vomiting

(4) Respiratory abnormalities (e.g., hyperventilation, Kussmaul's respiration)

e. Hyperphosphatemia arises from decreased phosphate excretion. It is generally not seen in ARF.

(1) As serum phosphate rises, hypocalcemia results from the formation of insoluble calcium phosphate complexes.

(2) The signs and symptoms relate to resultant hypocalcemia and metastatic soft-tissue calcification.

(3) Manifestations of hypocalcemia include:

(a) Neuromuscular irritability, cramps, spasms, and tetany

(b) Hypotension

(c) Soft-tissue calcification

(d) Mental status changes (e.g., confusion, mood changes, loss of intellect and memory)

(e) Hyperactive deep-tendon reflexes and Trousseau's and Chvostek's signs

(f) Abdominal cramps

(g) Stridor and dyspnea

f. Hyponatremia results from dilution and intravascular fluid shifts during the diuretic phase of ARF. Physical findings include lethargy, weakness, seizures, cognitive impairment, and possible reduction in level of consciousness.

g. Intravascular volume depletion, suggesting **prerenal failure,** may cause:

(1) Flat jugular venous pulses when the patient lies supine

(2) Orthostatic changes in blood pressure and pulse

(3) Poor skin turgor and dry mucous membranes

h. Other findings suggesting **prerenal failure** include:

(1) An abdominal bruit, possibly indicating renal artery stenosis

(2) Increased paradoxus, suggesting pericardial tamponade

(3) Increased jugular venous pressure, pulmonary rales, and a third heart sound, signaling CHF

i. Postrenal failure caused by obstructed urinary flow may manifest itself in:

(1) A suprapubic or flank mass

(2) Bladder distention

(3) Costovertebral angle tenderness

(4) Prostate enlargement

2. Diagnostic test results

a. Urinalysis includes an examination of sediment; identification of proteins, glucose, ketones, blood, and nitrites; and measurement of urinary pH and urine-specific gravity (concentration) or osmolality (dilution). Prior administration of fluids, diuretics, and changes in urinary pH may confound accurate diagnosis, using urinalysis.

(1) Urinary sediment examination

(a) Few casts and formed elements are found in prerenal ARF.

(b) Pigmented cellular casts and renal tubular epithelial cells appear with ATN.

(c) Red blood cell and white blood cell casts generally reflect inflammatory disease.

(d) Large numbers of broad white cell casts suggest chronic renal failure.

(2) The presence of blood in the urine **(hematuria)** or proteins **(proteinuria)** indicates renal dysfunction.

(3) Urine-specific gravity ranges from 1.010–1.016 in ARF.

(4) Urine osmolality typically rises in prerenal ARF due to increased secretion of antidiuretic hormone.

b. Measurement of urine sodium and **creatinine levels** can help classify ARF.

(1) In **prerenal** ARF, the urine creatinine concentration **increases,** and urine sodium level **decreases.**

(2) In **intrarenal** ARF resulting from ATN, the urine creatinine concentration **decreases,** and the urine sodium level **increases.**

c. Creatinine clearance, an index of the **glomerular filtration rate (GFR),** allows estimation of the number of functioning nephrons; decreased creatinine clearance indicates renal dysfunction. A timed urine collection should be used to calculate GFR in acute renal failure.

d. Blood chemistry provides an index of renal excretory function and body chemistry status. Findings typical of ARF include:

(1) Increased blood urea nitrogen (BUN)

(2) Increased serum creatinine concentration

(3) Possible increase in hemoglobin and hematocrit values due to dehydration

(4) Abnormal serum electrolyte values

(a) Serum potassium level above 5 mEq/L

(b) Serum phosphate level above 2.6 mEq/L (4.8 mg/dl)

(c) Serum calcium level below 4 mEq/L (8.5 mg/dl), reflecting hypocalcemia. (The serum calcium level must be correlated with the serum albumin level. Each rise or fall of 1 g/dl of serum albumin beyond its normal range is responsible for a corresponding increase or decrease in serum calcium of approximately 0.8 mg/dl. A below-normal serum albumin level may result in a deceptively low serum calcium level.)

(d) Serum sodium level below 135 mEq/L, reflecting hyponatremia

(5) Abnormal arterial blood gas values [pH below 7.35, bicarbonate concentration (HCO^{-3}) below 22], reflecting metabolic acidosis

e. Renal failure index (RFI) is the ratio of urine sodium concentration to the urine-to-serum creatinine ratio. The RFI helps determine the etiology of ARF. Typically, the RFI is less than 1 in prerenal ARF or acute glomerulonephritis (a cause of intrarenal ARF). The RFI is greater than 2 in postrenal ARF and in other intrarenal causes of ARF.

f. Electrocardiography (ECG) may show evidence of hyperkalemia—that is, tall, peaked T waves; widening QRS complexes; prolonged PR interval, progressing to decreased amplitude and disappearing P waves; and, ultimately, ventricular fibrillation and cardiac arrest.

g. Radiographic findings
  (1) Ultrasound may detect upper urinary tract obstruction.
  (2) Kidney, ureter, or **bladder radiography** may reveal:
    (a) Urinary tract calculi
    (b) Enlarged kidneys, suggesting ATN
    (c) Asymmetrical kidneys, suggesting unilateral renal artery disease, ureteral obstruction, or chronic pyelonephritis
  (3) Radionuclide scan may reveal:
    (a) Bilateral differences in renal perfusion, suggesting serious renal disease
    (b) Bilateral differences in dye excretion, suggesting parenchymal disease or obstruction as the cause of ARF
    (c) Diffuse, slow, dense radionuclide uptake, suggesting ATN
    (d) Patchy or absent radionuclide uptake, possibly indicating severe, acute glomerulonephritis
  (4) Computed tomography (CT) scan may provide better visualization of an obstruction.
h. Renal biopsy may be performed in selected patients when other test results are inconclusive.

E. Treatment objectives

  1. Correct reversible causes of ARF, preventing or minimizing further renal damage or complications.
    a. Discontinue nephrotoxic drugs; remove other nephrotoxins through dialysis or gastric lavage for poisonings.
    b. Treat underlying infection.
    c. Remove any urinary tract obstructions.

  2. Correct and maintain proper fluid and electrolyte balance. Match fluid, electrolyte, and nitrogen intakes to urine output.

  3. Treat body chemistry alterations, especially hyperkalemia and metabolic acidosis, when present. Treatment may include renal dialysis.

  4. Improve urine output.

  5. Treat systemic manifestations of ARF.

F. Therapy

  1. Conservative management alone may suffice in uncomplicated ARF.
    a. Fluid management
      (1) Fluid intake should match fluid losses. **Sensible losses** (i.e., urine, stool, tube drainage) and **insensible losses** (i.e., skin, respiratory tract) of 500–1000 mL/day should be included in fluid balance calculations.
      (2) Volume overload should be avoided to minimize the risk of hypertension and CHF.
      (3) The patient should be weighed daily to determine fluid volume status.
    b. Dietary measures
      (1) Because catabolism accompanies renal failure, the patient should receive a **high-calorie, low-protein diet.** Such a diet helps to:
        (a) Reduce renal workload by decreasing production of end products of protein catabolism that the kidneys cannot excrete
        (b) Prevent ketoacidosis
        (c) Alleviate manifestations of uremia (e.g., nausea, vomiting, confusion, fatigue)
      (2) If edema or hypertension is present, sodium intake should be restricted.
      (3) Potassium intake must be limited in most patients. Fruits, vegetables, and salt substitutes containing potassium should be limited or avoided.

  2. Management of body chemistry alterations
    a. Treatment of hyperkalemia
      (1) Dialysis may be used to treat acute, life-threatening hyperkalemia (see II F 7).
      (2) Calcium chloride or calcium gluconate
        (a) Mechanism of action and therapeutic effects. Calcium chloride or calcium gluconate replaces and maintains body calcium, counteracting the cardiac effects of acute hyperkalemia.

    (b) Administration and dosage. When used to reverse hyperkalemia-induced cardiotoxicity, calcium chloride is given intravenously, as 5–10 mL of a 10% solution (1.4 mEq Ca^{2+}/mL) administered over 2 minutes. Doses of up to 20 mL of a 10% solution are safe when given slowly. Another 10–20 mL of a 10% solution placed in a larger fluid volume and administered slowly may follow the initial dose. Calcium gluconate is administered as 10 mL of a 10% solution (1 g) over 2–5 minutes. This may be repeated a second time.

    (c) Precautions and monitoring effects

        (i) Intravenous (IV) calcium is contraindicated in patients with ventricular fibrillation or renal calculi.

        (ii) The infusion rate should not exceed 0.5 mL/min. Patients should remain recumbent for about 15 minutes after infusion.

        (iii) The ECG should be monitored during calcium gluconate therapy.

        (iv) Calcium gluconate should not be mixed with solutions containing sodium bicarbonate because this can lead to precipitation.

        (v) Adverse effects include hypotension, tingling sensations, and renal calculus formation.

    (d) Significant interactions. Calcium may cause increased digitalis toxicity when administered concurrently with digitalis preparations.

(3) Sodium bicarbonate may be given as an emergency measure for severe hyperkalemia or metabolic acidosis.

    (a) Mechanism of action and therapeutic effect. IV sodium bicarbonate restores bicarbonate that the renal tubules cannot reabsorb from the glomerular filtrate and increases arterial pH. This results in a shift of potassium into cells and reduces serum potassium concentration.

    (b) Onset of action is 15–30 minutes.

    (c) Administration and dosage

        (i) Sodium bicarbonate is administered intravenously.

        (ii) The dosage is calculated as follows:
[50% of body weight (kg)] $\times$ [desired arterial bicarbonate (HCO^{-3}) − actual HCO^{-3}]
One ampule (50 mEq) may be given intravenously over 5 minutes.

    (d) Precautions and monitoring effects

        (i) To avoid sodium and fluid overload, sodium bicarbonate must be given cautiously. Half of the patient's bicarbonate deficit is replaced over the first 12 hours of therapy.

        (ii) Sodium bicarbonate may precipitate calcium salts in IV solutions and should not be mixed in the same infusion fluid.

        (iii) Arterial blood gas values and serum electrolyte levels should be monitored closely during sodium bicarbonate therapy.

(4) Regular insulin with dextrose

    (a) Mechanism of action and therapeutic effect. The insulin causes an intracellular shift of potassium. The combination of insulin with dextrose deposits potassium with glycogen in the liver, reducing the serum potassium.

    (b) Onset of action is 15–30 minutes.

    (c) Administration and dosage. Regular insulin (10 units in 500 mL of 10% dextrose) is administered intravenously over 60 minutes.

    (d) Precautions and monitoring effects

        (i) The serum glucose level should be monitored during therapy.

        (ii) The patient should be assessed for signs and symptoms of fluid overload.

(5) Sodium polystyrene sulfonate (SPS)

    (a) Mechanism of action. SPS is a potassium-removing resin that exchanges sodium ions for potassium ions in the intestine (1 g of SPS exchanges 0.5–1 mEq/L of potassium). The SPS is distributed throughout the intestines and excreted in the feces.

    (b) Therapeutic effect. Administered as an adjunctive treatment for hyperkalemia, SPS reduces potassium levels in the serum and other body fluids.

    (c) Onset of action of orally administered SPS is 2 hours; effects are seen in 1 hour when SPS is administered as a retention enema.

    (d) Administration and dosage

        (i) SPS is usually administered orally, although it may be given through a nasogastric tube. The oral dose is 15–30 g in a suspension of 70% sorbitol, administered every 4–6 hours until the desired therapeutic effect is achieved.

   (ii) When oral or nasogastric administration is not possible due to nausea, vomiting, or paralytic ileus, SPS may be given by retention enema. The rectal dose is 30–50 g in 100 mL of sorbitol as a warm emulsion, administered deep into the sigmoid colon every 6 hours. Administration may be done with a rubber tube that is taped in place or via a Foley catheter with a balloon inflated distal to the anal sphincter.

  (e) Precautions and monitoring effects

    (i) The patient's serum electrolyte levels should be monitored closely during SPS therapy. Sodium, chloride, bicarbonate, and pH should be monitored in addition to potassium.

    (ii) SPS therapy usually continues until the serum potassium level drops to between 4 and 5 mEq/L.

    (iii) The patient should be assessed regularly for signs of potassium depletion, including irritability, confusion, cardiac arrhythmias, ECG changes, and muscle weakness.

    (iv) SPS exchanges sodium for potassium, so sodium overload may occur during therapy. Patients with hypertension or CHF should be closely monitored.

    (v) For oral administration, SPS should be mixed only with water or sorbitol. Orange juice, which has a high potassium content, should not be used because it decreases the effectiveness of the SPS. For rectal administration, SPS should be mixed only with water and sorbitol, never with mineral oil.

    (vi) Adverse effects of SPS include constipation, fecal impaction with rectal administration, nausea, vomiting, and diarrhea.

    (vii) SPS should not be used as the sole agent in the treatment of severe hyperkalemia; other agents or therapies should be used in conjunction with this agent.

  (f) Significant interactions. Magnesium hydroxide and other nonabsorbable cation-donating laxatives and antacids may decrease the effectiveness of potassium exchange by SPS and may cause systemic alkalosis.

b. Treatment of metabolic acidosis. Sodium bicarbonate may be given if the arterial pH is below 7.35 [see I F 2 a (3)].

c. Treatment of hyperphosphatemia

  (1) IV calcium is first-line therapy for severe life-threatening hyperphosphatemia. Calcium reduces the serum phosphorus concentration by chelation.

  (2) Oral calcium salts bind dietary phosphorus in the GI tract.

  (3) Sevelamer is a non-ionic polymer that binds dietary phosphorus in the GI tract.

  (4) Dialysis may be used to treat acute, life-threatening hyperphosphatemia accompanied by acute hypocalcemia (see II F 7). It is also performed when volume overload is present.

  (5) Aluminum hydroxide (an aluminum-containing antacid)

    (a) Mechanism of action and therapeutic effect. Aluminum binds excess phosphate in the intestine, thereby reducing phosphate concentration.

    (b) Onset of action is 6–12 hours.

    (c) Administration and dosage. Aluminum hydroxide is administered orally as a tablet or suspension. For the treatment of hyperphosphatemia, 0.5–2 or 15–30 mL of suspension is administered three or four times daily with meals.

    (d) Precautions and monitoring effects

      (i) Aluminum hydroxide may cause constipation and anorexia.

      (ii) Serum phosphate levels should be monitored because aluminum hydroxide can cause phosphate depletion.

      (iii) Aluminum hydroxide can cause calcium resorption and bone demineralization.

d. Treatment of hypocalcemia. Immediate treatment is necessary if the patient has severe hypocalcemia, as evidenced by tetany.

  (1) Calcium gluconate [see I F 2 a (2)]

    (a) Mechanism of action and therapeutic effect. This drug replaces and maintains body calcium, raising the serum calcium level immediately.

      (b) Administration and dosage. When used to reverse hypocalcemia, calcium gluconate is administered intravenously in a dosage of 1–2 g over a period of 10 minutes, followed by a slow infusion (over 6–8 hours) of an additional 1 g.

      (c) Precautions, monitoring effects, and significant interactions [see I F 2 a (2) (c), (d)]

    (2) Oral calcium salts. Calcium carbonate, chloride, gluconate, or lactate may be given by mouth when oral intake is permitted or if the patient has relatively mild hypocalcemia. The usual adult dosage is 4–6 g/day given in three or four divided doses.

  e. Treatment of hyponatremia

    (1) Moderate or asymptomatic hyponatremia may require only **fluid restriction.**

    (2) Sodium chloride may be given for severe symptomatic hyponatremia (i.e., a serum sodium level below 120 mEq/L).

      (a) Mechanism of action and therapeutic effect. Sodium chloride replaces and maintains sodium and chloride concentration, thereby increasing extracellular tonicity.

      (b) Administration and dosage

        (i) A 3% or 5% sodium chloride solution may be administered by slow IV infusion. The amount of solution needed is calculated from the following equation:

(Normal serum sodium level − actual serum sodium level) × total body water

        (ii) Typically, 400 mL or less is administered.

      (c) Precautions and monitoring effects

        (i) Hypertonic sodium chloride must be administered very slowly to avoid circulatory overload, pulmonary edema, or central pontine demyelination.

        (ii) Serum electrolyte levels must be monitored frequently during therapy.

        (iii) Excessive infusion may cause hypernatremia and other serious electrolyte abnormalities and may worsen existing acidosis. Infusion rates should not exceed 0.5 mEq/kg/hr.

3. Management of systemic manifestations

  a. Treatment of fluid overload and edema. As water and sodium accumulate in extracellular fluid during ARF, fluid overload and edema may occur. **Diuretics** and dopamine may be given to reduce fluid volume excess and edema. Treatment should be initiated as soon as possible after oliguria begins. **Mannitol** or a **loop diuretic** may be used; thiazide diuretics are avoided in renal failure because they are ineffective when creatinine clearance is less than 25 mL/min, and they may worsen the patient's clinical status.

    (1) Step 1. Loop (high-ceiling) diuretics. These agents include **furosemide, bumetanide, torsemide** and **ethacrynic acid.** Loop diuretics are more potent and faster-acting than thiazide diuretics.

      (a) Mechanism of action and therapeutic effects. Loop diuretics inhibit sodium and chloride reabsorption at the loop of Henle, promoting water excretion.

      (b) Onset of action for an oral dose is 1 hour; several minutes for an IV dose. Duration of action for an oral dose is 6–8 hours; 2–3 hours for an IV dose.

      (c) Administration and dosage

        (i) Furosemide, the **most commonly used** loop diuretic, usually is administered intravenously in patients with ARF to hasten the therapeutic effect. The dose is titrated to the patient's needs; the usual initial dose is 1–1.5 mg/kg. If the first dose does not produce a urine output of 10–15 mL within 20–30 minutes, a dose of 2–3 mg/kg is administered; if the desired response still does not occur, a dose of 3–6 mg/kg is administered 20–30 minutes after the second dose.

        (ii) Bumetanide may be given to patients who are unresponsive or allergic to furosemide. The usual dosage, administered intravenously or intramuscularly in the treatment of ARF, is 0.5–1 mg/day; however, some patients may require up to 20 mg/day. A second or third dose may be given at intervals of 2–3 hours. When bumetanide is given orally, the dosage is 0.5–2 mg/day, repeated up to two times, if necessary, at intervals of 2–3 hours.

        (iii) Ethacrynic acid is **less commonly used** to treat ARF because ototoxicity (sometimes irreversible) is associated with its use. It may be given intravenously (slowly over several minutes) in a dose of 50–100 mg. The usual oral dosage is 50–200 mg/day; some patients may require up to 200 mg twice daily. Ethacrynic acid can be safely given to patients who may have a sulfonamide allergy, which would preclude them from therapy with furosemide or torsemide.

(iv) Torsemide may also be given to patients unresponsive to or allergic to furosemide. The usual dose is 20 mg, administered intravenously. Doses may be increased by doubling up to 200 mg; 10–20 mg of torsemide is equipotent to 40 mg of furosemide or 1 mg bumetanide. Torsemide offers better bioavailability compared to other loop diuretics; however, it is considerably more expensive.

(d) Precautions and monitoring effects

(i) Loop diuretics must be used cautiously because they may cause overdiuresis leading to orthostatic hypotension, fluid and electrolyte abnormalities, including volume depletion and dehydration, hypocalcemia, hypokalemia, hypochloremia, hyponatremia, hypomagnesemia, and transient ototoxicity, especially with rapid IV injection.

(ii) Serum electrolyte levels should be monitored frequently and the patient assessed regularly for signs and symptoms of electrolyte abnormalities.

(iii) Blood pressure and pulse rate should be assessed during diuretic therapy.

(iv) GI reactions include abdominal pain and discomfort, diarrhea (with furosemide and ethacrynic acid), and nausea (with bumetanide).

(v) Blood glucose levels should be monitored in diabetic patients receiving loop diuretics because these agents may cause hyperglycemia and impaired glucose tolerance.

(vi) Patients who are allergic to sulfonamides may be hypersensitive to bumetanide and furosemide.

(vii) Furosemide and ethacrynic acid may cause agranulocytosis.

(e) Significant interactions

(i) Aminoglycoside antibiotics may potentiate ototoxicity when administered with any loop diuretic.

(ii) Nonsteroidal anti-inflammatory drugs (NSAIDs) may hamper the diuretic response to furosemide and bumetanide; **probenecid** may hamper the diuretic response to bumetanide.

(iii) Ethacrynic acid may potentiate the anticoagulant effects of **warfarin.**

(2) Step 2. Mannitol, an osmotic diuretic, is a non-reabsorbable polysaccharide.

(a) Mechanism of action and therapeutic effect. Mannitol increases the osmotic pressure of the glomerular filtrate; fluid from interstitial spaces is drawn into blood vessels, expanding plasma volume and maintaining or increasing the urine flow. This drug may be given to prevent ARF in high-risk patients, such as those undergoing surgery or suffering from severe trauma or hemolytic transfusion reactions.

(b) Onset of action is 15–30 minutes. Duration of action is 3–4 hours.

(c) Administration and dosage. Mannitol is available in solutions, ranging from 5%–25%. For the treatment of oliguric ARF or the prevention of ARF, the usual initial dose is 12.5–25 g, administered intravenously; the maximum daily dosage is 100 g, administered intravenously. The exact concentration of the solution is determined by the patient's fluid requirements.

(d) Precautions and monitoring effects

(i) Mannitol is contraindicated in patients with anuria, pulmonary edema or congestion, severe dehydration, and intracranial hemorrhage (except during craniotomy).

(ii) Mannitol may cause or worsen pulmonary edema and circulatory overload. If signs and symptoms of these problems develop, the infusion should be stopped.

(iii) Other adverse effects of mannitol include fluid and electrolyte abnormalities, water intoxication, headache, confusion, blurred vision, thirst, nausea, and vomiting.

(iv) Vital signs, urine output, daily weight, cardiopulmonary status, and serum and urine sodium and potassium levels should be monitored during mannitol therapy.

(v) Mannitol solutions with undissolved crystals should not be administered.

4. Dialysis. If the above strategies fail, hemodialysis or peritoneal dialysis may be necessary in ARF patients who develop anuria, acute fluid overload, severe hyperkalemia, metabolic acidosis, or a BUN level above 100 mg/dl. For a discussion of dialysis, see II F 7.

II. CHRONIC KIDNEY DISEASE

A. **Definition.** Chronic kidney disease (CKD) is the progressive, irreversible deterioration of renal function. Usually resulting from long-standing disease, CKD sometimes derives from ARF that does not respond to treatment.

B. **Classification and pathophysiology**

1. CKD is defined as kidney damage or GFR <60 mL/min/1.73 m² for ≥3 months. Kidney damage is defined as pathological abnormalities or markers of damage, including abnormalities in blood or urine tests or imaging studies. CKD has recently been reclassified as stages I–V to denote the severity of renal impairment. Generally, CKD, if left untreated, progresses at a predictable, steady rate from stage I through stage V.
   a. **Stage 1** is defined as kidney damage with a normal or increased GFR. The corresponding GFR in stage I CKD is usually >90 mL/min/1.73 m².
   b. **Stage 2** is defined as kidney damage or a mildly decreased GFR (60–89 mL/min/1.73 m²).
   c. **Stage 3** signifies moderate reductions in GFR (30–59 mL/min/1.73 m²).
   d. **Stage 4** connotes a GFR of 15–29 mL/min/1.73 m².
   e. **Stage 5** is kidney failure or a GFR of <15 mL/min/1.73 m².

2. As CKD progresses, nephron destruction worsens, leading to deterioration in the kidneys' filtration, reabsorption, and endocrine functions.

3. Renal function typically does not diminish until about 75% of kidney tissue is damaged. Ultimately, the kidneys become shrunken, fibrotic masses.

C. **Etiology. Causes of CKD in adults include:**

1. Diabetic nephropathy

2. Hypertension

3. Glomerulonephritis

4. Polycystic kidney disease

5. Long-standing vascular disease (e.g., renal artery stenosis)

6. Long-standing obstructive uropathy (e.g., renal calculi)

7. Exposure to nephrotoxic agents

D. **Clinical evaluation**

1. **Physical findings.** Signs and symptoms, which vary widely, do not appear until renal insufficiency progresses to renal failure.
   a. **Metabolic abnormalities** include loss of the ability to maintain sodium, potassium, and water homeostasis, leading to hyponatremia or hypernatremia, based on relative sodium or water intake. Hyperkalemia is uncommon until end-stage disease. Fluid overload, edema, and CHF may become a problem unless fluid intake is closely managed. As renal failure progresses, the inability to excrete acid and maintain buffer capacity leads to metabolic acidosis (see I D 1 b, d, g, h). Calcium and phosphate metabolism is altered due to hyperparathyroidism.
   b. **Neurological manifestations** include short attention span, loss of memory, and listlessness. As CKD progresses, these advance to confusion, stupor, seizures, and coma. Neuromuscular findings include peripheral neuropathy; pain, itching, and a burning sensation, particularly in the feet and legs. Patients may appear intoxicated. If dialysis is not started after these abnormalities occur, motor involvement begins, including loss of deep-tendon reflexes, weakness, and finally, quadriplegia.
   c. **Cardiovascular problems** include arterial hypertension, peripheral edema, CHF, and pulmonary edema. Uremic pericarditis is now increasingly infrequent as a result of early dialysis.
   d. **GI manifestations** include hiccups, anorexia, nausea, vomiting, constipation, stomatitis, and an unpleasant taste in the mouth. CKD patients have an increased incidence of ulcers, pancreatitis, and diverticulosis.
   e. **Respiratory problems** include dyspnea when CHF is present, pulmonary edema, pleuritic pain, and uremic pleuritis.

    f. Integumentary findings typically include pale yellowish, dry, scaly skin; severe itching; uremic frost; ecchymoses; purpura; and brittle nails and hair.

    g. Musculoskeletal changes range from muscle and bone pain to pathological fractures and calcifications in the brain, heart, eyes, joints, and vessels. Soft-tissue calcification and renal osteodystrophy may occur.

    h. Hematological disturbances include anemia. The signs and symptoms of anemia arise from lack of erythropoietin and reduced life span of red blood cells, including:

        (1) Pallor of the skin, nail beds, palms, conjunctivae, and mucosa

        (2) Abnormal bruising or ecchymoses, and uremic bleeding due to platelet inactivation

        (3) Dyspnea and angina pectoris

        (4) Extreme fatigue

2. Diagnostic test results

    a. Creatinine clearance may range from 0–90 mL/min, reflecting renal impairment.

    b. Blood tests typically show:

        (1) Elevated BUN and serum creatinine concentration

        (2) Reduced arterial pH and bicarbonate concentration

        (3) Reduced serum calcium level

        (4) Increased serum potassium and phosphate levels

        (5) Possible reduction in the serum sodium level

        (6) Normochromic, normocytic anemia (hematocrit 20%–30%)

    c. Urinalysis may reveal glycosuria, proteinuria, erythrocytes, leukocytes, and casts. Specific gravity is fixed at 1.010.

    d. Radiographic findings. Kidney, ureter, and bladder radiography, IV pyelography, renal scan, renal arteriography, and nephrotomography may be performed. Typically, these tests reveal small kidneys (less than 8 cm in length).

E. Treatment objectives

1. Improve patient comfort and prolong life.

2. Treat systemic manifestations of CKD.

3. Correct body chemistry abnormalities.

F. Therapy. Management of the CKD patient is generally conservative. Dietary measures and fluid restriction relieve some symptoms of CKD and may increase patient comfort and prolong life until dialysis or renal transplantation is required or available (see I F 1 a, b).

1. Treatment of edema. Angiotensin-converting enzyme (ACE) inhibitors and **diuretics** may be given to manage edema and CHF and to increase urine output.

    a. ACE inhibitors—captopril, enalapril, lisinopril, fosinopril—are widely used to delay progression of CKD because they help preserve renal function and typically cause fewer adverse effects than other antihypertensive agents (see Chapter 39). They also decrease proteinuria and nephrotic syndrome.

    b. Diuretics. An osmotic diuretic, a loop diuretic, or a thiazide-like diuretic may be given.

        (1) Osmotic and loop diuretics. See I F 3 a (1), (2) for information on the use of these drugs in renal failure.

        (2) Thiazide-like diuretics. Metolazone is the most commonly used thiazide diuretic in CKD.

            (a) Mechanism of action and therapeutic effect. Metolazone reduces the body's fluid and sodium volume by decreasing sodium reabsorption in the distal convoluted tubule, thereby increasing urinary excretion of fluid and sodium.

            (b) Administration and dosage. Metolazone is given orally at 5–20 mg/day; the dose is titrated to the patient's needs. Due to its long half-life, metolazone may be given every other day. Furosemide and metolazone act synergistically. Combination use is common, and metolazone should be administered 30 minutes before furosemide to achieve the optimal diuretic effect.

            (c) Precautions and monitoring effects

                (i) Metolazone should not be given to patients with hypersensitivity to sulfonamide derivatives, including thiazides.

                (ii) To avoid nocturia, the daily dose should be given in the morning.

                (iii) Metolazone may cause hematological reactions, such as agranulocytosis, aplastic anemia, and thrombocytopenia.

(iv) Fluid volume depletion, hypokalemia, hyperuricemia, hyperglycemia, and impaired glucose tolerance may occur during metolazone therapy.

(v) Metolazone may cause hypersensitivity reactions, including vasculitis and pneumonitis.

(d) **Significant interactions**

(i) **Diazoxide** may potentiate the antihypertensive, hyperglycemic, and hyperuricemic effects of metolazone.

(ii) **Colestipol** and **cholestyramine** decrease the absorption of metolazone.

2. **Treatment of hypertension. Antihypertensive agents** may be needed if blood pressure becomes dangerously high as a result of edema and the high renin levels that occur in CKD. Antihypertensive therapy should be initiated in the lowest effective dose and titrated according to the patient's needs.

a. **ACE inhibitors—captopril, enalapril, lisinopril, fosinopril**—as above in II F 1 a (see also Chapter 39).

b. **Dihydropyridine calcium-channel blockers,** including **amLodipine** and **felodipine,** have similar effects and may be used instead of ACE inhibitors.

c. **β-Adrenergic blockers,** including **propranolol** and **atenolol,** reduce blood pressure through various mechanisms (see Chapter 39).

d. **Other antihypertensive agents** are sometimes used in the treatment of CKD, including α-adrenergic drugs, **clonidine,** and vasodilators, such as **hydralazine** (see Chapter 39).

3. **Treatment of hyperphosphatemia** involves administration of a phosphate binder, such as aluminum hydroxide or calcium carbonate (see I F 2 c).

4. **Treatment of hypocalcemia**

a. **Oral calcium salts** [see I F 2 d (2)]

b. **Vitamin D**

(1) **Mechanism of action and therapeutic effect.** Vitamin D promotes intestinal calcium and phosphate absorption and utilization and, thus, increases the serum calcium concentration.

(2) **Choice of agent.** For the treatment of hypocalcemia in CKD and other renal disorders, **calcitriol** (vitamin D_3, the active form of vitamin D) is the preferred vitamin D supplement because of its greater efficacy and relatively short duration of action. Other single-entity preparations include dihydrotachysterol, ergocalciferol, and calcifediol. Newer vitamin D analogues include doxercalciferol and paricalcitol.

(3) **Administration and dosage.** Calcitriol is given orally or via IV; the dose is titrated to the patient's needs (0.5–1 mg/day may be effective).

(4) **Precautions and monitoring effects**

(a) Vitamin D administration may be dangerous in patients with renal failure and must be used with extreme caution.

(b) Vitamin D toxicity may cause a wide range of signs and symptoms, including headache, dizziness, ataxia, convulsions, psychosis, soft-tissue calcification, conjunctivitis, photophobia, tinnitus, nausea, diarrhea, pruritus, and muscle and bone pain.

(c) Vitamin D has a narrow therapeutic index, necessitating frequent measurement of BUN and serum urine calcium and potassium levels.

5. **Treatment of other systemic manifestations of CKD**

a. **Treatment of anemia** includes administration of iron (e.g., ferrous sulfate), folate supplements, and erythropoietin.

(1) Severe anemia may warrant transfusion with packed red blood cells.

(2) Erythropoietin stimulates the production of red cell progenitors and the production of hemoglobin. It also accelerates the release of reticulocytes from the bone marrow.

(a) An initial dose of erythropoietin is 50–100 U/kg intravenously or subcutaneously three times a week. The dose may be adjusted upward to elicit the desired response.

(b) Erythropoietin works best in patients with a hematocrit below 30%. During the initial treatment, the hematocrit increases 1%–3.5% in a 2-week period. The target hematocrit is 33%–35%. Maintenance doses are titrated based on hematocrit after this level is reached.

(c) Erythropoietin therapy should be temporarily stopped if hematocrit exceeds 36%. Additional side effects include hypertension in up to 25% of patients. Headache and malaise have been reported.

(d) The effects of erythropoietin are dependent on a ready supply of iron for hemoglobin synthesis. Patients who do not respond should have iron stores checked. This includes serum iron, total iron-binding capacity, transferrin saturation, and serum ferritin. Iron supplementation should be increased as indicated.

(3) Darbepoeitin is a new erythropoietin analogue. Its advantage is a prolonged plasma half-life, thus allowing it to be administered once weekly or biweekly.

(4) Intravenous iron products may be given to replete iron stores. This route is preferred to oral supplementation due to low oral bioavailability and GI intolerance. Iron dextran is commonly used; however, it is associated with hypotension and anaphylaxis. Newer iron products include sodium ferric gluconate and iron sucrose, which are better tolerated and can be infused more rapidly compared to iron dextran. Patients with severe iron deficiency may receive up to a total of 1 g of an iron preparation over several days. The rate of infusion depends on the preparation used.

b. Treatment of GI disturbances
(1) Antiemetics help control nausea and vomiting.
(2) Docusate sodium or methylcellulose may be used to prevent constipation.
(3) Enemas may be given to remove blood from the GI tract.
c. Treatment of skin problems. An antipruritic agent, such as diphenhydramine, may be used to alleviate itching.

6. Management of body chemistry abnormalities (see I F 2)

7. Dialysis. When CKD progresses to end-stage renal disease and no longer responds to conservative measures, long-term dialysis or renal transplantation is necessary to prolong life.

a. Hemodialysis is the preferred dialysis method for patients with a reduced peritoneal membrane, hypercatabolism, or acute hyperkalemia.
(1) This technique involves shunting of the patient's blood through a dialysis membrane-containing unit for diffusion, osmosis, and ultrafiltration. The blood is then returned to the patient's circulation.
(2) Vascular access may be obtained via an arteriovenous fistula or an external shunt.
(3) The procedure takes only 3–8 hours; most patients need three treatments a week. With proper training, patients can perform hemodialysis at home.
(4) The patient receives heparin during hemodialysis to prevent clotting.
(5) Various complications may arise, including clotting of the hemofilter, hemorrhage, hepatitis, anemia, septicemia, cardiovascular problems, air embolism, rapid shifts in fluid and electrolyte balance, itching, nausea, vomiting, headache, seizures, and aluminum osteodystrophy.

b. Peritoneal dialysis is the preferred dialysis method for patients with bleeding disorders and cardiovascular disease.
(1) The peritoneum is used as a semipermeable membrane. A plastic catheter inserted into the peritoneum provides access for the dialysate, which draws fluids, wastes, and electrolytes across the peritoneal membrane by osmosis and diffusion.
(2) Peritoneal dialysis can be carried out in three different modes.
(a) Intermittent peritoneal dialysis is an automatic cycling mode lasting 8–10 hours, performed three times a week. This mode allows nighttime treatment and is appropriate for working patients.
(b) Continuous ambulatory peritoneal dialysis is performed daily for 24 hours with four exchanges daily. The patient can remain active during the treatment.
(c) Continuous cyclic peritoneal dialysis may be used if the other two modes fail to improve creatinine clearance. Dialysis takes place at night; the last exchange is retained in the peritoneal cavity during the day, then drained that evening.
(3) Advantages of peritoneal dialysis include a lack of serious complications, retention of normal fluid and electrolyte balance, simplicity, reduced cost, patient independence, and a reduced need (or no need) for heparin administration.
(4) Complications of peritoneal dialysis include hyperglycemia, constipation, and inflammation or infection at the catheter site. Also, this method carries a high risk of peritonitis.

8. Renal transplantation. This surgical procedure allows some patients with end-stage renal disease to live normal and, in many cases, longer lives.
a. Histocompatibility must be tested to minimize the risk of transplant rejection and failure. Human leukocyte antigen (HLA) type, mixed lymphocyte reactivity, and blood group types are determined to assess histocompatibility.

b. Renal transplant material may be obtained from a living donor or a cadaver.
c. Three types of graft rejection can occur.
  (1) Hyperacute (immediate) rejection results in graft loss within minutes to hours after transplantation.
    (a) Acute urine flow cessation and bluish or mottled kidney discoloration are intra-operative signs of hyperacute rejection.
    (b) Postoperative manifestations include kidney enlargement, fever, anuria, local pain, sodium retention, and hypertension.
    (c) Treatment for hyperacute rejection is immediate nephrectomy.
  (2) Acute rejection may occur 4–60 days after transplantation.
  (3) Chronic rejection occurs more than 60 days after transplantation.
    (a) Signs and symptoms include low-grade fever, increased proteinuria, azotemia, hypertension, oliguria, weight gain, and edema.
    (b) Treatment may include alkylating agents, cyclosporine, antilymphocyte globulin, and corticosteroids. In some cases, nephrectomy is necessary.
d. Complications include:
  (1) Infection, diabetes, hepatitis, and leukopenia, resulting from immunosuppressive therapy
  (2) Hypertension, resulting from various causes
  (3) Cancer (e.g., lymphoma, cutaneous malignancies, head and neck cancer, leukemia, colon cancer)
  (4) Pancreatitis and mental and emotional disorders (e.g., suicidal tendencies, severe depression, brought on by steroid therapy)

STUDY QUESTIONS

Directions: Each of the numbered items or incomplete statements in this section is followed by answers or by completions of the statement. Select the **one** lettered answer or completion that is **best** in each case.

Questions 1–5

A 48-year-old black man has a history of mild to severe hypertension. His hypertension has been poorly controlled with enalapril and hydrochlorothiazide. On prior visits, his blood pressure control has varied and seems to correspond with a lack of compliance with his treatment regimen. The patient states that he occasionally forgets his pills or does not take them when he is feeling "okay." The patient's history does not include diabetes mellitus or heart disease. He completed a 14-day course of clarithromycin for an upper respiratory infection in the past month and has returned to the clinic for follow-up review of the infection and his hypertension therapy.

On this visit, the patient complains of dizziness, loss of energy, increased frequency of urination, and edema of the lower extremities. His physical examination reveals an overweight man with a standing blood pressure of 175/100 mm Hg moderate edema of the ankles, and a slight third heart sound. Laboratory results include blood urea nitrogen (BUN) of 45 mg/dl, serum creatinine concentration of 3.7 mg/dl, serum calcium of 5.3 mg/mL, serum potassium of 6.3 mg/mL, and a hematocrit of 25. Serum iron, total iron-binding capacity, transferrin saturation, and serum ferritin are normal. Microscopic urine and chemical analyses reveal mild proteinuria and a specific gravity of 1.010.

1. The history, physical examination, laboratory values, and current signs and symptoms suggest that the patient has which of the following conditions?

(A) Acute renal failure brought on by a nephrotoxic drug (clarithromycin, enalapril)
(B) Acute renal failure resulting from renal obstruction by a kidney stone
(C) Acute renal failure precipitated by severe dehydration
(D) Chronic renal failure resulting from hypertension

2. Treatment of the patient's fluid retention and edema should begin with all of the following EXCEPT

(A) restriction of fluid intake
(B) therapy with furosemide or metolazone
(C) treatment of hypertension using a β-blocker or angiotensin-converting enzyme inhibitor
(D) digitalis glycoside therapy if congestive heart failure is present
(E) hemodialysis

3. The most likely cause of the anemia seen in this patient is

(A) urinary blood loss
(B) vitamin B_{12} deficiency
(C) iron deficiency
(D) decreased red cell life span and a deficiency of erythropoietin

4. This patient's symptoms seemed to appear suddenly and may result from his history of uncontrolled hypertension. Which statement best describes hypertension?

(A) A major cause of chronic renal failure
(B) A major cause of acute renal failure
(C) A major cause of both chronic and acute renal failure
(D) Only seen in patients whose renal failure has caused excessive fluid retention

5. When should peritoneal dialysis or hemodialysis be considered to treat this patient's renal failure?

(A) As soon as possible to prevent further complications resulting from decreased renal function
(B) Only when renal function has decreased to a point where fluid and electrolyte status cannot be maintained using conservative measures
(C) On an intermittent basis as the situation demands
(D) Only if the patient is a kidney transplant candidate

6. Acute renal failure (ARF) may be caused by all of the following EXCEPT

(A) acute tubular necrosis (ATN) due to drug therapy (e.g., aminoglycosides, contrast media)
(B) severe hypotension or circulatory collapse
(C) decreased cardiac output, as from congestive heart failure
(D) hemolysis and myoglobinuria
(E) hyperkalemia

7. Life-threatening cardiac arrhythmias due to hyperkalemia should be treated with

(A) calcium chloride or calcium gluconate intravenously
(B) digoxin or other digitalis preparations
(C) loop diuretics to rapidly eliminate potassium
(D) sodium polystyrene sulfonate (SPS)

8. Aluminum hydroxide is used to treat hyperphosphatemia associated with renal failure. Chronic use of aluminum hydroxide may cause all of the following conditions EXCEPT

(A) phosphate depletion
(B) calcium resorption and bone demineralization
(C) anorexia and constipation
(D) fluid retention

9. The diuretic of choice for the initial treatment of a patient with either acute or chronic renal failure (ARF, CKD) whose creatinine clearance is below 25 mL/min is

(A) hydrochlorothiazide
(B) bumetanide
(C) furosemide
(D) ethacrynic acid

10. Erythropoietin is used commonly to treat the anemia associated with chronic renal failure (CKD). Which of the following conditions limits the effectiveness of erythropoietin?

(A) A patient's allergy to erythropoietin
(B) Depletion of iron stores, requiring oral or parenteral supplementation
(C) The ineffectiveness of erythropoietin, as 30% of patients do not respond
(D) The anemia of chronic renal failure is not due to a lack of erythropoietin, so erythropoietin will not ameliorate.

ANSWERS AND EXPLANATIONS

1. The answer is D *[II D 1]*.
The fluid and electrolyte status of the patient described in the case, combined with the urine-specific gravity, lack of crystals or casts in the urine, and the complaint of fatigue, suggest chronic renal failure resulting from uncontrolled hypertension or an unknown cause. The antibiotic therapy (clarithromycin) and antihypertensive drug (enalapril) are not nephrotoxic, and the patient's blood pressure and fluid status do not indicate a prerenal cause.

2. The answer is E *[II F 1, 2]*.
All of these measures are indicated as initial therapy for the treatment of edema and fluid retention due to chronic renal failure except hemodialysis, which should be reserved until more conservative measures are tried.

3. The answer is D *[II D 1 h]*.
There is no evidence of frank blood loss. The decreased hematocrit and the clinical signs indicate the anemia of chronic renal failure due to the shortened red blood cell life span. Decreased erythropoietin is the cause.

4. The answer is A *[II C 2]*.
Systemic long-standing high blood pressure is the second most common cause of chronic renal failure (CKD). Only malignant hypertension can cause acute renal failure (ARF), which is not common. High blood pressure is common after substantial renal damage has occurred in both CKD and ARF, but it does not occur as the first or only manifestation.

5. The answer is B *[II F 7]*.
Dialysis should be considered when the patient's renal function has decreased to a point where conservative measures are ineffective. Peritoneal dialysis and hemodialysis have associated complications and morbidity, so intermittent or early use of these therapies is not indicated. Patients can be maintained on dialysis for extended periods, so eligibility for transplant is not required.

6. The answer is E *[I B 1–3]*.
Hyperkalemia is a sign of acute and chronic renal failure, resulting from the decreased renal function and changes in acid–base balance.

7. The answer is A *[I F 2 a]*.
Intravenous calcium chloride or gluconate is used to treat potassium-induced arrhythmias. Digoxin is not indicated. Loop diuretics and sodium polystyrene sulfonate (SPS) do not have a significant enough effect on potassium in a short period to treat a life-threatening arrhythmia. SPS and loop diuretics, along with dialysis, may be considered to remove potassium in the short term, preventing the recurrence of arrhythmias.

8. The answer is D *[I F 2 c (5) (d) (i–iii)]*.
Common effects of the sustained use of aluminum-containing antacids include phosphate depletion, calcium resorption, bone demineralization, anorexia, and constipation. Fluid retention does not result from the use of antacids containing aluminum hydroxide.

9. The answer is C *[I F 3 a (1) (c)]*.
Furosemide is the diuretic of choice for the initial treatment of a patient with either acute or chronic renal failure (ARF, CKD) whose creatinine clearance is below 25 mL/min. A thiazide diuretic has little effect at a creatinine clearance below 25 mL/min. Bumetanide, torsemide, and ethacrynic acid are appropriate only if the patient is allergic to furosemide or if repeated doses of furosemide are ineffective.

10. The answer is B *[II F 5 a (2) (d)]*.
Erythropoietin is widely used and highly effective in treating the anemia associated with chronic renal failure (CKD). Few reports of patients refractory to erythropoietin therapy have appeared in medical literature. However, the depletion of iron stores will not allow the formation of red blood cells, even in the presence of appropriate amounts of erythropoietin. All CKD patients receiving erythropoietin require some iron supplementation, and most patients require parenteral iron to achieve sufficient supplies to continue developing hemoglobin over the term of their illness.

Cancer Chemotherapy

Janet Espirito
Judy Chase

I. PRINCIPLES OF ONCOLOGY. The term cancer refers to a heterogeneous group of diseases.

A. Characteristics of cancer cells. Cancer cells are also referred to as tumors, or neoplasms. Tumors arise from a single abnormal cell, which continues to divide indefinitely. Uncontrolled growth, ability to invade local tissues, and ability to spread, or **metastasize**, are characteristics of cancer cells.

1. **Carcinogenesis.** The mechanism of how cancers occur is thought to be a multistage, multifactorial process that involves both genetic and environmental factors.
    a. **Initiation.** The first step involves the exposure of normal cells to a carcinogen, producing genetic damage to a cell.
    b. **Promotion.** The environment becomes altered to allow preferential growth of mutated cells over normal cells. The mutated cells become cancerous.
    c. **Progression.** Increased proliferation of cancer cells allows for invasion into local tissue and metastasis.

2. **Types of cancer.** Tumors can be benign or malignant. **Benign** tumors are generally slow growing, resemble normal cells, are localized, and are not harmful. **Malignant** tumors often proliferate more rapidly, have an atypical appearance, invade and destroy surrounding tissues, and are harmful if left untreated. Malignant cancers are further categorized by the location from where the tumor cells arise.
    a. Solid tumors. **Carcinomas** are tumors of epithelial cells. These include specific tissue cancers (e.g., lung, colon, breast). **Sarcomas** include tumors of connective tissue such as bone (e.g., osteosarcoma) or muscle (e.g., leiomyosarcoma).
    b. Hematological malignancies. **Lymphomas** are tumors of the lymphatic system and include Hodgkin's and non-Hodgkin's lymphomas. **Leukemias** are tumors of blood-forming elements and are classified as acute or chronic, myeloid or lymphoid.

B. Incidence. Cancer is the **second leading cause of death** in the United States. The lifetime probability of developing cancer is greater than 30%. The estimated incidences of new cancers and cancer-related deaths by site are illustrated in Figure 55-1. The most common cancers are breast, prostate, lung, and colorectal. The leading cause of cancer death is due to lung cancer.

C. Etiology. Many factors have been implicated in the etiology of cancer. These factors are listed below.

1. **Viruses,** including Epstein-Barr virus (EBV), hepatitis B virus (HBV), and human papillomavirus (HPV)

2. **Environmental and occupational exposures,** such as ionizing and ultraviolet radiation and exposure to chemicals, including vinyl chloride, benzene, and asbestos

3. **Life-style factors,** such as high-fat, low-fiber diets and tobacco and ethanol use

4. **Medications,** including alkylating agents and immunosuppressants

5. **Genetic factors,** including inherited mutations, cancer-causing genes (oncogenes), and defective tumor-suppressor genes

D. Detection and **diagnosis** are critical for the appropriate treatment of cancer. Earlier detection may improve response to treatment.

1. **Warning signs** of cancer have been outlined by the American Cancer Society.
    a. **C**hange in bowel or bladder habits
    b. **A** sore that does not heal

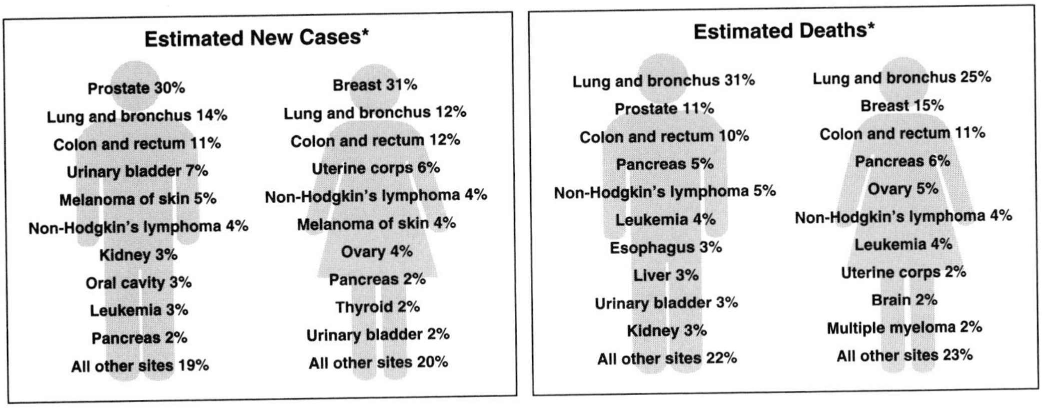

Figure 55-1. Cancer incidence and deaths. Leading cancer sites for estimated new cases and deaths by gender in the United States, 2002 estimates. *Excludes basal and squamous cell skin cancers and in situ carcinomas except urinary bladder. [Adapted from Jemal A, Thomas A, Murray T, et al. Cancer Statistics, 2002. *CA Cancer J Clin* 2002;52:23–47.]

    c. Unusual bleeding or discharge

    d. Thickening or lump in the breast or elsewhere

    e. Indigestion or difficulty swallowing

    f. Obvious change in a wart or mole

    g. Nagging cough or hoarseness

  2. Guidelines for screening asymptomatic people for the presence of cancer have been established by the American Cancer Society, the National Cancer Institute, and the United States Preventive Health Services Task Force. Since many cancers do not produce signs or symptoms until they have become large, the goal of screening is to detect cancers early, when the disease is curable, and reduce mortality. The different guidelines have slightly varied recommendations for age and frequency of screening procedures. Table 55-1 lists the American Cancer Society recommendations for screening.

  3. Tumor markers are biochemical indicators of the presence of neoplastic proliferation detected in serum, plasma, or other body fluids. These tumor markers may be used initially as screening tests, to reveal further information after abnormal test results, or to monitor the efficacy of therapy. Elevated levels of these markers are not definitive for the presence of cancer, as levels can be elevated in other benign and malignant conditions, and false-positive results do occur. Examples of some commonly used markers include:

    a. Carcinoembryonic antigen (CEA) for colorectal cancer

    b. Alpha-fetoprotein (AFP) for hepatocellular carcinoma

    c. Prostate-specific antigen (PSA) for prostate cancer

  4. Tumor biopsy. The definitive test for the presence of cancerous cells is a biopsy and pathological examination of the biopsy specimen. Several types of procedures are used in the pathological analysis of tumors, including evaluating the morphological features (appearance) of the tissue and cells, looking for cell-surface markers, and cytogenetic evaluation for specific chromosomal abnormalities.

  5. Imaging studies, such as x-rays, computed tomography (CT) scans, magnetic resonance imaging (MRI), or positron emission tomography (PET), may be used to aid in the diagnosis or location of a tumor and to monitor response to treatment.

  6. Other laboratory tests commonly used for cancer diagnosis include complete blood counts (CBCs) and blood chemistries.

E. Staging is the categorizing of patients according to the extent of their disease. The stage of the disease is used to determine prognosis and treatment. Two different staging systems are widely employed for the staging of neoplasms.

Table 55-1. Recommendations for Cancer Screening

Cancer Site	Population	Starting Age	Tests or Procedures
Breast	Women	20+ 20+ 40+	Breast self-examination Clinical breast examination Mammography
Colorectal	Men and Women	50+ 50+ 50+ 50+	Fecal occult blood test (FOBT) Flexible sigmoidoscopy Colonoscopy Double contrast barium enema
Prostate	Men	50+ 50+	Digital rectal examination (DRE) Prostate-specific antigen (PSA)
Cervix	Women	18+ 18+	Pap (Papanicolaou) test Pelvic examination

American Cancer Society recommendations for the early detection of cancer in average-risk, asymptomatic people. [Adapted from Smith RA, Cokkinides V, von Eschenbach AC, et al. American Cancer Society guidelines for the early detection of cancer. *CA Cancer J Clin* 2002;52:8–22.]

    1. TNM classification

        a. T indicates tumor size and is classified from 0–4, with 0 indicating the absence of tumor.

        b. N indicates the presence and extent of regional lymph node spread and is classified from 0–3, with 0 indicating no regional lymph node involvement and 3 indicating extensive involvement.

        c. M indicates the presence or absence of distant metastases and can be classified as only 0 for absence or 1 for presence of distant metastases.

        d. For example, T2N1M0 indicates a moderate-sized tumor with limited nodal disease and no distant metastases.

    2. AJCC staging, developed by the American Joint Committee on Cancer, denotes cancers as stages 0–IV. An assigned TNM translates into a stage. A high number indicates larger tumors with extensive nodal involvement and/or metastasis. Generally, high numbers also indicate a worse prognosis. There are specific staging criteria for each tumor type.

  F. Survival depends on the tumor type, the extent of disease, and the therapy received. Although some patients are free of all detectable disease, not all patients are cured. Oncologists prefer to use the term **complete response** or **remission** to indicate a patient with no evidence of disease after treatment. This is not a synonym for cure. For some slow-growing tumors, these disease-free periods may extend for 10–15 years after the initial remission. However, a number of patients who have achieved complete remission may relapse.

II. CELL LIFE CYCLE. Knowledge of the cell life cycle and cell cycle kinetics is essential to the understanding of the activity of chemotherapy agents in the treatment of cancer (Figure 55-2).

  A. Phases of the cell cycle

    1. M phase, or **mitosis,** is the phase in which the cell divides into two daughter cells.

    2. G$_1$ phase, or **postmitotic gap,** is where RNA and the proteins required for the specialized functions of the cell are synthesized.

    3. S phase (follows G$_1$) is the phase in which DNA synthesis and replication occurs.

    4. G$_2$ phase, or the **premitotic** or **postsynthetic gap,** is the phase in which RNA and the enzymes topoisomerase I and II are produced to prepare for duplication of the cell.

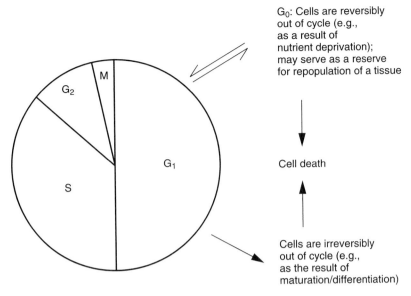

G$_0$: Cells are reversibly
out of cycle (e.g.,
as a result of
nutrient deprivation);
may serve as a reserve
for repopulation of a tissue

Cell death

Cells are irreversibly
out of cycle (e.g.,
as the result of
maturation/differentiation)

Figure 55-2. The cell cycle. Diagrammatic representation of the cell growth cycle, emphasizing the relationship between proliferating cell populations. [Reprinted with permission from Lenhard MJ Jr. et al. (eds.). *The American Cancer Society's Clinical Oncology*. Atlanta: American Cancer Society, 2001.]

   5. **G$_0$ phase,** or **resting phase,** is the phase in which the cell is not committed to division. Cells in this phase are generally not very sensitive to chemotherapy. Some of these cells may reenter the actively dividing cell cycle. In a process called **recruitment,** some chemotherapy regimens are designed to enhance this reentry by killing a large number of actively dividing cells.

 B. **Cell growth kinetics.** Several terms describe cell growth kinetics.

   1. **Cell growth fraction** is the proportion of cells in the tumor dividing or preparing to divide. As the tumor enlarges, the cell growth fraction decreases because a larger proportion of cells may not be able to obtain adequate nutrients and blood supply for replication.

   2. **Cell cycle time** is the average time for a cell that has just completed mitosis to grow and again divide and again pass through mitosis. Cell cycle time is specific for each individual tumor.

   3. **Tumor doubling time** is the time for the tumor to double in size. As the tumor gets larger, its doubling time gets longer because it contains a smaller proportion of actively dividing cells due to restrictions of space, nutrient availability, and blood supply.

   4. The **gompertzian growth curve** illustrates these cell growth concepts (Figure 55-3).

 C. **Tumor cell burden** is the number of tumor cells in the body. Because of the large number of cells required to produce symptoms and be clinically detectable (approximately 10^9 cells), the tumor may be in the plateau phase of the growth curve by the time it is detected. The **cell kill hypothesis** states that a certain percentage of tumor cells will be killed with each course of cancer chemotherapy. As tumor cells are killed, cells in G$_0$ may be recruited into G$_1$, resulting in tumor regrowth. Thus, repeated cycles of chemotherapy are required to achieve a complete response or remission (Figure 55-4). The percentage of cells killed is dependent on the chemotherapy dose. In theory, the tumor burden would never reach absolute zero since only a percentage of cells are killed with each cycle. Less than 10^4 cells may depend on elimination by the host's immune system.

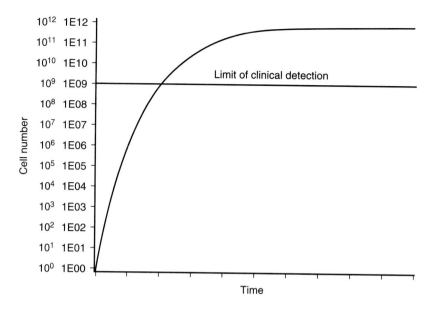

Figure 55-3. The gompertzian growth curve. During the early stages of its development, a tumor's growth is exponential. But as a tumor enlarges, the growth slows. By the time a tumor becomes large enough to cause symptoms and be clinically detectable, the majority of its growth has already occurred and is no longer exponential. [Reprinted with permission from Lenhard MJ Jr. et al. eds. *The American Cancer Society's Clinical Oncology.* Atlanta: American Cancer Society, 2001.]

D. Chemotherapeutic agents may be classified according to their **reliance on cell cycle kinetics** for their cytotoxic effect. Combinations of chemotherapy agents that are active in different phases of the cell cycle may result in a greater cell kill. A cell cycle classification of some commonly used chemotherapeutic agents is listed below.

1. **Phase-specific agents** are most active against cells that are in a specific phase of the cell cycle. These agents are most effective against tumors with a high growth fraction. Theoretically, by administering these agents as continuous intravenous infusions or by multiple repeated doses, it may increase the likelihood of hitting the majority of cells in the specific phase at any one time. Therefore, these agents are also considered schedule-dependent agents. Examples:
   a. M phase: mitotic inhibitors (e.g., vinca alkaloids, taxanes)
   b. G_1 phase: asparaginase, prednisone
   c. S phase: antimetabolites
   d. G_2 phase: bleomycin, etoposide

2. **Phase-nonspecific agents** are effective while cells are in the active cycle but do not require that the cell be in a particular phase. These agents generally show more activity against slow-growing tumors. They may be administered as single bolus doses, since their activity is independent of the cell cycle. These drugs are also considered dose-dependent agents. Examples include alkylating agents and antitumor antibiotics.

3. **Cell cycle–nonspecific agents** are effective in all phases, including G_0. Examples include carmustine, lomustine, and radiation.

III. CHEMOTHERAPY

A. Objectives of chemotherapy

1. A **cure** may be sought with aggressive therapy for a prolonged period of time to eradicate all disease. For leukemias, this curative approach may consist of remission induction, at-

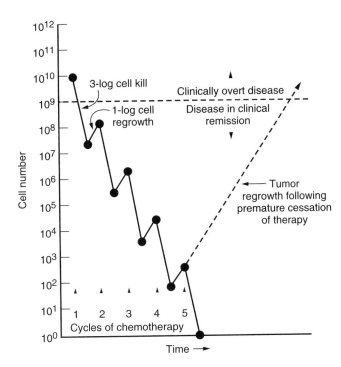

Figure 55-4. Chemotherapy and tumor cell survival. Relationship between tumor cell survival and chemotherapy administration. The exponential relationship between chemotherapy drug dose and tumor cell survival dictates that a constant proportion, not number, of tumor cells is killed with each cycle of treatment. In this example, each cycle of drug administration results in 99.9% (3 log) cell kill, and 1 log of cell regrowth occurs between cycles. The broken line indicates what would occur if the last cycle of therapy was omitted. Despite complete clinical remission of disease, the tumor would ultimately recur. [Reprinted with permission from Lenhard MJ Jr. et al. eds. *The American Cancer Society's Clinical Oncology.* Atlanta: American Cancer Society, 2001.]

tempting the maximal cell kill, followed by consolidation therapy to eradicate all clinically undetectable disease and to lower the tumor cell burden below 10^3, where host immunological defenses may keep the cells in control.

2. If the goal is **palliation,** chemotherapy may be given to decrease tumor size, control growth, and reduce symptoms. Palliative therapy is usually given when complete eradication of the tumor is considered unlikely or the patient refuses aggressive therapy.

3. **Adjuvant** chemotherapy is given after more definitive therapy, such as surgery, to eliminate any remaining disease or undetected micrometastasis.

4. **Neoadjuvant** chemotherapy is given to decrease the tumor burden before definitive therapy, such as surgery or radiation.

5. **Salvage** chemotherapy is given as an attempt to get a patient into remission, after previous therapies have failed.

B. **Chemotherapy dosing** may be based on **body weight,** body surface area (**BSA**), or area under the concentration versus time curve (**AUC**). BSA is most frequently used because it provides an accurate comparison of activity and toxicity across species. In addition, BSA correlates with cardiac output, which determines renal and hepatic blood flow and, thus, affects drug elimination.

C. **Dosing adjustments** may be required for kidney or liver dysfunction in order to prevent toxicity.

D. Combination chemotherapy is usually more effective than single-agent therapy.

1. When combining chemotherapy agents, factors to consider include:
   a. Antitumor activity
   b. Different mechanisms of action
   c. Minimally overlapping toxicities

2. The reasons for administering combination chemotherapy include:
   a. Overcoming or preventing resistance
   b. Cytotoxicity to resting and dividing cells
   c. Biochemical enhancement of effect
   d. Rescue of normal cells

3. **Dosing** and **scheduling** of combination regimens are important, as they are designed to allow recovery of normal cells. These regimens generally are given as short courses of therapy in cycles.

4. **Acronyms** often are used to designate chemotherapy regimens. For example, CMF refers to a combination of cyclophosphamide, methotrexate, and fluorouracil used in the treatment of breast cancer.

E. Administration

1. **Routes** of administration vary, although intravenous (IV) administration is employed most commonly.

2. Other administration techniques include oral, subcutaneous, intrathecal, intra-arterial, intraperitoneal, intravesical, continuous IV infusion, bolus IV infusion, and hepatic artery infusion.

3. Drugs that may be given **intrathecally** are methotrexate and cytarabine. Drugs should not be administered by the intrathecal route without specific information supporting intrathecal administration. Deaths have occurred when vincristine and other drugs have been administered by the intrathecal route. Caution should be used in the preparation and delivery of drugs to be used in this manner.

4. Products with different formulations, including liposomal or pegylated agents (e.g., liposomal doxorubicin, pegfilgrastim), are being used to decrease frequency of administration and/or reduce toxicities.

F. Response to chemotherapy is defined in a number of ways and does not always correlate with patient survival.

1. **Complete response (CR)** indicates disappearance of all clinical, gross, and microscopic disease.

2. **Partial response (PR)** indicates a greater than 50% reduction in tumor size, lasting a reasonable period of time. Some evidence of disease remains after therapy.

3. **Response rate (RR)** is defined as CR plus PR.

4. **Stable disease** indicates tumor that neither grows nor shrinks significantly (<25% change in size).

5. **Progression** or **no response** after therapy is defined by a greater than 25% increase in tumor size or the appearance of new lesions.

G. Factors affecting response to chemotherapy

1. **Tumor cell heterogeneity.** Large tumors have completed multiple cell divisions, resulting in several mutations and genetically diverse cells.

2. **Drug resistance.** The **Goldie-Coldman hypothesis** states that genetic changes are associated with drug resistance, and the probability of resistance increases as tumor size increases. The hypothesis assumes that at the time of diagnosis, most tumors possess resistant clones. The most well-studied mechanism of resistance involves the mdr (multidrug resistance) gene, which codes for membrane-bound P-glycoprotein. P-glycoprotein serves

as a channel through which cellular toxins (i.e., chemotherapeutic agents) may be excreted from the cell.

3. **Dose intensity** is defined as a specific dose delivered over a specific period of time. Occasionally, the full dose cannot be given or a cycle is delayed due to complications or toxicities. Suboptimal doses have resulted in reduced response rates and survival.

4. **Patient-specific factors** such as poor functional status, impaired organ function, or concomitant diseases may compromise how a chemotherapy regimen is given and affect how the patient responds to treatment.

IV. CLASSIFICATION OF CHEMOTHERAPEUTIC AGENTS

A. **Alkylating agents** were the first group of antineoplastic agents. The prototype of this class is mechlorethamine, or **nitrogen mustard,** which was researched as a chemical warfare agent. Alkylating agents cause cross-linking and abnormal base pairing of DNA strands, which inhibit replication of the DNA. This mechanism is known as **alkylation.** These are phase-nonspecific agents. Examples of alkylating agents and their toxicities are listed in Table 55-2.

B. Most of the **antitumor antibiotics** are obtained from organisms of the *Streptomyces* genus. These agents may act by either alkylation (mitomycin) or **intercalation.** Intercalation is the

Table 55-2. Cancer Chemotherapeutic Agents by Mechanism of Action and Toxicities

Drug	Toxicities
Alkylating Agents	
Altretamine (hexamethylmelamine)	Nausea and vomiting, myelosuppression, paresthesias, CNS toxicity
Busulfan	Myelosuppression, pulmonary fibrosis, aplastic anemia, skin hyperpigmentation
Carmustine (BCNU)	Delayed myelosuppression, nausea and vomiting, hepatotoxicity
Chlorambucil	Myelosuppression, pulmonary fibrosis, hyperuricemia
Carboplatin	Myelosuppression, nausea and vomiting, peripheral neuropathy, ototoxicity
Cisplatin	Nephrotoxicity, nausea and vomiting, peripheral neuropathy, myelosuppression, ototoxicity
Cyclophosphamide	Myelosuppression, hemorrhagic cystitis, immunosuppression, alopecia, stomatitis, SIADH
Dacarbazine (DTIC)	Myelosuppression, nausea and vomiting, flu-like syndrome, hepatotoxicity, alopecia, flushing
Estramustine	Myelosuppression, ischemic heart disease, thrombophlebitis, hepatotoxicity, nausea and vomiting
Ifosfamide	Myelosuppression, hemorrhagic cystitis, somnolence, confusion
Lomustine (CCNU)	Delayed myelosuppression, nausea and vomiting, hepatotoxicity, neurotoxicity
Mechlorethamine	Myelosuppression, nausea and vomiting, phlebitis, gonadal dysfunction
Melphalan	Myelosuppression, anorexia, nausea and vomiting, gonadal dysfunction
Oxaliplatin	Sensory peripheral neuropathy, nausea and vomiting, diarrhea, mucositis, transaminase elevations, alopecia
Procarbazine	Myelosuppression, nausea and vomiting, lethargy, depression, paresthesias, headache, flu-like syndrome
Streptozocin	Renal toxicity, nausea and vomiting, diarrhea, altered glucose metabolism, liver dysfunction
Temozolamide	Myelosuppression, nausea and vomiting, fatigue, headache, peripheral edema
Thiotepa	Myelosuppression, nausea and vomiting, mucositis, skin rashes

(Continued on next page)

Table 55-2. *Continued*

Drug	Toxicities
Antitumor Antibiotics	
Bleomycin	Pneumonitis, pulmonary fibrosis, fever, anaphylaxis, hyperpigmentation, alopecia
Dactinomycin	Stomatitis, myelosuppression, anorexia, nausea and vomiting, diarrhea, alopecia
Daunorubicin	Myelosuppression, cardiotoxicity, stomatitis, alopecia, nausea and vomiting
Doxorubicin	Myelosuppression, cardiotoxicity, stomatitis, alopecia, nausea and vomiting
Epirubicin	Myelosuppression, nausea and vomiting, cardiotoxicity, alopecia
Idarubicin	Myelosuppression, nausea and vomiting, stomatitis, alopecia, cardiotoxicity
Mitomycin C	Myelosuppression, nausea and vomiting, anorexia, alopecia, stomatitis
Mitoxantrone	Myelosuppression, cardiotoxicity, alopecia, stomatitis, nausea and vomiting
Valrubicin	(For intravesical bladder administration) Urinary frequency, dysuria, hematuria, bladder spasm, incontinence, cystitis
Antimetabolites	
Capecitabine	Diarrhea, stomatitis, nausea and vomiting, hand-foot syndrome, myelosuppression
Cladribine (2Cda)	Myelosuppression, fever, rash
Cytarabine (Ara-C)	Myelosuppression, nausea and vomiting, diarrhea, stomatitis, hepatotoxicity, fever, conjunctivitis, CNS toxicity
Fludarabine	Myelosuppression, nausea and vomiting, fever, malaise, pulmonary infiltrates
Floxuridine	Hepatotoxicity, gastritis, mucositis
5-Fluorouracil	Stomatitis, myelosuppression, diarrhea, nausea and vomiting, cerebellar ataxia
Gemcitabine	Myelosuppression, fever, flu-like syndrome, rash, mild nausea and vomiting
Hydroxyurea	Myelosuppression, mild nausea and vomiting, rash
6-Mercaptopurine	Myelosuppression, nausea and vomiting, anorexia, diarrhea, cholestasis
Methotrexate	Mucositis, myelosuppression, pulmonary fibrosis, hepatotoxicity, nephrotoxicity, diarrhea, skin erythema
Pentostatin	Nephrotoxicity, CNS depression, myelosuppression, nausea and vomiting, conjunctivitis
6-Thioguanine	Myelosuppression, hepatotoxicity, stomatitis
Mitotic Inhibitors	
Docetaxel	Myelosuppression, fluid retention, hypersensitivity, paresthesias, rash alopecia
Paclitaxel	Myelosuppression, peripheral neuropathy, alopecia, mucositis, anaphylaxis, dyspnea
Vinblastine	Myelosuppression, paralytic ileus, alopecia, nausea, stomatitis
Vincristine	Peripheral neuropathy, paralytic ileus, SIADH
Vinorelbine	Peripheral neuropathy, myelosuppression, nausea and vomiting, hepatic dysfunction
Topoisomerase Inhibitors	
Etoposide	Myelosuppression, nausea and vomiting, diarrhea, fever, hypotension with infusion, alopecia
Irinotecan	Myelosuppression, diarrhea, nausea and vomiting, anorexia
Teniposide	Myelosuppression, nausea and vomiting, alopecia, hepatotoxicity, hypotension with infusion
Topotecan	Myelosuppression, fever, flu-like syndrome, nausea and vomiting
Enzymes	
Asparaginase	Allergic reactions, nausea and vomiting, liver dysfunction, CNS depression, hyperglycemia
Pegasparaginase	Hypersensitivity reactions, hepatotoxicity, fever, nausea and vomiting
Protein Tyrosine Kinase Inhibitor	
Imatinib mesylate (STI-571)	Myelosuppression, hepatotoxicity, fluid retention, nausea, diarrhea

Table 55-2. *Continued*

Drug	Toxicities
Miscellaneous	
Tretinoin (all-*trans* retinoic acid, ATRA)	Leukocytosis, arrythmias, headache, nausea and vomiting, scaling of skin, ATRA syndrome (fever, dyspnea, weight gain, pulmonary infiltrates)
Arsenic trioxide	Arrythmias, hyperleukocytosis, nausea and vomiting, diarrhea, abdominal pain, APL differentiation syndrome (fever, dyspnea, weight gain, pulmonary infiltrates)
Hormonal Agents	
Adrenocorticoids	
Dexamethasone	Fluid retention, hyperglycemia, hypertension, infection
Methylprednisolone	
Prednisone	
Estrogens	
Diethylstilbestrol	Fluid retention, feminization, uterine bleeding, nausea and vomiting, thrombophlebitis
Estradiol	
Progestins	
Medroxyprogesterone	Weight gain, fluid retention, feminization, cardiovascular effects
Megesterol acetate	
Antiestrogens	
Fulvestrant	Hot flashes, nausea and vomiting, altered menses
Tamoxifen	
Toremifene	
Aromatase Inhibitors	
Aminoglutethimide	Rash, electrolytes disturbance, drowsiness, nausea, anorexia
Anastrozole	
Exemestane	
Letrozole	
Androgens	
Testosterone	Masculinization, amenorrhea, gynecomastia, nausea, water retention, changes in libido, skin hypersensitivity, hepatotoxicity
Methyltestosterone	
Fluoxymesterone	
Antiandrogens	
Bicalutamide	Hot flashes, decreased libido, impotence, diarrhea, nausea and vomiting, gynecomastia, hepatotoxicity
Flutamide	
Nilutamide	
LHRH Analogues	
Leuprolide	Hot flashes, menstrual irregularity, sexual dysfunction, edema
Goserelin	

process by which the drug slides between DNA base pairs and inhibits DNA synthesis. These are phase-nonspecific agents. Examples of antitumor antibiotics and their toxicities are listed in Table 55-2.

C. **Antimetabolites** are structural analogues of naturally occurring substrates for biochemical reactions. They inhibit DNA synthesis by acting as false substitutions in the production of nucleic acids. These are S phase-specific agents. Examples of antimetabolites and their toxicities are listed in Table 55-2.

D. **Mitotic inhibitors.** The vinca alkaloids arrest cell division by preventing microtubule formation. The taxanes promote microtubule assembly and stabilization, thus prohibiting cell division. These are M phase-specific agents. Examples of these agents and their toxicities are listed in Table 55-2.

E. **Topoisomerase inhibitors** inhibit the enzymes topoisomerase I or topoisomerase II. The topoisomerases are necessary for DNA replication and RNA transcription. These are G_2 phase-specific agents. Examples of these agents and their toxicities are listed in Table 55-2.

F. Enzymes. Asparaginase (see Table 55-2) is an enzyme that causes the degradation of the essential amino acid asparagine to aspartic acid and ammonia. Unlike normal cells, tumor cells lack the ability to synthesize asparagine. This is a G_1 phase-specific agent.

G. Protein tyrosine kinase inhibitors. Imatinib mesylate (see Table 55-2) is a selective tyrosine kinase inhibitor that causes apoptosis or arrest of growth in cells expressing the BCR-ABL oncoprotein. BCR-ABL is the product of a specific chromosomal abnormality (Philadelphia chromosome), which is present in virtually all patients with chronic myelogenous leukemia (CML). It is the first approved antineoplastic agent designed to have targeted enzyme activity.

H. Other **miscellaneous** agents are listed in Table 55-2.

  1. **Tretinoin (all-*trans* retinoic acid, ATRA)** is a retinoid derived from vitamin A, used for a specific form of acute leukemia known as acute promyelocytic leukemia (APL), to help cells differentiate into functionally mature cells.

  2. **Arsenic trioxide** is an antineoplastic arsenic compound used for APL that may induce selective apoptosis of APL cells.

I. Hormones are a class of heterogeneous compounds that have varying effects on cells. Table 55-2 contains a list of some of the most commonly used hormonal agents in cancer therapy.

J. Biological response modifiers alter or enhance the patient's immune system to fight cancer or to lessen the side effects of the cancer treatment. Examples are listed in Table 55-3.

Table 55-3. Biological Agents Used in Oncology

Cytokine	Indications	Toxicity
Interferon-α 2a, 2b (Roferon-A^R, Intron A)	Malignant melanoma, chronic myelogenous leukemia, hairy-cell leukemia, Kaposi's sarcoma, chronic hepatitis B and C, follicular lymphoma	Flu-like syndrome, anorexia, depression, fatigue
Interleukin-2 (Aldesleukin) (Proleukin)	Renal cell carcinoma, malignant melanoma	Chills, fever, dyspnea, pulmonary congestion, edema, nephrotoxicity, hypotension, mental status changes, anemia, thrombocytopenia, diarrhea, nausea and vomiting
Interleukin-11 (Oprelvekin) (Neumega)	Thrombocytopenia	Fluid retention, peripheral edema, dyspnea, tachycardia, atrial arrythmias, dizziness, blurred vision
Filgrastim (G-CSF) (Neupogen)	Decrease incidence/duration of neutropenia, hematopoietic stem-cell mobilization	Bone pain, fever, malaise
Pegfilgrastim (Neulasta)	Decrease incidence/duration of neutropenia	Bone pain, fever, malaise
Sargramostim (GM-CSF) (Leukine)	Acceleration of myeloid recovery, BMT failure or engraftment delay, induction for acute myelogenous leukemia, hematopoietic stem cell mobilization, myeloid reconstitution after bone marrow transplant	Bone pain, arthralgia/myalgia, chills, fever, rash, first-dose reaction (hypotension, tachycardia, dyspnea)
Epoetin alfa (Erythropoietin) (Epogen, Procrit)	Anemia associated with chronic renal failure, cancer chemotherapy or HIV treatments, reduction of blood transfusions in surgery patients	Hypertension, headache, arthralgias
Darbepoetin alfa (Aranesp)	Anemia associated with chronic renal failure, chronic renal insufficiency, cancer- and chemotherapy-associated anemia	Hypertension, myalgia, headache, fever, tachycardia, nausea

Table 55-3. *Continued*

Monoclonal Antibody	Indications	Toxicity
Alemtuzumab (Campath^R)	B-cell chronic lymphocytic leukemia	Infusion-related fevers, chills, rash, hypotension, shortness of breath, nausea and vomiting, opportunistic infections, neutropenia, thrombocytopenia
Gemtuzumab ozogamicin (Mylotarg^R)	Acute myeloid leukemia	Infusion-related fever, chills, nausea and vomiting, headache, hypotension, myelosuppression, hepatotoxicity, hypersensitivity
Ibritumomab tiuxetan (Zevalin^R)	Non-Hodgkin's lymphoma	Infusion-related fevers, chills, rigors, hypersensitivity, hypotension, myelosuppression
Rituximab (Rituxan^R)	Non-Hodgkin's lymphoma	Hypersensitivity, infusion-related fevers, chills, rigors, hypotension
Trastuzumab (Herceptin^R)	Breast cancer	Infusion-related fevers, chills, cardiac dysfunction including dyspnea, cough, peripheral edema, nausea and vomiting, hypersensitivity, hypotension, diarrhea

Immunotoxin	Indications	Toxicity
Deneleukin diftotox (Ontak^R)	Cutaneous t-cell lymphoma	Acute hypersensitivity including hypotension, dyspnea, rash, chest pain, tachycardia, vascular leak syndrome, dizziness, nausea and vomiting, diarrhea

1. **Cytokines** are soluble factors secreted or released by cells, which affect the activity of other cells and/or the secreting cell itself. These agents generally act as regulatory or hematopoietic growth factors.

2. **Monoclonal antibodies** are recombinant antibodies designed to identify cancer-specific antigens, bind to the antigens on the patient's cancer cells, and allow the patient's immune system to eliminate those cells. Some monoclonal antibodies are being conjugated to antitumor agents or radioisotopes (e.g., gemtuzumab ozogamicin, ibritumomab tiuxetan) to help target cytotoxic therapy to the tumor cells.

3. **Immunotoxins.** Denileukin diftitox is a fusion protein composed of diptheria toxin and interleukin-2 (IL-2). It is designed to direct the cytocidal action of diptheria toxin to cells with the IL-2 receptor on their surface. This form of therapy is able to bypass the need for a functioning immune system, which may be defective in many cancer patients.

V. TOXICITIES OF CHEMOTHERAPY AGENTS.
Chemotherapeutic agents are most toxic to rapidly proliferating cells. The tissues most commonly affected are those of the mucous membranes, skin, hair, gastrointestinal (GI) tract, and bone marrow. Of these, bone marrow toxicity can be the most life threatening.

A. **Bone marrow suppression** is the **most common** dose-limiting **side effect** of cancer therapy.

  1. **Complications**
     a. **Infections.** White blood cells are most affected due to their short life span (6–12 hours). A significant decrease in the white blood cell count, particularly a neutrophil count <500/mm³ **(neutropenia),** predisposes the patient to development of serious infections. The usual signs and symptoms of infection may be absent, and fever may be the only indicator **(febrile neutropenia). Colony-stimulating factors (e.g., G-CSF, GM-CSF)** may be used to stimulate neutrophil production and lessen the degree and duration of neutropenia.

    b. Bleeding. Platelets have an intermediate life span of 5–10 days. Decreased platelets **(thrombocytopenia)** can also occur from chemotherapy, which can lead to bleeding and may require platelet transfusions.

    c. Anemia and **fatigue** secondary to cancer chemotherapy may also occur. It generally does not occur as quickly as other bone marrow toxicities because of the long life span of red blood cells (about 120 days). **Human recombinant erythropoietin** (e.g., epoetin alfa, darbepoetin alfa) may be used to increase hemoglobin, decrease transfusion requirements, and decrease fatigue.

2. The **time course** of myelosuppression varies with the chemotherapy regimen. In general, the onset of myelosuppression is 7–10 days after the chemotherapy has been administered. The lowest point of the counts, called the **nadir**, is usually reached in 10–14 days. Recovery of counts usually occurs in 2–3 weeks.

3. A patient's counts must be sufficiently **recovered** before receiving subsequent chemotherapy cycles. Generally, the neutrophil count must be greater than 1,500/mm^3 and the platelet count greater than 100,000/mm^3 before receiving additional chemotherapy.

4. The extent of myelosuppression is related to the **chemotherapy agents** used and **doses** given. Drugs that can cause severe myelosuppression include carmustine, cytarabine, daunorubicin, doxorubicin, and paclitaxel.

5. Some chemotherapy agents cause little or no myelosuppression. These include asparaginase, bleomycin, and vincristine.

B. Dermatological toxicity

1. **Alopecia** is the loss of hair associated with chemotherapy. Not all agents cause alopecia, and hair loss may be partial or complete. Chemotherapy agents that commonly cause alopecia include cyclophosphamide, doxorubicin, mechlorethamine, and paclitaxel.

2. Drugs associated with necrosis of tissue are called **vesicants. Local necrosis** may result from **extravasation** of vesicant chemotherapy drugs outside the vein during their administration. Vesicant agents include dactinomycin, daunorubicin, doxorubicin, idarubicin, mechlorethamine, mitomycin, vinblastine, vincristine, and vinorelbine.

    a. Most vesicant extravasations produce **immediate pain** or **burning.** However, a delayed reaction may occur hours or weeks later. Significant tissue injury, including ulceration or necrosis, may require plastic surgery intervention.

    b. The **treatment** of extravasations varies depending on the vesicant. Heat or cold packs and chemicals such as hyaluronidase or dimethyl sulfoxide (DMSO) may be used.

3. Cancer chemotherapy can also cause **skin changes** such as dryness and sensitivity to sunlight. Examples are fluorouracil and methotrexate.

C. GI toxicities are frequently experienced by patients receiving chemotherapy.

1. **Nausea** and **vomiting** are often the most distressing toxicities from the patient's perspective. However, this side effect can generally be prevented, or better controlled, with the use of currently available antiemetics.

    a. Severe vomiting can result in dehydration, electrolyte imbalances, and esophageal tears and may cause the patient to discontinue therapy.

    b. Nausea and vomiting may be **acute, delayed,** or **anticipatory** in nature. Antiemetics should be used prophylactically to prevent the occurrence of nausea and vomiting, particularly with chemotherapeutic agents that have a high emetogenic risk.

    c. Table 55-4 lists **commonly used chemotherapeutic agents** and their emetogenic potential on a scale of 1–5. The emetogenic potential of combinations of chemotherapy agents can be estimated by identifying the most emetogenic agent in the combination. The contribution of the other agents can then be evaluated by using the following guidelines: (1) Level 1 agents do not contribute to the emetogenicity of the regimen. (2) Adding one or more level 2 agents increases the emetogenicity to one level higher than the most emetogenic agent in the combination. (3) Adding level 3 or 4 agents increases the level of emetogenicity by one level per agent.

    d. The occurrence of nausea and vomiting is influenced by the emetogenicity of the chemotherapeutic agent or combination of agents, the chemotherapeutic dose, the method of administration, and individual patient characteristics.

Table 55-4. Emetogenic Potential of Cancer Chemotherapeutic Agents

Level 5 Very Highly Emetogenic	Level 4 Highly Emetogenic	Level 3 Moderately Emetogenic	Level 2 Low Emetic Risk	Level 1 Very Low Emetic Risk
Carmustine >250 mg/m^2	Carmustine ≤ 250 mg/m^2	Carboplatin	Docetaxel	Asparaginase
Cisplatin ≥ 50 mg/m^2	Cisplatin <50 mg/m^2	Cyclophosphamide ≤ 750 mg/m^2	Etoposide	Bleomycin
Cyclophosphamide ≥ 1500 mg/m^2	Cyclophosphamide 750–1500 mg/m^2	Cytarabine <1000 mg/m^2	Fluorouracil	Capecitabine
Dacarbazine	Cytarabine >1000 mg/m^2	Daunorubicin	Gemcitabine	Chlorambucil
Mechlorethamine	Dactinomycin	Doxorubicin ≤ 60 mg/m^2	Irinotecan	Fludarabine
Streptozocin	Doxorubicin >60 mg/m^2	Idarubicin	Methotrexate 50–250 mg/m^2	Hydroxyurea
	Lomustine	Ifosfamide	Mitomycin	Methotrexate ≤ 50 mg/m^2
	Methotrexate >1000 mg/m^2	Methotrexate 250–1000 mg/m^2	Paclitaxel	Melphalan
	Procarbazine	Mitoxantrone	Thiotepa <15 mg/m^2	Rituximab
	Temozolomide		Topotecan	Thioguanine
	Thiotepa ≥ 15 mg/m^2			Trastuzumab
				Vinblastine Vincristine Vinorelbine

2. **Stomatitis** is a generalized inflammation of the oral mucosa or other areas of the GI tract. Because of the rapid turnover of epithelial cells in the GI tract, this is a common site of toxicity.
   a. **Signs** and **symptoms** include erythema, pain, dryness of the mouth, burning or tingling of the lips, ulcerations, and bleeding.
   b. Chemotherapy agents associated with stomatitis include capecitabine, fluorouracil, and methotrexate.
   c. **Time course.** Stomatitis usually appears within a week after the offending agent is administered, and resolves in 10–14 days.
   d. **Consequences** of stomatitis include infection of the ulcerated areas, inability to eat, pain requiring opioid analgesics, and subsequent decreases in chemotherapy doses.
   e. **Amifostine** is a cytoprotective agent that may be used to reduce the incidence of radiation-induced xerostomia in head and neck cancer treatment.

3. Other GI toxicities include **diarrhea** (e.g., irinotecan, fluorouracil), **constipation** (e.g., vincristine), **anorexia,** and **taste changes.**

D. **Tumor lysis syndrome (TLS)** may occur in hematological malignancies such as leukemia and lymphoma, where there is a high tumor cell burden or rapidly growing tumors. Due to the spontaneous lysis of cells from treatment with chemotherapy, cell lysis causes release of intracellular products, including uric acid, potassium, and phosphate, which can lead to renal failure and cardiac arrythmias. This may be prevented by giving intravenous hydration, by alkalinizing the urine, and by giving agents such as **allopurinol** or **rasburicase** (Elitek) to decrease uric acid.

E. **Chills** and **fever** may occur after the administration of some chemotherapy and biological agents. This fever generally can be differentiated from fever due to infection because of its temporal relationship to chemotherapy administration. This reaction is commonly associated with bleomycin, cytarabine monoclonal antibodies, and IL-2.

F. **Pulmonary toxicity** is generally irreversible and may be fatal.

1. **Signs** and **symptoms** are shortness of breath, nonproductive cough, and low-grade fever. In some cases, the risk of pulmonary toxicity increases as the cumulative dose of the drug increases (e.g., bleomycin).

2. Chemotherapeutic agents associated with pulmonary toxicity include bleomycin, busulfan, carmustine, and mitomycin.

G. **Cardiac toxicity** may manifest as an acute or chronic problem.

1. **Acute changes** are generally transient electrocardiograph abnormalities that may not be clinically significant.

2. **Chronic cardiac toxicity** is irreversible congestive heart failure. **Risk factors** include chest irradiation and high cumulative doses of cardiotoxic chemotherapy.

3. Chemotherapy agents that are associated with chronic cardiotoxicity include daunorubicin, doxorubicin, epirubicin, idarubicin, and mitoxantrone. **Dexrazoxane** is a cardioprotective agent that may be used with doxorubicin to help prevent or lessen its toxic effects to the heart.

H. **Hypersensitivity reactions** may occur with any chemotherapy agent. Life-threatening reactions, including anaphylaxis, appear to be more common with asparaginase, carboplatin, cisplatin, etoposide, paclitaxel, and teniposide.

I. **Neurotoxicity** may occur with systemic or intrathecal chemotherapy.

1. Vincristine is associated with **autonomic** and **peripheral** neuropathies. Patients may experience gait disturbances, numbness and tingling of hands and feet, and loss of deep-tendon reflexes. Intrathecal administration of vincristine results in fatal neurotoxicity.

2. **Peripheral neuropathy** and **ototoxicity** are common dose-limiting toxicities of cisplatin. **Sensory** neuropathies, causing tingling or numbing of the hands and feet, may be associated with capecitabine, oxaliplatin, and paclitaxel.

3. High doses of cytarabine may produce **cerebellar toxicity** that manifests initially as loss of eye–hand coordination and may progress to coma.

4. **Arachnoiditis** has been associated with intrathecal administration of cytarabine and methotrexate.

J. **Hemorrhagic cystitis** is a bladder toxicity that is seen most commonly after administration of cyclophosphamide and ifosfamide. **Acrolein,** a metabolite of these agents, is thought to cause a chemical irritation of the bladder mucosa, resulting in bleeding. Preventive measures include aggressive hydration with subsequent frequent urination, and the administration of the uroprotectant mesna. **Mesna** acts by binding to acrolein and preventing it from contacting the bladder mucosa.

K. **Renal toxicity** may manifest by elevations in serum creatinine and blood urea nitrogen (BUN), as well as electrolyte abnormalities. Nephrotoxicity is associated with cisplatin, ifosfamide, methotrexate, and streptozocin. **Amifostine** may be used to protect the kidneys from the nephrotoxic effect of cisplatin.

L. **Hepatotoxicity** may manifest as elevated liver function tests, jaundice, or hepatitis. Asparaginase, cytarabine, mercaptopurine, and methotrexate are known to cause hepatic toxicity.

M. **Secondary malignancies,** such as solid tumors, lymphomas, and leukemias, may occur many years after chemotherapy or radiation. Antineoplastic agents known to possess a high carcinogenic risk include cyclophosphamide, etoposide, melphalan, and mechlorethamine.

N. Chemotherapy may cause **infertility,** which may be temporary or permanent. Cyclophosphamide, chlorambucil, mechlorethamine, melphalan, and procarbazine are associated with a significant incidence of infertility in males and females.

VI. OTHER THERAPEUTIC MODALITIES

A. Surgery may be diagnostic (biopsy, exploratory laparotomy, "second-look") or therapeutic (tumor debulking or removal). Surgery is often combined with chemotherapy and/or radiation.

B. Radiation therapy involves high doses of ionizing radiation directed at the cancerous tissue. Radiation may be combined with surgery and/or chemotherapy. Depending on the area of the body being irradiated, **adverse reactions** may include stomatitis, nausea and vomiting, diarrhea, and myelosuppression.

C. Hematopoietic stem-cell transplantation involves intravenous infusion of stem cells from a compatible donor to a recipient following high-dose chemotherapy. It is used for treatment of diseases involving the bone marrow or immune system, and to allow for administration of high-dose chemotherapy or radiation for tumors resistant to standard doses. Stem cells can be obtained from bone marrow or peripheral blood.

1. In **autologous** transplants, stem cells are obtained from the patient, preserved, and later reinfused into the same patient. **Allogeneic** transplants involve two separate individuals. Cells are obtained from a matched donor and then infused into a separate patient.

2. Transplant-related complications include hepatic venoocclusive disease (VOD), acute and chronic graft versus host disease (GVHD), infection, and pulmonary complications.

STUDY QUESTIONS

Directions: Each of the numbered items or incomplete statements in this section is followed by answers or completions of the statement. Select the **one** lettered answer or completion that is **best** in each case.

1. The top four most commonly diagnosed cancers include all of the following EXCEPT

(A) lung
(B) prostate
(C) colon and rectum
(D) thyroid
(E) breast

2. Which statement regarding phase-specific chemotherapeutic agents is correct? They

(A) are most effective in one phase of the cell cycle
(B) are effective in all phases of the cell cycle
(C) are only effective in G_0 phase
(D) include the alkylating agents
(E) include the antitumor antibiotics

3. Body surface area (BSA) is used in calculating chemotherapy doses because

(A) BSA is an indicator of tumor cell mass
(B) BSA correlates with cardiac output
(C) BSA correlates with gastrointestinal transit time
(D) the National Cancer Institute requires that BSA be used
(E) the Food and Drug Administration (FDA) requires that BSA be used

4. The rationale for combination chemotherapy includes all of the following EXCEPT

(A) biochemical enhancement of effect
(B) rescue of normal cells
(C) overcoming or preventing resistance
(D) biochemical nullification of effect
(E) cytotoxic to both resting and dividing cells

5. All of the following chemotherapy agents can be administered intrathecally EXCEPT

(A) methotrexate
(B) cytarabine
(C) hydrocortisone
(D) thiotepa
(E) vincristine

6. Which of the following chemotherapeutic agents is classified as an alkylating agent?

(A) Cyclophosphamide
(B) Etoposide
(C) Mechlorethamine
(D) Paclitaxel
(E) Cyclophosphamide and mechlorethamine

7. Which of the following chemotherapy agents acts by intercalation?

(A) Vincristine
(B) Paclitaxel
(C) Doxorubicin
(D) Vincristine and paclitaxel
(E) Topotecan

8. How do antimetabolites exert their cytotoxic effect?

(A) Inhibiting DNA synthesis by sliding between DNA base pairs
(B) Inhibiting RNA synthesis by sliding between RNA base pairs
(C) Acting as false metabolites in the microtubules
(D) Acting as false substitutions in the production of nucleic acids
(E) Promoting microtubule assembly and stabilization

9. All of the following chemotherapy agents work through affecting microtubule function EXCEPT

(A) docetaxel
(B) vinblastine
(C) mitoxantrone
(D) vincristine
(E) vinorelbine

10. Hormonal agents that are useful in the treatment of cancer include

(A) tamoxifen
(B) prednisone
(C) flutamide
(D) tamoxifen and flutamide
(E) tamoxifen, prednisone, and flutamide

11. When does the neutrophil nadir associated with chemotherapy agents generally occur?

(A) During administration of the chemotherapy
(B) 1–2 days after therapy
(C) 10–14 days after therapy
(D) 1 month after therapy
(E) When the platelet count begins to rise

12. Stomatitis is characterized by all of the following signs and symptoms EXCEPT

(A) headache
(B) erythema
(C) bleeding
(D) ulcerations
(E) dryness of mouth

13. Which of the following statements describes hemorrhagic cystitis? It

(A) is caused by excretion of tumor cell breakdown products
(B) is associated with ifosfamide or cyclophosphamide administration
(C) is caused by the administration of mesna
(D) can be prevented or treated with acrolein
(E) can be treated with G-CSF

14. All of the following chemotherapy agents are vesicants EXCEPT

(A) doxorubicin
(B) mechlorethamine
(C) vincristine
(D) methotrexate
(E) idarubicin

15. Match each of the following toxicities to the agent most likely to cause the toxicity.

(A) Cardiotoxicity   (1) Vincristine
(B) Hypersensitivity   (2) Irinotecan
(C) Diarrhea   (3) Doxorubicin
(D) Pulmonary toxicity   (4) Paclitaxel
(E) Constipation   (5) Bleomycin

ANSWERS AND EXPLANATIONS

1. The answer is D *[I B].*
Prostate cancer is the most common cancer in men, breast cancer is the most common cancer in women, followed by lung, then colon and rectum for both men and women.

2. The answer is A *[II D 1, 2, 3].*
Phase-specific agents are most active in one specific phase of the cell cycle. These agents have no activity against cells in G_0, the resting phase. Examples of phase-specific agents include the mitotic inhibitors, asparaginase, the antimetabolites, and etoposide.

3. The answer is B *[III B].*
BSA correlates with cardiac output, which determines renal and hepatic blood flow and, thus, affects drug elimination.

4. The answer is D *[III D 2].*
Combination chemotherapy has been developed to have maximal cytotoxicity to tumor cells and minimal toxicity to normal cells. The drugs are dosed and scheduled such that maximal cell kill occurs, while sparing normal cells as much as possible. Combination regimens often contain agents with different spectrums of toxicity.

5. The answer is E *[III E 3].*
Intrathecally administered vincristine is fatal. All syringes of vincristine must be labeled "Fatal if given intrathecally. For intravenous use only."

6. The answer is E *[IV A 1].*
Cyclophosphamide and mechlorethamine are nitrogen mustards, a subgroup of the alkylating agents. Etoposide is a topoisomerase II inhibitor, and paclitaxel is a mitotic inhibitor.

7. The answer is C *[IV B 1].*
Doxorubicin is an antitumor antibiotic that inhibits DNA synthesis by intercalation. Vincristine and paclitaxel are mitotic inhibitors that act on microtubule assembly. Topotecan inhibits topoisomerase I.

8. The answer is D *[IV C].*
Antimetabolites are structural analogues of naturally occurring substrates for biochemical reactions. They inhibit DNA synthesis by acting as false substitutions in the production of DNA.

9. The answer is C *[IV D].*
Docetaxel is a taxane, which works by promoting microtubule assembly and stabilization, resulting in inhibition of cell division. Vincristine, vinblastine, and vinorelbine are vinca alkaloids, which work by preventing microtubule formation. Mitoxantrone is an antitumor antibiotic that works by DNA intercalation.

10. The answer is E *[VI, Table 55-2].*
Tamoxifen is an antiestrogen used in the treatment of breast cancer. Prednisone is used for its antilymphocytic properties in the treatment of non-Hodgkin's lymphoma. Flutamide is an antiandrogen used in the treatment of prostate cancer.

11. The answer is C *[V A 2].*
Bone marrow suppression, particularly of the neutrophils, usually is the most profound 10–14 days after chemotherapy.

12. The answer is A *[V C 2].*
Stomatitis, or mucositis, is an inflammation of the mucous membranes, particularly the oral mucosa. Although the symptoms generally are limited to the mouth and throat, stomatitis may affect any part of the gastrointestinal tract, potentially causing diarrhea and anal fissures.

13. The answer is B *[V J].*
Hemorrhagic cystitis results from irritation of the lining of the bladder by acrolein, a metabolite of ifosfamide and cyclophosphamide. Mesna may be used to inactivate the acrolein, thus preventing hemorrhagic cystitis.

14. The answer is D *[V B 2].*
Vesicant chemotherapy agents may cause local necrosis if extravasated outside the vein. Doxorubicin, idarubicin, mechlorethamine, and vincristine are all classified as vesicants.

15. The answers are A-3, B-4, C-2, D-5, E-1 *[V C 3, E, F, G].*
Cardiotoxicity is associated with cumulative doses of doxorubicin and other antitumor antibiotics. Hypersensitivity from paclitaxel may be due to its Cremophor diluent. Severe diarrhea, requiring treatment with atropine, is associated with irinotecan. Pulmonary toxicity is associated with cumulative doses of bleomycin. Severe constipation and paralytic ileus is associated with the use of vincristine.

56
Pain Management
Alan F. Kaul

I. INTRODUCTION

A. Definitions

1. **Pain** is an unpleasant sensory and emotional experience that usually is associated with structural or tissue damage. It is a subjective, individual experience that has physical, psychological, and social determinants. There is no objective measurement of pain. In the United States alone, recurrent or persistent pain is experienced by more than 75 million individuals.

2. **Acute pain** lasts less than 30 days and occurs following muscle strains and tissue injury, such as trauma or surgery. The pain is usually self-limiting, decreasing with time as the injury heals. It is described as a linear process with a beginning and an end. Increased autonomic nervous system activity often accompanies acute pain, causing tachycardia, tachypnea, hypertension, diaphoresis, and mydriasis. Increased anxiety also may occur.

3. **Chronic pain** is persistent or episodic pain of a duration or intensity that adversely affects the function or well-being of the patient. Some define it as lasting more than 6 months. **Chronic nonmalignant pain** may be a complication of acute injury where the healing process does not occur as expected or may be caused by a disease such as a rheumatological disorder like osteoarthritis, rheumatoid arthritis, or fibromyalgia. The elderly are more likely to experience chronic pain because of the increased prevalence of degenerative disorders in this age group. The pain is constant, does not improve with time, and is described as a cyclic process (vicious cycle). Compared to acute pain, there is no longer autonomic nervous system stimulation so the patient may not "appear" in pain. Instead, the patient may be depressed, suffer insomnia, weight loss, and sexual dysfunction and may not be able to cope with the normal activities of daily living, including family and job-related activities.

4. **Chronic cancer pain** occurs in 60%–90% of patients with cancer. Its characteristics are similar to those of chronic nonmalignant pain. In addition to depression, fear, anger, and agony may be prominent occurrences. The etiology of chronic cancer pain can be related to the tumor or cancer therapy or can be idiosyncratic. Tumor causes of pain include bone metastasis, compression of nerve structures, occlusion of blood vessels, obstruction of bowel, or infiltration of soft tissue.

5. **Breakthrough pain** is the intermittent, transitory increase in pain that occurs at a greater intensity over baseline chronic pain. It may have temporal characteristics, precipitating factors, and predictability.

B. Principles of management

1. **Comprehensive pain assessment** should determine the characteristics of the patient's pain complaint, clinical status, and pain management history.
   a. Assessment of the pain complaint should include chronology and symptomatology of the presenting complaint such as information about onset, location, intensity, duration, quality, distribution, provocative factors, temporal qualities, severity, and pain history.
   b. Assessment of clinical status should include the extent of underlying trauma or disease. Also, the patient's physical, psychological, and social conditions should be determined.
   c. Assessment of pain management history includes drug allergies, analgesic response, onset, duration, and side effects.

2. **Appropriate pain management targets** should be established.
   a. The primary pain management goal is to improve patient comfort.
   b. For acute pain management, improved comfort can aid the healing and rehabilitation process.
   c. For chronic pain, the specific objectives are to break the pain cycle (i.e., erase pain memory) and minimize breakthrough pain.
   d. Other targets for chronic pain management include improvement of general well-being, sleep, outlook, self-esteem, activities of daily living, support, and mobility.

3. **Individualized pain management regimens** should be determined and initiated promptly.
   a. The optimal analgesic regimen, including dose, dosing interval, and mode of administration, should be selected.
   b. Additional pharmacological adjuncts and nonpharmacological therapies should be added if needed.
   c. The most common regimens for acute pain include intermittent (as needed) dosing, patient-controlled analgesia (PCA), or epidural infusions with narcotic or nonnarcotic agents.
   d. Although the practice is controversial, narcotic use usually is minimized or avoided for chronic nonmalignant pain. Nonnarcotic analgesics and nonpharmacological management usually are maximized.
   e. For chronic cancer pain, an individualized around-the-clock analgesic regimen is established, using a long-acting analgesic. An intermittent, as-needed regimen for breakthrough pain, using a short-acting analgesic, is also determined.

4. **Monitoring** the pain management regimen and **reassessment** of the patient's pain should occur on a continuous, timely basis. Any changes in analgesic, dose, dosing interval, or method of administration should be noted in the patient's medical record and carried out in a timely fashion.

II. ANALGESICS

A. **Nonnarcotic analgesics** include aspirin; other salicylates; acetaminophen; nonsteroidal anti-inflammatory drugs (NSAIDs); selective, cyclooxygenase (COX)-2 inhibitors; disease-modifying antirheumatic drugs (DMARDs); and tumor-necrosis factor (TNF)-α inhibitors (Table 56-1). Aspirin products, acetaminophen, and some low-dose NSAIDs such as ibuprofen, ketoprofen, and naproxen sodium are available for use without a prescription.

1. **Mechanism of action.** Salicylates and NSAIDs are prostaglandin inhibitors and prevent peripheral nociception by vasoactive substances such as prostaglandins and bradykinins. Most NSAIDs inhibit both COX-1, which produces prostaglandins that are believed to be cytoprotective of the stomach lining, and COX-2, which produces prostaglandins responsible for pain and inflammation. Newer COX-2 selective inhibitors like celecoxib, valdecoxib, and rofecoxib do not inhibit COX-1. Etanercept, a TNF-α, acts by binding or capturing excess TNF, one of the dominant cytokines or proteins that play an important role in the inflammatory response. The exact mechanism of action of acetaminophen and leflunomide, a novel drug used to treat rheumatoid arthritis, are not known.

2. **Therapeutic effects**
   a. The peripherally acting, nonnarcotic analgesics have several effects in common. These effects distinguish these agents from narcotic analgesics.
      (1) They are antipyretic.
      (2) They are anti-inflammatory (except acetaminophen).
      (3) There is a ceiling effect to the analgesia.
      (4) They do not cause tolerance.
      (5) They do not cause physical or psychological dependence.
   b. The efficacy of nonnarcotics is compared to aspirin. Most drugs are comparable to aspirin; however, several NSAIDs have shown a superior effect to 650 mg of aspirin.
      (1) Diflunisal (500 mg)
      (2) Ibuprofen (200–400 mg)
      (3) Naproxen sodium (550 mg)
      (4) Ketoprofen (25–50 mg)
   c. The newer classes of drugs have not been compared to aspirin.

3. **Clinical use**
   a. Generally, the nonnarcotic analgesics are used orally to manage mild to moderate pain.
      (1) They are particularly suited for acute pain of skeletal muscle (orthopedic) or oral (dental) origin.
      (2) They are used to treat pain and inflammation associated with osteoarthritis and rheumatoid arthritis.
      (3) They are used in chronic malignant pain and can have an additive effect with narcotic analgesics.
      (4) They also may be effective in managing pain due to bone metastases.

Table 56-1. Nonnarcotic Oral Analgesics and Nonsteroidal Anti-Inflammatory Drugs (NSAIDs)

Drug	Adult Dose Range (mg)	Dosing Interval (hr)	Maximum Dose/Day (mg)
Para-aminophenol derivatives			
Acetaminophen	325–1000	4–6	4000
Salicylates			
Aspirin	325–1000	4–6	4000
Choline magnesium trisalicylate	1000–1500	12	3000
Diflunisal	250–1000	8–12	1500
Salsalate	500–1000	8	3000
Arylpropionic acid derivatives			
Fenoprofen	200	4–6	3200
Flurbiprofen	50–100	6–12	300
Ibuprofen	300–800	6–8	3200
Ketoprofen	12.5–75	6–8	300
Naproxen	200–500	12	1250
Naproxen sodium	275–550	12	1375
Oxaprazocin	600–1200	12	1200
Heteroaryl acetic acid derivatives			
Diclofenac	25–75	6–12	200
Ketorolac (intramuscular)	15–60	6	120
Ketorolac (oral)	10	4–6	40
Tolmetin	200–600	6–8	1800
Indole and indene acetic acid derivatives			
Etodolac	200–400	6–12	1200
Indomethacin	25–50	8–12	200
Sulindac	150–200	12	400
Antranilic acid derivatives (fenamates)			
Meclofenamate	50–100	4–6	400
Mefanamic acid	250–	6	1000
Alkanone derivatives			
Nabumetone	1000–	12–24	2000
Enolic acid derivatives (oxicams)			
Piroxicam	20	24	20
Meloxicam	7.5–15	24	15
Cyclooxygenase (COX)-2 selective inhibitors			
Celecoxib	100–200	12–24	400
Rofecoxib	12.5–50	24	50
Valdecoxib	10–20	12–24	40
Disease-modifying antirheumatic drugs (DMARDs)			
Leflunomide	20	24	20*
Biological response modifiers (tumor-necrosis factor-α inhibitors)			
Etanercept	25 SC injection	84	25 twice weekly

*Excludes loading dose of 100 mg/day for 3 days.

SC = subcutaneous.

   b. The NSAID ketorolac is administered intramuscularly and is useful in moderate to severe pain, particularly in cases where narcotics are undesirable (e.g., with drug addicts, excessive narcotic sedation, respiratory depression).
   c. Patients may vary in their response and tolerance to nonnarcotic analgesics. If a patient does not respond to the maximum therapeutic dose, then an alternate NSAID should be tried. Likewise, if a patient experiences side effects with one drug, then another agent should be tried.
   d. Several drugs (e.g, diflunisal, choline magnesium trisalicylate, naproxen, celecoxib, valdecoxib, rofecoxib, leflunomide, etanercept) have long half-lives and, therefore, may be administered less frequently. Rofecoxib, with a 17-hour half-life, may be administered once daily.

e. The cost of nonnarcotic analgesics is highly variable and should be considered when an agent is selected. Pharmacotherapy with the newer classes of drugs such as the COX-2 inhibitors are more expensive, and pharmacotherapy with leuflunomide or TNF-α inhibitor is significantly more expensive than older agents.

4. **Adverse effects**
   a. **Gastrointestinal (GI) effects.** Most nonnarcotic analgesics cause GI symptoms secondary to prostaglandin inhibition. At normal doses, acetaminophen and choline magnesium trisalicylate produce minimal GI upset. Because of their mechanism of action, the COX-2 inhibitors have a GI toxicity similar to placebo. Etanercept has not been associated with GI side effects, whereas leuflunomide has been associated with nausea and diarrhea.
      (1) The most common GI symptom is dyspepsia, but ulceration, bleeding, or perforation can occur.
      (2) Patients most predisposed to severe GI effects include the elderly, patients with a history of ulcers or chronic disease, and those who smoke or use alcohol.
      (3) To minimize GI effects, the lowest possible analgesic dose should be used. Aspirin, available as enteric-coated products, may minimize GI upset. Combination therapy with a GI "protectant" (e.g., antacid, H_2-antagonist, sucralfate, misoprostol) may be needed.
   b. **Hematological effects.** Most nonnarcotic analgesics inhibit platelet aggregation. The effect is produced by reversible inhibition of prostaglandin synthetase. Aspirin is an irreversible inhibitor. Acetaminophen and choline magnesium trisalicylate lack antiplatelet effects. Etanercept has not been associated with hematological side effects.
      (1) The effect of the NSAIDs correlates to the presence of an effective serum concentration.
      (2) Use of anticoagulants (e.g., heparin, warfarin) is relatively contraindicated in combination with aspirin or NSAIDs.
   c. **Renal effects.** NSAIDs can produce renal dysfunction. Selective COX-2 inhibitors are not devoid of this effect. Etanercept has not been shown to affect renal function.
      (1) The mechanism of NSAID-induced renal dysfunction includes prostaglandin inhibition, interstitial nephritis, impaired renin secretion, and enhanced tubular water/sodium reabsorption.
      (2) Many risk factors have been implicated, including congestive heart failure (CHF), chronic renal failure (CRF), cirrhosis, dehydration, diuretic use, and atherosclerotic disease in elderly patients.
      (3) Renal dysfunction is commonly manifested as abrupt onset oliguria with sodium/water retention. The effect reverses after discontinuation of the NSAID.
   d. **Miscellaneous effects**
      (1) Even in normal doses, acetaminophen can cause hepatotoxicity in those patients with liver disease or chronic alcoholism. Hepatotoxicity has also been reported with the use of all NSAIDs, including the COX-2 selective inhibitors. Leflunomide has also been shown to cause transient elevations in liver function tests.
      (2) Some patients exhibit acute hypersensitivity reactions to aspirin. Manifestations include either a rhinitis or asthma presentation or a true allergic reaction (e.g., urticaria, wheals, hypotension, shock, syncope). A cross-sensitivity to other NSAIDs may develop.
      (3) Some NSAIDs produce central nervous system (CNS) effects, including impaired mentation, headaches, and attention deficit disorder.
      (4) Leflunomide has been associated with weight loss, alopecia, rash, and anemia. It is classified as a pregnancy category X drug.
      (5) Etanercept has been associated with reactions at the injection site, autoantibody production, and serious infections including sepsis.
      (6) The long-term effects of the COX-2 inhibitors on the CNS, renal, and reproductive system are still uncertain. These drugs are contraindicated in those patients hypersensitive to sulfonamides, aspirin, or NSAIDs. Celecoxib is the only selective COX-2 inhibitor contraindicated in patients with sulfonamide allergy.

5. **Drug interactions.** Salicylates have two clinically significant drug interactions.
   a. **Oral anticoagulants.** Aspirin should be avoided in anticoagulated patients. Aspirin inhibits platelet function and can cause gastric mucosal damage. This significantly increases the risk of bleeding in anticoagulated patients. Also, doses of more than 3 g/day of aspirin produce hypoprothrombinemia. Choline magnesium trisalicylate or acetaminophen should be used if a nonnarcotic is needed in an anticoagulated patient.

b. Methotrexate. Salicylates may enhance the toxicity of methotrexate. The primary mechanism is blockage of methotrexate renal tubular secretion by salicylates. The resultant methotrexate toxicity has been reported as pancytopenia or hepatotoxicity. Salicylates should be avoided in patients receiving methotrexate.

B. Narcotic analgesics include the opioid drugs (Table 56-2). Because of their abuse potential, opioids are classified as controlled drugs. Special regulations control their prescribing.

1. Mechanism of action
   a. Endogenous opiates afford the body self–pain-relieving mechanisms. These endogenous peptides include the endorphins, enkephalins, and dynorphins.
   b. Exogenous opiates are classified as agonists (stimulate opiate receptors), antagonists (displace agonists from opiate receptors), and mixed opiates (agonist–antagonist or partial agonist actions).
   c. Opiate receptors are located in the brain and spinal cord. Several types of opiate receptors have been identified, including μ, κ, δ, σ, and ε.
   d. Stimulation of μ receptors produces the characteristic narcotic (morphine-like) effects.
      (1) Analgesia
      (2) Miosis
      (3) Euphoria
      (4) Respiratory depression
      (5) Sedation
      (6) Physical dependence
      (7) Bradycardia
   e. The specific mechanism (central and spinal) of opiate agonist is alteration of the effects of nociceptive neurotransmitters, possibly norepinephrine or serotonin.

2. Clinical use
   a. Opioid analgesics are used for the management of moderate to severe pain (acute or chronic pain) of somatic or visceral origin.
   b. The use of narcotics should be individualized for each patient. The optimal analgesic dose varies from patient to patient. Each analgesic regimen should be titrated by increasing the dose up to the appearance of limiting adverse effects. Changing to another analgesic should only occur after an adequate therapeutic trial.

Table 56-2. Some Commonly Used Opioid Analgesics (Doses Equivalent to 10 mg IM/SC Morphine*)

Drug	Parenteral Dose (mg)	Oral Dose (mg)	Duration (hr)
Morphine	10	60	4–7
Morphine (CR)	NA	NA	12–24
Hydromorphone	1.3	7.5	4–6
Oxymorphone	1	–	4–6
Levorphanol	2	4	4–7
Methadone	10	20	4–6
Meperidine	75	300	3–6
Fentanyl	0.1	–	1–2
Fentanyl transdermal	NA	NA	48–72
Codeine	130	200	4–6
Hydrocodone*	–	5–10	4–5
Dihydrocodeine*	–	32	4–5
Oxycodone*	–	5–10	4–5
Oxycodone (CR)	–	NA	12–24
Propoxyphene	–	65–100	4–6
Nalbuphine	10	–	4–6
Butorphanol	2	–	4–6
Dezocine	10	–	4–7

*Doses for moderate pain not necessarily equivalent to 10 mg morphine.

CR = controlled release; IM = intramuscular; NA = not applicable; SC = subcutaneous.

c. The appropriate route of administration should be selected for each patient.
   (1) Oral administration is the preferred route, particularly for patients with chronic, stable pain. Controlled-release morphine and oxycodone tablets are available for convenience in controlling continuous pain, particularly in those patients with cancer.
   (2) Intramuscular and subcutaneous administration are very commonly used in the postoperative period. Fluctuations in absorption may occur, particularly in elderly or cachectic patients.
   (3) Intravenous (IV) bolus administration has the most rapid, predictable onset of effect.
   (4) IV infusion is used to titrate pain relief rapidly, particularly in those patients with unstable chronic pain. Morphine is most commonly used, often with supplemental IV bolus doses for breakthrough pain. A mechanical infusion device is necessary.
   (5) IV PCA is most often used for acute postoperative pain. It produces prompt analgesia with minimal side effects because small doses (e.g., 1–2 mg morphine) are delivered at frequent intervals (e.g., every 10 minutes). It allows patient control of pain management. Morphine and meperidine are the most commonly used agents. A mechanical infusion device and properly trained patient and staff are necessary.
   (6) Epidural and **intrathecal administration** are used for acute postoperative pain and early management of chronic cancer pain. All drugs used epidurally or intrathecally must be preservative free because of the neurotoxicity of parabens and benzyl alcohol when administered via these routes. Intrathecal doses are generally 1/10 of the corresponding drug's epidural dose.
      (a) Low opiate doses stimulate spinal opiate receptors and reduce the amount of narcotic reaching the brain. This results in delayed or minimal effects such as sedation, nausea, and respiratory depression. The opiate distribution that causes such effects is dependent on the site of spinal injection, water solubility of the opiate, and volume infused. For example, after lumbar administration of a more water-soluble opiate (morphine), severe respiratory depression can be observed 12–24 hours after initial dosing.
      (b) Local side effects of intrathecal opiate administration are itching and urinary retention. Depending on the opiate used and the type of pain being treated, intermittent doses or continuous infusions (via a mechanical infusion device) can be used (Tables 56-3 and 56-4).
   (7) Rectal administration is an alternative for patients unable to take oral narcotics. Generally, poor absorption results in an unreliable analgesic response. It is an unacceptable route of administration for many patients.
   (8) Transdermal administration is an alternative for patients with chronic pain who are unable to take oral narcotics. A controlled-release patch is available for fentanyl.

Table 56-3. Epidurally Administered Preservative-Free Opioids (Intermittent Dosing)

Drug	Dose (mg)	Onset of Action (min)	Time to Peak Effect (min)	Duration of Action (hr)
Morphine	5–10	25	60	12–24
Fentanyl	0.1	5–10	20	6
Meperidine	50–100	5–10	15–30	7
Hydromorphone	1	10–15	20	12
Buprenorphine	0.3	30	40–60	8–9

Table 56-4. Epidurally Administered Preservative-Free Opioids (Continuous Infusion)

Drug	Initial Bolus Dose (mg)	Infusion Concentration (mg/mL)	Rate (mg/hr)
Morphine	2	0.05–0.25	0.2–1.5
Fentanyl	0.05–0.1	0.005–0.025	0.02–0.15
Meperidine	50–100	10–20	5–20
Hydromorphone	0.5–1	0.02–0.05	0.15–0.3

Slow onset requires additional analgesia when starting treatment. The duration of analgesia is 48–72 hours per patch. A slow reduction of effect follows removal of the patch and requires 24–36 hours of monitoring.

d. Patients who have chronic pain or acute pain that is constant throughout the day should receive regularly scheduled (around-the-clock) doses of narcotics.

(1) Long-acting opiates (e.g., controlled-release morphine and oxycodone) are preferable.

(2) A supplement given as needed may be necessary to manage breakthrough pain, for which short-acting opiates (e.g., immediate-release morphine, hydromorphone) are preferable. If frequent supplements are required, then the around-the-clock regimen should be adjusted based on morphine equivalents (see Table 56-2).

e. Although the analgesia and side effects of opiates are qualitatively similar, individual patients may respond differently. Analgesic selection is based on:

(1) Patient's past analgesia experience

(2) Need for a rapid onset of effect

(3) Preference for a long (or short) duration of action

(4) Preference for a particular mode of delivery

(5) Preference for a particular dosage form

(a) Controlled-release morphine or oxycodone for a long duration of action (8–12 hours) may be preferable to opiates with long half-lives (e.g., methadone, levorphanol), which can accumulate and cause overdose symptoms (e.g., respiratory depression).

(b) Transdermal fentanyl can be used for patients who are unable to swallow.

(c) Rectal suppositories can be used for patients who are unable to swallow. They are available for morphine, hydromorphone, and oxymorphone.

(d) Concentrated hydromorphone injection (10 mg/mL) can be used for cachectic patients who require subcutaneous injections and in those patients whose injection volumes must be minimized.

(6) Individual sensitivity to side effects, which includes nausea, euphoria, sedation, and respiratory depression.

(a) Partial agonists or mixed agonist–antagonists may be preferable for acute pain management in patients at risk for respiratory depression secondary to opiate agonists. These agents should not be used in patients who have received chronic doses of opiates because withdrawal symptoms will occur.

(b) Epidural administration may be preferable for critically ill patients at risk for respiratory depression secondary to systemic narcotic administration.

3. Adverse effects. All narcotics can produce a variety of side effects that range from bothersome to life-threatening.

a. Constipation occurs as a result of decreased intestinal tone and peristalsis. There is a patient variability, but generally most patients experience constipation after several days of therapy. Constipation may be more bothersome with certain types of opiates (e.g., codeine). It may occur sooner and be more problematic in hospitalized or bedridden patients or in patients who have received anesthesia or drugs with anticholinergic effects. Prophylaxis with a laxative/stool softener combination (e.g., bisacodyl/docusate) and dietary counseling are warranted in patients who need chronic opiate therapy.

b. Nausea and **vomiting** occur due to central stimulation of the chemoreceptor trigger zone. It is more problematic with one-time or intermittent parenteral dosing for acute pain. Occasionally, patients require concomitant therapy with an antiemetic (e.g., hydroxyzine, prochlorperazine); however, these agents may add to the sedative effects of opiates.

c. Sedation is a dose-related effect but sometimes is enhanced by concomitant use of other drugs with sedating effects (e.g., benzodiazepines, antiemetics). Most chronic pain patients become tolerant to this effect, but occasionally the addition of a CNS stimulant, such as dextroamphetamine or methylphenidate, is needed. Patients starting therapy with narcotics should be warned about driving or operating machinery. Sedation may be a sign of excessive dosing or accumulation. However, sedation should not be confused with physiological sleep in those patients who have pain control difficulties. Patients in pain often develop insomnia. When pain is brought under control by appropriate narcotic titration, the patient initially may sleep for several hours.

d. Respiratory depression is the most serious adverse effect accompanying narcotic overdose. Respiratory depression may be a sign of an excessive dose, accumulation of long half-lived opiates (e.g., methadone, levorphanol), or accumulation of active morphine metabolites in renal failure patients.

      (1) Respiratory rate should be carefully monitored in patients receiving IV or epidural opiates, in neonates, in elderly patients, and in patients receiving other drugs that cause respiratory depression.

      (2) The opiate antagonist, naloxone, is administered intravenously to reverse life-threatening respiratory depression. Use of naloxone in an opiate-dependent patient (e.g., a chronic cancer pain patient) can precipitate opiate withdrawal.

    e. Anticholinergic effects, such as dry mouth and urinary retention, can be bothersome for some patients.

    f. Hypersensitivity reactions, such as itching due to histamine release, can occur secondary to opiate use, particularly with epidural or intrathecal administration. Wheals sometimes occur at the site of morphine injection. These reactions do not represent true allergy.

    g. CNS excitation, such as myoclonus and other seizure-like activity, can be produced with the use of meperidine in renal failure. These symptoms have also been observed in patients with normal renal functions who receive high doses of meperidine (e.g., more than 800 mg/day of intramuscular meperidine). The accumulation of the metabolite normeperidine is the cause.

4. Drug interactions

    a. Narcotics have additive CNS depressant effects when used in combination with other drugs that also are CNS depressants (e.g., alcohol, anesthetics, antidepressants, antihistamines, barbiturates, benzodiazepines, phenothiazines).

    b. Narcotics, particularly meperidine, can cause severe reactions such as excitation, sweating, rigidity, and hypertension in patients receiving monoamine oxidase (MAO) inhibitors. Meperidine should be avoided and other narcotics started at lower doses in patients being treated with MAO inhibitors.

5. Tolerance means that increasing doses of opiate are needed to maintain analgesia. Tolerance usually develops to the analgesic, sedative, and euphoric effects of opioids, but not to the pupillary-constricting and constipating effects. This is usually observed as a decreasing duration of analgesia in chronic pain patients. The addition of an NSAID may help delay or provide adequate analgesia in tolerant patients.

6. Dependence. The use of opiates for chronic pain may result in physical dependence, such that the abrupt discontinuation of the opiate results in the development of withdrawal symptoms.

    a. Withdrawal symptoms include anxiety, irritability, insomnia, chills, salivation, rhinorrhea, diaphoresis, nausea, vomiting, GI cramping and diarrhea, and piloerection.

      (1) The appearance and intensity of withdrawal symptoms vary according to the half-life of the opiate. For example, the withdrawal symptoms after discontinuation of chronic methadone may take several days to develop and may be less intense as compared to withdrawal from morphine due to its shorter half-life.

      (2) The development of tolerance may be associated with withdrawal symptoms.

      (3) The use of naloxone or a partial agonist–antagonist such as pentazocine in a patient receiving chronic opiate therapy produces acute withdrawal.

    b. The development of physical dependence seen in chronic pain patients is not the same as psychological dependence or addiction. Also, the drug-seeking behavior observed in many acute pain patients (i.e., from postoperative pain) is not a sign of addiction, but rather a need for adequate pain relief. Studies suggest that the addictive rates for long-term treatment of noncancer pain are low in patients without a prior history of addiction. The analgesic needs of this type of patient should be reassessed and usually necessitates increasing the dose of opiate, changing to a longer duration drug, changing to a PCA, or adding an analgesic adjunct.

C. Tramadol is an oral, centrally acting analgesic with weak opiate activity. It has not been placed in a controlled drug schedule.

    1. Mechanism of action

      a. Tramadol is a synthetic aminocyclohexanol that binds to opiate receptors, inhibiting norepinephrine and serotonin.

      b. The analgesic effects are partially antagonized by naloxone.

    2. Clinical use

      a. Tramadol is used for moderate to moderately severe pain.

b. The recommended dosage is 50–100 mg every 4–6 hours, up to a maximum of 400 mg/day.

c. At maximum dosage, tramadol appears no more effective than acetaminophen–codeine combinations.

3. Adverse effects

a. GI effects include nausea, constipation, and dry mouth.

b. CNS effects include dizziness, headache, sedation, and seizures (overdose).

c. Diaphoresis

4. Drug interactions

a. Tramadol can increase the sedative effect of alcohol and hypnotics.

b. Tramadol inhibits monoamine uptake and should not be used with MAO inhibitors.

c. Tramadol used with SSRIs and other agents that increase serotonergic activity can cause "serotonin syndrome," which is characterized by irritability, anxiety, CNS excitation, and myoclonus.

D. Miscellaneous agents

1. Capsaicin, a component of red peppers, causes the release of substance P from sensory nerve fibers, resulting in prolonged cutaneous pain transmission, histamine release, and erythema because of reflex vasodilation. Repeated local application depletes the peripheral sensory C-nerve fiber of substance P, resulting in pain inhibition. Topical capsaicin cream 0.025% or 0.075% has been shown to be useful in treating joint pain and tenderness in patients with arthritis. Other uses may include treating diabetic neuralgia, reflex sympathetic dystrophy, trigeminal neuralgia, notalgia paresthetica, psoriasis and psoralen (P) and long-wave ultraviolet radiation (UVA)-induced skin pain, and postherpetic neuralgia. Local toxicity may include burning, stinging, erythema, pruritus, and superficial skin ulcers.

2. Glucosamine sulfate and chondroitin sulfate have been used with increasing frequency in the treatment of degenerative joint disease. Glucosamine sulfate appears to act as a substrate for and stimulant to the biosynthesis of glucosaminoglycans and hyalouronic acid for forming proteoglycans found in the structural matrix of joints. Chondroitin sulfate provides additional substrates for the formation of healthy joint matrix. Short-term side effects associated with glucosamine include GI problems, drowsiness, skin reactions, and headache. Further research is needed to validate their roles.

E. Analgesic adjuncts. Other classes of drugs affect nonopiate pain pathways and may be useful in certain types of pain (e.g., neurogenic pain). These drugs often are used with other analgesics, and some may help manage narcotic side effects (Table 56-5).

Table 56-5. Analgesic Adjuncts

Class	Drugs	Indications
Tricyclic antidepressants	Amitriptyline, desipramine, doxepin, imipramine	Neurogenic pain; chronic pain complicated by depression or insomnia
Anticonvulsants	Carbamazepine, clonazepam, phenytoin, valproate, gabapentin	Lancinating neurogenic pain (e.g., trigeminal neuralgia, phantom limb pain, posttrauma neurogenic pain)
Neuroleptics	Fluphenazine, haloperidol, prochlorperazine	Refractory neurogenic pain; pain complicated by delirium or nausea (prochlorperazine)
Corticosteroid	Dexamethasone	Pain from neural infiltration; pain associated with bony metastases
Antihistamine	Hydroxyzine	Pain complicated by anxiety or nausea
Benzodiazepines	Alprazolam, lorazepam	Pain complicated by anxiety or muscle spasm
Amphetamines	Dextroamphetamine, methylphenidate	For excessive opiate-induced sedation in chronic pain patients

F. Nonpharmacological pain management. Other therapeutic modalities for pain management include cognitive behavioral interventions and physical methods. These modalities are appropriate for interested patients, patients experiencing anxiety with their pain, patients who have incomplete relief from analgesic therapy, and patients who need to avoid or reduce analgesic use (e.g., those with chronic nonmalignant pain).

1. **Cognitive behavioral interventions** include education and instruction, simple relaxation, biofeedback, and hypnosis.

2. **Physical methods** include acupuncture, physical therapy, compression gloves, orthotic devices, heat and cold applications, massage, exercise, rest, immobilization, and transcutaneous electrical nerve stimulation (TENS).

STUDY QUESTIONS

Directions: Each of the numbered items or incomplete statements in this section is followed by answers or by completions of the statement. Select the **one** lettered answer or completion that is **best** in each case.

1. An emaciated 69-year-old man with advanced inoperable throat cancer is hospitalized for pain management. He is receiving a morphine solution (40 mg orally) every 3 hours for pain. He complains of dysphagia and the frequency with which he must take morphine. An appropriate analgesic alternative for this patient would be

(A) changing to a controlled-release oral morphine
(B) increasing the dose of the oral morphine solution
(C) changing to intramuscular methadone
(D) changing to transdermal fentanyl
(E) decreasing the frequency of oral morphine administration

Questions 2 and 3
A 52-year-old woman with a diagnosis of ovarian cancer presents with complaints of pain. Her pain was reasonably well-controlled with two capsules of oxycodone every 4 hours until 2 weeks ago, at which point she was hospitalized for pain control. She was placed on meperidine (75 mg) every 3 hours but still complained about pain. Her meperidine dosage was increased to 100 mg every 2 hours.

2. At this dosage of meperidine, the patient is likely to experience

(A) excellent pain relief
(B) respiratory depression
(C) worsening renal function
(D) myoclonic seizures
(E) excessive sedation

3. An appropriate next step in this patient's therapy would be to

(A) add a nonsteroidal anti-inflammatory drug (NSAID)
(B) discontinue the meperidine and convert her to a controlled-release oral morphine or oxycodone
(C) continue the present meperidine dosage because she will eventually get relief
(D) decrease the meperidine dose to avoid side effects
(E) consider hypnosis or relaxation techniques

4. A 20-year-old victim of a motor vehicle accident is 3 days postsurgery for orthopedic and internal injuries. He has been in severe pain and was placed on a regimen of intramuscular morphine (5–10 mg) every 4 hours as needed for pain. A pain consultant starts the patient with a 20-mg intravenous morphine loading dose and then begins a continuous intravenous morphine infusion with as-needed morphine boosters. Two hours after this regimen is started, the patient is asleep. The nurse is concerned and calls the physician. The physician should

(A) call for a psychiatric consult
(B) administer naloxone
(C) examine the patient and reconfirm the dosage and monitoring parameters
(D) add an injectable nonsteroidal anti-inflammatory drug (NSAID)
(E) add an amphetamine

5. Potential adverse effects associated with aspirin include all of the following EXCEPT

(A) gastrointestinal ulceration
(B) renal dysfunction
(C) enhanced methotrexate toxicity
(D) cardiac arrhythmias
(E) hypersensitivity asthma

6. All of the following facts are true about non-steroidal anti-inflammatory drugs (NSAIDs) EXCEPT

(A) they are antipyretic
(B) there is a ceiling effect to their analgesia
(C) they can cause tolerance
(D) they do not cause dependence
(E) they are anti-inflammatory

7. Which of the following narcotics has the longest duration of effect?

(A) Methadone
(B) Controlled-release morphine
(C) Levorphanol
(D) Transdermal fentanyl
(E) Dihydromorphone

Directions: The questions below contain three suggested answers, of which **one or more** is correct. Choose the answer

A	if **I only** is correct
B	if **III only** is correct
C	if **I and II** are correct
D	if **II and III** are correct
E	if **I, II, and III** are correct

8. Agents that are safe to use in a patient with bleeding problems include

I. choline magnesium trisalicylate
II. acetaminophen
III. ketorolac

9. Cyclooxygenase-2 selective inhibitors block the following:

I. Production of cytoprotective prostaglandins
II. Tumor-necrosis factor-α
III. Production of prostaglandins responsible for pain and inflammation

10. Leflunomide has been associated with

I. diarrhea
II. alopecia
III. anemia

ANSWERS AND EXPLANATIONS

1. The answer is D *[II B 2 c (8)]*.
Patients with throat cancer often cannot take oral analgesics. The patient described in the question is also having pain difficulties with an every–3-hour regimen. Transdermal fentanyl is a good alternative because, after titration, excellent analgesia can be produced without using oral or parenteral agents. Also, the frequency of analgesic use may be decreased when titration has occurred.

2–3. The answers are: 2-D *[II B 3 g]*, **3-B** *[II B 2 c (1), d (1)]*.
Myoclonic seizures can occur after frequent, high-dose meperidine due to the accumulation of the metabolite, normeperidine. Both oxycodone and meperidine have short durations of effect. In the chronic pain patient, an around-the-clock regimen, using a controlled-released oral morphine, would be an appropriate alternative. With titration, the patient should have good pain relief with an every 8- to 12-hour regimen.

4. The answer is C *[II B 3 c]*.
A patient suffering from pain cannot sleep properly. When the pain is adequately controlled, the patient may sleep initially for many hours. This usually is not oversedation due to the narcotic. These patients should be monitored closely (e.g., respiratory rate), and other sedating drugs should be eliminated. Usually, no other intervention is needed.

5. The answer is D *[II A 4]*.
Aspirin has several adverse effects and drug interactions. However, cardiac arrhythmias are not induced by aspirin.

6. The answer is C *[II A 2]*.
Unlike the opiates, nonsteroidal anti-inflammatory drug (NSAID) use is not associated with the development of tolerance.

7. The answer is D *[Table 56-2]*.
Transdermal fentanyl is a controlled-release dosage form that is effective for up to a 72-hour period. All of the other drugs listed in the question are effective for periods of 1–8 hours.

8. The answer is C (I, II) *[II A 4 b]*.
Unlike aspirin and nonsteroidal anti-inflammatory drugs (NSAIDs), acetaminophen and choline magnesium trisalicylate lack antiplatelet effects. Therefore, they are safe to use for patients with bleeding problems.

9. The answer is B (III) *[II A 1]*.
Cyclooxygenase (COX)-2 selective inhibitors by definition selectively block prostaglandins responsible for pain and inflammation. They cause fewer gastrointestinal problems than nonselective nonsteroidal anti-inflammatory drugs (NSAIDs) because they are believed not to block COX-1, which protects the stomach lining.

10. The answer is E (all) *[II A 4 a, d 4]*.
Leflunomide has been associated with weight loss, diarrhea, nausea, alopecia, rash, anemia, and transient elevations in liver function tests.

57
Nutrition and the Hospitalized Patient

Robert A. Quercia
Kevin P. Keating
Maria Evasovich

I. NUTRITIONAL PROBLEMS IN HOSPITALIZED PATIENTS

A. Incidence. It has been estimated that 30%–50% of patients admitted to hospitals have some degree of malnutrition. As many as 75% of patients undergo a deterioration of nutritional status while hospitalized.

B. Definitions

1. **Malnutrition** is a pathological state, resulting from a relative or absolute deficiency or excess of one or more essential nutrients.

2. **Marasmus** is a chronic disease that develops over months or years as a result of a deficiency in total caloric intake. Depletion of fat stores and skeletal protein occurs to meet metabolic needs. Marasmic patients are generally not hypermetabolic and are able to preserve their visceral protein compartment as determined by measurements of serum albumin, prealbumin, and transferrin.
   a. Marasmus is a well-adapted form of malnutrition, and despite a cachectic appearance, immunocompetence, wound healing, and the ability to handle short-term stress are generally well preserved.
   b. Nutritional support in these patients should be initiated cautiously because aggressive repletion can result in severe metabolic disturbances, such as hypokalemia and hypophosphatemia.

3. **Kwashiorkor** is an acute process that can develop within weeks and is associated with visceral protein depletion and impaired immune function. It is due to poor protein intake with adequate to slightly inadequate caloric intake; thus, patients usually appear well nourished. A hypermetabolic state (e.g., trauma, infection) combined with protein deprivation can rapidly develop into a severe kwashiorkor malnutrition characterized by hypoalbuminemia, edema, and impaired cellular immune function.
   a. In hospitalized patients, the development of kwashiorkor has been implicated in poor wound healing, gastrointestinal (GI) bleeding, and sepsis.
   b. Aggressive nutritional support to replete protein stores and decrease morbidity and mortality is indicated when the diagnosis of kwashiorkor is made.

4. **Mixed marasmic kwashiorkor** is a severe form of protein–calorie malnutrition that usually develops when a marasmic patient is subjected to an acute hypermetabolic stress, such as trauma, surgery, or infection.
   a. This condition results in depletion of fat stores, skeletal muscle protein, and visceral protein.
   b. Because of the marked immune dysfunction that develops in this state, vigorous nutritional support is indicated.

II. NUTRITIONAL ASSESSMENT AND METABOLIC REQUIREMENTS

A. Nutritional assessment. The most commonly used tools for nutritional assessment are discussed below.

1. **Subjective global assessment (SGA)** relies heavily on the patient's history.
   a. SGA takes into account:
      (1) Recent weight change

(2) Diet history

(3) Type and length of symptoms affecting nutritional status (e.g., nausea, vomiting, diarrhea)

(4) Functional status

(5) Metabolic demands of the current disease process

(6) Gross physical signs

(a) Status of subcutaneous fat

(b) Evidence of muscle wasting

(c) Presence or absence of edema and ascites

b. Patients are then classified as being well nourished or moderately or severely malnourished.

2. Prognostic nutritional index (PNI) is derived from a formula that attempts to quantify a patient's risk of developing operative complications based on a variety of markers of nutritional status.

$$PNI(\%) = 158 - 16.6\,(ALB) - 0.78\,(TSF) - 0.20\,(TFN) - 5.8\,(DH)$$

where ALB is the serum albumin (g/dl); TSF is the triceps skin-fold thickness (mm); TFN is the serum transferrin (mg/dl); and DH is the delayed hypersensitivity skin-test reactivity graded 0 (nonreactive), 1 (<5 mm induration), or 2 ($\geq$5 mm induration).

a. Predicted risk of complications: low risk (PNI <40%), intermediate risk (PNI = 40%–49%), high risk (PNI $\geq$50%)

b. Serum markers (i.e., albumin, transferrin) are indicators of visceral protein status.

c. Delayed hypersensitivity reaction is an indicator of immune competence.

d. PNI is of value in predicting the potential for complications in stable patients scheduled to undergo elective surgery.

3. Body composition analysis assesses nutritional status by measuring and comparing the ratios of various body compartments.

a. Bioelectrical impedance. The resistance to an electrical current is used to calculate lean body mass. The equipment is relatively inexpensive and easy to use. The results are inaccurate in critically ill patients and patients with fluid and electrolyte abnormalities.

b. Dual energy x-ray absorptiometry. The differential attenuation of x-rays is used to measure fat and lean body mass. The equipment is expensive, and results are affected by hydration status.

c. Total body potassium estimates lean body mass by using a whole body counter to measure a potassium isotope concentrated in lean tissue. This method of body composition analysis is impractical and available at only a few centers.

d. Total body water estimates lean body mass from deuterium total body water measurements. This technique is clinically impractical.

e. In vivo neutron activation analysis. Unlike other techniques, this analysis divides the body into several compartments. This technique requires a significant dose of radiation and is available at only a few research centers.

4. Tests of physiological function attempt to quantitate malnutrition based on the decrease in muscle strength caused by amino acid mobilization.

a. Maximum voluntary grip strength is measured with isokinetic dynamometry. The results correlate well to total body protein. This test requires patient cooperation.

b. Electrical stimulation of the ulnar nerve measures contractile function of the adductor pollicis muscle. This technique does not require voluntary patient effort and is inexpensive and easy to do. Its prognostic reliability is still under evaluation.

B. Metabolic requirements

1. Energy requirements are determined as **nonprotein calories (NPCs).** It is important to avoid excess calories to minimize complications of nutrient delivery and to optimize nutrient metabolism. Energy requirements can be determined by the following three methods.

a. Indirect calorimetry or measured energy expenditure (MEE) is the most accurate method of determining caloric requirements. Oxygen (O_2) consumption and carbon dioxide (CO_2) production are measured directly. Energy expenditure is related directly to oxygen consumption and is calculated from these measurements. A respiratory quotient (RQ) can also be obtained from an MEE and is defined as the ratio of the amount of CO_2 produced to that of O_2 consumed during the course of oxidation of body fuels.

The oxidation of carbohydrate results in an RQ of 1.0; that is, as much CO_2 is produced as O_2 is consumed. The oxidation of fat produces significantly less CO_2 and results in an RQ of 0.7. Normal mixed substrate oxidation results in an RQ of 0.8–0.9. The provision of excess carbohydrate calories causes their conversion to fat (lipogenesis). Lipogenesis produces significantly more carbon dioxide than oxidation does. This can result in an RQ >1.0, which is consistent with overfeeding. The determination of RQ can, therefore, indicate patterns of substrate utilization.

  b. Estimated energy expenditure (EEE) first requires the calculation of the **basal energy expenditure (BEE)** from the **Harris-Benedict equation;** the BEE is then multiplied by appropriate stress and activity factors.
  (1) Men: BEE = 66.5 + [13.8 x wt (kg)] + [5 x ht (cm)] − [6.8 x age (years)]
  (2) Women: BEE = 655 + [9.6 x wt (kg)] + [1.8 x ht (cm)] − [4.7 x age (years)]
  (3) Stress factors: uncomplicated surgery 1.00–1.05, peritonitis 1.05–1.25, and sepsis or multiple trauma 1.25–1.5
  (4) Activity factors: bed rest 0.95–1.10 and ambulation 1.10–1.30
  c. Simple nomogram. The least accurate method of estimating caloric requirements, this technique is based on the patient's weight in kilograms. It is useful when the other methods cannot be used. Patients with mild to moderate degrees of stress require approximately 25–30 kcal/kg/day, whereas the severely stressed patient (e.g., a patient with major burns) may require 35 kcal/kg/day or more.

2. **Protein (nitrogen) requirements** can be determined by a number of techniques, but nitrogen balance determinations and nomograms appear to be the most practical.
  a. Nitrogen balance techniques. The practitioner determines the patient's nitrogen output and develops a nutritional support program in which the protein administered results in a nitrogen input that exceeds losses.
  (1) Nitrogen balance = 24-hour nitrogen intake − 24-hour nitrogen output.
  (2) A 24-hour nitrogen intake = 24-hour total protein intake, divided by 6.25 (approximately 16% of protein is comprised of nitrogen).
  (3) A 24-hour nitrogen output = [24-hour urine urea nitrogen (UUN) x 1.25] + 2, where 1.25 accounts for nonurea urine nitrogen losses (e.g., ammonia, creatinine) and 2 accounts for nonurine nitrogen losses (e.g., skin, feces). Total urinary nitrogen (TUN) determinations are currently available in some centers. Because TUN is a more accurate method of assessing urinary nitrogen losses, it should be used when available in place of a 24-hour UUN x 1.25 when calculating a nitrogen balance.
  (4) A positive nitrogen balance of 3–6 g is the goal.
  (5) This method cannot be used in renally impaired patients.
  b. Nomogram method. This method estimates protein needs based on lean body weight. Protein requirements are 1.5–2.0 g protein/kg/day for hospitalized patients.
  c. Nonprotein calorie to nitrogen (NPC:N) ratio. An NPC:N ratio of 125–150:1 generally has been recommended for the mildly to moderately stressed patient to achieve optimal nitrogen retention and protein synthesis. In the severely stressed patient, some studies indicate that ratios as low as 85:1 may be effective.

3. **Essential fatty acids (EFAs)** are those polyunsaturated fatty acids that cannot be synthesized by humans. EFAs affect immune responses by influencing energy production, eicosanoid synthesis, and cell membrane fluidity. They also affect levels of arachidonic acid in lymphycytes [especially monocytes, macrophages, and polymorphonuclear neutrophils (PMNs)]. Linoleic acid, an omega-6 polyunsaturated fatty acid (PUFA), is the principal EFA for humans. α-Linolenic acid, an omega-3 PUFA, also cannot be synthesized in vivo; its metabolic significance in humans continues to be investigated. It might be a conditionally essential fatty acid.
  a. Deficiency states of **linoleic acid** are characterized by diarrhea, dermatitis, and hair loss.
  b. The currently available lipid emulsions have a high linoleic acid content.
  c. Providing 4%–7% of a patient's caloric requirements as linoleic acid from lipid emulsion prevents the development of essential fatty acid deficiency.

4. **Vitamins** are essential for proper substrate metabolism. Accepted daily allowances for oral administration have been established, but there is no consensus on recommendations for intravenous (IV) administration.
  a. Vitamin A (fat soluble). Normal stores can last up to a year but are rapidly depleted by stress. Vitamin A has essential functions in vision, growth, and reproduction. Recommended oral intake is 2500–5000 IU/day. IV requirements are 2800–8000 IU/day secondary to binding of the IV form to glass and plastic.

b. Vitamin D (fat soluble). In conjunction with parathormone and calcitonin, vitamin D helps to regulate calcium and phosphorous homeostasis. Recommended intake is 100–400 IU/day. IV requirements are 200–400 IU/day.

c. Vitamin E (fat soluble) appears to function as an antioxidant, inhibiting the oxidation of free unsaturated fatty acids. Recommended daily oral allowances are 12–15 IU/day. Suggested IV requirements are 2.1–60 IU/day. The presence of polyunsaturated fatty acids increases the requirement for vitamin E, which needs to be considered with the use of lipid system parenteral nutrition (PN).

d. Vitamin K (fat soluble) plays an essential role in the synthesis of clotting factors. The suggested oral intake is 0.7–2.0 mg/day.

e. Vitamin B_1 (thiamine) [water soluble] functions as a coenzyme in the phosphogluconate pathway and as a structural component of nervous system membranes. The development of its deficiency state (i.e., acute pernicious beriberi with high output cardiac failure) is well described in patients on PN receiving inadequate thiamine replacement. A prolonged deficiency state can cause Wernicke's encephalopathy. Recommended doses are 0.5 mg/1000 oral calories/day and 3–21 mg/day in PN.

f. Vitamin B_2 (riboflavin) [water soluble] functions as a coenzyme in oxidative phosphorylation. Essentially, no intracellular stores are maintained. Oral requirements are 1.3–1.7 mg/day. IV requirements are 3.6–7.5 mg/day.

g. Vitamin B_3 (niacin) [water soluble] functions as a coenzyme in oxidative phosphorylation and biosynthetic pathways. Pellagra is the well-described deficiency state. Oral requirements are 14.5–19.8 mg/day. IV requirements are 40–140 mg/day.

h. Vitamin B_5 (pantothenic acid) [water soluble]. The functional form of vitamin B_5 is coenzyme A, which is essential to all acylation reactions. Oral requirements are 5–10 mg/day. IV requirements are 10–29 mg/day.

i. Vitamin B_6 (pyridoxine) [water soluble] functions as a coenzyme in a variety of enzymatic pathways. Deficiency states are accentuated by some medications, including isoniazid, penicillamine, and cycloserine. Oral requirements are 1.5–2.0 mg/day. IV requirements are 4.0–6.3 mg/day.

j. Vitamin B_7 (biotin) [water soluble] functions in carboxylation reactions. It is synthesized by intestinal flora; therefore, deficiency states are rare. IV requirements are 60 mg/day.

k. Vitamin B_9 (folic acid) [water-soluble] is involved in a variety of biosynthetic reactions and amino acid conversions. Folate cofactors are necessary for purine and pyrimidine (DNA) synthesis. Stores usually last 3–6 months; however, rapid depletion is seen with metabolic stress. Deficiency of vitamin B_{12} causes deficiency in folate. A megaloblastic anemia is classic in the deficiency state. Deficiency of folic acid in a pregnant mother can cause neural tube defects in the fetus. Oral requirements are 200–400 μg/day. For pregnant women, the daily recommended dose is 600 μg/day.

l. Vitamin B_{12} (cyanocobalamin) [water soluble] has a variety of metabolic and biosynthetic functions. Because of large stores, deficiency states can take years to develop. Megaloblastic (pernicious) anemia is one manifestation of deficiency. Another manifestation of deficiency is peripheral neuropathy because B_{12} is responsible for biosynthesis of the insulation sheet on nerves called myelin. Oral requirements are 2 μg/day. IV requirements are 0.5–1.0 μg/day.

5. Trace mineral deficiency may develop during PN because of reduced intake, increased use, decreased plasma binding, or increased excretion.

a. Iron is necessary for hemoglobin and myoglobin production and is a necessary cofactor in a variety of enzymatic reactions. Deficiency is classically demonstrated by a hypochromic, microcytic anemia as well as by the development of immune deficiency. Oral requirements are 16–18 mg/day. IV requirements are 0.5–1.0 mg/day.

b. Zinc is necessary for DNA and RNA synthesis and is a necessary cofactor in a variety of enzymatic reactions. Zinc deficiency results in impaired wound healing, growth retardation, hair loss, dermatitis, diarrhea, anorexia, and glucose intolerance. Patients at high risk for developing zinc deficiency are those with long-term steroid therapy, malabsorption syndromes, fistulas, sepsis, and major surgery. Oral requirements are 10–15 mg/day. IV requirements are 2.5–4.0 mg/day.

c. Copper is necessary for heme synthesis, electron transport, and wound healing. Deficiency that develops during PN usually manifests as anemia, leukopenia, and neutropenia. Oral requirements are 30 μg/kg/day. IV requirements are 20 μg/kg/day (0.5–1.5 mg/day).

d. Manganese is involved in protein synthesis and possibly glucose use. Oral requirements are 0.7–22 mg/day. IV requirements are 2–10 μg/kg/day (0.1–0.8 mg/day).

e. **Selenium** is important in antioxidant reactions. Deficiency during PN has been associated with muscle pain and cardiomyopathy. IV requirements are 20–40 μg/day.

f. **Iodine** is a component of the thyroid hormones. Deficiency manifests as a goiter. Recommended intake is 1 μg/kg/day.

g. **Chromium** is important in glucose use and potentiates the effect of insulin. Signs of deficiency include hyperglycemia and abnormal glucose tolerance. Oral requirements are 70–80 μg/day. IV requirements are 0.14–0.2 μg/kg/day (10–15 μg/day).

h. **Molybdenum** is essential to xanthine oxidase. Oral requirements are 2.0 μg/kg/day.

III. METHODS OF SUPPORT

A. PN is also called **total parenteral nutrition (TPN)** and **hyperalimentation.** It is used to meet the patient's nutritional requirements when the enteral route cannot accomplish this.

1. **Indications.** When the enteral route cannot be used because of dysfunction or disease states (e.g., acute pancreatitis, inflammatory bowel disease, complete bowel obstruction), PN is instituted.

2. **Initiation** of PN should be undertaken within 1–3 days in moderately to severely malnourished patients when the inadequacy of enteral support is anticipated for more than 5–7 days. In healthy or mildly malnourished patients, PN should be initiated within 5–7 days if enteral support has not been initiated.

3. **Routes of administration**
   a. **A central venous route** is used with hypertonic PN formulations (i.e., dextrose concentrations greater than 10%). Most commonly, dextrose concentrations of 25% are used centrally, and the osmolarity exceeds 2000 mOsm/L. Such highly osmolar solutions must be infused into a large-diameter central vein (e.g., superior vena cava), where they are rapidly diluted by high flow rates.
   b. **A peripheral venous route** can be used when the dextrose concentration is 10% or less. Solutions with 10% dextrose, amino acids, electrolytes, and trace minerals have a resulting osmolarity of 900–1000 mOsm/L. Higher osmolarity is associated with a higher incidence of thrombophlebitis. The major reason for use of the central venous PN rather than the peripheral route is the development of thrombophlebitis. Maintaining the osmolality of the peripheral PN solution below 900 mOsm/kg and preferably between 600 and 800 mOsm/kg with intravenous lipid emulsion administered concurrently over 24 hours minimizes the incidence of thrombophlebitis. Also, the development of new peripheral fine-bore catheters made from polyurethane or silicone has been shown to be significantly less thrombogenic. In addition, the use of low-dose heparin (1 unit/mL) and hydrocortisone (5 mg/L) delivered in the PN solutions has been shown to protect against thrombophlebitis. Recently, glyceryl trinitrate patches (5 mg), when applied over the area where the tip of the catheter is expected to lie, have been shown to significantly reduce peripheral PN infusion failure caused by phlebitis. With the use of this new catheter technology and new techniques for infusion, it is now feasible to administer peripheral PN in selected patients for short-term therapy (7–10 days) with a low incidence of peripheral vein thrombophlebitis.

4. **NPC sources**
   a. **Dextrose monohydrate** is the form of dextrose used for parenteral administration. It yields 3.4 kcal/g. It is the component in PN formulas that contributes the most to osmolarity. It is available commercially in concentrations up to 70%.
   b. **IV lipids** are commercially available as 10% or 20% emulsions derived from soybean oil (Intralipid) or a combination of soybean oil and safflower oil (Liposyn II).
      (1) Both the 10% and 20% emulsions are isotonic (280 and 340 mOsm/L, respectively) and can be administered via the peripheral vein with a low incidence of phlebitis; these emulsions provide 1.1 and 2.0 kcal/mL, respectively. They contain 1.2% egg yolk phospholipids as the emulsifying agent and 2.25%–2.5% glycerol to make the emulsions isosmotic.
      (2) Lipid emulsions can be given as part of the daily NPC requirement or 2–3 times per week to prevent essential fatty acid deficiency. Both types of lipid emulsion contain particles of 0.4–0.5 μm, which prevents the use of 0.22 μm bacterial retention filters.

5. **Protein (nitrogen) source. Synthetic crystalline amino acids** are currently used as the nitrogen source in PN formulations.
   a. These formulations are available commercially in concentrations of 3.5%, 5.5%, 7%, 8.5%, 10%, 11.4%, and 15%.
   b. These formulations yield 4 kcal/g.
   c. These solutions generally contain a mixture of free essential and nonessential L-amino acids.
   d. Specialized amino acid formulations are available for specific disease states.

6. **Systems of PN**
   a. **Glucose system PN**
      (1) **Definition.** The glucose system PN is a parenteral formulation in which dextrose is used exclusively as the NPC source. Nitrogen is provided as crystalline amino acids. Electrolytes, vitamins, and trace minerals are added to the formulation as needed.
      (2) **Administration.** The glucose system PN formulations usually have dextrose concentrations of 25% or greater and must be administered by the central venous route. These formulations are also referred to as two-in-one formulations because the dextrose and amino acids are usually mixed in one container with electrolytes, vitamins, and trace minerals.
         (a) Because of the high dextrose concentration, initial administration should be at low hourly rates (e.g., 50 mL/hr) and increased gradually over 24 hours to avoid hyperglycemia (>200 mg/dl).
         (b) To avoid reactive hypoglycemia (<70 mg/dl), discontinuation should be gradual over several hours.
         (c) Lipid emulsions should be administered for **essential fatty acid replacement** in a dose that provides 4%–7% of required calories as linoleic acid. This can be accomplished by the administration of 250 mL of 20% or 500 mL of 10% emulsion, two to three times weekly.
   b. **Lipid system PN**
      (1) **Definition.** The lipid system PN is a parenteral formulation in which lipid is administered daily to provide a substantial proportion of the NPC. Nitrogen is provided as crystalline amino acids. Electrolytes, vitamins, and trace minerals are added to the formulation as needed.
      (2) **Administration.** The lipid system PN is administered peripherally when the dextrose concentration is less than or equal to 10% and centrally when the dextrose concentration is more than 10%.
         (a) **Piggyback method.** The solution with amino acids, dextrose, electrolytes, trace minerals, and vitamins is infused concurrently with a separate bottle of lipid emulsion through a Y site on the intravenous administration set.
         (b) **Total nutrient admixture method** (TNA, three-in-one, all-in-one). Lipids, amino acids, dextrose, electrolytes, trace minerals, and vitamins are mixed in one container and administered by the central or peripheral route, depending on dextrose concentration.
            (i) **Advantages** include simplification of administration and decreased training time for home PN patients.
            (ii) **Disadvantages** include the inability to inspect for particulate matter in the opaque admixture, the inability to use 0.22-μm bacterial retention filters, and stability problems.
            (iii) Because the presence of lipid emulsion in TNAs obscures the presence of a precipitate and may present a life-threatening hazard to patients, the Food and Drug Administration (FDA) suggests that the piggyback method be used to administer lipid emulsion. If a TNA is deemed medically necessary, then specific admixture guidelines recommended by the FDA should be followed. Also, a particle filter (i.e., 1.2 micron) should be used with TNA administration.
         (c) **Lipid dosage**
            (i) Lipid calories should not exceed 60% of total daily calories, including protein calories.
            (ii) Maximum dosage of lipids for adults is 2.5 g/kg/day.
            (iii) Baseline and weekly serum triglycerides must be monitored in patients on lipid system PN.

(3) Adverse effects of lipids are uncommon. The most frequent adverse effects include fever, chills, sensation of warmth, chest pain, back pain, vomiting, and urticaria (overall incidence less than 1%). Severe hypoxemia has been reported with rapid infusion of lipid emulsion.

7. Additives

a. Electrolytes. PN formulations must include adequate amounts of sodium, magnesium, calcium, chloride, potassium, phosphorus, and acetate. The intracellular "anabolic" electrolytes—potassium, magnesium, and phosphate—are essential for protein synthesis. Requirements vary widely, depending on a patient's fluid and electrolyte losses; renal, hepatic, and endocrine status; acid–base balance; metabolic rate; and type of PN formula used. The electrolyte composition of the PN formula must be adjusted to meet the needs of the individual patient.

b. Vitamins and trace minerals. Vitamins are usually added to PN solutions in the form of commercially available multivitamin preparations. Currently, there are two multiple vitamins for infusion formulas available (MVI-12, Infuvite Adult). MVI-12 meets the guidelines of the National Advisory Group of the American Medical Association (NAG-AMA). Infuvite Adult meets the newly amended requirements of the FDA for adult parenteral multivitamins. The new FDA requirements are based on the prior multivitamin formulation recommended by the NAG-AMA but with increased dosages of vitamins B_1, B_6, C, and folic acid and the addition of vitamin K. Because of stability problems, one vial of MVI-12 contains vitamins A, D, E, B_1, B_2, B_3, B_5, B_6, and C. Infuvite Adult contains the same vitamins in one vial plus vitamin K. The second vial for both preparations contains vitamins B_{12}, biotin, and folic acid. Trace minerals may be added individually or as a commercially available multielement preparation. Precise requirements for trace minerals have yet to be determined.

c. Insulin may be required for patients receiving PN formulations (especially glucose system PN) to maintain blood glucose levels less than 200 mg/dl. If insulin is required, it is best provided by the addition of an appropriate amount of regular insulin to the PN formulation at the time of admixture. Although a small amount of insulin (5–10 units per bag) may be adsorbed to the container and tubing, such losses can be overcome by appropriate titration of the dose. The addition of insulin to the PN formulation has the advantage of changes in the rate of PN infusion being automatically accompanied by appropriate changes in the rate of insulin infusion.

d. Miscellaneous drugs. A number of medications have been successfully admixed with PN formulations for continuous infusion. The H_2-receptor antagonists are the most common drugs used in this way. The routine addition of medications to PN formulations remains controversial because of:

(1) Questions of stability over the wide range of PN component concentrations

(2) Possible **therapeutic inadequacy** or toxicity secondary to PN rate changes and loss of peak and trough levels

(3) Increased **potential for waste** with dose changes

8. Complications with the use of PN can be serious and potentially life-threatening but can be avoided by careful management. Complications can be divided into mechanical, infectious, and metabolic.

a. Mechanical complications generally relate to the central venous catheter or its placement and include pneumothorax, catheter occlusion, and venous thrombosis.

b. Infectious complications usually are related to the central venous catheter. This line-related sepsis is secondary to multiple catheter manipulations, contamination during insertion, or contamination during routine maintenance. Hyperglycemia and IV lipids also have been implicated. Maintaining blood sugars less than 200 mg/dl has been shown to significantly reduce septic complications in certain subsets of patients.

c. Metabolic complications are the most common. These include hyperglycemia, hypoglycemia, hypokalemia, hypomagnesemia, hypophosphatemia, metabolic acidosis, respiratory acidosis, prerenal azotemia, and zinc deficiency. A transient self-limited hepatic dysfunction is also seen with long-term PN.

B. Enteral nutrition (EN). Use of the GI tract to achieve total nutritional support or partial support in combination with the parenteral route should be attempted whenever possible in the face of inadequate oral intake. Theoretical advantages include maintenance of normal digestion, absorption, and gut mucosal barrier function.

1. **Contraindications** to EN include complete intestinal obstruction, high-output intestinal fistulas, severe acute pancreatitis, severe acute inflammatory bowel disease, and severe diarrhea.

2. **Routes of administration.** Tube feedings can be administered via nasogastric, nasoduodenal, nasojejunal, gastrostomy, and jejunostomy tubes.

3. **EN formulations** can be classified as being standard (complete) or modular.
   a. **Standard formulas** generally contain carbohydrates, fats, vitamins, trace minerals, and a nitrogen source. They are further classified according to their nitrogen source.
      (1) **Monomeric** formulas contain crystalline amino acids as their nitrogen source. These formulas are usually marketed commercially for specific indications (e.g., ileus, pancreatitis, hepatic coma).
      (2) **Short-chain peptide** formulas contain di- and tripeptides from hydrolyzed protein or de novo synthesis as their nitrogen source. They are currently marketed for the metabolically stressed patient.
      (3) **Polymeric** formulas contain either intact proteins or protein hydrolysates as their nitrogen source. Most patients can be managed with these formulas.
   b. **Modular formulas** consist of separate modules of specific nutrients that can be combined or administered separately. They are used for supplemental use or to custom design an EN formula to meet a specific clinical situation.
      (1) **Carbohydrate** modules differ in the type of carbohydrate present (e.g., polysaccharides, disaccharides, monosaccharides).
      (2) **Protein** modules contain either intact protein, hydrolyzed protein, or crystalline amino acids.
      (3) **Fat** modules contain either long-chain triglycerides (LCTs) prepared from vegetable oils or medium-chain triglycerides (MCTs) prepared from coconut oil. MCTs are more water soluble and more easily absorbed than LCTs. (Bypassing the intestinal lacteal and lymphatic system, MCTs are transported directly to the portal system.) MCTs are, however, relatively expensive and contain no essential fatty acids.

4. **Complications.** The two **most common** complications of EN are diarrhea and improper tube placement.
   a. **Diarrhea** in patients receiving EN is usually secondary to concomitant administration of medication (e.g., antibiotics and sorbitol-containing liquids). Infectious etiologies should be eliminated (e.g., *Clostridium difficile*), after which antidiarrheal medications may be beneficial. Reducing the rate or concentration may also be effective.
   b. A **feeding tube improperly placed** into the tracheobronchial tree can have disastrous consequences. Tube feedings should never be initiated without radiological verification of tube position.
   c. **Aspiration**

IV. MONITORING SUPPORT

A. **PN.** In addition to appropriate general medical and nursing care, patients receiving PN initially require daily and weekly laboratory monitoring to assess nutritional progress and metabolic status.

1. **Electrolytes**
   a. Initially, **potassium, sodium,** and **chloride** should be determined daily. Potassium is used intracellularly; thus, hypokalemia is not an uncommon finding.
   b. **Calcium, magnesium,** and **phosphate** are primarily intracellular electrolytes, serum levels of which become depleted during protein synthesis. Serum levels generally do not fall as rapidly as potassium; therefore, monitoring two to three times a week is recommended initially until the patient is stabilized, then weekly thereafter.
   c. **Bicarbonate** should be monitored to assess acid–base balance. Hyperchloremic metabolic acidosis may develop in patients on PN. This imbalance can be corrected by providing the potassium and sodium as acetate (converted to bicarbonate in the serum) rather than as the chloride salt. After initial correction, provision of one-half the sodium and potassium requirements as the acetate salt and one-half as the chloride salt may be beneficial.

2. **Serum glucose** should be monitored daily, particularly in central glucose systems. Maintaining a blood glucose concentration between 100–200 mg/dl is generally recommended.

3. **Weights** obtained on a daily or every-other-day–basis track optimum lean body weight gain of $\frac{1}{4}$–$\frac{1}{2}$ lb/day. Weight gain in excess of $\frac{1}{2}$ lb/day generally indicates fluid overload or fat deposition.

4. **Visceral proteins** (e.g., albumin, prealbumin, transferrin) are important indicators of the adequacy of nutritional support.
   a. **Albumin** is useful in the initial assessment of nutritional status, but its long half-life (18–21 days) limits its utility as a short-term marker of nutritional repletion.
   b. **Prealbumin** has a short half-life (2–3 days) and is a more sensitive and early indicator of the adequacy of nutritional support. Its serum value is falsely elevated in renal failure.
   c. **Transferrin** has an intermediate half-life (7–10 days), which makes weekly monitoring useful. Transferrin may be falsely elevated in iron-deficiency states.

5. **Serum creatinine** and **blood urea nitrogen (BUN)** should be obtained at least weekly. Evidence of renal impairment may require modification of the PN formula. Elevation of the BUN in the absence of renal impairment may be secondary to the PN formula (e.g., excess nitrogen, low NPC:N ratio) and appropriate adjustments need to be made.

6. **Liver function tests** [aspartate aminotransferase (AST), alanine aminotransferase (ALT), alkaline phosphatase, lactate dehydrogenase (LDH), and bilirubin] require baseline and periodic monitoring because of potential toxicity from the PN formulation (i.e., fatty infiltration of the liver). Abnormal liver function studies may necessitate changes in the PN formulation.

7. **Serum triglycerides** should be measured for a baseline and weekly thereafter for patients on lipid system PN. It is not necessary to monitor triglycerides on a weekly basis for patients receiving lipids two to three times per week for essential fatty acid replacement.

8. **Twenty-four–hour UUN** should be obtained weekly to determine nitrogen balance for patients in whom nitrogen requirements are uncertain. These are usually highly stressed, severely ill, or injured patients in an intensive care unit (ICU) setting.

9. **Serum iron** levels should be obtained weekly to determine deficiency and to allow appropriate interpretation of serum transferrin levels.

B. **EN** generally requires less intense laboratory monitoring. Specific laboratory guidelines for monitoring EN support vary from institution to institution.

V. SUPPORT OF SPECIFIC STATES

A. Conditionally essential nutrients

1. **Glutamine.** Because of its instability, glutamine is currently not a component of commercially available standard PN amino acid solutions and is found in free form in relatively few EN formulas. It is known to be used as a primary fuel source by enterocytes and may exert a trophic effect on the gut mucosa. It is most widely used as a PN component for bone marrow transplant patients and short gut syndrome. Glutamine-containing dipeptides that are stable and highly soluble are being investigated as a source of glutamine in PN. At present, glutamine must be added to the PN solution at the time of compounding. Optimum PN dose, contraindications, and EN necessity in free form are controversial and require further investigation.

2. **Arginine** has been shown experimentally and clinically to enhance immune function. EN formulas enriched with arginine are available commercially. Optimum dose has yet to be determined.

3. **Antioxidant formulations.** Oxidant production occurs as part of the normal inflammatory response and has been implicated in reperfusion injury. The body also produces antioxidant defenses to limit oxidant damage to healthy tissue. These defenses rely on adequate intake of dietary nutrients, such as the sulfur-containing amino acids, vitamin E, vitamin C, selenium, and zinc. Several investigators believe provision of these nutrients should be an early priority in critically ill patients. Optimum doses remain controversial.

4. **Tyrosine, cysteine,** and **taurine** are either absent or present in low concentrations in commercially available PN formulas. They are believed to be conditionally essential amino acids by some investigators.

5. **Omega-3 polyunsaturated fatty acids** are derived from fish oils and are currently found in some EN formulations. These fatty acids have been shown experimentally to enhance immune response, protect against tumor growth, and inhibit some of the proinflammatory effects of omega-6 fatty acids. In addition, they have been shown to lower cardiovascular risk factors by decreasing platelet activation, lowering blood pressure, and reducing triglycerides. However, well-controlled clinical trials in humans are needed to confirm the beneficial effects of immunomodulation seen in animal models.

B. **Nutritional support for renal failure.** The goal of nutritional support in acute renal failure (ARF) is to meet the patient's NPC requirements while minimizing volume, protein load, and potential electrolyte imbalance.

1. **PN formulations** used in ARF are low-nitrogen, high-caloric density formulas (e.g., 2% amino acid/47% dextrose), resulting in NPC:N ratios of approximately 500:1.

2. **Commercial renal failure formulations** (e.g., Nephramine, RenAmin, Aminosyn RF), containing primarily essential amino acids, have shown no clinical advantage over less expensive, low-concentration standard amino acid formulations.

3. **Standard glucose system formulations** (4.25% amino acid/25% dextrose) can generally be used in renal failure patients who are being dialyzed on a regular basis. This formulation is particularly useful in severely malnourished patients because it can provide adequate protein to attain positive nitrogen balance, which is not possible with renal failure PN.

4. **Monitoring transferrin** is a more sensitive and accurate visceral protein marker compared to albumin and prealbumin for assessing nutritional progress in these patients.

5. **Enteral formulations** that are low in nitrogen and calorie dense (1.7–2.0 NPC/mL) are available for patients with renal failure.

C. **Nutritional support for hepatic failure.** Patients with hepatic failure have altered protein metabolism, resulting in decreased serum levels of branched-chain amino acids (i.e., leucine, isoleucine, valine) and increased levels of aromatic amino acids (i.e., phenylalanine, tyrosine, tryptophan), methionine, and glutamine. A similar amino acid profile can exist in the cerebrospinal fluid (CSF) and is thought to contribute to hepatic encephalopathy. Fluid and electrolyte disturbances are frequently associated with hepatic failure as well.

1. **PN formulations** enriched in branched-chain amino acids (36%) and low in aromatic amino acids (e.g., Hepatamine) improve mental status in patients with altered serum amino acid profiles and hepatic encephalopathy. However, studies have not demonstrated definitive clinical differences in morbidity and mortality with these expensive formulations compared to standard formulas.

2. **Adequate NPC** with a 20–40 g/day protein load (e.g., 2% amino acid/25% dextrose) is an alternative approach to the use of hepatic failure amino acid formulations. Protein load can be liberalized slowly as long as mental status does not deteriorate.

3. **EN formulations** (e.g., Hepatic-Aid II) enriched with branched-chain amino acids and low in aromatic amino acids are commercially available for patients with hepatic failure.

D. **Nutritional support for respiratory failure.** The type and amount of substrate administered as NPC can have an impact on a patient's ventilatory status. Overfeeding with resultant lipogenesis and increased carbon dioxide production can be a cause of respiratory acidosis and/or increased minute ventilation and, therefore, should be avoided. Even in the presence of appropriate amounts of NPC administered as carbohydrate, the normal carbon dioxide load generated by glycolysis may be excessive for the patient with underlying pulmonary dysfunction [e.g., chronic obstructive pulmonary disease (COPD)].

1. **PN lipid system formulations** (e.g., 4.25% amino acid/15% dextrose with daily lipid emulsion), where the lipid component constitutes 40%–50% of the total NPC, may be beneficial in reducing the ventilatory demands in respiratory failure patients because lipolysis generates less carbon dioxide than glycolysis.

2. **EN formulations** containing similar amounts of fat can be prepared from standard EN formulas with the use of lipid modules (i.e., MCT oil, corn oil). More expensive commercial pulmonary formulas are also available.

3. **Oxepa,** a low-carbohydrate enteral formula containing antioxidants, eicosapentaenoic acid, and gamma linolenic acid, is currently available for adult respiratory distress syndrome (ARDS). It modulates the phospholipid fatty acid composition of inflammatory cell membranes, decreases the synthesis of the proinflammatory eicosanoids of lung injury, and attenuates endotoxin-induced increases in pulmonary microvascular protein permeability. Limited studies have shown some improvement in cardiopulmonary hemodynamics and respiratory gas exchange in ARDS.

E. **Nutritional support for cardiac failure.** The goal in these patients is to meet metabolic needs while restricting fluid and sodium intake.

1. **PN formulations** that provide protein and calories in as high a concentration as possible is the goal of nutritional therapy. This can be accomplished with both central glucose or lipid system PN formulations (e.g., 5% amino acid/35% dextrose; 7% amino acid/21% dextrose/20% lipid emulsion).

2. **Serum electrolyte monitoring** and **adjustment** are imperative in cardiac failure patients receiving PN, particularly when potent diuretics are used concurrently.

3. **EN formulations** with high nutrient density are available for oral supplementation or tube feedings. Infusion of enteral tube feedings should begin at one-third to one-half the strength, with a gradual increase in concentration, while maintaining a slow infusion rate (30–50 mL/hr) to avoid rapid increases in fluid load, cardiac output, heart rate, and myocardial oxygen consumption.

F. **Nutritional support in pancreatitis.** Severe acute pancreatitis is a hypercatabolic state that without nutritional support renders the patient a poor surgical candidate and at increased risk of infection. The goal of nutritional support in severe acute pancreatitis is to "rest" the pancreas by limiting exocrine stimulation while providing adequate nutrition.

1. **PN** is generally favored over EN to achieve this goal in the early phases of pancreatitis. Lipid system PN has been shown to be safe and effective when administered to these patients, provided there is no concurrent hyperlipidemia; in fact, it may be valuable in the patient with recalcitrant hyperglycemia.

2. **EN,** using chemically defined (elemental), low-fat formulas administered into the jejunum, results in minimal pancreatic stimulation and has been used safely in these patients.

G. **Nutritional support in stress/critical care.** In hypermetabolic critically ill patients, alterations in substrate utilization, the development of conditional nutrient deficiencies, and modulation of the immune response provide the rationale for specific nutritional formulations.

1. In critical illness, branched-chain amino acids (i.e., isoleucine, leucine, valine) are released from skeletal muscle for protein synthesis and as an energy substrate. PN formulations enriched in branched-chain amino acids (45%) [e.g., Freamine HBC, BranchAmin, Aminosyn-HBC] have been made available with the rationale that, being the preferred fuel source in this patient population, it would enhance protein synthesis, decrease protein catabolism, and improve the patient's clinical outcome. However, these more expensive branched-chain amino acid formulations have not been shown to favorably influence clinical outcomes in critically ill patients.

2. Enteral formulations are currently being produced (e.g., Impact, Perative) with varying amounts of the conditionally essential nutrients of critical illness and immunomodulatory substrates (e.g., omega-3 polyunsaturated fatty acids, arginine, glutamine). Clinical studies of the ability of these formulas to improve outcomes in critical illness have been mixed.

H. **Nutritional support in pregnancy.** Nutritional support in pregnancy can have a significant impact on fetal outcome. Weight gain throughout pregnancy is the primary indicator of the adequacy of the nutritional state of mother and child. A weight gain of approximately 11.5–16.0 kg should be the desired goal in women with normal prepregnancy body mass index. PN and EN have both been used successfully during pregnancy, with both modalities demonstrating adequate maternal weight gain, appropriate fetal growth, and term delivery. The calories required to achieve appropriate weight gain throughout the entire pregnancy per the World

Health Organization recommendations are an additional 300 kcal/day above the estimated basal energy expenditure (based on the pregravid weight) during all trimesters. The recommended daily protein intake during a normal pregnancy is approximately 1 g/kg/day. This amount represents the normal recommended daily allowance for females plus an additional 10 g/day. In pregnant patients with moderate to severe stress, both calories and protein requirements need to be adjusted in the same manner as for other hypermetabolic nonpregnant patients.

1. PN glucose system and lipid system formulations can both be used successfully to meet the nutrient requirements of pregnant patients. PN is most commonly used during pregnancy in patients with severe hyperemesis gravidarum.

2. Essential fatty acids (EFAs) are required by both mother and fetus. They are necessary for prostaglandin synthesis and normal fetal lipid development. The provision of at least 4.5–7.0% of calorie requirements as EFAs has been estimated to meet the minimum requirements during pregnancy.

3. The daily vitamin requirements in a normal pregnancy based on the 1999 Dietary Reference Intakes (DRI) can be met with the parenteral vitamin infusion Infuvite®Adult. If MVI-12 is used as the parenteral vitamin preparation, an additional 200 mcg of folic acid and 65 mcg of vitamin K need to be added to the daily PN formulation in order to meet the daily DRI requirements.

4. Prealbumin appears to be the preferred biochemical marker to assess protein status in pregnancy since albumin is falsely depressed and transferrin is falsely elevated in pregnant patients.

5. EN may be useful during pregnancy for patients with less severe hyperemesis gravidarum. The composition of polymeric formulas should be adequate for meeting the nutritional requirements of most pregnant patients.

6. Blood glucose levels should be kept at approximately 100 mg/dl during prolonged continuous PN or EN infusion since chronically elevated maternal glucose levels can result in fetal anomalies, increased risk of miscarriages, and stillbirth.

VI. TECHNICAL ASPECTS OF PN PREPARATIONS

A. PN formula preparation is performed **aseptically** in the pharmacy under a laminar flow hood that filters the air, removing airborne particles and microorganisms.

B. **Compatibility** of the various components of PN formulations is determined by several factors, including their concentration, solution pH, temperature, and the order of admixture. The **most common** compatibility concern is in regards to the addition of calcium and phosphate salts to PN solutions.

C. Following admixture of the various components, the PN solution should be **visually inspected** for precipitate or particulate matter. After labeling and final checking, the PN solution should be refrigerated until delivery to the nursing unit.

D. A statistically valid, continuous **sterility testing program** should be an essential component of quality control in preparing PN solutions.

VII. HOME PARENTERAL NUTRITION (HPN) has become a widely accepted and useful technique for provision of complete nutritional requirements in the home setting. When used appropriately, this modality benefits the patient medically and psychologically, with a decreased cost to the health-care system.

A. **Indications** for HPN include short bowel syndrome, severe inflammatory bowel disease, radiation enteritis, enterocutaneous fistulae, and selected malignancies.

B. **Candidate selection** requires a multidisciplinary approach to determine if the patient and family can assume the responsibility and training needed for safe and successful HPN.

C. Administration. HPN is infused through a central venous Silastic catheter (e.g., Hickman, Broviac), which allows for prolonged PN with low clotting and infection rates. The PN solution is generally infused over a 12- to 15-hour period at night. This type of cycling program allows the patient to be free from the infusion pump during the day, allowing for a more normal lifestyle.

D. Clinical monitoring and follow-up are done periodically, depending on the needs of the individual patient. Long-term HPN patients generally are seen by the physician on a monthly basis after initial stabilization.

VIII. MISCELLANEOUS

A. Soluble fiber is present in some commercially available EN formulas. This fiber is fermented by normal large intestinal flora to short-chain fatty acids that are used by colonocytes as a fuel source. These short-chain fatty acids also seem to have a trophic effect on the large intestinal mucosa.

B. Growth factors. The use of recombinant human growth hormone, insulin-like growth factor, and anabolic steroids, in combination with nutritional support to improve nitrogen balance and reduce hospital length of stay in select patient populations, is currently under investigation. To date, recombinant growth hormone (Humatrope) is available for nutritional support in children with cystic fibrosis, sickle cell anemia, and thalassemia and in adults with acquired immune deficiency syndrome (AIDS)-related cachexia.

STUDY QUESTIONS

Directions: Each of the numbered items or incomplete statements in this section is followed by answers or by completions of the statement. Select the **one** lettered answer or completion that is **best** in each case.

1. A 32-year-old well-nourished man involved in a motor vehicle accident was admitted to the surgical intensive care unit with multiple long bone fractures and abdominal injuries with no nutritional support for 4 days. This patient is most likely

(A) suffering from moderate to severe kwashiorkor malnutrition
(B) at low risk for hospital-acquired infection and other complications
(C) not suffering from protein or calorie malnutrition
(D) suffering from severe marasmus malnutrition
(E) not a candidate for aggressive nutritional support

2. A patient in the intensive care unit on a ventilator was placed on a glucose system parenteral nutrition (PN) formulation providing 2040 kcal/day and 98 g protein/day. A measured energy expenditure (MEE) and respiratory quotient (RQ) were subsequently obtained, with a resultant MEE of 2038 kcal and an RQ of 1.1. Which of the following is correct based on the above information?

(A) The patient is receiving adequate glucose calories, and an adjustment in the program is not necessary.
(B) The daily protein intake has to be decreased to reduce the patient's RQ.
(C) The PN formulation should be switched to a lipid system formulation to reduce the carbon dioxide load.
(D) The patient is retaining oxygen from the glucose calories in the PN formulation.
(E) Lipid emulsion should be added to the current PN formulation to enhance lipogenesis.

3. Total nutrient admixture (TNA)

(A) is more complicated to administer for home parenteral nutrition (PN) patients
(B) should be filtered with a 1.2-micron filter
(C) consists of glucose, amino acids, electrolytes, and trace minerals mixed in one container
(D) is the method recommended by the Food and Drug Administration (FDA) to administer lipid system PN
(E) can be visualized for particulate matter

4. The calorie requirements of a moderately hypermetabolic hospitalized patient are best estimated by utilizing the

(A) nomogram method
(B) nitrogen balance method
(C) estimated energy expenditure (EEE) method
(D) prognostic nutritional index (PNI)
(E) subjective global assessment method

5. Lipid system parenteral nutrition (PN)

(A) can be administered by peripheral vein if the glucose concentration is less than 15%
(B) requires daily serum triglyceride monitoring
(C) is contraindicated in patients with elevated carbon dioxide levels
(D) requires daily lipid administration to provide a portion of the patient's nonprotein calorie requirements
(E) can be administered with a maximum lipid dosage of 4.5 g/kg/day

6. Commercial parenteral nutrition (PN) formulations for hypermetabolic critically ill patients

(A) are enriched in branched-chain amino acids and contain low concentrations of aromatic amino acids
(B) contain primarily essential amino acids
(C) have not demonstrated a positive clinical outcome benefit in this patient population
(D) are the preferred PN formulation used in this clinical setting
(E) are enriched with arginine to enhance immune function

7. Which of the following methods of parenteral nutritional support would be most appropriate in a severely protein calorie malnourished patient with acute renal failure?

(A) 2% amino acid/47% dextrose
(B) 4.25% amino acid/25% dextrose
(C) 4% essential amino acid/47% dextrose
(D) 4.25% amino acid/25% dextrose with dialysis on a regular basis
(E) 2% amino acid/47% dextrose/20% lipid emulsion

8. Which of the following statements regarding the monitoring of nutritional support is true?

(A) Prealbumin is not the optimal marker to follow for short-term nutritional progress.
(B) Transferrin is falsely depressed in patients with iron deficiency.
(C) Albumin is falsely elevated in renal failure.
(D) A positive nitrogen balance of 3-6 g of nitrogen daily is optimal.
(E) A weight gains of $1^1/_2$–2 lb/day is indicative of optimal lean body weight gain.

9. Patients with end-stage liver disease

(A) generally have increased levels of branched-chain amino acids and decreased levels of aromatic amino acids
(B) should be placed on a low-branched chain, high aromatic amino acids parenteral nutrition (PN) solution
(C) can tolerate 20–40 g protein/day with a 2% standard amino acid PN solution
(D) require glutamine-enriched amino acid solutions
(E) can tolerate standard glucose system formulations 4.25% amino acid/25% dextrose with regular dialysis

Questions 10–12
A 67-year-old white female presented to the attending physician with a 3-month history of progressive difficulty swallowing and a 10-kg weight loss. She is currently 160 cm tall and weighs 50 kg. She has just undergone a distal esophagectomy and proximal gastrectomy for distal esophageal cancer. At the time of surgery, she had a feeding jejunostomy tube inserted.

10. The dieticians who are adept at using the Harris-Benedict equation have gone home for the day, and the surgeon calls you for your best guess at what the hourly goal rate for this patient should be utilizing isotonic enteral formula, which provides 0.85 nonprotein calories (NPCs)/mL. Your answer should be

(A) 65 mL/hr
(B) 75 mL/hr
(C) 85 mL/hr
(D) 95 mL/hr
(E) 50 mL/hr

11. The enteral formulation the surgeon has selected is enriched with fish oils. He is hoping this additive will

(A) prevent diarrhea
(B) prevent dermatitis
(C) prevent hyperglycemia
(D) improve immune function
(E) improve neurological function

12. On the fifth postoperative day, the feeding jejunostomy tube becomes clogged and unusable. The patient will be NPO an additional 5 days to ensure the integrity of her surgical anastamosis. The most appropriate course at this time is

(A) start the patient on a lipid-based peripheral parenteral nutrition program
(B) keep the patient NPO and without parenteral nutritional support
(C) have a central venous catheter inserted, and initiate a lipid-based parenteral nutrition program
(D) start the patient on a glucose-based peripheral parenteral nutritional program
(E) have a central venous catheter inserted, and start the patient on a high branched-chain amino acid parenteral program

Questions 13–14
RJ is a 28-year-old pregnant woman. She is in the ninth week of her pregnancy and is diagnosed with hyperemesis gravidarum. Her pregravid weight was 57 kg, and her height is 5′5″. She has lost 7 kg (12.3%) during her pregnancy. She was placed on a central glucose PN program.

13. Which one of the following represents the best estimate of her daily caloric requirements?

(A) 1675 kcal
(B) 1790 kcal
(C) 2261 kcal
(D) 2062 kcal
(E) 1925 kcal

14. MVI-12 is used as the parenteral vitamin preparation in the PN formulation. Which of the following vitamin(s) need to be supplemented in the daily PN formulation in order to meet the daily requirements during pregnancy?

(A) Vitamin K
(B) Thiamine (B_1)
(C) Folic acid
(D) (A) + (C)
(E) Pyridoxine (B_6)

ANSWERS AND EXPLANATIONS

1. The answer is A *[I B 3].*
A hypermetabolic state (e.g., trauma, infection) combined with protein deprivation can rapidly develop into a severe kwashiorkor malnutrition characterized by hypoalbuminemia, edema, and impaired cellular immune function.

2. The answer is C *[V D 1].*
Even in the presence of appropriate amounts of nonprotein calories (NPCs) administered as carbohydrate, the normal carbon dioxide load generated by glycolysis may be excessive for the patient with underlying pulmonary dysfunction. Parenteral nutrition (PN) lipid system formulations, in which the lipid component constitutes 40%–50% of the total NPCs, may be beneficial in reducing the ventilatory demands in respiratory failure patients because lipolysis generates less carbon dioxide than glycolysis.

3. The answer is B *[III A 6 b (2) (b) (iii)].*
A particle filter (i.e., 1.2 micron) should be used with total nutrient admixture (TNA) administration.

4. The answer is C *[II B 1].*
Energy requirements are determined as nonprotein calories by indirect calorimetry, estimated energy expenditure, and the simple nomogram method. The nomogram method is the least accurate method of estimating caloric requirements.

5. The answer is D *[III A 6 b (1)].*
The lipid system parenteral nutrition (PN) is a formulation in which lipid is administered daily to provide a substantial portion of the nonprotein calories (NPCs).

6. The answer is C *[V G 1].*
Parenteral nutrition (PN) formulations enriched in branched-chain amino acids have been made available with the rationale that, being the preferred fuel source in this patient population, it would enhance protein synthesis, decrease protein catabolism, and improve the patient's clinical outcome. However, these more expensive branched-chain amino acid formulations have not been shown to favorably influence clinical outcomes in critically ill patients.

7. The answer is D *[V B 3].*
Standard glucose system formulations (4.25% amino acid/25% dextrose) can generally be used in renal failure patients who are being dialyzed on a regular basis. This formulation is particularly useful in severely malnourished patients because it can provide adequate protein to attain positive nitrogen balance, which is not possible with renal failure parenteral nutrition (PN).

8. The answer is D *[II B 2 a (4)].*
A positive nitrogen balance of 3–6 g is the goal.

9. The answer is C *[V C 2].*
Adequate nonprotein calories (NPCs) with a 20–40 g/day protein load (e.g., 2% amino acid/25% dextrose) is an alternative approach to the use of hepatic failure amino acid formulations.

10–12. The answers are: 10-B *[II B 1 c],* **11-D** *[V A 5],* **12-A** *[III A 3 b].*
Use the nomogram of 30 kcal/kg to determine the nonprotein calories (NPCs)/day, and divide that by the NPCs/mL of the enteral formula to determine the volume of formula per day, which is divided by 24 hours to yield the hourly goal rate.

Omega-3 polyunsaturated fatty acids are derived from fish oils and are currently found in some enteral formulations. These fatty acids have been shown experimentally to enhance immune response.

With the use of new catheter technology and new techniques for infusion, it is now feasible to administer peripheral parenteral nutrition (PN) in selected patients for short-term therapy (7–10 days) with a low incidence of peripheral vein thrombophlebitis. This method of PN administration avoids the potential of more serious complications associated with central venous route administration.

13–14. The answers are: 13-A *[V H],* **14-D** *[V H 3].*
The estimated basal energy expenditure is calculated using the pregravid weight in the Harris-Benedict equation. An additional 300 kcal/day is added to the basal energy expenditure to provide the required calories per day during pregnancy.

An additional 200 mcg of folic acid and 65 mcg of vitamin K need to be added to the daily PN formulation when MVI-12 is used as the parenteral vitamin preparation to meet the daily requirements during pregnancy.

58
Immunosuppressive Agents in Organ Transplantation

David I. Min

I. ORGAN TRANSPLANTATION

A. Definition: Replacement of a diseased vital organ with a viable organ from a living or cadaver donor. Solid organ transplantation has become the therapy of choice for many patients with end-organ failure (i.e., heart, liver, lung, and kidney disease). However, it generally requires immunosuppression to overcome the immunological barrier between donor and recipient, except in syngenic (i.e., twins) or autologous transplantation.

B. Classification

1. Solid organ transplantation
   a. Life–saving transplantation (e.g., heart, heart–lung, lung, and liver transplantation). There is no alternative life-sustaining method available
   b. Non–life-saving transplantation (i.e., kidney, pancreas, and cornea transplantation). There are alternative life-sustaining methods available, such as dialysis or external insulin injection. In these cases, transplantation will improve the patient's quality of life or long-term survival significantly.

2. Bone marrow transplantation is used mainly for hematological malignancy or aplastic anemia.

II. GRAFT REJECTION

A. Transplant immunology (see Chapter 8)

1. Graft rejection. The body's immune system recognizes the allograft (transplanted organ) as a foreign antigen, and it initiates the immune response to remove or destroy the transplanted graft. This reaction is called "rejection." The degree of the reaction depends on the genetic similarities or differences between the organ of the donor and the immune system of the recipient.

2. Histocompatibility. The antigen determining the compatibility between the donor and the recipient is called a **histocompatibility antigen,** the gene being located on chromosome 6. In many transplants (e.g., bone marrow or kidney transplant), this histocompatibility matching is an important factor for determining the long-term survival of the graft. However, more selective, potent immunosuppression may alleviate the importance of tissue matching between donor and recipient (exception: in bone marrow, the tissue matching is still important).

3. Other factors. Another group of substances that also plays an important role is the **ABO blood group system** of red blood cells. The donor and recipient must be ABO-compatible; otherwise, immediate graft destruction occurs. Some patients may have preformed antibody for unspecified donors because of multiple blood transfusions or other reason. In this case, patients may destroy the transplanted organ immediately. To detect the preformed antibody, the recipient's serum will be tested immediately before the transplantation (cross-match).

B. Types of graft rejection

1. Types of graft rejection according to the time course
   a. Hyperacute rejection. Immediate destruction (within minutes or hours) of the transplant organ by a preformed antibody or complement system. Today, this is extremely rare. It occurs only in an ABO-mismatched organ or a cross-match positive (preformed antibody) organ. There is no adequate treatment available.
   b. Acute rejection occurs within a few days to several months after transplantation. It is mediated by T-lymphocyte (cell-mediated immunity), and this rejection can be reversible by steroids or antibody therapy such as muromonab/CD3 or antithymocyte globulin.

    c. Chronic rejection occurs several months to several years after transplantation. This re-action is mediated by B-lymphocyte (antibody), and there is no adequate treatment available.

  2. Graft versus host, host versus graft. In most solid organ transplants, rejection occurs as the host immune system rejects or attacks the transplant organ (host versus graft). However, in bone marrow transplant, the host is generally immune deficient and the transplanted graft is immune competent, which attracts host tissues (graft versus host).

III. PROPHYLAXIS AND TREATMENT OF GRAFT REJECTION (Table 58-1)

  A. Calcineurin inhibitors

    1. Cyclosporine (e.g., Neoral, Sandimmune, Gengraf)
      a. Mechanism of action. Cyclosporine binds an intracellular receptor, cyclophiline. This complex inhibits calcineurin, an intracellular phosphatase, which involves activation of

Table 58-1. Current Immunosuppressive Agents Used in Organ Transplantation

Classification	Drug	Usual Initial Dose	Major Side Effects	Monitoring
Calcineurin inhibitors	Cyclosporine Tacrolimus (FK506)	10 mg/kg/day 0.1–0.3 mg/kg/day	Nephrotoxicity Neurotoxicity	Blood concentrations and serum creatinine concentrations
Antimetabolites	Azathioprine	1.5–3 mg/kg/day	Bone marrow suppression	WBC count
	Mycophenolate mofetil	1 g twice daily	Same as above	Same as above
	Methotrexate	15 mg/m² on day 1, 10 mg/m²/day on days 3, 6, and 11	Same as above	Same as above
mTOR inhibitor	Sirolimus	6–15 mg loading dose and 2–5 mg once daily	Hyperlipidemia, leukopenia and thrombocytopenia	Blood concentrations and WBC, platelet, and lipid profile
Alkylating agent	Cyclophosphamide	3–4 mg/kg/day for 4 days, followed by reduction to 1 mg/kg/day for treatment of rejection	Hemorrhagic cystitis	WBC count
Antibody products	Muromonab/CD3 (OKT3)	5 mg daily for 7–14 days	Cytokine release syndromes (flu-like syndrome)	Signs and symptoms, CD3+ cell count
	Antithymocyte globulin	15–20 mg/kg/day for 7–14 days (Atgam) or 1.5 mg/kg/day for 7–14 days (Thymoglobulin)	Leukopenia and thrombocytopenia	T-cell count
	Daclizumab	1 mg/kg (max. 100 mg), on day 0, and every 2 weeks for a total of 5 doses	No significant side effects reported	No special monitoring required
	Basiliximab	For adults, 2 doses of 20 mg each (day 0 and day 4)	No significant side effects reported	No special monitoring required
Corticosteroids	Prednisone or methylprednisolone	500 mg IV on the day of surgery and rapidly tapering to 10 mg daily at 1 month	Fluid retention, psychosis, cataracts, osteonecrosis	Signs and symptoms

the promoter region for the gene-encoding cytokine, such as interleukin-2. This results in inhibiting T-cell activation in the early stage of immune response to a foreign antigen such as a graft.

b. **Dosing and monitoring.** Cyclosporine pharmacokinetics is unpredictable, and many factors such as age, time after transplant, different oral formulation (Neoral or Sandimmune), or drugs affect it. Oral bioavailability is about 30%. Generally, 10 mg/kg/day of oral cyclosporine is used in solid organ transplantation and adjusted according to the blood levels. Serum creatinine should be monitored with the blood levels of cyclosporine. The blood levels are useful in the clinical monitoring.

c. **Side effects. Nephrotoxicity** is the major side effect. Neurotoxicity and hepatotoxicity are also common. Numerous drug interactions have been reported (Table 58-2).

2. **Tacrolimus (Prograf)**

   a. **Mechanism of action.** It is very similar to cyclosporine (III A 1 a).

   b. **Dosing and monitoring.** Tacrolimus pharmacokinetics is also variable, and oral bioavailability is about 25%. Blood levels are useful in clinical monitoring.

   c. **Side effects. Nephrotoxicity** is the major side effect. Neurotoxicity and gastrointestinal (GI) toxicity are more common than with cyclosporine.

B. **Antimetabolites**

1. **Azathioprine (Imuran)**

   a. **Mechanism of action.** It is converted to 6-mercaptopurine in the body and is a non-specific purine synthesis inhibitor. It interferes with DNA and RNA synthesis so that it may reduce both cell-mediated and humoral immune responses.

   b. **Dosage and monitoring.** An initial dose of 3–5 mg/kg/day is administered preoperatively. Immediately after transplantation, the dose is usually tapered to a maintenance dose of 1–3 mg/kg/day or titrated to the patient's white blood cell (WBC) count. The WBC count is generally maintained greater than 3000/mm^3.

   c. **Side effects. Bone marrow suppression** (leukopenia, thrombocytopenia) is the major side effect. In addition, xanthine oxidase inhibitor allopurinol inhibits azathioprine me-

Table 58-2. Major Drug Interactions of Cyclosporine and Tacrolimus with Other Drugs and Their Management

Drugs	Mechanism	Effects	Management
Antiepileptic drugs Phenytoin Phenobarbital Carbamazepine	Increased metabo-lism by inducing cytochrome P450 enzyme	Cyclosporine or tacrolimus trough levels drop within 48 hr after initiation of these drugs	Increase cyclosporine dose or tacrolimus with frequent monitoring of blood levels
Rifampin or isoniazid	Same as above	Same as above	Same as above
Azole antifungal agents Ketoconazole Fluconazole Itraconazole	Inhibition of liver cytochrome P450 enzyme by these drugs	Significant increase of cyclosporine or tacrolimus levels	Reduce cyclosporine or tacrolimus dose with frequent monitoring of levels
Macrolide antibiotics Erythromycin Josamycin	Inhibition of liver and GI cytochrome P450 enzyme	Increase AUC ($\times$2) and cyclosporine or tacrolimus trough levels ($\times$ 2–3)	Same as above
Calcium-channel blockers Verapamil Diltiazem Nicardipine	Same as above	Same as above	Reduce cyclosporine or tacrolimus dose, or use nifedipine or isradipine
Grapefruit juice	Inhibition of GI cytochrome P450 enzyme	Increase AUC and peak concentrations of cyclosporine and possibly tacrolimus, and increase variability of blood levels	Avoid grapefruit juice

tabolism. When these drugs are used concurrently, the azathioprine dose should be reduced by 80%. Otherwise, the patient may develop severe leukopenia due to azathioprine overdose.

  2. **Mycophenolate mofetil (CellCept)**
     a. **Mechanism of action.** In the body, it is converted to mycophenolic acid, which inhibits *de novo* purine synthesis pathway by inhibiting inosine dehydrogenase. As a result, it inhibits DNA and RNA synthesis in the immune cells.
     b. **Dosing and monitoring.** A dose of 2 g/day is administered as two divided doses. The WBC and GI symptoms should be monitored.
     c. **Side effects. Bone marrow suppression** (leukopenia, thrombocytopenia) is the major side effect, as in azathioprine. In addition, GI side effects are more common than with azathioprine.

  3. **Methotrexate.** This agent is used mainly in autoimmune disease and preventing graft versus host disease in bone marrow transplant (BMT) patients.
     a. **Mechanism of action.** It prevents dihydrofolic acid from converting to tetrahydrofolic acid by inhibiting the enzyme dihydrofolate reductase. As a result, DNA and protein synthesis are inhibited.
     b. **Dosing and monitoring.** Dosage regimens in BMT patients usually consist of 15 mg/m^2/day on day 1 after transplant and 10 mg/m^2/day on days 3, 6, and 11 with other agents such as cyclosporine.
     c. **Side effects. Bone marrow suppression** (leukopenia, thrombocytopenia) is the major side effect as in azathioprine. In addition, diarrhea and mucositis are common.

C. **mTOR (mammarian Target of Rapamycin) inhibitor** is the alkylating agent mainly used for BMT patients. Rarely is it used as a substitute agent for azathioprine in solid organ transplantation.

  1. **Sirolimus (Rapamune)**
     a. **Mechanism of action.** Sirolimus binds intracellular receptor, FKBP-12 (FK binding protein-12). This complex inhibits the mTOR, which is a key regulatory kinase. This results in inhibiting T-cell activation in a later stage of immune response to foreign antigen such as a graft.
     b. **Dosing and monitoring.** A dose of 2–10 mg/day is administered as a once-daily dose. Usually, a loading dose of 6–15 mg with a maintenance dose of 2–5 mg once daily is used. Blood levels are useful in clinical monitoring. The serum lipid profile, WBC count, and GI symptoms should be monitored.
     c. **Side effects. Hyperlipidemia** is the major side effect. In addition, leukopenia, thrombocytopenia, and GI side effects are common.

D. **Alkylating agent. Cyclophosphamide** is the alkylating agent mainly used for BMT patients. Rarely, it is used as a substitute agent for azathioprine in solid organ transplantation.

  1. **Mechanism of action.** It is converted to the active metabolite phosphoramide mustard in the liver, which inhibits the cross-linking of DNA, leading to cell death.

  2. **Dosing and monitoring.** Doses of cyclophosphamide up to 3–4 mg/kg/day for 4 days followed by a reduction to 1 mg/kg/day to treat graft rejection. The dosage should be titrated to maintain a WBC count greater than 4000/mm^3.

  3. **Side effects. Hemorrhagic cystitis** and **bone marrow suppression** (leukopenia, thrombocytopenia). In addition, nausea, vomiting, and diarrhea are common.

E. **Antibody products**

  1. **Muromonab CD3 (Orthoclone OKT3)** is the first therapeutic mouse monoclonal antibody produced for use in humans.
     a. **Mechanism of action.** OKT3 is a mouse IgG2α immunoglobulin that binds to the CD3 structure on T-lymphocytes. Once OKT3 is bound to the CD3 region of T cells, they lose the antigen recognition function and cannot initiate the rejection process.
     b. **Dosing and monitoring.** The dosage is 5 mg/day intravenously for 7–14 days for prevention or treatment of rejection. The CD3+ lymphocyte counts are monitored, and it is desirable that CD+ cell be maintained at less than 30/mm^3.
     c. **Side effects.** With the first few doses, the patient will develop severe flu-like symptoms such as fever, chills, nausea, vomiting, and headache. The OKT3 stimulates T cells, and

these symptoms are caused by abrupt release of cytokines such as interleukin-1, tumor-necrosis factor-a, and interleukin-6 from opsonized T cells (cytokine release syndrome). It requires premedications such as acetaminophen, diphenhydramine, and corticosteroids to reduce these side effects before OKT3 injection.

2. **Antithymocyte globulin (Thymoglobulin, Atgam)**
   a. **Mechanism of action.** It is a purified polyclonal immunoglobulin from rabbits (Thymoglobulin) or horses (Atgam), which binds to the human T cells. However, it may have cross-reactivity against the red blood cells, platelets, and granulocytes.
   b. **Dosing and monitoring.** The dosage is 1.5 mg/kg (Thymoglobulin) or 15–20 mg/kg (Atgam) infusion daily through a central line for 7–14 days for prevention or treatment of rejection. The T-lymphocyte counts are monitored and maintained less than 100/mm³.
   c. **Side effects.** Antithymocyte globulin may cause fever, chills, erythema, leukopenia, thrombocytopenia, and anaphylactic reaction or serum sickness.

3. **Daclizumab (Zenapax)**
   a. **Mechanism of action.** It is a molecularly engineered humanized immunoglobulin active against interleukin-2 receptor (CD25, or Tac) that binds to block the interleukin-2 receptor on the surface of activated T-lymphocytes, thus preventing T-cell activation and proliferation.
   b. **Dosing and monitoring.** It is indicated only for the prevention of acute rejection. The usual recommended dosage is 1 mg/kg (max. 100 mg) within 24 hours posttransplantation and every 2 weeks up to 8 weeks (a total of 5 doses).
   c. **Side effects.** Based on results of clinical trials, no specific safety monitoring is required with daclizumab.

4. **Basiliximab (Simulect)**
   a. **Mechanism of action.** It is a chimeric (murine/human) monoclonal antibody (IgG1κ), produced by recombinant DNA technology, that binds to block the interleukin-2 receptor on the surface of activated T lymphocytes, and as a result, it prevents T-lymphocyte activation, thus preventing acute rejections.
   b. **Dosing and monitoring.** It is indicated only for the prevention of acute rejection. The usual recommended dosage for the adult patient is 2 doses of 20 mg each at day 0 and day 4 after kidney transplantation. No special monitoring is required.
   c. **Side effects.** Based on results of clinical trials, no cytokine release syndromes have been noticed.

F. **Corticosteroids. Prednisone** and **methylprednisolone** are the major corticosteroid products used for transplant patients.

   1. **Mechanisms of action.** Corticosteroids have multiple pharmacological effects in various cells. Corticosteroids bind with intracellular glucocorticoid receptors, which results in altering DNA and RNA translation. As a result, corticosteroids cause a rapid and profound drop in circulating T lymphocytes. They have potent anti-inflammatory effects by inhibiting arachidonic acid release and macrophage phagocytosis.

   2. **Dosing and monitoring.** They are used in both preventing and treating graft rejection and acute graft versus host disease. In general, prophylactic doses in solid organ transplantation are in the range of 1–2 mg/kg/day and tapered over months to 0.1–0.3 mg/kg/day. In the case of treatment, the dosage is 500 mg of methylprednisolone IV for 3–5 days or 1–2 mg/kg/day of oral prednisone, which should be tapered rapidly.

   3. **Side effects.** In the long-term, corticosteroids cause more troubling side effects. They include psychological disturbances (i.e., euphoria, depression), adrenal axis suppression, hypertension, sodium and water retention, myopathy, impaired wound healing, increased appetite, osteoporosis, hyperglycemia, and cataracts.

IV. COMPLICATIONS OF IMMUNOSUPPRESSION

A. **Infections**

   1. **Risk.** Transplant patients have a high risk of acquiring an infection due to patient factors such as diabetes mellitus, hepatitis, or uremia. In addition, immunosuppressive agents can cause various effects, such as leukopenia, lymphopenia, or T-cell dysfunction, which inhibit adequate immune response to the infection.

2. **Time course.** The risk of infection is greatest during the first 3 months after transplantation, when higher doses of immunosuppression are used, and again after a rejection episode is treated. This risk correlates with the overall level of immunosuppression.

3. **Types of infections** include bacterial, fungal, viral, and protozoan.

4. **Prevention**
   a. **Trimethoprim-sulfamethoxazole.** One single- or double-strength tablet daily for 6 months significantly reduces *Pneumocystis carinii* pneumonia and bacterial urinary tract infection. After 6 months, three times a week is effective.
   b. **Cytomegalovirus (CMV) infection.** High doses of acyclovir (800 mg qid for normal renal function, with doses adjusted according to renal function), oral ganciclovir (1 g tid for normal renal function, with doses adjusted according to renal function), intravenous ganciclovir, or high-titer CMV immunoglobulin are effective in reducing the incidence of CMV infection and invasive CMV disease.
   c. **Nystatin solution or clotrimazole troche** reduce oral candidiasis.

B. **Increased risk of malignancy**

1. **Cause.** Continuous immunosuppression interferes with normal immune surveillance and function for malignancy. In addition, some of the immunosuppressive drugs may be directly carcinogenic or activate oncogenic virus, such as Epstein-Barr virus (EBV).

2. **Characteristics.** Cancers that occur most frequently in the general population (e.g., lung, breast, colon) are not increased among transplant patients. However, various cancers uncommon in the general population are often more prevalent in transplant patients: lymphomas, squamous cell carcinomas of the lip and skin, Kaposi's sarcoma, other sarcoma.

3. **Posttransplant lymphoproliferative diseases (PTLDs).** The incidence of lymphoma appears to correlate with the intensity of immunosuppression. It is especially well documented that T-cell specific agents, including OKT3, cyclosporine, and tacrolimus, increase the incidence of lymphoproliferative diseases.

4. **Treatment.** In case of nonvital organ transplant, immunosuppression should be reduced or stopped. If EBV-related lymphoma occurs, acyclovir or ganciclovir therapy appears to be effective; the B-cell–specific monoclonal antibody, Rituximab, is also used.

C. **Hypertension.** Many immunosuppressive agents cause hypertension. Cyclosporine and tacrolimus clearly increase the arterial blood pressure and steroids may exacerbate hypertension after transplantation from fluid and sodium retention. Treatment usually requires the use of multiple agents, including diuretics and calcium-channel blockers.

STUDY QUESTIONS

Directions: Each of the numbered items or incomplete statements in this section is followed by answers or by completion of the statement. Select the **one** lettered answer or completion that is **best** in each case.

1. A 55-year-old patient with type II diabetes mellitus received a cadaveric renal transplant 2 years ago. He was maintained on cyclosporine 200 mg twice daily, mycophenolate mofetil 1 g twice daily, and prednisolone 10 mg daily, and his serum creatinine was 1.5 mg/dl. Recently, he had developed an upper respiratory infection, and his physician started erythromycin 500 mg three times daily for 1 week. Five days later, his creatinine level rose to 2.6 mg/dl, with a cyclosporine trough level of 550 ng/mL (therapeutic range 100–200 ng/mL). What is the likely cause of his renal function deterioration at this time?

(A) Erythromycin is a nephrotoxic drug.
(B) Erythromycin has synergistic nephrotoxicity with cyclosporine.
(C) He may have an acute graft rejection.
(D) Erythromycin inhibits cyclosporine metabolism and increases cyclosporine blood concentrations, resulting in renal toxicity.

2. All of the following are correct regarding infection prophylaxis in an organ transplant patient EXCEPT

(A) trimethoprime-sulfamethoxazole for *Pneumocytis carinii* pneumonia prophylaxis
(B) nystatin for fungal infection
(C) oral acyclovir for herpes simplex
(D) clotrimazole troche for sore throat

3. All of the following are correct regarding daclizumab (Zenapax) EXCEPT

(A) it is a humanized monoclonal antibody
(B) it is a monoclonal antibody directing to interleukin-2 receptor in T cells
(C) It is indicated only for the prevention of acute rejection.
(D) it requires premedications before its administration due to severe side effects

4. All of the following are side effects of long-term steroid use EXCEPT

(A) osteonecrosis
(B) hyperglycemia
(C) leukopenia
(D) fluid retention

5. All of the following are complications of antimetabolites such as mycophenolate mofetil EXCEPT

(A) leukopenia
(B) increased risk of cytomegalovirus infection
(C) renal dysfunction
(D) thrombocytopenia

ANSWERS AND EXPLANATIONS

1. The answer is D *[Table 58-2].*
This patient's renal dysfunction is likely caused by cyclosporine toxicity due to a drug interaction. Erythromycin is a cytochrome P450 enzyme inhibitor, which inhibits various drugs' metabolisms, including that of cyclosporine, tacrolimus, and theophylline. When erythromycin is started in the patient taking cyclosporine or tacrolimus, cyclosporine or tacrolimus blood levels should be monitored carefully with serum creatinine concentrations, and the dosage of cyclosporine or tacrolimus should be adjusted according to the blood concentrations. Because this patient had good renal function for 2 years and high cyclosporine levels, it is unlikely for him to have an acute graft rejection at this time.

2. The answer is D *[IV A 4].*
Clotrimazole troche is used to prevent oral fungal infection (candidiasis).

3. The answer is D *[III E 3 c].*
The daclizumab is a humanized monoclonal antibody that directs to the interleukin-2 (IL-2) receptor on the T cells. Interleukin-2 is T-cell growth factor, which initiates T-cell proliferation. The daclizumab opsonizes this IL-2 receptor, which prevents T-cell growth and proliferation, which is essential for the graft rejection process. Unlike OKT3 or antithymocyte globulin, it does not show any serious side effects, so it does not require premedications such as acetominophen, diphenhydramine, and corticosteroids before its administration.

4. The answer is C *[IV F 3].*
All except for leukopenia (reduced WBC count) are long-term complications of steroid therapy. The steroid therapy generally increases WBC count.

5. The answer is C *[III B 1, 2].*
Mycophenolate mofetil or azathioprine may cause bone marrow suppression, which manifests itself as leukopenia and thrombocytopenia. These also cause general immunosuppression, which increases the risk of opportunistic infections such as cytomegalovirus infection and cancer. Antimetabolites do not cause renal dysfunction.

59

Outcomes Research and Pharmacoeconomics

Peter K. Wong
Alan H. Mutnick

I. GENERAL CONCEPTS

A. Outcomes research (OR) is the study of health-care interventions (treatment modalities such as drug therapies, surgery, palliative therapy, etc.), care delivery processes, and health-care quality that are evaluated to measure the extent to which optimal and desirable outcomes can be reached. Normally, the purpose of OR is to assess the value of a program or therapy in question.

1. The **ECHO model** provides a framework for comprehensive evaluation of outcomes. Three areas of outcomes identified by Kozma & Reeder are economic outcomes, clinical outcomes, and humanistic outcomes.

2. **Outcomes research methodologies** include retrospective chart review, prospective clinical trials, observational studies, and computer modeling studies.

3. **Examples of outcomes measures**
   a. Economic outcomes include acquisition costs associated with care, labor cost–associated with care, costs to treat adverse drug reactions, costs of treatment failure, costs of hospital readmission, and costs of emergency room and clinic visits.
   b. Clinical outcomes include length of hospital stay, adverse drug reactions, hospital readmission, and death.
   c. Humanistic outcomes include patient satisfaction, functional status as measured by a validated instrument, and quality-of-life assessment.

B. Pharmacoeconomics (PE), a division of health economics, is designed to provide decision makers with information about the value of the different pharmacotherapies. According to Bootman, Townsend & McGhan, PE research identifies, measures, and compares the costs (resources consumed) and consequences (clinical, economic, and humanistic) of pharmaceutical products and services.

II. COST

A. Definitions

1. **Total cost**—all expenses that are directly and indirectly necessary to provide a product or service

2. **Average cost**—the average cost per unit of output (total cost divided by quantity)

3. **Fixed cost**—costs that do not vary with the quantity of output for a short-run production (e.g., rent, fixtures, fixed salary, depreciation, administrative costs)

4. **Variable cost**—costs that vary with the level of output (e.g., wages, supplies)

5. **Marginal cost**—the extra cost of producing *one extra* unit of output

6. **Incremental cost**—additional costs when comparing one alternative to another

7. **Direct cost**—costs directly related to producing/providing a specific quantity of services or output (e.g., salary, drug cost and supply cost for the provision of pharmacy services)

8. **Indirect cost**—costs that are allocated to the area(s) that produce/provide a specific quantity of services or output (e.g., overhead cost)

9. **Allowable cost**—a cost that is eligible to claim for purposes of reimbursement as necessary and relevant to the delivery of a unit of output

10. **Opportunity cost**—the cost of the benefit of pursuing an alternative course of action

11. **Operating cost**—any cost that supports the operations to provide the output

B. Cost and charge

1. The term cost has a different meaning, depending on the different perspectives for the analysis. The following examples show such differing perspectives.

2. Providers may include hospitals, and then the term cost means the total costs for providing the specific service(s).

3. Payors may include insurance companies, and then the term cost means the price that they have to pay to obtain the service (i.e., charges by providers).

4. Today, in many instances, charges do not equal the payment to providers. Depending on the contractual terms, many providers receive only a percentage of the charges for payment. These are called discounted charges.

5. Contractual terms are rarely reviewed and vary with different insurance carriers. This creates additional confusion as to the costs associated for various services or therapies.

6. A recognizable way to resolve these hurdles is to use the ratio of cost-to-charge (RCC) for the cost estimation. Multiply the RCC with the patient's charge to yield the estimated cost. RCC can be obtained from the individual hospital's Centers for Medicare & Medicaid Services (CMS) yearly cost report.

C. Basic steps in assessing cost

1. Define the units of service or output

2. Determine the number of service or output units provided

3. Determine cost drivers of these units of service or output

4. Calculate total costs, direct or indirect, related to the provision of this output or service

5. Calculate the average cost and incremental cost

III. ELEMENTS OF A GOOD STUDY

A. **Sound objective(s).** The study has defined objective(s) and answerable question(s).

B. **Perspective(s).** There is a defined perspective(s) for analysis (e.g., patient, payor, provider, society). In many cases, study perspective determines the cost-effectiveness of an intervention. Most of the published PE guidelines suggest that societal perspective be considered as an additional perspective for analysis.

C. **Patient population** chosen must be within the scope of analysis. Patient selection criteria that are too stringent pose a threat to external validity. Patient selection criteria that are too liberal are a threat to internal validity. Consideration is also given to comorbidity and multiple treatment modalities.

D. **Possible comparators and their effectiveness.** All relevant alternatives for comparison are identified. The Canadian PE Guidelines also state that no treatment is considered as an alternative.

E. **Metrics for costs and consequences.** Measures chosen for costs and consequences can affect the results of the analysis. Biases could be introduced into the analysis if units of measures are not clearly defined. This may pose a problem with a multicountry study in the aggregation of the final costs and consequences because currency exchange rates may fluctuate from time to time.

F. **Inclusion of relevant costs and consequences in the analysis** are based on the perspective chosen. The computation of costs and consequences should be transparent to readers. The key is reproducibility. Readers should be able to use the published computation methods with the local data to validate the findings.

G. A valid data source. Depending on the design of the study, data can come from clinical trials, observational studies, health-care claim databases, chart reviews, and epidemiological data. Each of the sources of these data were designed for some other purpose than economic analysis. Limitations are listed under section VIII.

H. Discounting for costs and consequences. Much discussion has been devoted to the appropriateness of discounting costs and consequences as well as the discount rate. The consensus at this time is to discount both costs and consequences. The discount rate normally is the opportunity cost of using resources. Many researchers have used the government bond rate. Regardless, the researcher must offer the justification for the chosen discount rate(s).

I. Incremental analysis provides an insight on the comparison for cost generated from one alternative to another alternative, and the additional benefit yielded from the increased cost.

J. Sensitivity analysis should include all the plausible values and their justification for the key parameters.

K. Time horizon of the analysis covers the full duration of treatment for the disease process. For example, the time horizon for the cholesterol-lowering agent's treatment should be the life span from the start day of treatment to the end of life.

L. Appropriateness and comprehensiveness of presentation and discussion of the study results. Similar to the clinical studies, the presentation of study results should not be biased. Interventional alternatives and study limitations must be addressed. Generalizability and applicability are also discussed.

IV. PHARMACOECONOMIC METHODOLOGIES

A. Cost of illness (COI) is the evaluation and assessment of the resources used in treating an illness. This technique is used to obtain the baseline cost information before the introduction of a new intervention. Costs are measured in terms of dollars. Like any PE analysis, the evaluator needs to define the analysis perspective. A different perspective will change the cost structure. For example, from a patient's perspective, the cost of illness will include the transportation to and from the treatment site. Time duration of the disease can be critical in determining the cost and may be a source of bias. No comparison is made in this type of analysis.

B. Cost-benefit analysis (CBA) is a tool used to determine priority for the resource allocation. The technique can be applied to the comparison of health-care programs and with non–health-care programs such as social welfare programs. For example, one can compare the cost and benefit of a coronary risk factor reduction program and the childhood immunization program and the domestic violence prevention program. This technique consists of identifying all of the benefits that accrue from the program and converting them into dollars in the year that they occur. The stream of costs and benefits are then discounted to present value at the selected discount rate. Net benefit is computed for each program and can then be compared with other programs.

C. Cost-minimization analysis (CMA). The underlying assumption for this type of analysis assumes that consequences are equivalent. Therefore, only cost is compared. The cheapest intervention will be chosen for implementation. Equivalent outcomes may not necessarily be equal. One needs to determine the key outcome of each comparator. For example, two drugs may have the equivalent therapeutic value but different side effect profiles. In such cases, consequences may not be equivalent, and this technique is not appropriate. CEA should be used instead.

D. Cost-effectiveness analysis (CEA) is a technique to assist the decision maker in identifying a preferred choice among possible alternatives within similar consequences (e.g., same therapeutic category) in terms of health improvement created (e.g., life year gained, clinical cures). It is not to be used to compare different consequences for each alternative, such as blood pressure reduction to degree of cholesterol lowering. Consequences can be intermediate outcomes or surrogate outcomes such as the reperfusion time of the vessel after thrombolytic therapy. Generally, the incremental cost of a program or an intervention from a specified perspective is compared to the incremental health effects. An example is the cost per unit of blood pressure reduction with each antihypertensive agent compared. The results of the analysis normally are stated in terms of cost per unit of effectiveness.

E. Cost-utility analysis (CUA). Unlike CEA, CUA measures the consequences in terms of the quality-adjusted life year (QALY) gained. The results of the analysis are normally expressed as a cost per QALY. The metric of QALY incorporates both the improvement in quantity of life, quality of life, and the preference (utility value) of the health state. There are three sources of obtaining utility values for health states in CUA: judgment to estimate the utility values, values from the literature, or values elicited from a sample of subjects. Common techniques for eliciting utility values are rating scale (visual analogue scale), standard gamble, and time trade-off. Five circumstances have been summarized that detail when CUA may be the appropriate technique to apply.

1. When quality of life is the only outcome

2. When quality and quantity of life are health outcomes

3. When the intervention affects both mortality and morbidity and a combined unit of outcome is desired

4. When the intervention being compared has a wide range of potential outcomes and a common unit of outcome is needed

5. When the objective is to compare a gold standard intervention that already has the cost per QALY. QALY is calculated by multiplying the utility values obtained for the specific health state with the quantity of life years spent in that specific health state. Comparison can then be made for the program and intervention.

F. Multiattribute utility theory (MAUT) or analysis (MAUA) is another technique frequently used in assessing utilities. In this situation, one is able to include several attributes, such as clinical effect and financial effect, as well as quality of life. One is able to preferentially weigh the decision based on what the priorities are for the decision maker and can apply the weights in order to identify the most preferable therapy, service, and so on. As evidenced from the following three examples, the individual's perspective will have a major impact on the final decision made, based on the varying levels of priority chosen for evaluation.

1. A physician may view clinical outcome to represent 70% of the decision, followed by patient's quality of life (20%), and lastly the costs (10%).

2. A hospital administrator may view the financial outcomes (70%) as a major priority, followed by the clinical outcome (20%), and lastly the quality of life (10%).

3. A patient with health insurance might view the clinical outcome (45%) and quality of life (45%) as the top priorities and have minimal concern for the financial outcomes (10%) of such a decision.

G. Willingness to pay (WTP) technique is used to assess the perceived value or benefit of a product and service. The WTP values can be obtained through two approaches: (1) indirect measurement, which examines in actual payments previous real-world decisions that involve trade-offs between money and expected outcomes, and (2) direct measurement, which uses survey methods to elicit stated dollar on the perceived benefits. In the second approach, researchers are seeking to provide background information sufficient to create within the respondent's mind a hypothetical market in which the person provides a judgment of the value of the proposed service. The challenge of using contingent valuation is to present within the questionnaire sufficient information organized clearly to allow this judgment to occur. Basic facts need to be given at the appropriate time. Unlike CBA, WTP takes into consideration the psychological aspects of the illness as well as the physical deterioration. The use of WTP as an outcome measure is theoretically consistent with welfare economics. It also provides a means to assign dollar values to health outcomes.

V. DECISION ANALYSIS is a systematic approach to decision-making under conditions of uncertainty. It is a tool to assist the decision makers to identify options that are available, to predict the consequences and value of each option based on the probabilities assigned to each option, and to make the decision in choosing the option that has the best payoff. Decision analysis can be incorporated into the pharmacoeconomic evaluation. Steps in performing a decision analysis are:

A. Identify and bound the decision. All the ground rules such as analysis perspective, comparators selection, time span, and decision rules are identified and clarified.

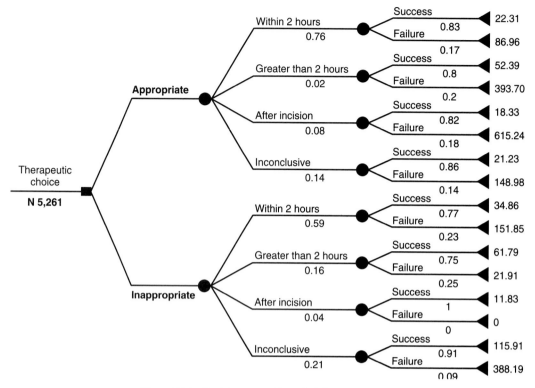

Figure 59-1. Decision tree with probabilities included.

B. **Develop a decision tree** (Figure 59-1). The decision maker will structure the decision in the form of a tree with branches from left to right. Each branch is a segment of a path that leads to an outcome. The process of setting up the tree helps the decision maker put the thought on paper and provides an evaluation for each option that occurs.

C. **Assess and assign probabilities.** Probability related to each branch is assessed and assigned. Probabilities can be obtained from the published literature, an expert panel, or clinical trials.

D. **Value outcomes.** For each of the outcome possibilities, assign a value. This can be in the form of monetary or utility values.

E. **Calculate the expected value.** Using the averaging-out and folding-back method, start from the right and work backward to the left, and calculate the expected value by multiplying the outcome value to each assigned probability (Figure 59-2).

F. **Choose the preferred course of action.** Depending on the ground rules set in the beginning of either optimization or minimization, choose the best course of action.

G. **Perform a sensitivity analysis.** Assign different values to all plausible outcomes and resolve decision tree to identify the robustmess of the data and/or results.

VI. **HEALTH-RELATED QUALITY OF LIFE (HRQOL).** While quality of life focuses on all aspects of life, HRQOL only focuses on a patient's nonclinical information such as functional status, well-being, perception of health, return to work from an illness, and other health outcomes that are directly impacted by health status. Standardized questionnaires are used to capture HRQOL data in a variety of research settings. Data are obtained either by telephone interview, self-administration, personal face-to-face interview, observation, or mail-in survey. These standardized questionnaires can also be divided into general health status instruments [e.g., Short-Form 36 (SF-36), Short-Form 12, Sickness Impact Profiles] or disease-specific instrument (e.g., McGill Pain Inventory, Beck Depression Scale, Functional Living Index—Cancer). The general health status instruments measure the global health status, whereas the disease-specific instruments target the disease-specific issues.

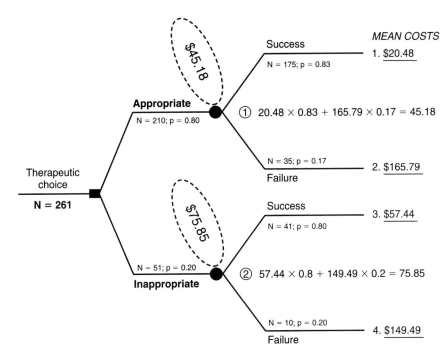

Figure 59-2. Completed decision tree after "averaging out and folding back."

A. SF-36 is the most frequently used general health status instrument. There are eight dimensions that include physical functions, social functions, emotional role, physical role, bodily pain, mental health, general health, and vitality.

B. Psychometric properties. Before using any instrument, the researcher must understand the psychometric properties of the chosen instrument. The psychometric properties consist of the reliability and validity information of the instrument. In addition, the sensitivity and specificity of the instrument are also important.

  1. Reliability is a measure of consistency. Can we reproduce the same score under the same conditions with the same individual? Statistical methods of measuring reliability are Cronbach's alpha, Pearson's r coefficient, and Kappa statistic.

  2. Validity is a measure of accuracy. Is the instrument measuring what it is supposed to measure? Types of validity are content validity, construct validity, criterion validity, and convergent/divergent validity.

  3. Use of the instrument. The psychometric properties preclude "mixing and matching" sections of established questionnaires or selection of a section of an established questionnaire for administration without recalibrating the instrument's psychometric properties.

VII. 1997 FDA MODERNIZATION ACT, SECTION 114, HEALTH CARE ECONOMIC INFORMATION

  A. Health care economic information provided to a formulary committee, or other similar entity, in the course of the committee or entity carrying out its responsibilities for the selection of drugs for managed care or other similar organizations, shall not be considered to be false or misleading under this paragraph if the health care economic information directly relates to an indication approved . . . for such drug and is based on competent and reliable scientific evidence.

  B. Health economic information means any analysis that identifies, measures, or compares the economic consequences including the costs of the represented health outcomes, or the use of a drug to the use of another drug, or to another health care intervention, or to no intervention.

C. Key concepts of the Act

1. A venue for the pharmaceutical industry to provide OR and/or PE research studies to decision makers

2. Economic information can be provided in the form of CMA, CBA, CUA, COI, and cost-quality of life.

3. Competent and reliable scientific information pertaining to an approved indication

4. Standard of competent and reliable scientific information has not been addressed.

VIII. PRACTICAL ISSUES IN INTERPRETING OUTCOMES RESEARCH AND PHARMACOECONOMIC STUDIES

A. Comparisons between economic study and randomized clinical trials (RCTs)

1. Economic studies are carried out in an observational environment, whereas RCTs depend on rigorous experimental design with strict inclusion/exclusion criteria.

2. RCTs rely on highly controlled and artificial clinical settings to demonstrate clinical efficacy. Clinical and economic end points of the study may not be the same. In addition, RCTs tend to have additional protocol costs (e.g., extra tests) and inflated benefits (e.g., medication compliance, appropriateness of utilization).

3. Economic studies have large sample sizes, while RCTs are limited to a relatively small sample size.

4. Economic studies are generalizable to the broader patient population, while RCTs are limited to those included within the stringent entry criteria, which might not represent the typical patient receiving the tested therapy.

B. Multiple countries' OR and PE studies

1. There are significant variations in physician practice patterns and care-delivery systems among different countries.

2. Different methods of funding health care and allocating health expenditures make it almost impossible to calculate costs.

3. Patients' variations and beliefs are different.

C. Budgetary constraints. Decision making should not be solely based on the information from the PE analysis because most published PE studies do not impose budgetary constraint as part of the analysis. Cost-effective does not equal affordable. In addition, one should also consider the implementation costs of the program. In many instances, implementation costs may exceed the benefits or effectiveness of the program.

D. Reproducibility

1. Often, due to journal space limitation, lengthy cost computations are eliminated from the published article. Such practice creates an impossible auditing mechanism for the derivation and computation of costs. Critical assessment of this section of the published article is necessary to ensure the validity and reliability of the results.

2. Modeling is an appropriate method when the disease and treatment in question has a lengthy time span and ethical dilemma of withdrawing treatment. However, assumptions and input values to these models are not transparent to readers.

3. Both issues make it almost impossible to reproduce the study results using the local data.

E. Limitations of claim data studies. Claim data are designed for billing purposes. There is no differentiation between comorbid conditions and complications in coding data. This can pose a problem in quality benchmark studies. In addition, coding practice may be different from one institution to another, a threat to reliability.

STUDY QUESTIONS

Directions: Each of the numbered items or incomplete statements in this section is followed by answers or by completions of the statement. Select the **one** lettered answer or completion that is **best** in each case.

1. The underlying assumption of cost-minimization analysis (CMA) is

(A) calculation of cost minimization ratio
(B) consequences are equivalent
(C) costs are equivalent
(D) no more than two comparators in any analysis

2. Which one of these statements is NOT true for the differences between economic studies and randomized clinical trials (RCTs)?

(A) Generalizability and applicability of the results differ between economic studies and RCTs.
(B) Clinical end point and economic end point are identical.
(C) RCTs tend to have inflated benefits and additional protocol-driven costs.
(D) Sample size of the economic study is normally larger than in the RCT.

3. In choosing an instrument to measure the health-related quality of life (HRQOL), attention should be paid to

(A) reliability and validity of the instrument
(B) sensitivity and specificity of the instrument
(C) length of the instrument
(D) all of the above

4. In choosing a study perspective, the current pharmacoeconomic (PE) guidelines have suggested which one of these perspectives to be included?

(A) Society
(B) Payors
(C) Patients
(D) Providers

5. When interpreting a multination economic clinical trial, what issue(s) need special attention?

(A) Cost computations
(B) Health-care funding and cost-allocating mechanisms?
(C) Patients' variations and beliefs
(D) All of the above

6. Which one of these pharmacoeconomic (PE) techniques does not address both cost and consequences?

(A) Cost-benefit analysis
(B) Cost-effectiveness analysis
(C) Cost-utility analysis
(D) Cost of illness

7. Which of the following would reflect an example of a clinical outcome indicator?

(A) Dollars spent treating acute myocardial infarction
(B) Resources utilized in diagnosing the presence of medical errors
(C) Duration of hospitalization and mortality versus discharge rate for ventricular fibrillation patients treated with amiodarone
(D) Functional capacity of patients treated with ramipril in the presence of cardiovascular risk factors

ANSWERS AND EXPLANATIONS

1. The answer is B *[IV C]*.
Cost-minimization analysis (CMA) assumes all consequences compared are equivalent. For this reason, only the cost of each alternative is compared. The least expensive alternative will be chosen.

2. The answer is B *[VIII A]*.
Clinical and economic end points are generally not equal. In the sequence of the study events, efficacy should come before effectiveness.

3. The answer is D *[VI]*.
All of the characteristics listed require attention.

4. The answer is A *[III B]*.
The societal perspective must be included. It is critical in the health-care environment to identify the perspective from which a decision is being made, and that perspective can result in a different decision. The decision to add a high-cost, moderately effective therapy for the treatment of hospitalized septic patients might be different if viewed from a hospital formulary committee (in-house budgetary concerns) as compared to the local community (saving lives at whatever expense).

5. The answer is D *[VIII B]*.
All of the issues stated need special attention and play a major role in developing multination economic evaluations to avoid carrying out a study, which when completed cannot be generalized to the broad patient population.

6. The answer is D *[IV A]*.
The cost of illness methodology is carried out as an assessment of the necessary resources, which will be utilized to treat a designated illness. Resources are measured in terms of dollars, and there are no comparator groups in the evaluation.

7. The answer is C *[I A 3]*.
Clinical outcomes include the following: length of hospital stay, adverse drug reactions, hospital readmission, and death. These are definable measures of a patient's response to a given treatment, such as amiodarone used for the treatment of ventricular fibrillation.

PRESCRIPTION DISPENSING INFORMATION AND METROLOGY

Prescriptions

PARTS OF THE PRESCRIPTION

A prescription is an order for medication for use by a patient that is issued by a physician, dentist, veterinarian, or other licensed practitioner who is authorized to prescribe medication or by their agent via a collaborative practice agreement. A prescription is usually written on a single sheet of paper that is commonly imprinted with the prescriber's name, address, and telephone number. A medication order is similar to a prescription, but it is written on the patient chart and intended for use by a patient in an institutional setting.

All prescriptions should contain accurate and appropriate information about the patient and the medication that is being prescribed. In addition, a prescription order for a **controlled substance** must contain the following information:

1. Date of issue
2. Full name and address of the patient
3. Drug name, strength, dosage form, and quantity prescribed
4. Directions for use
5. Name, address, and Drug Enforcement Agency (DEA) number of the prescriber
6. Signature of the prescriber

A written prescription order is required for substances listed in **Schedule II.** Prescriptions for controlled substances listed in **Schedule II** are **never** refillable. Any other prescription that has no indication of refills is not refillable.

Prescriptions for medications that are listed in Schedules III, IV, and V may be issued either in writing or orally to the pharmacist. If authorized by the prescriber, these prescriptions may be refilled up to five times within 6 months of the date of issue. If the prescriber wishes the patient to continue to take the medication after 6 months or five refills, a new prescription order is required.

THE PRESCRIPTION LABEL

In addition to the name of the patient, the pharmacy, and the prescriber, the prescription label should accurately identify the medication and provide directions for its use.

The label for a prescription order for a controlled substance must contain the following information:

1. Name and address of the pharmacy
2. Serial number assigned to the prescription by the pharmacy
3. Date of the initial filling
4. Name of the patient
5. Name of the prescriber
6. Directions for use
7. Cautionary statements as required by law*

AUXILIARY LABELS

Auxiliary, or cautionary, labels provide additional important information about the proper use of the medication. Examples include "Shake Well" for suspensions or emulsions; "For External Use Only" for

---

*The label of any drug that is listed as a controlled substance in Schedule II, III, or IV of the Controlled Substances Act must contain the following warning: **CAUTION: Federal law prohibits the transfer of this drug to any person other than the patient for whom it was prescribed.**

topical lotions, solutions, or creams; and "May Cause Drowsiness" for medications that depress the central nervous system. The information contained on auxiliary labels should be brought to the attention of the patient when the medication is dispensed. The pharmacist should place only appropriate auxiliary labels on the prescription container because too many labels may confuse the patient.

BEFORE DISPENSING THE PRESCRIPTION

Double-check the accuracy of the prescription.
Provide undivided attention when filling the prescription.

1. Check the patient information (e.g., name, address, date of birth, telephone number).
2. Check the patient profile (e.g., allergies, medical conditions, other drugs, including over-the-counter medications).
3. Check the drug (e.g., correct drug name, correct spelling, appropriate drug for the patient's condition), and verify that there are no known drug interactions. **Always verify the name of the drug. Beware of drug names that look alike (see table).**
4. Check the dosage, including the drug strength, the dosage form (e.g., capsule, liquid, modified release), the individual dose, the total daily dose, the duration of treatment, and the units (e.g., mg, mL, tsp, tbsp).
5. Check the label. Compare the drug dispensed with the prescription. Verify the National Drug Code (NDC) number. Ensure that the information is accurate, that the patient directions are accurate and easily understood, and that the auxiliary labels are appropriate.
6. **Provide patient counseling. Be sure that the patient fully understands the drug treatment as well as any precautions.**

Examples of Drugs with Similar Names

Brand name	Celebrex	Cerebyx	Celexa
Generic name	Celecoxib capsules	Fosphenytoin sodium injection	Citalopram HCl
Manufacturer	Searle	Parke-Davis	Forest
Indication	Osteoarthritis and rheumatoid arthritis	Prevention and treatment of seizures	Major depression

Common Abbreviations

Considerable variation occurs in the use of capitalization, italicization, and punctuation in abbreviations. The following list shows the abbreviations that are most often encountered by pharmacists.

A, aa., or aa	of each	**mcg, mcg., or μg**	microgram
a.c.	before meals	**mEq**	milliequivalent
ad	to, up to	**mg or mg.**	milligram
a.d.	right ear	**ml or mL**	milliliter
ad lib.	at pleasure, freely	**μl or μL**	microliter
a.m.	morning	**℔**	minim
amp.	ampule	**N&V**	nausea and vomiting
ante	before	**Na**	sodium
aq.	water	**N.F.**	National Formulary
a.s.	left ear	**No.**	number
asa	aspirin	**noct.**	night, in the night
a.u.	each ear, both ears	**non rep.**	do not repeat
b.i.d.	twice a day	**NPO**	nothing by mouth
BP	British Pharmacopoeia	**N.S., NS, or N/S**	normal saline
BSA	body surface area	**1/2 NS**	half-strength normal saline
c. or c̄	with	**O**	pint
cap. or caps.	capsule	**o.d.**	right eye, every day
cp	chest pain	**o.l. or o.s.**	left eye
D.A.W.	dispense as written	**OTC**	over the counter
cc or cc.	cubic centimeter	**o.u.**	each eye, both eyes
comp.	compound, compounded	**oz.**	ounce
dil.	dilute	**p.c.**	after meals
D.C., dc, or disc.	discontinue	**PDR**	*Physicians' Desk Reference*
disp.	dispense	**p.m.**	afternoon, evening
div.	divide, to be divided	**p.o.**	by mouth
dl or dL	deciliter	**Ppt**	precipitated
d.t.d.	give of such doses	**pr**	for the rectum
DW	distilled water	**prn or p.r.n.**	as needed
D5W	dextrose 5% in water	**pt.**	pint
elix.	elixir	**pulv.**	powder
e.m.p.	as directed	**pv**	for vaginal use
et	and	**q.**	every
ex aq.	in water	**q.d.**	every day
fl or fld	fluid	**q.h.**	every hour
fl oz	fluid ounce	**q. 4 hr.**	every four hours
ft.	make	**q.i.d.**	four times a day
g or Gm	gram	**q.o.d.**	every other day
gal.	gallon	**q.s.**	a sufficient quantity
GI	gastrointestinal	**q.s. ad**	a sufficient quantity to make
gr or gr.	grain	**R**	rectal
gtt or gtt.	drop, drops	**R.L. or R/L**	Ringer's lactate
H	hypodermic	**℞**	prescription
h. or hr.	hour	**s. or s̄**	without
h.s.	at bedtime	**Sig.**	write on label
IM	intramuscular	**sol.**	solution
inj.	injection	**S.O.B.**	shortness of breath
IV	intravenous	**s.o.s.**	if there is need (once only)
IVP	intravenous push	**ss. or ss**	one-half
IVPB	intravenous piggyback	**stat.**	immediately
K	potassium	**subc, subq, or s.c.**	subcutaneously
l or L	liter	**sup. or supp**	suppository
lb.	pound	**susp.**	suspension
μ	Greek mu	**syr.**	syrup
M	mix	**tab.**	tablet
m² or M²	square meter	**tal.**	such, such a one

tal. dos.	such doses	**U or u.**	unit
tbsp. or T	tablespoonful	**u.d. or ut dict.**	as directed
t.i.d.	three times a day	**ung.**	ointment
tr. or tinct.	tincture	**U.S.P. or USP**	United States Pharmacopoeia
tsp. or t.	teaspoonful	**w/v**	weight/volume
TT	tablet triturates		

Metrology

THE METRIC, APOTHECARY, AND AVOIRDUPOIS SYSTEMS

Metric system

1. Basic units

Mass = g or gram
Length = m or meter
Volume = L or liter
1 cc (cubic centimeter) of water is approximately equal to 1 mL and weighs 1 g.

2. Prefixes

kilo-	10^3, or 1000 times the basic unit
hekto-	10^2, or 100 times the basic unit
deka-	10, or 10 times the basic unit
deci-	10^{-1}, or 0.1 times the basic unit
centi-	10^{-2}, or 0.01 times the basic unit
milli-	10^{-3}, or 0.001 times the basic unit
micro-	10^{-6}, or one-millionth of the basic unit
nano-	10^{-9}, or one-billionth of the basic unit
pico-	10^{-12}, or one-trillionth of the basic unit

Examples of these prefixes include milligram (mg), which equals one-thousandth of a gram, and deciliter (dl), which equals 100 mL, or 0.1 L.

Apothecary system

1. Volume (fluids or liquid)

60 minims (℔) = 1 fluidrachm or fluidram (f ℥) or (℥)
8 fluidrachms (480 minims) = 1 fluidounce (f ℥ or ℥)
16 fluidounces = 1 pint (pt or 0)
2 pints (32 fluidounces) = 1 quart (qt)
4 quarts (8 pints) = 1 gallon (gal or C)

2. Mass (weight)

20 grains (gr) = 1 scruple (℈)
3 scruples (60 grains) = 1 drachm or dram (℥)
8 drachms (480 grains) = 1 ounce (℥)
12 ounces (5760 grains) = 1 pound (lb)

Avoirdupois system

1. Volume

1 fluidrachm = 60 min.
1 fluid ounce = 8 fl. dr.
= 480 min.
1 pint = 16 fl. oz.
= 7680 min.

```
1 quart  = 2 pt.
         = 32 fl. oz.
1 gallon = 4 qt.
         = 128 fl. oz.
```

2. Mass (weight)

The grain is common to both the apothecary and the avoirdupois systems.

```
437.5 grains (gr)  = 1 ounce (oz)
16 ounces (7000 grains)  = 1 pound (lb)
```

CONVERSION

Exact equivalents

Exact equivalents are used for the conversion of specific quantities in pharmaceutical formulas and prescription compounding.

1. Length

```
1 meter (m) = 39.37 in.
 1 inch (in) = 2.54 cm.
```

2. Volume

```
       1 ml = 16.23 minims (℥)
       1 ℥ = 0.06 mL
       1 f ʒ = 3.69 mL
       1 f ℥ = 29.57 mL
       1 pt = 473 mL
1 gal (U.S.) = 3785 mL
```

3. Mass

```
       1 g = 15.432 gr
       1 kg = 2.20 lb (avoir.)
       1 gr = 0.065 g or 65 mg
1 oz (avoir.) = 28.35 g
1 ℥ (apoth.) = 31.1 g
1 lb (avoir.) = 454 g
1 lb (apoth.) = 373.2 g
```

4. Other equivalents

```
 1 oz (avoir.) = 437.5 gr
 1 ℥ (apoth.) = 480 gr
 1 gal (U.S.) = 128 fl ℥
1 fl ℥ (water) = 455 gr
 1 gr (apoth.) = 1 gr (avoir.)
```

Approximate equivalents

Physicians may use approximate equivalents to prescribe the dose quantities using the metric and apothecary systems of weights and measures, respectively. Household units are often used to inform the patient of the size of the dose. In view of the almost universal practice of using an ordinary household teaspoon to administer medication, a teaspoon may be considered 5 mL. However, when accurate measurement of a liquid dose is required, the USP recommends the use of a calibrated oral syringe or dropper.

```
 1 fluid dram = 1 teaspoonful
              = 5 mL
4 fluidounces = 120 mL
8 fluidounces = 1 cup
              = 240 mL
      1 grain = 65 mg
        1 kg = 2.2 pounds (lb)
```

Surface Area Nomograms
Body Surface Area of Adults and Children[a]

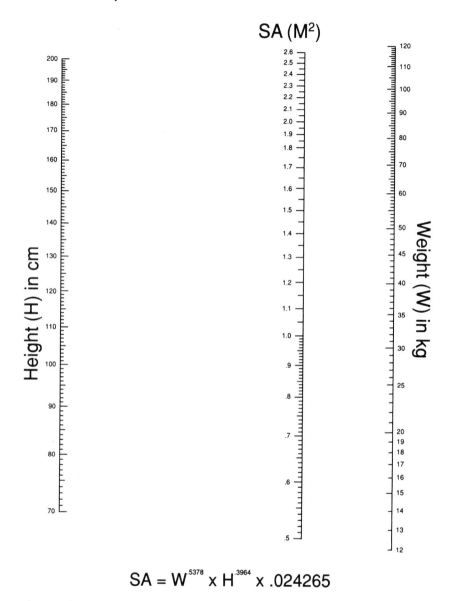

$$SA = W^{.5378} \times H^{.3964} \times .024265$$

Nomogram showing the relation among height, weight, and surface area in adults and children. To use the nomogram, align a ruler with the height and weight on the two lateral axes. The point at which the ruler intersects the center line shows the surface area. (Reprinted with permission from Haycock GB, Schwartz GJ, Wisotsky DH. Geometric method for measuring body surface area: a height–weight formula validated in infants, children, and adults. *J Pediatr* 1978;93:62–66.)

Body Surface Area of Infants*

SA (M²)

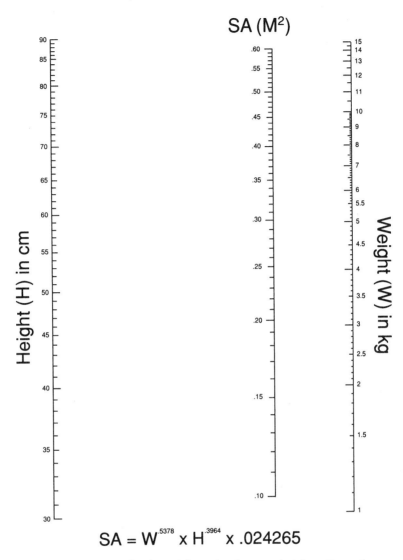

$$SA = W^{.5378} \times H^{.3964} \times .024265$$

Nomogram showing the relation among height, weight, and surface area in infants. To use the nomogram, align a ruler with the height and weight on the two lateral axes. The point at which the ruler intersects the center line shows the surface area. (Reprinted with permission from Haycock GB, Schwartz GJ, Wisotsky DH. Geometric method for measuring body surface area: a height–weight formula validated in infants, children, and adults. *J Pediatr* 1978;93: 62–66.)

COMMON PRESCRIPTION DRUGS AND OVER-THE-COUNTER PRODUCTS

The FDA Approved Drug Products With Therapeutic Equivalence Evaluation: The *Orange Book*

The United States Food and Drug Administration (FDA) publishes the book, *Approved Drug Products With Therapeutic Equivalence Evaluation,* often known as the *Orange Book.* An electronic version of the *Orange Book* is available on the Internet at http://www.fda/cder/ob. This book is also reproduced by the United States Pharmacopeial Convention, Inc., in the publication, USP DI, Volume III, *Approved Drug Products and Legal Requirements.*

These texts, which are published annually, identify the prescription and nonprescription products that are formally approved by the FDA on the basis of safety and effectiveness. They also provide the FDA's therapeutic equivalence evaluations for approved multiple-source prescription drug products.

The *Orange Book* is a drug product selection guide for pharmacists to use when dispensing a generic drug product as a substitute for the brand-name equivalent. A few drug products that were on the market before 1938 received a "grandfathered" FDA approval. These products are assumed to be safe and effective because of their long usage (e.g., digoxin tablets, phenobarbital tablets). These older products do not have therapeutic equivalence ratings at this time.

The *Orange Book* uses various codes to indicate therapeutic equivalence. The first letter "A" designates drug products that the FDA considers therapeutically equivalent to a pharmaceutically equivalent drug product. These products can be safely substituted. The first letter "B" designates drug products that, for various reasons, the FDA does not consider bioequivalent to the pharmaceutically equivalent drug product.

Therapeutic Equivalence Evaluation Codes

A Codes

Drug products that the FDA considers therapeutically equivalent to other pharmaceutically equivalent products

AA	Products in conventional dosage forms that do not present bioequivalence problems
AB	Products that meet necessary bioequivalence requirements
AN	Solutions and powders for aerosolization
AO	Injectable oil solutions
AP	Injectable aqueous solutions, and in certain instances, intravenous nonaqueous solutions
AT	Topical products

B Codes

Drug products that the FDA does not consider therapeutically equivalent to other pharmaceutically equivalent products at this time

B*	Drug products that require further FDA investigation and review to determine therapeutic equivalence
BC	Extended-release dosage forms (capsules, injectables, and tablets)
BD	Active ingredients and dosage forms that have documented problems with bioequivalence
BE	Delayed-release oral dosage forms
BN	Products in aerosol–nebulizer drug-delivery systems
BP	Active ingredients and dosage forms that have potential problems with bioequivalence
BR	Suppositories or enemas that deliver drugs for systemic absorption
BS	Drug products that have drug standard deficiencies
BT	Topical products that have bioequivalence issues
BX	Drug products for which the data are insufficient to determine therapeutic equivalence

Drug Class Symbols

The following symbols indicate the drug class of products under the Controlled Substances Act of 1970. They apply to all drug products in which they appear. These symbols are intended for use only as a guide. Check the manufacturer's label for definitive information.

C-I	Drug substances that have a high potential for abuse and have no accepted medical use in the United States. Examples include heroin, peyote, LSD, mescaline, and psilocybin.
C-II	Drug substances that have a high potential for abuse, but have a currently acceptable medical use in drug treatment. Prescriptions must be written in ink or typewritten and signed by the practitioner. Verbal prescriptions must be confirmed in writing within 72 hours and may be given only in a genuine emergency. No renewals are permitted. Examples include morphine, amphetamines, and barbiturates.
C-III	Drug substances that have some potential for abuse. Prescriptions may be oral or written. Up to 5 renewals are permitted in 6 months.
C-IV	Drug substances that have a low potential for abuse. Prescriptions may be oral or written. Up to 5 renewals are permitted in 6 months.
C-V	Drug substances that are subject to state and local regulation. The potential for abuse is low. A prescription may be required.
Rx	Drug substances that are available by prescription only, but are not classified as controlled substances.

Top 200 Prescription Drugs by Trade Name

The following list contains the top 200 brand-name prescription drugs dispensed through independent, chain, food store, mass merchandiser, and deep discount pharmacies. Rankings are based on total number of prescriptions for January to December 2001, as measured by Scott-Levin's Source Prescription Audit. Insulin products are included in the tally.

Rank	Product	Rank	Product
1	Lipitor	29	Accupril
2	Synthroid	30	Pravachol
3	Premarin Tabs	31	Neurontin
4	Norvasc	32	Lanoxin
5	Prilosec	33	Wellbutrin SR
6	Zoloft	34	Prinivil
7	Zithromax Z-Pak	35	Ultram
8	Claritin	36	Flonase
9	Paxil	37	Singulair
10	Celebrex	38	Glucotrol XL
11	Glucophage	39	Coumadin Tabs
12	Prevacid	40	Levaquin
13	Vioxx	41	Amoxil
14	Augmentin	42	Effexor XR
15	Zocor	43	Diflucan
16	Zestril	44	Flovent
17	Ortho Tri-Cyclen	45	Lotensin
18	Prempro	46	Nasonex
19	Levoxyl	47	Zithromax, Oral Suspension
20	Allegra	48	Plavix
21	Ambien	49	K-Dur 20
22	Zyrtec	50	Lotrel
23	Prozac	51	Cozaar
24	Celexa	52	Avandia
25	Toprol XL	53	Depakote
26	Viagra	54	Claritin D, 24-hr.
27	Fosamax	55	Diovan
28	Cipro	56	Risperdal

(Continued on next page)

Rank	Product	Rank	Product
57	Claritin D, 12-hr.	116	Miacalcin Nasal
58	Adderall	117	Nasacort AQ
59	Humulin N	118	Detrol
60	Xalatan	119	Endocet
61	Allegra-D	120	Biaxin XL
62	Oxycontin	121	Tequin
63	Klor-Con	122	Loestrin Fe 1/20
64	Altace	123	Relafen
65	Actos	124	Tobradex
66	Serevent	125	Seroquel
67	Zyprexa	126	Humalog
68	Evista	127	Atrovent Inhalation
69	Monopril	128	Phenergan Suppositories
70	Aciphex	129	Adalat CC
71	Protonix	130	Proventil HFA
72	Veetids	131	Tussionex
73	Hyzaar	132	Loestrin Fe 1.5/30
74	Amaryl	133	Aricept
75	Combivent	134	Alphagan
76	Flomax	135	Zithromax
77	Ortho-Novum 7/7/7	136	Lo/Ovral 28
78	Cefzil	137	Patanol
79	Levothroid	138	Coreg
80	Dilantin Kapseals	139	Apri
81	Zestoretic	140	Lotrisone
82	Ceftin	141	Azmacort
83	Alesse-28	142	Rhinocort Aqua
84	Roxicet	143	Ditropan XL
85	Diovan HCT	144	Pepcid
86	Ortho-Cyclen	145	Differin
87	Biaxin	146	Low-Ogestrel
88	Imitrex Oral	147	Atacand
89	Humulin 70/30	148	Prinzide
90	Serzone	149	Climara
91	Valtrex	150	Demadex
92	Macrobid	151	Ciloxan
93	Digitek	152	Estratest Tabs
94	Concerta	153	Humulin R
95	Necon 1/35	154	Benzamycin
96	Claritin RediTabs	155	Duragesic
97	Glucovance	156	Lamisil Oral
98	Baycol	157	Topamax
99	Avapro	158	Cardizem CD
100	Bactroban	159	Guaifenex PSE
101	Glucophage XR	160	Proscar
102	Triphasil	161	Omnicef
103	Mircette	162	Zanaflex
104	Skelaxin	163	Prometrium
105	Lescol	164	Mobic
106	Zyrtec Syrup	165	Vasotec
107	Remeron	166	Desogen
108	Nexium	167	Ocuflox
109	Tricor	168	Premphase
110	Tiazac	169	Xenical
111	Plendil	170	Niaspan
112	Trivora-28	171	Estratest HS
113	Advair Diskus	172	Estrostep Fe
114	Elocon	173	MetroGel Vaginal
115	Vicoprofen, Non-Injectable	174	Detrol LA

Rank	Product	Rank	Product
175	Accolate	188	Zaroxolyn
176	Actonel	189	Sonata
177	Univasc	190	Cosopt
178	Procardia XL	191	Axid
179	Covera-HS	192	Nizoral Shampoo
180	Zantac	193	Zovia 1/35
181	Lac-Hydrin	194	Terazol 7
182	Thyroid, Armour	195	Avelox
183	Asacol	196	Avalide
184	Lotensin HCT	197	Rhinocort
185	Claritin Syrup	198	Xanax
186	Cardura	199	Accutane
187	Femhrt	200	Meridia

Source: Scott-Levin's Source Prescription Audit (SPA).

Reprinted with permission from *The Drug Topics Red Book*, Thomson Medical Economics: Montvale, NJ, 2002.

Top 200 Prescription Drugs by Generic Name

The following list contains the top 200 generic prescription drugs dispensed through independent, chain, food store, mass merchandiser, and deep discount pharmacies. Rankings are based on total number of prescriptions for January to December 2001, as measured by Scott-Levin's Source Prescription Audit.

Rank	Product	Rank	Product
1	Hydrocodone/APAP	33	Isosorbide Mononitrate
2	Atenolol	34	Albuterol Nebulizer Solution
3	Amoxicillin	35	Methylprednisone Tablets
4	Furosemide Oral	36	Allopurinol
5	Albuterol Aerosol	37	Estradiol Oral
6	Alprazolam	38	Clonidine
7	Hydrochlorothiazide	39	Fluoxetine
8	Propoxyphene-N/APAP	40	Penicillin VK
9	Cephalexin	41	Doxazosin
10	Triamterene w/HCTZ	42	Folic Acid
11	Ibuprofen	43	Temazepam
12	Acetaminophen w/Codeine	44	Oxycodone w/APAP
13	Prednisone Oral	45	Hydroxyzine
14	Trimox	46	Meclizine HCl
15	Lorazepam	47	Metronidazole Tablets
16	Metoprolol Tartrate	48	Gemfibrozil
17	Amitriptyline	49	Promethazine Tablets
18	Ranitidine HCl	50	Terazosin
19	Trimethoprim/Sulfate	51	Triamcinolone Acetonide Topical
20	Naproxen	52	Cartia XT
21	Cyclobenzaprine	53	Spironolactone
22	Clonazepam	54	Metoclopramide
23	Trazodone HCl	55	Minocycline
24	Diazepam	56	Bisoprolol/HCTZ
25	Verapamil SR	57	Nifedipine ER
26	Glyburide	58	Propranolol HCl
27	Enalapril	59	Promethazine/Codeine
28	Potassium Chloride	60	Acyclovir
29	Carisoprodol	61	Glipizide
30	Doxycycline	62	Captopril
31	Warfarin	63	Butalbital/APAP/Caffeine
32	Medroxyprogesterone Tablets		*(Continued on next page)*

Rank	Product	Rank	Product
64	Clindamycin Systemic	121	Nystatin/Triamcinolone
65	Diltiazem CD	122	Phenytoin Sodium Extended
66	Nortriptyline	123	Ibuprofen Liquid
67	Tamoxifen	124	Guaifenesin Rx
68	Methylphenidate	125	Diphenoxylate w/Atropine
69	Tetracycline	126	Isosorbide Dinitrate
70	Albuterol Oral Liquid	127	Diphenhydramine Tablets
71	Cimetidine	128	Colchicine
72	Benzonatate	129	Promethazine DM
73	Phenobarbital	130	Docusate Sodium
74	Naproxen Sodium	131	Cefactor
75	Nitroglycerin	132	Hydroxyzine Pamoate
76	Phenazopyridine HCl	133	Pentoxifylline
77	Ferrous Sulfate	134	Labetalol
78	Aspirin, Enteric-Coated	135	Estropipate
79	Hyoscyamine	136	Carbidopa/Levodopa
80	Guaifenesin/Pseudoephedrine	137	Baclofen
81	Buspirone HCl	138	Ketoconazole Topical
82	Quinine Sulfate	139	Gentamicin Ophthalmic
83	Phentermine	140	Amiodarone
84	Methocarbamol	141	Dexamethasone Oral
85	Propranolol LA	142	Glyburide Micronized
86	Diclofenac Sodium	143	Prednisolone Acetate Ophthalmic
87	Dicyclomine HCl	144	Clorazepate Dipotassium
88	Nitroquick	145	Erythromycin Ophthalmic
89	Doxepin	146	Bumetanide, Non-Injectable
90	Carbamazepine	147	Polymyxin B/Trimethoprim
91	Famotidine	148	Cardec DM
92	Ery-Tab	149	Nitrofurantoin Macrocrystals
93	Indomethacin	150	Ipratropium Bromide
94	Methotrexate	151	Sodium Fluoride
95	Nystatin Systemic	152	Guaifenesin LA
96	Indapamide	153	Quintex PSE
97	Hydrocortisone Topical Rx	154	Clotrimazole/Betamethasone
98	Imipramine HCl	155	Timolol Maleate GFS
99	Diltiazem SR	156	Tobramycin Ophthalmic
100	Neomycin/Polymyxin/HC	157	Haloperidol
101	Guiatuss AC	158	Cefadroxil
102	Acetaminophen	159	Sulfatrim Pediatric
103	Theophylline SR	160	Hydrocortisone Valerate
104	Prednisolone Oral	161	Erythromycin Ethylsuccinate
105	Digoxin	162	Octicair
106	Benztropine	163	Piroxicam
107	Prochlorperazine Maleate	164	Timolol Maleate Ophthalmic
108	Atenolol Chlorthalidone	165	Clotrimazole Topical
109	Chlorhexidine Gluconate	166	Nifedipine
110	Levothyroxine	167	Chlordiazepoxide w/Clidinium
111	Hydroxychloroquine	168	Chlordiazepoxide HCl
112	Fluocinonide	169	HycoClear Tuss
113	Nadolol	170	Prenatal Plus
114	Nystatin Topical	171	Promethazine VC w/Codeine
115	Etodolac	172	Butalbital Compound
116	Lithium Carbonate	173	Triazolam
117	Oxybutynin Chloride	174	Bupropion
118	Clobetasol	175	Hydralazine
119	Clindamycin Topical	176	Nifedical XL
120	Multivitamins w/Fluoride, Chewable	177	Cyproheptadine

Rank	Product	Rank	Product
178	Erythromycin Topical	190	Guanfacine HCl
179	Tretinoin	191	Ketorolac Oral
180	Erythromycin Base	192	Lactulose
181	Orphenadrine Citrate	193	Lindane
182	Dipyridamole	194	Sulfasalazine
183	Sulindac	195	Methadone HCl, Non-Injectable
184	Butalbital Compound w/Codeine	196	Azathioprine
185	Phenobarbital/Belladonna	197	Promethazine VC
186	Morphine Sulfate, Non-Injectable	198	Enulose
187	Promethazine Liquid	199	Hemorrhoidal HC
188	Theochron	200	Cheratussin AC
189	Lonox		

Source: Scott-Levin's Source Prescription Audit (SPA).

Reprinted with permission from *The Drug Topics Red Book*, Thomson Medical Economics: Montvale, NJ, 2002.

Top OTC Drugs

The following list contains the Top OTC drugs by pharmacist recommendation in specific therapeutic classes.

Trade Name	Generic
Abreva	docosanol
Actifed	pseudoephedrine HCl (PSE), triprolidine HCl, acetaminophen (APAP)
Advil	ibuprofen
Afrin	oxymetazoline HCl
Aleve	naproxen sodium
ALternaGEL	aluminum hydroxide
Anusol	various formulations
Azo Standard	phenazopyridine hydrochloride
Bayer Aspirin	acetylsalicylic acid (ASA, aspirin)
Ben-Gay	methyl salicylate, menthol, and camphor
Benadryl Oral	diphenhydramine HCl (DPH), pseudoephedrine HCl (PSE), acetaminophen (APAP)
Betadine	povidine-iodine
Bonine	meclizine HCl
Bufferin	acetylsalicylic acid (ASA, aspirin) with buffers
Caladryl	pramoxine HCl, camphor with calamine or zinc acetate
Calcium	
Campho-Phenique	camphor, phenol, bacitracin zinc, neomycin sulfate, polymyxin B sulfate, lidocaine
Cepastat	phenol
Chlor-Trimeton	chlorpheniramine maleate (CPH), pseudoephedrine sulfate (PSE)
Chloraseptic	benzocaine and menthol or phenol
Citrucel	methylcellulose
Colace	docusate sodium
Compound W	salicylic acid
Comtrex	pseudoephedrine HCl (PSE), chlorpheniramine maleate (CPH), dextromethorphan HBr (DXT), acetaminophen (APAP), guaifenesin (GUA)
Contac	pseudoephedrine HCl (PSE), chlorpheniramine maleate (CPH), dextromethorphan HBr (DXT), acetaminophen (APAP), diphenhydramine HCl
Cortaid	hydrocortisone
Debrox	
Delsym	dextromethorphan polistirex
Dramamine and Dramamine II	dimenhydrinate or meclizine HCl

(Continued on next page)

Trade Name	Generic
Drixoral	pseudoephedrine sulfate (PSE), dexbrompheniramine maleate (DXB), acetaminophen (APAP)
Dulcolax	bisacodyl
Duofilm	salicylic acid
Emetrol	phosphorated carbohydrates
Excedrin	acetaminophen, aspirin, caffeine, diphenhydramine citrate
Femstat 3	butoconazole nitrate
FiberCon	polycarbophil calcium
Gas-X	simethicone, calcium carbonate
Gaviscon	aluminum hydroxide, magnesium trisilicate
Gyne-Lotrimin	clotrimazole
Imodium A-D	loperamide HCl
Kank-A	benzocaine, cetylpyridinium chloride
Kaopectate	bismuth subsalicylate
Lactinex	lactobacillus
Lamisil AT	terbinafine hydrochloride
Listerine	thymol, eucalyptol, methyl salicylate, and menthol
Lotrimin AF	clotrimazole or miconazole nitrate
Maalox/Maalox Plus	aluminum hydroxide, magnesium hydroxide, calcium carbonate, magnesium carbonate, simethicone
Metamucil	psyllium hydrophilic mucilloid
Midol/Midol PMS	pamabrom, pyrilamine maleate, acetaminophen, caffeine, ibuprofen
Monistat Vaginal	miconazole nitrate, tioconazole
Motrin IB	ibuprofen
Mylanta	aluminum hydroxide, magnesium (hydroxide and carbonate), calcium carbonate, simethicone
Mylanta Gas	simethicone
Mylicon Drops	simethicone
Myoflex	trolamine salicylate
Naphcon A	pheniramine maleate, naphazoline HCl
Nasalcrom	cromolyn sodium
Neo-Synephrine	phenylephrine HCl or oxymetazoline HCl
Neosporin	polymyxin B sulfate, neomycin, bacitracin, pramoxine HCl
Nicoderm CQ	nicotine Transdermal
Nicorette	nicotine Polacrilex
Nix	permethrin
Nizoral Shampoo	ketoconazole
NoDoz	caffeine
NyQuil	pseudoephedrine HCl (PSE), chlorpheniramine maleate (CPH), dextromethorphan HBr (DXT), acetaminophen (APAP), doxylamine succinate
Ocean	sodium chloride
Opcon A	pheniramine maleate, naphazoline HCl
OralBalance	glucose oxidase, lactoperoxidase, lysozyme
Orudis KT	ketoprofen
Pamprin	pamabrom, pyrilamine maleate, acetaminophen, magnesium salicylate
Pedia Care	pseudoephedrine HCl (PSE), chlorpheniramine maleate (CPH), dextromethorphan HBr (DXT)
Pepcid-AC	famotidine
Pepcid Complete	famotidine, calcium carbonate, magnesium hydroxide
Pepto Bismol	bismuth subsalicylate
Peri-Colace	docusate sodium and casanthranol
Phillips' MOM	magnesium hydroxide
Pin-X	pyrantel pamoate
Preparation H	shark liver oil, petrolatum, mineral oil, phenylephrine HCl
Primatine	epinephrine, ephedrine, guaifenesin
RID	pyrethrins

Trade Name	Generic
Robitussin (Adult)	guaifenesin (GUA)
Rogaine	minoxidil
Senokot	standardized senna concentrate with or without docusate
Sinutab	pseudoephedrine HCl (PSE), acetaminophen (APAP), chlorpheniramine maleate (CPH), guaifenesin
Sominex	diphenhydramine HCl
Sucrets	hexylresorcinol, dyclonine HCl, or dextromethorphan HBr
Sudafed	pseudoephedrine HCl (PSE), dextromethorphan HBr (DXT), acetaminophen (APAP), chlorpheniramine HCl (CPH), guaifenesin (GUA)
Tagamet HB 200	cimetidine
Tums	calcium carbonate
Tavist	clemastine fumarate, pseudoephedrine HCl, acetaminophen
Tears Naturale	hydroxypropyl methylcellulose, Dextran 70, white petrolatum, mineral oil
TheraFlu	pseudoephedrine HCl (PSE), chlorpheniramine maleate (CPH), acetaminophen (APAP), dextromethorphan HBr (DXT)
Tinactin	tolnaftate
Triaminic Oral	chlorpheniramine maleate (CPH), pseudoephedrine HCl (PSE) dextromethorphan HBr (DXT), guaifenesin (GUA) All formulations are alcohol-free.
Tylenol	acetaminophen (APAP)
Tylenol Allergy & Sinus	pseudoephedrine HCl (PSE), chlorpheniramine maleate (CPH), acetaminophen (APAP), doxylamine succinate
Tylenol Cold and Flu (Adult)	pseudoephedrine HCl (PSE), chlorpheniramine maleate (CPH), dextromethorphan HBr (DXT), acetaminophen (APAP), doxylamine succinate
Unisom	doxylamine succinate or diphenhydramine HCl
Visine	tetrahydrozoline HCl, oxymetazoline HCl, naphazoline HCl, pheniramine maleate
Vitamin A	retinol, retinoic acid, beta carotene, retinal, retinaldehyde; retinyl esters are all in the vitamin A family
Vitamin B Complex	vitamins B1 (thiamine), B2 (riboflavin), B3 (niacin), B5 (pantothenic acid), B6 (pyridoxine), B12 (cyanocobolamin), biotin, choline, folic acid, inositol, para-aminobenzoic acid
Vitamin C	ascorbic acid
Vitamin E	alpha-tocopherol
Zantac 75	ranitidine hydrochloride
Zostrix	capsaicin

Used with permission from *Nonprescription Drug Cards*. 4th ed. Sigler and Flanders, 2003.

APPENDIX **C**

REFERENCE CHARTS FOR PATIENT COUNSELING

Drugs That Should Not Be Crushed

Pharmacists may frequently encounter patients who, for one reason or another, cannot swallow tablets or capsules. When an alternative liquid formulation is not available, pulverizing the solid dosage form before administration may serve as a quick, safe solution to the problem.

However, not all pharmaceutical products may be crushed before administration. A variety of slow-release formulations can deliver dangerous immediate doses of their active ingredients if the integrity of the delivery system is destroyed, and enteric-coated products must remain intact in order to prevent their dissolution in the stomach.

Listed below are various slow-release as well as enteric-coated products which should not be crushed or chewed. Slow-release (sr) represents products that are controlled-release, extended-release, long-acting, and timed-release. Enteric-coated (ec) represents products that are delayed-release.

In general, capsules containing slow-release or enteric-coated particles may be opened and their contents administered on a spoonful of soft food. Instruct patients not to chew the particles, though. (Patients should, in fact, be discouraged from chewing any medication unless it is specifically formulated for that purpose.)

This list should be not considered all-inclusive. Generic and alternate brands of some products may exist. Tablets intended for sublingual or buccal administration (not included in this list) should also be administered only as intended, in an intact form.

Drug	Type of Release[a]	Drug	Type of Release
Abletex PSE	sr	Aquatab C	sr
Accuhist LA	sr	Aquatab D	sr
Aciphex	ec	Aquatab DM	sr
Adalat CC	sr	Aquatab-D	sr
Adderall XR	sr	Dose Pack	
Aerolate III	sr	Arthrotec	ec
Aerolate Jr	sr	Asacol	ec
Aerolate SR	sr	Ascocid-1000	sr
Aggrenox	sr	Ascocid-500-D	sr
Aleve Cold	sr	Ascriptin Enteric	ec
& Sinus		ATP	ec
Aleve Sinus &	sr	Atrohist	sr
Headache		Pediatric	
Allegra-D	sr	Azulfidine	ec
Allerx	sr	Entabs	
Allerx-D	sr	Bayer 8-Hour	sr
Allfen	sr	Extended	
Allfen-DM	sr	Release	
Alophen	ec	Bayer Arthritis	ec
Alterra	sr	Pain Regimen	
Amfed TD	sr	Bayer Aspirin	ec
Amibid DM	sr	Regimen	
Amibid LA	sr	Biaxin XL	sr
Amidal	sr	Bidex	sr
Aminoxin	ec	Bidex-DM	sr
Ami-Tex PSE	sr	Biohist LA	sr
Anatuss LA	sr	Bisac-Evac	ec
Aquabid-DM	sr	Biscolax	ec

Drug	Type of Release	Drug	Type of Release
Boca-Tex PSE	sr	Depakote	ec
Bontril Slow-Release	sr	Depakote ER	sr
		Depakote Sprinkles	ec
Bromadrine TR	sr	Desal II	sr
Bromfed	sr	Despec SR	sr
Bromfed-PD	sr	Detrol LA	sr
Bromfenex	sr	Dexaphen SA	sr
Bromfenex PD	sr	Dexatrim	sr
Bufferin Low Dose	ec	Dexedrine Spansules	sr
Caffedrine	sr	D-Feda II	sr
Calan SR	sr	Diamox Sequels	sr
Carbatrol	sr	Dilacor XR	sr
Cardene SR	sr	Dilantin Kapseals	sr
Cardizem CD	sr		
Cardizem SR	sr	Dilatrate-SR	sr
Carox Plus	sr	Diltia XT	sr
Cartia XT	sr	Dimetane Extentabs	sr
Catemine	ec		
Ceclor CD	sr	Disophrol Chronotab	sr
Ceclor CDpak	sr		
Cemill 1000	sr	Ditropan XL	sr
Cemill 500	sr	Donnatal Extentabs	sr
Cevi-Bid	sr		
Chlor-Phen	sr	Doryx	ec
Chlor-Trimeton Allergy	sr	Drexophed SR	sr
		Drituss GP	sr
Chlor-Trimeton Allergy Decongestant Tablets	sr	Drixomed	sr
		Drixoral	sr
		Drixoral Plus	sr
		Drixoral Sinus	sr
Choledyl SA	sr	Drize-R	sr
Claritin-D	sr	Drysec	sr
Claritin-D 24 Hour	sr	Dulcolax	ec
		Duradryl Jr	sr
Coldec TR	sr	Durasal II	sr
Compazine Spansule	sr	Duratuss	sr
		Duratuss G	sr
Concerta	sr	Duratuss GP	sr
Correctol	ec	Dura-Vent/DA	sr
Cotazym-S	ec	Dylaxol	ec
Covera-HS	sr	Dynabac	ec
Creon 10	ec	Dynabac D5-Pak	ec
Creon 20	ec	Dynacirc CR	sr
Creon 5	ec	Dynahist-ER Pediatric	sr
C-Tym	sr		
Cystospaz-M	sr	Dynex	sr
D.A. II	sr	Easprin	ec
Dairycare	ec	EC Naprosyn	ec
Dallergy	sr	Ecotrin	ec
Dallergy Jr	sr		
D-Amine-SR	sr	Ecotrin Adult Low Strength	ec
Deconamine SR	sr		
Decongest II	sr	Ecotrin Maximum Strength	ec
De-Congestine	sr		
Deconomed SR	sr		
Deconsal II	sr		
Defen-LA	sr		

(Continued on next page)

Drug	Type of Release	Drug	Type of Release
Ecpirin	ec	Guaimax-D	sr
Ed A-Hist	sr	Guaipax PSE	sr
Ed K+10	sr	Guai-Vent/PSE	sr
Effexor-XR	sr	Gua-SR	sr
Efidac 24 Chlorpheniramine	sr	Guiadrine DM	sr
Efidac 24 Pseudoephedrine	sr	Guiadrine G-1200	sr
Empro	sr	Guiadrine GP	sr
Endal	sr	Guiadrine PSE	sr
Entercote	ec	Guiatex II SR	sr
Entex LA	sr	Guiatex PSE	sr
Entex PSE	sr	H 9600 SR	sr
Entocort EC	ec	Halfprin	ec
Eryc	ec	Histade	sr
Ery-Tab	ec	Hista-Vent DA	sr
Eskalith-CR	sr	Histex CT	sr
Eudal SR	sr	Histex SR	sr
Extendryl Jr	sr	Humavent LA	sr
Extendryl SR	sr	Humibid DM	sr
Extress-60	sr	Humibid LA	sr
Feen-A-Mint	ec	Humibid Pediatric	sr
Femilax	ec	Iberet-500	sr
Femitrol	ec	Iberet-Folic-500	sr
Fenesin	sr	Icaps TR	sr
Fenesin DM	sr	Imdur	sr
Fero-Folic 500	sr	Inderal LA	sr
Fero-Grad-500	sr	Indocin SR	sr
Ferro-Sequels	sr	Iobid DM	sr
Ferro-Time	sr	Iofed	sr
Ferrous Fumarate DS	sr	Iofed PD	sr
Fetrin	sr	Ionamin	sr
Flagyl ER	sr	Iosal II	sr
Fleet Bisacodyl	ec	Iotex PSE	sr
Folitab 500	sr	Isoptin SR	sr
Fumatinic	sr	K-10	sr
Genacote	ec	K-8	sr
GFN/PSE	sr	Kadian	sr
Giltuss TR	sr	Kaon-Cl 10	sr
Glucophage XR	sr	K-Dur 10	sr
Glucotrol XL	sr	K-Dur 20	sr
GP 500	sr	Klor-Con 10	sr
G-Phed	sr	Klor-Con 8	sr
G-Phed-PD	sr	Klor-Con M10	sr
Guaifed	sr	Klor-Con M20	sr
Guaifed-PD	sr	Klotrix	sr
Guaifenex DM	sr	Kronofed-A	sr
Guaifenex G	sr	Kronofed-A-JR	sr
Guaifenex GP	sr	K-Tab	sr
Guaifenex LA	sr	Lescol XL	sr
Guaifenex PSE 120	sr	Levbid	sr
Guaifenex PSE 60	sr	Levsinex	sr
		Lexxel	sr
Guaifenex-Rx	sr	Lipram 4500	ec
Guaifenex-Rx DM	sr	Lipram-CR10	ec
		Lipram-CR20	ec

Drug	Type of Release	Drug	Type of Release
Lipram-PN10	ec	Norpace CR	sr
Lipram-PN16	ec	Omnihist L.A.	sr
Lipram-PN20	ec	Oramorph SR	sr
Lipram-UL12	ec	Oruvail	sr
Lipram-UL18	ec	Oxycontin	sr
Lipram-UL20	ec	Palgic-D	sr
Liquibid	sr	Palipase	ec
Liquibid 1200	sr	Palipase MT 16	ec
Liquibid-D	sr	Palipase MT 20	ec
Lithobid	sr	Palpeon DR 10	ec
Lodine XL	sr	Palpeon DR 20	ec
Lodrane 12 Hour	sr	Paltrase MT 20	ec
Lodrane LD	sr	Pancrease	ec
Mag Delay	sr	Pancrease MT 10	ec
Mag-SR	sr	Pancrease MT 16	ec
Mag-Tab SR	sr	Pancrease MT 20	ec
Maxifed	sr	Pancrecarb MS-4	ec
Maxifed DM	sr	Pancrecarb MS-8	ec
Maxifed-G	sr	Pancrelipase 16,000	ec
Maxovite	sr		
Medent DM	sr	Pancrelipase 20,000	ec
Medent LD	sr		
Med-Rx	sr	Pancron 10	ec
Med-Rx DM	sr	Pancron 20	ec
Mega-C	sr	Pangestyme CN-10	ec
Melfiat	sr		
Mescolor	sr	Pangestyme CN-20	ec
Mestinon Timespan	sr		
		Pangestyme EC	ec
Metadate CD	sr	Pangestyme MT16	ec
Metadate ER	sr		
Methylin ER	sr	Pangestyme UL12	ec
Micro-K	sr		
Micro-K 10	sr	Pangestyme UL18	ec
Miraphen PSE	sr		
Modane	ec	Pangestyme UL20	ec
MS Contin	sr		
Muco-Fen	sr	Panmist DM	sr
Muco-Fen 1200	sr	Panmist JR	sr
Muco-Fen DM	sr	Panmist LA	sr
Multi-Ferrous Folic	sr	Pannaz	sr
		Papacon	sr
Multiret Folic-500	sr	Para-Time SR	sr
Nalex-A	sr	Paser	or
Naprelan	sr	Pavacot	sr
Nasabid SR	sr	PCE Dispertab	or
Nasatab LA	sr	Pentasa	sr
Nd Clear	sr	Pentopak	sr
Nexium	ec	Pentoxil	sr
Niacin Time-Release	sr	Pharmadrine	sr
		Phendiet-105	sr
Niaspan	sr	Plendil	sr
Nifedical XL	sr	Poly Hist Forte	sr
Nitrocot	sr	Poly-Vent	sr
Nitrogard	sr	Poly-Vent JR	sr
Nitroglyn E-R	sr	Prehist D	sr
Nitro-Time	sr	Prelu-2	sr
Norflex	sr		

(Continued on next page)

Drug	Type of Release
Prevacid	ec
Prilosec	ec
Procanbid	sr
Procardia XL	sr
Profen Forte	sr
Profen Forte DM	sr
Profen II	sr
Profen II DM	sr
Prohist-8	sr
Prolex PD	sr
Prolex-D	sr
Pronestyl-SR	sr
Propan	sr
Protid	sr
Protonix	ec
Protuss-DM	sr
Proventil Repetabs	sr
Prozac Weekly	ec
Pseubrom	sr
Pseubrom-PD	sr
Pseudochlor	sr
Pseudocot-C	sr
Pseudocot-G	sr
Pseudo-G	sr
Pseudo-G/PSI	sr
Pseudo-PD	sr
Pseudovent	sr
Pseudovent Ped	sr
Q-Bid DM	sr
Q-Bid LA	sr
Quadra-Hist D	sr
Quadra-Hist D Ped	sr
Quibron-T/SR	sr
Quinaglute Dura-Tabs	sr
Quindal	sr
Quinidex Extentabs	sr
Regiprin	ec
Reliable Gentle Laxative	ec
Resbid	sr
Rescon	sr
Rescon JR	sr
Rescon MX	sr
Rescon-ED	sr
Respa-1st	sr
Respa-DM	sr
Respa-GF	sr
Respahist	sr
Respaire-120 SR	sr
Respaire-60 SR	sr
Ribo-2	ec
Rinade-BID	sr
Ritalin-SR	sr
Rodex Forte	sr
Rondamine	sr

Drug	Manufacturer	Type of Release
Rondec-TR		sr
Sam-E		ec
Sam-E		ec
Sinemet CR		sr
Sinuvent PE		sr
Slo-Niacin		sr
Slow Fe		sr
Slow Fe With Folic Acid		sr
Slow-Mag		sr
Spacol T/S		sr
S-Pak		sr
S-Pak DM		sr
St. Joseph Pain Reliever		ec
Stahist		sr
Stamoist E		sr
Sudafed 12 Hour		sr
Sudal 60/500		sr
Sudal DM		sr
Sular		sr
Superoxide Dismutase (SOD)		ec
Sureprin 81		ec
Symax-SR		sr
Tarka		sr
Tegretol-XR		sr
Tenuate Dospan		sr
Theo-24		sr
Theochron		sr
Theo-Time		sr
Thiamilate		ec
Thorazine Spansule		sr
Tiazac		sr
Time-Hist		sr
Toprol XL		sr
Totalday		sr
Touro Allergy		sr
Touro CC		sr
Touro DM		sr
Touro EX		sr
Touro LA		sr
T-Phyl		sr
Tranxene SD		sr
Trental		sr
Trinalin Repetabs		sr
Tussafed-LA		sr
Tussi-Bid		sr
Tylenol Arthritis		sr
Ultrabrom		sr
Ultrabrom PD		sr
Ultrase		ec
Ultrase MT12		ec
Ultrase MT18		ec
Ultrase MT20		ec
Uniphyl		sr
Urimax		ec
Urocit-K 10		sr

Drug	Type of Release	Drug	Type of Release
Urocit-K 5	sr	Voltaren	ec
Vanex Forte-D	sr	Voltaren-XR	sr
V-Dec-M	sr	We Mist LA	sr
Veracolate	ec	Wellbutrin SR	sr
Verelan	sr	Westrim LA	sr
Verelan PM	sr	Wobenzym N	ec
Versacaps	sr	Xiral	sr
Videx EC	ec	YSP Aspirin	ec
Vitamin C Timed-Release	sr	Zaptec PSE	sr
		Zephrex LA	sr
Vitamin C/Rose Hips	sr	Zorprin	sr
		Zyban	sr
Vitelle Irospan	sr	Zymase	ec
Vivotif Berna	ec	Zyrtec-D	sr
Volmax	sr		

^aec, enteric-coated; or, other; sr, slow-release.

Reprinted with permission from *The Drug Topics Red Book*. Thomson Medical Economics: Montvale, NJ, 2002.

Sugar-Free Products

Listed below, by therapeutic category, is a selection of drug products that contain no sugar. When recommending these products to diabetic patients, keep in mind that many may contain sorbitol, alcohol, or other sources of carbohydrates. This list should not be considered all-inclusive. Generics and alternate brands of some products may be available. Check product labeling for a current listing of inactive ingredients.

Product

ANALGESICS
Actamin Maximum Strength Liquid
Aminofen Tablet
Aminofen Max Tablet
Aspirtab Tablet
Aspirtab Max Tablet
Back Pain-Off Tablet
Backprin Tablet
Buffasal Tablet
Buffasal Max Tablet
Dyspel Tablet
Febrol Liquid
Medi-Seltzer Effervescent Tablet
Ms.-Aid Tablet
Non-Aspirin Pain Relief Elixir
PMS Relief Tablet
Silapap Children's Elixir
Sureprin 81 Tablet

Product

ANTACIDS/ANTIFLATULENTS
Almag Chewable Tablet
Alcalak Chewable Tablet
Aldroxicon I Suspension
Aldroxicon II Suspension
Baby Gasz Drops
Diabeti-Gest Tablet
Dimacid Chewable Tablet
Diotame Chewable Tablet
Diotame Liquid
Gas-Ban Chewable Tablet
Mallamint Chewable Tablet
Mylanta Gelcaplet
Neutralin Tablet
Pepto-Bismol Liquid
Pepto-Bismol Chewable Tablet
Riopan Plus Suspension
Riopan Suspension
Titralac Chewable Tablet
Titralac Plus Chewable Tablet
Tums E-X Chewable Tablet

(Continued on next page)

Product

ANTIASTHMATIC/RESPIRATORY AGENTS
Elixophyllin-GG Liquid
Jay-Phyl Syrup
Ventolin Syrup

ANTIDIARRHEALS
Diasorb Liquid
Diarrest Tablet
Di-Gon II Tablet
Donnagel Liquid
Imogen Liquid
Pepto-Bismol Liquid
Pepto-Bismol Chewable Tablet

BLOOD MODIFIERS/IRON PREPARATIONS
Diatx Fe Tablet
Iberet Liquid
I.L.X. B-12 Elixir
Irofol Liquid
Irofol Drops
Nephro-Fer Tablet
Niferex Elixir

CORTICOSTEROIDS
Prelone Syrup

COUGH/COLD/ALLERGY PREPARATIONS
Accuhist DM Pediatric Drops
Accuhist LA Tablet
Accuhist Pediatric Drops
Anaplex DM Syrup
Anaplex HD Syrup
Atuss EX Liquid
Biodec DM Drops
Biodec DM Syrup
Bromophed DX Syrup
B-Tuss Liquid
Carbofed DM Syrup
Carbofed DM Drops
Cepacol Sore Throat Children's Liquid
Cetafen Cold Tablet
Cheratussin DAC Liquid
Codal-DM Syrup
Codotuss Liquid
Coldonyl Tablet
Co-Tussin Liquid
Cotuss-V Syrup
Cytuss HC Syrup
D-Care Cough Syrup
Decorel Forte Tablet
Despec Liquid
Despec-SF Liquid
Diabetic Tussin Allergy Relief Liquid
Diabetic Tussin Allergy Relief Gelcaplet
Diabetic Tussin C Expectorant Liquid
Diabetic Tussin Children's Liquid
Diabetic Tussin Cold & Flu Gelcaplet
Diabetic Tussin DM Liquid
Diabetic Tussin DM Maximum Strength Liquid
Diabetic Tussin DM Maximum Strength Softgel

Product

Diabetic Tussin EX Liquid
Diabe-Tuss DM Liquid
Dimetapp Allergy Children's Elixir
Diphen Capsule
Double-Tussin DM Liquid
Duraganidin DM Liquid
Durahistine DM Syrup
Echotuss-HC Syrup
Endal Expectorant Liquid
Endal HD Liquid
Endal HD Plus Liquid
Endotuss-HD Syrup
Enplus-HD Syrup
Entex Syrup
Entex HC Syrup
Exo-Tuss Syrup
Gani-Tuss NR Liquid
Gani-Tuss-DM NR Liquid
Genecof-HC Liquid
Genecof-XP Liquid
Genedel Syrup
Genedotuss-DM Liquid
Genexpect DM Liquid
Genexpect-PE Liquid
Genexpect-SF Liquid
Giltuss Liquid
Giltuss HC Syrup
Giltuss Pediatric Liquid
Giltuss TR Tablet
Guai-Co Liquid
Guaicon DMS Liquid
Guai-DEX Liquid
Guiatuss AC Syrup
Guiatuss AC Syrup
Guiatuss DAC Syrup
Halotussin AC Liquid
Halotussin DAC Liquid
Hayfebrol Liquid
H-C Tussive Syrup
Histex PD Liquid
Histinex HC Syrup
Histinex PV Syrup
Hydro PC Syrup
Hydron KGS Liquid
Hydro-Tussin DM Elixir
Hydro-Tussin HC Syrup
Hydro-Tussin HD Liquid
Hyphen-HD Syrup
Hytuss Tablet
Hytuss 2X Capsule
Iofen-C NF Liquid
Iofen-DM NF Liquid
Iofen-NF Liquid
Iophen DM Liquid
Iotussin HC Liquid
Jaycof Expectorant Syrup
Jaycof-HC Liquid
Jaycof-XP Liquid
Kentuss Syrup

Product

Kita LA Tos Liquid
Levall 5.0 Liquid
Lodrane Liquid
Marcof Expectorant Syrup
M-Clear Syrup
M-End Liquid
Mytussin AC Cough Syrup
Mytussin DAC Syrup
Nalex DH Liquid
Nalex-A Liquid
Nalspan Senior DX Liquid
Neotuss S/F Liquid
Neotuss-D liquid
Norel DM Liquid
Nycoff Tablet
Onset Forte Tablet
Orgadin Liquid
Orgadin-Tuss Liquid
Orgadin-Tuss DM Liquid
Organidin NR Liquid
Organidin NR Tablet
Palgic-DS Syrup
Pancof HC Liquid
Pancof XP Liquid
Panmist DM Syrup
Pediatex Liquid
Pediatex DM Liquid
Pediatex-D Liquid
Phanasin Syrup
Phanasin Diabetic Choice Syrup
Phanatuss Syrup
Pneumotussin 2.5 Syrup
Poly-Tussin Syrup
Poly-Tussin DM Syrup
Poly-Tussin HD Syrup
Poly-Tussin XP Syrup
Pro-Cof Liquid
Pro-Cof D Liquid
Profen II DM Solution
Prolex DH Liquid
Prolex DM Liquid
Protuss Liquid
Protuss-D Liquid
Robafen DAC Syrup
Robitussin-DAC Syrup
Romilar AC Liquid
Romilar DM Liquid
Rondec Syrup
Rondec DM Syrup
Rondec DM Drops
Ru Tuss-DM Syrup
Scot-Tussin Allergy Relief Formula Liquid
Scot-Tussin DM Liquid
Scot-Tussin DM Cough Chasers Lozenge
Scot-Tussin Expectorant Liquid
Scot-Tussin Original Liquid
Scot-Tussin Senior Liquid

Product

Siladryl Allergy Liquid
Siladryl DAS Liquid
Sildec Syrup
Sildec Drops
Sildec-DM Syrup
Sildec-DM Liquid
Silexin Syrup
Silexin Tablet
Siltussin DAS Liquid
Siltussin DM DAS Cough Formula Syrup
Siltussin SA Syrup
S-T Forte 2 Liquid
Super Tussin DM Liquid
Supress DX Pediatric Drops
Suttar-SF Syrup
Tricodene Syrup
Trispec-PE Liquid
Tussafed Syrup
Tussafed-EX Pediatric Drops
Tussafed-HC Syrup
Tussaphen DM Syrup
Tuss-DM Liquid
Tuss-ES Syrup
Tussi-Organidin DM NR Liquid
Tussi-Organidin DM-S NR Liquid
Tussi-Organidin NR Liquid
Tussi-Organidin-S NR Liquid
Tussi-Pres Liquid
Tussirex Liquid
Vicks Dayquil Multi- Symptom Liquicap
Vicodin Tuss Expectorant Syrup
Vi-Q-Tuss Syrup
Vitussin Expectorant Syrup
Vortex Syrup
Z-Cof DM Syrup
Zyrtec Syrup

FLUORIDE PREPARATIONS
D-Care Baking Soda Toothpaste
D-Care Tartar Control Toothpaste
Fluorabon Tablet
Fluor-A-Day Tablet
Fluor-A-Day Lozenge
Flura-Loz Tablet
Lozi-Flur Lozenge
Sensodyne w/Fluoride Gel
Sensodyne w/Fluoride Tartar Control Toothpaste
Sensodyne w/Fluoride Toothpaste

LAXATIVES
Citrucel Powder
Fiber Ease Liquid
Fibro-XL Capsule
Konsyl Easy Mix Formula Powder
Konsyl-Orange Powder
Metamucil Smooth Texture Powder
Reguloid Powder

(Continued on next page)

Product

MISCELLANEOUS
Acidoll Capsule
Alka-Gest Tablet
Bicitra Solution
Colidrops Pediatric Drops
Cytra-2 Solution
Cytra-K Solution
Cytra-K Crystals
Melatin Tablet
Neutra-Phos Powder
Neutra-Phos-K Powder
Polycitra-K Solution
Polycitra-LC Solution
Questran Light Powder
Rhogam Solution

MOUTH/THROAT PREPARATIONS
Benloz Extra Strength Lozenges
Cepacol Maximum Strength Spray
Cepacol Sore Throat Lozenges
Cheracol Sore Throat Spray
Cylex Lozenges
Diabetic Tussin Cough Drops
Diabetirinse Solution
Fisherman's Friend Lozenges
Fresh N Free Liquid
Isodettes Sore Throat Spray
Larynex Lozenges
Medikoff Drops
N'Ice Lozenges
Ocusurg Powder
Oragesic Solution
Orasept Mouthwash/ Gargle Liquid
Robitussin Lozenges
Sepasoothe Lozenges
Spritz Mouthwash Powder
Thorets Maximum Strength Lozenges
Throtoceptic Spray
Vademecum Mouthwash & Gargle Concentrate

POTASSIUM SUPPLEMENTS
Cena K Liquid
Kaon Elixir
Kaon-CI 20% Liquid
Kay Ciel Powder
Klor-Con/25 Powder
Klor-Con/EF Tablet
Rum-K Liquid

VITAMINS/MINERALS/SUPPLEMENTS
Action-Tabs Made For Men
Adaptosode For Stress Liquid
Adaptosode R+R For Acute Stress Liquid
Amino Acid Complex Tablet
Aminoplex Powder
Aminostasis Powder
Aminotate Powder
B-C-Bid Caplet
Bevitamel Tablet
Biosode Liquid

Product

Biotect Plus Caplet
Bugs Bunny Complete Chewable Tablet
Bugs Bunny w/Extra Vitamin C Chewable Tablet
Bugs Bunny w/Iron Chewable Tablet
C & M Caps-375 Capsule
Calbon Tablet
Cal-Cee Tablet
Cal-Mint Chewable Tablet
Carox Plus Tablet
Cevi-Bid Tablet
Cholestratin Tablet
Chromacaps Tablet
Chromium K6 Tablet
Combi-Cart Tablet
Complete 2000 Capsule
Daily Herbs Formulas
D-Care Meal
    Replacement
D-Care Snack
Delta D3 Tablet
Detoxosode Liquid
DHEA Capsule
Diatx Tablet
Diet System 6 Gum
Diucaps Capsule
DI-Phen-500 Capsule
Electrotab Tablet
Endorphenyl Capsule
Enfagrow Oatmeal
Enterex Diabetic Liquid
Essential Nutrients Plus Silica Tablet
Evolve Softgel
Ex-L Tablet
Extress Tablet
Eyetamins Tablet
Fem Cal Tablet
Folacin-800 Tablet
Foltx Tablet
Gram-O-Leci Tablet
Hemovit Tablet
Herbal Slim Complex Capsule
Legatrin GCM Formula Tablet
Lynae Calcium/Vitamin C Chewable Tablet
Lynae Chondroitin/ Glucosamine Capsule
Lynae Ginse-Cool Chewable Tablet
Mag-Caps Capsule
Mag-Ox 400 Tablet
Mag-SR Tablet
New Life Hair Tablet
Nutrisure OTC Tablet
O-Cal Fa Tablet
Plenamins Plus Tablet
Powermate Tablet
Prostaplex Herbal Complex Capsule
Prostatonin Capsule
Protect Plus Liquid
Protect Plus Softgel
Quintabs-M Tablet
Re/Neph Liquid
Releaf For PMS Tablet

Product

Replace Capsule
Replace w/o Iron Capsule
Resource Arginaid Powder
Ribo-100 T.D. Capsule
Samolinic Softgel
Sea Omega 30 Softgel
Sea Omega 50 Softgel
Strovite Forte Syrup
Sunnie Tablet
Sunvite Tablet
Sunvite Platinum Tablet
Suplevit Liquid
Theraplex Liquid

Product

Triamin Tablet
Triamino Tablet
Tums Calcium For Life PMS Tablet
Ultramino Powder
Uro-Mag Capsule
Vitalize Liquid
Vitamin C/Rose Hips Tablet
Vitrum Jr Chewable Tablet
Xtramins Tablet
Yohimbe Power Max 1500 For Women Tablet
Yohimbized 1000 Capsule
Ze-Plus Softgel

Reprinted with permission from *The Drug Topics Red Book*. Thomson Medical Economics: Montvale, NJ, 2002.

Alcohol-Free Products

The following is a selection of alcohol-free products grouped by therapeutic category. The list is not comprehensive. Generic and alternate brands may exist. Always check product labeling for definitive information on specific ingredients.

Product

ANALGESICS
Acetaminophen Infants Drops
Actamin Maximum Strength Liquid
Advil Children's Suspension
Aminofen Tablet
Aminofen Max Tablet
APAP Elixir
Aspirtab Tablet
Aspirtab Max Tablet
Buffasal Tablet
Buffasal Max Tablet
Demerol Hydrochloride Syrup
Dolono Elixir
Dolono Infants Drops
Dyspel Tablet
Genapap Children Elixir
Genapap Infant's Drops
Motrin Children's Suspension
Silapap Children's Elixir
Silapap Infant's Drops
Tempra 1 Drops
Tempra 2 Syrup
Tylenol Children's Suspension
Tylenol Infant's Drops

ANTIASTHMATIC AGENTS
Dilor-G Liquid
Dy-G Liquid
Elixophyllin-GG Liquid

ANTICONVULSANTS
Zarontin Syrup

ANTIVIRAL AGENTS
Epivir Oral Solution

Product

COUGH/COLD/ALLERGY PREPARATIONS
Accuhist Pediatric Drops
Allergy Relief Medicine Children's Elixir
Anaplex DM Syrup
Anaplex HD Syrup
Andehist DM Drops
Andehist DM Syrup
Atuss DM Liquid
Atuss EX Liquid
Atuss G Liquid
Atuss MS Syrup
Biodec DM Drops
Biodec DM Syrup
Bromaline Solution
Bromaline DM Elixir
Bromanate Elixir
Bron-Tuss Liquid
B-Tuss Liquid
Carbatuss Liquid
Carbofed DM Drops
Carbofed DM Syrup
Cepacol Sore Throat Children's Liquid
Chlor-Trimeton Allergy Syrup
Codal-DH Syrup
Codal-DM Syrup
Codotuss Liquid
Coldonyl Tablet
Complete Allergy Elixir
Co-Tussin Liquid
Cotuss-V Syrup
Creomulsion Complete Syrup
Creomulsion Cough Syrup
Creomulsion For Children Syrup
Creomulsion Pediatric Syrup

(Continued on next page)

Product

Cytuss HC Syrup
D-Care Cough Syrup
Dehistine Syrup
Deltuss Liquid
Despec Liquid Labs
Diabetic Tussin Allergy Relief Liquid
Diabetic Tussin Allergy Relief Tablet
Diabetic Tussin C Expectorant Liquid
Diabetic Tussin Children's Liquid
Diabetic Tussin Cold & Flu Tablet
Diabetic Tussin DM Liquid
Diabetic Tussin DM Maximum Strength Liquid
Diabetic Tussin DM Maximum Strength Capsule
Diabetic Tussin EX Liquid
Diabe-Tuss DM Syrup
Dimetapp Allergy Children's Elixir
Dimetapp Cold & Fever Children's Suspension
Dimetapp Decongestant Pediatric Drops
Double-Tussin DM Liquid
Duraganidin DM Liquid
Durahistine DM Syrup
Echotuss-HC Syrup
Endagen-HD Syrup
Endal HD Syrup
Endal HD Plus Syrup
Endotuss-HD Syrup
Enplus-HD Syrup
Entex Syrup
Entex HC Syrup
Exo-Tuss
Father John's Medicine Plus Drops
Friallergia DM Liquid
Friallergia Liquid
Gani-Tuss NR Liquid
Gani-Tuss-DM NR Liquid
Genahist Elixir
Giltuss HC Syrup
Giltuss Liquid
Giltuss Pediatric Liquid
Guai-Co Liquid
Guaicon DMS Liquid
Guai-Dex Liquid
Guaifed Syrup
Guiatuss CF Syrup
Halotussin Syrup
Hayfebrol Liquid
H-C Tussive Syrup
Histex Liquid
Histex PD Drops
Histex PD Liquid
Histinex HC Syrup
Histinex PV Syrup
Hycomal DH Liquid
Hydone Liquid
Hydramine Elixir
Hydro-Tussin DM Elixir
Hydro-Tussin HC Syrup
Hydro-Tussin HD Liquid
Hyphen-HD Syrup
Iodal HD Liquid

Product

Iofen-C NF Liquid
Iofen-DM NF Liquid
Iofen-NF Liquid
Iophen DM Liquid
Iotussin HC Liquid
Jaycof Expectorant Syrup
Jaycof-HC Liquid
Jaycof-XP Liquid
Kentuss Syrup
KG-Dal HD Plus Syrup
Kita La Tos Liquid
Levall Liquid
Levall 5.0 Liquid
Lodrane Liquid
Marcof Expectorant Syrup
M-Clear Syrup
Medi-Brom Elixir
M-End Liquid
Motrin Cold Children's Suspension
Mytussin-PE Liquid
Nalex DH Liquid
Nalex-A Liquid
Nalspan Senior DX Liquid
Neotuss S/F Liquid
Neotuss-D Liquid
Norel DM Liquid
Nucofed Syrup
Nycoff Tablet
Orgadin Liquid
Orgadin-Tuss Liquid
Orgadin-Tuss DM Liquid
Organidin NR Liquid
Palgic-DS Syrup
Pancof HC Liquid
Pancof XP Liquid
Panmist DM Syrup
Panmist-S Syrup
Pediacare Cold + Allergy Children's Liquid
Pediacare Cough-Cold Liquid
Pediacare Decongestant Infants Drops
Pediacare Decongestant Plus Cough Drops
Pediacare Multi-Symptom Liquid
Pediacare Nightrest Liquid
Pedia-Relief Liquid
Pediatex Liquid
Pediatex-D Liquid
Phanasin Syrup
Phanatuss Syrup
Pharmasin Syrup
Pharmatuss DM Syrup
Phena-S Liquid
Pneumotussin 2.5 Syrup
Poly-Tussin Syrup
Poly-Tussin DM Syrup
Poly-Tussin HD Syrup
Poly-Tussin XP Syrup
Primsol Solution
Pro-Cof Liquid
Profen II DM Liquid
Prolex DH Liquid

Product

Prolex DM Liquid
Protuss Liquid
Protuss-D Liquid
Q-Tussin PE Liquid
Robitussin Cough & Congestion Liquid
Robitussin DM Syrup
Robitussin PE Syrup
Robitussin Pediatric Drops
Robitussin Pediatric Cough Syrup
Robitussin Pediatric Night Relief Liquid
Romilar AC Liquid
Romilar DM Liquid
Rondec Syrup
Rondec DM Drops
Rondec DM Syrup
Scot-Tussin Allergy Relief Formula Liquid
Scot-Tussin DM Liquid
Scot-Tussin Expectorant Liquid
Scot-Tussin Original Syrup
Scot-Tussin Senior Liquid
Siladryl Allergy Liquid
Siladryl DAS Liquid
Sildec Liquid
Sildec Syrup
Sildec-DM Drops
Sildec-DM Syrup
Siltussin DAS Liquid
Siltussin DM Syrup
Siltussin DM DAS Cough Formula Syrup
Siltussin SA Syrup
S-T Forte 2 Liquid
Sudatuss DM Syrup
Sudatuss-2 Liquid
Sudatuss-SF Liquid
Super Tussin DM Liquid
Triaminic Infant Decongestant Drops
Trispec-PE Liquid
Tussafed Syrup
Tussafed-EX Syrup
Tussafed-EX Pediatric Liquid
Tussafed-HC Syrup
Tuss-DM Liquid
Tuss-ES Syrup
Tussi-Organidin DM NR Liquid
Tussi-Organidin DM-S NR Liquid
Tussi-Organidin NR Liquid
Tussi-Organidin-S NR Liquid
Tussi-Pres Liquid
Tussirex Liquid
Tussirex Syrup
Tylenol Allergy-D Children's Liquid
Tylenol Cold Children's Liquid
Tylenol Cold Infants Drops
Tylenol Cold Plus Cough Children's Liquid
Tylenol Flu Children's Suspension
Tylenol Flu Night Time Max Strength Liquid
Tylenol Sinus Children's Liquid
Vanex-HD Syrup
Vicks 44E Pediatric Liquid
Vicks 44M Pediatric Liquid

Product

Vicks Dayquil Multi-Symptom Liquicap
Vicks Dayquil Multi-Symptom Liquid
Vicks Nyquil Children's Liquid
Vicodin Tuss Expectorant Syrup
Vi-Q-Tuss Syrup
Vitussin Expectorant Syrup
Vortex Syrup
Z-Cof DM Syrup

EAR/NOSE/THROAT PRODUCTS
4-Way Saline Moisturizing Mist Spray
Ayr Baby Saline Spray
Bucalsep Solution
Bucalsep Spray
Cheracol Sore Throat Spray
Diabetirinse Solution
Fresh N Free Liquid
Glandosane Solution
Gly-Oxide Liquid
Isodettes Sore Throat Spray
Lacrosse Mouthwash Liquid
Larynex Lozenges
Listermint Liquid
Nasal Moist Gel
Orajel Baby Liquid
Orajel Baby Nighttime Gel
Orasept Mouthwash/ Gargle Liquid
Spritz Mouthwash Powder
Tanac Liquid
Tech 2000 Dental Rinse Liquid
Throto-Ceptic Spray
Zilactin Baby Extra Strength Gel

GASTROINTESTINAL AGENTS
Agoral Liquid
Baby Gasz Drops
Colace Liquid
Colidrops Pediatric Drops
Diarrest Tablet
Imogen Liquid
Kaodene NN Suspension
Kaopectate Advanced Formula Suspension
Kaopectate Children's Liquid Suspension
Liqui-Doss Liquid
Mylicon Infants' Suspension
Neoloid Liquid
Neutralin Tablet
Senokot Children's Syrup

HEMATINICS
Feostat Suspension
Irofol Liquid

MISCELLANEOUS
Cytra-2 Solution
Cytra-K Solution
Emetrol Solution
Emetrol Solution
Fluorinse Solution
Rum-K Liquid

(Continued on next page)

Product

PSYCHOTROPICS
Thorazine Syrup

TOPICAL PRODUCTS
Aloe Vesta 2-N-1 Antifungal Ointment
Fleet Pain Relief Pads
Fresh & Pure Douche Solution
Handclens Solution
Klenz Kloth Pads
Lid Wipes-SPF Pads
Neutrogena Acne Wash Liquid
Neutrogena Antiseptic Liquid
Neutrogena Clear Pore Gel
Neutrogena T/Derm Liquid
Neutrogena Toner Liquid
Podiclens Spray
Propa PH Foaming Face Wash Liquid
Sea Breeze Foaming Face Wash Gel
Stri-Dex Pad
Stri-Dex Maximum Strength Pad
Stri-Dex Sensitive Skin Pad
Stri-Dex Super Scrub Pad

Product

VITAMINS/MINERALS/SUPPLEMENTS
Adaptosode For Stress Liquid
Adaptosode R+R For Acute Stress Liquid
Biosode Liquid
Detoxosode Products Liquid
Genesupp-500 Liquid
Genetect Plus Liquid
Multi-Delyn w/Iron Liquid
Poly-Vi-Sol Drops
Poly-Vi-Sol w/Iron Drops
Protect Plus Liquid
Soluvite-F Drops
Strovite Forte Syrup
Suplevit Liquid
Theragran Liquid
Theraplex Liquid
Tri-Vi-Sol Drops
Tri-Vi-Sol w/Iron Drops
Vitafol Syrup
Vitalize Liquid
Vitamin C/Rose Hips Tablet, Extended Release

Reprinted with permission from *The Drug Topics Red Book.* Thomson Medical Economics: Montvale, NJ, 2002.

Drugs That May Cause Photosensitivity

The drugs in this table are known to cause photosensitivity in some individuals. Effects can range from itching, scaling, rash, and swelling to skin cancer, premature skin aging, skin and eye burns, cataracts, reduced immunity, blood vessel damage, and allergic reactions. The list is not all-inclusive, and shows only representative brands of each generic. When in doubt, always check specific product labeling. Individuals should be advised to wear protective clothing and to apply sunscreens while taking the medications listed below.

Generic	Brand
Acetazolamide	Diamox
Acitretin	Soriatane
Alendronate	Fosamax
Alitretinoin	Panretin
Amiloride/ hydrochlorothiazide	Moduretic
Amiodarone	Cordarone, Pacerone
Amitriptyline	Elavil
Amitriptyline/ chlordiazepoxide	Limbitrol
Amitriptyline/perphenazine	Etrafon, Etrafon-Forte, Triavil
Amoxapine	
Anagrelide	Agrylin
Atenolol/chlorthalidone	Tenoretic
Atorvastatin	Lipitor
Aurothioglucose	Solganal
Azatadine/pseudoephedrine	Rynatan, Trinalin
Azithromycin	Zithromax
Benazepril	Lotensin
Benazepril/ hydrochlorothiazide	Lotensin HCT

Generic	Brand
Bendroflumethiazide/ nadolol	Corzide
Bexarotene	Targretin
Bismuth/metronidazole/ tetracycline	Helidac
Bisoprolol/ hydrochlorothiazide	Ziac
Brompheniramine/ dextromethorphan/ pseudoephedrine	Bromfed-DM, Dimetane-DX
Bupropion	Wellbutrin, Zyban
Candesartan/ hydrochlorothiazide	Atacand HCT
Capecitabine	Xeloda
Captopril	Capoten
Captopril/ hydrochlorothiazide	Capozide
Carbamazepine	Carbatrol, Tegretol, Tegretol-XR
Carbinoxamine/ pseudoephedrine	Palgic-D, Palgic-DS, Pediatex-D
Carvedilol	Coreg
Celecoxib	Celebrex

Generic	Brand
Cetirizine	Zyrtec
Cevimeline	Evoxac
Chlorhexidine gluconate	Hibistat
Chlorothiazide	Diuril
Chlorpheniramine/ hydrocodone/ pseudoephedrine	Tussend
Chlorpheniramine/ phenylephrine/pyrilamine	Rynatan
Chlorpromazine	Thorazine
Chlorpropamide	Diabinese
Chlorthalidone	Thalitone
Chlorthalidone/clonidine	Combipres
Cidofovir	Vistide
Ciprofloxacin	Cipro
Citalopram	Celexa
Clemastine	Tavist
Clozapine	Clozaril
Cromolyn sodium	Gastrocrom
Cyclobenzaprine	Flexeril
Cyproheptadine	Periactin
Dacarbazine	DTIC-Dome
Dantrolene	Dantrium
Demeclocycline	Declomycin
Desipramine	Norpramin
Diclofenac potassium	Cataflam
Diclofenac sodium	Voltaren, Voltaren-XR
Diclofenac sodium/ misoprostol	Arthrotec
Diflunisal	Dolobid
Dihydroergotamine	D.H.E. 45
Diltiazem	Cardizem, Tiazac
Diphenhydramine	Benadryl
Divalproex	Depakote
Doxepin	Sinequan
Doxycycline hyclate	Doryx, Periostat, Vibra-Tabs, Vibramycin
Doxycycline monohydrate	Monodox
Enalapril	Vasotec
Enalapril/felodipine	Lexxel
Enalapril/ hydrochlorothiazide	Vaseretic
Enalaprilat	Vasotec I.V.
Enoxacin	Penetrex
Epirubicin	Ellence
Erythromycin/sulfisoxazole	Pediazole
Estazolam	ProSom
Estradiol	Gynodiol
Ethionamide	Trecator-SC
Etodolac	Lodine
Felbamate	Felbatol
Fenofibrate	Tricor
Floxuridine	Sterile FUDR
Flucytosine	Ancobon
Fluorouracil	Efudex
Fluoxetine	Prozac, Sarafem
Fluphenazine	Prolixin
Flutamide	Eulexin

Generic	Brand
Fluvastatin	Lescol
Fluvoxamine	Luvox
Fosinopril	Monopril
Fosphenytoin	Cerebyx
Furosemide	Lasix
Gabapentin	Neurontin
Gatifloxacin	Tequin
Gemfibrozil	Lopid
Gentamicin	Garamycin
Glatiramer	Copaxone
Glimepiride	Amaryl
Glipizide	Glucotrol
Glyburide	DiaBeta, Glynase, Micronase
Glyburide/metformin HCl	Glucovance
Griseofulvin	Fulvicin P/G, Grifulvin, Gris-PEG
Haloperidol	Haldol
Hexachlorophene	pHisoHex
Hydralazine/ hydrochlorothiazide	Apresazide
Hydrochlorothiazide	HydroDIURIL, Hyzaar, Microzide, Oretic
Hydrochlorothiazide/ fosinopril	Monopril HCT
Hydrochlorothiazide/ irbesartan	Avalide
Hydrochlorothiazide/ lisinopril	Prinzide, Zestoretic
Hydrochlorothiazide/ losartan potassium	Hyzaar
Hydrochlorothiazide/ methyldopa	Aldoril
Hydrochlorothiazide/ moexipril	Uniretic
Hydrochlorothiazide/ propranolol	Inderide
Hydrochlorothiazide/ quinapril	Accuretic
Hydrochlorothiazide/ spironolactone	Aldactazide
Hydrochlorothiazide/ telmisartan	Micardis HCT
Hydrochlorothiazide/ timolol	Timolide
Hydrochlorothiazide/ triamterene	Dyazide, Maxzide
Hydrochlorothiazide/ valsartan	Diovan HCT
Hydroflumethiazide	Diucardin
Hypericum	Kira, St. John's Wort
Hypericum/vitamin B_1/ vitamin C/kava-kava	One-A-Day Tension & Mood
Ibuprofen	Motrin
Imipramine	Tofranil

(Continued on next page)

Generic	Brand	Generic	Brand
Indapamide	Lozol	Pimpinella major	Burnet
Interferon alfa-2b, recombinant	Intron A	Piroxicam	Feldene
		Polymyxin B/trimethoprim	Polytrim
Interferon alfa-n3 (human leukocyte derived)	Alferon-N	Polythiazide	Renese
		Polythiazide/prazosin	Minizide
Interferon beta-1a	Avonex	Porfimer sodium	Photofrin
Interferon beta-1b	Betaseron	Pravastatin	Pravachol
Irbesartan/ hydrochlorothiazide	Avalide	Prochlorperazine	Compazine, Compro
Isoniazid/pyrazinamide/ rifampin	Rifater	Promethazine	Phenergan
		Protriptyline	Vivactil
Ketoprofen	Orudis, Oruvail	Pyrazinamide	Pyrazinamide
Lamotrigine	Lamictal	Quetiapine	Seroquel
Leuprolide	Lupron	Quinapril	Accupril
Levamisole	Ergamisol	Quinidine gluconate	Quinaglute, Quinidine
Lisinopril	Prinivil, Zestril		
Lomefloxacin	Maxaquin	Quinidine sulfate	Quinidex
Loratadine	Claritin	Rabeprazole sodium	Aciphex
Loratadine/ pseudoephedrine	Claritin-D	Ramipril	Altace
		Riluzole	Rilutek
Losartan	Cozaar	Risperidone	Risperdal
Lovastatin	Mevacor	Ritonavir	Norvir
Maprotiline	Ludiomil	Rizatriptan	Maxalt, Maxalt-MLT
Mefenamic acid	Ponstel		
Meloxicam	Mobic	Ropinirole	Requip
Meperidine/promethazine	Mepergan	Ruta graveolens	Rue
Mesalamine	Pentasa	Saquinavir	Fortovase
Methazolamide	Neptazane	Saquinavir mesylate	Invirase
Methotrexate	Trexall	Selegiline	Eldepryl
Methoxsalen	Uvadex, Oxsoralen	Sertraline	Zoloft
Methyclothiazide	Enduron	Sibutramine	Meridia
Metolazone	Mykrox, Zaroxolyn	Sildenafil	Viagra
Minocycline	Dynacin, Minocin	Simvastatin	Zocor
Mirtazapine	Remeron	Somatropin	Serostim
Moexipril	Univasc	Sotalol	Betapace, Betapace AF
Moxifloxacin	Avelox		
Nabumetone	Relafen	Sparfloxacin	Zagam
Nalidixic acid	NegGram	Sulfamethoxazole/ trimethoprim	Bactrim, Septra
Naproxen	Naprosyn, EC-Naprosyn	Sulfasalazine	Azulfidine
Naproxen sodium	Anaprox, Naprelan	Sulfisoxazole	Gantrisin Pediatric
Naratriptan	Amerge	Sulindac	Clinoril
Nefazodone	Serzone	Sumatriptan	Imitrex
Nifedipine	Procardia	Tacrolimus	Prograf, Protopic
Nisoldipine	Sular	Tazarotene	Tazorac
Norfloxacin	Noroxin	Tetracycline	Achromycin
Nortriptyline	Pamelor	Thalidomide	Thalomid
Ofloxacin	Floxin	Thioridazine hydrochloride	Mellaril
Olanzapine	Zyprexa, Zyprexa Zydis	Thiothixene	Navane
		Tiagabine	Gabitril
Olsalazine	Dipentum	Topiramate	Topamax
Oxaprozin	Daypro	Triamcinolone	Azmacort
Oxcarbazepine	Trileptal	Triamterene	Dyrenium
Oxytetracycline	Terramycin	Trifluoperazine	Stelazine
Paroxetine	Paxil	Trimipramine	Surmontil
Pastinaca sativa	Parsnip	Trovafloxacin	Trovan
Pentosan polysulfate	Elmiron	Valacyclovir	Valtrex
Pentostatin	Nipent	Valproate	Depacon
Perphenazine	Trilafon	Valproic acid	Depakene
Pilocarpine	Salagen	Venlafaxine	Effexor

Generic	Brand	Generic	Brand
Verteporfin	Visudyne	Ziprasidone	Geodon
Vinblastine		Zolmitriptan	Zomig
Zalcitabine	Hivid	Zolpidem	Ambien
Zaleplon	Sonata		

Reprinted with permission from *The Drug Topics Red Book*. Thomson Medical Economics: Montvale, NJ, 2002.

Drug–Alcohol Interactions

The following information was extracted from PharmaCIS™, the new *Clinical Integration System for Drug Utilization Review*™ from Red Book Database Services. The PharmaCIS database modules cover the full range of Omnibus Reconciliation Act requirements for drug utilization review, including the production of leaflets for patient education and screening for drug–drug interactions, previous allergies, therapeutic duplication, and improper dosing.

For further information on integrating PharmaCIS into an existing pharmacy system, contact your system vendor or Red Book Database Services at 800-722-3062.

Products are listed alphabetically, with summary warning statements given for each interaction. Degrees of onset and severity are indicated as follows. Onset: 1 = rapid (within 24 hours); 2 = delayed (after 24 hours). Severity: 1 = major (possibly life-threatening or potential permanent damage); 2 = moderate (may exacerbate the patient's condition); 3 = minor (little, if any, clinical effect).

Product	Interaction	Onset	Severity
Acetaminophen	Concurrent use of Ethanol and Acetaminophen may result in an increased risk of hepatotoxicity.	2	2
Acetophenazine	Concurrent use of Acetophenazine and Ethanol may result in increased central nervous system depression and an increased risk of extrapyramidal reactions.	1	2
Acitretin	Concurrent use of Acitretin and Ethanol may result in a prolonged risk of teratogenicity.	2	1
Alfentanil	Concurrent use of Ethanol and Alfentanil may result in decreased therapeutic effects for alfentanil.	2	2
Alprazolam	Concurrent use of Ethanol and Alprazolam may result in increased sedation.	1	2
Amitriptyline	Concurrent use of Ethanol and Amitriptyline may result in enhanced CNS depression and impairment of motor skills.	1	2
Amobarbital	Concurrent use of Ethanol and Amobarbital may result in excessive CNS depression.	1	2
Amoxapine	Concurrent use of Ethanol and Amoxapine may result in Ethanol enhanced drowsiness; impairment of motor skills.	1	2
Amprenavir	Concurrent use of Amprenavir and Ethanol may result in an increased risk of propylene glycol toxicity (seizures, tachycardia, lactic acidosis, renal toxicity, hemolysis).	2	1
Aprobarbital	Concurrent use of Aprobarbital and Ethanol may result in excessive CNS depression.	1	2
Aspirin	Concurrent use of Ethanol and Aspirin may result in increased gastrointestinal blood loss.	1	2
Bupropion	Concurrent use of Bupropion and Ethanol may result in an Ethanol increased risk of seizures.	2	1
Butabarbital	Concurrent use of Butabarbital and Ethanol may result in excessive CNS depression.	1	2
Butalbital	Concurrent use of Butalbital and Ethanol may result in excessive CNS depression.	1	2
Cefamandole	Concurrent use of Ethanol and Cefamandole may result in disulfiram-like reactions.	2	1
Cefmenoxime	Concurrent use of Ethanol and Cefmenoxime may result in disulfiram-like reactions.	1	1

(Continued on next page)

Product	Interaction	Onset	Severity
Cefoperazone	Concurrent use of Ethanol and Cefoperazone may result in l disulfiram-like reactions.	2	1
Cefotetan	Concurrent use of Ethanol and Cefotetan may result in disulfiram-like reactions.	2	1
Chloral hydrate	Concurrent use of Ethanol and Chloral Hydrate may result in increased sedation.	1	3
Chloral hydrate	Concurrent use of Ethanol and Chlordiazepoxide may result in increased sedation.	1	2
Chlorpromazine	Concurrent use of Ethanol and Chlorpromazine may result in increased sedation.	1	2
Chlorpropamide	Concurrent use of Ethanol and Chlorpropamide may result in disulfiram-like reactions.	1	1
Cimetidine	Concurrent use of Ethanol and Cimetidine may result in increased ethanol concentrations.	1	3
Cisapride	Concurrent use of Cisapride and Ethanol may result in increased blood levels of ethanol.	1	2
Clomipramine	Concurrent use of Ethanol and Clomipramine may result in enhanced drowsiness; impairment of motor skills.	1	2
Clorazepate	Concurrent use of Ethanol and Clorazepate may result in increased sedation.	1	2
Cocaine	Concurrent use of Ethanol and Cocaine may result in increased heart rate and blood pressure.	1	2
Codeine	Concurrent use of Ethanol and Codeine may result in increased sedation.	1	2
Cycloserine	Concurrent use of Cycloserine and Ethanol may result in an increased risk of seizures.	1	1
Desipramine	Concurrent use of Ethanol and Desipramine may result in enhanced drowsiness; impairment of motor skills.	1	2
Diazepam	Concurrent use of Ethanol and Diazepam may result in increased sedation.	1	2
Dimethindene	Concurrent use of Dimethindene and Ethanol may result in increased sedation.	1	2
Diphenhydramine	Concurrent use of Ethanol and Diphenhydramine may result in increased sedation.	1	2
Disulfiram	Concurrent use of Ethanol and Disulfiram may result in ethanol intolerance.	1	1
Dothiepin	Concurrent use of Ethanol and Dothiepin may result in enhanced drowsiness; impairment of motor skills.	1	2
Doxepin	Concurrent use of Ethanol and Doxepin may result in enhanced drowsiness; impairment of motor skills.	1	2
Eterobarb	Concurrent use of Eterobarb and Ethanol may result in excessive CNS depression.	1	2
Ethopropazine	Concurrent use of Ethopropazine and Ethanol may result in increased central nervous system depression and an increased risk of extrapyramidal reactions.	1	2
Flunitrazepam	Concurrent use of Flunitrazepam and Ethanol may result in excessive sedation and psychomotor impairment.	1	2
Fluphenazine	Concurrent use of Fluphenazine and Ethanol may result in increased central nervous system depression and an increased risk of extrapyramidal reactions.	1	2
Fomepizole	Concurrent use of Fomepizole and Ethanol may result in the reduced elimination of both drugs.	2	2
Fosphenytoin	Concurrent use of Fosphenytoin and Ethanol may result in decreased phenytoin serum concentrations, increased seizure potential, and additive CNS depressant effects.	1	2
Furazolidone	Concurrent use of Ethanol and Furazolidone may result in disulfiram-like reactions.	1	1
Gliclazide	Concurrent use of Ethanol and Gliclazide may result in prolonged hypoglycemia, disulfiram-like reactions.	1	1

Product	Interaction	Onset	Severity
Glipizide	Concurrent use of Ethanol and Glipizide may result in prolonged hypoglycemia, disulfiram-like reactions.	1	1
Glutethimide	Concurrent use of Ethanol and Glutethimide may result in increased sedation.	1	2
Glyburide	Concurrent use of Ethanol and Glyburide may result in prolonged hypoglycemia, disulfiram-like reactions.	1	1
Griseofulvin	Concurrent use of Griseofulvin and Ethanol may result in disulfiram-like reactions (nausea, vomiting, diarrhea, flushing, tachycardia, hypotension).	1	1
Hydrocodone	Concurrent use of Ethanol and Hydrocodone may result in increased sedation.	1	2
Hydromorphone	Concurrent use of Hydromorphone and Ethanol may result in increased sedation.	1	2
Imipramine	Concurrent use of Ethanol and Imipramine may result in enhanced drowsiness; impairment of motor skills.	1	2
Insulin	Concurrent use of Ethanol and Insulin may result in increased hypoglycemia.	1	2
Insulin lispro	Concurrent use of Ethanol and Insulin lispro may result in increased hypoglycemia.	1	2
Isoniazid	Concurrent use of Ethanol and Isoniazid may result in decreased isoniazid concentrations and disulfiram-like reactions.	2	1
Isotretinoin	Concurrent use of Ethanol and Isotretinoin may result in a disulfiram-like reaction.	1	1
Kava	Concurrent use of Kava and Ethanol may result in increased central nervous system depression.	1	2
Ketoconazole	Concurrent use of Ethanol and Ketoconazole may result in disulfiram-like reactions (flushing, vomiting, increased respiratory rate, tachycardia).	1	1
Lofepramine	Concurrent use of Ethanol and Lofepramine may result in enhanced drowsiness; impairment of motor skills.	1	2
Lorazepam	Concurrent use of Ethanol and Lorazepam may result in increased sedation.	1	2
Meperidine	Concurrent use of Meperidine and Ethanol may result in increased sedation.	1	2
Mephobarbital	Concurrent use of Mephobarbital and Ethanol may result in excessive CNS depression.	1	2
Meprobamate	Concurrent use of Ethanol and Meprobamate may result in increased sedation.	1	2
Mesoridazine	Concurrent use of Mesoridazine and Ethanol may result in increased central nervous system depression and an increased risk of extrapyramidal reactions.	1	2
Metformin	Concurrent use of Metformin and Ethanol may result in an increased risk of lactic acidosis.	2	2
Methadone	Concurrent use of Ethanol and Methadone may result in increased sedation.	1	2
Methohexital	Concurrent use of Methohexital and Ethanol may result in excessive CNS depression.	1	2
Methotrexate	Concurrent use of Ethanol and Methotrexate may result in increased hepatotoxicity.	2	2
Methotrimeprazine	Concurrent use of Methotrimeprazine and Ethanol may result in increased central nervous system depression and an increased risk of extrapyramidal reactions.	1	2
Metronidazole	Concurrent use of Ethanol and Metronidazole may result in disulfiram-like reactions (flushing, increased respiratory rate, tachycardia) or sudden death.	1	1
Mirtazapine	Concurrent use of Mirtazapine and Ethanol may result in psychomotor impairment.	1	2
Morphine	Concurrent use of Ethanol and Morphine may result in increased sedation.	1	2

(Continued on next page)

Product	Interaction	Onset	Severity
Moxalactam	Concurrent use of Ethanol and Moxalactam may result in disulfiram-like reactions.	2	1
Nefazodone	Concurrent use of Ethanol and Nefazodone may result in an increased risk of CNS side effects.	1	3
Nilutamide	Concurrent use of Ethanol and Nilutamide may result in an increased risk of ethanol intolerance (facial flushing, malaise, and hypotension).	1	3
Nitroglycerin	Concurrent use of Ethanol and Nitroglycerin may result in hypotension.	1	2
Nortriptyline	Concurrent use of Ethanol and Nortriptyline may result in enhanced drowsiness; impairment of motor skills.	1	2
Olanzapine	Concurrent use of Olanzapine and Ethanol may result in excessive central nervous system depression.	1	2
Oxycodone	Concurrent use of Ethanol and Oxycodone may result in increased sedation.	1	2
Paraldehyde	Concurrent use of Paraldehyde and Ethanol may result in metabolic acidosis.	2	2
Paroxetine	Concurrent use of Ethanol and Paroxetine may result in an increased risk of impairment of mental and motor skills.	1	3
Pentazocine	Concurrent use of Pentazocine and Ethanol may result in increased sedation.	1	2
Pentobarbital	Concurrent use of Ethanol and Pentobarbital may result in excessive CNS depression.	1	2
Perphenazine	Concurrent use of Perphenazine and Ethanol may result in increased central nervous system depression and an increased risk of extrapyramidal reactions.	1	2
Phenelzine	Concurrent use of Phenelzine and Ethanol may result in hypertensive urgency or emergency.	1	2
Phenobarbital	Concurrent use of Ethanol and Phenobarbital may result in excessive CNS depression.	1	2
Phenytoin	Concurrent use of Phenytoin and Ethanol may result in decreased phenytoin serum concentrations, increased seizure potential, and additive CNS depressant effects.	1	2
Pipotiazine	Concurrent use of Pipotiazine and Ethanol may result in increased central nervous system depression and an increased risk of extrapyramidal reactions.	1	2
Primidone	Concurrent use of Primidone and Ethanol may result in excessive CNS depression.	1	2
Procarbazine	Concurrent use of Ethanol and Procarbazine may result in disulfiram-like reactions and increased sedation.	1	1
Prochlorperazine	Concurrent use of Prochlorperazine and Ethanol may result in increased central nervous system depression and an increased risk of extrapyramidal reactions.	1	2
Promazine	Concurrent use of Promazine and Ethanol may result in increased central nervous system depression and an increased risk of extrapyramidal reactions.	1	2
Propiomazine	Concurrent use of Propiomazine and Ethanol may result in increased central nervous system depression and an increased risk of extrapyramidal reactions.	1	2
Propoxyphene	Concurrent use of Propoxyphene and Ethanol may result in additive central nervous system depressant effects.	1	2
Protriptyline	Concurrent use of Ethanol and Protriptyline may result in enhanced drowsiness; impairment of motor skills.	1	2
Quetiapine	Concurrent use of Quetiapine and Ethanol may result in potentiation of the cognitive and motor effects of alcohol.	1	2
Secobarbital	Concurrent use of Secobarbital and Ethanol may result in excessive CNS depression.	1	2
Sertraline	Concurrent use of Ethanol and Sertraline may result in an increased risk of impairment of mental and motor skills.	1	3

Product	Interaction	Onset	Severity
Sodium oxybate	Concurrent use of Sodium Oxybate and Ethanol may result in increased sedation.	1	2
Sulfamethoxazole	Concurrent use of Ethanol and Cotrimoxazole may result in disulfiram-like reactions (flushing, sweating, palpitations, drowsiness).	1	1
Temazepam	Concurrent use of Ethanol and Temazepam may result in impaired psychomotor functions.	1	2
Thiethylperazine	Concurrent use of Thiethylperazine and Ethanol may result in increased central nervous system depression and an increased risk of extrapyramidal reactions.	1	2
Thiopental	Concurrent use of Thiopental and Ethanol may result in excessive CNS depression.	1	2
Thioridazine	Concurrent use of Thioridazine and Ethanol may result in increased central nervous system depression and an increased risk of extrapyramidal reactions.	1	2
Tizanidine	Concurrent use of Tizanidine and Ethanol may result in an increased risk of tizanidine adverse effects (excessive CNS depression).	1	2
Tolazamide	Concurrent use of Ethanol and Tolazamide may result in prolonged hypoglycemia, disulfiram-like reactions.	1	1
Tolazoline	Concurrent use of Tolazoline and Ethanol may result in disulfiram-like reactions.	2	1
Tolbutamide	Concurrent use of Ethanol and Tolbutamide may result in prolonged hypoglycemia, disulfiram-like reactions.	1	1
Tramadol	Concurrent use of Ethanol and Tramadol may result in an increased risk of excessive CNS depression.	1	2
Tranylcypromine	Concurrent use of Tranylcypromine and Ethanol may result in hypertensive urgency or emergency.	1	2
Triazolam	Concurrent use of Ethanol and Triazolam may result in increased sedation.	1	2
Trifluoperazine	Concurrent use of Trifluoperazine and Ethanol may result in increased central nervous system depression and an increased risk of extrapyramidal reactions.	1	2
Triflupromazine	Concurrent use of Triflupromazine and Ethanol may result in increased central nervous system depression and an increased risk of extrapyramidal reactions.	1	2
Trimethoprim	Concurrent use of Ethanol and Cotrimoxazole may result in disulfiram-like reactions (flushing, sweating, palpitations, drowsiness).	1	1
Trimipramine	Concurrent use of Ethanol and Trimipramine may result in enhanced drowsiness and impairment of motor skills.	1	2
Valerian	Concurrent use of Valerian and Ethanol may result in increased sedation.	1	2
Venlafaxine	Concurrent use of Ethanol and Venlafaxine may result in an increased risk of CNS effects.	1	3
Verapamil	Concurrent use of Ethanol and Verapamil may result in enhanced ethanol intoxication (impaired psychomotor functioning).	1	2
Warfarin	Concurrent use of Ethanol and Warfarin may result in increased or decreased international normalized ratio (INR) or prothrombin time.	2	2
Zaleplon	Concurrent use of Zaleplon and Ethanol may result in impaired psychomotor functions.	1	2
Zolpidem	Concurrent use of Ethanol and Zolpidem may result in increased sedation.	1	2

Onset: 1 = Rapid (within 24 hours)
2 = Delayed (after 24 hours)
Severity: 1 = Major (possible life-threatening or potential permanent damage)
2 = Moderate (may exacerbate patient's condition)
3 = Minor (little if any clinical effect)
Reprinted with permission from *The Drug Topics Red Book*. Thomson Medical Economics: Montvale, NJ, 2002.

Drug–Tobacco Interactions

Product	Interaction	Onset	Severity
Fluvoxamine	Concurrent use of Fluvoxamine and Tobacco may result in increased fluvoxamine metabolism.	2	3
Imipramine	Concurrent use of Imipramine and Tobacco may result in decreased imipramine concentrations.	2	2
Nortriptyline	Concurrent use of Nortriptyline and Tobacco may result in decreased nortriptyline concentrations.	2	2
Oral contraceptives	Concurrent use of Oral Contraceptives, Combination and Tobacco may result in an increased risk of cardiovascular disease.	2	3
Pentazocine	Concurrent use of Pentazocine and Tobacco may result in decreased pentazocine concentrations.	2	2
Propoxyphene	Concurrent use of Propoxyphene and Tobacco may result in decreased propoxyphene concentrations.	2	2
Theophylline	Concurrent use of Theophylline and Tobacco may result in decreased theophylline concentrations.	2	2
Tolbutamide	Concurrent use of Tolbutamide and Tobacco may result in decreased tolbutamide concentrations.	2	2
Warfarin	Concurrent use of Tobacco and Warfarin may result in increased or decreased international normalized ratio (INR) or prothrombin time.	2	2

Onset: 1 = Rapid (within 24 hours)
2 = Delayed (after 24 hours)
Severity: 1 = Major (possible life-threatening or potential permanent damage)
2 = Moderate (may exacerbate patient's condition)
3 = Minor (little if any clinical effect)
Reprinted with permission from *The Drug Topics Red Book*. Thomson Medical Economics: Montvale, NJ, 2002.

Use-In-Pregnancy Ratings

The U.S. Food & Drug Administration's Use-in-Pregnancy rating system weighs the degree to which available information has ruled out risk to the fetus against the drug's potential benefit to the patient. Following is a listing of drugs (by generic name) for which ratings are available.

X

CONTRAINDICATED IN PREGNANCY

Studies in animals or humans, or investigational or post-marketing reports, have demonstrated fetal risk which clearly outweighs any possible benefit to the patient.

Acitretin
Atorvastatin Calcium
Bicalutamide
Biperiden Hydrochloride
Cerivastatin Sodium
Clomiphene Citrate
Danazol
Demecarium Bromide
Desogestrel/Ethinyl Estradiol
Diclofenac Sodium/Misoprostol

Dienestrol
Dihydroergotamine Mesylate
Estazolam
Estradiol
Estrogens, Conjugated
Estrogens, Conjugated/
    Medroxyprogesterone Acetate
Estrogens, Esterified
Estrogens, Esterified/
    Methyltestosterone
Estropipate
Ethinyl Estradiol
Ethinyl Estradiol/Ethynodiol
    Diacetate
Ethinyl Estradiol/Levonorgestrel
Ethinyl Estradiol/Norethindrone
Ethinyl Estradiol/Norethindrone
    Acetate
Ethinyl Estradiol/Norgestimate
Ethinyl Estradiol/Norgestrel
Finasteride
Fluorouracil

Fluvastatin Sodium
Follitropin Alpha
Follitropin Beta
Gonadotropin, Chorionic
    (Profasi)
Goserelin Acetate
Interferon Alfa-2B/Ribavirin
Isotretinoin
Leflunomide
Leuprolide Acetate
Levonorgestrel
Lovastatin
Medroxyprogesterone Acetate
Megestrol Acetate
Menotropins
Mestranol/Norethindrone
Methyltestosterone
Misoprostol
Nafarelin Acetate
Norethindrone
Norethindrone Acetate
Norgestrel

Oxandrolone
Oxymetholone
Plicamycin
Pravastatin Sodium
Raloxifene Hydrochloride
Ribavirin
Simvastatin
Stanozolol
Tazarotene
Testosterone
Testosterone Enanthate
Thalidomide
Triazolam
Urofollitropin
Vitamin A Palmitate
Warfarin Sodium
Yohimbine Hydrochloride

D

POSITIVE EVIDENCE OF RISK

Investigational or postmarketing data show risk to the fetus. Nevertheless, potential benefits may outweigh the potential risk.

Alitretinoin
Alprazolam
Altretamine
Amiodarone Hydrochloride
Amlodipine Besylate/Benazepril Hydrochloride*
Anastrozole
Atenolol
Atenolol/Chlorthalidone
Azathioprine
Azathioprine Sodium
Benazepril Hydrochloride*
Benazepril Hydrochloride/ Hydrochlorothiazide*
Busulfan
Candesartan Cilexetil*
Capecitabine
Captopril*
Carbamazepine
Carboplatin
Carmustine
Cladribine
Clonazepam
Cytarabine Liposome
Dactinomycin
Daunorubicin Citrate Liposome
Daunorubicin Hydrochloride
Demeclocycline Hydrochloride
Divalproex Sodium
Docetaxel
Doxorubicin Hydrochloride
Doxorubicin Hydrochloride Liposome

Doxycycline Calcium
Doxycycline Hyclate
Doxycycline Monohydrate
Enalapril Maleate*
Enalapril Maleate/Felodipine*
Enalapril Maleate/ Hydrochlorothiazide
Enalaprilat*
Floxuridine
Fludarabine Phosphate
Flutamide
Fosinopril Sodium*
Fosphenytoin Sodium
Gemcitabine Hydrochloride
Hydrochlorothiazide/Irbesartan*
Hydrochlorothiazide/Lisinopril*
Hydrochlorothiazide/Losartan Potassium*
Hydrochlorothiazide/Moexipril Hydrochloride*
Hydrochlorothiazide/Valsartan*
Idarubicin Hydrochloride
Ifosfamide
Irbesartan*
Lisinopril*
Lithium Carbonate
Lithium Citrate
Lorazepam
Losartan Potassium*
Mechlorethamine Hydrochloride
Melphalan
Mephobarbital
Mercaptopurine
Methimazole
Midazolam Hydrochloride
Minocycline Hydrochloride
Mitoxantrone Hydrochloride
Moexipril Hydrochloride*
Neomycin Sulfate/Polymyxin B Sulfate
Nicotine
Paclitaxel
Pentobarbital Sodium
Pentostatin
Perindopril Erbumine*
Potassium Iodide
Procarbazine Hydrochloride
Quinapril Hydrochloride*
Ramipril*
Streptomycin Sulfate
Tamoxifen Citrate
Telmisartan
Thioguanine
Thiotepa
Tobramycin (Inhalation)
Tobramycin Sulfate
Topotecan Hydrochloride
Toremifene Citrate
Trandolapril*
Trandolapril/Verapamil Hydrochloride*

Tretinoin (Oral)
Valproate Sodium
Valproic Acid
Valsartan*
Vinblastine Sulfate
Vincristine Sulfate
Vinorelbine Tartrate

C

RISK CANNOT BE RULED OUT

Human studies are lacking, and animal studies are either positive for risk or are lacking as well. However, potential benefits may outweigh the potential risk.

Abacavir Sulfate
Abciximab
Acetaminophen/Butalbital
Acetaminophen/Butalbital/ Caffeine
Acetaminophen/Caffeine/ Chlorpheniramine Maleate/ Hydrocodone Bitartrate/ Phenylephrine Hydrochloride
Acetaminophen/Codeine Phosphate
Acetaminophen/Hydrocodone Bitartrate
Acetaminophen/Oxycodone Hydrochloride
Acetaminophen/Pentazocine Hydrochloride
Acetazolamide
Acetic Acid/Oxyquinoline Sulfate/Ricinoleic Acid
Acyclovir (Topical)
Adapalene
Adenosine
Alatrofloxacin Mesylate
Albendazole
Albumin, Human
Albuterol
Albuterol Sulfate
Albuterol Sulfate/Ipratropium Bromide
Alclometasone Dipropionate
Aldesleukin
Alendronate Sodium
Allopurinol Sodium
Alprostadil
Alteplase, Recombinant
Amantadine Hydrochloride
Amifostine
Aminohippurate Sodium
Aminosalicylic Acid
(Continued on next page)

Amlodipine Besylate
Amlodipine Besylate/Benazepril
 Hydrochloride*
Amoxicillin/Clarithromycin/
 Lansoprazole
Amphetamine &
 Dextroamphetamine Mixture
Amprenavir
Amylase/Cellulase/
 Hyoscyamine Sulfate/Lipase/
 Phenyltoloxamine Citrate/
 Protease
Amylase/Cellulase/Lipase/
 Protease
Amylase/Lipase/Protease
Anagrelide Hydrochloride
Antihemophilic Factor IX
 Complex (Human)
Antihemophilic Factor IX
 Complex (Recombinant)
Antihemophilic Factor VIIa
 (Recombinant)
Antihemophilic Factor VIII
 (Human)
Antihemophilic Factor VIII
 (Human)/Von Willebrand
 Factor Complex (Human)
Antihemophilic Factor VIII
 (Recombinant)
Antihemophilic Factor VIII:c
 (Human)
Anti-Inhibitor Coagulant
 Complex
Antipyrine/Benzocaine
Anti-Thymocyte Globulin
Antivenin (Latrodectus Mactans)
Apraclonidine Hydrochloride
Asparaginase
Aspirin/Carisoprodol
Aspirin/Carisoprodol/Codeine
 Phosphate
Aspirin/Methocarbamol
Atovaquone
Atropine Sulfate/Benzoic Acid/
 Hyoscyamine Sulfate/
 Methenamine/Methylene
 Blue/Phenyl Salicylate
Atropine Sulfate/Difenoxin
 Hydrochloride
Atropine Sulfate/Diphenoxylate
 Hydrochloride
Atropine Sulfate/Hyoscyamine
 Sulfate/Phenobarbital/
 Scopolamine Hydrobromide
Azelastine Hydrochloride
Bacillus of Calmette & Guerin,
 Live
Becaplermin
Beclomethasone Dipropionate
Beclomethasone Dipropionate
 Monohydrate

Benazepril Hydrochloride*
Benazepril Hydrochloride/
 Hydrochlorothiazide*
Bendroflumethiazide/Nadolol
Benzocaine
Benzonatate
Benzoyl Peroxide
Benzoyl Peroxide/
 Erythromycin
Bepridil Hydrochloride
Betamethasone Dipropionate,
 Augmented
Betamethasone Dipropionate/
 Clotrimazole
Betaxolol Hydrochloride
Bethanechol Chloride
Biperiden Lactate
Bisoprolol Fumarate
Bisoprolol Fumarate/
 Hydrochlorothiazide
Botulinum Toxin Type A
Brinzolamide
Budesonide
Bupivacaine Hydrochloride
Bupivacaine Hydrochloride/
 Epinephrine Bitartrate
Buprenorphine Hydrochloride
Butabarbital/Hyoscyamine
 Hydrobromide/
 Phenazopyridine
 Hydrochloride
Butorphanol Tartrate
Calcitonin, Salmon
Calcitriol
Calcium Acetate
Candesartan Cilexetil*
Captopril*
Carbachol
Carbetapentane Tannate/
 Chlorpheniramine Tannate/
 Ephedrine Tannate/
 Phenylephrine Tannate
Carbetapentane Tannate/
 Chlorpheniramine Tannate/
 Phenylephrine Tannate
Carbidopa/Levodopa
Carvedilol
Celecoxib
Chloramphenicol
Chloroprocaine Hydrochloride
Chlorothiazide
Chlorothiazide Sodium
Chlorothiazide/Methyldopa
Chloroxine
Chlorpheniramine Maleate/
 Methscopolamine Nitrate/
 Phenylephrine Hydrochloride
Chlorpheniramine Maleate/
 Pseudoephedrine
 Hydrochloride

Chlorpheniramine Polistirex/
 Hydrocodone Polistirex
Chlorpheniramine Tannate/
 Phenylephrine Tannate/
 Pyrilamine Tannate
Chlorpropamide
Chlorthalidone/Clonidine
 Hydrochloride
Choline Magnesium Trisalicylate
Cidofovir
Cilastatin Sodium/Imipenem
Cilostazol
Ciprofloxacin
Ciprofloxacin Hydrochloride
Ciprofloxacin Hydrochloride/
 Hydrocortisone
Citalopram Hydrobromide
Clarithromycin
Clobetasol Propionate
Clofibrate
Clonidine
Clonidine Hydrochloride
Clotrimazole (Oral)
Codeine Phosphate/Guaifenesin
Codeine Phosphate/
 Phenylephrine Hydrochloride/
 Promethazine Hydrochloride
Codeine Phosphate/
 Promethazine Hydrochloride
Colistimethate Sodium
Corticorelin Ovine Triflutate
Corticotropin, Repository
Cosyntropin
Crotamiton
Cyclosporine
Cytomegalovirus Immune
 Globulin Intravenous, Human
Dacarbazine
Daclizumab
Dantrolene Sodium
Dapsone
Deferoxamine Mesylate
Delavirdine Mesylate
Denileukin Diftitox
Desonide
Desoximetasone
Dexamethasone Sodium
 Phosphate
Dexamethasone Sodium
 Phosphate/Neomycin Sulfate
Dexamethasone/Neomycin
 Sulfate/Polymyxin B Sulfate
Dexamethasone/Tobramycin
Dexrazoxane
Dextroamphetamine Sulfate
Dextromethorphan
 Hydrobromide/Guaifenesin
Dextromethorphan
 Hydrobromide/Guaifenesin/
 Phenylpropanolamine
 Hydrochloride

Dextromethorphan
Hydrobromide/Promethazine
Hydrochloride
Dextrose/Milrinone Lactate
Dextrose/Vancomycin
Hydrochloride
Dichlorphenamide
Diflorasone Diacetate
Diflunisal
Digoxin
Digoxin Immune Fab (Ovine)
Diltiazem Hydrochloride
Dinoprostone
Diphtheria Toxoid/Haemophilus
B Conjugate Vaccine/
Pertussis Vaccine/Tetanus
Toxoid
Diphtheria Toxoid/Pertussis
Vaccine, Acellular/Tetanus
Toxoid
Diphtheria Toxoid/Tetanus
Toxoid
Dirithromycin
Disopyramide Phosphate
Donepezil Hydrochloride
Dorzolamide Hydrochloride
Dorzolamide Hydrochloride/
Timolol Maleate
Doxazosin Mesylate
Dronabinol
Dyphylline
Dyphylline/Guaifenesin
Efavirenz
Enalapril Maleate*
Enalapril Maleate/Felodipine*
Enalapril
Maleate/Hydrochlorothiazide
Enalaprilat*
Epinephrine
Epinephrine Hydrochloride
Epoetin Alfa
Erythromycin Ethylsuccinate/
Sulfisoxazole Acetyl
Esmolol Hydrochloride
Ethiodized Oil
Ethionamide
Etidronate Disodium
Etodolac
Felbamate
Felodipine
Fenofibrate
Fentanyl
Fentanyl Citrate
Ferrous Fumarate/Folic Acid/
Intrinsic Factor/Vitamin B12/
Vitamin C
Ferrous Fumarate/Folic Acid/
Vitamins, Multi
Fexofenadine Hydrochloride
Fexofenadine Hydrochloride/
Pseudoephedrine

Hydrochloride
Filgrastim (G-CSF)
Flecainide Acetate
Fluconazole
Flucytosine
Flumazenil
Flunisolide
Flucinolone Acetonide
Fluocinonide
Fluorometholone
Fluorometholone Acetate
Fluorometholone/Sulfacetamide
Sodium
Flurandrenolide
Fluticasone Propionate
Fluvoxamine Maleate
Foscarnet Sodium
Fosinopril Sodium*
Furosemide
Gabapentin
Ganciclovir
Ganciclovir Sodium
Gemfibrozil
Gentamicin Sulfate
Glimepiride
Glipizide
Globulin, Immune
Glyburide
Gonadotropin, Chorionic
(Novarel)
Guaifenesin
Guaifenesin/Hydrocodone
Bitartrate
Guaifenesin/Hydrocodone
Bitartrate/Pseudoephedrine
Hydrochloride
Guaifenesin/Pseudoephedrine
Hydrochloride (Duratuss,
Zephrex)
Haemophilus B Conjugate
Vaccine
Haemophilus B Conjugate
Vaccine/Hepatitis B,
Recombinant Vaccine
Halcinonide
Haloperidol Decanoate
Halothane
Hemin
Heparin Sodium
Hepatitis A Vaccine, Inactivated
Hepatitis B Immune Globulin
Hepatitis B Vaccine–
Recombinant
Hexachlorophene
Homatropine Methylbromide/
Hydrocodone Bitartrate
Homeopathic Product
Hydrochlorothiazide/Irbesartan*
Hydrochlorothiazide/Lisinopril*
Hydrochlorothiazide/Losartan
Potassium*

Hydrochlorothiazide/
Methyldopa
Hydrochlorothiazide/
Metoprolol Tartrate
Hydrochlorothiazide/Moexipril
Hydrochloride*
Hydrochlorothiazide/
Propranolol Hydrochloride
Hydrochlorothiazide/
Spironolactone
Hydrochlorothiazide/Timolol
Maleate
Hydrochlorothiazide/
Triamterene
Hydrochlorothiazide/
Valsartan*
Hydrocodone Bitartrate/
Ibuprofen
Hydrocortisone
Hydrocortisone Acetate
Hydrocortisone Acetate/
Neomycin Sulfate/Polymyxin
B Sulfate
Hydrocortisone Acetate/
Pramoxine Hydrochloride
Hydrocortisone Butyrate
Hydrocortisone Probutate
Hydrocortisone Valerate
Hydrocortisone/Iodoquinol
Hydrocortisone/Neomycin
Sulfate/Polymyxin B Sulfate
Hydroflumethiazide
Hydromorphone Hydrochloride
Hydroquinone
Hyoscyamine
Hyoscyamine Sulfate
Ibutilide Fumarate
Imiglucerase
Indinavir Sulfate
Indocyanine Green
Influenza Virus Vaccine
(Subvirion)
Influenza Virus Vaccine
(Whole-Virus)
Interferon Alfa-2A
Interferon Alfa-2B
Interferon Alfacon-1
Interferon Alfa-N3
Interferon Beta-1A
Interferon Beta-1B
Interferon Gamma-1B
Irbesartan*
Iron Dextran
Isoniazid/Pyrazinamide/
Rifampin
Isosorbide Dinitrate
Isosorbide Mononitrate (Ismo)
Isradipine
Itraconazole
Ivermectin
(Continued on next page)

Japanese Encephalitis Virus
  Vaccine
Ketoconazole
Ketorolac Tromethamine
Labetalol Hydrochloride
Lamivudine
Lamivudine/Zidovudine
Lamotrigine
Latanoprost
Levalbuterol Hydrochloride
Levamisole Hydrochloride
Levofloxacin
Levorphanol Tartrate
Lisinopril*
Losartan Potassium*
Lyme Disease Vaccine
  (Recombinant OSPA)
Mafenide Acetate
Measles/Mumps/Rubella
  Vaccine
Mebendazole
Mefenamic Acid
Mefloquine Hydrochloride
Meningitis Vaccine
Mepivacaine Hydrochloride
Metaproterenol Sulfate
Metaraminol Bitartrate
Methamphetamine
  Hydrochloride
Methenamine Mandelate/
  Sodium Acid Phosphate
Methocarbamol
Methoxsalen
Metoprolol Succinate
Metoprolol Tartrate
Metyrosine
Mexiletine Hydrochloride
Midodrine Hydrochloride
Milrinone Lactate
Mirtazapine
Modafinil
Moexipril Hydrochloride*
Mometasone Furoate
Monobenzone
Morphine Sulfate
Mumps Virus Vaccine
Muromonab-Cd3
Mycophenolate Mofetil
Mycophenolate Mofetil
  Hydrochloride
Nabumetone
Nadolol
Nalidixic Acid
Naloxone Hydrochloride/
  Pentazocine Hydrochloride
Naphazoline Hydrochloride
Naratriptan Hydrochloride
Natamycin
Nefazodone Hydrochloride
Neostigmine Methylsulfate
Niacin

Nicardipine Hydrochloride
Nifedipine
Nilutamide
Nimodipine
Nisoldipine
Nitroglycerin
Norfloxacin
Nystatin
Ofloxacin
Olanzapine
Olopatadine Hydrochloride
Olsalazine Sodium
Omeprazole
Oprelvekin
Orphenadrine Citrate
Oxaprozin
Oxymorphone Hydrochloride
Palivizumab
Pamidronate Disodium
Pancrelipase
Paricalcitol
Paroxetine Hydrochloride
Pegademase Bovine
Pegaspargase
Penbutolol Sulfate
Pentoxifylline
Perindopril Erbumine*
Phentermine Hydrochloride
Phenylephrine Hydrochloride
Phenylephrine Hydrochloride/
  Promethazine Hydrochloride
Phytonadione
Pilocarpine Hydrochloride
Pimozide
Pioglitazone Hydrochloride
Pirbuterol Acetate
Piroxicam
Plasma Protein Fraction
Pneumococcal Vaccine
Podofilox
Polio Vaccine, Inactivated
Polyethylene Glycol
Polyethylene Glycol/
  Potassium Chloride/
  Sodium
Polyethylene Glycol/Potassium
  Chloride/Sodium
  Bicarbonate/Sodium
  Chloride/Sodium Sulfate
Polymyxin B Sulfate/
  Trimethoprim Sulfate
Polythiazide/Prazosin
  Hydrochloride
Potassium Acid Phosphate
Potassium Chloride
Potassium Citrate
Potassium Phosphate/Dibasic
  Sodium Phosphate/Monobasic
  Sodium Phosphate
Potassium Phosphate/Sodium
  Phosphate

Pralidoxime Chloride
Pramipexole Dihydrochloride
Prazosin Hydrochloride
Prednicarbate
Prednisolone Acetate
Prednisolone Acetate/
  Sulfacetamide Sodium
Prednisolone Sodium Phosphate
Procainamide Hydrochloride
Promethazine Hydrochloride
Propafenone Hydrochloride
Proparacaine Hydrochloride
Propranolol Hydrochloride
Protamine Sulfate
Proteinase Inhibitor (Human),
  Alpha 1
Protirelin
Pyrazinamide
Pyrimethamine
Quetiapine Fumarate
Quinapril Hydrochloride*
Quinidine Gluconate
Quinidine Sulfate
Rabies Immune Globulin
Rabies Vaccine
Ramipril*
Repaglinide
Reteplase, Recombinant
Rho (D) Immune Globulin
Rifampin
Rifapentine
Riluzole
Rimantadine Hydrochloride
Rimexolone
Risedronate Sodium
Risperidone
Rituximab
Rizatriptan Benzoate
Rocuronium Bromide
Rofecoxib
Ropinirole Hydrochloride
Rosiglitazone Maleate
Rubella Virus Vaccine
Rubeola Virus Vaccine
Salicylsalicylic Acid
Salmeterol Xinafoate
Sargramostim
Scopolamine
Selegiline Hydrochloride
Sermorelin Acetate
Sertraline Hydrochloride
Sevelamer Hydrochloride
Sibutramine Hydrochloride
Sodium Polystyrene Sulfonate
Somatrem
Somatropin, E-Coli Derived
Spironolactone
Stavudine
Streptokinase
Succimer
Succinylcholine Chloride

Sulconazole Nitrate
Sulfabenzamide/Sulfacetamide/
  Sulfathiazole
Sulfacetamide Sodium
Sulfacetamide Sodium/Sulfur
Sulfamethoxazole/Trimethoprim
Sulfanilamide
Sumatriptan
Sumatriptan Succinate
Tacrine Hydrochloride
Tacrolimus
Telmisartan*
Terazosin Hydrochloride
Terconazole
Tetanus Immune Globulin
Tetanus Toxoid
Theophylline
Thiabendazole
Thrombin
Thyrotropin Alfa
Tiagabine Hydrochloride
Tiludronate Disodium
Timolol Maleate
Tizanidine Hydrochloride
Tocainide Hydrochloride
Tolcapone
Tolmetin Sodium
Tolterodine Tartrate
Topiramate
Tramadol Hydrochloride
Trandolapril*
Trandolapril/Verapamil
  Hydrochloride*
Tretinoin (Topical)
Triamcinolone Acetonide
Triamterene
Trientine Hydrochloride
Triethanolamine Polypeptide
  Oleate
Trifluridine
Trimethoprim
Trimipramine Maleate
Trovafloxacin Mesylate
Tuberculin
Typhoid Vaccine
Typhoid Vi Polysaccharide
  Vaccine
Valrubicin
Valsartan*
Varicella Virus Vaccine
Vecuronium Bromide
Venlafaxine Hydrochloride
Verapamil Hydrochloride
Vitamin B12
Yellow Fever Vaccine
Zalcitabine
Zaleplon
Zidovudine
Zileuton
Zolmitriptan

B

NO EVIDENCE OF RISK IN HUMANS

Either animal findings show risk while human findings do not, or, if no adequate human studies have been done, animal findings are negative.

Acarbose
Acebutolol Hydrochloride
Acrivastine/Pseudoephedrine
  Hydrochloride
Acyclovir (Oral)
Acyclovir Sodium
Amiloride Hydrochloride
Amiloride Hydrochloride/
  Hydrochlorothiazide
Amlexanox
Amoxicillin
Amoxicillin/Clavulanate
  Potassium
Amphotericin B Lipid Complex
Amphotericin B Liposome
Ampicillin Sodium/Sulbactam
  Sodium
Amylase/Lipase/Protease
  (Pancrease)
Antithrombin III (Human)
Aprotinin
Azelaic Acid
Azithromycin Dihydrate
Aztreonam
Basiliximab
Brimonidine Tartrate
Bupropion Hydrochloride
Butenafine Hydrochloride
Cabergoline
Carbenicillin Indanyl Sodium
Cefaclor
Cefadroxil
Cefamandole Nafate
Cefazolin Sodium
Cefdinir
Cefepime Hydrochloride
Cefixime
Cefoperazone Sodium
Cefotaxime Sodium
Cefotetan Disodium
Cefoxitin Sodium
Cefpodoxime Proxetil
Cefprozil
Ceftazidime
Ceftazidime Sodium
Ceftibuten
Ceftizoxime Sodium
Ceftriaxone Sodium
Cefuroxime Axetil
Cefuroxime Sodium

Cephalexin
Cetirizine Hydrochloride
Chlorhexidine Gluconate
Ciclopirox Olamine
Cimetidine
Cimetidine Hydrochloride
Clavulanate Potassium/
  Ticarcillin Disodium
Clindamycin Hydrochloride
Clindamycin Phosphate
Clopidogrel Bisulfate
Clotrimazole (Topical)
Clozapine
Cromolyn Sodium
Cyclobenzaprine Hydrochloride
Cyproheptadine Hydrochloride
Dalteparin Sodium
Danaparoid Sodium
Desflurane
Desmopressin Acetate
Diclofenac Potassium
Diclofenac Sodium
Didanosine
Diphenhydramine
  Hydrochloride
Dipyridamole
Dobutamine Hydrochloride
Dolasetron Mesylate
Dornase Alpha
Doxapram Hydrochloride
Edetate Calcium Disodium
Emedastine Difumarate
Enoxaparin Sodium
Epinephrine/Lidocaine
  Hydrochloride
Epoprostenol Sodium
Eptifibatide
Erythromycin
Erythromycin Ethylsuccinate
Erythromycin Stearate
Etanercept
Ethacrynate Sodium
Ethacrynic Acid
Etidocaine Hydrochloride
Famotidine
Fenoldopam Mesylate
Ferric Sodium Gluconate
Flavoxate Hydrochloride
Fosfomycin Tromethamine
Glatiramer Acetate
Glucagon Hydrochloride
Glycopyrrolate
Gonadorelin Hydrochloride
Guaifenesin/Pseudoephedrine
  Hydrochloride (Guaifed)
Guanfacine Hydrochloride
Hydrochlorothiazide
Ibuprofen
Imiquimod

(Continued on next page)

Indapamide
Infliximab
Insulin Lispro, Human
Ipratropium Bromide
Isosorbide Mononitrate
(Monoket, Imdur)
Ketoprofen
Lactulose
Lansoprazole
Lepirudin
Levocarnitine
Lidocaine
Lidocaine Hydrochloride
Lidocaine/Prilocaine
Lindane
Lodoxamide Tromethamine
Loracarbef
Loratadine
Loratadine/Pseudoephedrine
Sulfate
Malathion
Meclizine Hydrochloride
Meropenem
Mesalamine
Metformin Hydrochloride
Methohexital Sodium
Methyldopa
Metoclopramide Hydrochloride
Metolazone
Metronidazole
Metronidazole Hydrochloride
Miglitol
Montelukast Sodium
Mupirocin
Mupirocin Calcium
Naftifine Hydrochloride

Nalbuphine Hydrochloride
Nalmefene Hydrochloride
Naloxone Hydrochloride
Naproxen
Naproxen Sodium
Nelfinavir Mesylate
Nitrofurantoin, Macrocrystals
Nitrofurantoin, Macrocrystals/
Nitrofurantoin Monohydrate
Nizatidine
Octreotide Acetate
Ondansetron
Ondansetron Hydrochloride
Orlistat
Oxiconazole Nitrate
Oxybutynin Chloride
Oxycodone Hydrochloride
Pemoline
Penicillin G Benzathine
Penicillin G Benzathine/
Penicillin G Procaine
Penicillin G Potassium
Pentosan Polysulfate Sodium
Pergolide Mesylate
Permethrin
Piperacillin Sodium
Piperacillin Sodium/
Tazobactam Sodium
Praziquantel
Progesterone
Propofol
Psyllium
Ranitidine Hydrochloride
Rifabutin
Ritonavir
Ropivacaine Hydrochloride

Saquinavir
Saquinavir Mesylate
Sildenafil Citrate
Silver Sulfadiazine
Sodium Fluoride
Somatropin, E-Coli Derived
(Genotropin)
Sotalol Hydrochloride
Sucralfate
Sulfasalazine
Tamsulosin Hydrochloride
Terbinafine Hydrochloride
Terbutaline Sulfate
Ticlopidine Hydrochloride
Tirofiban Hydrochloride
Tobramycin (Ophthalmic)
Torsemide
Trastuzumab
Ursodiol
Valacyclovir Hydrochloride
Vancomycin Hydrochloride
Zafirlukast
Zolpidem Tartrate

A

**CONTROLLED STUDIES
SHOW NO RISK**

*Adequate, well-controlled
studies in pregnant women
have failed to demonstrate risk
to the fetus.*
Levothyroxine Sodium
Liothyronine Sodium

---

* Category C or D depending on the trimester the drug is given.
Reprinted with permission from *The Drug Topics Red Book*. Thomson Medical Economics: Montvale, NJ, 2002.

Drugs Excreted in Breast Milk

The following is a selection of drug products that can be excreted in breast milk. The list is not comprehensive. Generics and alternate brands of some products may exist. When recommending drugs to pregnant or nursing patients, always check product labeling for specific precautions.

Accolate	Alesse	Asacol	Azulfidine	Cafergot
Accuretic	Alfenta	Astramorph/PF	Bactramycin	Calan
Achromycin	Aloprim	Ativan	Bactrim	Capoten
Actiq	Altace	A/T/S	Benadryl	Capozide
Adalat	Ambien	Augmentin	Bentyl	Captopril
Adderall	Anaprox	Avalide	Betapace	Carbatrol
Aggrenox	Ancef	AVC	Bicillin	Cardizem
Aldactazide	Androderm	Axid	Blocadren	Cataflam
Aldactone	Apresoline	Axocet	Brethine	Catapres
Aldomet	Aralen	Azactam	Brevicon	Catapres-TTS
Aldoril	Arthrotec	Azathioprine	Brontex	Ceclor

Cefizox
Cefobid
Cefotan
Ceftin
Celexa
Ceptaz
Cerebyx
Ceredase
Cipro
Claforan
Claritin
Claritin-D
Cleocin
Clorpres
Clozaril
Codeine
CombiPatch
Combipres
Combivir
Compazine
Cordarone
Corgard
Cortisporin
Cortone
Corzide
Cosopt
Coumadin
Covera-HS
Crinone
Cystospaz
Cystospaz-M
Cytotec
Cytoxan
Dalalone D.P.
Dapsone
Daraprim
Darvon
Darvon-N
Decadron
Decadron-LA
Deconsal II
Demerol
Demulen
Depacon
Depakene
Depakote
Depo-Provera
Desogen
Desoxyn
Desyrel
Dexedrine
DextroStat
D.H.E. 45
Diabinese
Diastat
Diflucan
Dilacor
Dilantin
Dilantin-125
Dilaudid
Dilaudid-HP
Diovan

Diprivan
Disalcid
Diucardin
Diuril
Dolobid
Dolophine
Doral
Doryx
Droxia
Duraclon
Duragesic
Duramorph
Duratuss
Duricef
Dyazide
Dyrenium
E.E.S.
EC-Naprosyn
Ecotrin
Effexor
Elavil
EMLA
E-Mycin
Enduron
Equanil
ERYC
EryPed
Ery-Tab
Erythrocin
Erythromycin
Esgic-plus
Eskalith
Estrostep
Ethmozine
Felbatol
Feldene
Fero-Folic
Fiorinal
Flagyl
Florinef
Floxin
Fluorescite
Fortaz
Furosemide
Galzin
Garamycin
Glucophage
Glyset
Guaifed
Guaifed-PD
Halcion
Haldol
Helidac
Hydrocet
Hydrocortone
HydroDIURIL
Iberet-Folic
Ifex
Imitrex
Imuran
Inderal
Inderide

Indocin
INFeD
Inversine
Isoptin
Kadian
Keflex
Keftab
Kefurox
Kefzol
Kerlone
Klonopin
Kutrase
Lamictal
Lamisil
Lamprene
Lanoxicaps
Lanoxin
Lariam
Lescol
Levbid
Levlen
Levlite
Levora
Levothroid
Levoxyl
Levsin
Levsin/SL
Levsinex
Lexxel
Lindane
Lioresal
Lithium
Lithobid
Lo/Ovral
Loestrin
Lomotil
Loniten
Lopressor
Lortab
Lotrel
Ludiomil
Lufyllin
Lufyllin-400
Lufyllin-GG
Luminal
Luvox
Macrobid
Macrodantin
Mandol
Marinol
Maxipime
Maxzide
Maxzide-25
Mefoxin
Mepergan
Meruvax II
Methergine
Methotrexate
MetroCream
MetroGel
MetroLotion
Mexitil

Mezlin
Micronor
Microzide
Midamor
Migranal
Miltown
Minizide
Minocin
Mircette
M-M-R II
Modicon
Moduretic
Monocid
Monodox
Mono-Gesic
Monopril
Morphine
MS Contin
MSIR
Myambutol
Mykrox
Mysoline
Naprelan
Naprosyn
Nascobal
Necon
NegGram
Nembutal
Neoral
Netromycin
Niaspan
Nicotrol
Nizoral
Norco
Nor-QD
Nordette
Norinyl
Noritate
Normodyne
Norpace
Norplant
Novantrone
Nubain
Nucofed
Nydrazid
Oramorph
Oretic
Ortho-Cept
Ortho-Cyclen
Ortho-Novum
Orudis
Ovcon
Ovral
Ovrette
Oxistat
OxyContin
OxyFast
OxyIR
Pacerone
Pamelor
Panlor SS
Paxil

PCE
Pediapred
Pediazole
Pediotic
Pentasa
Pepcid
Periostat
Persantine
Pfizerpen
Phenergan
Phenobarbital
Phrenilin
Pipracil
Plan B
Platinol-AQ
Ponstel
Pravachol
Premphase
Prempro
Prevacid
Preven
PREVPAC
Prinzide
Procanbid
Prograf
Proloprim
Prometrium
Pronestyl
Propofol
Prosed/DS
Provera
Prozac
Pseudoephedrine
Pulmicort
Pyrazinamide
Quibron
Quibron-T
Quibron-T/SR
Quinaglute
Quinidex
Quinine
Reglan
Renese
Requip
Reserpine
Restoril
Retrovir
Ridaura
Rifadin
Rifamate
Rifater
Rimactane
RMS
Robaxisal
Rocaltrol
Rocephin
Roferon A
Roxanol
Roxanol-T
Salflex
Sandimmune

(Continued on next page)

Sansert	Tarka	Tol-Tab	Uni-Dur	Xanax
Seconal	Tavist	Toprol-XL	Uniphyl	Zagam
Sectral	Tazicef	Toradol	Uniretic	Zantac
Sedapap	Tazidime	Trandate	Uroqid-Acid	Zarontin
Semprex-D	Tegretol	Tranxene	Valium	Zaroxolyn
Septra	Tegretol-XR	Tranxene-SD	Vanceril	Zestoretic
Sinequan	Tenoretic	Trental	Vancocin	Ziac
Slo-bid	Tenormin	Trilafon	Vantin	Zinacef
Solganal	Tenuate	Trileptal	Vascor	Zithromax
Soma	Testoderm	Tri-Levlen	Vaseretic	Zoloft
Sonata	Thalitone	Trilisate	Vasotec	Zonalon
Sporanox	Theo-24	Tri-Norinyl	Verelan	Zonegran
Stadol	Theo-Dur	Triostat	Vermox	Zosyn
Stelazine	Theo-X	Triphasil	Versed	Zovia
Streptomycin	Thorazine	Trivora	Vibramycin	Zovirax
Stromectol	Tiazac	Trizivir	Vibra-Tabs	Zyban
Symmetrel	Timolide	Trovan	Vicodin	Zydone
Syn-Rx	Timoptic	Tylenol	Viramune	Zyloprim
Synthroid	Timoptic-XE	Tylenol with	Visken	Zyrtec
Tagamet	Tobi	Codeine	Voltaren	
Tambocor	Tofranil	Ultram	Voltaren-XR	
Tapazole	Tolectin	Unasyn	Wellbutrin	

Reprinted with permission from *The Drug Topics Red Book*. Thomson Medical Economics: Montvale, NJ, 2002.

Dietary Considerations

Potassium and Tyramine Content of Foods
Potassium Content of Foods
High-Potassium Foods

Fruits	Vegetables	Other Foods
Apricot	Artichokes	Bran/Bran products
Avocado	Beans, dried	Coffee (limit 2 cups/day)
Banana	Broccoli	Chocolate
Cantaloupe	Brussels Sprouts	Coconut
Casaba	Celery	Granola
Dates	Escarole	Ice Cream (limit 1 cup/day)
Dried fruits	Endive	Molasses
Figs	Greens (swiss chard, collard,	Nuts/seeds
	dandelion, mustard, beet)	
Honeydew	Kale	Orange flavored pop
Mango	Kohlrabi	Salt substitutes/like salt
Nectarine	Lentils	Snuff/chewing tobacco
Orange	Legumes	Tea (limit 2 cups/day)
Papaya	Lima Beans	
Plums	Mushrooms	
Prunes	Parsnips	
Raisins	Potatoes (french fries, baked, sweet)	
Rhubarb	Salt-free vegetable juice	
Juice of these fruits	Tomatoes	

Low-Potassium Foods

Fruits	Vegetables	Other Foods
Apples	Alfalfa sprouts	Rice
Blackberries	Asparagus	Noodles
Blueberries	Beans, green or wax	Bread & bread products
Boysenberries	Bean sprouts	Cereals
Cherries	Beets	Cake
Cranberries	Cabbage	Cookies

Fruits	Vegetables	Other Foods
Gooseberries	Carrots	Pies (no chocolate or high-potassium fruit)
Grapes	Cauliflower	
Loganberries	Corn	
Mandarin oranges	Cucumber	
Pears	Eggplant	
Pineapple	Lettuce	
Raspberries	Mixed vegetables	
Strawberries	Okra	
Tangerines	Onions	
Watermelon	Parsley	
Juice of these fruits	Peas	
	Radishes	
	Rutabagas	
	Squash (summer, zucchini)	

© 2001 National Kidney Foundation, Inc. Reprinted with permission.
Reprinted with permission from *The Drug Topics Red Book.* Thomson Medical Economics: Montvale, NJ, 2002.

Tyramine Content of Foods

Food	Allowed	Minimize Intake	Not Allowed
Beverages	Milk, decaffeinated coffee, tea, soda	Chocolate beverage, caffeine-containing drinks, clear spirits	Acidophilus milk, beer, ale, wine, malted beverages
Breads/cereals	All except those containing cheese	None	Cheese bread and crackers
Dairy products	Cottage cheese, farmers or pot cheese, cream cheese, ricotta cheese, all milk, eggs, ice cream, pudding (except chocolate)	Yogurt (limit to 4 oz per day)	All other cheeses (aged cheese, American, Camembert, cheddar, Gouda, gruyere, mozzarella, parmesan, provolone, romano, Roquefort, stilton)
Meat, fish, and poultry	All fresh or frozen	Aged meats, hot dogs, canned fish and meat	Chicken and beef liver, dried and pickled fish, summer or dry sausage, pepperoni, dried meats, meat extracts, bologna, liverwurst
Starches— potatoes/rice	All	None	Soybean (including paste)
Vegetables	All fresh, frozen, canned, or dried vegetable juices except those not allowed	Chili peppers, Chinese pea pods	Fava beans, sauerkraut, pickles, olives, Italian broad beans
Fruit	Fresh, frozen, or canned fruits and fruit juices	Avocado, banana, raspberries, figs	Banana peel extract
Soups	All soups not listed to limit or avoid	Commercially canned soups	Soups which contain broad beans, fava beans, cheese, beer, wine, any made with flavor cubes or meat extract, miso soup
Fats	All except fermented	Sour cream	Packaged gravy
Sweets	Sugar, hard candy, honey, molasses, syrups	Chocolate candies	None
Desserts	Cakes, cookies, gelatin, pastries, sherbets, sorbets	Chocolate desserts	Cheese-filled desserts
Miscellaneous	Salt, nuts, spices, herbs, flavorings, Worcestershire sauce	Soy sauce, peanuts	Brewer's yeast, yeast concentrates, all aged and fermented products, monosodium glutamate, vitamins with Brewer's yeast

NATIONAL AND STATE BOARDS OF PHARMACY CONTACT INFORMATION

This appendix contains the most recent contact information for the national and state boards of pharmacy. A current listing of contact information for state boards of pharmacy is maintained at the National Association of Boards of Pharmacy website, www.napb.com. In addition, contact information for all the pharmacy schools in the United States can be found at the American Association of Colleges of Pharmacy website, www.aacp.org.

NATIONAL ASSOCIATION OF BOARDS OF PHARMACY

Carmen A. Catizone
Executive Director
700 Busse Highway
Park Ridge, IL 60068-2402
847-698-6227, Fax: 847-698-0124
www.nabp.net

STATE BOARDS OF PHARMACY

Alabama
Jerry Moore, RPh
Executive Director
1 Perimeter Park South, Suite 425S
Birmingham, AL 35243
205-967-0130, Fax: 205-967-1009
e-mail: rphbham@bellsouth.net
www.albop.com

Alaska
Barbara Roche
Licensing Examiner
PO Box 110806
Juneau, AK 99811
907-465-2589
www.decd.state.ak.us/occ/ppha.htm

Arizona
Llyn A. Lloyd, RPh
Executive Director
4425 W Olive Avenue, Suite 140
Glendale, AZ 85302
623-463-2727
e-mail: vsevilla@azsbp.com
www.pharmacy.state.az.us

Arkansas
Charles S. Campbell
Executive Director
101 East Capitol Avenue, Suite 218
Little Rock, AR 72201
501-682-0190, Fax: 501-682-0195
e-mail: charlie.campbell@mail.state.ar.us
www.state.ar.us/asbp

California
Patricia Harris
Executive Officer
400 R Street, Suite 4070
Sacramento, CA 95814
916-445-5014, Fax: 916-327-6308
e-mail: patricia_harris@dca.ca.gov
www.pharmacy.ca.gov

Colorado
Susan L. Warren
Program Administrator
1560 Broadway, Suite 1310
Denver, CO 80202
303-984-7750 ext. 313, Fax: 303-894-7764
e-mail: pharmacy@dora.state.co.us
www.dora.state.co.us/pharmacy

Connecticut
Michelle Sylvestre
Drug Control Agent and Board Administrator
State Office Building, Room 110
165 Capitol Avenue
Hartford, CT 06106
860-713-6070, Fax: 860-713-7242
e-mail: michelle.sylvestre@po.state.ct.us
www.ctdrugcontrol.com/rxcommission.htm

Delaware
David W. Dryden, RPh, Esq.
Executive Secretary
PO Box 637
Dover, DE 19903
302-739-4798, Fax: 302-739-3071
e-mail: gbunting@state.de.us
www.professionallicensing.state.de.us

District of Columbia
Graphelia Ramseur
Health Licensing Specialist
825 N Capitol St NE, Room 2224
Washington, DC 20002
202-442-4775, Fax: 202-442-9431
http://dchealth.de.gov/

Florida
John D. Taylor, RPh
Executive Director
4052 Bald Cypress Way, Bin #C04
Tallahassee, FL 32399-3254
850-245-4292
e-mail: mqa_pharmacy@doh.state.fl.us
www.doh.state.fl.us/mqa

Georgia
Anita O. Martin
Executive Director
237 Coliscum Dr
Macon, GA 31217-3858
478-207-1686
www.sos.state.ga.us/plb/pharmacy/

Guam
Teresita Villagomez
Acting Administrator
PO Box 2816
Hagatna, GU 96932
671-735-7406, Fax: 671-735-7413
e-mail: tlgvillagomez@dphss.gcvguam.net

Hawaii
Lee Ann Teshima
Executive Officer
PO Box 3469
Honolulu, HI 96801
808-586-2698, Fax: 808-586-2874
e-mail: pharmacy@dcca.state.hi.us
www.state.hi.us/dcca/pvl/

Idaho
R. K. Markuson, RPh
Executive Director
PO Box 83720
Boise, ID 83720-0067
208-334-2356, Fax: 208-334-3536
www.state.id.us/bop

Illinois
Judy Cullen
Pharmacy Coordinator
Illinois Department of Professional Regulation
320 West Washington Street, Third Floor
Springfield, IL 62786
217-785-0800
www.dpr.state.il.us/

Indiana
Joshua Bolin
Director
402 West Washington Street, Room 041
Indianapolis, IN 46204
317-234-2067
e-mail: hpb4@hpb.state.in.us
www.in.gov/hpb/boards/isbp/

Iowa
Lloyd K. Jessen, RPh, JD
Executive Secretary/Director
400 SW Eighth Street, Suite E
Des Moines, IA 50309-4688
515-281-5944, Fax: 515-281-4609
e-mail: debbie.jorgensen@ibpe.state.ia.us
www.state.ia.us/ibpe

Kansas
Susan Linn
Executive Director
900 Jackson Street SW, Room 513
Landon State Office Building
Topeka, KS 66612-1231
785-296-4056, Fax: 785-296-8420
e-mail: pharmacy@ink.org
www.accesskansas.org/pharmacy

Kentucky
Michael A. Moné, RPh, JD
Executive Director
23 Millcreek Park
Frankfort, KY 40601
502-573-1580, Fax: 502-573-1582
e-mail: pharmacy.board@mail.state.ky.us

Louisiana
Malcolm J. Broussard
Executive Director
5615 Corporate Boulevard, 8E
Baton Rouge, LA 70808
225-925-6496
www.labp.com

Maine
Geraldine Betts
Board Administrator
35 State House Station
Augusta, ME 04333
207-624-8603, Fax: 207-624-8637
Hearing Impaired: 207-624-8563
e-mail: kelly.l.mclaughlin@state.me.us
www.maineprofessionalreg.org

Maryland
LaVerne George Nasea
Executive Director
4201 Patterson Avenue
Baltimore, MD 21215
410-764-4755, Fax: 410-358-6207
e-mail: mdbop@dhmh.state.md.us
www.dhmh.state.md.us/pharmacyboard/

Massachusetts
Charles R. Young
Executive Director
239 Causeway Street
Boston, MA 02113
617-727-9953
e-mail: charles.r.young@state.ma.us
www.state.ma.us/reg/boards/ph

Michigan
Melanie Brim
Licensing Manager
611 West Ottawa, First Floor
PO Box 30670
Lansing, MI 48909-8710
517-373-9102, Fax: 517-373-2179
www.michigan.gov/cis/0,1607,7-154-
    10568_17671_17688-42779--,00.html

Minnesota
David E. Holmstrom, RPh, JD
Executive Director
2829 University Avenue SE, Suite 530
Minneapolis, MN 55414
612-617-2201, Fax: 612-617-2212
e-mail: david.holmstrom@state.mn.us
www.phcybrd.state.mn.us

Mississippi
Leland McDivitt
Executive Director
PO Box 24507
Jackson, MS 39225-4507
601-354-6750, Fax: 601-354-6071
www.mbp.state.ms.us

Missouri
Kevin E. Kinkade, RPh
Executive Director
PO Box 625
Jefferson City, MO 65102
573-751-0091
e-mail: kkinkade@mail.state.mo.us
www.ecodev.state.mo.us/pr/pharmacy

Montana
Rebecca Deschamps, RPh
Executive Director
111 North Jackson
PO Box 200513
Helena, MT 59620-0513
406-841-2356, Fax: 406-841-2343
e-mail: dlibspdha@state.mt.us
http://discoveringmontana.com/dli/bsd/license/
    bsd_boards/pha_board/board_page.htm

Nebraska
Becky Wisell
Executive Secretary
PO Box 94986
Lincoln, NE 68509-4986
402-471-2115
www.hhs.state.ne.us

Nevada
Keith W. MacDonald, RPh
Executive Secretary
555 Double Eagle Court, Suite 1100
Reno, NV 89521
775-850-1440
e-mail: pharmacy@govmail.state.nv.us
http://nvbop.glsuite.us/renewal/glsweb/
    homeframe.aspx

New Hampshire
Paul G. Boisseau, RPh
Executive Director
57 Regional Drive
Concord, NH 03301-8518
603-271-2350, Fax: 603-271-2856
e-mail: nhpharmacy@nhsa.state.nh.us
www.state.nh.us/pharmacy/

New Jersey
Debora C. Whipple
Executive Director
PO Box 45013
Newark, NJ 07101
973-504-6450, Fax: 973-648-3355
e-mail: askconsumeraffairs@dca.lps.state.nj.us

New Mexico
Jerry Montoya
Chief Inspector/Director
1650 University Boulevard NE, Suite 400-B
Albuquerque, NM 87102
505-841-9102, Fax: 505-841-9113
e-mail: joseph.montoya@state.nm.us
www.state.nm.us/pharmacy

New York
Lawrence H. Mokhiber, RPh
Executive Secretary
89 Washington Avenue, Second Floor W
Albany, NY 12234-1000
518-474-3817 ext. 130, Fax: 518-473-6995
www.nysed.gov/prof/pharm.htm

North Carolina
David R. Work, RPh
Executive Director
PO Box 459
Carrboro, NC 27510-0459
919-942-4454, Fax: 919-967-5757
e-mail: drw@ncbop.org
www.ncbop.org

North Dakota
Howard C. Anderson, Jr, RPh
Executive Director
PO Box 1354
Bismarck, ND 58502-1354
701-328-9535, Fax: 701-258-9312
e-mail: ndboph@btinet.net

Ohio
William T. Windsley
Executive Director
77 South High Street, Room 1702
Columbus, OH 43215-6126
614-466-4143, Fax: 614-752-4836
e-mail: exec@bop.state.oh.us
www.state.oh.us/pharmacy/

Oklahoma
Bryan H. Potter, RPh
Executive Director
4545 North Lincoln Boulevard, Suite 112
Oklahoma City, OK 73105-3488
405-521-3815, Fax: 405-521-3758
e-mail: pharmacy@oklaosf.state.ok.us
www.pharmacy.state.ok.us

Oregon
Gary A. Schnabel
Executive Director
State Office Building, Suite 425
800 NE Oregon Street, #9
Portland, OR 97232
503-731-4032, Fax: 503-731-4067
e-mail: pharmacy.board@state.or.us
www.pharmacy.state.or.us

Pennsylvania
Melanie Zimmerman
Executive Secretary
124 Pine Street
PO Box 2649
Harrisburg, PA 17105-2649
717-783-7156, Fax: 717-787-7769
e-mail: pharmacy@pados.dos.state.pa.us
www.dos.state.pa.us/bpoa/phabd/mainpage.htm

Puerto Rico
Magda Bouet Graña
Executive Director
Department of Health, Board of Pharmacy
Call Box 10200
Santurce, PR 00908
787-725-8161, Fax: 787-725-7903

Rhode Island
Catherine A. Cordy
Chief of the Board
3 Capitol Hill, Room 205
Providence, RI 02908
401-222-2837, Fax: 401-222-2158
e-mail: dianet@doh.state.ri.us

South Carolina
LeeAnn Bundrick
Interim Administrator
100 Centerview Drive, Suite 306
Columbia, SC 29211-1927
803-896-4700, Fax: 803-896-4596
e-mail: funderbm@mail.llr.state.sc.us

South Dakota
Dennis M. Jones, RPh
Executive Secretary
4305 South Louise Avenue, Suite 104
Sioux Falls, SD 57106
605-362-2737, Fax: 605-362-2738
e-mail: dennis.jones@state.sd.us
www.state.sd.us/dcr/pharmacy

Tennessee
Kendall M. Lynch
Director
Second Floor, Davy Crockett Tower
500 James Robertson Parkway
Nashville, TN 37243
615-741-2718, Fax: 615-741-2722
e-mail: klynch@mail.state.tn.us
www.state.tn.us/commerce/pharmacy

Texas
Gay Dodson, RPh
Executive Director
333 Guadalupe, Suite 3-600
Box 21
Austin, TX 78701-3942
512-305-8000, Fax: 512-305-8082
e-mail: geninfo@tsbp.state.tx.us
www.tsbp.state.tx.us

Utah
Diana L. Baker
Bureau Director
Division of Occupational and Professional
    Licensing
PO Box 146741
Salt Lake City, UT 84114-6741
801-530-6179, Fax: 801-530-6511
e-mail: dbaker@utah.gov
www.commerce.state.ut.us/dopl/dopl1.htm

Vermont
Peggy Atkins
Board Administrator
26 Terrace Street, Drawer 09
Montpelier, VT 05609-1106
802-828-2875, Fax: 802-828-2465
e-mail: cpreston@sec.state.vt.us
www.vtprofessionals.org

Virgin Islands
Lydia T. Scott
Executive Assistant
Commissioner of Health
Roy L. Schneider Hospital
48 Sugar Estate
St. Thomas, VI 00802
340-774-0117 ext. 5078, Fax: 340-777-4001

Virginia
Elizabeth Scott Russell, RPh
Executive Director
6606 West Broad Street, 4th Floor
Richmond, VA 23230-1717
804-662-9911, Fax: 804-552-9313
e-mail: scotti.russell@dhp.state.va.us
www.dhp.state.va.us/pharmacy/default.htm

Washington
Donald H. Williams, RPh
Executive Director
PO Box 47863
Olympia, WA 98504-7863
360-236-4825, Fax: 360-586-4359
e-mail: don.williams@doh.wa.gov
http://wws2.wa.gov/doh/hpqa-
      licensing/HPS4/Pharmacy/default.htm

West Virginia
William T. Douglass, Jr
Executive Director
232 Capitol Street
Charleston, WV 25301
304-558-0558, Fax: 304-558-0572
e-mail: wdouglass@wvbop.com

Wisconsin
Deanna Zychowski
Director
1400 East Washington
PO Box 8935
Madison, WI 53708
608-266-2812, Fax: 608-267-0644
e-mail: web@drl.state.wi.us
www.state.wi.us/agencies/drl

Wyoming
James T. Carder
Executive Director
1720 South Poplar Street, Suite 4
Casper, WY 82601
307-234-0294, Fax: 307-234-7226
e-mail: wypharmbd@wercs.com
http://pharmacyboard.state.wy.us

BUDGETING FOR DRUG
INFORMATION RESOURCES

A. Basic Library

References	Cost*
American Hospital Formulary Service (AHFS) Drug Information	$ 175.00
Drug Facts and Comparisons	$ 180.00
Handbook on Injectable Drugs	$ 170.00
Handbook of Non-Prescription Drugs	$ 129.00
Martindale: The Complete Drug Reference	$ 470.00
Nonprescription Product Therapeutics	$107.00
Physicians' Desk Reference	$ 90.00
Remington's Pharmaceutical Sciences	$ 99.00
USP DI (three-volume set)	$ 397.00

B. Additional Resources

References	Cost*
Drug–Drug Interaction	
• *Drug Interactions Analysis & Management*	$ 180.00
• *Drug Interaction Facts*	$ 72.00
• *Evaluations of Drug Interactions*	$ 240.00
Herbal	
• *PDR for Herbal Medicines*	$ 60.00
• *The Review of Natural Products*	$ 80.00
Internal Medicine	
• *Cecil Textbook of Medicine*	$ 139.00
• *Harrison's Principles of Internal Medicine*	$ 125.00
Pediatrics	
• *Pediatric Dosage Handbook*	$ 40.00
• *The Harriet Lane Handbook*	$ 40.00
Pharmacokinetics	
• *Applied Biopharmaceutics and Pharmacokinetics*	$ 55.00
• *Clinical Pharmacokinetics Pocket Reference*	$ 53.00
• *Concepts in Clinical Pharmacokinetics*	$ 79.00
• *Therapeutic Drug Monitoring*	$ 33.00
Pharmacology	
• *Goodman and Gilman's The Pharmacological Basis of Therapeutics*	$ 125.00
Pregnancy/Breast-feeding	
• *Drugs in Pregnancy and Lactation*	$ 140.00
Therapeutics	
• *Applied Therapeutics: The Clinical Use of Drugs*	$ 157.00
• *Pharmacotherapy: A Pathophysiologic Approach*	$ 194.00
• *Textbook of Therapeutics: Drug and Disease Management*	$ 157.00

C. CD-ROM Computer Systems/Programs

	Cost*
AHFS first WEB	$ 2,990.00
Clinical Pharmacology Internet Monograph Service	$ 145.00
Clinical Reference Library (Lexi–Comp) online	$ 350.00
CliniTrend Software	$ 688.00
DataKinetics Software	$ 688.00
eFacts Drug Facts and Comparisons online	$ 360.00
eFacts Drug Interaction Facts online	$ 180.00
Iowa Drug Information System (CD-ROM)	$ 4,400.00
IPA (SilverPlatter)	$ 472.00
Medline (SilverPlatter) Internet only (1966+)	$21,000.00
MedTeach Software	$ 549.00
Micromedex >200 licensed bed facility	
Diseasedex	$13,200.00
Drugdex System	$15,598.00
Poisindex System	$15,477.00
Other Micromedex Databases	
CareNotes System	$10,285.00
Drug–Reax	$ 1,738.00
Kinetidex	$ 3,960.00
Martindale: The Complete Drug Reference	$ 1,848.00
PDR	$ 6,358.00
P&T Quik	$ 1,525.00
Reprorisk	$ 2,893.00

D. Major Online Vendors

Dialog
EBSCO Information Services
Gale Group
National Library of Medicine
Ovid Technologies, Inc.
OCLC First Search
SilverPlatter

*Costs are approximate and are based on 2002 figures.

Index

In this index, page numbers in *italics* designate figures; page numbers followed by the letter "t" designate tables; *see also* cross-references designate related topics or more detailed lists of subtopics.

Biotechnologic products, 208–223
  antisense drugs, 219
  approved therapies and vaccines,
      209–216t
  gene therapy, 219
  glycoproteins, 218–219
  immunoglobulin (Ig), 217, 217t, 218t
  proteins and peptides, 217
  recombinant human granulocyte
      colony-stimulating factor, 217–218
  terminology, 208, 216–217
Biotin, 1132
Biotransformation (process), 115
Biotransformation pathways
  oxidation, 362–364, 365t
  phase II (conjugation) reactions,
      364–366, 367t
  phase I reactions, 362–364, 366t
  reduction, 364, 366t
Biperiden, *234*
Birth defects, anticonvulsants in,
    279–280
Bisacodyl, 609
Bismuth subsalicylate, 614–615
  in *H. pylori* infection, 1024t
  in peptic ulcer disease, 1024–1025
Bisoprolol, 773, 795t
Bites, snake, 462–463
Bitolerol, 968t
Bivalirudin, 327, 328
Black cohosh (*Cimicifuga racemosa*),
    643
Blastogenesis, pharmacokinetics in,
    678
Bleeding, in bone marrow suppression,
    1108
Blepharitis (eyelid inflammation), 546
Blood-brain barrier, 114
Blood flow, effective renal (ERBF), 123
Blood glucose meters, 528
Blood glucose self-monitoring,
    527–528, 1048–1049
Blood pressure, 762–764, *764* (see also
    Hypertension; Hypotension)
  renin-angiotensin-aldosterone system
      and, 762–764
  sympathetic baroceptors and, 762
Blood pressure monitors, for patient
    use, 526
Blood urea nitrogen (BUN), 1082,
    1089, 1137
Boards of pharmacy
  national, 1208
  state, 1208–1212
Body (bodies)
  basal, 163
  inclusion, 164
Body compartments, in children,
    674–675
Body composition analysis, 1130
Body mass index (BMI), 575
Body surface area (BSA), 12
  adults and children, *1168*
  chemotherapy dosing and, 1101
  infants, *1169*
Boiling point, 33–34
Boils, in ear, 537
Bolus injection, 118, *119,* 119–121
Bond(s)
  hydrogen, 149, *149*
  peptide, *153*
Bonding
  hydrogen, 154
  hydrophobic, 150
Bone marrow suppression, by cancer
    chemotherapy, 194, 1107–1108

Bottle feeding, ear disorders and, 538
Bottle method, of emulsification, 49
Botulinum toxin, recombinant, 214t
Braces, orthopedic, 529–530
Bradykinesia, 909, *910*
Brain, imaging, 404–405 (see also un-
    der Radiopharmaceuticals)
BRAT diet, 613
Breakpoint concentrations, 820
Breast feeding
  diarrhea and, 613
  gastric emptying and, 673–674
Breast imaging, 407
Breast milk
  drug excretion in, 681, 682,
      1204–1206t
  drugs affecting production, 681–682
Bretylium
  as antiarrhythmic, 753, 754, 755, 756
  precautions and interactions,
      755–756
Bromocriptine, 916t, 917–919
  adverse effects, 281
  pharmacology, 281
Bronchitis, chronic, 979–985 (see also
    Chronic obstructive pulmonary
    disease)
Bronchoconstriction, paradoxical, 966
Buccal administration, 81
Buccal and sublingual tablets, 64, 65
Budesonide, 971t
Buffer(s)
  defined, 37
  ocular, 546
Buffer action, 37
Buffer capacity, 37
Buffer salts, 41
Bulk-forming laxatives, 607–608
Bumetanide, 771, 795t, 1086
Bundle of His, 737, *738,* 745
Buprenorphine, 1121t
Burns, chemical, of eye, 546
Burow's solution (aluminum acetate),
    in poison ivy, 570
Buspirone, *275*
  adverse effects, 277
  pharmacology, 277
  therapeutic indications, 277
Butabarbital, 276t
Butanediol fermentation, 166
Butenafine, 828t, 850
Butoconazole, 828t, 850–851
Butorphanol, *284284,* 1120t
Butyric acid fermentation, 167
Butyrophenones, 269, *270*

C

Calcineurin inhibitors, in graft rejec-
    tion, 1147t, 1147–1148
Calcium (Ca)
  as digoxin agonist, 793
  parenteral preparations, 512
  serum tests, 704
Calcium carbonate
  in gastroesophageal reflux disease
      (GERD), 621
  thyroid function tests and, 1066t
Calcium-channel blockers, *314,*
    314–315, 318, 319t, 320
  adverse effects, 321
  in angina pectoris, 721t, 722
  as antiarrhythmics, 756–757
  drug interactions, 753, 755, 756–757
  in heart failure, 798
  in hypertension, 768t, 779–780
  in post-thrombolytic therapy, 732

in renal failure, 1090
  toxicity, 458
Calcium gluconate, in renal failure,
    1085–1086
Calcium hydroxide solution, 46
Calcium polycarbophil, 614
Calcium salts, in renal failure, 1086
Calendar method of contraception, 634
Caloric restriction, 577
Campath-1, 220
Campylobacter pylori (see Helicobac-
    ter pylori)
Cancer (see also Cancer chemother-
    apy)
  American Cancer Society screening
      guidelines, 1097, 1098t
  American Cancer Society warning
      signs, 1096–1097, 1098t
  colorectal, 616
  epidemiology, 1096, *1097*
  gastric, 1013
  immunosuppression and risk of, 1151
  oral, 544
  skin, 564–565, 566
  staging, 1097–1098
    AJCC staging, 1097
    TNM classification, 1097
  therapy
    hematopoietic stem cell transplanta-
        tion, 1111
    pharmaceutical (see Cancer
        chemotherapy)
    radiation, 1111
    surgical, 1111
  types, 1096
Cancer chemotherapy, 1096–1115,
    1101 (see also Chemotherapeutic
    agents)
  administration, 1102
  cell growth kinetics, 1099, *1100*
  cell life cycle, 1098–1100, *1099,*
    1100
  dosing systems, 1101
  response factors, 1102–1103
Candidiasis, 1151
  oral (thrush), 544
  vaginal, 632
Canes, 524
Canker sores (recurrent aphthous ul-
    cers; recurrent aphthous stomati-
    tis), 542–543
Capping, of tablets, 64
Capreomycin, 828t, 862
Capsaicin, 993, 1124
Capsule, bacterial, 163
Capsules
  compounding of, 103t, 103–104
  as dosage form, 58–60
  formulation of, 86
  hard gelatin, 59–60
  quality control, 94
  sizes, 103, 103t
  soft gelatin, 60
Captopril, 778, 795t
Carbamazepine, *279*
  drug interactions, 752, 833, 861
Carbamide peroxide
  in cerumen impaction, 536
  in tooth whiteners, 540
Carbapenems, 825t, 831
Carbenicillin, 826t, 836, 837
Carbenicillin indanyl, 826t
Carbidopa, 916t, 916–917
  pharmacology, 281
  structure, *280*
Carbohydrate counting, 1038–1039